T0195397

Fifth Edition

OCCUPATIONAL THERAPY WITH OLDER ADULTS

STRATEGIES FOR THE OTA

Fifth Edition

OCCUPATIONAL THERAPY WITH OLDER ADULTS

STRATEGIES FOR THE OTA

Helene L. Lohman, OTD, OTR/L, FAOTA
Professor
Department of Occupational Therapy
School of Pharmacy and Health Professions
Creighton University
Omaha, Nebraska

Amy L. Shaffer, Ed. D, COTA/L
Program Director
Occupational Therapy Assistant Program
Chattahoochee Technical College
Marietta, Georgia

Patricia J. Watford, OTD, MS, OTR/L
Assistant Professor
Low Vision Rehabilitation
Department of Occupational Therapy
College of Allied Health Sciences
Augusta University
Augusta, Georgia

ELSEVIER

Elsevier
3251 Riverport Lane
St. Louis, Missouri 63043

OCCUPATIONAL THERAPY WITH OLDER ADULTS:
STRATEGIES FOR THE OTA, FIFTH EDITION

ISBN: 978-0-323-82410-1

Copyright © 2024 by Elsevier, Inc. All rights reserved.

"OTR" is a certification mark of the National Board for Certification in Occupational Therapy, Inc., which is registered in the United States of America. "COTA" is a certification mark of the National Board for Certification in Occupational Therapy, Inc., which is registered in the United States of America. "NBCOT" is a service and trademark of the National Board for Certification in Occupational Therapy, Inc., which is registered in the United States of America.

NBCOT did not participate in the development of this publication and has not reviewed the content for accuracy. NBCOT does not endorse or otherwise sponsor this publication, and makes no warranty, guarantee, or representation, expressed or implied, as to its accuracy or content. NBCOT does not have any financial interest in this publication, and has not contributed any financial resources.

Notice

Practitioners and researchers must always rely on their own experience and knowledge in evaluating and using any information, methods, compounds, or experiments described herein. Because of rapid advances in the medical sciences, in particular, independent verification of diagnoses and drug dosages should be made. To the fullest extent of the law, no responsibility is assumed by Elsevier, authors, editors, or contributors for any injury and/or damage to persons or property as a matter of products liability, negligence or otherwise, or from any use or operation of any methods, products, instructions, or ideas contained in the material herein.

Previous editions copyrighted 2019, 2012, 2004, and 1998.

Content Strategist: Lauren Willis
Content Development Manager: Somodatta Roy Choudhury
Content Development Specialist: Akanksha Marwah
Publishing Services Manager: Deepthi Unni
Project Manager: Nayagi Anandan
Book Designer: Ryan Cook

Printed in India

Last digit is the print number: 9 8 7 6 5 4 3 2

I dedicate this book to my students, who over the years have inspired me to be the best educator in all areas I teach. To my late parents, Mira Lee and Henry Goldstein, and my late in laws Caroline Camp and Benedict Lohman, who exemplified living a full meaningful life. To my late dear husband Michael, for all the love and support he gave me over the years as well as his sisters who continue to be a family support. Finally, I dedicate this book to my sons Ben and Lee, to Robbe, Alice, Terri, Vikki, Jules and to all my friends who are like family.

Helene

My contributions in this book are dedicated to Mrs. Gail Walker, OTA (retired), whose enthusiastic teachings laid the foundation for the OTA that I am, and continue to inspire me to share what I have learned by teaching others. To my parents, who taught me at a young age, the value that older adults added to our lives, the importance of working hard and learning new things, and the need to proofread and use spell check—every time! To my husband, who supports my desire to have a passion project, and appreciates the opportunities it gives him to indulge in his. God gave me you!

Amy

I would like to dedicate this book to my grandparents, Hoke & Nettie Wilcox and Sydney & Doris Wigmore, for their spunk and zest for life that instilled my deep love of older adults. To my parents, Hoke & Joyce Wilcox, who made me the person I am. To my sweet husband Ron, my wonderful children Sarah and Mitchell, my sister Suzann, and my brother Hoke, Jr. for their support and encouragement during this process. To the older adult clients I have had over the years, who have taught me so much more than I ever taught them. And most of all to God for His amazing grace and mercies that are truly new every morning.

Patty

Shadows and Sunlight

I remember being young and wild,
Although my body forgets and betrays me.
I peer out of this aging body
With a mind that still knows
Who, when, where and how.
When did fifty
Or even sixty seem like young?
Birthdays only serve as a yardstick for the outside.
How can you measure what I feel on the inside?

My heart tears seeing friends disappear
Into places I only fear.
My memories of yesteryear seem crystal clear.
I close my eyes and feel myself running in the breeze.
The crowds along the college track applauding my triumph,
When the sound of my therapist
Cheering my toddling in a walker wakes me.
I laugh out loud
And people shake their heads as if I am half crazed.
So many losses totaling into this single moment.

The respect I had as a working man
Still fills my chest with pride.
My dearest Rosalie leaving me on Earth so quickly.
Our dreams of travel and leisurely walks are gone.
Saying goodbye to my neighborhood of 43 years,
To move into a room with a stranger.
Overhearing the hushed voices of my son and daughter
As they discuss the exorbitant costs of my care outside my door.
Then the frustrated voices in deciding who will take Dad home.

How did the tables get turned so fast?
Ironically my children become my caretakers now.
How can I express to those I love,
Do not grieve for my losses so deeply.
As I still intend to live
As best I can,
As much as you will allow me.
Keep open the windows of possibilities.
Do not shut the door of life just yet.

Yolanda Griffiths

Contributors to the Fifth Edition

Tonya Bartholomew, OTR/L
Gottsche Therapy Rehabilitation and Wellness
Powell, Wyoming

Lea C. Brandt, PhD, OTD, MA, OTR/L
Director, MU Center for Health Ethics
Associate Professional Practice Professor
Department of Medicine
School of Medicine
University of Missouri
Columbia, Missouri

Sue Byers-Connon, MS, COTA/L, ROH
Instructor OTA Program (Retired)
Mt. Hood Community College
Gresham, Oregon

Carolyn Ciccotello, COTA/L
Certified Occupational Therapy Assistant
Sugar Hill, Georgia

Bryan Clever, COTA/L, ATP, CRTS
Pediatric/CRT Project Manager
Friends of Disabled Adults and Children (FODAC)
Stone Mountain, Georgia

Kimberly Collins, MS, OTR/L, CPAM
Outpatient Director of Rehabilitation
Aegis Therapies
Duluth, Georgia

Kelli L. Coover, PharmD, BCGP
Associate Professor and Vice Chair
Assistant Director of Experiential Education
Department of Pharmacy Practice
School of Pharmacy and Health Professions
Creighton University
Omaha, Nebraska

Brenda M. Coppard, PhD, OTR/L, FAOTA
Professor of Occupational Therapy
Associate Dean for Assessment
School of Pharmacy and Health Professions
Creighton University
Omaha, Nebraska

Sharon Cosper, Ed. D, OTR/L
Vice Chair/Associate Professor
Department of Occupational Therapy
College of Allied Health Sciences
Augusta University
Augusta, Georgia

Michele A. Faulkner, PharmD, FASHP
Medical Science Liaison
Alexion AstraZeneca Rare Disease
Omaha, Nebraska

Yolanda Griffiths, OTD, OTR/L, FAOTA
Professor
Department of Occupational Therapy
College of Pharmacy and Health Sciences
Drake University
Des Moines, Iowa

Meghan V. Hall, MHS, OTR/L
Assistant Professor
Director of the Low Vision Clinic
Department of Occupational Therapy
College of Allied Health Sciences
Augusta University
Augusta, Georgia

Stephanie Johnson, MHS, OTR/L
Associate Professor
Department of Occupational Therapy
College of Allied Health Sciences
Augusta University
Augusta, Georgia

Evelyn Z. Katz, BSOT, BFA, OT/L
Occupational Therapist (Retired)
Low Vision Rehabilitation Consultant
Omaha, Nebraska

Pamalyn Kearney, EdD, MS, OTR/L, FAOTA
Chair and Program Director
Department of Occupational Therapy
College of Allied Health Sciences
Augusta University
Augusta, Georgia

Brenda Kornblit Kennell, OTR/L FAOTA
Program Chair (Retired)
Occupational Therapy Assistant Program
Central Piedmont Community College Central Campus
Charlotte, North Carolina

Mallory Rosche, MHS, OTR/L
Assistant Professor
Clinical Director of the Occupational Therapy Low Vision Clinic
Department of Occupational Therapy
College of Allied Health Sciences
Augusta University
Augusta, Georgia

Betsy B. McDaniel, MS, COTA/L
Department of Rehabilitation Sciences Division Chair
Occupational Therapy Assistant Program Director
Middle Georgia State University
Cochran, Georgia

Sara Munzesheimer, OTD, OTR/L
Occupational Therapist
University of Miami Hospital
Miami, Florida

René Padilla, PhD, OT, FAOTA
Vice Provost for Global Engagement
Creighton University
Omaha, Nebraska

Angela Patterson, OTD, OTR/L, FNAP
Associate Professor
Department of Occupational Therapy
Director Master of Science in Rehabilitation
Director Master of Science in Occupational Therapy
School of Pharmacy and Health Professions
Creighton University
Omaha, Nebraska

Angela M. Peralta, OTA
Occupational Therapy Assistant
Jewish Community Center
Staten Island, New York

Sherrell Powell, OTR/L
Professor Emeritus
Occupational Therapy Assistant Program
LaGuardia Community College
City University of New York, New York

Barbara Jo Rodrigues, MS, OTR/L
Director of Acute Care Therapy
Dominican Hospital
Santa Cruz, California

Michelle Rudolf, OTD, OTR/L
Occupational Therapist
Littleton, Colorado

Christina-Marie K. Sleight OTD, OTR/L
Staff Therapist
Sprouts Therapy
Waipio, Hawaii

Laura Smith, MS, OTR/L
Director
Occupational Therapy Assistant Program
Wallace State Community College
Hanceville, Alabama

Kaisa Syväoja OTD, OTR/L
Assistant Professor
Department of Occupational Therapy
School of Health Sciences
The College of Saint Scholastica
Duluth, Minnesota

Janistres Teemer, OTD, OTR/L
Occupational Therapist
Northside Cherokee Hospital
Canton, Georgia

Andrea Thinnes, OTD, OTR/L, FNAP
Associate Professor
Department of Occupational Therapy
School of Pharmacy and Health Professions
Creighton University
Omaha, Nebraska

Laurie Vera, MHS, OTR/L
Academic Fieldwork Coordinator/Assistant Professor
Department of Occupational Therapy
College of Allied Health Sciences
Augusta University
Augusta, Georgia

Student Contributors From Augusta University

Students were in the Master of Occupational Therapy Program and were members of Pi Theta Epsilon Honor Society at Augusta University in Augusta, Georgia at the time of contributing to this book, and titles may have changed.

Rebekah Bauknight, OTS

Mary Beth Brewster, OTS

Shelby Cannon, OTS

Morgan Glaze, OTS

Jenny Grant, OTS

Emily Holton, OTS

Cassidy Long, OTS

Brette Moore, OTS

Emma Morris, OTS

Olivia Parker, OTS

Kristian Taylor, OTS

Meghan Williams, OTS

Student Contributors From Creighton University

Students were in the Doctor of Occupational Therapy Program and were members of Pi Theta Epsilon Honor Society at Creighton University in Omaha, Nebraska at the time of contributing to this book, and titles may have changed.

Jenna Ackerman, OTS

Claire Beglcy, OTS

Alicia Dovin, OTS

Stephany Freed, OTS

Ellie Leonard, OTS

Kayshe Miles, OTS

McKenzie Osborn, OTS

Paige Peitzmeier, OTS

Sara Spellerberg, OTS

Sarah Synek, OTS

Preface

Occupational Therapy Assistants (OTAs) continue to be a significant part of the occupational therapy workforce treating older adults. The most recent American Occupational Therapy Association (AOTA) workforce and salary survey report[1] states that skilled nursing facilities, which primarily service older adults, continue to be the number one employer of OTAs. Furthermore, the US Department of Labor's Bureau of Labor Statistics (BLS)[2] projected employment of OTAs to increase by 34% or more between 2020 and 2030, much faster than the average growth rate of 7% for all professions. This trend has much to do with the growth of the older adult population. The need for OTAs to possess a strong knowledge base that will allow them to provide the best care possible, and to confidently represent the profession remains as high a priority as when we prepared the first through fourth editions of this text. Therefore, we have sought to include the most up-to-date information possible to support OTAs as they work with older adults in various practice areas. Information in this book, especially about public policy, was current at the time of writing.

Based on reader feedback, we retained the conceptual organization of the previous editions. The first section, Concepts of Aging, presents foundational concepts related to the experience of older adults. A general discussion of aging trends, concepts, and theories is followed by a discussion of occupational therapy professional beliefs, including an introduction to the fourth edition of the *Occupational Therapy Practice Framework*.[3] The second section, Occupational Therapy Intervention With Older Adults, includes updated OT strategies that consider the principles presented in Section 1. We begin Section 2 with issues related to all older adults with such topics as cultural diversity, OT theories applied to older adults, ethical aspects, and working with caregivers. We conclude Section 2 with chapters dedicated to strategies applicable to the work with older adults who have specific medical conditions.

As we prepared this fifth edition, we remain committed to the goals that guided us in the previous editions:

■ We wanted the project to acknowledge the reality of life experience of older adults and be respectful of them as active, occupational people. We changed the term "elder" to "older adult" to reflect the most commonly accepted term this population uses to describe themselves.

■ We continued to emphasize the importance of collaboration between the Occupational Therapist (OT) and Occupational Therapy Assistant (OTA). Our own collaboration as an editorial team continues to be a vivid example to us of the richness of such collaboration. Following feedback from OTA leaders, we changed the titles "COTA" to "OTA" and "OTR/L" to "OT" to be more inclusive of all occupational therapy practitioners. We do, however, continue to support the contribution of national certification to maintaining high standards of competent practice to provide consumers high-quality services.

■ We wanted to produce a comprehensive text for both OTA students and practicing OTAs who wish to refresh their knowledge and for OTs who are committed to the development of the OTA/OT partnership.

■ We wanted to highlight the important contribution OTAs make to the life of older adults.

■ We updated and integrated available research evidence for effectiveness of intervention to enhance justification for services and advocacy for meeting the needs of older adults. This research can be found in the section titled "Evidence Nuggets," based on research of current practice. We continue to emphasize that occupational therapy practitioners should stay current with research to provide evidence-based practice. This emphasis on research evidence is highlighted by the guideposts for the "Centennial Vision 2025" of the American Occupational Therapy Association.[1]

■ We endeavored to create a book that acknowledged the diversity of older adults across the United States and is more inclusive of a variety of older adult populations.

■ We included technology resources for many chapters in our new section "Tech Talk."

■ We added video clips to several chapter resources encouraging a multimedia approach to learning concepts.

■ We emphasized the illustration of principles and strategies through case studies and narratives using the language of the fourth edition of the *Occupational Therapy Framework*[3] (OTPF-4) so that readers can easily relate their learning to real-life situations.

■ We updated chapters and added new material, including the updated OTPF-4 and Code of Ethics, health policy, health management with chronic conditions, telehealth, universal precautions, an expanded view of the definition of cultural diversity, and more robust mobility and wellness sections.

■ We continued to ground the suggested strategies in traditional OT philosophy and practice and emphasized the kind of reasoning that should be a part of all OT intervention regardless of the professional level.

It remains our hope that this text will enhance readers' knowledge so that they can contribute to the improvement of life satisfaction of older adults wherever they encounter them.

Helene L. Lohman, OTD, OTR/L, FAOTA
Amy L. Shaffer, Ed. D, COTA/L
Patricia J. Watford, OTD, MS, OTR/L

REFERENCES

1. The American Occupational Therapy Association. 2019 *AOTA workforce and salary survey;* 2019. Bethesda, MD: AOTA Press.
2. Bureau of Labor Statistics, U.S. Department of Labor. *Occupational Outlook Handbook, Occupational Therapy Assistants and Aides; 2022.* Retrieved from https://www.bls.gov/ooh/healthcare/occupational-therapy-assistants-and-aides.htm
3. American Occupational Therapy Association. *Occupational therapy practice framework: Domain and process, 4th ed.* Am J Occup Ther. 2020;74(Suppl. 2):1-87. 7412410010. DOI: 10.5014/ajot.2020.74S2001
4. American Occupational Therapy Association. *AOTA unveils Vision 2025; 2016.* Retrieved from https://www.aota.org/AboutAOTA/vision-2025.aspx.

Acknowledgments

As was true in previous editions, writing a book is not a simple process that one person can undertake alone. We wish to acknowledge many people for their contributions to this project:

- Lauren Willis, Akanksah Marwah, Nayagi Anandan and all other editorial support from Elsevier for their patience and guidance.
- René Padilla and Sue Byers-Connon for their exemplary work on previous editions and their help in tying up loose ends for this edition.
- Janistres Teemer for her contributions in updating each chapter's PowerPoint presentation for the Evolve Website.
- Laura Smith for updating/developing test questions that require critical thinking skills to translate knowledge from words to application for the Evolve Website.
- Caroline Ciccotello for her work in defining the Glossary contents.
- The contributing authors for their hard work.
- Pi Theta Epsilon OT students from Augusta University and Creighton University who contributed in updating references and constructing Evidence Nuggets.
- OT Students: Alexis Gordon, Mia Marrow, Jaya Pitts, and their loved ones who graciously agreed to appear in photographs.
- Contributing photographers for this edition, Fitz Johnson, Amanda Caldwell, and Johnny Barfield, who kindly shared their captured moments.
- Yolanda Griffiths for the moving poem that appears for the fifth time at the beginning of this book.
- The administrators and faculty of the Department of Occupational Therapy, College of Allied Health Sciences at Augusta University, for their support and encouragement.
- The administrators and faculty of the Department of Occupational Therapy, School of Pharmacy and Health Professions at Creighton University for their support and encouragement.
- Helene Lohman for her unending support mentoring two new editor team members.

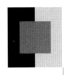

Contents

CONTENTS

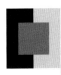

Video TOC

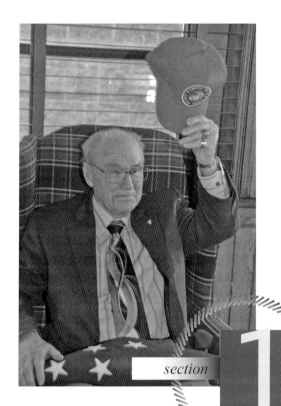

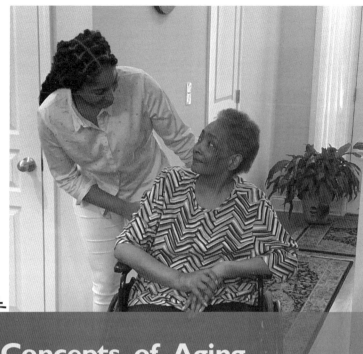

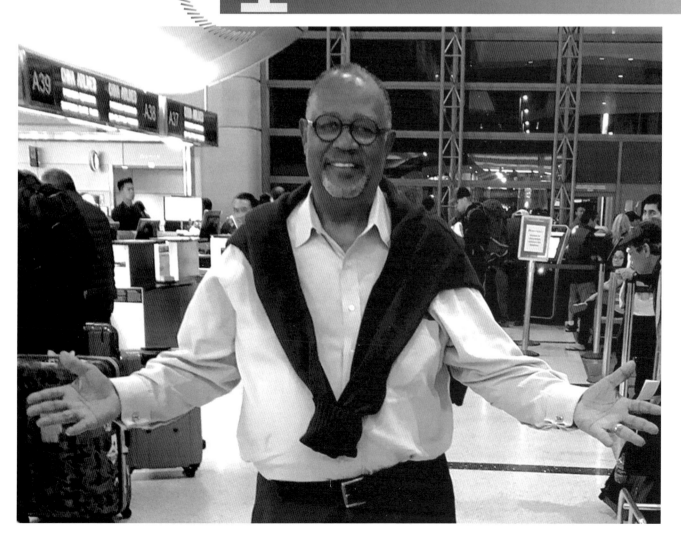

chapter 1

Aging Trends and Concepts

HELENE L. LOHMAN

(PREVIOUS CONTRIBUTIONS FROM EMILY PENINGTON AND ELLEN SPERGEL)

KEY TERMS

ageism, aging in place, cohort, chronic illness, demography, generational cohorts (Traditionalists, Baby Boomers, Generation X, Generation Y), geriatrics, gerontology, health, illness, intergenerational, mid old, old, trends, young old

CHAPTER OBJECTIVES

1. Define relevant terminology regarding older adults.
2. Describe the relationship between aging and illness.
3. Discuss components of health and chronic illness.
4. Discuss a client-centered approach.
5. Describe the three stages of aging (young old, middle old, old old), and define their differences.
6. Explain the effects of growth of the elder population in society.
7. Discuss the effects of an increasingly large number of older adult women in society.
8. Examine the problems and needs of the oldest old populations—that is, those older adults 85 years and older, including the centenarians.
9. Describe living arrangements of older adults and living trends, such as aging in place.
10. Discuss the significance of economic trends on older adults.
11. Relate implications of demographical data for occupational therapy practice.
12. Discuss current trends affecting older adults in America and implications for occupational therapy practice.
13. Describe the importance of intergenerational contact for occupational therapy intervention.
14. Explain the importance of understanding generational cohorts for intervention.
15. Describe the concept of "ageism" in today's society and the effect of the views of the American youth culture on aging.

Jacob is a 25-year-old occupational therapy assistant (OTA) practicing in a skilled nursing facility (SNF). He provides daily occupational therapy intervention 5 days a week. Most of the older adults are in some stage of recovery from an acute illness and are participating in occupational therapy to regain functional abilities. Many of the older adults are quite frail and some have cognitive impairments. As a student, Jacob observed Chris, an OTA working in an independent living facility. Chris was part of a team providing wellness programming for older adults. Most of Chris's clients were quite active at the facility and in the community. Jacob especially enjoyed watching Chris lead Tai Chi groups with the residents. On weekends, Jacob visits his grandparents, both of whom are 75 years of age and independent, active members of the community. One spring break, Jacob had the opportunity to accompany his grandfather to an AARP advocacy meeting. He was proud to watch his grandfather and others ask probing questions that reflected critical thinking about policy issues. Jacob often thinks about his

grandparents, the older adults at the AARP meeting and the independent living facility, as well as the SNF residents. He contemplates about who are the typical older adults.

Julia is a 20-year-old occupational therapy assistant student in an OTA program. As one of her course requirements, class members participate in intergenerational book discussion groups at an independent living facility. The specific readings focus the discussions on intergenerational values and beliefs. Julia is surprised to identify generational differences and similarities. The eldest of the participants discuss the influences that post-World War II (post-WWII) and the Korean War had on their lives. Some of the younger older adults talk about the influence of the Vietnam War, Woodstock, the civil rights, and women's movements had on their generation. Her instructors also participate in the groups. Depending on their age cohort, some of them discuss coming of age in the 1970s and 1980s and the influence of the media, technology, being "latchkey" children, and how the

Internet changed their lives. They describe vivid memories of the Challenger Space Shuttle disaster. Julia and some of her classmates often comment on the strong influence that technology has had on their generation and how they cannot imagine a world without the Internet. Most of the generations commonly share the effects of the terrorist attacks on September 11, 2001 and the COVID pandemic. Jessica notes that within each generation there are a variety of perspectives based on individual life experiences. These lively discussions have increased each participant's awareness of intergenerational commonalities and differences, as well as the individual uniqueness of each group member. The discussions have created a strong bond among the group members. Julia feels that as a result of participating in the intergenerational book discussion group, she will be more comfortable working with older adults in a clinical practice.

Julia has a strong desire to go into practice with older adults. She remembers helping her grandmother recover from a stroke. When she studied the content about older adults in her course work, Julia was surprised to learn of the diversity among the older population. She realized that, just as her OTA class represents diversity among age groups and cultural groups, so does the older adult population. She also recognized misconceptions she had about the elder generations. Some were based on clinical observations at a SNF and informal observations from visits to her grandmother. One misconception was that all older adults are sick and frail. Another misconception was that most older adults have cognitive impairments. Through her participation in course experiences with older adults in community settings, Julia learned that many older adults are healthy and active, especially the younger generation of older adults (those 65–75 years of age). Julia also learned that cognitive impairment affects a small portion of the older population, primarily the oldest of the old (those 85 years and older).[1]

OTAs may easily acquire a skewed image of the older population, especially in a skilled nursing home facility, which is the largest practice area for OTAs.[2] Older adults in skilled nursing facilities tend to be representative of a sicker, older, and frailer older population. Older adults in skilled nursing facilities often have circulatory, cognitive, and neurological disorders, and most residents require assistance with activities of daily living (ADL).[3] In reality, only 1.2 million people, 65 years and older adults, reside in institutions with the majority being 85 years or older.[3,4] Occupational therapy practice continues to change with a movement toward community-based practice, where the majority of older adults reside. Therefore, OTAs must have a broader perspective about older adults to work effectively with a diverse, continuously changing older population. This chapter provides relevant background information as it relates to occupational therapy practice and to the overall older adult population.

DEFINITIONS

The term *gerontology* comes from the Greek terms *geron* and *lojas*, which mean "study of old men." Gerontology is often thought of as the study of the aged and can include the aging process in humans and animals. The field of gerontology is broad and encompasses the historical, philosophical, religious, political, psychological, anthropological, and sociological issues of the older population. The term *geriatrics* is often used to describe medical interventions with the older adults. In occupational therapy practice, geriatrics sometimes refers to an area of clinical specialty. The term *cohort* refers to "a component of the population born during a particular period and identified by period of birth so that its characteristics can be ascertained as it enters successive time and age periods."[5] In gerontological literature, the older generation may also be referred to as the *elder* (or *aged*) *cohort* compared to younger cohorts.

HEALTH, ILLNESS, AND WELL-BEING

Although health, illness, and well-being are familiar terms, they require expanded definitions for occupational therapy practice in geriatrics. One part of a definition for health is "functioning optimally without evidence of disease or abnormality."[5] Few older adults would be considered healthy with this general definition. However, a theory of well-being can be developed if health is considered the most favorable level of functioning for a person's age and condition. Many individuals have chronic illnesses to which they have adjusted and are able to live optimally. These people should be considered as being in a state of well-being. For example, to live optimally, individuals with lifelong disabilities, such as multiple sclerosis, need health care system services such as occupational therapy home evaluations for environmental adaptations even though they are not ill. These individuals do not think of themselves as ill and may resent being labeled as "patients" and placed in this role by health care professionals.

The biological systems of older adults may change. Some changes that result in disease or dysfunction may be treated through medication or surgery. Other biological changes, such as decreased balance, can be handled with environmental adaptations such as installing brighter lights in stairwells and removing loose rugs and electrical cords from traffic areas in the home. Some sensory changes can be partially resolved with glasses and hearing aids. These biological and sensory changes should not be thought of as illnesses. These are changes that older adults adjust to and incorporate into their daily lives.

Chronic Illness

Many medical conditions of older adults are chronic—that is, they cannot be cured, but they can be managed. The physician may not cure heart disease, but the pain and debilitating consequences can be managed for years with medications, diet, exercise, surgery, and technology. OTAs can provide ideas to help older adults manage their chronic conditions to maintain involvement in occupations (see Chapter 5). In these cases, it could be said that, although the disease has not been cured, the older adult's life has been extended in a qualitatively meaningful way.

Most older adults have a minimum of one and often multiple chronic conditions. Recent data indicate the most prevalent conditions for older adults over 65 years of age are hypertension (58.5% men, 55.7% women), arthritis (50.5%), heart disease (29.1%), cancer (25.8%), and diabetes (21.5%).[6] The incidence of chronic illness may be greater in minority older adult groups than in white older adults. Blacks and Hispanics over age 65 report higher levels of diabetes than Whites. Hypertension is more prevalent among Blacks than Whites.[6]

The following examples illustrate the way one older adult learns to adapt to a chronic illness. Henry has osteoarthritis and needs assistance with some ADL functions. He continues to maintain his apartment and values his independence. He takes frequent breaks to rest while performing housekeeping tasks. Because of his decreased endurance, he uses a lightweight upright vacuum, which also helps reduce upper extremity strain. Henry has an active social life outside of his home. He maintains mobility in the community by taking a bus to activities. Osteoarthritis is a disease that cannot be cured, however, most OTAs would say that Henry is not sick.

Miriam is 89 years old. She lives with her 97-year-old husband in the same house that they moved into after they got married. She has a chronic blood condition called thrombocytopenia, along with osteoporosis and hearing loss. She has been admitted several times to the hospital for complications related to the thrombocytopenia. After she returns home and when she gets her energy back, she resumes her normal routine of managing cooking, housework, and walking every morning for 3 miles around the neighborhood. Through her walks, she has met many of her younger neighbors and established friendships. Miriam desires to stay in her home, and she enjoys residing in an intergenerational community. Again, with this example, most OTAs would say that Miriam is not sick.

Some health care practitioners may dismiss an older adult's complaints with comments such as, "It's your age; it's your problem; what do you expect from me? I can't cure you." They are likely to overlook important ways to treat and reduce symptoms that may increase the length and quality of the older adult's life. Generally, health professionals are educated to cure illness, and some may be less knowledgeable about illness management. Thus, some health care practitioners feel uncomfortable treating older adults who cannot be cured, and in response, they develop a dismissive approach.

The alternative to a dismissive approach is a collaborative therapeutic relationship, or what has been referred to in occupational therapy literature as client-centered therapy.[7] With this approach, emphasized in the fourth edition of the *Occupational Therapy Practice Framework: Domain and Process*,[7] occupational therapists (OTs) and OTAs partner with their clients to help determine therapy goals and intervention activities. They spend time getting to know clients by hearing their stories through formal and informal interview techniques, assessments such as the Canadian Occupational Performance Measure (COPM)[8], and developing an occupational profile.[7] An occupational profile helps gain a better understanding of the older adult's personal history, viewpoints, and meaningful contexts.[7] Older adults are central to the management of their own health and well-being. By using a client-centered approach, older adults identify meaningful occupational activities and thus are more invested in interventions selected by practitioners.[7]

A partnership involves the OT, OTA, and the older adult working together to help determine meaningful intervention goals that enhance the older adult's quality of life. The following example illustrates this partnership.

Sadie is an 86-year-old widow with arthritis and living in senior citizen housing. Her daily life is a balance of self-maintenance, simple meal preparations, visits with neighbors in the community recreation room, telephone calls to family members, and watching television. Sadie has reported to her primary care physician decreasing vision, weakness, and joint pain. She displays general anxiety and depression. She comments to her physician, "I think that I belong in a nursing home. I'm old, and I'm having difficulty taking care of myself."

Placing Sadie in a nursing home may manage some of her medical conditions, as well as provide care and social opportunities. However, the interprofessional medical team can also evaluate additional supports to maintain independent living in the community if that is what Sadie really desires. For Sadie, the physician adjusts drug dosages to manage her arthritis and orders an occupational therapy evaluation and intervention. The OT and OTA decide to first screen Sadie using the COPM to help develop her occupational profile to obtain a clearer picture of her concerns. With the COPM, Sadie mentions that she would really like to remain home and identifies her main concerns as having difficulties with meal preparation and reading the newspaper. Both concerns are related to her low vision. In addition, she has difficulty getting dressed because of arthritis. On the basis of this information, the OT, OTA, and Sadie collaborate to develop the following intervention recommendations:

- A kitchen evaluation for suggestions on adaptations for low vision
- A lighted magnifier to improve visual function with reading
- Arthritis education that includes joint protection and mobilization, energy conservation, work simplification, and adaptive devices to improve dressing

The occupational therapy interventions suggested in the example of Sadie may result in improved functional abilities in many areas of her life and may help decrease her anxiety about independent living. As with Sadie's story, a client-centered approach can address an older adult's chronic conditions, interests, and desires. Like Sadie, it is not unusual for older adults to have multiple chronic conditions, often accompanying acute conditions. When managed properly, all interventions work smoothly to improve the older adult's independent status and occupational well-being.

With any condition, older adults may need to adjust to a different functional status with changed occupational roles. However, the accumulation of medical conditions does not necessarily lead to decreased function and increased disability. Despite the "graying of America,"[9] older adults are experiencing less disability and are living longer and better with the right combination of behavioral, genetic, and even personality factors[10] as well as support from others.

Societal Trends and Chronic Conditions

It is beneficial for OTAs to be aware of a larger societal trend toward focusing on chronic conditions. Increasingly, policy and major reports are addressing people with chronic conditions because they access more health care services, account for the largest percentage of health care spending, and require more family and caregiver support.[11] Exemplifying these larger societal trends is the implementation of primary care models to address the chronic conditions of the older adult population. Occupational therapy practitioners are important contributors toward older adult primary care needs on interprofessional teams because of our holistic background and focus on occupational engagement.[12] Possibilities for practitioner's contribution to primary care practices are endless. Home safety and fall prevention are just a couple examples.[12] OTAs are encouraged to access the many resources that AOTA has developed regarding primary care as well as chronic conditions on the AOTA website.

THE STAGES OF AGING

What age constitutes "old age"? The federally mandated age to collect Social Security varies between 65 and 67 years based on year of birth. The age that most retirement communities set as the minimum for their residents is 55 years. At age 50 years, one can join the AARP, and by age 40 years, Americans are protected by the Age Discrimination in Employment Act. The third stage of aging, called senescence, which social gerontologists define as a stage of biological decline, begins at age 30 years.

One definition of old age classifies 65–74 years of age as young old, 75–84 as middle old, and 85 and greater as old old.[13] This may help OTAs think of old age in terms of occupational role performance and expectations. However, OTAs should use this classification as a guideline because every person ages differently, and every older adult does not fit neatly into one of these three categories. Socioeconomic factors, societal changes, cultural factors, and personality considerations can largely influence the way each older adult approach aging. As the Baby Boomers continue to enter the aging population, these categories may change and, ultimately, this generational cohort may change how aging is defined as they desire to stay youthful. Along with maintaining youthful attitudes, their life expectancy has increased.[10] Yet as the following discussion indicates, Baby Boomers will also inevitably experience changes with an aging body.

Young Old (65–74 Years of Age)

Older adults who are young old may be recently retired and enjoying the results of their years of employment, their essential role as grandparents, and their continuing role as parents in the growth of their adult children. They have increased leisure time to pursue interests and to develop new ones. They may choose to do volunteer work with a community service, return to school, or travel. Some older adults, however, because of economic incentive or other personal reasons, will decide to remain in the workforce.[14] Others, because of family circumstances, may reassume the role of raising children with their grandchildren. The young old must often cope with chronic conditions such as osteoarthritis, hypertension, and cardiovascular disease. However, these chronic conditions are often managed medically and usually do not represent a major barrier to functioning or satisfactory occupational role performance.

Middle Old (75–85 Years of Age)

In the middle old period of life, more changes may be evident. These older adults may make modifications in their occupational role performance. They may reduce or simplify their lives in various ways, including resting during the day, volunteering less, traveling less, and limiting distance of trips. They may rely more on social systems such as Meals on Wheels, public transportation, and family for some assistance with ADLs (Fig. 1.1). OTAs may provide interventions when necessary. The frequent loss of significant others brings affective stressors and additional role changes (see Chapter 2 for a discussion of specific theories explaining the stages of aging).

Old Old (85 Years of Age and Older)

During the old old period of life, older adults may reflect on the meaning of their lives, the quality of their relationships, and their contributions to society. They may think about the losses they are experiencing and about their own deaths. This may be a time of peace and generosity; older adults in the old old period of life may find it meaningful to give valued objects to loved ones who will treasure them. Conversely, it can be a period of fear and anger resulting from unresolved conflicts. Resolution of these

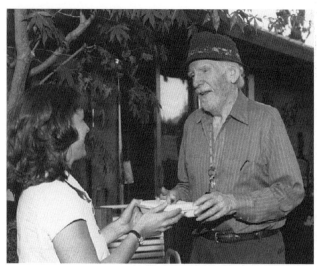

FIG. 1.1 Lifestyle adaptations for older adults. Some older adults may use Meals on Wheels to maintain nutrition and remain in their own homes.

conflicts can make this the most spiritual and fulfilling period for older adults. Personal growth and reflection continue throughout life.

This time in an older adult's life is usually a period of further systemic change affecting the sensory, motor, cardiac, and pulmonary systems. Chronic conditions impair self-maintenance capacities, and adults in the old old stage may need personal assistance with bathing, mobility, dressing, and money management that OTAs and others can provide. If these older adults live independently, they may need some family member support. As previously discussed, older adults may have multiple chronic conditions and require more health care and caregiver support.

An alternative health care delivery option to help frail older adults primarily in the middle old and old old age group is a national demonstration project called Program for All-Inclusive Care of the Elderly (PACE).[15] PACE addresses older adults' preventive, acute, and long-term health care needs, providing medical and support services to help keep older adults in their homes and communities after they have been certified to need skilled nursing home care. PACE is financially supported by monthly capitation payments from Medicare and Medicaid or by private pay. In general, the goal of the project is to demonstrate that older adults remain independent longer when their health care delivery system is sensitive and responsive to their medical, rehabilitative, social, and emotional needs. This project provides alternative models of long-term care such as adult day care, primary health care, rehabilitation, home care, transportation, housing, nutritional services, social services, and hospitalization. An interdisciplinary team manages care management. OTs and OTAs are important team members with their strong skills of prevention, adaptation, and restoration of function.

PACE has been demonstrated to reduce inpatient hospitalizations, improve certain aspects of quality of care, and decrease mortality rates. And while the PACE project incurs higher Medicaid costs initially, over time the cost is consistent with that of care for comparison enrollees.[16] PACE may be one answer to the ethical and economic dilemmas regarding ways to meet the increasing needs of elders as they live longer in a health care climate of declining resources and advancing technology.

DEMOGRAPHICAL DATA AND THE GROWTH OF THE AGED POPULATION

Demography is "the study of populations, especially with reference to size, density, fertility, mortality, growth rate, age distribution, migration, and vital statistics."[5] Demographic data clearly suggest that the aged population is growing. This growth is often referred to in the literature as "the graying of America." The portion of the older population that consists of those 65 years or older comprises 16% of the total US population. This population is expected to continue growing; "the older population is beginning to burgeon again as more than one-third (41%) of the 'baby boom' generation is now age 65 and older" (p. 4).[4] The older generation is projected to be 21.6% of the total population by the year 2040.[4] Minority older populations also are growing rapidly and are projected to represent 34% of the older population by the year 2040 compared to 19% of the older population in 2008.[4] Future generations of older adults will be more ethnically and racially variant than the current older population. By 2060, the older white population is projected to decline from 76.5% to 55% of the total older population. The growth of the minority populations will be greatest among Hispanics, who are projected to account for 21% of the older population in 2060.[6] Many factors contribute to this significant population growth, including a declining mortality rate, advances in medicine and sanitation, and enhanced technology. Other factors are improved diet, increased awareness of risk factors for disease, and elevated health expectancy with better chronic illnesses management.[10] Fig. 1.2 illustrates the growth of the older population.

Accompanying the "graying of America" is a growth of the female aged population. For every 100 men older than 65 years, there are 125 women. This ratio increases with age. There are 181 women for every 100 men in the 85 years and older age group.[4] Women, though, are much more likely to live with a disability, which is often defined as "a lack of ability to perform activity,"[5] such as ADLs, and indicates a need for occupational therapy intervention.

About 31% of women older than 65 years are widows, and there are more than three times as many widows as widowers.[4] These statistics have broad sociocultural implications. A major consequence for some older women with the loss of a spouse is an increased risk for poverty.

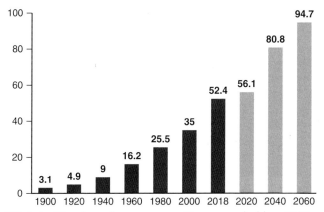

FIG. 1.2 Number of persons age 65 years and older: 1900–2060 (numbers in millions). *(From Administration on Aging: Profile of Older Americans: 2019, Department of Health and Human Services.)*

In 2018, older women had a higher poverty rate (9.7%) as compared to older men (8.1%), and a higher percentage of older individuals living alone were more likely to be poor (17.3%) than those living with families.[4] Hispanic women who lived alone experienced the highest poverty rates at 37.8%.[4]

The Aging of the Aged Population

The fastest growing segment of the older adult population is the 85 years and older cohort. As of 2018, adults older than 85 years numbered 6.5 million, and their size is projected to increase to 14.4 million by 2040.[6] The 85 years and older cohorts have their own unique needs for services in the home and in the community because they may have more difficulty with physical and social functioning.[17] The 85 years and older cohorts are at risk for health problems such as cardiovascular disease, osteoporosis, dementia, and vision and hearing problems, and the rising rate of obesity in the aging population will only increase these health risks.[17] The risk for serious injuries from falling rises as aging progresses because the number of risk factors increases.[17] Risk factors for falls can include issues such as having a chronic condition, decreased reaction time and other cognitive changes, decreased visual acuity, or environmental factors such as poor lighting in the home.[17] (Refer to Chapter 14 for more information about falls.) In addition, the risk for severe cognitive impairment is much greater in the 85 years and older age group. Approximately, 23% of men and 24% of women aged 85 years and older experience dementias, including Alzheimer's disease, compared to 4% of men and 2% of women between 65 and 74 years of age.[6] The prevalence of Alzheimer's disease is increasing with a trend toward more older adults having the condition.[1] Not surprisingly, the 85 years and older group uses a large amount of health, financial, and social services provided by public policies such as Medicare.[6] The current older adult population, one of many groups of Americans who can qualify for Medicaid, spends the highest amount of Medicaid funds.[18] This large usage of federal money, along with concerns about increasing costs, may have future implications for continual modifications of public policies.

The 85 years and older age cohort is more likely to be institutionalized compared to their younger age cohorts. Although only 1.2 million of the 65 years and older population reside in institutional settings, the amount increases from 1% of people ages 65–74 to 7% for those 85 years and older.[4] The need for long-term care is anticipated to increase as this age group grows, especially for those with no living children or those living alone without other supports.[19]

Although there are more older adults among the 85 years and older population than in any age cohort who live in nursing homes and other long-term care facilities, the majority still reside in the community.[19] Living in the community presents challenges because of the need for assistance with ADL functions for some older adults.[4] ADLs include bathing, toileting, dressing, personal hygiene and grooming, eating, and getting around the house. Instrumental activities of daily living (IADL) include preparing meals, shopping, managing money, using a telephone, doing housework, caring for others, and taking medication.[7]

Many older adults require a support system to have assistance with ADLs. Currently, nearly half (44%) of women 75 years and older live by themselves in households, and only 49% of women (and 72% of men) 65 years and older live with a spouse.[4] Many members of this age cohort also live with family members such as adult children who help with ADL functions. The majority of care in the community is informally provided by family members, usually spouses and adult daughters.[19] A future trend that may influence the type of caregiving needed for some members of the Baby Boom generation as they become the older adult generation is a larger percentage of couples that are childless or unmarried. These Baby Boomers should plan ahead and learn about community resources before they need them.[20]

Another important factor to consider is that some older adults, particularly the old old age group, have relatively minimal formal education. However, the education level of all older adults is increasing.[6] The number of older adults completing a high school education increased from 23.5% in 1965 to 86.4% in 2018. Approximately 29.3% of older adults have a baccalaureate degree or higher level of graduate education.[6] Knowing the educational level of their clients will help OTAs adjust or determine the instruction or training. (Refer to Chapter 5 for a discussion of health literacy, which influences education.)

The Oldest of the Old: The Centenarians

An even older and more quickly growing group of older adults are the centenarians, or those older adults living

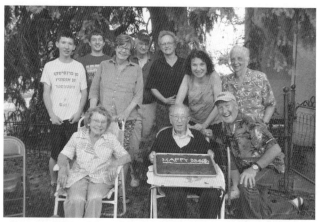

FIG. 1.3 This older adult celebrates his 100.5 birthday surrounded by family and friends. *(Courtesy Michael Lohman.)*

beyond 100 years. Between 1980 and 2010, this population increased by 65.8% (Fig. 1.3).[21] Researchers are fascinated about factors contributing to this longevity. Lifestyle, genes, environment, social connections, resiliency, and adaptability are researched contributors to longevity.[10,22] Of these factors, environmental influences on lifestyle appear to strongly affect longevity, although further research is warranted.[22] Debate as to whether centenarians represent a model of successful aging is ongoing, as portions of this population experience more years of age-related illness and severely compromised physical health due to their longevity, while others do not live with age-related ailments for extended periods of time. This population appears to be minimally impacted by cognitive impairment.[21] Centenarians mainly experience a rapid decline in health status in their final years of life.[23] Centenarians tend to escape or delay chronic illnesses during their lifetimes,[10,22] but may also be at risk of higher social isolation and experience more social dysfunction than younger cohorts.[21]

LIVING ARRANGEMENTS

OTAs working in geriatric practice need to consider the older adult's home environment because housing problems can negatively affect the older adult's physical and psychological well-being.[6] Age influences living arrangements. More than half of people over age 65 live with spouses and 28% of older adults live alone.[4] The majority of older adults living alone are women who outlive their husbands.[4]

There are a variety of living options available for older adults. For older adults with few economic resources, low-income housing is available. However, the number of units is limited, and there may be long waiting lists or lottery systems for applicants. Continuing Care Residential Communities and Life-Care Community Housing are other alternatives for older adults with low incomes. In some cases, residents are required to contribute all of their assets. Residents have contracts for housing,

supportive services, and often a continuum of services that include health and nursing facilities.

Assisted living facilities are a growing and dynamic living option for older adults and adults with disabilities and have been available in the United States since the mid-1980s.[24] In assisted living facilities, older adults receive person-centered care management and supportive services to enable maximal independence in a homelike setting. Assisted living residents need some help to remain independent but do not require the same level of 24-hour care provided in nursing home facilities.[24] More than 50% of assisted living residents are 85 years or older and the majority are women.[24] Residents of assisted living facilities typically need assistance with some ADLs, with bathing and walking being the two most common.[24] Most residents use private funds to finance assisted living.[24] However, some older adults can receive help to finance assisted living through Medicaid in some states. However, Medicare, the major insurer of older adults, does not cover assisted living facility costs or any long-term care.[24] The growth of assisted living is attributed to the increase in the aged population and the desire of older adults to have their own home and not go into nursing homes.[25] There is significant variability in the types of assisted living facilities, and this variability, as well as the expensive costs for residents, are areas of discussion.[25] Additionally, because there are no federal regulations for assisted living facilities and inconsistency in the way that states regulate them,[25] it would be beneficial for OTAs who practice in them to learn their state regulations.

Board and care homes, personal care, adult day care, adult foster care, family care, and adult congregate living facilities are other alternative care options in the community. Board and care homes service older adults, many of whom have been deinstitutionalized. Adult day care is a community-based group program designed to meet the needs of functionally impaired older adults. This structured, comprehensive program delivers a variety of health, social, and related support services in a protective setting during any part of the day but provides less than 24-hour care. Adult foster homes are family homes or other facilities that offer residential care for older or physically disabled residents not related to the provider by blood or marriage. Adult congregate living facilities provide seniors with high-rise living accommodations with innovative service delivery options such as team laundry, cleaning, shopping, congregate meals, and home-delivered meals. Home health services are available but are usually restricted to more acute episodic needs and require some level of homebound restrictions for reimbursement by Medicare (see Chapter 6). Private agencies can provide home caregiving support, such as with meal prepar, but for a cost. For those older adults with assets, retirement communities are another living option and include a variety of services such as leisure activities, congregate meals, laundry, transportation, and possibly health care.

Aging in Place

Aging in place, or living independently in one's current household or community with adequate support for as long as possible,[26] is a trend expected to influence present and future older generations A high percentage of adults aged 50 and older (nearly 80%), and Baby Boomers in particular, desire to age in place according to research by the AARP.[27,28] Aging in place can be perceived as involving more than just an older adult's home, including also the broader community considering the accessibility and availability of services, amenities, and transportation.[26] Taking into account the broader community addresses an older adult's context and environment as is discussed in the OTPF-4.[7] Older adults desire affordable housing, well-kept and convenient health care facilities, parks, and streets with easy-to-read traffic signs.[28]

Goals of aging in place include allowing older adults a good quality of life by enabling them to stay in their homes, participate in their communities, and modify their homes to permit aging in place.[26] Aging in place is so valued by older adults that they are willing to consider other living options such as home sharing, accessory dwelling units (second smaller home on the same property), or villages with services.[28]

Along with aging in place is the phenomenon of Naturally Occurring Retirement Communities (NORC), which are apartments or communities of single-family homes comprising older adult populations that remain in their home and age together.[29] Older adults living in NORCs can work together to provide enough resources to help the residents maintain a high quality of life.[29] Some health care professionals are choosing to become Certified Aging in Place Specialists (CAPS). With this certification developed by the National Association of Home Builders Remodelers Council (NAHB) along with AARP, health care practitioners are trained in understanding the specific needs of older adults for home modification to promote older adults aging in their home residence for longer.[30]

Another growing trend within the concept of aging in place is universal design, an approach that focuses on creating built environments and products that are accessible and usable by all people regardless of physical, cognitive, or sensory impairments.[31] Within a home environment, some universal design principles include no-step entrances, wider doorways, and curb-less showers. These standards are being encouraged in new construction homes and projects.[31] According to research conducted by AARP, only about 1% of homes in the United States have five key features that ensure accessibility which include no-step entry to the home, living spaces all on the first floor, outlets and light switches at reachable heights, hallways and doors that are wider, and door handles and faucets that are levers.[31] Given this and the large number of older adults that desire to remain in their homes as they age, home modifications become necessary to allow aging in place to be possible.

Aging in place is also sometimes perceived as a market-driven concept where older adults in a facility receive various levels of care. Thus, older adults might start out on an independent living unit and, when their functional status changes, then move to an assisted living unit and eventually to a skilled nursing unit or even a memory care unit, all in the same facility. This is referred to as Continuing Care Retirement Communities (CCRC).[29] OTAs working in these facilities can provide intervention as the resident's functional status changes.

For those older adults who desire to remain in their homes and communities, support services such as adult day care, meal programs, senior centers, and transportation services can help them age in place.[29] If they can afford home support services from a private company, that too may enable them to age in place. Aging in place is a trend that occupational therapy practitioners should pay close attention to follow.

Financial Aspects of Living Arrangements

Most of these discussed living options require adequate financial assets and good retirement planning because long-term care is costly. In 2020, the national average cost for living in an assisted living apartment was $4300 per month or approximately $51,600 a year.[32] Nursing home yearly costs vary across the country with an average cost of $255 daily or almost $93,075 yearly for a semiprivate room and an average cost of $290 daily or approximately $105,850 annually for a private room.[32] As discussed, Medicare does not cover long-term care.[33] Some older adults have shifted their finances to qualify for Medicaid, a program that provides some long-term care coverage for the indigent. However, the Deficit Reduction Act of 2005 now imposes a period of ineligibility for older adults who give away assets or resources to qualify for Medicaid.[34]

Most federal funds for older adults go for institutional care rather than home and community services. However, there has been a movement toward care in the community financially supported by the Centers for Medicare and Medicaid (CMS) which was expedited with the Coronavirus pandemic.[35] Some states operate under the Money Follows the Person (MFP) programs that aid in transitioning individuals from institutions such as nursing homes to community and home-based care, a more cost-effective option and typically preferred by older adults.[35] Other options for funding community services besides Medicaid were provided in the Older Americans Act (see Chapter 6).

Long-term care insurance is an alternative to help people plan for their future long-term care needs. Plans differ but usually cover a variety of long-term care supports such as assisted living, nursing home, meal services, respite services, and home health. Coverage is usually based on the policy's eligibility criteria of either having difficulty with a set number of ADLs or having a cognitive impairment.[33] Generally, it is more financially advantageous to purchase a plan when one is younger, which results in lower premiums.[33]

Findings from a study by AP-NORC regarding long-term care found that about 36% of respondents over 40 years of age were very or extremely confident in their ability to pay for long-term care in the future, which demonstrates a trend of increasing confidence.[36] One-third of the respondents in this study reported no planning for their future long-term care.[36] Additionally, one-fourth of the study participants were not familiar with the fact that Medicare does not cover long-term care.[36] Given these findings, education regarding long-term care planning and long-term care insurance will continue to be a subject of significant discussion as more Baby Boomers age and enter the older adult cohort.

Finally, recent data on community-resident older adults age 65 or older suggest that 34% reported having some sort of disability ranging from difficulty with hearing, vision, cognition, ambulation, self-care, and independent living.[4] These data highlight the need for occupational therapy intervention in any of the discussed settings.

ECONOMIC FACTORS

Most older adults are not impoverished. Data suggest that medium-income older adults account for 30% and high-income older adults account for 40% of the total older adult population.[6] However, the economic status of the older adult population has been variable. The poverty rate in the 1960s was almost 30% for older adults aged 65 and older.[6] Since the early 2000s, however, the poverty rate has been significantly reduced and continues to remain fairly stable, hovering around 9%–10% for those older adults aged 65 and older.[6] The current poverty rate for the older adult population is approximately 10%.[4,6] Several factors influence an older adult becoming at risk for poverty, including reduced working hours, the rising cost of housing and health expenses, and loss of preretirement savings.[37,38] General risk indicators of becoming impoverished after retirement are work history, occupational type, retirement savings, and preretirement income.[39]

Older women have a greater poverty rate than older men. Approximately 9.7% of older women are below the poverty line compared to 8.1% of older men.[4] The economic statuses of older men and women differ due to many factors. When they were younger, older women were generally housewives, took time off from work for caregiving or worked only occasionally at paid employment, often resulting in lower wages. This resulted in fewer Social Security benefits and smaller, or no, pensions leading to lower retirement savings for women in general. Additionally, older women who are not married as a result of being widowed, divorced, or never married are more likely to be impoverished due to the lack of a second income during retirement.[40] Older women in minorities are especially at risk for poverty due to lower lifetime earnings and accruing fewer assets during their working years.[41]

Although there are differences across ethnic groups in rates of poverty, a wide economic disparity exists between white older adults and older adults of minority groups. Approximately 7.3% of white older adults are poor compared to 18.9% of Black older adults, 11.7% of Asian older adults, and 19.5% of Hispanic older adults.[4] Older Hispanic women living alone have the highest poverty rate at 37.8%.[4] Due to being at risk for lower lifetime wages as well as fewer retirement savings and assets, older adult minorities rely more heavily on social security than whites as they age.[42]

Public policy influences the older population's economic status. Social Security provides retirement income for older adults, and Supplemental Security Income delivers some financial support for lower income older adults.[42] Social security is a significant source of income for those over 65 years of age.[6] Overall, these public policies have proven to be antipoverty measures for older adults, with a study suggesting that social security helped 35% of the older adult population stay above the poverty line.[42]

Changes are projected to occur because of concerns related to the economic solvency of Social Security. Amendments to the Social Security Act in 1983 gradually increased the age in which upcoming generations of older adults can start receiving Social Security.[43] The current social security retirement age for those born in 1955 is 66 years and 2 months; it will eventually increase to 67 years for those born after 1960.[43] Early retirement benefits can still be taken at age 62; however, there is a reduction of the benefits, if taken early.[43] The economic solvency of Social Security is related to an increasing aging population with fewer tax dollars in the federal budget to pay for benefits with social security currently projected to only be able to pay 75% of its benefits beginning in 2033.[43] Discussed reforms are higher payroll taxes, benefit cuts, or privatizing retirement funds. Social Security reform will be an important discussion throughout the rest of this century, as the population continues to age.

Changes in Medicare and Medicaid policy will also continue to affect the economic status of the older population, especially if older adults are required to pay more money for health care. These programs which finance the health care and some long-term care (Medicaid) of older adults are highly scrutinized. This is due to these program's ties to the US economy and the increasing numbers of baby boomers becoming eligible for Medicare each year. At the time of this writing, with the Affordable Care Act, some positive benefits for Medicare beneficiaries were improved coverage for preventive services, such as annual physicals. Yet cost changes have occurred with other areas of Medicare, such as for therapy payment in skilled nursing facilities with the Patient-Driven Payment Model (PDPM), which focuses on value and the more complex patients rather than volume of care.[44] Other factors such as the increasing costs of health care and the general state of the American economy also influence the economic status of older adults. For example, after the events of September 11, 2001, and in 2008, the stock market took a downswing, which decreased many retirement funds, and the long-range impact of the Coronavirus pandemic on the economic status of older adults (see Chapter 6 for a discussion about public policy) remains to be seen.

ADDITIONAL TRENDS AND THE INFLUENCE OF AGING TRENDS ON OCCUPATIONAL THERAPY PRACTICE

OTAs working with older adults need to be aware of aging trends. This section discusses three additional trends that affect older adults and their possible influence on OTA practice. One growing trend is older adults raising grandchildren. Reasons for this phenomenon vary and can result from parental substance abuse, parental neglect or abuse, teen pregnancy, divorce, incarceration, deportation due to immigration status, illness, death or disability, and the increasing number of single-parent families.[45] Grandparents in a parenting role can range in age from their 30s to 70s and even older.[45,46] Approximately 7.5 million children in the United States are living with a grandparent and grandparents are the primary caregivers for about 2.5 million children.[47] Grandparents raising grandchildren occur in all socioeconomic, racial, ethnic, and geographic groups.[47,48] However, grandparent-headed households are more likely to be living in poverty than other family units.[45,48]

Grandparents raising children can experience major challenges. For example, some older adults may be dealing with their own health or financial issues along with the stresses of caregiving, which can cause feelings of anger, guilt, or resentment.[45] It can be difficult to learn to set limits as they did with their children and the cultural differences between generations can contribute to stress.[45] However, some grandparents in a parenting role may find it rewarding to provide a sense of stability and predictability for their grandchildren.[45] OTAs working with older adults raising grandchildren need to be sensitive to the stress and demands, as well as the enjoyment and rewards of this parenting role.

An aging trend that can be observed is an increase in older adults remaining in the workforce. In 2019, 20.2% of older adults aged 65 and older remained working or were seeking employment.[4] In a 2017 survey conducted by the Employee Benefit Research Institute (EBRI), 14% of the workers surveyed reported that their decision for retirement age had increased in the past year.[49] The primary reasons for this retirement age increase included, being unable to afford retirement, lack of trust in social security, as well as mounting health care costs.[49] The 2022 EBRI Retirement Confidence Survey (RCS) reported that 70% workers anticipate working for pay during retirement; however, only 27% of retirees report that they have worked for pay during retirement.[49,50] Many of those retirees who work for pay report doing so for positive reasons, such as staying active and involved, or for the enjoyment of employment.[49] However, some do report having financial reasons for working, such as wanting to buy extra items, needing to meet expenses, or seeing a decrease in their personal savings or investments.[49]

The percentages of older adults remaining employed have varied over the past 40 years with the greatest percentage occurring in the 1960s. Since the late 1990s, the percentage of older adults remaining in the workforce has gradually increased,[6] and projections are for a continual growth of older adults in the workforce through 2024, especially as the Baby Boomer generation ages.[51] Since the increase in older adults participating in the workforce beginning in the 1960s, the gap between older men and women who are a part of the labor force has narrowed with only a 12% difference.[6] Many older workers choose to work into their later years because of healthier lifestyles and longer life expectancies, as well as having more education.[51] Additionally, public policy changes, such as the 1983 amendments with the Social Security Act and concerns over social security solvency, will influence the next generation of older adults to remain in the workforce. These amendments allow increases in payment if retirement is delayed between ages 65 and 69 and, as discussed earlier, full Social Security benefits will be extended until a person is 67 years old.[43] The Age Discrimination in Employment Act of 1967 and its amendments along with the removal of required retirement laws also help older workers remain in the workforce.

The influence of an aging labor force on OT practice remains to be seen. However, innovative therapists may identify new areas of practice to ensure continual success of older adults in the workforce.

A third trend influencing older adults is the increased use of technology including computers, smartphones, and other technology products. A survey conducted by the AARP reports that approximately 91% of individuals over the age of 50 use a computer.[52] This same survey reports that 94% recognize the benefits of technology such as decreasing isolation and providing telemedical support.[52] Older adults who desire more intergenerational contact can communicate through email, Facebook, and instant messaging. Furthermore, computers can assist older adults with making purchases, which is a helpful benefit for those who are homebound. Computers have also become an educational source of lifelong learning by providing opportunities for older adults to take classes and watch how-to tutorials about various topics. As indicated by the AARP survey, 23% of older adults are taking online classes to work toward a degree or certificate.[52] In addition to computer usage, more than 80% of older adults ages 50–64 have a smartphone that they use regularly, which is comparable to the general population.[52]

While many older adults own many technology devices and regularly use them, according to Pew research, only 26% of older adults age 65 or older reported feeling very confident in their ability to navigate technology.[53] Some older adults have physical challenges that interfere with their ability to utilize technology. Adaptive computer programs aid older adults with disabilities. For example, voice recognition programs help older adults who have arthritis and difficulty with keyboarding. Older adults with low vision can benefit from many computer programs geared for their visual needs or they can increase font sizes on their smartphones and other handheld technology devices. OTAs can suggest computer resources in the community, such as state sites supported by the Assistive Technology Act, which provides computer training or libraries. They can recommend appropriate software and apps to assist older adults with functional concerns and can make adaptations to allow computer usage. (Options for software and apps will be suggested throughout this book.)

In summary, these three highlighted trends are examples from many trends influencing older adults. As the older generation continues to grow and as society continues to change, it will be paramount that OTAs remain aware of aging trends and consider them in terms of society and OT practice.

Implications for Occupational Therapy Practice

Due to the growth of the older population, as the Baby Boomer generation continues to age, the need for OTs and OTAs to work with them will increase. The effects of the demographics, issues, and trends discussed in this chapter on OT practice remain to be seen. However, it can be assumed that, in the future, dilemmas related to limited resources will affect the practice arena. In the coming years, as the Baby Boomer cohort reaches 85 years of age, there may be increased burdens on families and society.[19] At this time, no one can predict whether there will be adequate funding and social services to meet the needs of the growing older population and whether there will be enough health care resources to address this population's health care needs. The increasing cost of health care,[54] the ever-changing economy, and the tenuous state of Social Security are current concerns that have future implications for the aged population. OT personnel will continue to be challenged to provide quality intervention in a cost-constrained environment. New models of OT care for older adults will evolve in the future, especially in community settings, where the majority of older adults reside. All OT practitioners should be at the front end of this evolution.

INTERGENERATIONAL CONCEPTS AND GENERATIONAL COHORTS

In today's society, same-age cohorts socialize, for the most part, among themselves and have minimal intergenerational contact. When they work in a SNF, OTAs may have little daily interaction with older adults in the community. OTAs provide intervention for older adults who are often two or three generations removed. Yet OTAs must have meaningful contact, either informally or formally, with both community and institutionalized older adults to work effectively with that population. Many benefits are mentioned in the literature about formal intergenerational programs. Some of these benefits include a better understanding of the older generation from a historical perspective and their values and beliefs,[55] increased positive views of older adults,[56,57] improved social skills and academic performance for youth, as well as improved socialization, well-being, health outcomes, and emotional support for older adults.[56,57] These formal intergenerational programs have been shown to be effective to help reconnect older adults to the larger community and reintegrate them into society.[58]

In recent literature, there has been significant discussion about generational cohorts referring to a group of "individuals who were born at a similar time" (p. X).[59] Other classical defining factors of generational cohorts are being from the same area and experiencing similar historical and social events.[60] Thus, generational cohorts experience comparable social and historical occurrences, including shifts in technological advancements, political changes, and social movements, that predispose them to related life perspectives.[59] From an OT standpoint, context, including both personal and environmental factors,[7] are some considerations with a population of generational cohorts. Current generations are divided into several groups, each with its own characteristics (Table 1.1). In reviewing this table, consider generational traits and historical/social factors that influenced the generational cohort that you are from as well as from the generations that you will work with as an OTA. Table 1.1 also emphasizes concepts about approaching interventions with the current older generations—the Traditionalist/Silent Generation and the newest older generation of the Baby Boomers. Some considerations when determining interventions are how each generation approaches work, reward, communication, learning, and authority. Contemplate how you can capitalize on the generational characteristics to maximize interventions. Also, while reading this discussion, keep in mind that there is individual variation in any generational cohort based on each individual's life experiences. Individuals born closer to the end or beginning of a generational cohort may take on traits from their own or the previous or next generational cohort. Therefore, ideas presented in this discussion should be viewed as general guidelines.

Consider the influence that post-WWII and the Korean War had on the current oldest older generation. That generation, the Traditionalists, or sometimes called the Silent Generation were born between 1925 and 1942. The younger members of this group came of age after the "Greatest Generation," the oldest members who experienced WWII as young adults. These younger Silent Generation members went through WWII as children, the

TABLE 1.1

Intergenerational Factors to Consider With Therapy With the Current Older Generational Cohorts

Generational cohort	Birth years	Historical and contextual influences	Sample characteristics	Elder generation as clients in therapy
Traditionalist (Veterans and Silent Generation)	1928–1945	Great Depression WWII Korean War Postwar building of America (GI Bill) Cold War	Appreciate hierarchal organizational structure "Chain of Command" Loyal Disciplined Value tradition and are conformers Formal in approach Articulate with writing and speaking	Respect of health care team Hard worker Adherence to intervention program Value formal communication with intervention and education Value compassionate approach Value in person communication (not technological-based)
Baby Boomer	1946–1964	Assassination of John F. Kennedy and Martin Luther King Jr. Cuban Missile Crisis Civil Rights Movement Disability Rights Movement Sexual Revolution Vietnam War Television First walk on the moon Watergate	Interactive and team players Strong work ethic and work identification Driven and ambitious High expectations of self and others Desire personal satisfaction and self-realization Value learning Value personal communication Idealistic	Work as a team in intervention (client-centered approach) Value in person communication Works hard Wants to be valued Wants to learn
Generation X	1965–1980	Fall of Berlin Wall Gulf War Challenger Space Shuttle disaster Latchkey children MTV Video games Seeding of Internet	Balance of work, family, and leisure Self-reliant Flexible and at ease with change Informal Focus on quality outcomes Desire support and encouragement Technologically strong part of their lives Value diversity Skeptical of institutions	
Generation Y (Millennial)	1981–1996	September 11 terrorist attacks Oklahoma City bombing Columbine school shooting Internet, cell phones "Baby on Board" generation	Balance of work, family, and leisure Technology large part of their lives Multitasking Success oriented Value recognition Optimistic Altruistic Politically active Social and participative Desire quick reward and feedback Educated generation Diverse generation that tolerates diversity	

Continued

TABLE 1.1

Intergenerational Factors to Consider With Therapy With the Current Older Generational Cohorts—cont'd

Generational cohort	Birth years	Historical and contextual influences	Sample characteristics	Elder generation as clients in therapy
Generation Z	1997–2012	Terrorism Facebook Economy crash Hurricane Katrina Public violence Unemployment Coronavirus Pandemic	Passionate about technology and interact in a digital world Racial and ethnic diversity Well educated May have underdeveloped social skills Like fast delivery, instant gratification Are kinesthetic learners Desire immediate practical information Value individualized learning and more independent in approach Cautious about emotional, physical, and financial safety More risk adverse	

Data from Chicca J, Shellenbarger T. Connecting with generation Z Approaches in nursing education. *Teaching and Learning in Nursing.* 2018;13(3):180–184; Fogg P. When generations collide. *The Chronicle of Higher Education.* 2008;54:B18–B20; Hammill G. Mixing and managing four generations of employees. *FDU Magazine online.* 2005. Retrieved from http://www.fdu.edu/newspubs/magazine/05ws/generations.htm; Fox, M. The coronavirus pandemic is a defining moment for Gen Z-here's how it's impacting their future. 2020. Retrieved from https://www.cnbc.com/2020/06/01/how-the-coronavirus-pandemic-is-shaping-the-future-for-gen-z.html/; Johnson SA, Romanello, ML. Generational diversity: Teaching and learning approaches. *Nurse Educator.* 2005;30(5):212–216; Mueller K. *Communication from the inside out: Strategies for the engaged professional.* Philadelphia: FA Davis; 2010; Pew Research Center. On the cusp of adulthood facing an uncertain future: What we know about Gen Z so far. 2020; retrieved from https://www.pewresearch.org/social-trends/2020/05/14/on-the-cusp-of-adulthood-and-facing-an-uncertain-future-what-we-know-about-gen-z-so-far-2/. Zemke R, Raines C, Filipczak B. Generational gaps in the classroom. *Training* 1999;36(11):48–54.

reconstruction of America post-WWII and the Cold War. The entire cohort are described as the silent generation as they worked hard maintaining the status quo and are not complainers (Fig. 1.4).[61] Based on these traits, older adults from the Silent Generation, in an intervention situation, may be very respectful and adherent to the suggestions of "the authorities" on the health care team. It will be important to ask these older adults how they want to be addressed because many from this generation embrace a formal communication style.[61] The Silent Generation values formality and conformity; therefore, OTAs should be particularly cognizant of their dress and language. Additionally, members of this generation desire a compassionate approach to health care and trust the expertise of the health care professional.[62] Some of them had experienced the Great Depression, or at least were aware of it because of their parent's descriptions, and may be frugal about spending their money, such as for adaptive equipment.

Now consider the Baby Boomer generation that came of age during a time in American history when there was much optimism, prosperity, and yet societal angst and turbulence. Growing up in a secure time post-WWII, Baby Boomers experienced the benefits of an expanding American society with many advances in science and technology. They also experienced the assassination of President Kennedy, Martin Luther King Jr., the Vietnam War, Cuban Missile Crisis, and related unrest. The defining events as the Baby Boomer came of age may have contributed to this generation's belief that their work could change the world and generate societal change.[63] Many societal changes were happening, such as the reformation of Congress to be more liberal, the Civil Rights Movement, and the Disability Rights Movement. Concurrently, the deinstitutionalization of people with mental illness or developmental disabilities was occurring. Growing up in such a prosperous time, many members of the Baby Boomer generation were more educated than those of previous generations.[64] Generational slogans developed during the youthful period of the Baby Boomers reflected their beliefs. The slogan "Make Love Not War" suggested the unrest of the time about the Vietnam War and the sexual revolution. "Don't Trust Anyone Over Thirty" reflected the distrust that the Baby Boomer generation had of people in authority and the previous generations.

According to generational cohort literature, the Baby Boomer generation based on their life experiences have a very different perspective from the present oldest aged

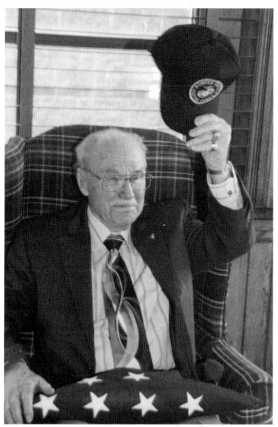

FIG. 1.4 This older adult from the Traditionalist generation, who was a prisoner of war during WWII, values his years of service. *(Courtesy Helene Lohman.)*

population, the Traditionalists/Silent generation. Baby Boomers value a team approach rather than the authoritative leadership approach that the Traditionalist/Silent Generation desires.[65] However, similar to the Traditionalists/ Silent Generation, Baby Boomers value hard work and are very driven in what they do, often thought of as achievers.[66] Baby Boomers desire personal gratification with life's occupations,[65] enjoy learning, and want to be valued.[66] Given their emphasis on hard work and dedication to establishing a career, the Baby Boomer generation has been known for their "workaholic" tendencies, working longer than 40-hour work weeks.[63,65] Recent research suggests that these hardworking characteristics of the Baby Boomer generation are translating into a desire to age productively, through participation in either paid or unpaid work.[67] Aging productively allows these older adults to feel more socially connected and useful and have an overall higher quality of life.[67] Additionally, research indicates that Baby Boomers want to age in place in their homes and remain in their own communities, or move to a community designed for their aging needs.[28]

OTAs contemplating intervention approaches with Baby Boomers, based on generational cohort theory, would recognize that older adults from this generation may need to be approached differently than older adults from the current generational cohort, the Traditionalists/ Silent Generation. With Baby Boomers, OTAs might strongly integrate a client-centered approach or a team partnership with intervention based on this generational cohort values about work and leadership. In addition, OTAs might recognize that Baby Boomers want in-depth education about their condition due to the value and emphasis they place on learning, understanding that they may have already researched their condition before therapy. The OT/OTA therapy team will have a strong role to play in helping older adults from the Baby Boomer generation who desire to age in place or perhaps help design homes in communities for them.

OTAs should familiarize themselves with the characteristics of all generations, including their own, because knowing these characteristics may help enhance a positive influence on intergenerational interactions. The exercise in Fig. 1.5 demonstrates that each generation may have certain values and attitudes that are influenced by similar generational experiences and historical events.[68] Yet each person has his or her own story to tell. This exercise can be completed as a group or individually. The exercise in Box 1.1 will help pull together concepts about working with the youngest aged population, the Baby Boomers.

AGEISM, MYTHS, AND STEREOTYPES ABOUT THE AGED

If you are a man and you are prejudiced against women, you will never know how a woman feels. If you are white and you are prejudiced against blacks, you will never know how a black person feels. But if you are young and you are prejudiced against the old, you are indeed prejudiced against yourself, because you, too, will have the honor of being old someday.

(Lewis, 1989)[69]

The World Health Organization defines ageism as "stereotyping and discrimination against individuals or groups on the basis of their age."[70] Ageism is a form of prejudice because it promotes general assumptions, or stereotypes, about a group of people. These assumptions are not true for all members of the older population and may change to some different expressions of ageism with the Baby Boomer population. Following are some stereotypes expressed with ageism:

- Older adults are useless because they cannot see, hear, or remember.
- Older adults are slow when they move about.
- Older adults are in ill health or are depressed.
- Older adults cannot learn new things.
- Older adults drain the economy rather than contribute to it; they are unproductive.
- Older adults are too old to remain part of the workforce.
- Older adults cannot perform or enjoy sexual activity.

Fill in the following lifelines with significant historical and personal events about yourself, someone from the generation 10 years older than you, one of your parents, and one of your grandparents. After filling in the lifeline, answer the questions below.
Refer to the following example:

Grandparent:

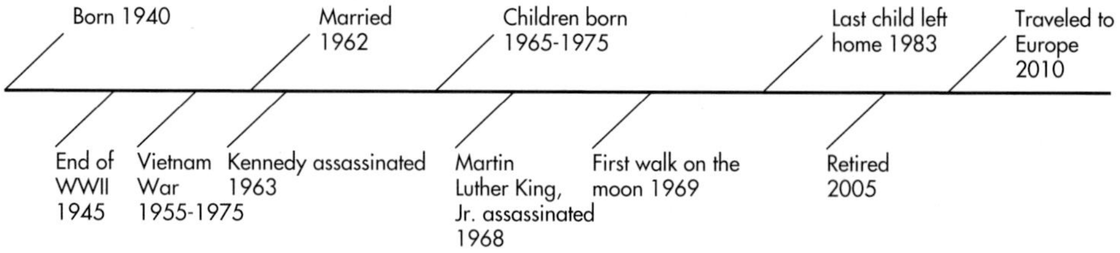

| Born 1940 | Married 1962 | Children born 1965-1975 | | Last child left home 1983 | Traveled to Europe 2010 |

End of WWII 1945 | Vietnam War 1955-1975 | Kennedy assassinated 1963 | Martin Luther King, Jr. assassinated 1968 | First walk on the moon 1969 | Retired 2005

Yourself:

Born

Someone 10 years older than you:

Born

Your parent (choose one):

Born

Your grandparent (choose one):

Born

Answer the following questions:
What significant intergenerational differences did you notice between your generation, your parents' generation, your grandparents' generation, and even the generation 10 years older than you? What are some of the significant values of each generation and how were they influenced by historical events? How might these similarities and differences between generations affect clinical treatment?

FIG. 1.5 Lifeline exercise. *(Adapted from Davis LJ, Kirkland M Rote: The role of occupational therapy with the elderly: Faculty guide. Rockville, MD: American Occupational Therapy Association; 1987, with permission.)*

- Older adults prefer being with and talking with other older adults.
- Older adults complain about all that is new.
- Older adults are rich; or older adults are poor.

Many of these statements have been challenged by research. With any stereotype, there may be a small element of truth for some members of the group. For example, it is true that older adults frequently need glasses as aging progresses; however, the need for glasses does not render an older adult useless. An unfortunate result of these myths is that some older adults may believe them. For example, whereas young persons may

Active Learning Exercises

You have been asked to be on a marketing committee to redesign an assisted living facility to meet the needs of the Baby Boomer generation. What will be your suggestions? Consider concepts of context and environment from the *Occupational Therapy Practice Framework,* fourth edition with this exercise.[7]

joke about becoming forgetful, older adults may seriously question their cognitive abilities if they have trouble remembering something as a result of the stereotype.

These stereotypes may develop as a result of fear of the unknown or from a lack of contact with the aged. American culture often focuses on youth. Youth is seen as beautiful, as something to aspire to and maintain at any cost. Young is sexy and old is not.

The medical system in the United States also has been focused on youth. The goal of this system has traditionally been to find a cure for all illnesses. This goal has prompted significant contributions to the world's health care; however, the belief in a cure for all illness may conflict with the care older adult's need. As with current knowledge about health care, some chronic illnesses of old age can be only managed, not cured.

In the health care system, references to ageism often occur as a response to a medical diagnosis. occupational therapy documentation that begins "This 91-year-old female was admitted with the diagnosis of total hip replacement" may trigger preconceived ideas based on age bias, such as the opinion that the client is too old for intervention. Readers of this type of documentation may question the benefits versus risks of surgery or occupational therapy intervention for this older adult.

In day-to-day interactions, language can encourage ageism. People working in the health care field may unintentionally be condescending when they refer to older adults as "dear" or "sweetie." This type of "elderspeak" can contribute to more negative images of aging and lead to worse functional health over time.[71] "Elderspeak" may also reinforce ideas of dependency and social isolation.[71] Simply referring to a person as "the older stroke patient in Room 570" dehumanizes the person. Stating that a person is incapable of doing a task because of being old or having some deficits without a true understanding of the person's functional abilities also promotes ageism.

The following story illustrates this concept of ageism. At an assisted living facility, there were several older adults who had mild to moderate cognitive deficits. The OTA knew each older adult as a human being and understood each person's identified meaningful occupations. For older adults who valued cooking, the OTA organized a cooking group followed by a party. She adapted the

activity so that all of the older adults would be successful. Before the cooking activity, the team leader expressed negative feelings because she felt that the older adults would be incapable of cooking. The team leader was surprised to observe that the cooking activity turned out to be beneficial and successful for the older adults. The team leader later honestly remarked that often times her feelings of being "protective" of the residents got in her way. Feeling protective of older adults promotes ageism. A protective attitude can encourage assumptions, such as older adults are incapable or older adults are like children. Sometimes staff working with older adults who have cognitive deficits and have regressed in their function can inadvertently talk to them in a childish manner.

Unprofessional actions also can reflect ageism. One OTA who had a very full day skipped an appointment with an older adult assuming that the older adult had a cognitive deficit and would not remember. Later that day, the older adult called the OTA to inquire about what happened. The OTA learned a hard lesson from that experience about her own ageism. As these stories illustrate, reflection often helps people realize their own stereotypical beliefs and attitudes. A way to be more aware of ageism and general attitudes is to record in a journal one's feeling about contact with older adults. Box 1.2 provides reflection questions about ageism that OTAs should ask themselves.

Perspectives are changing as illustrated in initiatives such as the International Classification of Functioning, Disability, and Health (ICF)[72] and *Healthy People 2030.*[73] The ICF is a tool to measure health and disability of individuals and populations.[72] The ICF focuses on the effect of disability rather than cause and considers not just the disease but also the environmental context in which people live.[72]

The Occupational Therapy Practice Framework, fourth edition, reflects some of the perspectives from the ICF. The *Framework* considers the intervention process within the broad "domain" of OT.[7] Similar to the ICF, the *Framework* considers the influence of context and environment on occupation. A person's context is constructed of both environmental and personal factors that include the person's natural physical surroundings, technology and products, relationships, attitudes, and features of the person's background. These contextual

Reflection Questions About Ageism

How did I respond to the elders I saw today?
Am I aware of any actions or language that I used that might promote ageism?
Am I aware of any actions or language that others used that might promote ageism?

factors are considered separate from a person's health condition or health state, such as age, gender, sexual orientation, and culture.[7] As Youngstrom[74] stated, "Occupational therapists [need] to understand their role within a larger societal and health context in order to position themselves in changing traditional areas and to take advantage of opportunities in emerging areas" (p. 607).

Healthy People 2030 envisions "a society in which all people achieve their full potential for health and well-being across the lifespan."[73] It is based on the following five goals: (1) "attain high quality, longer lives free of preventable disease, disability, injury, and premature death; (2) eliminate health disparities, achieve health equity and attain health literacy to improve the health and well-being for all; (3) create social and physical environments that promote attaining the full potential for health and well-being for all; (4) promote healthy development, healthy behaviors and well-being across all life stages; and (5) engage leadership, key constituents, and the public across multiple sectors to take action and design policies that improve the health and well-being of all."[73] All goals affect the older adult population.

Many aspects of American society, including housing, employment, and recreational resources, are geared toward youth. However, that focus is slowly changing with the emergence of the senior citizen as a powerful political and economic force and with the growth of the aged population. Who knows what changes the next generation of entering older adults of Baby Boomers will bring to society?

CASE STUDY

Peter and Alice, both 68 years old, have been married for 46 years and raised four children. They live in the home they built 35 years ago to accommodate their growing family. Responsibilities of raising children, getting them to and from their activities, and Peter's work schedule left little time to think about their distant future. Retirement, possible illness/accidents, or financial needs were not concerns. The "future" seemed like a long way away; however, much to their surprise, the future they put off planning for became a reality. Although they had had many conversations about retiring during the past 3 years, due to financial reasons, they both remain in the workforce. Peter has a manual labor job and worries about the physical toll it is beginning to take on his body. Alice returned to work as an office manager for a small company when their youngest child was in the fourth grade. Initially, she worked part time so she could be home when the children were home from school and during the summer. She eventually moved to working full time.

Both Peter and Alice feel that they are among the oldest employees and seem to have nothing in common with their younger colleagues. They often comment to each other about differing values, respect, and work ethics. They have heard comments from the younger employees about their age, lack of speed, and abilities. They also worry that they will be the first to be let go if layoffs occur. Financially, they remortgaged their home several times to help defray costs of college and weddings and, as a result, find themselves with a mortgage

payment. They have talked about moving to a smaller house, but their real desire is to stay in the home they built. One of the children recently proposed moving in with them to help defray costs. This would mean two more adults and three young children living together. Peter and Alice have apprehensions regarding how a multigenerational household can be cohesive. Currently, Peter is able to keep up with the outside maintenance. However, he has noticed it is becoming more difficult as he needs to take breaks before completing tasks like cutting the lawn. He does not express this change in status to anyone. Alice also enjoys the outdoors and loves to garden but has found she can no longer bend safely to pull weeds or plant new flowers. She has also noticed that her hands are a "little stiff," and it has become harder to complete everyday tasks like dusting and vacuuming as well as opening small containers or tight lids. Alice experienced a fall about a year ago but because she was not injured, she did not tell anyone.

Peter and Alice belong to a card club, have good friends, occasionally go out to eat or to a movie, and enjoy attending family events. They wonder if they will ever be like many of their friends who are now enjoying a well-deserved retirement.

■ CASE STUDY QUESTIONS

1 Identify some interventions that could be used in the work environments of Peter and Alice for multigenerational understanding/tolerance.
2 Identify some interventions that would help Alice participate in ADLs/IADLS.
3 State some recommendations that could be made for Peter and Alice to "age in place."
4 Give examples of the advantages and disadvantages to multigenerational cohabitation.

■ CHAPTER REVIEW QUESTIONS

1 Define the terms gerontology, geriatrics, and cohort.
2 What is the relationship between aging and illness?
3 What is a client-centered approach? How might it affect client care?
4 What considerations should be taken for managing clients with chronic illnesses?
5 What factors are related to the significant population growth of the older adult generation?
6 What is a result of more widows than widowers among the older adult population?
7 What are some of the needs of the 85 years and older generation?
8 What does the OTA need to know about the educational level of any older adult for intervention?
9 What age group has the highest poverty rate and why?
10 How has public policy influenced the economic status of older adults?
11 What are some implications of the demographical data for future occupational therapy practice?
12 How do you think the three discussed trends (grandparents raising children, aging workforce, and increased computer usage) can affect occupational therapy practice?

13 How do you keep abreast of aging trends?

14 What is ageism? Provide examples of it in today's culture. How do you think expressions of ageism might differ or stay the same with the Baby Boomers?

15 What were misconceptions you had about growth of the aged population, minority older adults, the old old (85 years and older), economic demographics, and living arrangements before reading this chapter?

16 What are some of your ideas about what will happen as the Baby Boomers are now part of the older generation?

REFERENCES

1. Alzheimer's Association. *2020 Alzheimer's Disease Facts and Figures*. 2020. Available at: https://www.alz.org/media/Documents/alzheimers-facts-and-figures.pdf.
2. American Occupational Therapy Association. *AOTA 2019 Workforce and Salary Survey*. Bethesda, MD: AOTA Press; 2019.
3. Harris-Kojetin L, Sengupta M, Lendon JP, Rome V, Valverde R, Caffrey C. Long-term care providers and services users in the United States, 2015–2016. National Center for Health Statistics. *Vital Health Stat 3*. 2019;(43).
4. US Department of Health and Human Services (DHHS). 2019 Profile of Older Americans. Accessed from https://acl.gov/sites/default/files.
5. Stedman TL. *Stedman's Medical Dictionary*. 28th ed. Baltimore: Lippincott Williams & Wilkins; 2006.
6. Federal Interagency Forum on Aging Related Statistics. *Older Americans 2020: Key Indicators of Well-Being*. 2016. Available at: https://agingstats.gov/docs/LatestReport/OA20_508_10142020.pdf.
7. American Occupational Therapy Association. Occupational therapy practice framework: domain and process – fourth edition. *Am J Occup Ther*. 2020;74:7412410010. doi:10.5014/ajot.2020.74S2001.
8. Law M, Baptiste S, Carswell A, et al. *Canadian Occupational Performance Measure*. 3rd ed. Ottawa, Ontario, Canada: CAOT Publications ACE; 1998.
9. Sade RM. The Graying of America: challenges and controversies. *J Law Med Ethics*. 2012;40(1):6-9. doi:10.1111/j.1748-720X.2012.00639.x.
10. *Longevity Research: Unraveling the Determinants of Healthy Aging and Longer Life Spans. Population Reference Bureau*. Available at: https://www.prb.org/todays-research-aging-healthy-aging-longer-life-spans/.
11. Holman HR. The relation of the chronic disease epidemic to the health care crisis. *ACR Open Rheumatol*. 2020;2(3):167-173. doi:10.1002/acr2.11114.
12. American Occupational Therapy Association. Role of occupational therapy in primary care. *Am J Occup Ther*. 2020;74(suppl 3): 7413410040p1-7413410040p16. doi:10.5014/ajot.2020.74S3001.
13. Little W, Vyrain S, Scaramuzzo G, et al. *Introduction to Sociology*. 2nd Canadian ed. BC campus; 2016.
14. Mather M, Jacobsen LA, Pollard KM. *Aging in the United States. Population Reference Bureau Population Bulletin [PDF file]*. 2015. Available at: https://www.prb.org/wp-content/uploads/2016/01/aging-us-population-bulletin-1.pdf.
15. National PACE Association. *PACE by the Numbers*. 2020. Available at: https://www.npaonline.org/sites/default/files/PDFs/4068_pace_infographic_update_dec2020.pdf.
16. Ghosh A, Orfield C, Robert S. *Evaluating PACE: A Review of the Literature*. Assistant Secretary for Planning and Evaluation (ASPE); 2014. Available at:
17. Jaul E, Barron J. Age-related diseases and clinical and public health implications for the 85 Years old and over population. *Front Public.*
18. *2017;5:335. doi:10.3389/fpubh.2017.00335. Available at: https://www.ncbi.nlm.nih.gov/pubmed/29312916.*
19. Paradise J. *Medicaid Moving Forward*. 2015. Available at: http://kff.org/health-reform/issue-brief/medicaid-moving-forward/.
19. Spillman B, Favreault M, Allen EH. *Family Structures and Support Strategies in the Older Population*. Urban Institute; 2020. Available at: https://www.urban.org/sites/default/files/publication/103486/family-structure-and-support-strategies-in-the-older-population.pdf.
20. Chris C. *Who Will Care for Us—The Aging, Childless, and Single Population?* Huffington Post; 2015. Available at: http://www.huffingtonpost.com/carol-marak/who-will-care-for-us---the-aging-childless-and-single-population_b_7890462.html.
21. Jopp D, Park M, Lehrfeld J, Paggi M. Physical, cognitive, social and mental health in near-centenarians and centenarians living in New York City: findings from the Fordham Centenarian Study. *BMC geriatrics* 16.1(2016):1-10.
22. Pignolo RJ. Exceptional human longevity. *Mayo Clin Proc*. 2019;94(1):110-124. doi:10.1016/j.mayocp.2018.10.005.
23. Andersen SL, Sebastiani P, Dworkis DA, et al. Health span approximates life span among many supercentenarians: compression of morbidity at the approximate limit of life span. *J Gerontol A Biol Sci Med Sci*. 2012;67A(4):395-405. doi:10.1093/gerona/glr223.
24. National Center for Assisted Living. *Assisted Living: A Growing Aspect of Long Term Care*. 2019. Available at: https://www.ahcancal.org/Advocacy/IssueBriefs/NCAL_Factsheet_2019.pdf.
25. National Center for Assisted Living (NCAL). *Assisted Living State Regulatory Review 2019*. 2019. Available at: https://www.ahcancal.org/Assisted-Living/Policy/Documents/2019_reg_review.pdf.
26. Guzman S, Viveiros J, Salmon E. *Housing Policy Solutions to Support Aging with Options*. AARP Policy Institute; 2017. Available at: https://www.aarp.org/content/dam/aarp/ppi/2017/06/housing-policy-solutions-to-support-aging-with-options.pdf.
27. Harrell R, Lynott J, Guzman S, Lampkin C. *What is Livable? Community Preferences of Older Adults*. AARP Public Policy Institute; 2014. Available at: https://www.aarp.org/ppi/issues/livable-communities/?migration=rdrct.
28. Binette J, Vasold K. *2018 Home and Community Preferences: A National Survey of Adults Age 18-Plus*. Washington, DC: AARP Research; 2018. Available at: https://doi.org/10.26419/res.00231.001.
29. Seniorresource.com. *Aging in Place*. 2016. Available at: http://www.seniorresource.com/ageinpl.htm.
30. Ageinplace.com. *Introduction to Certified Aging in Place Specialists (CAPS)*. n.d. Available at: http://ageinplace.com/aging-in-place-professionals/certified-aging-in-place-specialists-caps/.
31. Guzman S, Viveiros J, Salomon E. *Expanding Implementation of Universal Design and Visitability Features in the Housing Stock*. AARP Public Policy Institute; 2017. Available at: https://www.aarp.org/content/dam/aarp/ppi/2017/06/expanding-implementation-of-universal-design-and-visitability-features-in-the-housing-stock.pdf.
32. Genworth Financial, Inc. *Genworth Cost of Care: Summary and Methodology*. 2020. Available at: https://pro.genworth.com/riiproweb/productinfo/pdf/131168.pdf.
33. American Health Insurance Plans. *Guide to Long-Term Care Insurance*. 2013. Available at: https://www.ahip.org/wp-content/uploads/2014/02/PRO_817_19_LTC_Guide_Update.pdf.
34. Gosselin J. Medicaid Planning. *Aging Well*. 2009;2(4):26. Available at: http://www.todaysgeriatricmedicine.com/archive/083109p26.shtml.
35. Centers for Medicare and Medicaid Services (CMS). *CMS Announces New Federal Funding for 33 States to Support Transitioning Individuals from Nursing Homes to the Community*. 2020. Available at: https://www.cms.gov/newsroom/press-releases/cms-announces-new-federal-funding-33-states-support-transitioning-individuals-nursing-homes.
36. NORC Center for Public Affairs Research. *Long-Term Care in America: Expectations and Preferences for Care and Caregiving*. 2016. Available at: https://www.longtermcarepoll.org/wp-content/uploads/2017/11/AP-NORC-Long-term-Care-2016_Trend_Report.pdf.

37. National Council on Aging. *Economic Security for Seniors Facts.* 2016. Available at: https://d2mkcg26uvg1cz.cloudfront.net/wp-content/uploads/NCOA-Economic-Security.pdf.

38 National Council on Aging. *Get the facts on economic security for seniors.* 2021. Assessed from https://www.ncoa.org/article/get-the-facts-on-economic-security-for-seniors.

39. Lee S, Sohn S, Rhee E, et al. *Consumption Patterns and Economic Status of Older Households in the United States Bureau of Labor Statistics.* 2014. Available at: http://www.bls.gov/opub/mlr/2014/article/consumption-patterns-and-economic-status-of-older-households.htm.

40. National Institute on Retirement Security. *Still Shortchanged: An Update on Women's Retirement Preparedness.* 2020. Available at: https://www.nirsonline.org/wp-content/uploads/2020/04/Still-Shortchanged-Final.pdf.

41 Justice in Aging. *Older women & poverty.* 2018. Accessed from https://justiceinaging.org/wp-content/uploads/2020/08/Older-Women-and-Poverty.pdf.

42. Shelton A. *Social Security: Who's Counting on It.* AARP Public Policy Institute; 2014. Available at: https://www.aarp.org/content/dam/aarp/research/public_policy_institute/econ_sec/2014/social-security-whos-counting-AARP-ppi-econ-sec.pdf.

43. National Academy of Social Insurance. *What is the Social Security Retirement Age.* n.d. Available at: https://www.nasi.org/learn/socialsecurity/retirement-age.

44. MedPac. *Skilled Nursing Facility Services. Report to Congress: Medicare Payment Policy.* 2020. Available at: http://www.medpac.gov/docs/default-source/reports/mar20_medpac_ch8_sec.pdf.

45. American Academy of Child & Adolescent Psychiatry. *Grandparents Raising Grandchildren.* 2017. Available at: https://www.aacap.org/AACAP/Families_and_Youth/Facts_for_Families/FFF-Guide/Grandparents-Raising-Grandchildren-077.aspx.

46 Legacy Project. *Grandparents today.* n.d. Accessed from https://www.legacyproject.org/guides/gptoday.html.

47. Generations United. *Grandfamilies: Strengths and Challenges.* 2020. Available at: http://www.grandfamilies.org/Portals/0/Documents/Grandfamilies-GeneralFactSheet%20%287%29.pdf.

48 Generations United. Reinforcing a strong foundation: Equitable supports for basic needs of grandfamilies. 2021. Accessed from https://www.gu.org/app/uploads/2021/12/2021-Grandfamilies-Report-Release.pdf

49. Employee Benefit Research Institute (EBRI). *2019 RCS Fact Sheet #2: Expectations About Retirement.* Retirement Confidence Survey; 2019. Available at: https://www.ebri.orrg/docs/default-source/rcs/2019-rcs/rcs_19-fs-2_expect.pdf?sfvrsn=2a553f2f_4.

50 Employee Benefit Research Institute (EBRI) 2022. *2022 Retirement confidence survey.* Accessed from https://www.ebri.org/docs/default-source/rcs/2022-rcs/2022-rcs-summary-report.pdf?sfvrsn=a7cb3b2f_12.

51. Toossi M, Torpey E. *Older workers: Labor Force Trends and Career Options.* Bureau of Labor Statistics; 2017. Available at: https://www.bls.gov/careeroutlook/2017/article/older-workers.htm.

52. Kakulla BN. *Older Americans' Technology Usage Keeps Climbing.* AARP Research; 2019. Available at: https://www.aarp.org/research/topics/technology/info-2019/2019-technology-trends-older-americans.html.

53. Anderson M, Perrin A. *Barriers to Adoption and Attitudes Towards Technology.* Pew Research Center; 2017. Available at: https://www.pewresearch.org/internet/2017/05/17/barriers-to-adoption-and-attitudes-towards-technology/.

54. Swagel P.L. *An Overview of the 2020 Long-Term Budget Outlook.* Congressional Budget Office; 2020. Available at: https://www.cbo.gov/system/files/2020-10/56677-NAHB-presentation.pdf.

55. Lohman H, Griffiths Y, Coppard B, et al. The power of book discussion groups in intergenerational learning. *Educ Gerontol.* 2003;29(2):103-116. doi:10.1080/713844284.

56. Golenko X, Radford K, Fitzgerald JA, Vecchio N, Cartmel J, Harris N. Uniting generations: a research protocol examining the impacts of an intergenerational learning program on participants and organisations. *Australas J Ageing.* 2020;39(3):e425-e435. doi:10.1111/ajag.12761.

57. Giraudeau C, Bailly N. Intergenerational programs: what can school-age children and older people expect from them? A systematic review. *Eur J Ageing.* 2019;16(3):363-376. doi:10.1007/s10433-018-00497-4.

58. Skropeta CM, Colvin A, Sladen S. An evaluative study of the benefits of participating in intergenerational playgroups in aged care for older people. *BMC Geriatr.* 2014;14:109. doi:10.1186/1471-2318-14-109.

59. Dimock M. *Defining Generations: Where Millennials End and Generation Z Begins.* Pew Research Center; 2019. Available at: https://www.pewresearch.org/fact-tank/2019/01/17/where-millennials-end-and-generation-z-begins/.

60. Ryder NB. The cohort as a concept in the study of social change. *Am Sociol Rev.* 1965;30(6):843-861. doi:10.2307/2090964.

61. Howe N. *The Silent Generation, "The Lucky Few" Part 3 of 7.* Forbes; 2014. Available at: https://www.forbes.com/sites/neil-howe/2014/08/13/the-silent-generation-the-lucky-few-part-3-of-7/?sh=597d077d2c63.

62. Hoonpongsimanont W, Sahota PK, Chen Y, et al. Physician professionalism: definition from a generation perspective. *Int J Med Educ.* 2018;9:246-252. doi:10.5116/ijme.5ba0.a584.

63. Bell JA. Five Generations in the nursing workforce. *J Nurses Prof Dev.* 2013;29(4):205-210. doi:10.1097/NND.0b013e31829aedd4.

64. Hoyt J. *The Baby Boomer Generation.* SeniorLiving.org; 2020. Available at: https://www.seniorliving.org/life/baby-boomers/.

65. Paterson T. Generational considerations in providing critical care education. *Crit Care Nurs Q.* 2010;33(1):67-74. doi:10.1097/CNQ.0b013e3181c8dfa8.

66. Cekada T. Training a multigenerational workforce. *Prof Saf.* 2012;57(3):40-44.

67. Akintayo T, Häkälä N, Ropponen K, Paronen E, Rissanen S. Predictive factors for voluntary and/or paid work among adults in their sixties. *Soc Indic Res.* 2016;128(3):1387-1404. doi:10.1007/s11205-015-1084-5.

68. Larson K, Stevens-Ratchford R, Pedretti L, et al, eds. *ROTE: The Role of Occupational Therapy 1996; 1996. ROTE: The Role of Occupational Therapy with the Elderly: Faculty Guide. Module I: Teaching Resources Gerontology in Theory and Practice.* Rockville, MD: American Occupational Therapy Association; 1996:71-79.

69. Lewis C. How the myths of aging impact rehabilitative care for the older person. *Occup Ther Forum.* 1989;10:1-11.

70. World Health Organization. *Ageing: Ageism.* World Health Organization; 2020. Available at: https://www.who.int/newsroom/questionsandanswers/item/ageingageism#:~:text=Ageism%20refers%20to%20the%20stereotypes,of%20their%20culture's%20age%20stereotypes.

71. Alden J, Toth-Cohen S. Impact of an educational module on occupational therapists' use of elderspeak and attitudes toward older adults. *Phys Occup Ther Geriatr.* 2015;33(1):1-16. doi:10.3109/02703181.2014.975884.

72. World Health Organization. *International Classification of Functioning, Disability, and Health (ICF).* 2015. Available at: http://www.who.int/classifications/icf/en/.

73. U.S. Department of Health and Human Services (DHHS). *Healthy People 2030 Framework.* 2018. Available at: https://health.gov/healthypeople/about/healthy-people-2030-framework.

74. Youngstrom MJ. The occupational therapy practice framework: the evolution of our professional language. *Am J Occup Ther.* 2002;56(6):607-608. doi:10.5014/ajot.56.6.607.

Biological and Social Theories of Aging

MICHELLE RUDOLF

(PREVIOUS CONTRIBUTIONS FROM MARLENE J. AITKEN)

KEY TERMS

genetic aging, nongenetic aging, programmed aging, nonprogrammed aging, senescence

CHAPTER OBJECTIVES

1. Identify the purpose and use of current theories of aging.
2. Discuss the biological theories of aging: genetic, non-genetic, programmed, and nonprogrammed theories.

3. Discuss the psychosocial theories of aging.
4. Understand the ways to apply the theories of aging to the care of older adults.

Alex is a certified occupational therapy assistant (OTA) employed in an assisted living facility that offers several levels of care. Her daily work involves treating older adults who have a variety of diagnosed conditions and the planning of occupation-based activities. Alex has observed that, although many of the older adults require rehabilitation, each reacts differently to illness and the aging process. At least once a week, Alex meets with Casey, a registered occupational therapist (OT), for a supervisory session in which they thoroughly discuss each person participating in occupational therapy (OT).

After reviewing the caseload during one particular session, Alex and Casey began a lively discussion about the complexities of aging. Alex noted that some of the older adults whom she treats as part of her caseload seem active and vigorous, whereas others seem withdrawn and lack energy to participate in therapeutic tasks. She also commented that some of the older adults seem older than their chronological ages, and others seem to be their age or younger. Casey encouraged Alex to review theories about aging to form a context in which to think about the older adults. The next week Alex and Casey discussed the application of the theories to their work with older adults who are part of their caseloads.

Research on aging consists of many different studies and perspectives. As a result, Alex's questions can be answered multiple ways regarding reasons for and differences in aging. Theories attempt to explain what is observed or experienced and why and how it is important—going beyond the data to the fundamental biological, social, or psychological processes.[1] Likewise, theories of aging attempt to explain how and why we age.[2] Therefore it is important for OTAs to understand several theories of aging because

one theory may not completely answer the questions regarding aging (senescence)—it may be a combination of theories.

Aging is fundamentally a biopsychosocial process involving three broad contributing factors: (a) social structural influences (gender, socioeconomic status, race, age, and cultural context), (b) individual influences (psychosocial and behavioral), and (c) biological influences (inflammatory and oxidative damage, damage to irreplaceable molecules and cells, and blood metabolic hormones) (p. 8)[1].

This chapter presents current biological, social, and psychological theories to provide insight on aspects of aging. (The physical and psychological changes that occur with the aging process are described in Chapters 3 and 4, respectively.)

BIOLOGICAL THEORIES OF AGING

Theory development is a dynamic process and, as research improves and progresses, theories may shift and change or be found to be irrelevant and dismissed.[3] The major biological theories of aging can be classified by one or more of four categories: genetic, relating to genes or deoxyribonucleic acid (DNA); nongenetic, biological but acquired aging; programmed, predetermined aging or essentially apoptosis (programmed cell death); and nonprogrammed or stochastic aging, randomly occurring changes that accumulate with time.[1,2,4,5] Theories may be hard to classify—genetic versus nongenetic and programmed versus nonprogrammed—because a theory may be primarily nongenetic but have genetic factors (e.g., free radical/oxidative stress theory) or may be nonprogrammed but have underlying unexplainable root causes (e.g., neuroendocrine theory). Sometimes, it is

TABLE 2.1

Biological Theories of Aging

Theory	Genetic/nongenetic, programmed/nonprogrammed	Key characteristics
Programmed aging (telomere shortening)	Genetic, programmed	Genetically influenced-limited cell divisions Telomere attrition
Mutation	Genetic, nonprogrammed	Accumulated errors of DNA/mtDNA Wear and tear components
Free radical/oxidative stress	Nongenetic, nonprogrammed	Accumulation of damage from highly reactive agents Wear and tear components
Neuroendocrine	Nongenetic, nonprogrammed	Hypothalamic dysregulation of homeostasis Hormone-influence deterioration
Wear and tear	Nongenetic, nonprogrammed	Accumulated damage Ineffective damage repair

Adapted from Bengtson VL, Bonder BR. Theories of aging: A multidisciplinary review for occupational and physical therapists. In: Bonder BR, Dal Bello-Haas V, eds. *Functional Performance in Older Adults*. 3rd ed. Philadelphia: FA Davis; 2009.

difficult to categorize a theory as either a cause or a consequence—fate or chance[4,6] (see Table 2.1).

Programmed Aging Theory

In 1882, Arthur Weismann first proposed that organisms live within a limited space and time as an explanation for aging and ultimately death.[7] Limited space means organisms have a size limit. Thus, a fly will never reach the size of a giraffe.[7] Limited time (death) is an evolutionary way to ensure resources are available for coming generations and organisms of reproductive age rather than being used by postreproductive individuals among the population.[2,7] Therefore, unlimited growth (size or lifespan) of a population would result in an exponential decrease of resources.[2,7] The premise of the programmed aging theories is that the human body has an inherited internal "genetic clock" that determines the aging process. This genetic clock may manifest as a predetermined or limited number of cell divisions rather than actual clock or calendar time, called the Hayflick limit (also known as replicative senescence or cellular senescence).[2,8] The Hayflick limit does not affect all cells in the body; germ cells (sperm or egg), stem cells, and cells in some tumors (cancer) seem to divide infinitely.[5,9] The Hayflick limit has been researched extensively and has been determined that telomere shortening explains the limited cell division first observed in somatic cells.[5,8,10,11] The theory of cellular aging explains why many older adults have one or multiple conditions related to decreased or impaired client factors (sensory, neuromusculoskeletal, cardiovascular, respiratory, digestive, metabolic, and reproductive) and why it is rare to find any of these impairments in young adults.[12]

Telomere Shortening (End-Underreplication) Theory

Telomeres are a sequence of DNA at the end of linear chromosomes that protect DNA from mutation and identify the DNA strand for replication.[5,11] Unlike circular DNA (e.g., bacterium) that has no end, linear DNA has ends, and it is from the end that DNA replication must occur for cell division.[10] Imagine the telomere end-cap is the alphabet in which each letter is repeated two times before the next letter (i.e., AABBCC … XXYYZZ), then the DNA code begins. When DNA is copied before cell division, the code reader (DNA polymerase) must first locate the strand via the telomere and attach, but it can only replicate after attaching. The result is a copied strand that is two letters shorter (i.e., BBCC … XXYYZZ). Thus the strand can only be copied 26 times before the alphabet (telomere) is gone. Without the telomere, the DNA polymerase cannot attach to begin DNA replication and ultimately carry out cellular division, meaning the cell can only divide a limited number of times.[5,11,13] The mechanism for telomere shortening is not completely understood, so it can be considered programmed.[13] Telomerase, an enzyme, was discovered to elongate telomeres, resulting in unlimited cell divisions or cellular immorality (e.g., germ, stem, and cancer cells).[5,11,14] Lack of telomerase activity in somatic cells helps to suppress malignancy.[5] So even if uncontrolled cellular growth occurs via mutations, the end-underreplication theory will ensure a limited number of divisions. End-underreplication theory is applicable on a cellular level, not organismal, but it could factor into the vitality and function of systems and/or organs resulting in change to overall health related to aging.[5,15]

Mutation Theory

Mutation is a genetic, nonprogrammed theory of aging in which stochastic (random) changes occur as a result of miscoding, translation errors, irradiation, UV light, and metabolic activity.[2] These mutations result in changes in the ribonucleic acid (RNA) or DNA code sequences or more commonly noted mitochondrial DNA (mtDNA).[13,16-18] Mitochondria are the power factory of the cell, creating adenosine triphosphate (ATP), and contain their own portion of the DNA code, which mainly codes for molecules needed to run the power factory.[5,16] The body has mechanisms in place to repair and/or remove mutations (cellular or mtDNA) and cells (e.g., apoptosis) that may negatively affect function or effectiveness; however, sometimes the mechanisms do not work properly or completely, and mutations accumulate or are carried over through cellular divisions.[13,19,20] The accumulation of mutations can alter the genetic sequence of a cell in such a way that the "safe guard" to control the proliferation of cellular growth is deactivated, resulting in unrestrained cell division, sometimes leading to tumorigenesis and/or cancer.[21,22] Mutations can also occur in the expression of the genetic code or the way that the code is read without directly changing the RNA or DNA sequence; the expression of the genetic code is the epigenome, and the mutations are epimutations.[23-25]

Free Radical/Oxidative Stress Theory

Free radical theory of aging studies the highly reactive, unstable atoms in living cells as they try to stabilize (pairing of unpaired electron[s]) and the damage caused to cells, proteins, lipids, and DNA (by altering their structures).[26-28] Free radicals happen naturally in the body and are usually associated with byproducts to cellular, enzymatic, and metabolic reactions; a key byproduct is reactive oxygen species (ROS).[29-31] A major manufacturer of ROS within the cell are mitochondria, which also sustain the most damage from the byproduct.[16,29,31] Accumulated damage of mitochondria is associated with system-wide dysfunction in relation to neuromuscular, cardiovascular, and other age-related declines as cells, tissue, and organs deteriorate.[16,32-34] One natural defense to free radicals and oxidative stress are antioxidants; however, too many antioxidants tend to increase oxidative stress and cellular damage while not enough hinders repair of free radical/oxidative damage and decreases overall function.[35,36] Bouzid[35] suggests that routine, moderate exercise can guard aging individuals from oxidative damage and improve antioxidant defense.[36] The direct effect of the free radical theory on aging and dysfunction continues to be studied, but it is clear that the presence of oxidative damage from free radicals increases through the life span.[28,35,36]

Neuroendocrine Theory

The neuroendocrine theory, or elevation theory of aging, suggests that the central nervous system, especially the hypothalamus, is the starting point for aging in the body.[5,6,37] "The vital processes under control of the hypothalamus include regulation of body temperature, nutrient intake and energy balance, sleep and wake cycle, sexual behavior, reproductive cyclicity, water and electrolyte balance, stress adaptation, … and growth" (p. 2).[4] The slow deterioration of the hypothalamus over the life span may activate a series of biochemical responses that might result in programmed death, or phenoptosis.[38] One example may be the decreased effectiveness of the immune system due to homeostasis-regulation issues stemming from the hypothalamus that could cause a person to become more susceptible to illness and disease resulting in death.[37] Prolonged stress can also affect the endocrine system and hormones, which may have negative physiological effects and result in advanced aging.[39] Olenski[40] stated the aging and mortality risk among elected officials was considerably higher than that of runner-up candidates (nonelected), which they suggest may be due to increased stress in office.

Wear and Tear Theory

Wear and tear from the environment are natural and expected with almost all living things and inanimate objects, but the body has repair mechanisms to decrease the accumulated damage.[5,6] Mutation theory and accumulated waste (e.g., free radical/oxidative stress theory) can be classified within wear and tear. The wear and tear theory can be studied in greater depth with identical (monozygotic) twins; identical twins are nature's natural clones in that they have identical genotypes (genetic information).[5,6,41,42] Identical genetic codes provide evidence for programmed aging as growth, disease, and death are sometimes similar between the individuals, but these factors rarely perfectly align (e.g., natural time of death varying between twins).[41-45] This lack of alignment affords support for nonprogrammed, external factors as having an effect on life span.[41-45]

PSYCHOSOCIAL THEORIES OF AGING

Longer life spans and an increasing population of older individuals in the United States resulted in greater attention to the aging process.[6,46] Understanding psychosocial theories of aging are important for health care professionals because people do not live life like programmed robots. Social factors influence how people live, age, and ultimately die.[1,47] In terms of OTA treatment of patients, it is important to consider the whole person during treatment—biological, psychological, and social.[12] Two patients of identical age may be receiving treatment for a broken hip—one occurred while hesitantly walking to the bathroom in the middle of the night while the other incident occurred during a night out dancing with friends. The patient who fell at home may have other ailments and be more reluctant to participate in life's activities due to accepting increasing frailty—disengagement theory— while the other patient may be eager to participate to return to prior level of function (PLOF)—activity theory.[12,47] Disengagement, activity, and continuity theories each focus on different aspects of aging (see Table 2.2). Psychosocial theories, like biological theories of aging, are not one-size-fits-all, instead they can be considered as

TABLE 2.2

Summary of Theories of Activity of Older Adults

Theory	Theorists	Constructs
Disengagement	Cumming and Henry (1961)	Older adults typically withdraw from previous activities in preparation for death.
Activity theory	Havighurst (1961)	Older adults maintain activity and do best when they are active and engaged.
Continuity theory	Atchley (1989)	Individuals in later life sustain previous beliefs, values, and characteristics.
		Older adults strive to retain previous activities.
		When previous activities cannot be sustained, older adults strive to replace those with activities that carry the same meanings.

Adapted from Bonder BR. Meaningful occupation in later life. In: Bonder BR, Dal Bello-Haas V, eds. *Functional Performance in Older Adults.* 3rd ed. Philadelphia: FA Davis; 2009.

possibilities along a continuum of engagement and disengagement.[48,49]

Disengagement Theory

Disengagement theory (social) illustrates the mutual process of a person withdrawing from social roles and responsibilities.[6,50] The mutual components include a person's withdrawal from society and society's withdrawal from the person.[6,51,52] A person may begin to reduce their responsibilities as they accept the natural and inevitable end of life[52]—"the ultimate disengagement" (p. 553).[51] Inward reflection and increasing preoccupation with self can result in decreasing involvement with others.[50] However, individual disengagement may be more than psychological—desiring to reduce the burden of loss after one's death—but also biological—illness and/or deterioration of health and physical abilities.[47,51,53] For example, an individual might decline attending an event due to vision or hearing loss, instead choosing to listen to a live broadcast or watch closed caption TV. As a person withdrawals from society, society withdrawals by "reassigning" their former roles and responsibilities, such as in the workforce.[47,52,54] Retirement can be perceived positively as a reduction of responsibility or negatively as a loss of purpose by the older individual (Fig. 2.1).[49]

While completing an interest checklist with the OTA, an older adult might indicate a sense of meaning found in former activities and roles with various social clubs or organizations. However, the older adult might claim that it is because of age that they are no longer participating (excluding biological factors).[12] Health care professionals should be aware of the consequences of involuntary disengagement.[47] Older adults may wish to continue an activity, but they withdraw because they believe that other people may think they are "too old," or it is socially expected to withdraw.[49] For example, it may be socially expected in some workplaces to retire at a certain age.[49] In terms of biological factors, a hospitalization or disability may remove the individual from a social circle or relationship. Either situation could result in depression, which is not

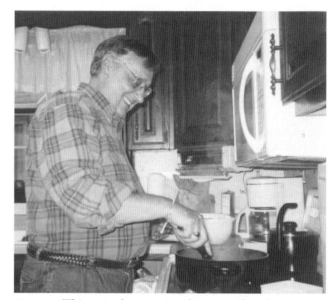

FIG. 2.1 This retired man enjoys his new role as he prepares the family meal.

normal in the aging process.[47,55,56] It has been studied that disengagement is different from isolation.[51,55] For older adults who think they are too old or unable to continue certain activities, the OTA could discuss doing activities that would be similar to former interests or suggest adaptations to the specific activity.[12] If older adults are interested in gardening, they could assist with the plants in and around their residence or start a personal window garden. Email or video chatting could be an appropriate adaptation if older adults are interested in communicating with friends or family, if forms of communication like handwriting have become difficult (Fig. 2.2). It is important to reassure older individuals that adaptations or increased time to complete an activity can be part of the normal aging process, as it is sometimes socially implied that such changes are the result of dementia.[56]

The disengagement theory, in its original proposal, is highly criticized for its assumption of universality, inevitability, and personal and social importance.[47,51] On the

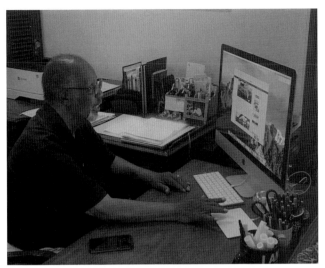

FIG. 2.2 This older adult embraces technology and enjoys using his computer to locate information about his interests. *(Courtesy Fitz Johnson.)*

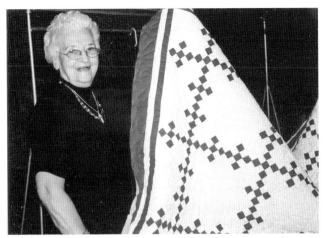

FIG. 2.3 This older adult gets satisfaction in making quilts for her family *(Courtesy Helene Lohman.)*

premise of universality, the disengagement theory states that withdrawal is successful disengagement—successful aging—as a person ages and individuals who remain engaged are "unsuccessful disengagers" (p. 555).[51] Disengagement theory is viewed as inevitable for every individual and considers that individuals living more than 80 years are perceived to be biologically and psychologically privileged.[50] In some societies or cultures, mainly non-Western, aging individuals receive honor, respect, and prestige.[47,51] Cumming[50] did not consider that individuals may find meaning and purpose in their engagements and therefore desire to remain engaged.[47,51,55]

Socioemotional Selectivity Theory

Carstensen and colleagues[57] proposed the socioemotional selectivity theory, which states that older adults shift their personal goals from obtaining knowledge to enhancing positive emotional relationships and activities—it is a quality-over-quantity approach.[49,56,57] This psychological theory attempts to explain "why the social exchange and interaction networks of older persons are reduced over time" (p. 35).[48] The important part about socioemotional selectivity is that it is positive and enlightening for the older adults not depressing and negative.[56] Reminiscence groups and other life review activities conducted as part of an intervention program by OTAs can be one way of helping older adults process the changes associated with aging; developing a video to leave for future generations may be one group activity.[56]

Activity Theory

Activity theory was proposed by Havighurst[58] as an alternative view of the disengagement theory to explain psychosocial aspects of aging. Activity theorists believe that disengagement is unnatural and not conducive to successful aging.[54,58] This theory implies that older adults need

and desire social activities and roles for satisfaction in life (Fig. 2.3).[47,59] Thus the activity theory embraces an anti-aging viewpoint and proposes that when some life roles and pursuits are lost, older adults should develop additional roles and pursuits as replacements.[54] For example, a retired teacher may seek a youth mentoring program at their local community center or church to continue their role of teaching. Activity theory has been greatly criticized as it focuses on quantity and amount of involvement in activities and roles and excludes older adults' physical well-being, past lifestyle, personality attributes, ability and personal meaning (Fig. 2.4).[47,48]

Continuity Theory

The premise of continuity theory is that older adults adapt to changes by using strategies to maintain continuity in their lives, both internal and external.[47,60] Internal continuity refers to the strategy of forming personal links between new experiences and memories of previous ones

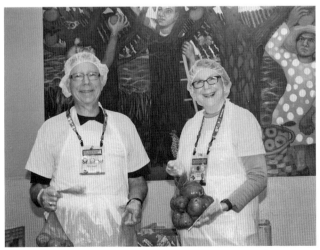

FIG. 2.4 This couple finds personal meaning in volunteering at their local food bank.

and external continuity refers to interacting with familiar people and living in familiar environments.[47,61] According to the continuity theory, a person's personality, behaviors, and preferences will remain similar into old age.[47,59] OTAs should remember this when attempting to get everyone involved in an activity; outgoing individuals will likely thrive with active group tasks while reserved individuals may prefer quiet, solitary activities.[47] Some older adults may welcome participation in physical activities such as bowling and walking (Fig. 2.5), and others may be content with listening to quiet music and reading (Fig. 2.6).

Health care and provided services should not be based on one theory but a combination of theories as they apply and are appropriate to our clients. For instance, it may be

FIG. 2.5   Through ongoing social interactions, older adults can maintain a positive self-concept (*Courtesy Fitz Johnson.*)

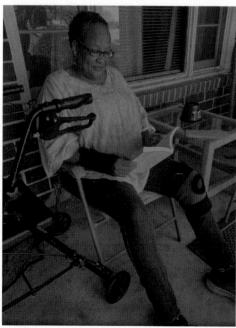

FIG. 2.6   This older adult enjoys a sedentary activity (*Courtesy Mia Marrow.*)

dangerous to allow an older adult to withdraw by considering it a normal function of aging or to push meaningless activity with a disinterested older adult. OTAs may want to discuss with older adults what activities have meaning to them and allow older adults to reminisce about past activities or perform client-centered assessments such as an interest checklist or the Canadian Occupational Performance Measure.[62] Occupational profiles can provide valuable information about the older adult. The information gleaned from the individual could give OTAs more insight into a selection of activities that are most appropriate.

The activity and continuity theories are compatible with OT as they present that performance of meaningful activities promotes competence, independence, and well-being. Kielhofner[63] states that human beings are occupational in nature; therefore occupation is vital for our well-being. The Model of Human Occupation incorporates this assumption and is a valuable theory of OT for aging.[63] What a person does depends on individual factors such as level of interest, values, personal causation, health, socioeconomic status, and prior occupations.

Life Span and Life Course Perspectives

Life span and life course perspectives present different angles to a "social-psychological study of the life cycle" (p. 464).[64] Life span perspective is a psychological approach that looks at the developmental changes throughout life and adaptations to cognitive, emotional, and behavioral factors.[56,64] Life course theory is considered a social perspective on collective, cultural, and historical factors that influence an individual from birth to death.[64,65] The overlap within these perspectives demonstrates that aging cannot be examined with a single-facet viewpoint, but interrelated approaches.[56]

Life span perspective

Key components of the life span approach are the lifelong view of development changes including causality for the changes—biological or environmental (external)—and the growth and decline of the individual throughout the life span.[66] Selective optimization with compensation (SOC) theory is a model for coping with loss within the life span perspective to optimize successful aging. "The model suggests that people adapt by *selecting* goals, *optimizing* the skills and abilities necessary for goal attainment, and *compensating* for lost competencies through replacement or substitution" (p. 7).[59] Selecting goals is usually a reduction for focus on quality and optimization versus quantity.[48,56,61] OTAs can help individuals examine and identify meaningful personal goals and best use the resources available to enhance goal obtainment.[12,56]

Life course perspective

Life course focuses on the life history of an individual to better understand the aging process.[6]

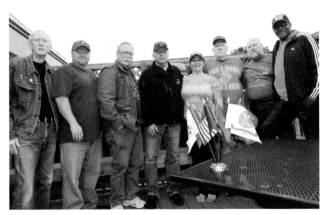

FIG. 2.7 This cohort of veterans enjoys spending time together socially as well as volunteering in their community.

In a life course approach to health, a person's life experiences inform understanding of their current health and overall status. These experiences may be individual, such as surviving polio, or may be specific to a cohort, such as those who grew up during the Great Depression. In the life course perspective, the term cohort refers to a group of people born during the same time period who experience certain historical and social changes at about the same age (p. 476)[47] (Fig. 2.7).

Older adults who experienced the Great Depression seem to have a different perception of the meaning of "poor." As a result, older adults may reject offers of help because they compare what little they had in the past with what they currently have, which seems sufficient. In addition, some older adults who are eligible for Social Security insurance may not accept it. This viewpoint may vary with subsequent generations of older adults. Please refer to Table 1.1 in Chapter 1 for more information about generational cohorts.

The life experiences that shape a person's life course are influenced through social structure, age-related trajectory (time frame), and the individual's interaction within society.[48,64] Social structure defines how a person functions in society (e.g., hierarchical education process, labor laws, family structure).[6,48,64] Age-related trajectory looks at time-sensitive roles and transitions that a person performs within society (e.g., schooling, parenthood, employment, retirement).[6,48,64] The individual's interaction within society examines the cohort in which a person relates (e.g., seeking marriage in relation to others seeking marriage).[6,48,64] Historical contexts are very important to the study of life courses (e.g., peace/war, cultural/religious tolerance, economic recession/depression).[64]

CONCLUSION

OT focuses on assessing a person's needs and wants, and it is the role of the OTA to integrate all the theories (biological, social, and psychological) into a client-centered approach that emphasizes client factors, performance skills, performance patterns, and context.[12]

CASE STUDY

Wilma is a 72-year-old widow. She has three adult children who live nearby and six grandchildren she sees on a regular basis. Recently, Wilma fell while standing on a chair to wash windows, resulting in a broken hip.

Wilma had surgery and remained in the hospital for 4 days secondary to unstable blood pressure. Once medically stable, she was transferred to a rehabilitation facility. During the initial care conference, the children dominated the conversation, answered all questions for their mother, and excluded her from any decisions regarding treatment and discharge.

Wilma is being followed by the rehabilitation team. Tayler, a OTA working with Wilma, noticed that in the past 2 days Wilma was not as engaged in treatment, appears withdrawn, and no longer verbalizes plans for discharge. Tayler communicates with the OT regarding Wilma's change in behavior. Additionally, she researches psychosocial theories of aging along with possible biological causes but cannot find an answer that fits the current situation. When Tayler goes to get Wilma for therapy, she notices that the room is dark and Wilma is in bed crying. She first asks for permission to enter the room and open the curtains, then expresses concern for Wilma and inquires about her feelings. Wilma tearfully confides that her children have decided to sell her home as they feel that she is no longer safe to live independently. They offered her two choices: (1) she can move to an assisted living facility, which they will help finance or (2) she can move in with the eldest child and his family. However, neither of these options is acceptable to Wilma; she feels that she does not have the "energy" to speak up for herself and make her wishes known.

Wilma is doing well in therapy. She follows hip precautions without incident; transfers to bed, toilet, and chair with stand-by assistance; and has a walker in her room for mobility. Her weight-bearing status has been upgraded to weight bearing as tolerated. Although Wilma has admitted to "missing" a dose of medication now and then, cognitively there is no immediate concern. Staff plans to provide and educate her about following a medication schedule. Taylor observed Wilma completing a light meal preparation activity and documented that Wilma is "safe" to return to previous cooking activities. Wilma participated in washing dishes, putting dishes in cupboards, folding laundry while standing, putting clothes on hangers, and placing them in the closet without difficulty. Energy conservation and work simplification techniques were taught, and Wilma was able to demonstrate a good understanding. She is scheduled for discharge at the end of the following week.

■ CASE STUDY QUESTIONS

1 Choose and explain how aging theories apply to Wilma.
2 Explain how psychosocial theories of aging affect Wilma's current level of function?
3 Explain concerns that should be raised related to Wilma's functioning in terms of biological theories of aging.
4 Give examples of interventions that will help Wilma reengage in meaningful occupations.
5 Illustrate how the OTA can be an advocate for Wilma.
6 Provide examples of how the OTA can help Wilma be an advocate for herself.

▉ CHAPTER REVIEW QUESTIONS

1 Scenario one: Ethel Shanas, a very famous gerontologist, once said that if you want to live a long time, you should choose your grandparents carefully. Which aging theory or theories support Dr. Shanas' suggestion?

2 Scenario two: Alex, the OTA introduced at the beginning of this chapter, decided to include reminiscence and life review as part of her therapeutic interventions with older adults in the nursing home. Which aging theory supports the selection of these activities?

3 Scenario three: The family of one of Alex's elderly clients is upset because the older adult insists on planning her own funeral and asking for specific clothes in which to be buried. In addition, she has made a list of all of her furniture and other property and has designated which of her children or grandchildren is to inherit these items. Although this client has accepted her terminal illness, her family has not. Which aging theory would Alex use to explain to the family what is happening with their relative?

4 Scenario four: Margaret's children decide to move her away from her current hometown to a new assisted living facility in the town where they reside. Since the move, Margaret seems more depressed and is having difficulty adapting to her new living arrangements. What aging theory explains her behavior?

5 The risk for having cancer increases significantly as people grow older. Use an aging theory to explain a possible reason for this.

6 Some older adults may become extremely depressed once they retire. What could you suggest, other than antidepressant medications, that may improve their outlook on life? Discuss the theory that supports your suggestion.

7 An 80-year-old man made headlines because he entered the Boston marathon. Why did this make the news? How do cultural age norms influence the persistence of ageism?

8 An 85-year-old woman with severe Parkinson's disease requested that, during her activities of daily living session, the OTA help her dress herself and put on makeup. The woman's doctor has suggested that she is "too old for rehab" and is thinking of discontinuing OT. Justify her intervention with a theory, and then explain how you would convince the doctor that it is important.

9 Give an example of the disengagement theory.

10 Give an example of the activity theory.

For additional video content, please visit Elsevier eBooks+ (eBooks.Health.Elsevier.com)

REFERENCES

1. Bengtson VL, Gans D, Putney NM, et al. Theories about age and aging. In: Bengston VL, Gans D, Pulney NM, et al., eds. *Handbook of Theories of Aging*. 2nd ed. New York, NY: Springer Publishing Co; 2009:3-23.

2. Goldsmith TC. *An introduction to Biological Aging Theory*. 2nd ed. Crownsville, MD: Azinet Press; 2014.

3. Gans D, Putney NM, Bengtson VL, et al. The future of theories of aging. In: Bengston VL, Gans D, Pulney NM, et al., eds. *Handbook of Theories of Aging*. 2nd ed. New York, NY: Springer Publishing Co; 2009:723-737.

4. Chen TT, Maevsky EI, Uchitel ML. Maintenance of homeostasis in the aging hypothalamus: The central and peripheral roles of succinate. *Front Endocrinol (Lausanne)*. 2015;6(7):1-11. doi:10.3389/fendo.2015.00007.

5. Sergiev PV, Dontsova OA, Berezkin GV. Theories of aging: an ever-evolving field. *Acta Naturae*. 2015;7(1):9-18.

6. Moody HR, Sasser JR. *Aging: Concepts and Controversies*. 8th ed. Los Angeles, CA: Sage Publications; 2015.

7. Weismann A. The duration of life [Shipley AE, Trans.]. In: Weismann A, Poulton EB, Schonland S, eds. *Essays Upon Heredity and Kindred Biological Problems, 1889*. Oxford: Clarendon Press; 1881:1-66.

8. Hayflick L, Moorhead PS. The serial cultivation of human diploid cell strains. *Exp Cell Res*. 1961;25:585-621.

9. López-Otín C, Blasco MA, Partridge L, et al. The hallmarks of aging. *Cell*. 2013;153:1194-1217. doi:10.1016/j.cell.2013.05.039.

10. Olovnikov AM. A theory of marginotomy: The incomplete copying of template margin in enzymic synthesis of polynucleotides and biological significance of the phenomenon. *J Theor Biol*. 1973;41(1):181-190.

11. Olovnikov AM. Telomeres, telomerase, and aging: origin of the theory. *Exp Gerontol*. 1996;31(4):443-448. doi:10.1016/0531-5565(96)00005-8.

12. American Occupational Therapy Association. Occupational therapy practice framework: domain and process, 3rd ed. *Am J Occup Ther*. 2014;68:S1-S48. doi:10.5014/ajot.2014.682006.

13. Trusina A. Stress induced telomere shortening: longer life with less mutations? *BMC Syst Biol*. 2014;8:27. doi:10.1186/1752-0509-8-27.

14. Greider CW, Blackburn EH. Identification of a specific telomere terminal transferase activity in Tetrahymena extracts. *Cell*. 1985;43(2 Pt 1):405-413. doi:10.1016/0092-8674(85)90170-9.

15. Dillin A, Karlseder J. Cellular versus organismal aging. In: Rudolph KL, ed. *Telomeres and Telomerase in Aging, Disease, and Cancer: Molecular Mechanisms of Adult Stem Cell Ageing*. Berlin: Springer; 2008:3-22.

16. Khrapko K, Turnbull D. Mitochondrial DNA mutations in aging. *Prog Mol Biol Transl Sci*. 2014;127:29-62. doi:10.1016/B978-0-12-394625-6.00002-7.

17. Li Z, Pearlman AH, Hsieh P. DNA mismatch repair and the DNA damage response. *DNA Repair (Amst)*. 2016;38:94-101. doi:10.1016/j.dnarep.2015.11.019.

18. Mandal PK, Blanpain C, Rossi DJ. DNA damage response in adult stem cells: pathways and consequences. *Nat Rev Mol Cell Biol*. 2011;12(3):198-202. doi:10.1038/nrm3060.

19. Gladyshev VN. The origin of aging: imperfectness-driven non-random damage defines the aging process and control of lifespan. *Trends Genet*. 2013;29(9):506-512. doi:10.1016/j.tig.2013.05.004.

20. Gladyshev VN. On the cause of aging and control of lifespan: heterogeneity leads to inevitable damage accumulation, causing aging; control of damage composition and rate of accumulation define lifespan. *Bioessays*. 2012;34(11):925-929. doi:10.1002/bies.201200092.

21. Frisan T. Bacterial genotoxins: the long journey to the nucleus of mammalian cells. *Biochim Biophys Acta*. 2016;1858(3):567-575. doi:10.1016/j.bbamem.2015.08.016.

22. Wickramasinghe VO, Venkitaraman AR. RNA processing and genome stability: cause and consequence. *Mol Cell*. 2016;61(4):496-505. doi:10.1016/j.molcel.2016.02.001.

23. Bird A. Perceptions of epigenetics. *Nature.* 2007;447(7143):396-398.

24. Jones MJ, Goodman SJ, Kobor MS. DNA methylation and healthy human aging. *Aging Cell.* 2015;14(6):924-932. doi:10.1111/acel.12349.

25. Moskalev AA, Aliper AM, Smit-McBride Z, et al. Genetics and epigenetics of aging and longevity. *Cell Cycle.* 2014;13(7):1063-1077. doi:10.4161/cc.28433.

26. Harman D. Aging: a theory based on free radical and radiation chemistry. *J Gerontol.* 1956;11:298-300. doi:10.1093/geronj/11.3.298.

27. Muller FL, Lustgarten MS, Jang Y, et al. Trends in oxidative aging theories. *Free Radic Biol Med.* 2007;43(4):477-503. doi:10.1016/j.freeradbiomed.2007.03.034.

28. Shringarpure R, Davies KJA. Free radicals and oxidative stress in aging. In: Bengston VL, Gans D, Pulney NM, et al., eds. *Handbook of Theories of Aging.* 2nd ed. New York, NY: Springer Publishing Co; 2009:229-243.

29. Hekimi S, Lapointe J, Wen Y. Taking a "good" look at free radicals in the aging process. *Trends Cell Biol.* 2011;21(10):569-576. doi:10.1016/j.tcb.2011.06.008.

30. Schöttker B, Brenner H, Jansen EH, et al. Evidence for the free radical/oxidative stress theory of ageing from the CHANCES consortium: a meta-analysis of individual participant data. *BMC Med.* 2015;13:1-15. doi:10.1186/s12916-015-0537-7.

31. Ziegler DV, Wiley CD, Velarde MC. Mitochondrial effectors of cellular senescence: beyond the free radical theory of aging. *Aging Cell.* 2015;14(1):1-7. doi:10.1111/acel.12287.

32. Akhmedov AT, Marín-García J. Mitochondrial DNA maintenance: an appraisal. *Mol Cell Biochem.* 2015;409(1-2):283-305. doi:10.1007/s11010-015-2532-x.

33. Gonzalez-Freire M, de Cabo R, Bernier M, et al. Reconsidering the role of mitochondria in aging. *J Gerontol A Biol Sci Med Sci.* 2015;70(11):1334-1342. doi:10.1093/gerona/glv070.

34. Zinovkina LA, Zinovkin RA. DNA methylation, mitochondria, and programmed aging. *Biochemistry (Mosc).* 2015;80(12):1571-1577. doi:10.1134/S0006297915120044.

35. Bouzid M, Filaire E, McCall A, et al. Radical oxygen species, exercise and aging: an update. *Sports Med.* 2015;45(9):1245-1261. doi:10.1007/s40279-015-0348-1.

36. Pingitore A, Pereira Lima GP, Mastorci F, et al. Exercise and oxidative stress: potential effects of antioxidant dietary strategies in sports. *Nutrition.* 2015;31(7/8):916-922. doi:10.1016/j.nut.2015.02.005.

37. Golub VV. Hypothalamus as a possible modulator of the rates of development and aging of mammals. *Russian J Gen Chem.* 2010;80(7):1425-1433. doi:10.1134/S1070363210070388.

38. Rzheshevsky AV. Decrease in ATP biosynthesis and dysfunction of biological membranes. Two possible key mechanisms of phenoptosis. *Biochemistry (Mosc).* 2014;79(10):1056-1068. doi:10.1134/S0006297914100071.

39. Ranabir S, Reetu K. Stress and hormones. *Indian J Endocrinol Metab.* 2011;15(1):18-22. doi:10.4103/2230-8210.77573.

40. Olenski AR, Abola MV, Jena AB. Do heads of government age more quickly? Observational study comparing mortality between elected leaders and runners-up in national elections of 17 countries. *BMJ.* 2015;351:h6424. doi:10.1136/bmj.h6424.

41. Christiansen L, Lenart A, Tan Q, et al. DNA methylation age is associated with mortality in a longitudinal Danish twin study. *Aging Cell.* 2016;15(1):149-154. doi:10.1111/acel.12421.

42. Ye K, Beekman M, Lameijer E, et al. Aging as accelerated accumulation of somatic variants: whole-genome sequencing of centenarian and middle-aged monozygotic twin pairs. *Twin Res Hum Genet.* 2013;16(6):1026-1032. doi:10.1017/thg.2013.73.

43. McGue M, Skytthe A, Christensen K. The nature of behavioural correlates of healthy ageing: a twin study of lifestyle in mid to late life. *Int J Epidemiol.* 2014;43(3):775-782. doi:10.1093/ije/dyt210.

44. Moayyeri A, Hart DJ, Snieder H, et al. Aging trajectories in different body systems share common environmental etiology: the Healthy Aging Twin Study (HATS). *Twin Res Hum Genet.* 2016;19(1):27-34. doi:10.1017/thg.2015.100.

45. Robert L, Labat-Robert J. Longevity and aging: role of genes and of the extracellular matrix. *Biogerontology.* 2015;16(1):125-129. doi:10.1007/s10522-014-9544-x.

46. Carnes B, Olshansky S, Hayflick L. Can human biology allow most of us to become centenarians? *J Gerontol A Biol Sci Med Sci.* 2013;68(2):136-142. doi:10.1093/gerona/gls142.

47. Hasworth SB, Cannon ML. Social theories of aging: a review. *Dis Mon.* 2015;61(11):475-479. doi:10.1016/j.disamonth.2015.09.003.

48. Bonder BR, Dal Bello-Haas V. *Functional Performance in Older Adults.* 3rd ed. Philadelphia: FA Davis; 2009.

49. Robinson OC, Stell AJ. Later-life crisis: towards a holistic model. *J Adult Dev.* 2015;22(1):38-49. doi:10.1007/s10804-014-9199-5.

50. Cumming E, Henry W. *Growing Old.* New York: Basic Books; 1961.

51. Hochschild AR. Disengagement theory: a critique and proposal. *Am Sociol Rev.* 1975;40(5):553-569.

52. Powell JL. *Aging, Culture and Society: A Sociological Approach.* Hauppauge, NY: Nova Science Publishers, Inc; 2013.

53. Johnson KJ, Mutchler JE. The emergence of a positive gerontology: from disengagement to social involvement. *Gerontologist.* 2014;54(1):93-100.

54. Powell JL. *Social Gerontology.* Hauppauge, NY: Nova Science Publishers, Inc; 2013.

55. Kuroda A, Tanaka T, Hirano H, et al. Eating alone as social disengagement is strongly associated with depressive symptoms in Japanese community-dwelling older adults. *J Am Med Dir Assoc.* 2015;16(7):578-585. doi:10.1016/j.jamda.2015.01.078.

56. Wernher I, Lipsky MS. Psychological theories of aging. *Dis Mon.* 2015;61:480-488. doi:10.1016/j.disamonth.2015.09.004.

57. Carstensen L, Fung H, Charles S. Socioemotional selectivity theory and the regulation of emotion in the second half of life. *Motiv Emot.* 2003;27(2):103-123.

58. Havighurst RJ. Successful aging. *Gerontologist.* 1961;1:8-13. doi:10.1093/geront/1.1.8.

59. Franklin NC, Tate CA. Lifestyle and successful aging: an overview. *Am J Lifestyle Med.* 2009;3(1):6-11. doi:10.1177/1559827608326125.

60. Atchley RC. A continuity theory of normal aging. *Gerontologist.* 1989;29(2):183-190. doi:10.1093/geront/29.2.183.

61. Nimrod G, Kleiber DA. Reconsidering change and continuity in later life: toward an innovation theory of successful aging. *Int J Aging Hum Dev.* 2007;65(1):1-22. doi:10.2190/Q4G5-7176-51Q2-3754.

62. Law M, Baptiste S, Carswell A, et al. *Canadian Occupational Performance Measure.* 5th ed. Ottawa, Canada: CAOT Publications ACE; 2014.

63. Kielhofner G. *A Model of Human Occupation: Theory and Application.* 4th ed. Baltimore: Lippincott Williams & Wilkins; 2007.

64. Mayer KU. The sociology of the life course and lifespan psychology: Diverging or converging pathways? In: Staudinger UM, Lindenberger U, eds. *Understanding Human Development: Dialogues with Lifespan Psychology.* Dordrecht, Netherlands: Kluwer Academic Publishers; 2003:463-481.

65. Barrett AE, Montepare JM. 'It's about time': Applying life span and life course perspectives to the study of subjective age. In: Diehl M, Wahl H, eds. *Annual Review of Gerontology and Geriatrics: Subjective Aging: New Developments and Future Directions.* Vol. 35. New York, NY: Springer Publishing Co; 2015:55-77.

66. Ryff CD. Life span and life course approaches to dermatological disease. *Curr Probl Dermatol.* 2013;44:1-16. doi:10.1159/000350007.

The Aging Process

SUE BYERS-CONNON

(WITH PREVIOUS CONTRIBUTIONS FROM DANIELLE LANCASTER BARBER, CLAUDELLE CARRUTHERS, JODI LANE, LISA WALKER, MIRTHA MONTEJO WHALEY)

KEY TERMS

primary aging, secondary aging, successful aging, function, occupational performance, environment

CHAPTER OBJECTIVES

1. Describe the aging process.
2. Explore the concepts of successful, primary, and secondary aging.
3. Discuss usual and pathological aging within the context of age-related physiological changes in the integumentary, cardiopulmonary, musculoskeletal, neurological, and sensory systems.
4. Explore how normal and abnormal age-related changes present in older adults within clinical case studies.

The process of aging is complex, multidirectional, and influenced by multiple contexts or environments.[1,2] Aging is a universal event that is inherent to the individual and occurs within biological and genetic parameters. We all age regardless of race, gender, ethnicity, or geographic location. The variability of the aging process among individuals, however, is not only dependent on a person's biological and genetic blueprint but also is highly influenced by other factors such as lifestyle choices and behaviors over the life span, proximal contexts or environments (i.e., family, friends, community, culture, etc.), which affect development, maturation, and function. Other factors are the distal contexts (i.e., the historical period within which we develop and the public policies and decisions), which indirectly affect the opportunities afforded us to participate in occupation or the barriers that keep us from reaching our maximum potential.[1]

AGING

The fact that we all age attests to the biological nature of aging, but although aging itself is universal, the process of aging, that is, the rate at which we age, varies both across individuals and even organ systems within the individual.[1,3] That we age differently explains the effect that environments, contexts, and lifestyle behaviors exert on each individual.[1,2] Aging is the sum total of our genetic and biological makeup combined with all of the lifestyle decisions, events, and exposures (whether by choice or otherwise) that we experience throughout the life span.[1] Despite arbitrary determinations as to when we become old, aging is really a lifelong process. In fact, aging is a chronic, progressive, and terminal event that begins at the moment of conception. Some authorities, however, would argue that aging begins at age 30 with the onset of decrements in physiological function and efficiency, and that changes that occur through childhood and young adulthood are the result of maturation and development, rather than aging. Baltes,[4] as early as 1987, and Kolling and Knopf,[3] as recently as 2014, cautioned against that type of differentiation, which has been long adopted by scholars and researchers because of its implications as to the perceived potential of older individuals of continuing to grow and develop throughout the life span.

Although throughout history there have been individuals who lived long past the life expectancy of their times, the increased life span of entire cohorts is a more recent occurrence, resulting from advances in public health and medicine during the 20th century.[5] In 2019, the worldwide age for life expectancy was 72.6 years compared to 72.3 years in 1950 within the healthiest country.[6] This increased longevity has created a growing interest in aging, propelling aging research, theories of aging, and a variety of new aging fields. As health care professionals, learning about the process of aging has implications on several levels. On a personal level, the more we know about aging, the better equipped we are to make lifestyle decisions that have a bearing on our own aging process. On another level, enhancing our knowledge of aging can provide us with useful tools to assist our loved ones through their own aging process, given that most of us are or will be involved as family caregivers of aging parents.

Last, as a result of the changing demographics and the growing numbers of aging consumers of health services, Occupational Therapy Assistants (OTAs) are likely to provide services to older adults. As such, there are several key issues to be aware of regarding services to an aging population.

The Institute of Medicine (IOM), in its report on the state of the health care workforce, identified serious gaps in knowledge of the aging process that potentially compromise the care provided to older persons. The IOM's report, *Retooling for an Aging America: Building the Health Care Workforce*, calls for actions to prepare competent health care practitioners to meet the health care needs of an aging population and improve the way in which care is delivered to the aging.[7] As a result, the Eldercare Workforce Alliance, a partnership of 35 national organizations, was founded in 2009 to address a shortage of qualified health care providers and caregivers.[6]

The Centers for Disease Control and Prevention's Healthy People initiative, currently known as *Healthy People 2030*,[8] establishes goals for the health of the nation and identified health indicators to track progress toward these goals. These include improving the health and wellness of the aging population, preventing injuries, reducing disabilities, addressing health disparities, paying attention to the environmental impact on health, health literacy, and health well-being.[8]

In the *Occupational Therapy Practice Framework: Domain and Practice*, Fourth Edition, the American Occupational Therapy Association[9] provides the blueprint for the delivery of occupational therapy services. These are the principles and procedures that guide our interventions by delineating the domains and process of occupational therapy practice.[9]

These key issues are important because occupational therapy is only one component of a large ecological system inextricably connected to the public's health. As a profession and as individual practitioners, we must understand that the effect of our services and the outcomes we achieve extend beyond the clinical environment or in patients' homes. Although we must be accountable to third-party payers and responsive to the fiscal requirements of our employers, we must also be cognizant that the extent and appropriateness of the services we deliver have a significant bearing on the health and functional status of not just our patients, but also on the health of our communities and our nation.

Successful, Primary, and Secondary Aging

Definitions and categories of aging abound in the literature and can be confusing, misleading, and even discriminatory in nature. Rowe and Kahn[10] proposed a definition of successful aging as an optimal state that could be attained by avoiding disease and disability, maintaining high cognitive and physical functioning, and continuing to be actively engaged with life. Despite its popularity and the substantial amount of research based on the concept of successful aging, that definition has been called to question by a number of researchers.[11]

Some of the criticisms are based on research findings that indicate that "successful aging," as defined by Rowe and Kahn[10] in their earlier work, describes the aging experience of a very narrow segment of the population. Others have objected to the use of a strictly quantitative research methodology in published studies because it fails to consider individuals' constructions of successful aging. Still others propose that the aging experience cannot be understood through the individual alone, but that it must consider the effect of contexts and environments on aging.[12] Labeling optimal or healthy aging as "successful" risks devaluing disabled individuals, institutionalized older adults, and those with chronic illnesses who, by default, age otherwise "unsuccessfully."

The concepts of primary and secondary aging define the aging process from a different perspective. Primary aging describes the normal, gradual changes in organ systems that, although annoying, are inevitable, experienced by everyone, and not associated with disease, impairment, or disability.[1] Some changes eventually become visible, as with the loss of moisture and elasticity of the skin that gives it a sagging, tired, and wrinkled appearance, or the changes in texture and color and even the loss of aging hair (Fig. 3.1). Others, such as changes in

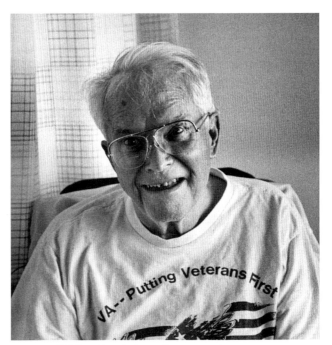

FIG. 3.1 With aging, hair tends to grow in a sparser pattern.

visual and auditory acuity, slowed mobility, and decline in strength,[1] may only be noticeable by the way in which an individual performs daily routines and/or the use of assistive devices such as eyeglasses and canes. Although primary aging changes manifest themselves later in life, they actually begin to take place much earlier, and it is estimated that organ systems begin to gradually lose function and efficiency at a rate of 1% per year after age 30.[1] Secondary aging changes are neither normal nor usual; are experienced by some individuals but not all; are associated with disease, injury, dysfunction, and impairment; and are frequently preventable through lifestyle changes.[2]

What is certain is that whether primary or secondary, normal or pathological, aging brings about changes. Baltes,[4] in his Life Span Perspective, proposed that aging is marked by a series of gains and losses requiring adaptation through a process of selection, compensation, and optimization. That is, as we age and experience changes in our ability to engage in valued occupations, we select domains of function and activities that are important to us and compensate for the losses by changing the task, changing the environment in which we perform the task, or changing the manner in which we perform it. Selection and compensation allow us to optimize our engagement in life through involvement in valued roles and occupations.[2] Optimal aging can then be viewed in terms of our successful adaptation and continued participation in life, a premise that Pizzi and Smith[13] propose is at the very core of occupational therapy: "Successful aging ... is having the physical, emotional, social and spiritual resources, combined with an ability to adapt to life changes, in order to engage in meaningful and important self-selected occupations of life as one ages" (p. 466).

AGING CHANGES

Older adults are not a homogeneous group, or wrinkled versions of their younger selves. Aging is marked by physiological, cognitive, and psychosocial changes that affect a person's occupational performance and quality of life. It stands to reason that if aging is the sum total of all we have experienced, consumed, and/or engaged in throughout our lives, individuals who through their lifestyles have built a physiological and cognitive reserve capacity will fare better as they age than will individuals who age with limited reserves.

Having knowledge of the aging process allows OTAs to discriminate between changes that are a normal part of the process and those that may be a sign of pathology. Such knowledge is basic to designing and implementing appropriate and client-centered occupational therapy interventions. Additionally, given the time constraints and demands imposed on practitioners today, there is a risk of becoming so focused on the diagnosis and presenting problem as to exclude signs and symptoms that should not be ignored. There is also the risk of allowing stereotypes

of aging to interfere with sound clinical reasoning. Being able to discriminate between what is usual or normal and what may be a manifestation of pathology allows the practitioner to design appropriate interventions, as well as to identify a potential problem and alert the appropriate health care professional(s) [i.e., the occupational therapist (OT), nurse, the physician of the older adult, etc.], so that the issue can be addressed before it becomes a serious threat to the older adult's well-being and quality of life.

INTEGUMENTARY SYSTEM

The integumentary system, consisting of the skin, hair, nails, sebaceous (oil), and sweat glands, has a protective and regulatory function and, indirectly, an aesthetic one as well. Smooth, healthy, and vibrant skin, hair, and nails are appreciated, sought after, and rewarded in our society. For the individual, the integrity and appearance of the integument have important implications in terms of self-appraisal, self-esteem, and self-confidence.

There are noticeable changes associated with primary aging. As we age, there is a decrease in the number of hair follicles, a slowing in the rate of growth of the follicles that remain, and a decrease in the production of melanin. These changes contribute to the loss, but, because hair also shields the scalp from the effects of the sun, the loss and thinning of hair also impair its protective function against exposure to sunlight.[14]

As the largest organ in the human body, the skin protects internal organs and serves as a barrier to infectious organisms and to noxious and injury-producing agents. The skin also prevents dehydration from the loss of water and is an important part of the immune system.[14,15] Through sensory receptors in the skin, we are able to detect temperature, pain, touch, and pressure. Through sweat glands and superficial blood vessels, the skin is able to cool the body and regulate its internal temperature.[15,16]

Loss of collagen and elastin, proteins that help the skin maintain its elasticity and tone, contribute to the thinning, sagging, and wrinkling of the skin, which we recognize as signs of aging. In primary aging, normal thinning of the epidermis combined with fragile capillaries and loss of fatty tissue increase the risk of bruising in older adults. These normal changes are further exacerbated in the presence of chronic conditions, such as diabetes, and the use of medications to treat these conditions. Changes precipitated by chronic conditions and medications are not normally experienced by all individuals and are associated with secondary aging.[17] These physiological and structural changes in the integumentary system make aging skin more vulnerable to injury and can increase the risk of adverse health outcomes for aging persons. As an example, fatty tissue, which normally cushions the skin, becomes thinner as we age. Aesthetically, this accounts for the structural changes in the face and the aged appearance of hands and feet (Fig. 3.2). Physiologically, the loss of fatty tissue increases the risk of injury to the skin and,

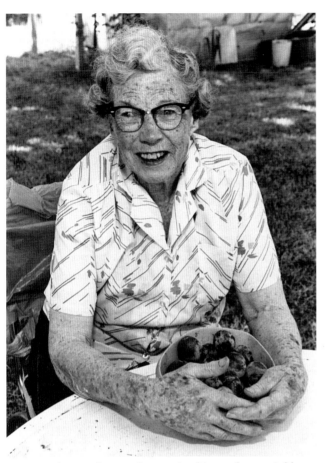

FIG. 3.2 As people age, changes in skin, such as wrinkles and bruises, become evident.

combined with a decrease in sweat production, interferes with the skin's ability to effectively regulate the body's internal temperature. Functionally, the loss of padding in the feet can cause pain and discomfort while walking[14] and can have implications as to the older adult's tolerance for footwear and even his or her activity level.

The sluggish replacement of epidermal cells and a decline in the production of melanin decrease the skin's ability to protect against exposure to the sun's ultraviolet rays and increase the risk of sunburn and skin cancer in older adults.[14] Blood supply to the skin, also reduced as we age, impairs wound healing and interferes with what is recognized as signs of inflammation, such as redness and swelling, which is the body's way to alert us of an infection or injury. Injuries to the skin caused by infection or sunburn may go unnoticed in older adults, and treatment may be delayed or not provided.

Inefficient temperature regulation as a result of the reduction in sweat glands and loss of fatty tissue increases the risk of heat stroke in older adults.[14] Loss of sensory receptors in the skin affects sensitivity to touch, temperature, and pain, making older adults more susceptible to cuts, abrasions, and burns. These changes in sensory receptors are also responsible for an increase in pain threshold and impaired pain localization in older adults and, as

in the case of injury to the skin, can preclude prompt intervention and treatment.

Nutrition and hydration play an important part in maintaining the integrity of the skin and other components of the integumentary system. The frailty and decreased resilience of aging skin are further compromised by the use of prescription and over-the-counter medications that make it more susceptible to the effects of sun exposure, more prone to bleeding, and less able to heal. OTAs need to be particularly cautious when working on transfers with older adults to prevent skin injuries. Avoiding and addressing pressure areas from orthotics and braces, from prolonged sitting and improper seating equipment, or from confinement to bed can prevent complications from wounds that endanger the health and well-being of older adults.

NEUROMUSCULOSKELETAL SYSTEM

Aging of the nervous system is characterized by morphological and biological changes, which have an effect on the integrity and function of other systems as well. Aging brains undergo atrophic changes, decreased weight, and enlargement of the ventricles with loss of adjacent white and gray matter, which affect the normal activity of nerve cells and their processes. Loss of neurons and dendritic changes and impaired nerve conduction velocity affect the neuron's ability to communicate with other nerve cells.[18]

These biochemical, structural, and metabolic alterations in the aging nervous system have an effect on sensory and motor function, coordination, reaction time, gait, and proprioception. However, despite their potential effect, research has not been able to clearly establish an association between these aging changes and specific declines in functional performance. One explanation that has been offered is that the older adult responds to nervous system changes in individual ways, so changes that would precipitate functional decline and even dementia in some will not have the same effect on others. Another explanation is that of neuroplasticity, the ability of the brain to reorganize and form new pathways to compensate for atrophic changes and neuronal losses so that functional performance is maintained. Yet another explanation has been that changes in the nervous system may not have implications for the functional performance of daily activities of young-old adults (75 years of age and younger) but that the effect is more significant in those age 75 and older.[19]

SKELETAL SYSTEM

Skeletal system changes resulting from primary aging are responsible for a decline in bone density, lowered skeletal resistance to stress, and loss of skeletal flexibility and mobility. Both men and women experience age-related changes in bone density, however, the change is most pronounced in women following menopause and is associated with a decrease in estrogen.[20] Structural and physiological changes in muscles contribute to a loss in strength. Weak postural muscles and loss of bone density and cartilage in the vertebrae are responsible for the "shortening" and stooped and round-shouldered posture (kyphosis) often seen in older adults.

Although some skeletal changes result from the wear and tear caused by normal aging, others are the result of disease processes or trauma. Degenerative changes in the joints are frequently caused by osteoarthritis (OA), a condition that affects about 50% of the population age 65 years and older.[21] Although OA generally involves weight-bearing joints such as the vertebrae, hips, and knees, it can also affect joints in the elbows, hands, and wrists. Osteoarthritic changes can cause pain and limited range of motion and consequently may have an effect on quality of life, but they are not life threatening and can be treated with medication, joint protection, surgery, therapy, and exercise.[21] Rheumatoid arthritis (RA) is a progressive autoimmune disease with onset in young adulthood or midlife.[22] RA initially presents with inflammation and pain in the metacarpophalangeal and interphalangeal joints of the hands and eventually progresses to other organs. Signs and symptoms include inflammation, pain, joint deformities, fatigue, and weight loss. RA severely impairs functional performance and quality of life.[22]

Osteoporosis is a disease that causes bone to become more porous and brittle and more prone to fracture.[20] Although the disease affects both genders, it is more prevalent in women and is associated with drops in estrogen levels experienced with menopause. The risk of osteoporosis is lessened by building up a reserve starting in young adulthood through a diet rich in calcium and vitamins and exercise that includes weight-bearing activities, which are essential for maintaining bone density.[2,20] Occupational therapy interventions have shown promise in helping adults with osteoporosis maintain physical health and engagement in valued activities.[23]

Hundreds of thousands of fibers (muscle cells) make up each of approximately 700 muscles in the human body.[24] These muscle fibers and the branches of motor nerves that innervate them form motor units (MUs) of varying sizes, depending on the work required of the muscle. At about age 30,[25] we begin to experience declines in physical strength, that can result in 3%–5% of muscle loss per decade.[26] The rate of decline increases around our 50s, and the decline in muscle can increase to 15% per decade.[25] It is common for individuals between 50 and 70 to have a 30% decline in muscle strength.[26,27] This decline in strength, which depending on the muscle, can range from 12% to 60%, is mainly due to physiological changes affecting muscle mass.[25] This age-associated loss of muscle mass (sarcopenia) involves decrements in both the number of muscle fibers and the size of the fibers, which affect the strength of the muscle contraction. However, research suggests it is the decrease in the number of fibers, rather than a change in their size, that accounts for the decline in

strength.[28] The muscle mass that is lost within the aging process is caused by the decline of motoneurons, and causes the size and number of muscle fibers to decrease.[28] Additionally, as motor neurons are lost, the remaining motor neurons provide compensatory innervations that causes a reduction in the functions of the muscle.[28]

Sarcopenia is responsible for functional declines in older persons[28] and is associated with physiological changes that increase the risk of disease in this population. Physiologically, as muscle mass declines, there is an increase in the deposition of fatty tissue (adiposity) in and around the muscle with a subsequent decline in basal metabolism, which increases the risk for obesity, malnutrition, dyslipidemia, and diabetes.[28,29] Functionally, changes in strength, motor control, and fatigability contribute to difficulties with balance, activities of daily living (ADL), and instrumental activities of daily living (IADL) performance in older adults. Research conducted by McGee and Mathiowetz[30] found an association between the strength of shoulder abductors and external rotators on IADL function and elbow extensors on the ability to shop for groceries. Unaddressed sarcopenia increases the risk for falls and fractures, frailty, and loss of independence, which can lead to a less-than-optimal quality of life.[31,32]

Older adults naturally compensate for changes in strength and functional capacity by avoiding tasks that require high levels of force and by performing tasks at a slower pace.[19] Compensation can be observed in gait patterns as well, with older adults typically taking shorter steps and walking at a slower pace, maintaining a smaller heel-to-ground angle while walking and exhibiting a wider stance.[19] The key in working with older adults is to encourage and maintain a reasonable level of activity and prevent hypokinesis because inactivity can accelerate the loss of strength and endurance and further compromise mobility, ADL, and IADL performance.

Improving muscle strength and endurance in older adults is crucial, and research indicates that exercise can reduce and even reverse the effects of sarcopenia.[28] OTAs working with older adults should ensure that interventions consider individual factors and preferences because there is evidence of the benefits of client-focused programs that improve ADLs and IADLs.[33] Community dwelling older adults should be encouraged to participate in personally valued occupations that incorporate physical activity such as gardening, grocery shopping, golfing, or mall walking.[33] OTAs should also take advantage of opportunities to educate older adults and their caregivers on the importance of proper nutrition and hydration in maintaining muscle strength, endurance, and overall health.

CARDIOPULMONARY SYSTEM

With age, the inner lining of the heart (endocardium) becomes fibrotic (more rigid and thick), fatty tissue builds up in the heart and surrounding area, and there is a decline in the number of pacemaker cells that regulate the rhythm of the cardiac contraction.[14] Changes in the elastin of the arterial walls cause the walls to become thicker and more rigid, due to the increase in collagen fibers and calcium within the arterial walls.[34] The increase in size and stiffness of arteries have been associated with the development of increased systolic and pulse pressure. These arterial changes can lead to the risk of experiencing a stroke and long-term cerebrovascular disease and mortality in individuals age 60 years and older.[34] Loss of elasticity in the arteries causes an increase in stiffness and also a rise in the development of cardiovascular disease.[35] Structural and physiological changes in the heart and cardiovascular system reduce the efficiency of the cardiac muscle and its ability to respond to sympathetic stimulation. As a result, the stroke volume, maximum heart rate, and cardiac output decrease. These cardiac changes, which seem to not have a significant effect on the organism at rest, are noticeably altered in response to external stress, as when the organism is challenged during physical exertion. As a result, and compared with younger adults, older adults have less endurance, tire more quickly, and experience shortness of breath in response to exercise.[14] Practitioners should take these changes into account when designing therapeutic interventions for older patients to ensure that exercises and activities meet specific goals and avoid unnecessary exertion.

In the pulmonary system, effective gas exchange is compromised by a decrease in lung volume associated with the loss of elasticity in the lungs and in the medium and small airways. Pulmonary function is further affected by neuromuscular and musculoskeletal changes that increase the effort required to breathe. These pulmonary changes include weakened respiratory and postural muscles, changes in the spine and ribs, and increased kyphosis, which affect the flexibility of the thoracic cage and prevent the normal movement of the chest wall, reducing the efficiency of the pulmonary system.[36-39]

IMMUNE SYSTEM

Immunosenescence is a term that refers to the changes in immune function that contribute to the increased susceptibility to disease in older adults. Recent research suggests that immunosenescence is not likely the result of primary aging,[40,41] but rather is due to secondary changes caused by environmental and lifestyle factors, even in healthy older adults free of chronic illnesses. Nutrition, exercise, and even medications taken over the life span can influence immune function as we age. Over time, the epithelial barriers of the skin and digestive tract break down, making us more susceptible to pathogens.[42] On a cellular level, immune cells such as T cells and B cells behave differently in the aging body. The ability of these cells to respond to the threat of foreign bodies is diminished, increasing the risk of acquiring infections such as influenza and pneumonia.[43] Immunosenescence not only affects the immune system's ability to protect against disease but also has a suppressant effect on vaccines, making them less effective in older adults. Older adults should consult with their physicians and keep their influenza, pneumonia, and any other suggested vaccinations up to date.[44] As a way of counteracting the effects of immunosenescence, physicians may recommend proper nutrition, vitamin and nutritional supplements, hormone therapy, or the administration of a higher dose of vaccines to boost their effectiveness.[41,43]

Given the effect of the aging immune system on its ability to protect against infections, OTAs should be aware of other factors that increase the risk of infection in older individuals. Hospitalized and institutionalized older adults are at risk of acquiring serious and sometimes fatal iatrogenic (caused by medical treatment) and nosocomial (facility acquired) infections such as methicillin-resistant *Staphylococcus aureus* (MRSA), *Clostridium difficile* (C-Diff), and vancomycin-resistant *Enterococcus* (VRE). OTAs should observe universal precautions and any other precautions, such as wearing masks, with older adults. OTAs must be alert for signs of possible infection, which they should report to the nurse, nurse practitioner, or physician so that proper assessment and treatment can be provided and preventable and life-threatening complications avoided.

COGNITION

As with the effect of aging on other bodily systems and physical abilities, one's cognitive abilities are influenced by both personal and environmental factors. Cognition is influenced by our genetic makeup, lifestyle choices, health status, and the external environments that have either provided opportunities for optimal development throughout our life span or have precluded us from achieving our optimal capacity. Just as reserve capacity in muscular strength varies across individuals based on their habitual level and types of activity, maintaining good intellectual functioning has been associated with factors such as achieving a high level of education and employment, having an intact family, engaging in activities that enhance cognitive abilities, enjoying good health, and having good sensory function.

In terms of age-related changes, research studies indicate that older adults experience a slowing in information processing and psychomotor speed, deficits in tasks requiring abstraction, set-shifting, and divided attention, and declines in fluid intelligence. The latter, contingent on the health of the central nervous system (CNS), reflects intellectual processes that affect numerical reasoning and logic. Fluid intelligence allows us to solve novel problems and "think on our feet" when presented with new situations. It represents intelligence that is not a product of learning and is not influenced by social or cultural factors. In contrast is crystallized intelligence, the knowledge accumulated through the life span.[45]

For older adults, executive function is crucial in setting and managing doctors' appointments, anticipating medication refills, anticipating and identifying hazards, and problem-solving their way out of situations, including those that may be potentially dangerous. Fluid abilities play an important part when faced with new situations, such as those patients often encounter in rehabilitation when they have to learn novel ways of doing routine activities, manage new medical and dietary regimes, or apply safety precautions.

Studies also indicate that factors such as physical illness, chronic conditions, depression, neurological damage, medication side effects, drug interactions, and the effects of surgery and anesthesia may also cause varying degrees of cognitive impairment.[46-48] Impairment of cognitive function is known to affect treatment and rehabilitation outcomes for older adults and increases their likelihood of institutionalization.

Differentiating between normal age-related alterations in cognition and abnormal changes in cognitive function is crucial in geriatric rehabilitation. Screening/assessing the cognitive status of older adults in occupational therapy is useful in establishing treatment plans based on ability to function, determining the type and extent of assistance needed, and addressing safety issues. Identification of cognitive impairment can lead to referrals for further evaluation, allow for treatment of reversible conditions, provide early intervention in cases of progressive decline, and assist with caregiver education.

Suitable screening and assessment instruments should be standardized, valid, and reliable and should explore the individual's capacity to problem-solve and to shift and divide attention. Conversing with a patient and/or observing the individual perform a familiar ADL can be misleading because people frequently retain social skills in the presence of a cognitive impairment, and ADL are overlearned activities and therefore not a good measure of ability to problem-solve, learn, and safely engage in ADL and IADL.

SENSORY SYSTEM

In our later years, almost every aspect of our sensory systems experiences a change in functioning. These changes can negatively affect social participation, occupational engagement, health, and overall quality of life.[49,50] When designing and implementing intervention activities for older adults, occupational therapy professionals should understand the nature and consequences of age-related sensory changes and how older adults typically respond to such changes.

Olfactory and Gustatory Systems

It is estimated that that more than 50% of older individuals that are 65–80 years old experience diminished olfaction due to impairment to the olfactory epithelium and a decrease in enzymes and nasal receptors.[51] It is unclear whether anatomical changes in the taste system are to blame

for changes in taste sensation, but it has been suggested that there may be a loss of taste buds or age-related changes to the taste cell membranes.[52] It is difficult to differentiate between primary and secondary changes to olfaction and taste. Like many other age-related changes, factors such as age, gender, and lifestyle are most commonly linked to chemosensory changes. Medical conditions, including neurological disorders such as Alzheimer's disease, endocrine disorders, nutritional deficiencies, cancer, and viruses, as well as medications taken, can all be contributors to alterations in taste and smell function.[52,53]

Age-related changes in the chemical senses of smell and taste are less apparent than many other sensory changes and therefore are typically less likely to be addressed. Impairment of chemical senses is really an issue of safety. Proper olfactory function alerts us to noxious odors that may themselves be detrimental to health or may indicate the presence of harmful gases such as methane. If the olfactory sense is impaired, an older adult may not realize that he or she has failed to turn off a gas stove or may not notice the smell of smoke. Impairment in taste may also pose a safety threat because an older adult with diminished taste may not realize when food is spoiled. Because these changes are not reversible, it is important that older adults learn to compensate for impairment of these senses.

Beyond concern for safety, changes in smell and taste function can affect quality of life.[51,53] Some studies have found that older adults with chemosensory impairments report changes in mood, functional impairments such as difficulties with cooking and preparing foods, and lowered enjoyment in other areas of life.[49,52] Additionally, changes in taste and smell can negatively affect social participation. In many cultures, occupations of preparing food and sharing meals are central and profoundly influence quality of life. Chemosensory impairments can lead to decreased engagement or enjoyment of such activities. Impairments in olfaction may also be a source of uncertainty or vulnerability for older adults because they may not be aware of personal body odor or the presence of dangerous fumes.[49]

Perhaps the most important issue regarding impairment in chemosensory functioning is the effect on physical health. Alterations in taste and smell have been found to be associated with decreased food intake and nutritional status.[54,55] The literature refers to this phenomenon as the "anorexia of aging." Many older adults experience a loss of appetite,[49,54,55] perhaps because it is the enticing aroma of food that stimulates hunger or because a decreased intake of food leads to reduced need for food or, as some research suggests, because older adults may experience changes in the digestive system that make them feel satiated sooner.[53,54]

The issue of excessive weight gain or loss is also of concern for older adults. Changes of taste and smell have been linked to a reduction in the consumption of nutrient-rich foods and overconsumption of foods high in fat, sugar, and salt.[56] Anorexia of aging has been linked to protein deficiencies that may contribute to impaired muscle function, impaired cognition, decreased bone mass, immune dysfunction, anemia, poor wound healing, and generally increased morbidity and mortality.[54]

There are several ways that OTAs can help remediate the negative consequences of olfactory and gustatory sensory impairments. The first is to educate older adults about proper nutrition and appropriate food intake. The next is to make adaptations to food by adding flavorings that enhance taste like pepper, herbs, or spices but not add excessive salt or sugar.[55] Collaborating with nutritionists and speech therapists whenever possible is recommended to address nutritional needs of older adults. Last, because the social and temporal contexts in which meals take place can influence food intake, OTAs may be able to ensure adequate nutritional intake by encouraging older adults to consume meals with others and by creating a socially enriching environment for mealtime.

Somatosensory and Kinesthetic Systems

Proprioception is the sense that makes us aware of our body's position in space and gives us information about the static position as well as the kinesthetic movement of our joints.[57] Somatosensory and kinesthetic senses are clinically tested through passive movement to determine whether individuals are able to detect changes in joint position.

Proprioceptive function in the lower extremities has been extensively researched and found to decline with age and to affect older adults' sensorimotor performance, particularly balance. Problems with balance not only increase older adults' risks for falling, but also may lead to restricted activity in response to a fear of falling, and ultimately contribute to further decline. Less research has been conducted on the effect of aging on upper extremity somatosensory and kinesthetic function, but there is evidence of an age-related decline that contributes to decreased coordination during tasks involving the upper extremities.[58] Research also suggests that declines in kinesthetic or motor memory, the ability to perceive and plan movement patterns, may contribute to difficulty in learning new motor tasks.[59]

Studies indicate that, compared with younger subjects, older adults experience more difficulty sensing joint movement and that this may result from the effect of changes in the central processing abilities.[60] There are also indications that age-related somatosensory and kinesthetic changes progress from distal to proximal joints. Exercises such as tai chi, with its slow and deliberate movements and a constant focus on monitoring motion, have been successful in improving position sense in older adults.[61]

As with other declines in function, older adults appear to compensate for these somatosensory changes by reducing the amplitude and the speed of their movements to maintain balance.[62] This type of compensation, mediated by the CNS, allows older individuals to remain functional.

Conversely, changes leading to the loss of integrity of the CNS interfere with this integrative function, leading to disability.[62]

SUMMARY

Aging is marked by physiological, sensory, cognitive, and psychosocial changes that affect a person's occupational performance and quality of life. The process of aging is universal in that all experience age-related changes, however, the rate at which people age varies both across individuals and even organ systems within the individual. Aging is the product of our genetic and biological makeup, our life's experiences, our lifestyle decisions and choices, and the effect of the contexts or environments of which we have been a part. Therefore, it stands to reason that individuals who, through their lifestyles, have built physiological and cognitive reserve capacity will fare better as they age than individuals who age with limited reserves.

This chapter explored two major categories of aging. Primary aging, the normal gradual changes in organ systems experienced by everyone and not associated with disease, impairment, or disability; and secondary aging, changes that are experienced by some individuals but not all, are associated with disease, injury, dysfunction, and impairment, and are frequently preventable through lifestyle changes.

Baltes' Life Span Perspective[4] proposes that aging is marked by a series of gains and losses (multi-directionality) requiring adaptation through a process of selection, compensation, and optimization. That is, as we experience changes in our ability to engage in valued occupations, we select domains of function and activities that are important to us and compensate for the losses by changing the task, changing the environment in which we perform the task, or changing the manner in which we perform it. Selection and compensation allow us to optimize our engagement in life through involvement in valued roles and occupations. Older adults compensate for changes in strength and functional capacity by avoiding tasks that require high levels of force and performing tasks at a slower pace. Compensation can be observed in gait patterns as well, that is, shorter steps, slower pace, and maintaining a wider stance when walking.

Having knowledge of the aging process allows OTs and OTAs to discriminate between changes that are a normal part of the process and those that may be a sign of pathology. This knowledge is basic to designing and implementing appropriate and client-centered occupational therapy interventions and proactively identifying abnormal conditions that may require treatment or referral to other professionals.

Musculoskeletal changes affect our strength and predispose us to conditions such as osteoporosis and OA. Sensory changes affect our ability to receive and process sensory stimulus and can lead to isolation, depression, and impaired quality of life. Cardiovascular and pulmonary changes, which seem to not have a significant effect on the organism at rest, are noticeably altered during physical exertion. As a result, and compared with younger adults, older adults have less endurance, tire more quickly, and experience shortness of breath in response to exercise. Practitioners should take these changes into account when designing therapeutic interventions for older patients to ensure that exercises and activities meet specific goals and avoid unnecessary exertion.

Immunosenescence not only affects the immune system's ability to protect against disease but also has a suppressant effect on vaccines, making them less effective in the older adult. Given the effect of aging on the immune system's ability to protect against infections, OTAs should be aware of other factors that increase the risk of infection in older individuals, observe universal precautions with all of their patients and residents, and be alert for signs of possible infection and report them to the nurse, nurse practitioner, or physician so that proper assessment and treatment can be provided and preventable and life-threatening complications avoided.

Information processing and psychomotor speed slow down with aging, and we experience deficits with tasks requiring abstraction, set-shifting, and divided attention. Fluid intelligence has an important function in dealing with new situations, such as those patients often encounter in rehabilitation when they have to learn novel ways of doing routine activities, manage new medical and dietary regimes, or apply safety precautions. Whereas fluid intelligence declines with normal aging, crystallized intelligence, the knowledge we accumulate, increases throughout the life span.

Age-related changes affecting smell and taste are less apparent and frequently not addressed. Taste and smell have a safety function in that they allow us to identify spoiled food and smell leaking gas or smoke. In terms of quality of life, they are important for food consumption, cooking, and social participation. Ultimately, these sensory impairments affect nutritional status, may lead to anorexia, and affect physical health.

Practitioners working with older adults should provide client-centered, occupation-based interventions. The key in working with older adults is to promote engagement in valued roles and occupations. Older adults should be encouraged to remain active and prevent hypokinesis because inactivity can accelerate the loss of strength and endurance and further compromise mobility, ADL and IADL performances, and increase the risk of falling.

CASE STUDY

Shirley is a 68-year-old married woman admitted to a skilled nursing facility (SNF) after a 3-day hospital stay for a left hip replacement secondary to a fall in her home. Tasha is the OTA working with Shirley. On reviewing Shirley's occupational therapy evaluation, Tasha noted that Shirley had been diagnosed with multiple sclerosis (MS) approximately 20 years earlier, had a history of osteoporosis and panic disorder, and had recently experienced several falls. At the time of evaluation, Shirley required moderate assistance with ADL and mobility.

Over the course of Shirley's 20-day stay at the SNF, Tasha found a client-centered approach to be helpful, especially in helping Shirley manage her increased anxiety and feelings of loss of control within her environment. Because Shirley's MS was affecting her ability to remember new information, Tasha included Shirley's husband when providing patient/caregiver education. Tasha also suggested placing a cue card on the front-wheeled walker listing the steps for incorporating total hip precautions during mobility as a memory aid for Shirley. Based on Shirley's goals to be more independent in ADLs, Tasha instructed her and her husband in the use of adaptive equipment for the lower extremities and provided them with resources for obtaining durable medical equipment for the bathroom in their community. Shirley called to arrange for a shower seat and bedside commode to be delivered to her home before discharge. In addition, Shirley also pursued ordering the adaptive equipment that Tasha had recommended through a local vendor and had the items sent to the SNF. As part of Shirley's plan of care to improve IADL performance, Tasha established a home exercise program to increase upper extremity strength and instructed both Shirley and her husband to promote compliance and safety.

In terms of IADLs, Tasha also spent several sessions focusing on Shirley's goal of improving function with simple meal preparation and laundry tasks. Tasha incorporated total hip precautions and energy conservation/work simplification techniques with the IADL tasks to prevent fatigue and reduce the risk of falling. Responding to Shirley's concerns about being able to manage safely at home, Tasha recommended a home visit to assess home safety. On her discharge from the facility, Shirley's anxiety and low frustration level had markedly diminished. Involving Shirley in the treatment plan allowed her to become independent in performing occupations that she valued. Use of the recommended adaptive and durable medical equipment facilitated her postsurgical recovery and improved her functional status while preventing undue fatigue and decreasing her risk for falls.

◼ CASE STUDY QUESTIONS

1. List the strategies used by the OTA to compensate for the primary and secondary aging process changes exhibited by the patient.
2. Identify possible negative outcomes if there had been no occupational therapy intervention.
3. What are the positive outcomes that were achieved?
4. Discuss the influence of a client-centered approach with the case study.

◼ CHAPTER REVIEW QUESTIONS

1. Explain the differences between primary and secondary aging.
2. Summarize primary and secondary changes, and describe possible functional implications of these changes for each of the following: cognitive, integumentary, cardiopulmonary, skeletal, muscular, neurological, and sensory systems.
3. Discuss why OTAs should have knowledge of sensory and physiological changes in older adults.

For additional video content, please visit Elsevier eBooks+ (eBooks.Health.Elsevier.com)

REFERENCES

1. Erber J. *Aging and Older Adulthood*. 4th ed. Belmont, CA: Thomson Learning; 2020.
2. Kail R, Cavanaugh J. *Human Development: A Lifespan View*. 8th ed. Belmont, CA: Thomson Learning; 2019.
3. Kolling T, Knopf M. Late life human development: boosting or buffering universal biological aging. *GeroPsych (Bern)*. 2014;27(3): 103-108. doi:10.1024/1662-9647/a000108.
4. Baltes P. Theoretical propositions of life-span developmental psychology: on the dynamics of growth and decline. *Dev Psychol*. 1987;23(5):611-626. doi:10.1037/0012-1649.23.5.611.
5. Mathers CD, Stevens GA, Boerma T, et al. Causes of international increases in older age life expectancy. *Lancet*. 2015;385(9967): 540-548. doi:10.1016/S0140-6736(14)60569-9.
6. Eldercare Workforce Alliance. *Who We Are*. 2020. Available at: https://eldercareworkforce.org/about/who-we-are/.
7. Institute of Medicine (US) Committee on the Future Health Care Workforce for Older Americans. *Retooling for an Aging America: Building the Health Care Workforce*. US: National Academies Press; 2008.
8. *Healthy People 2030* [Internet]. Washington, DC: U.S. Department of Health and Human Services, Office of Disease Prevention and Health Promotion. Available at: https://health.gov/healthypeople.
9. American Occupational Therapy Association Commission on Practice. Occupational therapy practice framework: domain and process, 4th ed. *Am J Occup Ther*. 2020;74(suppl 2):7412410010p1-7412410010p87. Available at: https://doi.org/10.5014/ajot.2020.74S2001.
10. Rowe JW, Khan RL. *Successful Aging*. New York: Pantheon; 1998.
11. Urtamo A, Jyväkorpi SK, Strandberg TE. Definitions of successful ageing: a brief review of a multidimensional concept. *Acta Biomed*. 2019;90(2):359-363. doi:10.23750/abm.v90i2.8376.
12. Eaton NR, Krueger RF, South SC, et al. Genes, environments, personality, and successful aging: toward a comprehensive developmental model in later life. *J Gerontol A Biol Sci Med Sci*. 2012; 480-488. doi:10.1093/gerona/gls090.
13. Pizzi M, Smith T. Promoting successful aging through occupation. In: Scaffa M, Reita T, Pizzi M, eds. *Occupational Therapy in the Promotion of Health and Wellness*. Philadelphia: FA Davis; 2010.
14. Sandmire D. The physiology and pathology of aging. In: Chop WC, Robnett RH, eds. *Gerontology for the Health Care Professional*. 4th ed. Philadelphia: FA Davis; 2020:153-188.
15. McLafferty E, Hendry C, Farley A. The integumentary system: anatomy, physiology and function of skin. *Nurs Stand*. 2012;27(3): 35-42. doi:10.7748/ns2012.10.27.7.35.c9358.
16. Framgen B, Frucht S. *Medical Terminology: A Living Language*. 7th ed. Upper Saddle River, NJ: Pearson; 2018.
17. United States Department of Health and Human Services, National Institute of Health, National Institute on Aging. *Health Information: Skin Care and Aging*. 2017. Available at: https://www.nia.nih.gov/health/skin-care-and-aging.
18. Dal Bellow-Hass V, MacIntyre NJ, Seng-lad S. Chapter 10: Neuromuscular and movement functions: muscle, bone, and joints. In: Bonder B, Dal Bellow-Hass V, eds. *Functional Performance in Older Adults*. 4th ed. Philadelphia: PA: F.A. Davis; 2018.
19. Dal Bellow-Hass V, MacIntyre NJ, Seng-lad S. Chapter 11: Neuromuscular and movement functions: coordination, balance, and gait. In: Bonder B, Dal Bellow-Hass V, eds. *Functional Performance in Older Adults*. 4th ed. Philadelphia: PA: F.A. Davis; 2018.
20. United States Department of Health and Human Services, National Institute of Health, Osteoporosis and Related Bone Diseases National Resource Center. *The Surgeon General's Report on Bone Health and Osteoporosis: What It Means to You*. 2019. Available at: https://www.bones.nih.gov/health-info/bone/SGR/surgeon-generals-report.
21. Arthritis Foundation. *Arthritis by The Numbers: Books of Trusted Facts & Figures*. 2019. Available at: https://www.arthritis.org/getmedia/e1256607-fa87-4593-aa8a-8db4f291072a/2019-abtn-final-march-2019.pdf.
22. Arthritis Foundation. *Rheumatoid Arthritis: Causes, Symptoms, Treatments and More*. n.d. Available at: https://www.arthritis.org/diseases/rheumatoid-arthritis.
23. Arbesman M, Mosley LJ. Systematic review of occupation- and activity-based health management and maintenance interventions for community-dwelling older adults. *Am J Occup Ther*. 2012;66: 277-283. doi:10.5014/ajot.2012.003327.
24. Marieb EN, Hoehn KN. Chapter 10: The muscular system. In: *Human Anatomy & Physiology*. 11th ed. San Francisco, CA: Pearson/Benjamin Cummings; 2019.
25. Besdine RW, Merck Manual. *The Aging Body: Changes in the Body with Aging*. Kenilworth, NJ: Merck & Company; 2019. Available at: https://www.merckmanuals.com/home/older-people%E2%80%99s-health-issues/the-aging-body/changes-in-the-body-with-aging.
26. Harvard Health Publishing. *Preserve Your Muscle Mass*. Harvard Medical School; 2016. Available at: https://www.health.harvard.edu/staying-healthy/preserve-your-muscle-mass.
27. AARP. *Your Muscles and Bones at 50+*. 2018. Available at: https://www.aarp.org/health/healthy-living/info-2018/muscle-strength-bone-health-aging.html#:~:text=On%20average%2C%20people%20lose%20about,people%20in%20their%2050s%20skip.
28. Larsson L, Degens H, Li M, et al. Sarcopenia: aging-related loss of muscle mass and function. *Physiol Rev*. 2019;99(1):427-511. Available at: https://doi.org/10.1152/physrev.00061.2017.
29. De Carvalho FG, Justice JN, Freitas EC, Kershaw EE, Sparks LM. Adipose tissue quality in aging: how structural and functional aspects of adipose tissue impact skeletal muscle quality. *Nutrients*. 2019;11(11):2553. doi:10.3390/nu11112553.
30. McGee C, Mathiowetz V. The relationship between upper extremity strength and instrumental activities of daily living performance among elderly women. *OTJR*. 2003;23(4):143-154. doi:10.1093/geronj/44.5.
31. Visser M, Schaap LA. Consequences of sarcopenia. *Clin Geriatr Med*. 2011;27(3):387-399. doi:10.1016/j.cger.2011.03.006.
32. Beaudart C, Zaaria M, Pasleau F, Reginster JY, Bruyère O. Health outcomes of sarcopenia: a systematic review and meta-analysis. *PLoS One*. 2017;12(1):e0196548. Available at: https://doi.org/10.1371/journal.pone.0169548.
33. Hunter EG, Kearney PJ. Occupational therapy interventions to improve performance of instrumental activities of daily living for community-dwelling older adults: a systematic review. *Am J Occup Ther*. 2018;72(4):7204190050p1-7204190050p9. Available at: https://doi.org/10.5014/ajot.2018.031062.
34. Izzo C, Carrizzo A, Alfano A, et al. The impact of aging on cardio and cerebrovascular diseases. *Int J Mol Sci*. 2018;19(2):481. doi:10.3390/ijms19020481.
35. Kohn JC, Lampi MC, Reinhart-King CA. Age-related vascular stiffening: causes and consequences. *Front Genet*. 2015;6:112. doi:10.3389/fgene.2015.00112.
36. Lowery EM, Brubaker AL, Kuhlmann E, et al. The aging lung. *Clin Interv Aging*. 2013;8:1489-1496. doi:10.2147/CIA.
37. Gonzalez J, Coast JR, Lawler JM, et al. A chest wall restriction to study effects on pulmonary function and exercise. *Respiration*. 1999;66(2):188-194. doi:10.1159/000029367.
38. Dean E. Cardiopulmonary and cardiovascular function. In: Bonder BR, Dal Bello-Haas V, eds. *Functional Performance in Older Adults*. 4th ed. Philadelphia: FA Davis Company; 2018:109-128.
39. Jeong I, Lim JH, Parks JS, Oh YM. Age-related changes in the gene expression profile of human lungs. *Aging (Albany NY)*. 2020;12(21):21391-21403. doi:10.18632/aging.103885.
40. Cannizzo ES, Clement CC, Sahu R, et al. Oxidative stress, inflam-aging and immunosenescence. *J Proteomics*. 2013;74(11):2313-2323. doi:10.1016/j.jprot.2011.06.005.

41. Dorrington MG, Bowdish DM. Immunosenescence and novel vaccination strategies for the elderly. *Front Immunol.* 2013;4:171. doi:10.3389/fimmu.2013.00171.

42. Man AL, Gicheva N, Nicoletti C. The impact of ageing on the intestinal epithelial barrier and immune system. *Cell Immunol.* 2014;289:112-118. doi:10.1016/j.cellimm.2014.04.001.

43. Montecino-Rodriguez E, Berent-Maoz B, Dorshkind K. Causes, consequences, and reversal of immune system aging. *J Clin Invest.* 2013;123(3):958-965. doi:10.1172/JCI64096.

44. Oviedo-Orta E, Ka-Fai Li C, Rappuoli R. Perspective on vaccine development for the elderly. *Curr Opin Immunol.* 2013;25:529-534. doi:10.1016/j.coi.2013.07.008.

45. Judge KS, Dawson NT. Cognitive function. In: Bonder BR, Dal Bella-Haas VD, eds. *Functional Performance in Older Adults.* 4th ed. Philadelphia: F.A. Davis Company; 2018:93-108.

46. Saraçlı Ö, Akca ASD, Atasoy N, et al. The relationship between quality of life and cognitive functions, anxiety and depression among hospitalized elderly patients. *Clin Psychopharmacol Neurosci.* 2015;13(2):194-200. doi:10.9758/cpn.2015.13.2.194.

47. Kanagaratnam L, Dramé M, Trenque T, et al. Adverse drug reactions in elderly patients with cognitive disorders: a systematic review. *Maturitas.* 2015;85:56-63. doi:10.1016/j.maturitas.2015.12.013.

48. Schulte PJ, Roberts RO, Knopman DS, et al. Association between exposure to anaesthesia and surgery and long-term cognitive trajectories in older adults: report from the Mayo Clinic Study of Aging. *Br J Anaesth.* 2018;121(2):398-405. doi:10.1016/j.bja.2018.05.060.

49. Croy I, Nordin S, Hummel T. Olfactory disorders and quality of life: an updated review. *Chem Senses.* 2014;39:185-194. doi:10.1093/chemse/bjt072.

50. Vreeken HL, van Nispen RMA, Kramer SE, van Rens GHMB. 'Dual Sensory Loss Protocol' for communication and wellbeing of older adults with vision and hearing impairment – A randomized controlled trial. *Front Psychol.* 2020;11:570339. doi:10.3389/fpsyg.2020.570339.

51. Attems J, Walker L, Jellinger KA. Olfaction and aging: a mini-review. *Gerontology.* 2015;61(6):485-490. doi:10.1159/000381619.

52. Seiberling K, Conley D. Aging and olfactory and taste function. *Otolaryngol Clin North Am.* 2004;37:1209-1228. doi:10.1016/j.otc.2004.06.006.

53. Malafarina V, Uriz-Otano F, Gil-Guerrero L, et al. The anorexia of ageing: physiopathology, prevalence, associated comorbidity and morality. A systematic review. *Maturitas.* 2013;74:293-302. doi:10.1016/j.maturitas.2013.01.016.

54. Visvanathan R. Anorexia of aging. *Clin Geriatr Med.* 2015;31:417-427. doi:10.1016/j.cger.2007.06.001.

55. Pilgrim AL, Robinson SM, Sayer AA, Roberts HC. An overview of appetite decline in older people. *Nurs Older People.* 2015;27(5):29-35. doi:10.7748/nop.27.5.29.e697.

56. Sergi G, Bany G, Pizzato S, Veronese N, Manzato E. Taste loss in the elderly: possible implications for dietary habits. *Crit Rev Food Sci Nutr.* 2017;57(17):3684-3689. doi:10.1080/10408398.2016.1160208.

57. Goble DJ, Coxon JP, Van Impe A, et al. The neural basis of central proprioceptive processing in older versus younger adults: an important sensory role for the right putamen. *Hum Brain Mapp.* 2012;33:895-908. doi:10.1016/j.neurobiolaging.2016.10.024.

58. Dunn W, Griffith JW, Sabata D, et al. Measuring change in somatosensation across the lifespan. *Am J Occup Ther.* 2015;69(3):1-10. doi:10.5014/ajot.2015.014845.

59. Ruffino C, Bourrelier J, Papaxanthis C, et al. The use of motor imagery training to retain the performance improvement following physical practice in the elderly. *Exp Brain Res.* 2019;237(4):1375-1382. doi:10.1007/s00221-019-05514-1.

60. Chiu SL, Chang CC, Dennerlein JT, Xu X. Age-related differences in inter-joint coordination during stair walking transitions. *Gait Posture.* 2015;42(2):152-157. Available at: https://doi.org/10.1016/j.gaitpost.2015.05.003.

61. Ruffino C, Bourrelier J, Papaxanthis C, et al. The use of motor imagery training to retain the performance improvement following physical practice in the elderly. *Exp Brain Res.* 2019;237(4):1375-1382. doi:10.1007/s00221-019-05514-1.

62. Gorgon EJR, Lazaro RT, Umphred DA. Aging and the central nervous system. In: Kauffman TL, Scott RW, Barr JO, et al., eds. *A Comprehensive Guide to Geriatric Rehabilitation.* China: Elsevier Health Sciences; 2014:22-33.

chapter 4

Psychological Aspects of Aging

YOLANDA GRIFFITHS AND ANDREA THINNES

KEY TERMS

adaptations, aging stereotypes, coping skills, learned helplessness, loss, occupational shifts, stressors

CHAPTER OBJECTIVES

1. Describe myths and facts about psychological aspects of aging.
2. Identify common stressors, changes, and losses to which older adults must adapt.
3. Discuss common emotional problems that may accompany losses.
4. Discuss coping skills and interventions that promote healthy transition with age.

Physical milestones measure a person's age in years, but indications of mental aging are less clear. Learning about the psychological aspects of aging enhances the occupational therapy assistant's (OTA's) ability to deal effectively and empathetically with older adults. This chapter explores key concepts about the psychology of aging that assist in understanding older adults and enhancing empathy when working with them.

MYTHS AND FACTS ABOUT AGING

The way older adults are perceived significantly affects the way they are treated. Stereotypes are rigid concepts, exaggerated images, and inaccurate judgments used to generalize about groups of people. Positive and negative stereotypes create false images of aging that can affect older adults. Western culture often perpetuates negative views of aging. Some older adults are empowered by positive stereotypes, while others are motivated to be an example of an active older adult to dispel the negative stereotypes. "Seniors who are well educated, maintain a high level of health, and live in a city environment that welcomes seniors may result in individuals who are more resistant to negative characterizations. Such seniors may be the best antidote to negative stereotypes."[1]

Buying into the erroneous beliefs and myths of aging produces a biased negative perception of older adults and colors objectivity when working with them. "Stereotypes about aging and the old, both negative and positive, have significant influence upon the older people themselves."[2] This is a form of ageism or discrimination against the aged and can deter from a realistic approach in working with older adults. "Negative aging stereotypes have the power to influence reactions toward older people, creating assumptions in the midst of others about their limited or poor abilities, judgment, and behaviors."[2] According to the National Poll on Healthy Aging, the majority of older adults experienced at the minimum of one type of ageism in their daily lives. This ageism occurred from exposure to messages or through interpersonal interactions.[3] Clarifying misperceptions about older adults is the first step in developing effective rapport when working with this population. Consider the following myths about the psychological aspects of aging.

Myth 1: Chronological Age Determines the Way an Older Adult Acts and Feels

Melissa, an OTA, receives a referral to see Simone, who is 89 years of age. Melissa has images of an older, cranky woman sitting in a chair with her head bowed, responding in a belligerent way about receiving treatment. Melissa enters the room of the assistive living center that Simone shares with her roommate, Julia. The room is filled with sports mementos, photos, and awards from both of their respective grandchildren. Julia taps Melissa's shoulder and says, "If you're looking for Simone, she's in the sun room teaching dance lessons. You have to get up pretty early to catch up with Simone, or she'll leave you in the dust!"

The aging process varies with each individual, and each person has different perceptions about it. Some older adults do believe that their minds will deteriorate along with their bodies. Personality, lived experiences, natural responses to actual losses, expected reactions to one's own aging process and death, and predictable emotional reactions to physical illness are separate aspects of aging. The truth is that older adults are in a time of transition, and they should be treated as individuals within their particular contexts, history, and circumstances. Refrain from generalizing that all older adults approach aging in the same way.

For example, the stereotype that older adults should avoid engaging in any strenuous exercise because their organs will fail or bones will break is a myth. Exercise is beneficial for most and dangerous for only a few older adults (Fig. 4.1). One study concluded "that in a general elderly population, moderate or high physical activity, compared with no physical activity, are independently associated with a lower risk of developing incident cognitive impairment after 2 years of follow-up."[4] Older adults should check with their physician for any limitations before they begin an exercise program, and recognize that the body does change in terms of stamina and flexibility with aging. It is not uncommon for older adults to start exercising later in life even if they have been inactive for years.[5] Recent research suggests that older adults can build muscle mass even if they had previously not worked out regularly.[6] From a therapeutic perspective, the older adult should:

- Be aware of the safety concerns of beginning to exercise
- Set realistic goals and expectations
- Warm up and stretch before exercising, and cool down and stretch following exercise
- Gradually progress to add more time or slightly more difficulty to the exercise routine

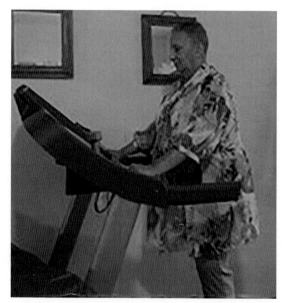

FIG. 4.1 This older adult remains physically active by regularly using the treadmill at her home. (*Courtesy Jaya Pitts.*)

- Consider strengthening as well as aerobic activity as exercise

OTAs should encourage older adults to take brisk walks, consider new activities such as tai chi or water aerobics, and enjoy life. Increased mobility, strength, and flexibility may lead to better overall health, a decrease in fall risk, and may delay the need for long-term care.

Myth 2: You Cannot Teach an Old Dog New Tricks

The applause is thunderous as the graduates walk across the stage. It is a very special day for both Emily and Eugenia Meyer as they receive their Bachelor of Science degrees in accounting. Eugenia Meyer is 68 years of age and Emily is her 24-year-old granddaughter. Eugenia had experienced a heart attack, and her granddaughter had been her caregiver during her rehabilitation. Eugenia often expressed regret about not finishing college, so Emily encouraged Eugenia to follow her dreams of furthering her education.

The potential of an older adult should not be underestimated. One delightful example of the passion for lifelong learning can be found in Douglas's story. Douglas, 74 years old, was married to his wife for 53 years when she died. He moved to a retirement community following his wife's death. After recovering from his loss, Douglas desired a new challenge. He decided to go back to school and earn a master's degree in theology. He was concerned about the pace of school, the technology, and the way others would view him, but the concerns did not stop him from trying. He first took a computer course for older adults and practiced his skills with his new friends at the retirement community. In his theology courses, he found that his younger colleagues valued his stories and the life experiences he shared.

Douglas is not out of the norm of the capabilities of the typically aging brain. The ability to learn does not decline with age. In fact, the current number of persons older than age 55 years in noncredit continuing education courses is continuing to grow. According to Findsen and Formosa,[7] the desire to learn and experience new things is great for older adults, despite the physical and intellectual challenges they face. Learning strategies and preferences may differ for older students and their younger classmates; however, the richness in experience that older adults bring to the classroom can be beneficial to all learners. "Many older adults want to participate in a learning process and become actively engaged in that process when it is interesting, relevant, and recognizes the experience they bring to the education context."[8]

Crystallized and fluid intelligence must be considered in an older adult learning environment. Crystallized intelligence comes from lived experiences from which older adults can tap into the wisdom gained. Fluid intelligence is new learning on the spot, such as in a classroom setting when learning a new concept.[7] There may be increased time needed by the older adult to grasp a new concept, technique, or skill. The OTA should remember that age-related changes in learning should be considered in the context that they occur and with regard to each individual, within a classroom setting, but also within the context of education when the older adult is a client of occupational therapy services and must be educated on a variety of things. Educational materials and presentation of the information must be modified to reflect the needs of the older adult learner.

Biological changes also may affect learning. For example, older adults may be unable to sit for long periods because of back or hip problems. Older adults may tire quickly and demonstrate decreased physical stamina. With increased use of computers, good ergonomics while using a computer station will decrease fatigue and neck or back stiffness associated with sustained computer use.

As a result of poor vision or hearing skills, older adults may not accurately process all sensory information. Older adults may need additional time to organize and process new information. People may quickly assume that an older adult is confused when the information recalled seems jumbled or inaccurate. Although there may be some cognitive decline with aging because of particular medical conditions, in many ways older adults may be better learners with more time given for learning and processing new information.[5] Older adults can integrate life experience and a broader perspective with new knowledge that younger persons often do not consider. The OTA can make an outstanding contribution by adjusting the environment or technique of completing a task to the capacities of the older adult to effectively utilize the skills and lived experience of the older adults.

Older adults who feel threatened by new situations may have poor self-confidence in learning situations that require decision-making and risk-taking. Older adults may avoid learning opportunities that may result in embarrassment, frustration, or conflict. In times of stress, older adults may be less flexible in problem-solving and rely on set ways and habits of dealing with situations. Ultimately, the older adult must want to learn, be willing to recognize any limitations, and explore other learning techniques, such as keeping the brain exercised with problem-solving tasks, crossword puzzles, board games, and "neurobic" exercises (see Chapter 3 for more information on cognitive changes with aging).

Myth 3: As You Age, You Naturally Become Older and Wiser

It was most disturbing to Jerry that he could not remember what he was doing sometimes. After all, Jerry was a former professor of chemistry and retired from teaching only last year. Now his body seemed slower, and his mind so forgetful. His forgetfulness started with little things like losing his keys and progressed to forgetting the road home after driving to the store. One day Jerry became upset after becoming confused in the grocery store parking lot, unable to recall the kind of car he owned. What was happening? His daughter feared that Jerry was experiencing early stages of Alzheimer's disease. Neither Jerry nor his daughter could understand why this was happening, especially because Jerry had always been so active and was only 63 years of age. Jerry had been an accomplished author and teacher and prided himself on his intellectual abilities.

Positive stereotyping can be as detrimental as negative stereotyping. Unrealistic expectations that older adults can and should continue to perform as they did when they were younger may cause an older adult to feel like a failure. Stating that all older adults will be wiser or that all older adults will become senile is not true. These contradictory statements prove that older adults should not be lumped into one homogeneous group.

Intelligence does not decline with age. Studies done in the 1920s by Bayley and Bradway[9] indicate that intelligence quotient (IQ) scores increase until the age of 20, then level off and remain unchanged until late in life. Continued intellectual stimulation promotes successful aging. Staying active socially and engaged in activities make an older adult less vulnerable to negative psychosocial situations.[10] With aging, it is important to determine which behaviors are caused by medical conditions versus personality traits or natural aging processes.[11]

Myth 4: Older Adults Are Not Productive, Especially at Work

Initially, all the young employees at the local burger place called the new employment program "adopt a geezer." Paul, the manager and owner of a thriving fast food restaurant located across from the high school, often came home and complained to his wife about the unreliability of many of the youth he hired to fill the shifts. Paul said that "it was as if the kids just wanted the paycheck and had no real concern about the quality of their work."

Paul's wife, Michelle, an OTA who worked 3 days a week at the senior citizen center, suggested a mutually beneficial program that would financially help older adults who were interested and capable of fulfilling a part-time position. Paul would be able to fill shifts open during the school day with steady, reliable help. To the amazement of the young employees, the older employees were efficient and demonstrated stamina. In fact, the young employees often remarked, "They're cool!"

The opportunity for young employees to work beside their older counterparts will continue to increase. Between 2010 and 2020, the number of workers age 55 years and older rose, but this is expected to slow through 2029. However, the number of workers age 65-and-older and 75-and-older is expected to continue to increase as baby boomers move into this age group.[12] Work is not only a social or leisure pursuit of older adults, but also a necessity to maintain a lifestyle they desire. The psychological adaptation to the new role of retiree can be either dreaded

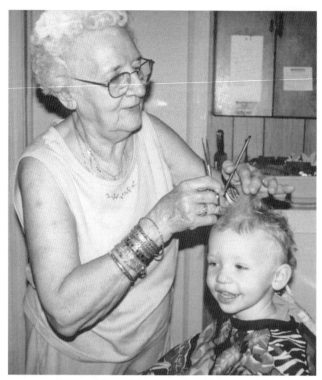

FIG. 4.2 Some older adults remain productive by using their talent and skills at work.

different line of work on a part-time basis to feel productive. According to a recent survey (N-1000) by the Voya Financial Group, 59% of employed baby boomers plan to work in their retirement.[13] Reasons for remaining in the workforce included finances and mental stimulation[14] (Fig. 4.2). With challenges in the economy about job security and possible discrimination against older adults in the workplace, older workers may feel vulnerable. "Nearly half of older concerned workers fear that their old age will hamper their job search." Many older workers fear that they could lose their job, with their age being a factor.[15]

After retirement, older adults often seek new areas of employment (Fig. 4.3A). According to the American Association of Retired Persons (AARP), among the older adults who plan to seek employment postretirement, about half will be looking for a job in a new field of interest.[16] Older adults are capable of learning new skills and effectively solving problems in new situations. OTAs can promote integration and participation of an older worker into a job successfully by looking at adaptations to the environment, supplies, and training required to fulfill the job description. For example, an older adult who would like to work in the reception area of an office may answer phones and greet customers but may need additional time and training in computer data entry needed for the job.

Retirement is sometimes a paradox when older adults may have time and energy but lack financial means to be active. Conversely, when older adults have the financial means and have retired from their jobs, they may desire socialization or interesting activities. According to Kielhofner,[17] older adults may be challenged in their activity choices by lack of transportation, finances, companions, or self-limiting fears. Gupta and Sabata state

or embraced. For some older adults, retirement is anticipated as a withdrawal from traditional, stressful workday events. They are capable of learning new skills and effectively solving problems in new situations. Upon retiring, many older adults engage in social activities, community service or volunteer work, or become employed in a

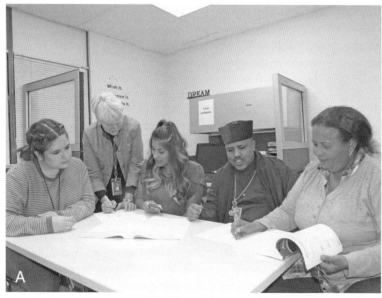
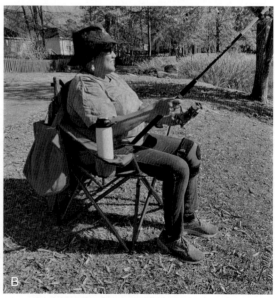

FIG. 4.3 (A) After retirement this older adult works in a new area of employment tutoring students. (B) With added leisure time, older adults can explore new interests and find more time for existing hobbies.

"training older adults in how to use technology can help reduce some of the fears that limit them from adopting technologies, including assistive technology in the workplace."[18] OTAs can help retired older adults create a plan for managing added leisure hours (Fig. 4.3B). Productive engagement can help older adults continue to be involved in their communities. Volunteering among older adults can stimulate social meaning in life through the positive psychosocial effects that it can provide through social participation in the community. It allows older adults to contribute to the common good that benefit all in society, while also promoting wellbeing through improvements in mental and physical health for themselves (Fig. 4.3A).[19]

Myth 5: Older Adults Become More Conservative as They Age

Organizing a neighborhood petition to get an overpass built over the busy street next to the elementary school was the last thing Elena thought she would be doing on her 80th birthday. Here she was in the midst of neighbors and community workers stacking flyers, affixing petition forms to clipboards, and filling out a shift schedule. For years, Elena had observed many close calls when children crossing the street were almost hit by automobiles. She thought, "I could never forgive myself if one of those kids got hurt, and I just sat here and watched from my front window."

Contrary to myth, many older adults are receptive to new ideas and accept fresh roles. In fact, many older adults become more politically active and even seek political office to initiate social change (Fig. 4.4). According to the continuity theory, adults perform consistent behaviors, such as learning continuously over their lifetime. Aging reflects this continuation of the patterns of their roles, responsibilities, and activities, which are influenced by one's individual personality.[20] Even though habits and preferences contribute to a consistency in personality, developmental psychologists note that personality may be influenced as individuals deal with crisis points in each phase of life and add to their repertoires of adaptive skills. According to Canja,[21] it is untrue that older adults do not want to be active, contributing members of society and that the later years of life should be reserved for idleness.

Myth 6: Older Adults Prefer Quiet and Tranquil Daily Lives

Jose looked around the reception area of Applewood Manor on his first day of work as an OTA. Only the sounds of a television murmuring the chant of a daily game show and the shuffling of residents down the hall broke the silence. The head nurse, Mrs. Kessler, walked up to Jose and said, "Isn't it wonderful how quiet and peaceful it is here? We work very hard to preserve a sense of tranquility in the sunset years of one's life."

Jose interviewed all of the residents during the week to determine activities he could develop based on their

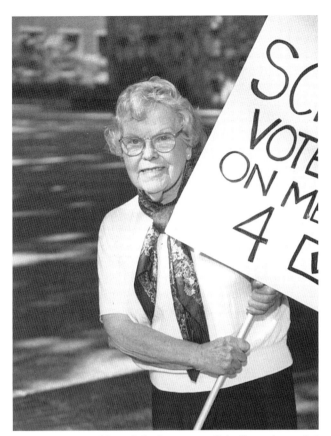

FIG. 4.4 Many older adults become politically active to initiate social change. *(Courtesy Michael Lohman.)*

interests. Not surprisingly, more than half of the residents wanted less sedentary activities than they currently were experiencing. Some even wanted organized sports like tennis. Other residents wanted a piano and perhaps a jazz hour scheduled.

Another incorrect generalization is that all older adults prefer a sedentary lifestyle. An older adult who has experienced a rather staid and uneventful life before retirement will not necessarily continue that type of lifestyle. Older adults may move in with their children's families, and their lives may become rather frenzied. Some pursue totally new interests that they may not have had time for earlier because of career and family demands. Many older adults continue with vibrant lifestyles and do not sit awaiting death. Staying active is a key to healthy psychological aging.

Myth 7: All Older Adults Become Senile

The expression "senior moment" infers an idea that as one ages, memory lapses become commonplace. Harry has always been a proud, independent man. He was decorated twice during his participation in the Korean War. After experiencing a heart attack, Harry adjusted to the many lifestyle changes that were suggested by the health care team. Today, Harry sighed as he walked with multiple pieces of paper toward the receptionist in the

Occupational Therapy department. This was the third stop in a confusing, maze-like journey inside the Veterans' Administration Hospital. The hospital was under reorganization again, and procedures for appointments had changed. Previously, Harry always called for an appointment, showed up characteristically 10 minutes early, and cheerfully greeted the young OTA who assisted with his treatments. Today, a young man at the front desk rattled off multiple instructions about the new procedures and handed Harry a photocopied map of the building along with a stack of new forms to be completed. Harry was still trying to understand the map when he asked the young man to slowly repeat the instructions. The young man repeated himself in a louder tone and pointed Harry in the direction of the elevators. The young man muttered, "These senile old guys."

When older adults appear confused or require more time to understand directions, misunderstandings often result. Getting older is not synonymous with feeble-mindedness or imbecility. Brain damage may be evident as a result of physical illness. However, senility is a label often used inaccurately to describe specific psychosocial disorders that older adults may be dealing with, such as depression, grief, anxiety, or dementia. People age at different rates. Evidence points to the connection between engagement in physical exercise, a leisure time activity, and the overall health of older adults.[22]

STRESSORS, LOSSES, AND EMOTIONS ASSOCIATED WITH AGING

Older adults often must deal with major life crises such as retirement, loss of spouse, economic changes, residence relocation, physical illness, loss of friends, and the reality of mortality. Box 4.1 lists these and other stresses that older adults may experience. There are predictable shifts that occur in occupational patterns across the life span in regard to developmental processes and life stages.[23] The significant occupational shifts or changes in meaningful activities associated with aging may include dealing with financial burden, emotional losses, variance in roles, adapting to different routines and habits, diminishing physical and mental performances, and challenges to adaptation.[23-25] Lieberman and Tobin[26] found that "events that lead to loss and require a major disruption to customary modes of behavior seem to be the most stressful for elders." Recent studies have attempted to measure other aspects of daily life and stress levels. Bellingtier and Neupert indicated that having a positive attitude toward aging resulted in better coping with daily stressors and conversely a negative attitude resulted in enhanced emotional responses to daily stressors.[27] OTAs must consider the ways various life events affect older adults to understand what motivates certain behaviors.

According to Kielhofner,[17] role changes can sometimes be involuntary, such as the unexpected death of a loved one, and older adults struggle with the loss or diminishment

---

BOX 4.1

Stressors That Affect Older Adults

- Slowing down
- World events
- Time with children and or grandchildren
- Decreased family members and or friends
- Concerns about own death
- Sleep habit changes
- Pain and or discomfort
- Life regrets
- Feeling that time is brief
- Concerns about decreasing mental faculties
- Money problems
- Health
- Caregiving
- Chronic illness
- Relocation

Data from: Anderson, G.O. Americans Age 50+ and Stress: An AARP Bulletin Poll, 2014. Retrieved 5/18/2021 from https://www.aarp.org/research/topics/health/info-2014/older-americans-and-stress-bulletin-poll.html and Stokes, S. Gordon, S.E. Common stressors experienced by the well elderly: Clinical implications. Journal of Gerontological Nursing; Thorofare, 29, 5, 2003: 38–46.

---

of accompanying roles. Older adults may need to adapt to shifts in occupational patterns possibly related to atypical or unpredictable life events and developmental aging. For example, unexpected economic demise of a company may lead to the unforeseen loss of a job and retirement funds. Such losses significantly affect a person's occupation, inherent roles, and habits.

NEED FOR SOCIAL SUPPORT

Pivotal to the ability of an older adult to cope with a major life change is the social support of family, friends, church members, and neighbors. Although stressors may not be avoided, social support can help older adults deal with losses.

The support an older adult receives with the death of a loved one often diminishes to a large extent after the funeral or mourning period. The reality of the loss may not occur until later when the older adult is alone. The survivor may grieve over the loss of finances and possible change in residence, social status, or role associated with the death of the loved one. OTAs can assist the surviving spouse in adjusting to new roles, habits, and routines, as well as developing a strong network of social support.

Loneliness is a form of emotional isolation. Older adults may experience increased social isolation with retirement as family members relocate or as friends move or die. Social interactions with pets, weekly church services, grocery shopping trips, or occasional visits from family members may not be emotionally fulfilling enough for an older adult. OTAs can assist in exploring and structuring more frequent or new areas of social interaction in the community. Community centers offer a variety of activities, such as cooking and art classes, trips to local attractions, and classes specifically designed for grandparents and grandchildren to attend together.

Older adults may become reclusive and socially paralyzed with anxiety as a result of increasing neighborhood violence. Intensifying anger is a common emotional problem experienced by many older adults as they feel a loss of control over their lives. Older adults may be viewed as cantankerous or verbally aggressive when in fact they may be using angry words to express feelings of helplessness. Anger also can be expressed based on fear and sadness over losses.

Other changes in environment such as new living arrangements, whether imposed or by choice, also may be a challenge for older adults. According to Kielhofner,[17] older adults develop habits sustained over a long period often in a stable environment; when the environment changes, demands to shift habits are stressful. The physical or mental ability to sustain previous habits in a new environment also may be diminished.

PHYSICAL ILLNESS

Older adults may need to cope with a chronic disease or a serious physical illness. A serious physical illness with a sudden onset may be more debilitating to the older adults in terms of independence and self-care. A chronic illness is no less stressful; however, the older adult may have adapted to the illness more gradually. Box 4.2 lists stressors associated with common physical illnesses of older adults.

Petra, an 81-year-old woman, who was legally blind, was receiving occupational therapy services in her home. She lived by herself in a cozy one-bedroom apartment. Petra was known to the home health care team to be quite rude; in fact, she had "fired" several home health nurses and therapists that had come to provide services in

BOX 4.2

Stressors Associated With Physical Illness Common to Older Adults

- Threat to life
- Loss of body integrity
- Change in self-concept
- Threat to future plans
- Change in social roles
- Change in routine activities
- Loss of autonomy
- Need to rapidly make critical decisions
- Loss of emotional equilibrium
- Physical discomfort
- Monotony and boredom
- Fear of medical procedures

Adapted from Davis L. Coping with illness. In: Davis L, Kirkland M, eds. *ROTE: The Role of Occupational Therapy with the Elderly*. Rockville, MD: American Occupational Therapy Association; 1988.

her home. The occupational therapist (OT) asked Rodney, an OTA that worked with her, to see Petra. Almost immediately after Rodney introduced himself, Petra told him she never met a health care worker that could think for themselves. She continued to insult his profession and his coworkers. Rodney tried to understand more about Petra and to find out reasons for her behavior. He learned from her past medical history that Petra's blindness had become progressively worse. In fact, she stopped leaving her home all together because she was embarrassed that she could not fix her hair and makeup the way she used to. Rodney took the time to speak to her about this and to offer suggestions for how he could assist her in being able to do those tasks again. He was the first person to look beyond her sarcastic remarks and rude exterior and notice that she was really scared and confronting her own mortality. Rodney continued to see Petra and work with her on coming to terms with her blindness and need for assistance. He felt that he made a difference in her life. He shared his experience with other members of the health care team so that they, too, could better understand Petra.

An older person copes with physical illness through a psychosocial process. A negative perception of the situation and a hopeless attitude will adversely affect the way a person deals with the illness. Schussler[28] pointed out that those who view a physical illness as a challenge were more emotionally healthy than those who view it as a punishment.

A grief process in dealing with any illness is to be expected. Five stages to the grief process originally identified by Kubler-Ross[29] continue to help health professionals better understand and help their clients: denial, anger, depression, bargaining, and acceptance.[30] This grief process may not be linear—that is, the older adult may become depressed and then become angry or deny the situation again before possibly accepting the illness.

An older adult's ability to adapt is contingent on physical health, personality, life experiences, stress, and level of social support.[11,31,32] To successfully deal with a chronic condition, an older adult should adopt the following important concepts:

- Recognize permanent changes such as diet, lifestyle, work habits, or exercise that may promote recovery
- Mentally deal with losses caused by the illness
- Accept a new self-image
- Identify and express feelings, such as anger, fear, and guilt
- Seek out and maintain social support from family and friends

OTAs can help an older adult deal with a chronic illness in the following ways:

- Reduce fears about the illness through education
- Listen and be sensitive to the feelings expressed verbally and nonverbally
- Provide encouragement

■ Assist in the development of creative, yet realistic ways for older adults to gain more control over their illnesses or losses associated with an illness

■ Identify ways to reduce stress and to promote social support

■ Surround the older adult who has moved to a facility as a result of an illness with familiar objects, which may help maintain a sense of continuity, provide comfort and security, and aid memory

LEARNED HELPLESSNESS

When older adults perceive that they have no control over a particular outcome or multiple stresses in their life, they may give up hope and become dependent on others to fulfill their needs.[32,33] A person with an external locus of control frequently feels powerless over decisions and actions, and the more this feeling is reinforced, the more likely it is that learned helplessness will occur. Older adults who experience loss of control also experience diminishing coping skills and are at risk for illness.[33] Health care workers and family members often contribute to a state of learned helplessness in the following ways:

■ Expecting older adults to be unable to do for themselves, and completing tasks for them, thereby promoting dependence

■ Imposing routines on older adults for the sake of the health care worker's convenience, such as giving them a bath at 2:00 p.m.

■ Showing a negative attitude by expressing condescending remarks about physical appearance or behaviors

■ Perpetuating the sick or institutional role by validating somatic complaints or disapproving decisions

Learned helplessness often results when the older adult believes a situation is permanent, and then depression and a marked lack of self-esteem follow. OTAs can encourage independence and self-care activities. As older adults regain a feeling of competence, learned helplessness can be reversed. Robnett and Chop[11] suggest giving choices and options as much as possible and to challenge the client to work at a greater level than currently functioning. The concept of the client advocating for themselves enhances personal control in everyday life and should be integrated into daily therapy. OTAs can empower older adults by creative problem-solving to assist them in being as independent as possible.

Sena is an 88-year-old woman who is in a skilled nursing facility after falling at home. Shannon, the OTA, works with her daily and is aware of what Sena can and cannot do physically by herself. She continues to be fed because she is just too tired. Shannon knows that she can feed herself, and may well be tired, but does not oblige her request. While documenting later that afternoon, Shannon sees Sena's son eating dinner with her, and he is feeding her with a spoon. The OTA observes the interaction but does not say anything to Sena's son. The next evening Shannon observes the same scenario and decides to address the situation with Sena's son and explain to him that his mother is capable of feeding herself. Shannon is respectful of him but talks to him about learned helplessness and what he can do to help his mother. The OTA must relinquish some of the power and control as a health care advocate and empower the older adult and their family members to engage in independent problem-solving. One of the key concepts in preventing learned helplessness is for the OTA to be aware of their own beliefs about aging and mortality and to consider stereotypes that may bias attitudes toward working with older adults.

CONCLUSION

Old age can be a time of self-reflection and exploration of new interests. It also can be a time of dealing with great losses and severe stress. Changes occur throughout the life span, and the way a person copes with changes and adapts to transitions ultimately determines their ability to psychologically cope with aging. Keeping active can help minimize the effects of the aging process. By clarifying assumptions and myths about aging, gaining awareness of the different stressors and losses associated with aging, and understanding the ways older adults cope with serious illnesses, OTAs can help them enhance their quality of life as they experience aging.

▌ TECH TALK: FOCUS ON PSYCHOSOCIAL HEALTH

NAME	PURPOSE	APPROX. COST	WHERE TO BUY
Calm App	App with resources for sleep hygiene, anxiety reduction, stress relief, and mindfulness	Free trial ~ $70/yr	Google Play IOS App Store get.calm.com
Down Dog	App providing guided yoga, Barre, meditation and other exercises for gentle physical activity and/or meditation	Free trial ~$49/yr	Google Play IOS App Store downdogapp.com
SuperBetter	SuperBetter is an app/website designed to use gaming to help users build social, mental, and emotional resilience in the face of any illness, injury, or health goal	$0	Google Play IOS App Store superbetter.com

CASE STUDY

Margaret, 79 years of age, sits in the sun porch clutching a pot of orchids. It is the last day she will enjoy this scene because today Margaret is moving to an assisted living facility in a town 260 miles away, which is close to her son, John. Margaret had lived in the same home for almost 35 years with her husband, Phillip. When Phillip died 2 years ago of pancreatic cancer, it was a shock almost too great for Margaret to bear. Phillip had been her rock. Margaret had been Phillip's primary caretaker while he was ill. During their 40-year marriage, Margaret and Phillip had traveled all over the world and shared lifelong interests, including cooking, golf, and cultivating orchids in their custom-built greenhouse. Margaret had been a volunteer with the children at the homeless shelter downtown until Phillip required her full-time care. The walls in their den were covered with awards and letters of appreciation for her work with the children. Now the house has been sold and many of her mementos have been packed up, sold, or given away.

Margaret had been an energetic high school history teacher and Phillip had been a chemist. They had two children, John and Karen. Karen is married and lives in London with her two daughters. Margaret and Phillip loved to travel to London to visit their grandchildren. John is recently divorced and is busy managing his new safety consulting company. Margaret has a beloved 9-year-old Labrador retriever named Henry, but she is unable to take Henry with her to the assisted living facility.

In the past 3 years, Margaret has been diagnosed with arthritis, vertigo, and early stages of dementia. Margaret fell 6 months ago and fractured her hip. She had begun to forget things such as paying bills, which caused her electricity to be turned off; leaving the stove on, which caused a small fire; and not remembering to take her medication regularly. John and Karen decided it was time to move their mother into a safer, more supervised environment. Margaret became depressed and less active after the decision was made. It seemed as if Margaret resigned herself to a situation beyond her control physically and socially. Margaret spent much of her time sleeping or sitting in the sun porch staring out the picture window. Moving to the new town meant saying goodbye to friends, relatives, and her beloved pet, as well as some memories of Phillip.

■ CASE STUDY QUESTIONS

1. Identify the losses Margaret has experienced.
2. Describe the stressors or emotional problems that may be related to these losses. What effect would Margaret's losses have on her occupations? Describe shifts in occupational patterns that are linked to the changes in her life. Consider changes in roles, habits, routines, relationships, work, and leisure interests and activities.
3. Discuss what the OTA could do to help Margaret deal with these losses in terms of attitude, education, and activities.

■ EXERCISES

The following are a few activities to help the OTA gain empathy and build rapport with older adults.

INTO AGING

"Into Aging" is a commercially available game that focuses on building empathy for those who are growing old. The manual describes the game as a way for players to increase awareness of older adults' problems by simulating experiences with similar problems, such as loss, isolation, powerlessness, dependency on others, and ageism. This game is available through Slack, Inc. (Thorofare, NJ).

ROLE PLAYING

Role playing is a useful activity for groups to understand aging-related issues. In preparation for the activity, each of the myths of aging discussed in the chapter should be written on index cards. Each small group will be given a set of index cards. Members of the groups then enact some of the myths and stereotypes associated with the psychological aspects of aging. Examples should be followed with a discussion of feelings and thoughts about the stereotype or myth. What misconceptions did you have about aging before the activity that was subsequently clarified? What concept or concern is still puzzling or requires further exploration? How can you use the information learned in the role play in occupational therapy practice?

STEREOTYPE EXERCISE

Every member of a group should list the first six or seven images that immediately come to mind with the term *older adult*. Group members should think about advertisements, movies, and personal experiences that influence their perceptions of older adults. All group members should share their images and explain the reasons the images are so vivid. Group members should discuss whether the images are realistic or stereotypical. Further discussion may involve how these stereotypes could bias the way an OTA would approach intervention with older adults or with caregivers. Group members should brainstorm different ways to change stereotypical images to make them more realistic.

Position yourself comfortably in a quiet room. You may sit in a comfortable chair or lie down. Take three deep breaths. As you exhale, clear your mind of any concerns, and concentrate on the directions. Give yourself permission to use the next 10–15 minutes to explore what it would feel like to be 75 years old.

Pretend that you are looking into a large mirror. Imagine your physical appearance at age 75 years. What physical changes have taken place? Do you need any assistance with self-care? What emotions are you experiencing as a result of these changes?

What changes have occurred in your living arrangements? Do you live alone? Identify any changes in lifestyle as a result of finances.

What have you accomplished in your life thus far? Do you regret any events? Do you regret not achieving certain goals? Are you satisfied with your life?

Remember what you have just experienced with the visual imagery. Now slowly count to 10. As you get closer to 10, you will become more awake and tuned to the sounds of the room you are in. When you reach 10, gently open your eyes.

Free write for the next 5 minutes. It may be poetry, prose, or just phrases of what you remember of your visual imagery trip to age 75. Reflect on what key concepts of aging were apparent in the imagery. Describe your feelings.

RESOURCES

Older adult resources for mental health and wellness are available through Wellness Reproductions and Publishing, LLC (a Guidance Channel Company). This company carries a wonderful collection of books, music CDs, games, products, and tools to help those who work with the elderly deal with stress, aging, caregiving, and other challenges of older adults.

■ CHAPTER REVIEW QUESTIONS

1 Does chronological aging determine psychological aging? Discuss your position.

2 Identify aspects of aging that may affect learning for older adults.

3 Coping with a serious illness can be especially stressful for an older adult. Discuss any resulting occupational shifts and what an OTA can do to help older adults understand change.

4 What is learned helplessness, and what can OTAs do to help older adults vulnerable to learned helplessness?

For additional video content, please visit Elsevier eBooks+ (eBooks.Health.Elsevier.com)

REFERENCES

1. Horton S, Baker J, Pearce W, et al. Immunity to popular stereotypes of aging? Seniors and stereotype threat. *Educ Gerontol*. 2010; 36(5):353-371. doi:10.1080/03601270903323976.

2. Bennett T, Gaines J. Believing what you hear: the impact of aging stereotypes upon the old. *Educ Gerontol*. 2010;35:435-445. doi:10.1080/03601270903212336.

3. National Poll on Healthy Aging. *Everyday Ageism and Health: Older Adults' Experiences with Everyday Ageism*. 2019. Available at: https://deepblue.lib.umich.edu/bitstream/handle/2027.42/156038/0192_NPHA-ageism-report_FINAL-07132020.pdf?sequence=3&isAllowed=y.

4. Etgen T, Sander D, Huntgeburth U, et al. Physical activity and incident cognitive impairment in elderly persons. *Arch Intern Med*. 2010;170(2):186-193. doi:10.1001/archinternmed.2009.498.

5. Tufts University. You can't teach an old dog new tricks and other myths about the aging process. *Tufts University Health & Nutrition Letter*. 2002;20:1-3.

6. McKendry J, Shad BJ, Smeuninx B, Oikawa SY, Wallis G, et al. Comparable rates of integrated myofibrillar protein synthesis between endurance-trained master athletes and untrained older individuals. *Front Physiol*. 2019;10:1084. doi:10.3389/fphys.2019.01084.

7. Findsen B, Formosa M. *Lifelong Learning in Older Adults: A Handbook on Older Adult Learning*. Vol. 7. Netherlands: Sense Publishers; 2011.

8. Anetzberger GJ. Community-based services. In: Bonder BR, Dal Bello-Haas V, eds. *Functional Performance in Older Adults*. 4th ed. FA Davis; 2018:383-396.

9. Teichner G, Wagner M. The Test of Memory Malingering (TOMM): normative data from cognitively intact, cognitively impaired, and elderly patients with dementia. *Arch Clin Neuropsychol*. 2009;24(3):455-464. doi:10.3233/NRE-151287.

10. Nilsson I, Nyqvist F, Gustafson Y, et al. Leisure engagement: medical conditions, mobility difficulties, and activity limitations - A later life perspective. *J Aging Res*. 2015;2015:1-8. doi:10.1155/2015/610154.

11. Robnett R, Chop W. *Gerontology for the Health Care Professional*. 3rd ed. Burlington, MA: Jones and Bartlett; 2015.

12. Dubina DS, Kim JL, Rollen E, Rieley MJ. *Projections Overview and Highlights, 2019-29*. Monthly Labor Review; 2020. Available at: https://www.bls.gov/opub/mlr/2020/article/pdf/projections-overview-and-highlights-2019-29.pdf.

13. Maulucci L. *New Voya Survey Finds Half of Employed Americans Plan to Work in Retirement as a result of COVID-19*. Voya Financial; 2020. Available at: https://www.voya.com/news/2020/09/new-voya-survey-finds-half-employed-americans-plan-work-retirement-result-covid-19.

14. Kiger P. *Many Say They Plan to Work Longer, Save More*. 2020. Available at: https://www.aarp.org/work/working-at-50-plus/info-2020/coronavirus-pandemic-retirement.html.

15. Perron R. *Ageism Could Hurt Job Prospects, Say Job-Insecure Older Workers*. AARP Research; 2021. Available at: https://www.aarp.org/research/topics/economics/info-2021/ageism-job-security-older-workers.html.

16. Kielhofner G. *A Model of Human Occupation: Theory and Application*. 4th ed. Baltimore: Lippincott Williams & Wilkins; 2008.

17. Anderson GO. *AARP Work and Jobs Study*. AARP Research; 2015. Available at: https://www.aarp.org/research/topics/economics/info-2015/aarp-post-retirement-career-study.html.

18. Gupta J, Sabata D. Maximizing occupational performance of older workers. *OT Pract*. 2010;15(7):CE 1-CE 8.

19. Gil-Lacruz M, Saz-Gil MI, Gil-Lacruz AI. Benefits of older volunteering on wellbeing: an international comparison. *Front Psychol*. 2019;10(2647):1-12. doi:10.3389/fpsyg.2019.02647.

20. Jett K. Theories and processes of aging. In: Touhy TA, Jett K, eds. *Ebersole and Hess' Toward Healthy Aging: Human Needs and Nursing Response*. 10th ed. St. Louis: Elsevier; 2020.

21. Canja E. Aging in the 21st century: myths and challenges. *Exec Speeches*. 2001;16:24-27.

22. Touhy TA. Mobility and aging. In: Touhy TA, Jett K, eds. *Ebersole and Hess' Toward Healthy Aging: Human Needs and Nursing Response*. 10th ed. St. Louis: Elsevier; 2020.

23. Royeen C. The human life cycle: paradigmatic shifts in occupation. In: Royeen C, ed. *The Practice of the Future: Putting Occupation Back into Therapy*. Bethesda, MD: American Occupational Therapy Association; 1995.

24. Pizzi MA, Smith TM. Promoting successful aging through occupation. In: Scaffa ME, Reitz SM, Pizzi MA, eds. *Occupational Therapy in the Promotion of Health and Wellness*. Philadelphia: FA Davis Company; 2010.

25. Metcalfe J. Metacognition of agency across the lifespan. *Cognition*. 2010;116(2):267-282. doi:10.1016/j.cognition.2010.05.009.

26. Lieberman MA, Tobin SS. Stress in the aged: concepts and issues. In: Lieberman MA, Tobin SS, eds. *The Experience of Old Age: Stress, Coping and Survival*. New York: Basic Books; 1983:3-19.

27. Bellingtier JA, Neupert SD. Negative aging attitudes predict greater reactivity to daily stressors in older adults. *J Gerontol B Psychol Sci Soc Sci*. 2018;73(7):1155-1159. doi.org/10.1093/geronb/gbw086.

28. Schussler G. Coping strategies and individual meanings of illness. *Soc Sci Med*. 1992;34:427-432. Available at: https://doi.org/10.1016/0277-9536(92)90303-8.

29. Kubler-Ross E. *On Death and Dying*. New York: Macmillan; 1969.

30. Kubler-Ross E, Kessler D. *On Grief and Grieving: Finding Meaning of Grief Through the Five Stages of Loss*. New York: Scribner; 2007.

31. Higgins L, Mansell J. Quality of life in group homes and older persons homes. *Br J Learn Disabil*. 2009;37(3):207-212. doi:10.1111/j.1468-3156.2009.00550.x.

32. Bretherton SJ, McLean LA. Interrelations of stress, optimism and control in older people's psychological adjustment. *Aust J Ageing*. 2014;34(2):103-108. doi:10.1111/ajag.12138.

33. Coudin G, Alexopoulos T. Help me! I'm old! How negative aging stereotypes create dependency among older adults. *Aging Ment Health*. 2010;14(5):516-523. doi:10.1080/13607861003713182.

Aging Well: Health Promotion and Health Management

PAMALYN KEARNEY, BETSY B. MCDANIEL, AND KAISA SYVÄOJA

KEY TERMS

health behaviors, Health Belief Model, health education, health literacy, health management, health promotion, occupational engagement, prevention, Recovery Model, rest, self-management, sleep, sleep hygiene, Social Cognitive Theory, Transtheoretical Model of Health Behavior Change

CHAPTER OBJECTIVES

1. Discuss the role(s) of occupational therapy practitioners to influence health management and healthy aging through programs and services for individuals, organizations, communities, and populations.
2. Describe health promotion activities that can be incorporated in practice with older adults.
3. Describe theories and models that guide health promotion program development for individuals, organizations, communities, and populations.
4. Explain the impact of health risks and their effects on older adult occupational engagement and participation.
5. Apply health literacy principles to the development of health management and health promotion materials.
6. Describe best practices for health management with older adults.
7. Describe the focus of intervention for older adults with chronic mental illness.

INTRODUCTION

Mr. and Mrs. Patel currently live in the home where they have lived for the past 40 years, a large two-story home on a wooded lot close to the university where they both taught prior to retirement. They have three children and seven grandchildren, with one daughter living nearby with her family. They have enjoyed relatively good health although Mr. Patel does have high blood pressure and osteoarthritis in his knees which occasionally results in activity limiting pain. Mrs. Patel's physician has told her that she is at an increased risk of developing diabetes due to her weight, body mass index, and waist to hip ratio. Both Mr. and Mrs. Patel enjoy swimming at the community pool, attending lectures and other special events at the university, and traveling. Recently they have begun to talk about selling their home and moving to a continuing care retirement community where they can continue to live independently but with fewer homeowner responsibilities, which have become progressively more difficult for them to manage.

Mr. and Mrs. Patel are part of the over 46 million older adults living in the United States today, a number which is anticipated to increase to almost 90 million by 2050.[1] They also reflect the growing diversity of this population.

The older adult population includes a mix of those who are healthy, those who are at risk for developing chronic conditions and diseases, and those who are living with conditions that impact their ability to fully participate in desired occupations. Occupational therapy practitioners, including occupational therapy assistants (OTAs), are uniquely positioned to support older adults to age well, to manage their health risks and health conditions, and to remain engaged. In this chapter, we will explore concepts of health promotion, health management, prevention and related concepts that OT practitioners can incorporate into their work with aging adults.

CONCEPTS OF HEALTH PROMOTION AND HEALTH MANAGEMENT IN OCCUPATIONAL THERAPY

The belief that occupation has the power to influence health and wellness has been a central belief of the profession of occupational therapy since its founding. Indeed, several founders of the National Society for the Promotion of Occupational Therapy (later renamed the American Occupational Therapy Association) were already engaged in or supportive of community-based programs that used occupation to facilitate a return to productive living for participants in 1917 when they met to form our national association.[2] By the 1940s, occupational therapists working in the community were being encouraged to use occupational therapy interventions to reduce adverse health conditions and prevent future illness within families and communities.[3] The American Occupational Therapy Association (AOTA) adopted an official position paper titled *Role of the Occupational Therapist in the Promotion of Health and Prevention of Disabilities* in 1978[4]; this document has been updated numerous times since, most recently in 2019. The most current version, *Occupational Therapy in the Promotion of Health and Well-Being*, calls on OT practitioners to be involved with health promotion and prevention programs. Three critical roles have been identified for OT practitioners: (1) promoting healthy lifestyles and occupations for all persons, (2) emphasizing occupation as a fundamental component of health promotion, and (3) providing occupation-based health promotion and prevention interventions to individuals and their families, communities, and populations.[5]

According to the World Health Organization's (WHO) Ottawa Charter for Health Promotion, "Health promotion is the process of enabling people to increase control over, and to improve, their health. To reach a state of complete physical, mental and social wellbeing, an individual or group must be able to identify and to realize aspirations, to satisfy needs, and to change or cope with the environment. Health is, therefore, seen as a resource for everyday life, not the objective of living. Health is a positive concept emphasizing social and personal resources, as well as physical capacities. Therefore, health promotion is not just the responsibility of the health sector but goes beyond healthy lifestyles to wellbeing."[6] The WHO's attention to health and well-being is further emphasized in Healthy People 2030, which includes the promotion of "healthy development, healthy behaviors, and well-being across all life stages"[7] as one of the overarching goals.

A related concept is that of health management. Health management includes "activities related to developing, managing, and maintaining health and wellness routines, including self-management, with the goal of improving or maintaining health to support participation in other occupations."[8] The Occupational Therapy Practice Framework (OTPF-4) identifies a variety of occupations within the broader category of health management, including social and emotional health promotion and maintenance, symptom and condition management, communication within the health care system, medication management, physical activity, nutrition management, and personal care device management.[8]

Older adults can benefit from a range of health promotion and health management strategies and interventions to improve their health and participation in occupations, and occupational therapy practitioners are well positioned to address these concerns. We will further explore health promotion and health management within occupational therapy practice in the following sections.

HEALTH PROMOTION AND HEALTH EDUCATION MODELS

The goal of health education and health promotion is to effect voluntary changes in health behaviors among individuals, populations, and communities.[9] Health behaviors are actions that affect health. Health behaviors can include actions that will have a positive effect on health such as exercising regularly and eating a well-balanced diet, and actions that increase the risk of disease such as smoking or leading a sedentary lifestyle. Viewing health behavior through the person-environment-occupational-performance (PEOP) model of OT will help the OT practitioner to recognize the complex interaction of individuals with their environment and the many influences of the individual, the environment, and the community on occupational performance in health behaviors.[10] However, knowledge of some of the most frequently used theories and models in health promotion and education can assist OT practitioners in developing health promotion interventions. This section will briefly discuss the Health Belief Model,[11] Social Cognitive Theory,[12] and the Transtheoretical Model of Health Behavior Change.[13]

The *Health Belief Model* attempts to predict and explain health behavior by understanding how a person's beliefs about health affect their health behaviors. There are several components of the health belief model that can help an OT practitioner to understand the factors that will contribute to an individual's perceived state of health or risk of disease and the probability that an individual will make a positive health behavior change:

- Individual perception of susceptibility to a health condition
- Perceived seriousness of the disease
- Perceived benefits of health action
- Perceived barriers to the health action
- Cues that promote action
- Perceived ability to perform the action[14]

Recognizing an individual's perception of a health condition and their likelihood of acquiring the condition helps the OT practitioner to choose the most appropriate health education intervention.

Social Cognitive Theory is another model that addresses the determinants of health behavior, or why people behave the way that they do regarding their health. This model emphasizes the importance of self-efficacy on health behavior. Self-efficacy, in this context, refers to an individual's belief in their own ability to perform the behavior required to influence health. Social Cognitive Theory promotes reinforcement and observational learning as important aspects of engaging in and changing health behaviors.[15] Role playing or providing opportunities to imitate the behavior of others is an effective way to increase self-efficacy in desired positive health behaviors.

When assessing individual health promotion needs, it is important to identify predisposing, reinforcing, and enabling factors that may affect the desired health behavior. Attitude and readiness to change will also affect health behavior. The *Transtheoretical Model of Health Behavior Change* (TTM) outlines five stages of health-related behavior change which can be used to identify an individual's readiness to change:

1. Precontemplation: individual does not recognize that there is a problem and has no intention of making a behavior change
2. Contemplation: the problem has been identified and the individual is motivated to make a behavior change to remedy the problem
3. Planning or preparation: individual is planning to make a behavior change soon, is discussing the planned change with family and friends, and is acquiring resources needed to make the change
4. Action: individual changes behavior and makes environmental changes needed to facilitate the change
5. Maintenance: individual is able to sustain the behavior change over time and incorporate it into permanent lifestyle[16]

Self-efficacy, as described in Social Cognitive Theory, is also a key construct in TTM. Belief that one can be successful in making positive health-related behavior changes can lead to better and longer lasting results.[17] OT practitioners using the TTM should design interventions that correspond with an individual's current stage of readiness for change to either bring the problem to the person's attention, assist the person to understand the need for change, and teach or provide opportunities to practice the skills, habits, and lifestyle behaviors needed to make and maintain the change.

PREVENTION AND HEALTH PROMOTION AMONG OLDER ADULTS

Prevention and health promotion are two public health concepts that OTAs working with older adults should be familiar with. Prevention refers to interventions that aim to minimize the burden of disease or injury and associated risk factors by taking steps to prevent them. Health promotion is a process that seeks to empower people to have more control over their own health. Health promotion includes increasing health literacy (which will be discussed in a later section of this chapter) and taking action to increase healthy behaviors.[18] Many common health problems older adults face can be prevented or postponed through prevention-focused health education efforts to minimize the risk of or complications from conditions such as injury from falls, adverse medication reactions, disuse syndrome (limited physical activity), depression, malnutrition, alcohol abuse, hypertension,

and osteoporosis.[19] The OTPF-4 has identified prevention and health promotion as OT intervention approaches, and prevention; health and wellness are identified potential outcomes of occupational therapy services.[8] This highlights the suitability of OT practitioners to partner with public health agencies in efforts to prevent conditions that limit quality of life in older adults.

Prevention and health promotion strategies are generally organized into three categories: primary, secondary, and tertiary. Each of these is further described in the following sections.

Primary Prevention

OT practitioners may represent the first line of primary prevention for well, homebound, or facility dwelling older adults. Primary prevention is defined as "education or health promotion strategies designed to help people avoid the onset and reduce the incidence of unhealthy conditions, diseases, or injuries. These attempts to identify, reduce, and eliminate risk factors for disease and injury may include modifying the physical and social environment."[5] Primary preventive efforts with older adults may consist of facilitation of lifestyle changes and the use of necessary medications to reduce the development of life-threatening conditions such as cardiovascular disease and stroke. Primary prevention programs may include improving nutrition, accident (including falls) prevention, increasing exercise, weight management, and smoking and alcohol cessation.[5] A critical primary prevention effort should be focused on the prevention of falls in older adults since accidents are one of the leading causes of death among people over 65, and current trends project that there will be seven fall-related deaths per hour by 2030 in this age group.[20] In this capacity, OTAs have the opportunity to influence change among older adults by increasing awareness of health risks that can lead to falls. In assisting older adults to increase physical activity through leisure education and participation, OTAs may help reduce the ill effects of a sedentary lifestyle or disuse syndrome. Many disabilities experienced later in life start with disuse and are preventable. Studies have demonstrated the long-reaching effects of regular exercise in the prevention of weakness and fatigue, which increase the potential for falls and interfere with independence in activities of daily living (ADL) functions. Exercise also assists in the prevention of obesity, thus reducing consequent hypertension and diabetes. In addition, exercise is related to improvements in the psychological well-being of older adults.[21-25] A three times weekly exercise program, regular participation in an activity such as walking or hiking (Fig. 5.1), or participation in a community-based exercise group for older adults (Fig. 5.2) can significantly reduce the potential for falls and significantly increase overall health and well-being, thus increasing meaningful participation in occupations.[26]

When developing interventions that involve exercise, it is important for the OTA to remember that participation

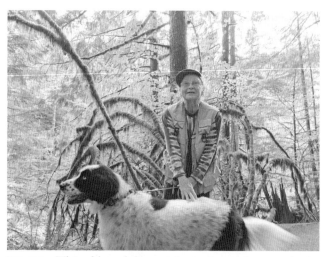

FIG. 5.1 This older adult participates in regular exercise by hiking with her pet.

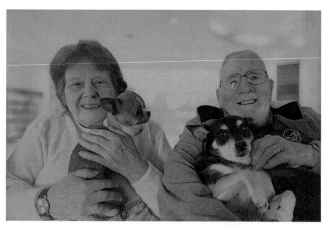

FIG. 5.3 Some older adults find caring for pets personally meaningful occupation. (*Courtesy Patty Watford.*)

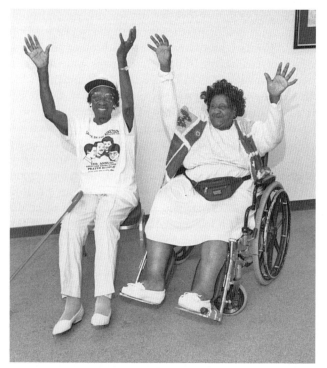

FIG. 5.2 Participating in a weekly community exercise program keeps these older adults physically active.

in meaningful activities produces better outcomes than rote exercise. Rote exercise involves the repetition of a particular movement, such as lifting a 10-lb dumbbell 10 times to develop strength, endurance, or skill. Personally meaningful occupations are intrinsically motivated or characteristic of activities that have a purpose in and of themselves, such as picking up a 10-lb infant or caring for a pet (Fig. 5.3). Designing interventions that encourage engagement in occupation to increase strength will potentially increase additional performance skills and client factors that rote exercise cannot. Consider the

many benefits of gardening compared to rote exercise. Participation in a gardening activity offers many potential physical (e.g., strength, endurance, balance), cognitive (e.g., problem solving, attending), and emotional (e.g., increased positive attitude, quality of life) benefits as well as a myriad of options for adaptation.[27,28] For example, gardening tasks can be completed outside or inside, alone or as a group activity, and might include planning and tending a garden (Fig. 5.4) or simply transplanting potted plants. Clients who enjoy gardening (intrinsic motivation) will also be much more likely to participate to their maximum capability and therefore realize more and longer-lasting gains than those who only participate in a rote exercise program for increasing upper body strength.[8] This demonstrates the core beliefs of occupational therapy regarding the positive relationship between occupation and health.[29]

Fall prevention is another critical aspect of primary prevention practices that OT practitioners can facilitate. A home or an institutional environmental assessment

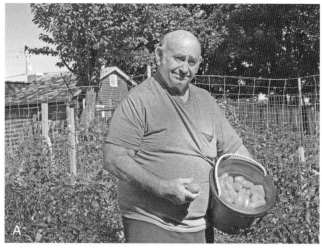

FIG. 5.4 Older adults often enjoy gardening tasks such as growing tomatoes.

may identify many fall hazards for older adults (see Chapter 14). A Matter of Balance is a well-researched fall prevention program that OTAs can implement in practice. The program uses a multimodal approach that addresses physical, social, and cognitive factors affecting a fear of falling.[30] The use of the *Home Safety Self-Assessment Tool* can contribute significant information to fall prevention.[31]

Secondary Prevention

Secondary prevention emphasizes "early detection and intervention after disease has occurred and is designed to prevent or disrupt the disability process."[32] An example of secondary prevention with older adults might include education and training regarding eating habits, activity levels, and the prevention of disabilities secondary to obesity. Early detection of hypertension and cancers may prevent early disability and mortality. Vision and hearing deficits are also preventable at times if detected early, as are breast and cervical cancers as well as depressive or substance use disorders. OTAs can contribute to early detection of serious conditions that contribute to disability and interfere with ADL and instrumental activities of daily living (IADL) functions through delivery of health promotion programs designed to inform older adults of the importance of recommended screening, such as the mammogram, Papanicolaou (Pap) test, colonoscopy and prostate cancer screening. Recommendations for health and risk screening of older adult populations can be different in some cases. For example, the Department of Health and Human Services does not provide specific suggestions for upper age limits of Pap testing but suggests recommending discontinuation after age 65 if the woman's previous regular screenings were consistently normal.[33] However, reduced access to health care and to culturally appropriate health care messages has increased the risk for cervical cancer and cervical cancer mortality in many groups including Hispanic and African American women as well as older white women living in rural areas.[34] OTAs should consider cultural and health literacy concepts when designing health promotion programs for secondary prevention to enhance success among the target population.

Research shows that women with disabilities are also significantly less likely than other women to receive screening and preventive services such as mammograms and Pap tests.[35] Because of the multiple and complex factors that contribute to health disparities among older adults, individuals with disabilities, and minority populations, health care providers at all levels should have an awareness of and a concern for the overall health of their clients. All health care providers should assume responsibility for encouraging and reminding older adult clients to schedule regular physical examinations.

Careful observation of functional capabilities may facilitate early detection of changes in the capabilities of older adults. OT practitioners can monitor loss or change of sensory capacity during routine interactions with clients (see Chapters 15 and 16). OTAs also may be instrumental in educating family members to monitor older adults for changes in mood or cognitive functioning that may influence independence in ADLs and IADLs. Changes in mood or cognition can be associated with poor nutrition or dehydration, which can be prevented or remediated (see Chapter 20). Changes also may indicate reactions to or side effects of medications or more serious physiological changes that require medical evaluation and attention (see Chapter 13).

Tertiary Prevention

Tertiary prevention refers to preventing the progression of existing conditions. It relates to functional assessment and rehabilitation both to reverse and to prevent progression of the burden of illness.[36] Tertiary prevention refers to services that are designed to prevent the progression of a condition, prevent further disability, and promote social opportunity.[5] An example of tertiary prevention initiated by the OT practitioner could be the treatment of a home-bound older adult who is experiencing limitations in ADLs and IADLs due to the pain of arthritis. The OTA would provide education about implementing the concepts of joint protection and energy conservation to prevent further deterioration of arthritic joints. In addition, joint mobility can be facilitated through regular participation in a hobby within the client's range of tolerance. Performing energy conservation activities may also provide the client with a sense of control over his or her daily routine. Control of pain and implementation of environmental adaptations and work simplification could assist the client and encourage greater involvement in meaningful occupations and engagement with others.

ROLE OF THE OCCUPATIONAL THERAPY ASSISTANT IN WELLNESS AND HEALTH PROMOTION

OT practitioners play a critical role in the promotion of health and prevention of disease among older adults. Health education is one strategy for implementing health promotion and disease prevention programs to help individuals and communities improve their health by increasing their knowledge or influencing their attitudes regarding their own health. Chronic illnesses that affect ADL and IADL functions are more often related to lifestyle, genetic predisposition, and environmental exposure than to age alone. Frequently, older adults need to change long-standing behaviors to prevent disability from developing or progressing. OT evaluation, intervention, and educational programs implemented by OTAs can foster such life-enhancing changes. The Occupational Profile can be used to determine the need for intervention through health education activities.

Health promotion strategies for older adults should focus on maintaining and increasing functional capacity,

BOX 5.1

Wellness Program for Elders

Program goals

- Enhance awareness of the positive effect of wellness on health at any age
- Promote awareness of the sensory changes that occur as aging progresses
- Improve knowledge of food consumption and effects on health
- Improve decision-making skills
- Encourage self-responsibility for health
- Encourage independence and environmental mastery
- Maximize a positive focus
- Heighten awareness of behaviors that inhibit health and perpetuate disease
- Encourage independence in self-care

Possible topics

- Personal nutrition
- Exercise: sitting, standing, low-impact aerobics
- Planning of health screenings, including annual screening for cancer
- Smoking cessation
- Activities: exploring interests
- Stress and effects on the heart
- Relaxation
- Responsibility for health
- Sensory loss and safety: eliminating hazards

Adapted from Glantz CH, Richman N. The wellness model in long-term care facilities. *Quest.* 1996;7:7–11.

maintaining or improving self-care, and preventing isolation.[37] Health promotion should also help older adults maintain functional autonomy as long as possible. Glantz and Richman (1996) proposed guidelines for the development of wellness programs for older adults with an emphasis on goals of "optimum achievement and maintenance of competence and independence" (Box 5.1).[38]

Hettinger (1996)[39] developed the following ABCs of the wellness model in occupational therapy, which may assist OTAs in encouraging their older clients to learn to improve and maintain their health:

- **A**ttitude that includes actively pursuing wellness and ADL that promote satisfaction and quality of life.
- **B**alancing productive activity, positive social support, emotional expression, and environmental interactions.
- **C**ontrolling health through education about behaviors that lead to wellness.

This model encourages OTAs to serve as mentors, coaches, and educators.

The *Well Elderly Study*, conducted at the University of Southern California, describes a successful model for OT wellness programming.[40] Results of this well-designed study validate that the lives of older adults living in an urban community can be enhanced through reactivation of interests and participation in meaningful occupations. The content of the program, based on input from older adults, provided detailed instructions about areas such as transportation, safety, social relationships, and finances. Interventions through education and self-discovery processes were offered in both individual and group contexts. A key outcome of the *Well Elderly Study* was the demonstrated importance and health-enhancing effects of reengaging elderly participants in meaningful occupations (Fig. 5.5). Elderly participants assigned to a group facilitated by occupational therapists (OTs) had better outcomes than those participants assigned to the control group or those participants of the group facilitated by a volunteer nonprofessional.[41] Overall, the program found that occupational therapy led groups offered a significant benefit to positive outcomes measures, and that therapy helped the elders improve health and functional ability necessary for community living.[42] The results of this program have been sustained over time and have led to an occupational therapy approach now known as Lifestyle Redesign.[40,43] OTAs can earn a digital badge from AOTA

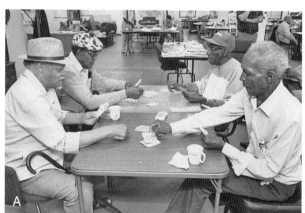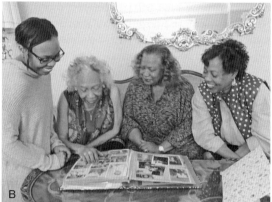

FIG. 5.5 It is important for older adults to participate in meaningful occupations, which can include activities such as (A) playing cards with friends and (B) reminiscing with family members.

in Lifestyle Redesign. The Lifestyle Redesign program has been expanded to include a variety of specialized focus areas such as diabetes management, pain management, and Parkinson's disease.

Health education empowers older adults to take increasing responsibility for their health. OTAs have many opportunities across practice domains to provide health education programs for this population. Health promotion can occur through individual or group education efforts.[5] OTAs can rely on their knowledge of group skills to facilitate discussion of materials and to encourage group development and cohesion. Generally, health-education topics for older adults will include activities to increase understanding of the benefits of physical activity, chronic disease management (including diabetes and arthritis), stroke prevention, immunization, osteoporosis, early detection of cancer and other major medical conditions, home safety, assistive devices, fall prevention, and sensory changes that occur with aging.[44] OTAs have the unique opportunity to demonstrate the distinct value of occupational therapy in health education programs by developing activities to increase occupational engagement with these topics. Traditional health education programs are designed to educate, but education without implementation is not very beneficial. Humans have the right to engage in occupations that contribute positively to their own well-being and the well-being of their communities.[45] Occupational therapy practitioners should design programs that offer opportunities for older adults to practice what they have learned in health promotion programs.

HEALTH RISKS AND THEIR EFFECTS ON OCCUPATIONAL ENGAGEMENT AND PARTICIPATION

As previously stated, the WHO defines health promotion as enabling a person to increase control of their health through social and environmental interventions that maintain health and quality of life and prevent the cause of poor health.[46] This suggests that health promotion is an active process by the older adult to understand their own health and how to maintain or promote positive health outcomes. It also makes the connection to the role of the physical and social environment in positively influencing this interaction. However, it is also critical to understand why an older person is in poor health and to address the primary causes as a way to improve health. Occupational therapy practitioners are important in this process as they are uniquely equipped to address current conditions and limitations to health through development of strategies to address root causes of illness or decreased occupational engagement as well as the ability to incorporate social and environmental interventions into care.

Providing older adults with education and resources on disease prevention and aging either in person or virtually increases self-efficacy which can have a positive impact on the aging process.[47] Allowing older adults to be active participants in their health care and giving relevant information enables them to become a part of their own health promotion. This may seem like a simple act but is a valuable first step to giving older adults control over their own health and wellness and can lead to increased independence of the person. Utilizing principles of occupational therapy when providing this education is beneficial to developing and fostering this relationship with the older adult. Providing education and resources to older adults aligns closely to prevention of illness, injury, or decreased occupational engagement. The interchange and collaboration with the occupational therapy practitioner is an empowering experience for the older adult.

Addressing social isolation is also of great importance when understanding health and wellness for older adults. There have been several studies that have examined the role of social isolation on health and its contributing factors. A variety of factors influence poor social participation for older adults including income, presence of depressive symptoms, and chronic conditions.[29,48,49] For many older adults, there is a desire for more social activities which illustrates the need to facilitate social interactions with older adults.[48] Factors that influenced positive social participation are living with a partner, good general health, and more physical activity or completion of household tasks.[49]

Occupational therapy practitioners must also consider other factors that impact quality of life, and health and wellness for older adults. As adults age, they may experience increasing limitations in ADL and IADL participation, with adults over the age of 75 experiencing the largest increase in limitations.[50] Both ADL and IADL are impacted; however, there is a higher rate of limitations with IADL participation. Both the risk of falls and actual incidence of falls increases, resulting in decreased engagement and participation in occupations. Predictors of decreased quality of life and overall occupational engagement include: female gender, comorbidities, poor nutrition, polypharmacy, decreased mobility, depression or dependency, poor economic conditions, and social isolation or sense of loneliness. Increased physical activity, lower rates of depressive symptoms, decreased obesity, and lower rate of alcohol abuse are associated with increased quality of life in older adults.[51]

A balance of positive and negative influencers is required for a person to be able to engage in meaningful activities and occupations. Spending time with friends and family, baking a cake, participating in a group exercise class, or gardening are just a few activities that may be meaningful to an older adult. An older adult who has good general health, is physically active, and is able to complete necessary ADL activities may find these activities and occupations easy to accomplish. However, if an older adult has chronic conditions, depressive symptoms, or economic barriers in their daily life, engagement in these activities and occupations may decrease or not exist.

Occupational therapy practitioners working with older adults use a variety of interventions to address health and wellness and health promotion. Incorporating health promotion into therapy sessions can be useful to many older adults. Effective interventions include enhancing or maintaining the ability to complete ADLs and IADLs, social participation, increasing physical engagement, education on health and aging and addressing overall life satisfaction. Older adults need to be able to continue to engage in their meaningful occupations and activities as well as interact with others. If an older adult is not able to find satisfaction and purpose in their daily activities and occupations, the older adult is not living to their fullest potential. When this occurs, there is a risk of increased dependency on others, decreased engagement, and decreased independence.

HEALTH MANAGEMENT AND CHRONIC CONDITIONS

Mrs. Simpson is a 70-year-old retired teacher. She has lived alone since her partner died following a myocardial infarction 6 years ago. Her daughter and four grandchildren live nearby. Mrs. Simpson has been diagnosed with fibromyalgia and Type 2 diabetes. Her pain keeps her from being as active as she would like and recently, she has been having difficulty with managing her blood glucose levels. When she is feeling well, she enjoys gardening, quilting, and playing cards with friends. While at the supermarket, she saw a flyer for an 8-week chronic disease self-management program being taught by a woman she knows from the community center and an occupational therapy assistant. She takes a flyer, planning to call for more information.

Older adults living with chronic conditions can benefit from health management interventions to help them to improve or maintain their overall health to support their ability to engage in meaningful occupations. These may include occupational therapy interventions to address healthy routines and habits that support health management, training in use of adaptive devices to support medication management, teaching energy conservation strategies, and more. One element of health management is self-management. The emphasis of self-management is on the individual, in collaboration with family and health care providers, taking charge of their own health and managing their chronic conditions and complications that arise from them, including treatments, symptom management (Fig. 5.6), and lifestyle changes necessary to maintain health, as well as managing any psychosocial, cultural, or spiritual effects of their chronic condition.[52,53] This process includes a variety of skills including goal setting and action planning, identifying and managing symptoms, identifying barriers to health and problem solving strategies to minimize their impact, behavior change for health management, lifestyle changes, coping with psychosocial impacts, and more.[54]

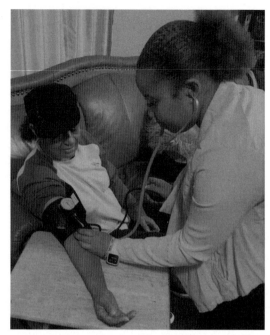

FIG. 5.6 An OTA assists an older adult in monitoring her blood pressure.

OTAs interested in incorporating health management and self-management into their interventions with older adults are encouraged to review AOTA's Chronic Conditions Evidence Based Practice Systematic Reviews and Research (https://www.aota.org). The National Council on Aging provides information on a variety of evidence-based chronic disease self-management programs (https://www.ncoa.org). OTAs can pursue training to become certified to deliver many of these programs within their communities.

AGING WELL WITH MENTAL ILLNESS (*PREVIOUS CONTRIBUTIONS FROM ANN BURKHARDT, SUE BYERS-CONNON)

Public health and aging trends in the United States indicate that approximately 20 percent of adults over age 65 will experience mental health concerns or develop a mental illness.[55] Older adults also experience mental health symptoms as a result of loss of functional capacity and diminishing social groups, although a formal diagnosis of mental illness might not be justified.[56] The most prevalent mental illness affecting this age group is depression.[57] Other common mental illnesses experienced in later life are dementia, anxiety disorders, depression leading to suicide, and substance abuse.[58] As technology in health care has improved, people with chronic mental illnesses are also living further into older age. Determining how chronic mental illness affects lifestyle over time is an ongoing discovery.

The population of adults aged 65 and older in the United States is growing rapidly. For the first time in US history, children are expected to be outnumbered by older adults by the year 2034.[59] By 2060, it is estimated that 94.7 million US residents will be over 65 years old.[59,60] The challenge that society now faces is managing health concerns for the aging masses. Health care financing often falls short of adequate dollars to spend on older adults living into later life. Historically, funding for intervention of mental illnesses has also fallen short when compared with funding for other general medical and surgical conditions. When persons age past 65, and when they age with chronic illnesses such as mental illnesses, the costs for their care can rise exponentially. Long-term use of antipsychotic medicines can affect a number of body functions. Neurological symptoms (such as tardive dyskinesia and parkinsonism), hematological concerns (such as pernicious anemia), and cognitive dysfunctions (such as dementia, delirium, and increased hallucinations) are some of the most devastating consequences of long-term antipsychotic use that affect functional ability. When people who have mental illness enter older age, they often need additional personal and environmental facilitators to enable them to remain safely in their communities. Some may require homecare with or without group housing, some may require skilled care with supervision and assistance, whereas some may require institutionalization.

Occupational therapy practitioners understand that aging well includes a healthy mind as well as a healthy body, making it imperative that mental health considerations in older age be acknowledged and addressed. Dementia is often thought of as a normal part of the aging process and thus it is not always treated aggressively. But cognitive decline is not an inevitable part of aging.[56] Healthy People 2030 has developed several Core Objectives to promote the needs of older adults with cognitive decline and dementia, and the public health sector is increasing efforts to educate the population regarding intervention options to alleviate or slow the progression of cognitive decline leading to dementia.[61] This presents growing opportunities for occupational therapy practitioners to promote the concepts of productive cognitive aging at the community level.

Occupational therapy practitioners frequently use the *Recovery Model* to address chronic mental health challenges among older adults. This model focuses on enabling people with mental illness to live a meaningful life in the community through the use of client-centered services.[62] Occupational therapy practitioners are uniquely qualified to provide mental health services that address an older adult's ability to function in a variety of occupations using occupation-based psychosocial, self-management, and environmental interventions.[63] Occupational therapy intervention for older adults with chronic or newly acquired mental illness should focus on:

- Engagement in occupation to foster recovery and achieve optimal levels of community participation, independence in daily life skills, quality of life, and sense of well-being

- Identification of and training in healthy habits, rituals, and routines to support wellness
- Training in coping strategies to alleviate stress, anxiety, and depression
- Environmental modifications for cognitive decline and physical comorbidities
- Family/caregiver education

NUTRITION AND OVERWEIGHT OR UNDERWEIGHT OLDER ADULTS

Balanced nutrition is essential to healthy aging, health maintenance and prevention of disease, obesity and malnutrition in older adults. Consuming a healthy diet is a challenge for many people in the United States for a variety of reasons including lack of knowledge to make healthy choices, access to healthy food options, and inability to afford healthy foods. In fact, one goal of Healthy People 2030 is to "improve health by promoting healthy eating and making nutritious foods available."[64] Occupational therapy practitioners working with older adults in nearly any area of practice have the opportunity to address nutrition as part of IADL interventions, including the activities of shopping, meal preparation, and nutrition management (Fig. 5.7). Occupational therapy practitioners can provide older adults with important information regarding balanced nutrition and encouragement to ensure a balanced intake of foods high in nutrients and low in saturated fats, refined sugars, and sodium.

Older adults are encouraged to follow dietary guidance similar to younger adults, with some special consideration due to the aging process and presence of chronic conditions. Older adults should obtain most of their daily intake via nutrient-dense foods and beverages, while staying within calorie limits. This includes a diet rich in fruits, vegetables, whole grains, dairy, and protein foods while also ensuring adequate hydration. Older adults generally fail to achieve recommended intake levels of

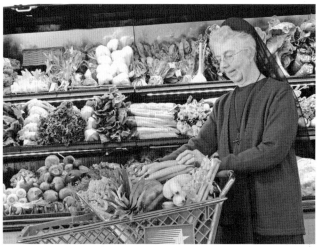

FIG. 5.7 Nutrition management can be addressed when working with older adults on the IADL of shopping.

fruits, vegetables, whole grains, and seafood-based protein as well as fluid intake.[65] Likewise, older adults should limit foods and drinks that include added sugars, saturated fats, and sodium as well as alcoholic beverages. Over 50% of older adults exceed recommended levels of added sugars, over 70% exceed recommended levels of sodium, and over 75% exceed recommended levels of saturated fats. Older adults may also feel the effects of alcoholic drinks more easily than younger adults and are recommended to limit consumption to no more than two alcoholic drinks per day for men or one alcoholic drink per day for women.[65]

Obesity is a concern for nearly 40% of US adults over the age of 60 and these numbers are anticipated to continue to increase in the future.[66] In addition, another one in three adults in the United States are overweight.[67] Obesity and becoming overweight is often the result of dietary excess, nutrient poor food choices, over consumption of added sugars and fats, as well as decreased physical activity; being overweight or obese can result in an increased risk of developing or worsening numerous chronic conditions, decreased physical functioning, increased risk of falling, and increased mortality risk. Malnutrition in older adults can also be multifactorial in etiology; the failure to consume adequate energy, nutrients, and fluids can result in a variety of complications including worsening health and health conditions as well as increased frailty (Box 5.2).[68] Insufficient hydration can further complicate this scenario as dehydration can impact digestion and absorption of nutrients during the digestion process.[65] While older adults who are malnourished often present as underweight and frail, it is also possible for

older adults who are overweight to also suffer from malnutrition due to consumption of a nutrient poor diet combined with decreased in physical activity.[68]

Occupational therapy practitioner assessment of factors associated with nutrition and weight is critical in developing client-centered interventions for older adults who are underweight or overweight. Issues that may affect eating and thus contribute to poor nutrition and underweight status include loss of teeth, low tolerance for textured foods, jaw pain when chewing, and medication side effects such as nausea, dry mouth, and fear of choking. Other issues that can impact recommended dietary intake include impaired cognition, loss of physical stamina and endurance for shopping and meal preparation, depression, vision loss, or pain.[68] Contextual factors may include decreased accessibility of the kitchen and dining areas, limited access to a grocery story with healthy food options, lack of transportation, or insufficient financial resources. Physical activity can be impacted by a range of factors including endurance, pain, psychosocial function, and context. Occupational therapy intervention strategies can be instrumental in helping older adults overcome barriers to adequate nutritional intake and physical activity to achieve healthy habits and behaviors.

REST AND SLEEP

Mr. Marshall has been seeing an occupational therapy practitioner to address difficulty sleeping. He has stated that he has difficulty falling asleep, staying asleep, and having energy throughout the day to complete basic tasks. At the initial evaluation, Mr. Marshall reported that he noticed that this has been getting worse over the past several years. He was widowed 3 years ago. Mr. Marshall continues to live in his own home independently but is feeling overwhelmed by the number of health care appointments that he is having to manage as well as the growing housework. Family is available to assist but live several hours away. Mr. Marshall shared that he is not moving as fast as he once did and is afraid of falling. Mr. Marshall had a heart valve replacement for a congenital abnormality 15 years ago but now has congestive heart failure and is not a candidate for a new valve replacement. Recent changes to his diuretic medication and heart medication have made him hypervigilant to changes in weight. He has difficulty getting in and out of bed due to lower back pain and has started to sleep in the recliner chair in the living room. He shares that it is easier to get out of and since he has to get up to use the bathroom several times a night, it just makes more sense. Mr. Marshall enjoyed working out previously and currently tries to do a few exercises but spends much of his time watching television and doing crossword puzzles. He has started napping in the afternoons and sometimes will sleep several hours at a time before dinner. Overall, Mr. Marshall appears to be well cared for but is showing some signs of anxiety when talking about everything that is a concern.

How would the occupational therapy practitioner address sleep and rest with this client using health promotion and health maintenance techniques?

BOX 5.2

Factors That Can Contribute to Insufficient Nutrition and Fluid Intake

- Sensory changes such as decreased taste or smell impact enjoyment of eating
- Changes in feelings of hunger or satiation
- Slowed gastric system
- Changes in dentition
- Dysphagia
- Medical conditions such as diabetes, cancer, renal disease, alcoholism, dementia, depression, anxiety
- Medications such as diuretics, antidepressants, antihypertensives, antibiotics
- Difficulty with community mobility to shop for food
- Lack of access to supermarket within community
- Difficulty with food preparation and other IADLs
- Financial status/low socioeconomic status
- Social isolation
- Psychosocial factors such as loneliness, stress, grief

Adapted from Evans C. Malnutrition in the elderly: A multifactorial failure to thrive. *The Permanente Journal.* 2005;9: 38–41. doi:10.7812/tpp/05-056

Rest and sleep is important for everyday function and engagement in daily occupations. For many older adults, this is something that becomes more challenging as a person grows older. This can be due to medications, pain, or feeling sick. Older adults continue to need the same amount of sleep as younger adults; however, their sleep patterns begin to change, going to bed earlier and waking earlier in the morning.[69] Due to the prevalence of rest and sleep concerns for older adults, it is imperative that OTAs address sleep problems with their clients.[70]

Occupational therapy practitioners use their background and understanding of sleep pathology and sleep disorders to address the effects of sleep insufficiency and sleep disorders on occupational performance and engagement. Occupational therapy practitioners approach sleep problems through the context of health maintenance and health promotion.[71] The interconnection of the environment, occupation, and person are important to understand when addressing rest and sleep using health maintenance or health promotion principles.

Community-dwelling older adults with insomnia concerns especially benefit from the use of the cognitive-behavioral interventions and educational techniques. These interventions can take place in person or via computer training and both have positive outcomes. Cognitive-behavioral interventions that incorporate sleep hygiene education, progressive relaxation, goal setting, development of a sleep schedule, and the use of a sleep diary are also beneficial.[72] These approaches coupled with self-relaxation, meditation, physical exercise, sleep hygiene education, and cognitive therapy can continue to lead to positive outcomes for community-dwelling older adults.[72] Therefore, for those older adults that are living in the community there are many beneficial intervention strategies that an Occupational therapy practitioner can use to address sleep-related concerns.

HEALTH LITERACY

When many people think of health literacy, their mind oftentimes goes to whether a person is able to read the materials provided. While this is an important detail to know about a person, health literacy includes much more. Healthy People 2030 has emphasized that health literacy is considered as two concepts: Personal Health Literacy and Organizational Health Literacy. "Personal Health Literacy is the degree to which individuals have the ability to find, understand, and use information and services to inform health-related decisions and actions for themselves and others." This differs from Organizational Health Literacy which "is the degree to which organizations equitably enable individuals to find, understand, and use information and services to inform health-related decisions and actions for themselves and others."[73] When Organizational Health Literacy is considered alongside Personal Health Literacy, the OTA understands that in order to address health literacy with a client they must not

only address the client's ability to locate, interpret, and utilize the information but also that they as an occupational therapy practitioner must be supporting the client through this process and developing resources and methods for assessing understanding that are appropriate for the client. Therefore, OTAs should possess the needed communication and education skills to help their clients understand, access and use health information and services and be able to develop of appropriate materials for a variety of clients.[74]

Health literacy is influenced by the person's native language or ability to read the written word, ability to communicate, age, cultural background or tradition, cognition and mental health status.[75,76] Low health literacy has been associated with increased hospitalizations and emergency treatment, decreased utilization of preventative health services, and poor ability to understand medication labels or take medications appropriately.[77] Low health literacy may also go undetected as a person may not want to appear incompetent. Good therapeutic relationships between client and the occupational therapy practitioner are important in fostering trust and ensuring dignity for everyone. For older adults, low health literacy can be especially problematic. An older adult may be wrongly assumed to be noncompliant or may be thought to have a cognitive impairment when the real problem is poor personal health literacy. An organization may also be failing to meet the needs of the older adult if materials are being provided in a way that is not relevant or appropriate for the person.

An OTA is educating an older adult with a recent hip replacement about their new hip precautions prior to discharge. The OTA is using correct but complex medical terms and relies on verbal and written instructions only. Later that day, the older adult is frequently breaking those precautions and the OTA is becoming frustrated with the older adult because they seemed to understand those precautions (i.e., nodding and smiling when asked if they understood) during their session together. The nursing staff are concerned that the older adult may have some cognitive limitations. However, if the care team is knowledgeable in health literacy, they would quickly realize that the noncompliance is not due to a cognitive impairment but low health literacy. If that same OTA would return and provide the education with the use of other visual aids (i.e., pictures, demonstrations), simple easy to understand language without medical jargon, and utilize a teach-back approach, that older adult may be able to not only demonstrate but understand and use the hip precautions correctly.

The era of technology and its frequent use in health care settings poses a new challenge of locating, accessing, and understanding health information online. Occupational therapy practitioners are uniquely capable of addressing this challenge by focusing on health management skills with the older adult. This is in line with the role of the occupational therapy practitioner and is well established in the scope of practice for the profession.[74] Older adults are able to gain necessary skills needed to properly find quality health information online, judge its trustworthiness, use online platforms to access information, and generally understand health information when provided with specific training in these areas. The occupational therapy practitioner can use several frameworks or models to assist with e-health literacy: the Health Literacy Model, the Health Literacy Skills Framework, and the e-Health Literacy Framework.[78] The use of a framework or model can assist the occupational therapy practitioner as they address health literacy concerns with an older adult by providing a structure in which to guide current and future encounters. The teach-back method serves as a beneficial tool to ensure that older adults with low health literacy are remembering the correct health information provided and are understanding the health information.[79] Teach-back methods can be used by the occupational therapy practitioner when they teach about precautions or safety procedures, educate a client or caregiver on a home program, or the goals of occupational therapy. Other strategies for ensuring understanding include: using personal pronouns, simple language, visual images, using an active voice, and relating it to familiar situations.[80]

OTAs who would like to improve their skills and knowledge on health literacy should consider accessing the following trainings and resources:

The National Institute on Aging provides a resource for health care providers when working with older adults (https://www.nia.nih.gov/health/doctor-patient-communication/talking-with-your-older-patient).

Centers for Disease Control and Prevention provide resources and trainings on health literacy (https://www.cdc.gov/healthliteracy/gettraining.html).

TOOLKIT for Making Written Material Clear and Effective (US Department of Health and Human Services Centers for Medicare & Medicaid Services) (https://www.cms.gov/Outreach-and-Education/Outreach/Written-MaterialsToolkit).

SUMMARY

In the United States, there is a growing recognition of the importance of health promotion and health management as necessary strategies to promote quality of life and occupational engagement for older adults. This will become even more critical as the number of adults over the age of 65, and the number of them living with chronic disease continues to rise through the first half of the 21st century. Occupational therapy practitioners can play a key role in facilitating the process of aging well for our aging population.

TECH TALK: FOCUS ON AGING WELL

NAME	PURPOSE	APPROX. COST	WHERE TO BUY
Rise	App designed to promote healthy sleep and develop sleep hygiene activities. Compatible with many wearables	Free trial ~$9.99/mo	Google Play IOS App Store Risescience.com
GoodRX	Website and app designed to locate prescription drug costs in user's area as well as discount coupons	$0 to ~$9.99/mo	Google Play IOS App Store Goodrx.com
LastPass	App designed to store and manage online/app passwords securely and in one place. Includes ability to look up passwords and autofill into websites and apps	$0	Google Play IOS App Store
First Aid: American Red Cross	Advice from the American Red Cross about how to handle every day emergencies	$0	Google Play IOS App Store

CHAPTER REVIEW QUESTIONS

1 Give examples of primary, secondary, and tertiary prevention functions of OTAs working with older adults.
2 Explain how health and occupation are interrelated.
3 Describe how an OTA might incorporate concepts of self-management into intervention implementation with an older adult client.
4 Describe the role of occupational therapy practitioners in wellness and health promotion program implementation.
5 Describe the impact of low health literacy on client outcomes.
6 What strategies might the OTA take to assess client understanding if low health literacy is suspected?

7 How would the occupational therapy practitioner address sleep and rest with the client described in that section, using health promotion and health maintenance techniques? Provide three examples of how to promote rest and sleep with an older adult.
8 Explain how an occupational therapy practitioner would use the teach-back method to increase the health literacy of an older adult client.
9 Describe the role of the occupational therapy practitioner in increasing occupational engagement and participation with an older adult. Provide three examples of interventions or activities that can increase this engagement and participation.
10 How do health risks impact health promotion and occupational engagement in older adults?

11 Describe the long-term effects of antipsychotic medications affecting many older adults aging with chronic mental illness.

12 Explain the focus of occupational therapy intervention for older adults with mental illness.

13 Define the Recovery Model as related to intervention for older adults with mental illness.

14 Describe the Health Belief Model.

15 Describe Social Cognitive Theory as related to health promotion.

16 Describe the Transtheoretical Model of Health Behavior Change.

REFERENCES

1. Rural Health Information. *Demographic Changes and Aging Population*. Available at: https://www.ruralhealthinfo.org/toolkits/aging/1/demographics.

2. Scaffa ME. Community-based practice: occupation in context. In: Scaffa ME, Reitz SM, eds. *Occupational Therapy in Community-Based Practice Settings*. Philadelphia, PA: F.A. Davis Company; 2014:1-18.

3. Reitz SM. Historical and philosophical perspectives of occupational therapy's role in health promotion. In: Scaffa ME, Reitz SM, Pizzi MA, eds. *Occupational Therapy in the Promotion of Health and Wellness*. Philadelphia, PA: F.A. Davis Company; 2010;1-21.

4. American Occupational Therapy Association. Role of the occupational therapist in the promotion of health and prevention of disabilities. *Am J Occup Ther*. 1979;33:50-51.

5. American Occupational Therapy Association. Occupational therapy in the promotion of health and well-being. *Am J Occup Ther*. 2020;74:7403420010. Available at: https://doi.org/10.5014/ajot.2020.743003.

6. World Health Organization. *The Ottawa Charter for Health Promotion*. 1986. Available at: https://www.who.int/teams/health-promotion/enhanced-wellbeing/first-global-conference.

7. U.S. Department of Health and Human Services. *Healthy People 2030 Framework*. 2018. Available at: https://health.gov/healthypeople/about/healthy-people-2030-framework.

8. American Occupational Therapy Association. Occupational therapy practice framework: domain and process. 4th ed. *Am J Occup Ther*. 2020;74(suppl 2):7412410010. Available at: https://doi.org/10.5014/ajot.2020.74S2001.

9. Sharma M. *Theoretical Foundations of Health Education and Health Promotion*. Burlington, MA: Jones & Bartlett Learning; 2020.

10. Reitz SM, Scaffa ME, Pizzi MA. Occupational therapy conceptual models for health promotion practice. In: Scaffa ME, Reitz SM, Pizzi MA, eds. *Occupational Therapy in the Promotion of Health and Wellness*. Philadelphia, PA: F.A. Davis Company; 2010;22-45.

11. Rosenstock IM, Strecher VJ, Becker MH. Social learning theory and the health belief model. *Health Educ Q*. 1988;15:175-183.

12. Bandura A. *Social Learning Theory*. Upper Saddle River, NJ: Prentice Hall; 1977.

13. Prochaska JO, DiClemente CC. Transtheoretical therapy: toward a more integrative model of change. *Psychother Theory Res Pract*. 1982;19:276-288.

14. Skinner CS, Tiro J, Champion VL. The health belief model. In: Glanz K, Rimer BK, Viswanath KV, eds. *Health Behavior: Theory, Research and Practice*. San Francisco, CA: John Wiley & Sons; 2015;75-94.

15. Merryman MB, Shank KH, Reitz SM. Theoretical frameworks for community-based practice. In: Scaffa ME, Reitz SM, eds. *Occupational Therapy in Community and Population Health Practice*. Philadelphia, PA: F.A. Davis; 2020:38-58.

16. Prochaska JO, Redding CA, Evers KE. The Transtheoretical Model and stages of change. In: Glanz K, Rimer BK, Viswanath KV, eds. *Health Behavior: Theory, Research and Practice*. San Francisco, CA: John Wiley & Sons; 2015;125-148.

17. Liu KT, Kueh YC, Arifin WN, Kim Y, Kuan G. Application of Transtheoretical Model on behavior changes, and amount of physical activity among university students. *Front Psychol*. 2018;9:2403. Available at: https://doi.org/10.3389/fpsyg.2018.02402.

18. World Health Organization. *Health Promotion and Disease Prevention Through Population-Based Interventions, Including Action to Address Social Determinants and Health Inequity*. Available at: http://www.emro.who.int/about-who/public-health-functions/health-promotion-disease-prevention.html.

19. Federal Interagency Forum on Aging-Related Statistics. *Older Americans 2020: Key Indicators of Well-Being*. 2020. Available at: https://www.agingstats.gov/docs/LatestReport/OA20_508_10142020.pdf.

20. Centers for Disease Control and Prevention. *Important Facts about Falls*. 2017. Available at: https://www.cdc.gov/homeandrecreationalsafety/falls/adultfalls.html.

21. Centers for Disease Control and Prevention. *How Much Physical Activity do Older Adults Need?* 2021. Available at: https://www.cdc.gov/physicalactivity/basics/older_adults/index.htm.

22. Kosteli MC, Williams SE, Cumming J. Investigating the psychosocial determinants of physical activity in older adults: a qualitative approach. *Psychol Health*. 2016;31:730-749. Available at: https://doi.org/10.1080/08870446.2016.1143943.

23. Langhammer B, Bergland A, Rydwik E. The importance of physical activity exercise among older people. *Biomed Res Int*. 2018;2018:7856823. Available at: https://doi.org/10.1155/2018/7856823.

24. Liu CJ, Chang WP, Chang MC. Occupational therapy interventions to improve activities of daily living for community-dwelling older adults: a systematic review. *Am J Occup Ther*. 2018;72:7204190060. Available at: https://doi.org/10.5014/ajot.2018.031252.

25. Macera CA, Cavanaugh A, Bellettiere J. State of the art review: physical activity and older adults. *Am J Lifestyle Med*. 2016;11:42-57. Available at: https://doi.org/10.1177/1559827615571897.

26. Guirguis-Blake JM, Michael YL, Perdue LA, Coppola EL, Beil TL. Interventions to prevent falls in older adults: updated evidence report and systematic review for the US Preventive Services Task Force. *JAMA*. 2018;319:1705-1716. Available at: https://doi.org/10.1001/jama.2017.21962.

27. Kumar P, Tiwari SC, Goel A, et al. Novel occupational therapy interventions may improve quality of life in older adults with dementia. *Int Arch Med*. 2014;7:26. Available at: https://doi.org/10.1186/1755-7682-7-26.

28. Scott TL, Masser BM, Pachana NA. Positive aging benefits of home and community gardening activities: older adults report enhanced self-esteem, productive endeavors, social engagement and exercise. *SAGE Open Med*. 2020;8:1-13. Available at: https://doi.org/10.1177/2050312120901732.

29. Prichard E, Barker A, Day L, Clemson L, Brown T, Haines T. Factors impacting the household and recreation participation of older adults living in the community. *Disabil Rehabil*. 2015;37:56-63. Available at: https://doi.org/10.3109/09638288.2014.902508.

30. Mazza NZ, Bailey E, Lanou AJ, Miller N. A statewide approach to falls prevention: widespread implementation of A Matter of Balance in North Carolina, 2014-2019. *J Appl Gerontol*. 2021;0733464821997212. Available at: https://doi.org/10.1177/0733464821997212.

31. Tomita MR, Saharan S, Rajendran S, Nochajski SM, Schweitzer JA. Psychometrics of the Home Safety Self-Assessment Tool (HSSAT) to prevent falls in community-dwelling older adults. *Am J Occup Ther*. 2014;68:711-718. Available at: https://doi.org/10.5014/ajot.2014.010801.

32. Pizzi MA. Health promotion for people with disabilities. In: Scaffa ME, Reitz SM, Pizzi MA, eds. *Occupational Therapy in the*

Promotion of Health and Wellness. Philadelphia, PA: F.A. Davis Company; 2010;376-396.

33. Centers for Disease Control and Prevention. *What Should I Know about Screening?* Available at: https://www.cdc.gov/cancer/cervical/basic_info/screening.htm.

34. Yu L, Sabatino SA, White MC. Rural–urban and racial/ethnic disparities in invasive cervical cancer incidence in the United States, 2010–2014. *Prev Chronic Dis.* 2019;16:180447. Available at: http://doi.org/10.5888/pcd16.180447.

35. Ramjan L, Cotton A, Algonso M, Peters K. Barriers to breast and cervical cancer screening for women with physical disability: a review. *Women Health.* 2016;56:141-156. Available at: https://doi.org/10.1080/03630242.2015.1086463.

36. Pizzi MA, Reitz SM, Scaffa ME. Health promotion and well-being for people with physical disabilities. In: Pendleton HM, Schultz-Krohn W, eds. *Pedretti's Occupational Therapy: Practice Skills for Physical Dysfunction.* St. Louis, MO: Elsevier; 2018:58-70.

37. Golinowska S, Groot W, Baji P, Pavlova M. Health promotion targeting older people. *BMC Health Serv Res.* 2016;16:345. Available at: https://doi.org/10.1186/s12913-016-1514-3.

38. Glantz CH, Richman N. The wellness model in long-term care facilities. *Quest.* 1996;7:7-11.

39. Hettinger J. The wellness connection. *OT Week.* 1996;10:12-13.

40. Jackson J, Carlson M, Mandel D, Zemke R, Clark F. Occupation in lifestyle redesign: the well elderly study occupational therapy program. *Am J Occup Ther.* 1998;52:326-334.

41. Dieterle C. Lifestyle redesign® programs. In: Scaffa ME, Reitz SM, eds. *Occupational Therapy in Community and Population Health Practice.* Philadelphia, PA: F.A. Davis Company; 2020:503-519.

42. Clark FA, Blanchard J, Sleight A, et al. *Lifestyle Redesign: The Intervention Tested in the USC Well Elderly Studies.* 2nd ed. Bethesda, MD: The American Occupational Therapy Association; 2015.

43. Mountain G, Chatters R. The "Lifestyle Matters" study: Results from a trial of an occupational therapy lifestyle intervention for older adults. *Am J Occup Ther.* 2016;70(4 suppl 1):7011515242. Available at: https://doi.org/10.5014/ajot.2016.70S1-RP304A.

44. Centers for Disease Control and Prevention. *Promoting Health for Older Adults.* Available at: https://www.cdc.gov/chronicdisease/resources/publications/factsheets/promoting-health-for-older-adults.htm.

45. Hammell KW. Opportunities for well-being; The right to occupational engagement. *Can J Occup Ther.* 2018;84:209-222. Available at: https://doi.org/10.1177/0008417417734831.

46. World Health Organization. *Health Promotion.* Available at: https://www.who.int/news-room/q-a-detail/health-promotion.

47. Behn L, Eklund K, Wilhelmson K, et al. Results from the RCT elderly persons in the risk zone. *Public Health Nurs.* 2015;33:303-315. Available at: https://doi.org/10.1111/phn.12240.

48. Hand C, Retrum J, Ware G, Iwasaki P, Moaalii G, Main DS. Understanding social isolation among urban aging adults: informing occupation-based approaches. *OTJR (Thorofare N J).* 2017;37:188-198. Available at: https://doi.org/10.1177/1539449217727119.

49. Robins LM, Hill KD, Finch CF, Clemson L, Haines T. The association between physical activity and social isolation in community-dwelling older adults. *Aging Ment Health.* 2018;22:175-182. Available at: https://doi.org/10.1080/13607863.2016.1242116.

50. Morbidity and Mortality Weekly Report. *QuickStats: Percentages of Adults with Activity Limitations by Age Group and Type of Limitation: National Health Review Survey, United States, 2014.* Centers for Disease Control and Prevention; 2016. Available at: https://www.cdc.gov/mmwr/volumes/65/wr/mm6501a6.htm.

51. Perez-Ros P, Martinez-Arnau FM, Tarazona-Santabalbina FJ. Risk factors and number of falls as determinants of quality of life of community-dwelling older adults. *J Geriatr Phys Ther.* 2018;42:63-72. Available at: https://doi.org/10.1519/JPT.0000000000000150.

52. American Occupational Therapy Association. *Fact Sheet: Occupational Therapy's Role with Chronic Disease Management.* 2015. Available at: https://www.aota.org/-/media/Corporate/Files/AboutOT/Professionals/WhatIsOT/HW/Facts/FactSheet_ChronicDisease-Management.pdf.

53. Richard AA, Shea K. Delineation of self-care and associated concepts. *J Nurs Scholarsh.* 2011;44:136-144. Available at: https://doi:10.1111/j.1547-5069.2012.01444.x.

54. Schulman-Green D, Jaser S, Martin F, et al. Processes of self-management in chronic illness. *J Nurs Scholarsh.* 2012;44:136-144. Available at: https://doi:10.1111/j.1547-5069.2012.01444.x.

55. Substance Abuse and Mental Health Services Administration. *Older Adults Living with Serious Mental Illness: The state of the Behavioral Health Workforce.* 2019. Available at: https://store.samhsa.gov/sites/default/files/d7/priv/pep19-olderadults-smi.pdf.

56. Mental Health America. *Position statement 35: Aging Well: Wellness and Psychosocial Treatment for the Emotional and Cognitive Challenges of Aging.* 2016. Available at: https://www.mhanational.org/issues/position-statement-35-aging-well-wellness-and-psychosocial-treatment-emotional-and-cognitive.

57. Centers for Disease Control and Prevention and National Association of Chronic Disease Directors. *The State of Mental Health and Aging in America Issue Brief 2: Addressing Depression in Older Adults: Selected Evidence-Based Programs.* Atlanta, GA: National Association of Chronic Disease Directors; 2009. Available at: https://www.cdc.gov/aging/pdf/mental_health_brief_2.pdf.

58. Centers for Disease Control and Prevention and National Association of Chronic Disease Directors. *The State of Mental Health and Aging in America Issue Brief 1: What Do the Data Tell Us?* Atlanta, GA: National Association of Chronic Disease Directors; 2008. Available at: https://www.cdc.gov/aging/pdf/mental_health.pdf.

59. United States Census Bureau. *An Aging Nation: Projected Number of Children and Older Adults.* 2019. Available at: https://www.census.gov/library/visualizations/2018/comm/historic-first.html.

60. United States Census Bureau. *Older People Projected to Outnumber Children for First Time in U.S. History.* 2019. Available at: https://www.census.gov/newsroom/press-releases/2018/cb18-41-population-projections.html.

61. Office of Disease Prevention and Health Promotion. *Older Adults. Healthy People 2030.* U.S. Department of Health and Human Services. Available at: https://health.gov/healthypeople/objectives-and-data/browse-objectives/older-adults.

62. Champagne T, Gray K. *Fact Sheet: Occupational Therapy's Role in Mental Health Recovery.* American Occupational Therapy Association; 2016. Available at: https://www.aota.org/-/media/corporate/files/aboutot/professionals/whatisot/mh/facts/mental%20health%20recovery.pdf.

63. American Occupational Therapy Association. *Occupational Therapy's Distinct Value: Mental Health Promotion, Prevention, and Intervention.* 2016. Available at: https://www.aota.org/-/media/Corporate/Files/Practice/MentalHealth/Distinct-Value-Mental-Health.pdf.

64. Office of Disease Prevention and Health Promotion. *Nutrition and Health Eating.* Healthy People 2030. U.S. Department of Health and Human Services. Available at: https://health.gov/healthypeople/objectives-and-data/browse-objectives/nutrition-and-healthy-eating.

65. U.S. Department of Agriculture and U.S. Department of Health and Human Services. *Dietary Guidelines for Americans, 2020-2025.* 9th ed. 2020. Available at: Dietaryguidelines.gov.

66. Batsis JA, Zagaria AB. Addressing obesity in aging patients. *Med Clin North Am.* 2018;102:65-85. doi:10.1016/j.mcna.2017.08.007.

67. National Institute of Diabetes and Digestive and Kidney Disease. *Overweight & Obesity Statistics.* Available at: https://www.niddk.nih.gov/health-information/health-statistics/overweight-obesity.

68. Bernstein M, Franklin R, Munoz R, Position of the Academy of Nutrition and Dietetics. Food and nutrition for older adults: promoting health and wellness. *J Acad Nutr Diet.* 2012;112:1255-1277. Available at: https://doi.org/10.1016/j.jand.2012.06.015.

69. National Institute on Aging. *A Good Night's Sleep*. Available at: https://www.nia.nih.gov/health/good-nights-sleep.
70. Leland NE, Marcione N, Niemiec SLS, Fogelberg KKD. What is occupational therapy's role in addressing sleep problems among older adults? *OTJR*. 2014;34:141-149. Available at: https://doi.org/10.3928/15394492-20140513-01.
71. American Occupational Therapy Association. *Fact Sheet: Occupational Therapy's Role with Sleep*. 2017. Available at: https://www.aota.org/About-Occupational-Therapy/Professionals/HW/Sleep.aspx.
72. Smallfield S, Elliott SJ. Occupational therapy interventions for productive aging among community-dwelling older adults. *Am J Occup Ther*. 2020;74:1-4. Available at: https://doi.org/10.5014/ajot.2020.741003.
73. U.S. Department of Health. *History of Health Literacy Definitions*. 2020. Available at: https://health.gov/our-work/healthy-people/healthy-people-2030/health-literacy-healthy-people-2030/history-health-literacy-definitions.
74. American Occupational Therapy Association. AOTA's societal statement on health literacy. *Am J Occup Ther*. 2011;65:S78-S79. Available at: https://doi.org/10.5014/ajot.2011.65S78.
75. Berkman ND, Sheridan SL, Donahue KE, Halpern DJ, Crotty K. Low health literacy and health outcomes: an updated systematic review. *Ann Intern Med*. 2011;155:97-107. Available at: https://doi.org/10.7326/0003-4819-155-2-201107190-00005.
76. Verney SP, Gibbons LE, Dmitrieva NO, et al. Health literacy, sociodemographic factors, and cognitive training in the ACTIVE study of older adults. *Int J Geriatr Psychiatry*. 2019;34:563-570. Available at: https://doi.org/10.1002/gps.5051.
77. Chesser AK, Woods NK, Smothers K, Rogers N. Health literacy and older adults: a systematic review. *Gerontol Geriatr Med*. 2016;2:1-13. Available at: https://doi.org/10.1177/2333721416630492.
78. Armstrong-Heimsoth A, Johnson ML, Carpenter M, Thomas T, Sinnappan A. Health management: occupational therapy's key role in educating clients about reliable online health information. *Open J Occup Ther*. 2019;7(4):1-12. Available at: https://doi.org/10.15453/2168-6408.1595.
79. Klingbeil C, Gibson C. The teach back project: a system-wide evidence-based practice implementation. *J Pediatr Nurs*. 2018;42:81-85. Available at: https://doi.org/10.1016/j.pedn.2018.06.002.
80. Pearce TS, Clark D. Strategies to address low health literacy in the older adult. *Top Geriatr Rehabil*. 2013;49:98-106. Available at: https://doi.org10.1097/TGR.0b013e31827e4820.

6

The Regulation of Public Policy for Older Adults

HELENE L. LOHMAN, KIMBERLY COLLINS, AND AMY L. SHAFFER

(PREVIOUS CONTRIBUTIONS FROM CORALIE H. GLANTZ AND NANCY RICHMAN)

KEY TERMS

advocacy, case mix groups (CMGs), Inpatient Rehabilitation Facility Patient Assessment Instrument (IRF-PAI), managed care, Medicare, Medicaid, Medicare Administrative Contractures (MACs), Minimum Data Set (MDS), Older Americans Act (OAA), Outcome and Assessment Information Set (OASIS), Omnibus Budget Reconciliation Act of 1987 (OBRA), Patient-Driven Groupings Model (PDGM), Patient-Driven Payment Model (PDPM), Section GG, skilled services, unskilled services

CHAPTER OBJECTIVES

1. Describe payment systems in different practice settings that influence occupational therapy (OT) practice.
2. Clearly define the role of the occupational therapy assistant (OTA) with regard to payment policy regulations.
3. Explain ways that input of the OTA into the various screening measurements and care plans is valuable for an integrated interprofessional team approach.
4. Express the importance of advocacy for the OT profession.
5. Explain how OTAs can become more aware of public policy trends and changes that affect practice.

Olivia is an occupational therapy assistant (OTA) who was invited to speak to a class of OTA students about public policy. Olivia begins her lecture by stating, "Today we are going to discuss the influence of public policies such as Medicare and Medicaid on OT practice." Olivia scans the faces of the students. They appear to look disinterested. She observes students checking their cell phones, using their computers to surf the Internet, and a few stifling yawns. "Okay," Olivia slowly states as she reorganized her thoughts, "I have decided to first share my story. In 2016, I was working for a rehabilitation company that contracted at several skilled nursing facilities in the area. I was making a very high salary for an OTA just out of school! I didn't think to question where that salary came from. Later, I realized that to pay my salary the contract company must have been getting money from somewhere and that money possibly came from charging large amounts to Medicare for patient interventions. "Anyway, one day in 2019, I was talking with your instructor about this upcoming lecture when she asked me if I had considered the effect of how the upcoming Patient-Driven Payment Model (PDPM) would change my practice in the SNF in which

I worked. 'No', I responded. 'I assume that my contract company will take care of me'. You see, I never paid much attention to public policy. I found that subject far removed from my life, and, frankly, I was not interested. I was only interested in caring for my patients. My ignorance about public policy ended up affecting me personally, because, shortly after that conversation the new PDPM regulations were instituted in skilled nursing facilities. I lost my job. The contract company reorganized because of the changes, and I was among several rehabilitation personnel who were laid off. In a blink of an eye, I went from earning over $50,000 a year to being on unemployment, which was difficult as a single mother."

Olivia pauses and looks around the classroom and observes a group of attentive students gazing back at her. Olivia continues, "I found myself reflecting about my career. What was I going to do? Should I enter another area of practice? The more I thought about it, I realized that my passion was in working with older adults. So I did a huge amount of networking and, within 6 months, I was lucky to be hired by a skilled nursing facility (SNF) as an in-house staff therapist. Practice had changed. Though patients still have an individualized treatment plan, instead of seeing most patients alone for about an hour, now many patients are participating in concurrent or group treatments. Individual treatment sessions are around 30 minutes, and I am expected to see approximately 10 patients in less than a 6-hour day. I had to learn about the PDPM and how it affects the therapy provided to the patients. It was difficult at first but, eventually, I adjusted and can see benefits of this new system with its focus on the complex patients and quality."

"Now I pay close attention to policy trends! I do not want to be surprised ever again! I have become involved in my state and national OT organizations, and I try to influence change by writing letters and making phone calls to the senators and congress people from my district. I even visited my representative while attending a conference in Washington, D.C. I never again want to be uninformed about public policy and its effect on practice. Practice will change again as the health care world is very fluid. I urge you to think beyond the classroom to how public policy can affect your lives as citizens and your professional practice." As Olivia continues with her lecture, the class is attentive.

As Emma, a member of the class, listens to the lecture, she feels overwhelmed. She begins thinking, *How can I ever learn all this material so I can apply it in practice? How can I become more aware of changes in public policy that affect practice?* These concerns bother her so much that she asks Olivia about them. Olivia answers, "I am glad that you ask those questions. When you are out in practice, this information will fall into place. Be sure to learn how documentation and billing are done in your practice setting, and don't be shy about asking any clarification questions. Also, for those of you going into practice settings that receive Medicare payment, be aware of the Centers for Medicare & Medicaid Services (CMS) website, which is a good resource, and there are many other resources online such as from the American Occupational Therapy Association (AOTA) that can help you."

A year later, Emma is employed as an OTA at an SNF. She is very excited and feels well equipped to work with the residents. As Emma prepares for her new job, she remembers the questions she asked Olivia and decides to review her course notes, study the policy and procedural manuals at the facility as well as online resources, and research anything she feels needs further clarification.

INTRODUCTORY CONCEPTS

Public policy develops from legislation at the federal and state levels and represents society's values at the time they are instituted (J. MacClain, personal communication, 1996). For example, the Medicare law, which resulted in a national health insurance plan for older adults, was enacted in 1965. Medicaid, a combined federal and state insurance program that addresses the health care needs of the indigent, was enacted in 1966. Both measures were enacted at a time when civil rights were valued by society and were reflected in many other government acts that passed around that time such as the Developmental Disabilities Act and the Vocational Rehabilitation Act.

The language of public policies is meant to be general. The specifics about each public policy are in its regulations. OTAs need to understand these regulations because these directives directly influence OT practice. OTAs also must have a direct understanding of how Medicare and Medicaid are regulated in any setting to ensure that interventions they provide are reimbursed by these third-party payers.

In this chapter, OTAs learn about significant payment sources and related public policies that they will work with in practice settings. Medicare, Medicaid, OBRA, and the Older Americans Act (OAA) are examples of such public policies. The intent of this chapter is to provide an introduction and overview of these key public policies that influence therapy practice and how they are regulated. New policies will continue to be enacted, and established policies can change based on societal needs and political climate. Therefore, not every specific detail of these changes will be or can be included. This chapter provides OTAs with a strong foundation for practice that they will need to keep updated with changes through resources provided. The chapter begins by discussing health care trends in the United States and then goes into specifics about federal public policies that influence OT practice. The chapter concludes with suggestions on ways to keep up with public policy trends as well as promote changes with public policy through advocacy.

HEALTH CARE TRENDS IN THE UNITED STATES: PAST, PRESENT, AND FUTURE

Health care in the United States is transforming rapidly as a result of a quickly changing society; and is moving away from a fee-for-service model in which payment is provided for each unit of care to payment based on aligning costs and quality outcomes.[1] Because health care is a large part of the gross national product with costs consistently increasing along with a growing aged population, ways to monitor these rising costs are discussed and addressed. Major entitlement programs that influence older adults such as Medicare, Medicaid, and Social Security are continually evaluated, discussed, and sometimes modified. A knowledge of these health care trends helps with understanding policies that develop. Besides these entitlement programs perhaps the most major recent law that has influenced health care in the United States was the Patient Protection and Affordable Care Act (ACA),[2] as amended by the Health Care Education Reconciliation Act of 2010,[3] or what has been nicknamed "Obamacare." This law was an attempt to overhaul a fragmented health care industry by making an insurance program with certain essential benefits, including occupational therapy, available for Americans. Although this law has been constantly challenged and modified it still remains intact at the time of this writing. As part of this law, many innovative types of approaches were introduced that influenced the provision of Medicare emphasizing coordinated cost-effective health care. One example of such initiatives was accountable care organizations (ACOs) that focus on managing the cost and quality of care of older adult patients with chronic conditions.[4] A key theoretical article that informed the ACA titled "The Triple Aim: Care, Health, and Cost" outlined the conceptual foundations behind the law.[5] Triple Aim refers to improvement of the health care system through a better health care experience, improvement of the overall health of populations, and reduced health care costs. The concepts discussed in this article are still relevant in today's health care environment.

Pushed forward by the ACA, and continuing to evolve in the health care environment, is the concept of providing services based on value (outcomes).[6,7] The Center for Medicare and Medicaid Services (CMS) defines value-based programs as those that "reward health care providers with incentive payments for the quality of care they give to people with Medicare."[8] An example of a value-based program introduced by CMS is the Hospital Readmission Reduction Program in which hospitals receive bonus payments for good performance and are fiscally penalized for unplanned readmissions within 30 days of discharge.[9] Research evidence indicates that occupational therapy practitioners have been successful in preventing hospital readmissions.[10]

This trend toward considering value affects many systems in the health care arena. In recent times, SNFs evolved from a prospective payment system called the Resource Utilization Groups (RUG-IV) in which a predetermined payment for therapy was based on the number of intervention minutes provided, to a daily rate considering complexity of care and quality indicators with the PDPM. A similar system was introduced in home health called the Patient-Driven Grouping Model (PDGM). These two systems reflect the current trend toward addressing quality of care along with function and patient characteristics (care needs).[11] OTAs can contribute to care in these settings by understanding the regulations and demonstrating value-based interventions that are patient centered, address quality metrics, and based on evidence. OTAs need to display care coordination with the patient/family, interprofessional team and across systems.[1] The PDPM and PDGM programs will be discussed in detail in this chapter.

Finally, modifications in the health care environment are happening very quickly to manage rising health care costs and based on the political agenda of the current Congress and President. Therefore, what is stated in this chapter is likely to change, and OTAs, more than ever, must be aware of modifications in the health care arena and how these modifications affect practice. The following sections describe public regulated sources.

PUBLIC REGULATED SOURCES

Public regulated sources include Medicare, Medicaid, federal and state employee health plans, the military, and the Veterans Administration. Medicare and Medicaid are often accessed by the older adult clients whom OTAs treat and are discussed in the following sections. Please refer to Table 6.1 for an overview of the Medicare system in which OTAs may work.

MEDICARE

Medicare, or Title 18 of the Social Security Act, was first implemented in 1966. As part of the Social Security Amendment of 1965, the Medicare program was created to establish a health insurance program to supplement those covered by the Federal Old Age, Survivors, and Disability Insurance (OASDI) benefits or Social Security. Originally, Medicare covered most people age 65 years and older. However, since then, the program has expanded to cover other groups of people, including those entitled to disability benefits for at least 24 months, those with end-stage renal disease, and those who elect to buy into the program.[12] Medicare is the largest entitlement program in the United States, and other insurance companies often follow the same standards as set up by Medicare.

Parts of the Medicare program and occupational therapy practice

Medicare is divided into four parts (A, B, C, and D).[12] Parts A, B, and C directly influence OT practice. Part A refers to (inpatient) hospital insurance. Although the term "hospital insurance" refers to Medicare Part A, it is easier to think of Part A coverage as inpatient coverage in many settings including hospitals, critical access hospitals, SNFs (not custodial or long-term care), hospice care, and some home health care. In the Medicare system patients are called "Beneficiaries" and they must meet certain conditions to get benefits.[13] OT practitioners follow Medicare beneficiaries under Part A in many settings (see Table 6.1). In most settings, therapy is included with a lump payment amount established in advance based on the anticipated resource use by the Medicare beneficiary or what is known as prospective payment system (PPS).[14] These rates can be based by time, such as a per diem or daily rate in SNF,[15] or per episode in home health.[16] Rates can also be established by a patient classification system such as with the diagnostic-related groups (DRGs) used in inpatient hospitals.[17]

Medicare Reimbursement under Part A as a PPS system was first instituted in inpatient acute hospital settings in 1983 based on a DRG patient classification system, and this system continues today.[17] PPS in each system (e.g., hospital, home health, SNF) is instituted differently, so OTAs will need to understand the specific system in which they work. For example, in inpatient hospitals, costs are bundled into the PPS rate. Most post-acute care settings have a specific screening tool, such as the Minimum Data Set (MDS) in SNFs. For an overview of

TABLE 6.1

Overview of the Medicare System

Parts	Part A	Part B	Part C	Part D
Facilities covered	Inpatient insurance	Medical insurance (Voluntary benefit)	Medicare advantage	Prescription drug coverage Individual voluntary coverage
Acute care hospital	X	X	X	
Hospice	X	X	X	
Long-term care hospital	X	X	X	
Inpatient rehabilitation facility	X	X	X	
Skilled nursing facility	X	X	X	
Home health agency	X	X	X	
Hospital outpatient		X	X	
Comprehensive outpatient rehabilitation facility		X	X	
Rehabilitation agency		X	X	
Partial hospitalization in hospital or community mental health center		X	X	
Inpatient psychiatric facility	X		X	
Physician's office		X	X	
Payment	A prospective payment system (PPS) or payment determined in advance is instituted differently in many of the listed systems	Medicare physician fee schedule		

Adapted from *AOTA guide to Medicare local coverage determinations.* Bethesda, MD: American Occupational Therapy Association. Retrieved from http://www.aota.org/-/media/corporate/files/secure/advocacy/reimb/news/archives/medicare/lcds/resources/lcd%20advocacy%20packet1.pdf

screening tools and payment systems for Part A in home health, inpatient rehabilitation facilities (IRFs), and SNFs, refer to Table 6.2.

Medicare Part B is the medical insurance that covers "doctors' services and outpatient care. It also includes some different medical services than Part A, or covers services with different regulations. These services include physical and occupational therapy, and some home health care."[18] Part B is a voluntary benefit, which is paid for by

monthly premiums. The cost of this premium continues to increase. It is important for OTAs to be aware that Medicare beneficiaries pay a deductible and 20% of their Part B costs unless they have purchased supplemental insurance.

Therapists can provide therapy and bill under Part B in many outpatient settings including physicians' offices, outpatient, home health services, assisted living, SNFs, and comprehensive outpatient rehabilitation facilities

TABLE 6.2

Screening Tools and Payment Specifics for Home Health, Inpatient Rehabilitation Facilities, and Skilled Nursing Facilities (Medicare Part A)

	Home health	Inpatient rehabilitation facilities	Skilled nursing facilities
Screening tool	Outcome and Assessment Information Set (OASIS)	Inpatient Rehabilitation Facility Patient Assessment Instrument (IRF-PAI)	Minimum Data Set (MDS 3.0)
Payment system	Prospective Payment System (PPS) based on Home Health Resource Groups (HHRGs)	PPS based on Case Mix Group (CMGs)	PPS based on Resource Utilization Categories (RUGs)

Adapted from CMS 2020.

(CORFs).[18] Certain regulations are required to be followed with Part B, such as the occupational therapist obtaining physician certification, and physician approval of the therapy plan. Therapy services are billed under a physician's fee schedule using the Physician's Current Procedural Terminology (CPT) codes, which can be revised. OTAs should pay attention to any revisions and learn any new codes for billing. For example, in 2017 a major revision changed the CPT evaluation codes to new codes identifying three levels of evaluation complexity (low, moderate, and high). These levels are determined by the client's occupational profile and client history, assessments of occupational performance, and clinical decision making.[19]

OTAs, in collaboration with the OT, decide how to code delivered interventions. Codes describe outcomes. They may be service codes that are billed once per day regardless of the amount of time spent in intervention delivery. Others can only be reported one time a day, but the code choice is also dependent on the amount of time spent in the service (evaluation/reevaluation). Service codes include evaluation, reevaluation, orthosis (orthotic) application, and most modalities. Timed codes are the majority of the codes applicable to intervention. Multiple units of timed codes can be delivered during a day of intervention. They are based on 15-minute units, and Medicare regulations guide how to calculate the units. For example, to report 1 unit, therapy practitioners provide skilled services with the client for between 8 and 22 minutes. This is also known as the 8-minute rule. Medicare requires that time be accurately recorded for timed codes. (Please refer to CMS Internet Manual 100.4, Chapter 5, Section 20.2 for more information.)

Healthcare Common Procedure Coding System (HCPCS) Level II are another type of coding used for "products, supplies, and services not included in the CPT codes, such as ambulance services and durable medical equipment, prosthetics, orthotics, and supplies."[20] Currently, Medicare beneficiaries who purchase Part B coverage have a therapy threshold, or set financial amount, per year that they can use for all of their outpatient rehabilitation costs (occupational therapy, physical therapy, and speech therapy). Service provided above the threshold requires a billing modifier confirming that the services are medically necessary, and the burden is on the therapist to provide appropriate documentation to support that claim ($2,150 in 2022).[21] The threshold for occupational therapy is one amount and physical therapy and speech therapy share the same amount. The AOTA advocated for adding an exception process to extend coverage for certain conditions that may warrant more therapy. With the exception process, a manual medical review is done on therapy services that exceed a set amount of money ($3,000 until 2028).[21]

Part C "are health plans offered by private companies approved by Medicare."[22] Part C or Medicare Advantage Plans includes the basic services covered by Parts A and B and comprise a variety of payment types such as managed care, fee for service, and medical savings accounts. Some plans offer more benefits than the traditional Medicare plans.

Medicare Part D is outpatient prescription drug coverage, an optional benefit. Although this part of the law does not directly influence OT practice, OTAs may want to read more about it on the CMS website. Older adults can purchase a Medicare supplement plan which can help cover some of the deductible or co-payments associated with Medicare.

General Guidelines for OT Payment and Intervention with Medicare

Table 6.3 overviews examples of justifiable therapy service. All therapy must be medically necessary and require the skilled intervention of a licensed therapy practitioner to be reimbursed. Professional therapy intervention should be developed according to client needs relative to the complexity and intensity of required intervention. Intervention plans should be based on function and must integrate the plan of care. Intervention should be reinforced by other disciplines, such as skilled nursing. The client's specific prior level of function, mobility, and safety in addition to self-care deficits are primary and essential indicators for professional intervention and must be reflected in assessments.[23] OTAs should understand and follow specific guidelines to receive payment and not have a claim denied. This includes understanding what and how to document the treatment delivered as well as the specific treatment interventions being skilled and necessary.

Skilled And Unskilled Therapy

The concept of skilled and unskilled therapy must be understood to obtain payment from Medicare for OT intervention. Skilled care involves specific guidelines. For example, in SNFs, Part A care is covered if performed under the supervision of a licensed professional, ordered by a physician, and provided on a daily basis. As in all Medicare settings, care "must be reasonable and necessary for the treatment of a patient's illness or injury" and "reasonable in terms of duration and quality."[24]

Examples of services that are unskilled and thus not reimbursable would be exercises that are repetitive in nature or passive exercises to maintain range of motion or strength that do not require the involvement of a skilled rehabilitation professional. Use of heat as a "palliative and comfort measure" and repetitive and routine (nonskilled) assistance in dressing, eating, or going to the toilet, and positioning in bed also would not be reimbursable (Table 6.4).[24]

Although a client's diagnosis is a valid factor in deciding the need for skilled services, it should never be the only consideration. The key issue is whether the skills of a therapist are needed for the required services. Skilled therapy services cannot be denied on the basis of diagnosis.

TABLE 6.3

Justification for Professional Therapy Service

Patient example	Justification
Barbara was admitted into an SNF to recuperate from hip replacement surgery. In addition, she was to learn to ambulate with a walker to perform her ADLs and work toward independently performing ADL functions, particularly dressing. Once Barbara learned these skills, she might return to her retirement home apartment and receive home health care to ensure her continued progress and safety.	A skilled client need to work on ADLs. The immediate or short-term potential for progress toward a less intensive or lesser skilled service area exists.
Barbara was depressed and the OTA primarily treated her for depression rather than the total hip replacement. However, intervention may be considered skilled if the OTA could demonstrate that the intervention was directly related to working with the client to safely perform ADL functions.	The philosophy and plan of intervention must realistically focus on achievement of outcomes for the specific phase of rehabilitation, such as being an inpatient in a skilled facility.
The OTA focuses on Barbara's intervention on going home with safety considerations.	Intervention also must focus on the plan for the next expected phase such as outpatient or home care.
During intervention, the OTA should address short-term deficits in safely performing ADL functions. The OT intervention should also take into account the performance component of the client's difficulty.	Intervention is expected to address the type and degree of deficits and effects of other problems in relation to the short-term or interim goals with problem solving.
The OTA would thoroughly document changes in Barbara's status and her motivational level.	The therapist must emphasize variances in the elder's response to intervention and new developments.

ADL, activities of daily living; *OTA*, occupational therapy assistant; *OT*, occupational therapy; *SNF*, skilled nursing facility.

TABLE 6.4

Skilled Occupational Therapy Services

Patient example	Justification
James: An 89-year-old client who recently had a stroke. Prior level of function was independent living at home. Because of hemianopsia and problem-solving difficulties, James requires moderate assistance with ADL functions that require use of upper and lower extremities. He is motivated to do OT intervention.	Identifiable functional deficits in performance areas which require moderate assistance with dressing and grooming upper and lower extremity Skilled expertise of the OTA for intervention with ADL functions Safety concerns
Patricia: A 72-year-old client who recently had a total hip replacement. She is unable to safely dress and requires education in hip safety precautions. The OTA provides instructions for lower extremity dressing and other ADL functions. Intervention includes teaching safety precautions.	Identifiable functional deficit in lower extremity dressing Skilled expertise of OTA for intervention with instructions in lower extremity dressing, ADLs, and hip safety precautions
Charles: A 92-year-old client who recently sustained a right wrist fracture. He is right-hand dominant. The client was independently performing ADL functions before his wrist was fractured. He now requires moderate assistance with ADL functions because of decreased range of motion (ROM) in the right upper extremity. The OTA provides a home ROM program and instruction in ADL functions.	Functional deficits with ADL (dressing, feeding, and grooming) caused by difficulty with the performance component of ROM Prior level of independence Skilled expertise of the OTA needed to teach home ROM program
Susan: A 72-year-old client has a long history of rheumatoid arthritis. Recently the condition has gotten worse and she can no longer dress herself for lower extremity. The OTA provides adaptive equipment and instructs Susan to dress self with the equipment in two sessions.	Skilled expertise of the OTA for working on ADLs Reasonable amount of intervention time Even though Susan will not necessarily improve with her rheumatoid arthritis condition (*Jimmo v. Sebelius* Settlement Agreement), therapy is justified for Susan's skilled need

Note: All services discussed in this table are under the direction of an occupational therapist. Although intervention is done by the OTA, the intervention plan needs to be established by the occupational therapist.
ADL, activities of daily living; *OTA*, occupational therapy assistant; *OT*, occupational therapy; *ROM*, range of motion.

SECTION ONE   CONCEPTS OF AGING

This was clarified in a CMS Program Memorandum as it relates to therapy services needed by individuals with a diagnosis of Alzheimer's disease or other dementias.[25] Before this memorandum, there had been many denials based on having the diagnosis of Alzheimer's disease. (Refer to the Internet *Medicare Benefit Policy Manual* Chapter 15[24] for more information about skilled and unskilled services.)

Further regulations as a result of a court case (*Jimmo v. Sebelious* approved in 2013) clarified that lack of improvement could not be the deciding factor for coverage. These revised Medicare regulations clearly state that therapy services can be provided to improve a patient's function but also to maintain or prevent deterioration of the patient's condition as long as there are skilled reasons for intervention.[26] Therapists should strive for improvement when it is appropriate, such as the provision of skilled therapy to improve an older adult's function post total hip replacement. Whereas for other situations, the skilled need might be to maintain or prevent deterioration of functional status for an older adult with rheumatoid arthritis.

It is important for therapy practitioners to provide interventions that are not only skilled but also meaningful and relevant. In recent years, AOTA joined the American Board of Internal Medicine and its *Choosing Wisely* initiative. This campaign is designed to spark dialogs between medical providers and their consumers in an effort to render care that is necessary, evidence based, and distinguished from care provided by other practitioners.[27] In 2018, AOTA identified five topics specific to the delivery of skilled occupational therapy services in its version of the *Choosing Wisely* campaign. Consumers should investigate these five topics, if they are implemented as interventions by their therapy practitioner. These topics include the use of pulleys with clients who have hemiplegic arms, the use of nonpurposeful activities in therapy sessions, the use of PAMs without a link to occupational performance, and the use of cognitive-based interventions without linking them to an individual's occupational performance.[28] AOTA added five additional topics for consumers to question if being implemented during occupational therapy treatment in 2021. These additional topics include initiation of occupational therapy interventions before completing occupational profile and setting collaborative goals, providing interventions for autistic persons to reduce or eliminate "restricted and repetitive patterns of behavior, activities, or interests" without understanding the meaning of the behavior to the person, using reflex integration programs with individuals with delayed primary motor reflexes without clear links to occupational outcomes, using slings for individuals with hemiplegic arms that place the arm in a flexor pattern for extended periods of time, and providing ambulation or gait training interventions that do not link to functional mobility.

Medicare Administrative Contractures

Currently the CMS contracts out vital program operational functions (e.g., claims processing and review, payments, provider and beneficiary services, appeals) to a set of contractors previously known as Medicare Administrative Contractors (MACs).[29] MACs determine local coverage determinations (LCDs). "An LCD is a decision by a Medicare administrative contractor (MAC) whether to cover a particular service."[30] Payment coverage from each MAC can vary, so it is important for OTAs to become familiar with their area MAC and pay attention to LCDs. OTAs should go to their MAC website to determine claims processing information, educational options, and any regulation changes.

Working With Medicare and Related Regulations In Different Payment Systems

OTAs work with Medicare beneficiaries in many different systems, including SNFs, home health, IRFs, hospital outpatient, CORFs, and rehabilitation agencies. Other settings include OT private practice, partial hospitalization programs, inpatient psychiatric facilities, and physicians' offices. In each therapy setting Medicare coverage will be different. OTAs need to be aware of the rules and regulations and follow the guidelines. This section will provide OTAs with resources to help better understand the various systems. In addition, some of the important aspects of a few systems in which they may practice (e.g., SNFs and inpatient rehabilitation) will be overviewed. The best resource for OTAs to understand the practice in different systems reimbursed by Medicare is the CMS website. As stated earlier, regulations change and OTAs need to stay current. The online CMS Manual System is organized by functional areas (e.g., eligibility, entitlement, claims processing, benefit policy, program integrity). The web-based manuals address coverage in many systems and are routinely updated. It is especially helpful to refer to the CMS Benefit Policy Manual, Chapter 15 (Covered Medical and other Health Services), Sections 220–230.[24] The outpatient regulations in this manual form the basis of coverage for all therapy services. Specific policies may differ by setting. Different policies concerning therapy services are found in other manuals. When a therapy service policy is specific to a setting, it takes precedence over documented general outpatient policies. Finally, keep in mind that all Medicare regulations are periodically reviewed and updated. The most current Medicare regulations will always be applied.[24] Table 6.5 overviews Medicare resources that OTAs can access to understand different systems in which they may work.

Working In Skilled Nursing Facilities

As of 2019, the largest employer of OTAs has been in SNFs.[31] Practice in SNFs is primarily influenced by the public policies of OBRA, Medicare, and Medicaid. OBRA, a landmark act of Congress, focuses on older adults'

TABLE 6.5

Medicare Resources Online

Resources	Information covered
100–01: Medicare General Information, Eligibility, and Entitlement Manual	Provides general information on program requirements
100–02: Medicare Benefit Policy Manuals	Discusses coverage criteria and guidelines for various Medicare settings
100–03: Medicare National Coverage Determinations (NCD) Manuals	Describes whether specific medical items, services, treatment procedures, or technologies can be paid for under Medicare
100–04: Medicare Claims Processing Manual	Provides all of the billing and claims processing information
Chapter 15 Section 220: Coverage of Outpatient Rehabilitation Therapy Services Under Medical Insurance	Provides specific coverage rules for outpatient therapy under Medicare Part B. The documentation in this section is considered by Medicare reviewers.
Chapter 15 Section 220-03: Documentation Requirements for Therapy Services	Provides information about documentation requirements

rights, quality of care, and quality of life in the nursing home setting. OBRA went into effect in October 1990 and was revised with final rules published in 1995.[32] Compliance with the OBRA regulation is necessary for a nursing facility to receive reimbursement from Medicare or Medicaid. The discrepancy between what is required for good care, rehabilitation, and dignity and what is funded can cause ethical and moral dilemmas for OTAs. Knowledge of the regulations that govern care can help the OTA advocate for the services patients need.

Minimum Data Set

The OBRA law was the impetus for developing the screening tool of the MDS, as it "called for the development of a comprehensive assessment tool to provide the foundation for planning and delivering care to nursing home residents."[33] Working in SNFs, OTAs need to be aware of the MDS because this screening tool identifies strengths and deficits recognized for further assessment. The MDS is a tool coordinated by nursing, although many sections of the MDS address areas within the scope of OT practice. For example, OTAs might be able to add input to the cognitive patterns section among others. Data from OT practitioners contribute to the section on self-cares in Section GG. The MDS has been revised, and, with the MDS 3.0, the resident is involved in the assessment process, and changes have been made in how data are collected for therapy.[34]

Under the regulations for the PPS for Medicare Part A, the MDS is also used to determine Medicare payment for those residents who meet the eligibility qualifications. OT intervention influences that payment system through functional scores. Even if no intervention has taken place, the data collection and resident interview may help OTAs give the necessary information to others on the interdisciplinary team. If OTAs are asked to complete any portion of the MDS assessment, they must certify accuracy of the section(s) they complete by noting their credentials and the date and indicating the portion of the assessment completed. The signature of a registered nurse is required to certify completion of the MDS assessment.

The Patient-driven Payment Model In Skilled Nursing Facilities

OTAs need to be aware of the changes to the PPS in SNFs because the effect on therapy delivery is monumental and SNF is a primary area of employment.[31] The PDPM went into effect on October 1, 2019 and replaced the previous PPS utilizing Resource Utilization Groups or RUGs, which had been utilized for 20 years. This change in the payment system shifts the focus of payment from the amount of therapy provided to patient-specific characteristics to determine the per diem or daily rate for each resident. In addition, PDPM includes a few other policy changes comprising concurrent and group therapy limits and changes to the MDS assessment schedule.[35]

The PDPM establishes the per diem rate utilizing five case-mix adjusted components and a variable per diem adjustment. The case-mix components are PT, OT, Speech Language Pathology (SLP), nursing, and non-therapy ancillary needs (e.g., medication, medical supplies). All these components allow the unique, individualized needs, characteristics, and goals of each resident to be captured when determining the per diem rate.[35] Under the PDPM, each resident is classified into a case-mix group (or group of patients with similar characteristics) for each of the case-mix adjusted components and each component utilizes different criteria as the basis for classification.[35]

Upon admission, each resident is assigned to one of 10 clinical categories based on their admitting SNF diagnosis (Table 6.6). These 10 clinical categories are then collapsed down to create four PT and OT clinical categories due to similar rehabilitative costs for PT and OT (Table 6.7). The functional score for the PT and OT component is based on the sum of scores for ten items including: two

TABLE 6.6

PDPM Clinical Categories

Major Joint Replacement or Spinal Surgery	Cancer
Nonsurgical Orthopedic/ Musculoskeletal	Pulmonary
Orthopedic Surgery (Except Major Joint Replacement of Spinal Surgery)	Cardiovascular and Coagulations
Acute Infections	Acute Neurological
Medical Management	Nonorthopedic Surgery

US Department of Health and Human Services. Patient Driven Payment Model. 2021. Retrieved from https://www.cms.gov/Medicare/Medicare-Fee-for-Service-Payment/SNFPPS/PDPM

bed mobility items, three transfer items, one eating item, one toileting item, one oral hygiene item, and two walking items. These items are often referred to as GG items because they are in the GG section of the MDS. The PT and OT clinical categories as well as functional status are utilized to assign residents to 1 of 16 case-mix groups for physical and occupational therapy. SLP has its own clinical criteria.[35]

TABLE 6.7

Collapsed Clinical Categories for PT and OT Classification

Major Joint Replacement or Spinal Surgery	Major Joint Replacement or Spinal Surgery
Nonorthopedic Surgery	Nonorthopedic Surgery and Acute Neurologic
Acute Neurologic	
Nonsurgical Orthopedic/ Musculoskeletal	Other Orthopedic
Orthopedic Surgery (Except Major Joint Replacement or Spinal Surgery)	
Medical Management	Medical Management
Acute Infections	
Cancer	
Pulmonary	
Cardiovascular and Coagulations	

US Department of Health and Human Services. Patient Driven Payment Model. 2021. Retrieved from https://www.cms.gov/Medicare/Medicare-Fee-for-Service-Payment/SNFPPS/PDPM

The last component to determine the per diem rate for each resident is the variable per diem adjustment schedule which applies an adjustment factor to the PT, OT, and nontherapy ancillary components based on the length of stay. This adjustment factor lowers the per diem rate by 2% for every 7 days after day 20.[35]

The other major policy change with the PDPM that effects therapy delivery is concurrent and group therapy limits. Concurrent therapy refers to when one therapist is working with two residents who are involved in different activities. Group therapy is when one therapist is working with four to six patients doing the same or similar activities.[36] PDPM introduces a combined limit of 25% for both concurrent and group therapy.[35]

Working in Home Health Care: The Patient Driven Grouping Model

The BBA of 1997,[37] as amended by the Omnibus Consolidated and Emergency Supplemental Appropriations Act of 1999,[38] called for the development and implementation of a PPS for Medicare home health services. The following discussion overviews the Medicare regulations for the home health system.

Eligibility for Medicare Part A home health services does not require a hospital stay as is mandated for Part A eligibility in SNFs. However, the older adult must be homebound, have a physician's referral, and require skilled services. Homebound means that it is not recommended that the person leave the home and leaving the home requires considerable effort and help.[39] Requirements for homebound is that the person either needs supportive devices along with assistance of another person or their condition is medically contraindicated to leave the home.[39] The older adult does not have to be bedridden.[39] However, leaving the home must be infrequent and for short time periods. Visiting a physician is an example of a legitimate reason to leave the home. With revisions of the law, home health eligibility has broadened to include "participating in therapeutic, psychosocial, or medical intervention in an adult day-care program" and "occasional absences from the home for nonmedical purposes, for example, an occasional trip to the barber, a walk around the block or a drive, attendance at a family reunion, funeral, graduation, or other infrequent or unique event."[16] A client does not qualify for Part A home health services based solely on the need for OT. Nursing, physical therapy, or speech-language pathology must first open the case. However, OT may be introduced along with these other services and may continue after the other services have ended.[16] Past legislative attempts by the AOTA to change these qualification regulations for eligibility as well as to make OT an initiating service have been unsuccessful, but AOTA continues to work on these issues. As a result of legislation that passed in 2020, the Consolidated Appropriations Act, 2021 (H.R. 133), the Home Health Flexibility Act: H.R. 3127/S.1725 allows occupational therapists to open a case by performing the initial and comprehensive assessments.[40]

The regulations for home health agencies (HHAs) are, of course, quite extensive. With assessment, the Outcome and Assessment Information Set (OASIS) is a key component of Medicare's partnership with the home care industry to foster and monitor improved home health care outcomes.[16] It represents core items of a comprehensive assessment for an adult home care patient and forms the basis for measuring patient outcomes for purposes of outcome-based quality improvement. Most data items in the OASIS were developed as systems of outcome measures for home health care. The items have use for outcome monitoring, clinical assessment, care planning, and other internal agency-level applications. OASIS data items encompass sociodemographic, environmental, support system, health status, and functional status attributes of adult patients. In addition, selected attributes of health service use are included. Refer to the Medicare online manuals listed in Table 6.5 for more information about current regulations on the CMS website.

The Bipartisan Budget Act of 2018 addressed several health care issues and established many requirements for home health payment reform which went into effect on January 1, 2020 resulting in the Patient-Driven Groupings Model (PDGM).[41] Mirroring the PDPM, the PDGM reduces the focus on the provision of therapy and instead relies heavily on the clinical characteristics and other patient information to improve the alignment of Medicare payments with patients' care needs. In addition, PDGM changes the payment structure to a national standardized 30-day payment rate if a period of care meets the minimum threshold of home health visits, which is then adjusted for case mix. The case mix adjustment utilizes information from the OASIS including clinical grouping based on diagnosis and functional impairment level in addition to other criteria obtained from Medicare. If the minimum number of visits is not met, the episode of care is paid by a per visit payment rate for the specific discipline providing care.[42]

Medicare in Inpatient Rehabilitation Facilities

OTAs employed in IRFs need to be informed about how the payment system works because there are very unique regulations for this area of practice. One of several admission regulations requires that 60% of patients have one of 13 qualifying diagnoses.[43] Examples of qualifying diagnoses are strokes and amputations. As in other health care settings (SNFs and inpatient hospitals), there are time limitations that influence therapy. In IRFs, OTAs and OTs provide intensive rehabilitation in 3-hour time blocks per day 5 days weekly along with physical therapists and speech language pathologists. Inpatient rehabilitation settings have a strong interprofessional team focus. Patients need to be able to tolerate this level of intensive therapy for continued stay on the unit.[43]

Similar to other settings, IRFs follow a PPS system for Medicare Part A beneficiaries. This PPS system establishes residents in one of numerous case mix groups (CMGs) based on a screening tool called the Inpatient Rehabilitation Facility Patient Assessment Instrument (IRF-PAI). The scoring from the IRF-PAI completed upon admission is used to assign a client to a CMG.[43] As in all postacute settings Section GG is used to evaluate function with self-cares and mobility as well contribute to the payment rate. In IRFs Section GG is part of the IRF-PAI.[44] OTAs can contribute functional information to the assessment process with Section GG, however they cannot complete sections of the IRF-PAI.

Medicare Regulations and OTA Practice

As illustrated in this chapter, health care in the United States is highly regulated, especially with Medicare. OTAs need to be aware of specific Medicare regulations that affect their practice. Medicare requires that OTAs be licensed by the states in which they practice and be supervised according to state laws. At the minimum, Medicare demands that OTAs have general supervision, except in private practice, which requires direct supervision. If supervision requirements in state law are stricter than the federal Medicare regulations, OTAs need to follow them. Each OTA should be aware of the state licensure laws and scope of practice for OT as regulations vary among states. The AOTA website provides resources on licensure requirements for all states.

Medicare services provided by the OTA are billed by his/her supervising OT. OTA services cannot be billed incident to a physician or nonphysician practitioner (NPP) or under their supervising name and National Provider Identifier (NPI) number. Medicare stipulates that OTAs cannot oversee the evaluation process, make clinical judgment/decisions about patient care, or develop/manage a skilled maintenance program in most settings. OTAs can contribute data or observations to the evaluation process.[24] Certification of a patient's plan of care is completed by the occupational therapist and signed off by physician, or nonphysician provider (NPP). Recertification for intervention is done when there are significant changes in function. Both the certification and recertification processes can involve OTA input through contributed data. OTAs can also contribute to documentation of parts of the progress reports but not sign off on the reports. In home health care, regulations specify that the OT not the OTA performs the initial assessment visit and 30-day reassessment visit. The OTA, under the supervision of the therapist, can perform maintenance therapy.[16] Chapters 7 and 15 of the Medicare Benefit Policy Manuals provide specific regulations regarding OT and OTA practice.[24]

As of this writing, changes are being implemented to the payment structure for Medicare services provided by OTAs. These changes were passed as part of the Bipartisan

Budget Act of 2018 (Pub. L. 115–123;132).[41] Though services provided by an occupational therapy practitioner have been reimbursed by Medicare at the same rate, beginning in January 2022, the payment for skilled OT services billed under Medicare Part B and provided by an OTA will be reduced to 85% for the same service payment when provided by a Registered Occupational Therapist.[45] This change was enacted to have the OTA/OT payment relationship mirror that of the physician/physician's assistant or nurse practitioner.[45]

MEDICAID

Medicaid is a health insurance "for low-income individuals and families who fit into an eligibility group that is recognized by federal and state law."[46] Because such a large portion of Medicaid dollars goes toward financing long-term care coverage and even more for people with disabilities, OTAs should become aware of this important public policy.[47] States must provide basic health services, including inpatient and outpatient hospital services, laboratory and x-ray examinations, nursing facility services, physician and nurse practitioner services, and family planning services. State administrations can choose to cover any of 30 or more optional services, including OT. States also have been required to ensure that descriptions of their services meet federal guidelines and that all Medicaid recipients are treated equally.[48]

In many states, the Medicaid program is administered as a managed care plan. Medicaid pays a high percentage of nursing care expenditures in the nursing home industry.[47] Trends with Medicaid have been toward more community-based care.[2,3,48,49] However, the degree of community emphasis varies among states because some have waiver programs and demonstration projects that involve broader funding for innovative programs and nontraditional care management. Thus, the Medicaid program varies considerably from state to state. Because of these variances, the OTA must access state information about their program and be an advocate for OT.

MANAGED CARE

Older adults may be in a managed care plan whether in Medicaid or Medicare Part C. Managed care organizations oversee the care given to consumers and often involve entire range of utilization control tools applied to manage the practice of physicians and others, regardless of practice setting. With Medicare Part C, care may be managed through a health maintenance organization (HMO) or preferred provider organization (PPO). Rates to managed care providers are capitated, meaning that a set rate is provided either per intervention or per condition. This payment may sometimes not be enough to include extensive therapy. The OT/OTA team needs to familiarize itself with the type of managed care services their clients are receiving, emphasize in documentation

the cost-efficient functional evidence-based intervention they provide, and advocate for services if there are any issues.

OTHER POLICIES THAT HELP OLDER ADULTS

This section of the chapter overviews other policies that can help older adults. The OAA which was reauthorized as the Supporting Older Americans Act of 2020 provides many community services and supports for older adults. In addition, trends with public policies aimed at telehealth usage will make health care easier to access for older adults.

Older Americans Act

In 1965, the OAA[50] was enacted to provide services for older adults. The premise of the OAA was that services delivered to older adults at least 60 years of age would enable them to remain in their homes and communities. Funding was established for nutrition programs, senior centers, transportation, housing, ombudsman, and legal services. Differences in these programs exist among states because administration is at the state level. In addition, more opportunity for OT involvement exists in some regions than in others. The original OAA was designed to foster independence, but rehabilitative services were not included. The act established the Administration on Aging, an agency specifically responsible for developing new social services for older adults.

In 2020, the Older American's Act was reauthorized and titled "The Supporting Older Americans Act of 2020." With this reauthorization financial support was provided toward informational services, nutritional programs (meals), disease prevention/health promotion, community, and workforce training for caregiving.[51] Unique to this reauthorization is the focus on caregivers through extending the RAISE Family Caregivers Act which will bring about a national strategy for caregiving support. The act fortified the National Family Caregiver Support Program, which provides respite care and training.[52] Addressing vulnerable older adults with the reauthorization continues with provisions for abuse/neglect. Relevant to therapy is the promotion of evidence-based programming with fall prevention and disease management programs. Furthermore, the act provides better access for older adults for assistive technology. This reauthorization has pertinent language directed toward social isolation of older adults.[52] The language of the act also suggests more education for older adults about infectious diseases and preventable diseases (e.g., sexually transmitted diseases) and assessments such as suicide risk and depression screens. OTAs should pay attention to policies such as the Supporting Older American's Act of 2020 because it can benefit their community dwelling clients. Furthermore, OTAs along with their occupational therapist partner, might consider developing creative programming with their local office on aging.

Telehealth

Telehealth is defined by the Health Resources Services Administration to include the use of electronic information and technology for communication in the support of long-distance delivery of health-related education, public health, and health administration.[53] Telehealth and its role in health care delivery have been evolving as technology use expands. The use of telehealth to deliver OT services to Medicare recipients was first introduced with a limited scope in 2014. At that time, telehealth was reserved for situations in which access to occupational therapy was less available, such as with remote or rural communities.

Each state is responsible for creating specific legislation in their respective practice acts for the delivery of occupational therapy using the telehealth practice model. As such, each practitioner is responsible for researching and following the state-specific regulations of the state in which OT service is delivered, and often the state in which the OT practitioner is residing (if different than the state of service delivery). In addition to state-specific regulations, each payer source (Medicare, Medicaid, health insurance companies, etc.) have specific regulations governing the provision of occupational therapy via telehealth.[54]

The provision of OT services using the telehealth model gained much traction with the 2020 COVID-19 Global Pandemic. In April 2020, CMS acquiesced and waived the requirements for the use of telehealth services for the provision of Occupational Therapy as a portion of the Coronavirus Aid, Relief, and Economic Security Act (CARES Act). At the time of this writing further legislation is in discussion for more permanent allocation of Medicare payment for telehealth.[55]

ADVOCACY FOR OLDER ADULTS

Health care is always in a state of flux that directly affects OT practice. To manage constant changes, advocacy is important to any profession. Involvement of OTAs in advocacy for older adults and the OT profession can make a difference and the AOTA's key documents emphasize this importance. As quoted in the mission statement for AOTA the association's mission is "to advance occupational therapy practice, education, and research through standard setting and **advocacy** on behalf of its members, the profession, and the public."[56] Membership in the association allows therapists access to numerous resources and supports the lobbyists who advocate on a national level for policies that benefit the profession. However, the lobbyist's voices would not be as effectively heard without the support of members of the profession. When issues come up about public policies that impact practice, occupational therapy practitioners should advocate with faxed or emailed letters or lobby directly with Congress to support the therapy stance. Advocacy can also take place with clients as reinforced by provisions discussed in the Occupational Therapy Code of Ethics.[57] As stated in Principle 4 Part L of the Occupational Therapy Code of Ethics, therapists should "provide information and resources to address barriers to access for persons in need of occupational therapy services[57] (Principle: Justice; key words: beneficence, advocate). Furthermore, Principle 4 Part M states that occupational therapy practitioners should "Report systems and policies that are discriminatory or unfairly limit or prevent access to occupational therapy.[57] (Principle: Justice; key words: discrimination, unfair, access, social justice)." OTAs should advocate for those clients who need and would benefit from therapy services, such as appealing denied coverage of services.

Every OTA and OT must encourage the benefits of occupational therapy and establish the role of the profession within society. OTAs must stay informed about all government decisions regarding health care (Table 6.8).

TABLE 6.8

Nonskilled Occupational Therapy Services

Example	Justification
Mary: A 69-year-old client diagnosed with right cerebral vascular accident. Previously, she performed all ADL functions independently. On initial evaluation, Mary was able to perform ADL functions independently, but slowly. Her status on initial evaluation was independent with ADL, although performance was slow.	Slow performance with ADL function is not significant enough to require the intervention of a skilled practitioner. The client will likely improve on her own over time without intervention.
Mark: A 75-year-old client diagnosed with rheumatoid arthritis. OT was ordered to provide an adapted pencil gripper to assist with writing. The OTA provided the gripper.	Intervention does not require the skilled expertise of the OTA. Anyone could provide an adapted pencil gripper.
David: A 74-year-old client diagnosed with Alzheimer's disease. He is dependent in feeding. The OTA monitors feeding three times a week for 2 weeks.	Intervention is routine therefore not requiring the skilled expertise of the OTA.

Note: All services discussed in this chart should have been under the direction of an occupational therapist. Although intervention is done by the OTA, the intervention plan needs to be established by the occupational therapist.
ADL, activities of daily living; *OTA*, occupational therapy assistant; *OT*, occupational therapy; *ROM*, range of motion.

One research study suggests that therapy practitioners primarily depend upon company resources to learn about Medicare regulation changes in SNF. The researchers recommend that therapy practitioners become more self-directed learners with policy changes using outside sources to critically consider other perspectives.[58]

The rapidly changing face of today's health care economy demands innovative and progressive responses from individuals. OTs and OTAs must be strong advocates for their profession and the clients that benefit from occupational therapy intervention by adjusting to change and adapting to new ways to deliver intervention. An example of a direct benefit of advocacy with CMS was the successful effort to get clarification of coverage for patients with the diagnosis of Alzheimer's disease.[59] Another example was the *Jimmo v. Sebelius* court case which confirmed that Medicare coverage is based on skilled need for therapy and not necessarily on improvement. Box 6.1 provides suggestions for ways that OTAs can become more involved with public policy and advocacy.

KEEPING UP WITH CHANGES

Let us return to Emma, the OTA discussed in the opening scenario. On the first day of her job, she meets with her boss, Sarah. After reviewing some of the documentation and billing aspects of the job, Sarah asks Emma how she will keep updated with the frequent changes in regulations related to payment provision. Sarah challenges Emma to research that question and come up with ideas the next day when they meet. That evening, Emma researches the CMS website and the AOTA website. She learns about and plans to follow postings on the CMS website called transmittals, which are used "to communicate new or changed policies, and/or procedures that are being incorporated into specific Centers for Medicare and Medicaid Services (CMS) program manual."[60] She finds manuals on the site that overview different Medicare regulations. Then she goes to the AOTA website. There, in the Advocacy and Policy section, she finds many resources to keep abreast with policy trends and practical suggestions for advocacy. She also finds the MAC site for her area and reads about regulation changes and looks at the LCDs. She searches further on the Internet and finds the AARP website that overviews extensive background related to public policy and advocacy. The next day when they meet again, Sarah is pleased to learn about Emma's efforts and states, "I hope that you take the initiative to keep current from now on, at least about this area of practice. In this rapidly changing health care environment, I expect all my employees to be proactive. I like to have monthly meetings where, along with our practice discussions, we educate and share about current health care changes and public policy."

BOX 6.1

Ways for Occupational Therapy Assistants to Advocate and Become Involved With Public Policy

1. On a clinical level, advocate for best client care by utilizing evidence-based practice and save costs by providing appropriate skilled interventions within a reasonable time period.
2. On a clinical level, address quality measures for the area of practice established by Medicare and articulate this in interprofessional team meetings (Quality reporting measures can be found on the CMS website).
3. Educate clients about their insurance coverage and advocate for them when appropriate, especially with treatment denials.
4. Be able and ready to articulate a clear definition of occupational therapy (OT) for the public; be visible.
5. Find a mentor who understands public policy.
6. Encourage "lunch and learn" work sessions about relevant policies and suggestions for advocacy that influence therapy practice.
7. Invite a Congress person to work.
8. Regularly access the American Occupational Therapy Association (AOTA) website, the Centers for Medicare and Medicaid Services (CMS) website, and their Medicare Administrative Contracture (MAC) website to keep abreast of public policy trends.
9. Be a member of state and local OT associations.
10. Serve on OT legislative task forces and committees on a state or national level with associations.
11. Become involved in advocacy groups in other associations related to therapy practice with older adults, such as the AARP and the Alzheimer's Association.
12. Read a variety of opinions on public web-based sites and in OT literature to keep up on trends. Access social media sites that support therapy.
13. Write and submit articles to professional and consumer publications about OT practice and public policy.
14. Write letters or visit people involved with public policy such as legislators, insurance executives, third-party payers, and case managers.
15. Learn the legislative process in your state and testify for relevant issues at public hearings.
16. Attend an AOTA Hill Day.
17. If questions or concerns cannot be answered or addressed on a local level, network with the legislative division of AOTA.

■ CHAPTER REVIEW QUESTIONS

1 What are the three parts of the "Triple Aim" and, based on reading the chapter, how can you see the Triple Aim being played out in the health care marketplace?

2 Name and describe the four parts of Medicare and those directly related to OT practice.

3 How is Medicare billed under Part B?

4 What is a Medicare Administrative Contracture (MAC), and how can it help inform practice?

5 Describe the current PDPM system used in skilled nursing facilities and how it influences therapy practice.

6 What is Medicaid and typically which clients access it in the health care system?

7 Is OT a required or optional benefit for Medicaid and how do you find out the benefits in your state?

8 What is the homebound status for clients in a home health care setting under Medicare Part A, and what are allowable reasons for leaving the home?

9 What is the current assessment system used in home health care?

10 What is the current assessment system used in inpatient rehabilitation settings?

11 How can OTAs access the Older Americans Act (OAA) for their clients?

12 How can OTAs be advocates for the OT profession?

13 How can OTAs stay aware of public policy changes that influence practice? What are you personally going to do?

REFERENCES

1. Laverdure P, Smiley J, Stotz N, Varland J. Student value MVPs. *OT Pract.* 2020;25(6):20-23.

2. Patient Protection and Affordable Care Act of 2010. Pub. L. 111-148, 124 Stat. 119.

3. The Health Care and Education Reconciliation Act of 2010. Pub. L. 111-152, 124 Stat. 1029.

4. Burns LR, Pauly MV. Accountable care organizations may have difficulty avoiding the failures of integrated delivery networks of the 1990s. *Health Aff.* 2012;31:2407-2416. doi:10.1377/hlthaff.2011.0675.

5. Berwick DM, Nolan TW, Whittington J. The triple aim: care, health and cost. *Health Aff.* 2008;27(3):759-769. doi:10.1377/hlthaff.27.3.759.

6. Peirce S. *The History of Value-Based Care.* 2018. Available at: https://www.elationhealth.com/healthcare-innovation-policy-news-blog/history-value/.

7. Abrams MK, Nuzum R, Zezza MA, et al. *The Affordable Care Act's Payment and Delivery System Reform: A Progress Report at 5 Years.* 2015. Available at: https://www.commonwealthfund.org/publications/issue-briefs/2015/may/affordable-care-acts-payment-and-delivery-system-reforms.

8. Centers for Medicaid and Medicare Services. *What Are the Value-Based Programs?* 2020. Available at: https://www.cms.gov/Medicare/Quality-Initiatives-Patient-Assessment-Instruments/Value-Based-Programs/Value-Based-Programs.

9. Centers for Medicaid and Medicare Services. *Hospital Readmission Reduction Program.* 2021. Available at: https://www.cms.gov/Medicare/Quality-Initiatives-Patient-Assessment-Instruments/Value-Based-Programs/HRRP/Hospital-Readmission-Reduction-Program.

10. Rogers AT, Bai G, Lavin RA, Anderson GF. Higher hospital spending on occupational therapy is associated with lower readmission rates. *Med Care Res Rev.* 2016. doi:10.1177/1077558716666981.

11. Gershman P, Kane J, Smith T. *SNF PPS: Patient Driven Payment Model.* Presented at: MLN Call: A Medicare Learning Network ® (MLN) Event; 2018. Available at: https://www.cms.gov/Outreach-and-Education/Outreach/NPC/Downloads/2018-12-11-SNF-PPS-PDPM.pdf.

12. US Department of Health and Human Services, Centers for Medicare & Medicaid Services. *What Is Medicare?* Available at: https://www.medicare.gov/what-medicare-covers/your-medicare-coverage-choices/whats-medicare.

13. US Department of Health and Human Services, Centers for Medicare & Medicaid Services. *Medicare part A. In: Medicare Program: General Information.* 2021. Available at: https://www.cms.gov/Medicare/Medicare-General-Information/MedicareGenInfo.

14. US Department of Health and Human Services, Centers for Medicare & Medicaid Services. *Prospective Payment Systems: General Information.* 2021. Available at: http://www.cms.gov/ProspMedicareFeeSvcPmtGen/.

15. US Department of Health and Human Services, Centers for Medicare & Medicaid Services. *Skilled Nursing Facilities PPS.* 2022. Available at: https://www.cms.gov/Medicare/Medicare-Fee-for-Service-Payment/SNFPPS/index.

16. US Department of Health and Human Services, Centers for Medicare & Medicaid Services. Chapter 7: Home health services. In: Centers for Medicare & Medicaid Services. Medicare Benefit Policy Manual. 2020. Available at: http://www.cms.gov/manuals/Downloads/bp102c07.pdf.

17. US Department of Health and Human Services, Centers for Medicare & Medicaid Services. *Acute inpatient PPS.* 2022. Available at: https://www.cms.gov/Medicare/Medicare-Fee-for-Service-Payment/AcuteInpatientPPS/index.html?redirect=/acuteinpatientpps/.

18. Department of Health and Human Services, Centers for Medicare & Medicaid Services. *Medicare Part B. In Medicare Program: General Information.* 2021. Available at: https://www.cms.gov/medicare/medicare-general-information/medicaregeninfo?redirect=/medicaregeninfo/03_part%20b.asp#TopOfPage%20Part%20B.

19. American Occupational Therapy Association (AOTA). *New Occupational Therapy Evaluation Coding Overview.* 2017. Available at: https://www.aota.org/~/media/Corporate/Files/Advocacy/Federal/Evaluation-Codes-Overview-2016.pdf.

20. US Department of Health and Human Services, Centers for Medicare & Medicaid Services. *Healthcare Common Procedure Coding System Level II Coding Procedures.* 2021. Available at: https://www.cms.gov/Medicare/Coding/MedHCPCSGenInfo/Downloads/2018-11-30-HCPCS-Level2-Coding-Procedure.pdf.

21. US Department of Health and Human Services, Centers for Medicare & Medicaid Services. *Your Medicare Coverage: Physical Therapy/Occupational Therapy/Speech-Language Pathology Services.* 2021. Available at: https://www.cms.gov/Medicare/Billing/Therapy Services.

22. US Department of Health and Human Services, Centers for Medicare & Medicaid Services. Section 4: Medicare advantage plans & other options. In: Medicare & You 2022. 2022. Available at: https://www.medicare.gov/Pubs/pdf/10050-Medicare-and-You.pdf.

23. Improving Medicare Post-Acute Care Transformation Act of 2014. H. R. 4994. Available at: https://www.congress.gov/bill/113th-congress/house-bill/4994.

24. US Department of Health and Human Services, Centers for Medicare & Medicaid Services. Chapter 15: Covered medical and other health services. In: Centers for Medicare & Medicaid Services. Medicare Benefit Policy Manual. 2022. Available at: https://www.cms.gov/Regulations-and-Guidance/Guidance/Manuals/downloads/bp102c15.pdf.

25. US Department of Health and Human Services, Centers for Medicare & Medicaid Services. *Program Memorandum Intermediaries/ Carriers: Medical Review of Services for Patients with Dementia.* Transmittal AB-01-135. 2001. Available at: https://www.cms.gov/ Regulations-and-Guidance/Guidance/Transmittals/downloads/ AB01135.pdf.

26. US Department of Health and Human Services, Centers for Medicare & Medicaid Services. *Jimmo v. Sebelius Settlement Agreement Fact Sheet.* 2013. Available at: https://www.cms.gov/Medicare/ Medicare-Fee-for-Service-Payment/SNFPPS/Downloads/Jimmo-FactSheet.pdf.

27. AOTA. *Choosing wisely: What is the Choosing Wisely initiative?* 2022. Available at: https://www.aota.org/practice/practice-essentials/evidencebased-practiceknowledge-translation/aotas-top-10-choosing-wisely-recommendations.

28. AOTA. *Five Things Patients and Providers Should Question.* 2021. Available at: https://www.choosingwisely.org/societies/american-occupational-therapy-association-inc/.

29. CMS. *What Is a MAC?* 2022. Available at: https://www.cms.gov/ Medicare/Medicare-Contracting/Medicare-Administrative-Contractors/What-is-a-MAC.

30. Medicare.gov. *Local Coverage Determination (LCD) Challenge.* n.d. Available at: https://www.medicare.gov/claims-appeals/local-coverage-determinations-lcd-challenge.

31. AOTA. *2019 Workforce and Salary Survey.* 2019. Available at: https://library.aota.org/AOTA-Workforce-Salary-Survey-2019/.

32. Omnibus Budget Reconciliation Act of 1987. Pub. L. No. 100-20, 101 Stat. 1330.

33. Continuity of Care Task Group. *MDS Long-Term Care.* n.d. Available at: http://continuityofcaretaskgroup.pbworks.com/w/ page/16430224/MDS%20Long%20Term%20Care.

34. US Department of Health and Human Services, Centers for Medicare & Medicaid Services. MDS 3.0 for nursing homes and swing bed providers. In: Nursing Home Quality Initiatives. 2022. Available at: http://www.cms.gov/NursingHomeQualityInits/25_NHQ-IMDS30.asp.

35. CMS. Medicare Learning Network ® Event. *SNF PPS: Patient Driven Payment Model.* Available at: https://www.cms.gov/Medicare/Medicare-Fee-for-Service-Payment/SNFPPS/Downloads/ MLN_CalL_PDPM_Presentation_508.pdf.

36. US Department of Health and Human Services, Center for Medicare and Medicaid Services. *Proposed Fiscal Year 2020 Payment and Policy Changes for Medicare Skilled Nursing Facilities.* 2019. Available at: https://www.cms.gov/newsroom/fact-sheets/proposed-fiscal-year-2020-payment-and-policy-changes-medicare-skilled-nursing-facilities-cms-1718-p.

37. Balanced Budget Act of 1997. Pub. L. 105-133, 111 Stat. 329.

38. Omnibus Consolidated and Emergency Supplemental Appropriations Act of 1999.

39. US Department of Health and Human Services, Centers for Medicare & Medicaid Services. *Medicare and Home Health Care.* 2020. Available at: https://www.medicare.gov/Pubs/pdf/10969-medicare-and-home-health-care.pdf.

40. AOTA. *Home Health Flexibility Act Enables Occupational Therapists to Open Medicare Home Health Cases.* 2021. Available at: https://www. aota.org/about/for-the-media/press-release-home-health-flexibility-act-enables-occupational-therapists-to-open-medicare-home-health-cases.

41. Bipartisan Budget Act of 2018, Pub. L. 115-123; 132 Stat. 64; February 9, 2018; H.R. 1892 (115th Congress). Available at: https:// www.congress.gov/bill/115th-congress/house-bill/1892/text.

42. US Department of Health and Human Services, Center for Medicare and Medicaid Services. *Home Health PPS.* 2021. Available at: https://www.cms.gov/Medicare/Medicare-Fee-for-Service-Payment/HomeHealthPPS/index.

43. Centers for Medicare and Medicaid Services. *Inpatient Rehabilitation Facility Prospective Payment System.* 2022. Available at: https:// www.cms.gov/Outreach-and-Education/Medicare-Learning-Network-MLN/MLNProducts/medicare-payment-systems. html#Inpatient2.

44. Strunk E. *Section GG Changes: What Do They Mean for Your Organization.* 2019. Available at: https://www.medbridgeeducation.com/ blog/2019/01/section-gg-changes-what-do-they-mean-for-your-organization/.

45. Department of Health and Human Services, Center for Medicare & Medicaid Services Physician Fee Schedule. *CY 2022 Physician Fee Schedule Final Rule.* 2022. Available at: https://www.cms.gov/ Medicare/Medicare-Fee-for-Service-Payment/PhysicianFeeSched.

46. Medicaid.gov. *National Medicaid and CHIP Program Information.* n.d. Available at: https://www.medicaid.gov/medicaid/national-medicaid-chip-program-information/index.html.

47. Paradise J. *Medicaid Moving Forward.* 2015. Available at: http://kff. org/health-reform/issue-brief/medicaid-moving-forward/.

48. Ryan J, Edwards B. Rebalancing Medicaid long-term services and supports. *Health Aff.* 2015. Available at: https://www.healthaffairs. org/do/10.1377/hpb20150917.439553/full/.

49. Medicaid.gov. *Long-Term Services & Supports.* 2016. Available at: https://www.medicaid.gov/medicaid/long-term-services-supports/ index.html.

50. The Older Americans Act of 1965. Pub. L. 89-73, 79 Stat. 218.

51. Marfeo E. The supporting older Americans Act of 2020: how policy connects with occupational therapy principles and practice. *Am J Occup Ther.* 2020;74(5):7405090010p1-7405090010p6. doi:10.5014/ajot.2020.745002.

52. AARP. *Older Americans Act Reauthorized for 5 Years.* 2020. Available at: https://www.aarp.org/politics-society/government-elections/ info-2020/oaa-reauthorization/.

53. Health Resources Services Administration. *Understanding Telehealth: What Is Telehealth?* 2021. Available at: https://telehealth.hhs. gov/patients/understanding-telehealth/?gclid=Cj0KCQiA88X_ BRDUARIsACVMYD9nCTFBhZ0-3UhdEcmJhckwqdn-zh04Az1iJfI9OskNzLmuNL_xIv90aAh7KEALw_wcB#what-is-telehealth.

54. American Occupational Therapy Association State Affairs Group. *Occupational Therapy and Telehealth: State Statutes, Regulations, and Regulatory Board Statements.* 2020. Available at: https://www.aota. org/-/media/Corporate/Files/Advocacy/State/telehealth/Telehealth-State-Statutes-Regulations-Regulatory-Board-Statements. pdf.

55. AOTA. *Medicare Telehealth Success.* 2020. Available at: https://www. aota.org/advocacy/issues/telehealth-advocacy/medicare-telehealth-success.

56. AOTA. *About AOTA.* 2021. Available at: https://www.aota.org/ about/mission-vision.

57. AOTA. *Occupational Therapy Code of Ethics.* 2020. Available at: http://www.ncbot.org/Downloads/practice%20act%20and%20 rules/code-of-ethics.pdf.

58. Sieck R, Lohman H, Stupica K, Minthorne-Brown L, Stoffer K. Awareness of Medicare regulation changes: occupational therapists' perceptions and implications for practice. *Phys Occup Ther Geriatr.* 2017;35(2):67-80. doi:10.1080/02703181.2017.1288672.

59. Charatan F. *Medicare Will Now Cover Some Treatments for Alzheimer' Disease.* Available at: https://www.bmj.com/content/324/7342/872.3.

60. US Department of Health and Human Services, Centers for Medicare & Medicaid Services. *Transmittals.* 2021. Available at: http:// www.cms.gov/Transmittals/.

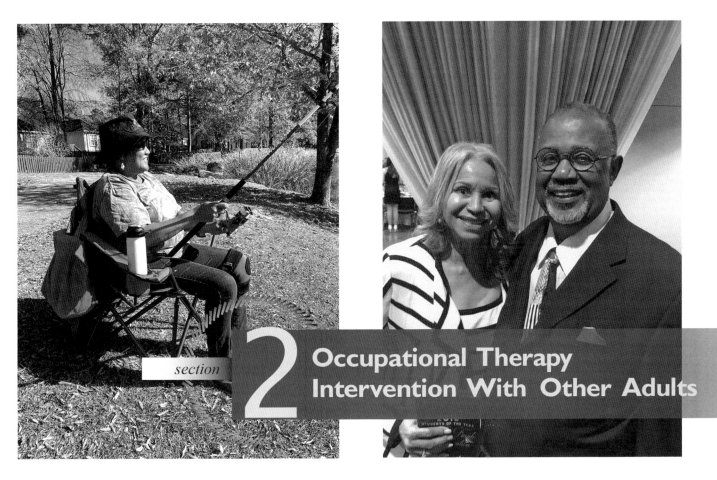

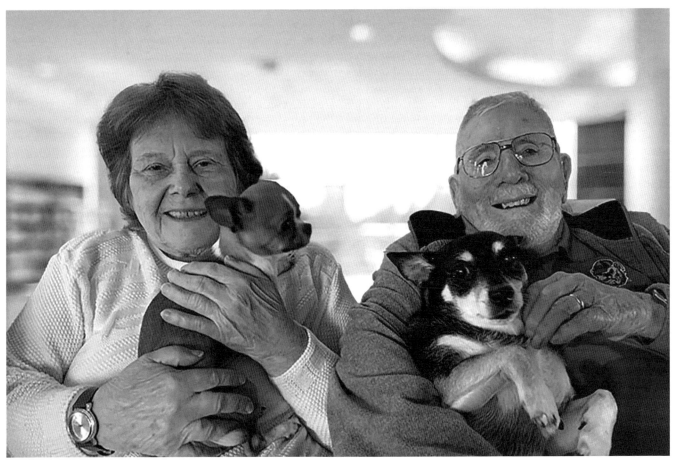

chapter 7

Occupational Therapy Models of Practice

ANGELA PATTERSON AND RENÉ PADILLA

KEY TERMS

assessment, cognition, context, clinical models of practice, culture, dysfunction, environment, function, habits, intervention, maturation, motor action, occupation, performance, play and leisure, roles, self-care, skills, subsystem, task, values, work

CHAPTER OBJECTIVES

1. Explain the importance and use of models of practice in occupational therapy intervention with older adults.
2. Briefly summarize the *Occupational Therapy Practice Framework: Domain and Process (4th ed.)* and four occupational therapy models of practice as they relate to aging, including the Facilitating Growth and Development Model,

the Cognitive Disabilities Model, and the Model of Human Occupation.
3. Demonstrate the ways occupational therapy assistants can incorporate theoretical principles into practice with older adults.

Amit was admitted to the rehabilitation center with a severe infection in the left knee. His status is 3 months post left knee replacement. Amit recently retired and is looking forward to leisure engagement. As an executive for a large firm, he and his family have lived in 10 different countries around the world. Now that all of his children have graduated from college, he was planning a peaceful life in a small town by the ocean where he and his wife could play golf every day, attend cultural events in a nearby city, and occasionally go deep-sea fishing. A few days after he was admitted to the rehabilitation center, he received news that his wife had fallen and fractured a hip. While preparing her for surgery at a different hospital, the doctors had discovered that she had a very aggressive cancer that had metastasized throughout her body. There was no hope for recovery, and she was discharged home under the care of her daughter and a hospice service. Amit spoke to his wife on the telephone twice a day, and often was tearful during his conversations with her. The purpose of Amit's inpatient rehabilitation was to become independent in his self-care and in his functional mobility with nonweight-bearing status on his left leg. The weight-bearing restrictions were expected to be necessary for at least 6 weeks while his infection cleared and he was able to have the hardware in his knee replaced again.

Elizabeth is a small, frail woman in her late 60s who has been living in a long-term care facility for more than a year. When she was in her late 20s, a train hit her automobile and she sustained a traumatic brain injury that resulted in her inability to speak and left hemiplegia. She had regained the ability to do her activities of daily living (ADLs) and to walk without assistance, although over the years she had suffered many falls because of poor balance. For more than 40 years she had lived with her sister. When her sister died, Elizabeth attempted to live on her own for some time but became ill with pneumonia. Her relatives insisted she live at a long-term care facility because they were not able to care for her. Because of another bout with pneumonia, Elizabeth is very weak and is unable to bathe and dress herself without assistance. She is also not able to walk.

Emilia was recently referred to an adult day center in the downtown area of a large city. Her Alzheimer's disease has progressed to the point where she needs 24-hour supervision. Emilia's husband has been working at a local bookstore to make some money to supplement his retirement income. Emilia and her husband were prisoners in a Nazi concentration camp in their youth, and in the past month Emilia has seemed to be reliving that experience, often becoming quite agitated and isolated while at the center.

Alejandro immigrated to the United States from Cuba nearly 40 years ago. Although he is in his early 70s, he continued to work running a family-owned restaurant until 5 days ago when he had a stroke. Because of his stroke, Alejandro seems unable to understand and speak in English and continually repeats the same two lines of a Spanish song whenever he does speak. He also is unable to hold himself in midline and does not seem aware of one side of his body. Nearly every day his room in the acute care hospital has been full of relatives and friends, many of whom bring food. Alejandro has a fever, and the doctors suspect he is having difficulty swallowing.

Amit, Elizabeth, Emilia, and Alejandro represent the diversity of people who seek occupational therapy intervention because they are not able to carry out the activities that are important to them in their daily lives. The occupational therapy assistant (OTA) needs tools to address all of these unique needs according to basic occupational therapy philosophy and theoretical principles. The occupational therapy programs for these individuals must consider the physical and cognitive limitations that affect their ability to care for themselves and must also consider the whole history of these individuals and the adjustments they may need because of dramatic changes in their environments. Amit's wife is dying, he is in inpatient rehabilitation, and his children no longer live at home. Elizabeth has been moved against her will from her familiar home to a long-term care facility where she knows no one. Emilia's mind has gradually replaced her physical surroundings for dreadful ones that reside in her memory, and Alejandro has gone from spending nearly all his waking hours at his business to a hospital room. Although the occupational therapy programs in their new environments must maintain a common thread that identifies them as "occupational therapy," they also should be flexible enough to provide individual meaningful activities for each client. Occupational therapy clinical models of practice are intended to connect professional philosophy and theory with daily practice.

OVERVIEW OF MODELS OF PRACTICE

This chapter provides an overview of multiple conceptual models in which occupation is described as the principal feature of any occupational therapy intervention. First, the *Occupational Therapy Practice Framework: Domain and Process (4th ed.) (OTPF-4)*[1] is reviewed, which articulates the general domain and process of intervention of the occupational therapy profession and gives the broadest look at how we might go about understanding Amit's life and current needs. Second, an overview of Llorens's[2] Facilitating Growth and Development Model is provided, which, although published over 4 decades ago, is still the only conceptual model that emphasizes a developmental perspective in the practice of occupational therapy with adult clients. This model can help us understand how to consider Elizabeth's stage in life. Third, the Cognitive

Disabilities Model (CDM)[3-5] is described, which helps us understand how cognitive process affects the performance of occupation and will be particularly useful in working with older adults such as Emilia, although it certainly also has applications for Amit, Elizabeth, and Alejandro. The Model of Human Occupation (MOHO)[6] is discussed as a model that makes an effort to assist practitioners to consider clients holistically. This model will help us understand older adults like Alejandro as people with dynamic abilities and needs who actively interact with their environments. Finally, to understand how a model of practice can apply to all four cases, the Kawa model is described. The Kawa model focuses on the cultural perspective of the client's occupational experiences with the environment and social groups as a collective through the use of a river metaphor.[7-9]

The common link in all forms of occupational therapy intervention is occupation. The philosophical base of occupational therapy practice includes the participation in meaningful occupations. Meaningful occupations influence healthy development and well-being supporting people's participation in life situations. Creating interventions focused on occupations individualized to the person's environment and context, promotes health, prevention, and adaptation.[10] Thus, the human is able to adapt to life's demands and become self-actualized. Dysfunction occurs when the human being's ability to adapt is impaired in some way. Occupational therapy intervention seeks to prevent and remediate dysfunction and facilitate maximal adaptation through the use of meaningful and purposeful activities to achieve their desired occupations.

Historically, the term *occupation* was described as the individual's active participation in self-care, work, and leisure,[11] which constitute the familiar activities people do in everyday context.[10] The person must use combinations of sensorimotor, cognitive, psychological, and psychosocial skills to perform these occupations.[12] Specific environments and different stages of life influence these occupations. Kielhofner[6] defined occupation as "the doing of work, play, or ADLs within a temporal, physical, and sociocultural context that characterizes much of human life." Today, the *OTPF-4* defines occupation as "everyday personalized activities that people do as individuals, in families, and with communities to occupy time and bring meaning and purpose to life."[1] Although the definition of occupational therapy has developed over the decades, occupational therapy fundamentally is focused on participation that brings meaning and achieves the goals not only of the individual, but also of the person, group, or population.

To understand the concepts of occupations and use them to facilitate function and adaptation, OTAs must have broad knowledge of the biological, social, and medical sciences in addition to occupational therapy theoretical premises. Occupational therapy models of practice provide organized frameworks for that knowledge, which allow the therapist to apply pertinent information to a specific client's problem. Thus, models of practice guide the therapist in creating individual intervention programs that are culturally meaningful and age-related and that facilitate development of sensorimotor, cognitive, psychological, and psychosocial skills. By using a practice model for guidance, the OTAs assisting the patients discussed earlier can ensure professional intervention programs that are tailored to meet the needs of each client.

Theorists have articulated many models of practice or approaches. Those presented here are certainly not the only ones that can provide guidance for occupational therapy intervention with older adults. For example, the Kinesiological Model,[13,14] also referred to as the *Biomechanical Approach*, provides insight into how older adults move based on mechanical principles of range of motion, muscle strength, and physical endurance. Concepts of this approach help us restore movement to an older adult after a stroke or apply hip precautions during participation in occupation after a hip replacement. Another example is the Sensory Integration Model,[15,16] which addresses dysfunctions that make it difficult for the brain to modulate sensory stimulation. Intervention guided by this model provides strategic sensory stimulation designed to organize the central nervous system and promote adaptive responses according to the person's neurological needs.

Occupational therapy models of practice do not offer concrete plans for improvement of function. Instead, these models suggest the use of various graded occupations that demand the development of performance abilities, thereby improving function. OTAs may use the information in the models of practice to formulate questions to assess the client's needs, interests, and meanings; select assessment tools; and accordingly design a unique intervention strategy. OTAs should be familiar with several models of practice because each model usually has a specific focus and does not address all dimensions of occupational functioning.

Occupational Therapy Practice Framework

The OTPF-4[1] represents the latest effort of the American Occupational Therapy Association (AOTA) to articulate language with which to describe the profession's focus. As such, the *OTPF-4* is intended to help occupational therapy practitioners analyze their current practice and consider new applications in emerging areas. In addition, the *OTPF-4* was developed to help the external stakeholders (interprofessional healthcare team, payers, educators, consumers, and others) understand the profession's emphasis on function and participation in social life.

The domain and process of a profession refers to the areas of human experience in which practitioners of the profession help others (Fig. 7.1). According to the *OTPF-4*, the focus of the occupational therapy profession is "the therapeutic use of everyday life occupations with persons, groups, or populations (i.e., the client) for the purpose of enhancing or enabling participation."[1] For occupational therapy, the breadth of meaningful everyday life activities

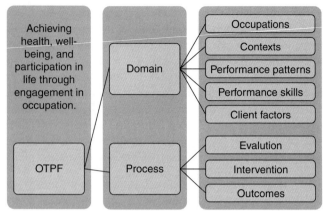

FIG. 7.1 The Occupational Therapy Practice Framework. *(Adapted from American Occupational Therapy Association. Occupational therapy practice framework: Domain and process. 4th ed. Am J Occup Ther. 2020;74:1-87; https://doi.org/10.5014/ajot.2020.74S2001.)*

is captured in the notion of "occupation." Occupational therapy practitioners help people actively engage in occupations that affect their health, well-being, and participation. These occupations and activities permit desired or needed participation in home, school, workplace, and community life. Notably, personal meaning and assigned value are emphasized as the central characteristics of occupation. These will vary among clients based on the "clients' needs, interests, and contexts."[1]

Engagement in occupation is interrelated to the aspects of the occupational therapy domain (Table 7.1). The *OTPF-4* describes engagement in individual occupations but also occupations that involve at least two individuals called co-occupations. Co-occupations happen in parallel or are shared typically requiring social interaction. Thus, the many types of occupations in which the client might engage should be addressed in occupational therapy intervention.

The *OTPF-4* has organized the many occupations in which a person, group, or population may engage into broad categories (Table 7.2). Engagement in these occupations depends on what "people need to do, want to do and are expected to do."[17] A client's intrinsic factors that influence occupational performance which the *OTPF-4* identifies as *client factors* are body structures and functions as well as values, beliefs, and spirituality. For example, to tie one's shoes (a dressing activity within the ADL area of occupation) one must, among many things, possess sufficient body functions supported by body structures and performance skills to maintain an erect posture while bending and reaching one's foot, and then one must manipulate the laces and pull on them with sufficient force to tighten them but not enough to break them (all examples of motor skills). This sequence of actions is carried out by using one's ability to plan and sequence events (examples of process skills).[1]

TABLE 7.1

Aspects of the Occupational Therapy Domain

Occupations	Contexts	Performance patterns	Performance skills	Client factors
Activities of daily living (ADLs) Instrumental activities of daily living (IADLs) Health management Rest and sleep Education Work Play Leisure Social participation	Environmental factors Personal factors	Habits Routines Roles Rituals	Motor skills Process skills Social interaction skills	Values, beliefs, and spirituality Body functions Body structures

Adapted from American Occupational Therapy Association. Occupational therapy practice framework: Domain and process. 4th ed. Am J Occup Ther. 2020;74:1-87; https://doi.org/10.5014/ajot.2020.74S2001.

TABLE 7.2

Occupations

Occupations	Types of occupations	Occupations	Types of occupations
Activities of daily living (ADLs)	Bathing, showering Toileting and toilet hygiene Dressing Eating and swallowing Feeding Functional mobility Personal hygiene and grooming Sexual activity	Rest and sleep	Rest Sleep preparation Sleep participation
Instrumental activities of daily living (IADLs)	Care of others Care of pets and animals Child rearing Communication management Driving and community mobility Financial management Home establishment and management Meal preparation and cleanup Religious and spiritual expression Safety and emergency maintenance Shopping	Education	Formal educational participation Informal personal educational needs or interests exploration (beyond formal education) Informal education participation
		Work	Employment interests and pursuits Employment seeking and acquisition Job performance and maintenance Retirement preparation and adjustment Volunteer exploration Volunteer participation
Health management	Social and emotional promotion and maintenance Symptom and condition management Communication with healthcare system Medication management Physical activity Nutrition management Personal care device management	Play	Play exploration Play participation
		Leisure	Leisure exploration Leisure participation
		Social participation	Community participation Family participation Friendships Intimate partner relationships Peer group participation

Adapted from American Occupational Therapy Association. Occupational therapy practice framework: Domain and process. 4th ed. Am J Occup Ther. 2020;74:1-87; https://doi.org/10.5014/ajot.2020.74S2001.

A fascinating feature of human occupation is that many combinations of performance skills are integrated and choreographed into automatic or semiautomatic performance patterns that enable one to function on a daily basis without demanding undue attention. After one has tied his or her shoelaces with sufficient frequency, he or she can often do it without thinking or looking at the laces because it has become a habit. Broader habits can be said to become organized into routines (e.g., one might dress in a certain way and take a particular route to get to work), and frequently routines correspond to the variety of roles in which one functions (e.g., because one is the supervisor of an office, one might routinely meet with employees each morning at a certain time). One's routine may be briefly interrupted when they take a day off of work to attend a religious service. A ritual that has an assigned "spiritual, cultural, or social meaning."[1] The *OTPF-4* notes that "occupational therapy practitioners who consider clients' past and present behavioral and performance patterns are better able to understand the frequency and manner in which performance skills and healthy and unhealthy occupations are, or have been, integrated into clients' lives."[1]

As stated earlier, the *OTPF-4* emphasizes the importance of considering the contexts (environmental and personal) in which a person engages in occupation. *Environmental factors* are the external physical and social surroundings in which the client's daily life occupations take place. *Personal factors* refer to the "internal influences affecting functioning and disability and are not considered positive or negative but rather reflect the essence of the person—"who they are."[1] Personal factors do not refer to a client's health condition or health state. Examples of personal factors are: cultural identification and cultural attitudes, age, gender, social background, sexual orientations, education, etc.[1] Older adults can have personal factors in common, as well as be very different. Best friends may be the same age, gender, education, and socioeconomic status but may differ in ethnicity, life experiences, and character traits.

A client's engagement in occupation and their performance may be determined by the occupational therapy practitioner's basic skill of activity selection. A person may not be able to meet the demands inherent in an activity (e.g., without a fair amount of conditioning, an older adult might not be able to climb up a mountain), or the person may find the demands too low (e.g., a champion chess player may find it quite boring to play Tic-Tac-Toe). Activity demands include such things as the objects used in the activity and the characteristics of these objects, space and social demands, required actions, and required body functions and structures. A well-matched activity improves a client's performance skills and performance patterns. For example, the activity of playing golf requires balls and golf irons; takes place on a golf course; is often played with others and therefore requires taking turns; involves a sequence of tasks from placing the ball, hitting

it, and then locating it in the distance; and requires the bodily functions of joint mobility and muscle power to swing the iron while not letting the iron fly away and harming someone standing nearby. Furthermore, playing golf involves the person's cardiovascular system while walking, vestibular functions while turning one's trunk and following through with the swing, and a variety of other body structures and functions. Interestingly, engagement in occupation is not only affected by these functions and structures, but also it may affect them in turn; for example, an older adult's cardiovascular and neuromuscular functions become conditioned while gradually increasing the time spent walking in a golf course. Identifying the demands of an activity and strategically utilizing them to facilitate participation is one of the primary skills of occupational therapy practitioners.[1]

The *OTPF-4* describes the occupational therapy process as consisting of three dynamic and interactive phases: evaluation, intervention, and outcomes.[1] Evaluation consists of four steps: (1) consultation and screening, (2) occupational profile, (3) analysis of occupational performance, and (4) synthesis of evaluation process. An initial consultation and screening determines if the client would benefit for occupational therapy services. The occupational profile is focused on a client interview to determine the client's history, experiences, daily living patterns, values, needs, beliefs, and so on. The profile consists, essentially, of understanding why the person is seeking services and what the person finds important and meaningful and, therefore, of high priority. Although obtaining contextual information is important throughout the whole occupational therapy process, it is particularly essential at the evaluation stage because it will provide the foundation for specific evaluations of occupational performance and certainly for the selection of intervention strategies later in the occupational therapy process.[1]

The analysis of occupational performance includes assessments to guide the identification of a client's strengths and weaknesses to determine occupational therapy intervention that addresses specific occupations. Following the analysis of occupational performance, the occupational therapy practitioner synthesizes the occupational profile and assessments to determine meaningful occupations attainable within the client's context supporting occupational engagement and activities for intervention. Selected goals for interventions will measure progress toward desired outcomes. Although it is the responsibility of the occupational therapist (OT) to initiate the evaluation process, both OTs and OTAs may contribute to the evaluation, following which the OT completes the analysis and synthesis of information for the development of the intervention plan.[1]

The intervention phase is centered around what the client finds most meaningful in life and of greatest priority. An intervention plan includes selecting the intervention approach, service delivery method, discharge plans, and referrals as appropriate. The occupational therapy practitioner implements the intervention plan and monitors the client's response. It is necessary to continually review intervention to progress toward desired outcomes. An ongoing collaboration among the OT, OTA, and client is indispensable to ensure that goals, intervention strategies, and progress are continually evaluated and adapted to meet the client's priorities.

An example of the first two phases of the occupational therapy process is if an older adult who has had a mild stroke states that he has assembled and collected fishing flies during his whole life, a detailed assessment of fine motor skills may be indicated to ascertain whether he has the necessary motor skills to manipulate the small pieces used in this meaningful occupation. Likewise, an analysis of any other areas of occupational performance that may negatively influence the person's engagement in meaningful occupation should be performed. Notably, barriers to participation in occupation may not necessarily reside in the client but may be located in the client's context. For example, although an older adult may like to tie fishing flies, his family may not make the materials available to him because they cannot imagine him going fishing any time soon. In this case, they may not understand the meaningfulness of the occupation of fly tying and therefore create a barrier for his participation in the occupation.

According to the *OTPF-4*, OTs and OTAs are catalysts in "achieving health, well-being and participation in life through engagement in occupation."[1] Phase 3 of the occupational therapy process outlines the responsibility of occupational therapy practitioners to ensure that their interventions lead to an actual outcome of participation in occupations and not simply to improve skills. Outcome measures are set early in the occupational therapy process and are continuously monitored.[1] In the example of the older adult who found tying fishing flies meaningful, it is not sufficient to help him develop the motor skills necessary to maintain this interest. The ultimate goal of occupational therapy is for the older adult to actually engage in fly tying in the most natural context possible. Thus instructing the older adult to exercise his fingers with elastic bands may contribute to his skills but cannot be the limit of occupational therapy intervention. Likewise, using fly fishing to develop dexterity can be considered insufficient intervention if the older adult never has the opportunity to use the product of his hands in a meaningful way. Outcome assessment information should be used to plan future interventions with the client and, ultimately, to review the effectiveness of the service program.

Amit: The OTPF-4 in Use

The *OTPF-4* can help us understand Amit's life situation and plan an intervention that best supports his participation in all areas of life. According to the *OTPF-4*, the evaluation phase should involve obtaining an occupational profile. By asking Amit about his current concerns related to engaging in occupations and daily life activities, as well as about his work history, life experiences, family traditions, and other personal facts, the occupational therapy practitioner discovers he has relied heavily on his wife to help with the family's transition while traveling from country to country. Amit now has a great sense of debt toward her and some guilt for having spent so much time working away from home. The physician has recommended that Amit not put any weight on his left leg for 6 weeks. Amit's main concern is that, because of his left knee infection, he will not be able to be of any assistance to his wife in her last weeks of life.

Understanding Amit's main concern will help us establish a collaborative relationship with him while we evaluate his performance skills and context. If, for example, we had proceeded to evaluate his ability to dress and bathe himself and assessed his endurance and joint range of motion without knowing about his concerns, we might have further reinforced his sense of uselessness and limited potential for social participation. Instead, we can now identify which activities he believes would be the most important for him to be able to do to convey caring for his wife. For Amit, these include being able to help her move in bed, get in and out of a bed and a chair, run errands for her and, if necessary, help her eat. Thus, we can proceed by evaluating his endurance, balance, and strength, all needed to help his wife move in bed or get in and out of a chair. We can help adapt the environment and teach him body mechanics to have the maximum leverage while moving his wife. We can further evaluate his ability to complete ADLs because he will need to be dressed to run errands outside of the home.

Naturally, there are many other areas for assessment and intervention with Amit. However, the previous illustrates how the central concern for him is related to an area of occupation rather than to a body structure. Occupational therapy intervention can still be organized to address many client factors, but the intervention is not likely to seem meaningful unless Amit is able to understand that it contributes to his primary concern.

Facilitating Growth and Development Model

The Facilitating Growth and Development Model views the occupational therapy practitioner's role as one "concerned with facilitating or promoting optimal growth and development in all ages of man."[2] An individual's growth and development may be threatened by disease, injury, disability, or trauma. The occupational therapy practitioner may be required to assist the individual in coping with illness, trauma, or disability, or to help with rehabilitation. The occupational therapy practitioner also may seek to prevent maladaptation and promote health maintenance.

The occupational therapy practitioner must understand the developmental tasks and adaptive skills usually mastered at different ages when utilizing the Facilitating Growth and Development Model. The model describes the belief that the human being "develops simultaneously in the areas of neurophysiological, physical, psychosocial and psychody-namic growth, and in the development of social language, daily living, sociocultural, and intellectual skills during the life span."[2] The way the individual integrates and organizes these areas of development to perform in work, education, play, self-care, and leisure activities during each stage of life is of primary concern to occupational therapy. In addition to understanding the individual's development, the occupational therapy practitioner must understand the ways illness, disease, trauma, and disability may threaten that development. Finally, OT addresses the environmental variables necessary to support the development and maintenance of the important adaptive skills cited by Llorens.[2]

The Facilitating Growth and Development Model synthesizes the work of numerous authors who have contributed to the understanding of human maturation.[2] The model includes descriptions of the adaptive skills mentioned during each life stage, including infancy to age 2 years, ages 2–3 years, ages 3–6 years, ages 6–11 years, adolescence, young adulthood, adulthood, and maturity. Each stage is built on the foundation of the stages that the person has completed (Table 7.3). This text, however, focuses on the last stage.

During the occupational therapy process, the OT and OTA team assess the client's development and determine potential disruptions in each performance skill area. The team analyzes this information to determine the effects on age-appropriate occupational performance in the areas of work, education, self-care, and play and leisure. The OT and OTA team may then devise intervention strategies that facilitate development of a specific skill needed for successful occupational performance (Table 7.4). Matching the client's needs with the right therapeutic activities requires careful analysis of inherent requirements of each activity.

Depending on the client's needs, selected activities may include sensory, developmental, symbolic, and daily life tasks. These activities are combined with the social interaction that is most beneficial for the client. Sensory activities are those that primarily influence the senses through human action, such as touching, rocking, running, and listening to sounds. Developmental activities involve the use of objects such as crafts and puzzles in play, learning, and skill development situations. The client develops specific performance skills by engaging in these types of activities. Symbolic activities are designed to help the client

TABLE 7.3

Characteristics of Maturity	
Neurophysiological and physical development	Possible alterations in sensory functions (visual, auditory, tactile, kinesthetic, gustatory, and olfactory), motor behavior (coordination of extremities), information processing (higher-level integration, including conceptualization and memory), and physical endurance
Psychosocial—ego integrity and maturity	Acceptance of life experiences and the life cycle
Psychodynamic	Coping with continued growth after middle age, decision making regarding growth or death (giving up on life), dealing with insincerity of friends and acquaintances, inner life trends toward survival, possible decrease in efforts to maintain false pride, often a reduction in defenses, more suspiciousness, and necessity of dealing with psychological deterioration
Sociocultural	Group affiliation: family, social, interest, civic
Social language development	Predominantly verbal use, some use of nonverbal behavior to communicate
Activities of daily living and developmental tasks	Adjustment to decreasing physical strength and health, adjustment to retirement and reduced income, adjustment to death of spouse, adjustment to one's own impending death, establishment of affiliations with own age group, and meeting of social obligations
Ego-adaptive skills	Ability to function independently; ability to control drives and select appropriate objects; ability to organize stimuli, plan, and execute purposeful motion; ability to obtain, organize, and use knowledge; ability to participate in primary group; ability to participate in a variety of relationships; ability to experience self as a holistic, acceptable object; ability to participate in mutually satisfying relationships oriented to sexual needs
Intellectual development	Possible neurophysiological and physical development alteration and return of egocentrism

Adapted from Llorens LA. *Application of a Developmental Theory for Health and Rehabilitation.* Rockville, MD: American Occupational Therapy Association; 1976.

TABLE 7.4

	Activity Analysis
Sensory aspects	How much touch and movement does the activity require?
	To what extent are visual perception skills used in the activity?
	Does the activity require auditory perception and discrimination?
	Are perception and discrimination of smells and taste involved in the activity?
Physical aspects	How much does the activity require bilateral movements of arms and legs?
	Does the activity require the use of both hands at the same time?
	Can the activity be completed with one hand?
	How much muscle strength and joint range of motion does the activity require?
	How much sitting, standing, and variability in position is necessary to complete the activity?
	Does the physical performance require much thought organization?
	Which fine and gross motor movements does the activity require?
	How much eye–hand coordination is needed for the activity?
	How much time, and what equipment is needed for the activity?
Psychodynamic aspects	Does the activity permit expression of feelings, thoughts, original ideas, and creativity?
	Is there opportunity for the constructive expression of hostility, aggression, expansiveness, organization, control, narcissism, expiation of guilt, dependence, and independence?
	How does the activity permit or require sex role identification?
Social aspects	How much contact and guidance from others are required to complete the activity?
	How much does the activity require the person to work alone or with others?
	How much socialization does the activity permit?
Attention and skill aspects	How much initiative and self-reliance does the activity require?
	Does the activity require technical skills?
	Are manipulative and creative abilities needed?
	Does the activity require persistence to complete?
	How much repeated motion is needed?
Practical aspects	How much noise and dirt are created during the activity?
	What materials and equipment are used, and what are their costs?
	Can waste or scrap material be used?

Data from Llorens LA. *Application of a Developmental Theory for Health and Rehabilitation.* Rockville, MD: American Occupational Therapy Association; 1976.

satisfy needs and elicit and cope with emotional responses. Examples include gouging wood and kneading clay, which may release muscle tension and help process anger. Another example of a symbolic activity is leading a group in a task, which may satisfy the client's need to be heard and feel competent. The emotional response from leading a group may be improved self-esteem. Daily life tasks, also called ADLs, include tasks such as brushing teeth, getting dressed, cooking, and cleaning. Finally, social interaction includes participation in dyads with the therapist or another person and groups. These activities encourage the development of sociocultural competence and language and intellectual skills.

According to the Facilitating Growth and Development Model, occupational therapy intervention should continue until the client reaches sufficient competence in performing the skills and activities described as developmentally appropriate. The OT and OTA team continually monitor and reevaluate the client's progress in improving, maintaining, or restoring areas of occupational performance and therefore clearly know when the client no longer requires specialized occupational therapy services.

Elizabeth: The Model in Use

Llorens's Developmental Model[2] can help give us a more complete picture of Elizabeth's life and occupational needs. She has lived for more than half her life with the disability that resulted from her traumatic brain injury. However, she has been relatively healthy and independent. She now is facing the neurophysiological and physical alterations that are normal with maturity but they seem to compound the occupational performance challenges brought by her disability. Her bouts with pneumonia have left her debilitated, and she has been moved to a long-term care facility.

According to Llorens's Developmental Model,[2] a life priority for Elizabeth is to accept life experiences and the life cycle, not to distinguish which of her problems are caused by her age and which by her traumatic brain injury. Of great importance will be for her to continue developing coping skills to deal with both her limitations in function and the changes in her environment now that she no longer lives with her sister. She has the opportunity to participate in a variety of relationships with fellow patients and staff. In addition, of great importance will be to stimulate her continued intellectual development. Although her ability to bathe and dress herself independently is important, that need should not overshadow the other needs she has as a developing human being.

Cognitive Disabilities Model

As its name indicates, the Allen's CDM is concerned with occupational therapy services that are designed for clients with cognitive impairments.[5] These impairments may be the result of psychiatric illness, medical diseases, brain traumas, or developmental disorders. Psychiatric illnesses such as depression and schizophrenia have associated cognitive impairments. Alzheimer's dementia and cerebrovascular accidents are examples of medical conditions that result in cognitive impairments, and traumatic head injuries are an example of trauma to the brain that can also result in a brain disorder. Brain dysfunction also may result from use of prescribed medications or other drugs. The cognitive impairment that results from these conditions may be short term or long lasting.

Assertions of the Allen's CDM are based on information from neuroscience, biology, psychology, and traditional occupational therapy theory.[5] According to this model, occupation is synonymous with voluntary motor action. Observing voluntary motor actions such as dressing, completing a craft, or preparing a simple meal is of primary interest to the occupational therapy practitioner because of the inferences that can be made about brain function. Voluntary motor actions are "behavioral responses to a sensory cue that are guided by the mind."[3] That is, voluntary motor actions occur as a consequence of the relation among the external physical environment of matter, which provides sensory cues; the internal mind, which provides purpose; and the body, which produces behavior in the form of motor activity. Observing a person's voluntary motor action gives the occupational therapy practitioner insight into the relation among these three domains. Each domain is further described by subclassifications.

Based on extensive research, the Allen's CDM proposes a categorization of six cognitive levels that describe the way an individual relates matter, behavior, and mind as demonstrated in performance of voluntary motor actions (Table 7.5).[3,5] Level 1 represents the greatest degree of impairment, and level 6 represents normal performance. As the CDM has evolved, each cognitive level has been expanded to include several subcategories or *modes*. Only the global characteristics of each level are described in this text. This model of practice may be used to describe client performance and to guide selection of activities or tasks that permit the client to function consistently at the greatest possible level. (Other chapters in this book describe conditions associated with older adults for whom the application of the CDM may be appropriate, including the aging process in Chapter 3; side effects of medication in Chapter 13; malnutrition and dehydration in Chapter 18; strokes in Chapter 19; Alzheimer's dementia in Chapter 20; and brain tumors in Chapter 24.)

Observing clients performing activities and tasks that are part of their daily routines is ideal during assessment because these activities are usually important to the client and caregivers. These activities allow the OT and OTA team to separate issues related to learning a new activity, which might not accurately convey the client's current cognitive performance. Consequently, task assessment should be preceded by information obtained from the client and caregivers regarding the client's most familiar tasks. After observing the client, the OT and OTA team can compare the performance with the characteristic behaviors for each cognitive level. The OT and OTA team must remember that a client may function at a variety of levels depending on familiarity with the task and the time of day. Knowledge of the client's optimal functional level helps the OT and OTA team design intervention strategies that maximize the client's abilities.

Several standardized tests may be used to determine cognitive level, including the Expanded Routine Task Inventory (RTI)[3,18] and the Allen Cognitive Levels (ACL) Test.[5,19] The RTI evaluates the individual's ability at each of the six levels to complete a variety of routine tasks along a physical scale, such as grooming, dressing, bathing, walking, exercising, feeding, toileting, taking medication, and using adaptive equipment; a community scale, such as housekeeping, obtaining and preparing food, spending money, doing laundry, traveling, shopping, telephoning, and taking care of a child; a communication scale, such as listening, talking, reading, and writing; and an employment scale, such as maintaining pace and schedule, following instructions, performing simple and complex tasks, getting along with coworkers, following safety precautions and responding to emergencies, and supervising and planning work. The ACL test helps determine cognitive level by assessing the response to verbal instructions and problem-solving techniques when a client is presented with a leather lacing project.[3] Based on the Allen's Cognitive Disability Theory, the large ACL was developed to compensate for visual loss in the older adult population, and the Cognitive Performance Test (CPT) was developed to provide a standardized, ADL-based instrument for the assessment of functional level in Alzheimer's dementia.[20]

Once the client's cognitive level has been determined, the occupational therapy intervention goals must be considered.[4] Allen states that participation in an occupation does not necessarily mean the client will improve.[3] The assumption that OT has led to a particular recovery may fail to recognize other possible reasons for recovery, including that the client may recover spontaneously without any intervention. Consequently, the purpose of occupational therapy intervention should be to document alterations and improvements in functional abilities, sustain current performance, and reduce pain and distress associated with the

TABLE 7.5

Allen Cognitive Levels

		Level 1	Level 2	Level 3	Level 4	Level 5	Level 6
Matter	Sensory cues	Automatic actions	Postural actions	Manual actions	Goal-directed actions	Exploratory actions	Planned actions
	Perceptibility	Awareness is at threshold of consciousness; Attends to cues that penetrate subliminal state	Responds to proprioceptive cues; Aware of own body and objects that come into contact with it	Responds to tactile cues; Aware of immediate external surfaces	Follows visible cues; Aware of concepts of color and shape of objects	Follows related cues; Aware of concepts of space and depth	Follows symbolic cues; Aware of intangible concepts
	Setting	Mainly internal	Within range of motion	Within arm's reach	Within visual field	Restricted to task environment	Expanded to potential task environments
	Sample	Responds to alerting stimuli	Copies demonstrated body action	Identifies material objects	Makes exact match of sample	Conceives tangible possibilities of variations	Conceives hypothetic ideas
Behavior	Motor actions	Actions are habitual and automatic and have little thought	Spontaneous actions are postural (bending and stretching)	Hands are used to manipulate material objects repetitively	Actions are goal directed but restricted to tangible environment	Possibilities are explored through motor action that causes a visible effect	Actions are preceded by pause to think and plan
	Tool use	Needs stimulation to use body parts in habitual tasks	Uses body parts spontaneously	Uses found objects by chance; success is accidental	Uses hand tools as a means to a concrete end	Uses hand tools to vary means and end	Creates tools; uses power tools
	Number	Completes one action at a time	Completes one action at a time	Completes one action at a time	Completes task one step at a time	Completes several steps at a time	Completes indefinite steps
	People	Attends to those who shout or touch	Attends to those who move	Attends to the object manipulation of others	Shares goals with others	Shares exploration with others	Shares plans and recognizes autonomy
	Directions	Understands single verbs; physical contact is needed for action	Understands pronouns and names of body parts; gross motor and guided movement	Understands names of material objects and actions on an object	Understands adjectives and adverbs; must see each step in a series	Understands prepositions and explanations; each step and potential errors must be demonstrated	Understands conjunction and conjectures; demonstration is not necessary
Mind	Attention	Attention is focused on subliminal cues; external attention is very transient	Attends to proprioceptive cues, to own body, and to movement	Attends to tactile cues, focuses attention on the immediate effects of own actions	Attends to clearly visible cues; focuses attention to complete a task, end product sustains attention	Attends to related visual cues; may seek novelty through variation, but must see effects first	Attends to symbolic cues, thinks before testing results
	Goal attainment	Is awake; completes very habitual behaviors (eating and drinking)	Chance body movement creates interesting results that may be repeated	Chance movement creates visible results that are repeated many times	Uses several movement schemes to achieve an end goal	Becomes aware of problems when they become visible; uses trial and error approach	Problems are solved covertly; images are used to test solutions
	Time	Attention is maintained for seconds at a time	Attention is directed for minutes at a time	Attention is directed for half an hour at a time	Attention is maintained for an hour at a time	Attention is maintained and goals are remembered for weeks at a time	Sense of past, present, and future is maintained

Data from Allen C. *Occupational Therapy for Psychiatric Diseases: Measurement and Management of Psychiatric Diseases.* Boston: Little Brown; 1985.

symptoms. Goals are not intended to improve cognitive level but to ensure consistency of performance at the safest and least restrictive level. The case of Ray illustrates this point.

Ray is a 70-year-old man with Alzheimer's dementia. An OT and OTA team determined that he is currently functioning at cognitive level 4, which means that Ray can spontaneously complete tasks when cues are clearly visible. A goal for Ray to live independently would not be appropriate because he does not deal with cues that are not within his field of vision and consequently can easily place himself in danger. Appropriate occupational therapy goals for Ray according to the Allen's CDM may include consistent initiation of daily self-care routines, initiation of laundry washing, consistent monitoring of Ray in unfamiliar environments, and provision by his caregivers of appropriate cues to maximize his performance.

Once the client's goals have been determined, the OTA may select a variety of activities that match the characteristics of the matter, mind, and behavior domains appropriate to the client's cognitive level. The OTA must be adept at analyzing a task to precisely know the way it requires matter, mind, and behavior to interact for the client to successfully perform a voluntary motor action. Tasks are selected by the degree of demand on the client to perform consistently at a particular cognitive level. The OT and OTA team evaluated Ray and determined he was at cognitive level 4. Consequently, he can understand basic goals of activities, can purposefully use objects placed within his field of vision, and is able to match examples of tasks demonstrated to him. To reinforce his ability to maintain a sense of accomplishment, the OTA may select a simple woodworking project for Ray. The OTA can place all materials for the project on a table in front of Ray and instruct him to sand the wooden pieces. Telling him to pick up the sandpaper, hold it so the grain comes in contact with the wood, and rub it against the wood is unnecessary. These steps would be obvious to Ray because the materials are in his field of vision. Once Ray completes the sanding, the OTA may instruct him in a similar way to glue the pieces together as shown in the sample, stain the finished project, and varnish it. Ray lacks the foresight to plan for potential problems; consequently, the OTA should demonstrate the amount of glue, stain, and varnish needed in addition to the application procedures.

Once the client is performing at a level that most consistently demonstrates remaining task abilities and the environment has been structured to compensate for the client's limitations, specialized occupational therapy services should be discontinued. Discharge considerations are determined at the beginning of occupational therapy intervention. The CDM specifically focuses on preparing the client for discharge to the least restrictive environment.[5] Therefore, the OTA must observe voluntary motor actions to understand the way each client interacts with the environment. The OT and OTA team should recommend that the client be discharged to the setting that best supports the client's task abilities.

Emilia: The Model in Use

Emilia's Alzheimer's disease has progressed to the point where there is a clear cognitive deficit. Therefore, the Allen's CDM is ideal to help us develop a suitable intervention plan. The first step is to determine the cognitive level at which Emilia is functioning. During the RTI, Emilia shows that she performs at cognitive level 4. This is consistent with her husband's report, which states that at home, Emilia follows his visible cues and seems to pay attention to only those objects within her immediate visual field. He notes that she does not seem able to find items she needs even though they are in plain view in the room. However, once she finds the item, she is able to use it correctly.

The occupational therapy program for Emilia should consist of activities at level 4 that encourage her to complete steps of repetitive tasks after they have been demonstrated for her. For her safety, the environment should be structured so that all of the items she needs are in plain view in front of her. She should be given one instruction at a time, and instructions should focus on the motor actions rather than on the abstract goal of projects. Examples of suitable projects include simple printing or painting tasks, woodworking kits with few and large pieces, and simple food preparation tasks that do not require use of a stove or other potentially dangerous appliances. For her safety, Emilia should never be left alone or unattended.

Model of Human Occupation

The MOHO was designed to better understand how people participate in daily occupations and their order and disorder (function and dysfunction). It is for use with any individual experiencing difficulties in performing an occupation. This model evolved from earlier research by Reilly[21] on occupational behavior. Using concepts from General Systems Theory, Open Systems Theory, and Dynamical Systems Theory, the MOHO gives an explanation for the way occupation is motivated, organized, and performed, thereby emphasizing the human system's spontaneous, purposeful, tension-seeking properties, and acknowledging its creative properties.[6] In addition, this model provides a view of the degree of intimacy between the environment and the performance of occupation.

Human beings maintain constant interaction with the environment and receive many types of input such as olfactory and sensory stimulation and behavior expectations. The individual uses that input in many ways (e.g., food becomes energy; sensory stimulation may translate to touch, pain, or temperature; and words are interpreted). This process is known as throughput. Part of the result of the process of input and throughput is that a behavior, or output, is produced. Finally, as the person performs the behavior, the experience of doing it and any results from it form the process of feedback, which becomes a new source of input into the system.[22] The MOHO explains occupation as the cumulative and highly dynamic expression of this interactive process. For example, in meal preparation, a grandparent preparing a family meal sees the food items (input), considers what recipe to use (throughput), prepares the food items (output), feels arm movement, and sees the result of the preparation (feedback). While seeing that feedback, the cook notices that the food is beginning to turn brown (input), decides it is burning (throughput), removes the pan from the stove (output), and experiences moving the pan until it is off of the stove (feedback). To further explain the dynamic interaction between the individual and the environment from which the occupation arises, the MOHO describes external and internal environments of the human being as composed of several subsystems.

According to the MOHO, the external environment offers opportunities for certain behaviors while requiring others. For example, the institution of church offers the volunteer prayer group leader a room in which to sit in a chair, speak, and write reflection. At the same time, the church requires from the volunteer the behavior of reading and presenting the Bible story. The volunteer may be replaced if they are not able to perform their tasks and gather people together. Providing opportunity and requiring behavior is a complementary relationship. The influence of this relationship comes from several sources in the environment, including the physical realm, such as objects and built or natural structures; the social realm, which includes the tasks deemed appropriate and desirable and the social groups sanctioning the behavior; the settings or spaces in which occupation occurs, such as home, neighborhood, school, workplace, and gathering, recreation, and resource sites; and the overall culture, such as values, norms, and customs, which affect the individual's life. In addition, cultural contexts, political forces, and socioeconomic conditions of the society in which a person lives influence the person's occupation by making resources available or restricting access to them. For example, a person in a wheelchair may not be able to access an entertainment venue if society does not mandate the presence of cut curbs, ramps, and elevators in public spaces. However, the presence of adapted environments will not make much difference if the person lacks the economic means to obtain a wheelchair in the first place (Fig. 7.2).

The earlier example of meal preparation can be used to further elaborate on external environment concepts. To perform this occupation, the grandparent requires several objects, including food ingredients and seasonings, a knife, some pans, and the stove. The processes of dicing, chopping, stirring, and frying the food are all tasks recognized as cooking. Because of health concerns, the cook may choose to prepare a meal consisting only of vegetables for his or her family (social group). The setting of the meal is the cook's home, where they can exercise creativity

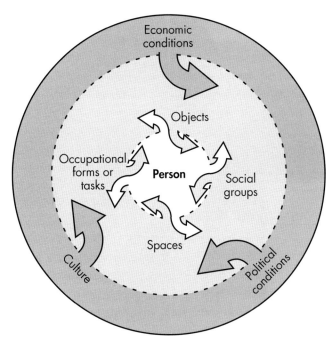

FIG. 7.2   External environment layers.

in preparing and seasoning the food and presenting the meal. In addition, the choice of vegetables only may be influenced by a cultural value that an athletic body is preferable to an obese one. If the grandparent were performing the occupation of cooking as the main task of their job at a restaurant, however, the objects, tasks, social group, setting, and possibly cultural expectations may present completely different opportunities and behavior expectations. There they might use industrial-size knives and tools, prepare large amounts of fried fish, be part of a team of cooks, and work in a restaurant that specializes in ethnic food.

The MOHO describes the individual's internal environment as composed of interrelated components, volition, habituation, and performance capacity (Fig. 7.3). Volition is responsible for guiding the individual through occupation choices throughout the day. According to this model, occupational choice is influenced by the individual's disposition about expected outcome and by self-knowledge, or awareness of the self as an active participant in the world. Both of these influences determine the way the individual anticipates, chooses, and experiences occupation. These concepts are illustrated by George and Pam, an older adult couple residing in a senior housing community. Every Saturday night they dress in their best clothes and walk to the common hall to play bridge with other members of their community. They choose to do this because they anticipate the pleasure of friends' company and because they believe they are capable bridge players. Helen, who lives in the same community as George and Pam, chooses not to play bridge. Although she is a champion player, she anticipates feeling out of place because she is a widow and does not have a regular partner.

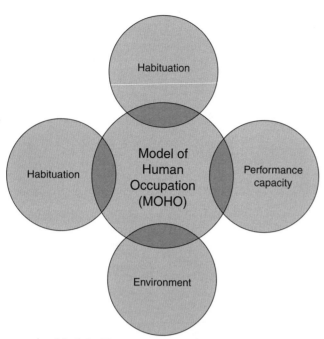

FIG. 7.3 Model of human occupation. *(Adapted from Taylor, R. R. (2017). Kielhofner's model of human occupation: Theory and application. 5th ed. Philadelphia, PA: Lippincott Williams & Wilkins.)*

Volition is composed of personal causation, values, and interests. Personal causation refers to the awareness individuals have of their abilities (i.e., knowledge of capacity) and to individuals' perceptions that they have control over their behavior (i.e., sense of efficacy). An individual is more likely to engage in an occupation he or she feels capable of doing. Values refer to the convictions people have that help them assign significance and standards of performance to the occupations they perform. Everyone has values that form the individual's views of life. These values elicit a sense of obligation to do what the individual believes is right. Finally, interests refer to the desire to find pleasure, enjoyment, and satisfaction in certain occupations. Interests may also be attractions that people feel toward certain occupations and preferences regarding ways that occupations are performed. For example, George, Pam, and Helen each has a sense of themselves as good or effective bridge players (personal causation). This sense was developed through experience over time, so that after playing as partners for more than 30 years, George and Pam have a specific playing style and are attracted to the opportunity to play bridge on Saturday nights rather than staying home and watching television (interest). Although Helen may have developed the same interest and personal causation, she believes that playing bridge is most meaningful with your spouse as your partner. Because she has no spouse, this value is sufficient to deter her from participating in the Saturday night games at the senior housing community.

In contrast to volition, which has to do with conscious choice and motivation of occupation, habituation has to do with the organization of occupations routines, patterns, and roles. ADLs are an example of a routine occupation. These routines require little deliberation because they are built on repetition. Habituation is composed of habits and internalized roles. Habits have to do with the typical way an individual performs a particular occupation and organizes it within a typical day or week and the unique style the individual brings to performance. For example, going to the common hall on Saturday night to play bridge is part of George and Pam's weekly routine. While playing bridge, both drink coffee. George typically puts one teaspoon of sugar in his cup before pouring in the coffee, and Pam pours her coffee first and then mixes in the sugar. During the game, George is talkative and Pam is quiet, but both break into song when they win the game.

Internalized roles refer to typical ways in which an individual relates to others. Roles are the identities and behaviors that people assume in various social situations. These roles are based on the individual's perceived expectations of others. Thus, roles involve obligations and rights of the individual in the various social contexts. According to the MOHO, the specific occupational behaviors that encompass a role, the style in which actions in a role occur, and the way an individual's roles are prioritized are of particular interest to the occupational therapy practitioner. George, Pam, and Helen each have an image of the role of bridge player. For George and Pam, this role includes the occupations of dressing nicely, walking to the common hall, playing by the rules, and sitting around a table conversing with others. Helen may view the role in a similar way, but she has the additional sense that the role of bridge player requires having one's spouse as partner. Because she is a widow, Helen has abandoned the role of bridge player. Conversely, George and Pam routinely enter this role on Saturday nights.

The final element of the human being's internal environment is the mind–brain–body performance capacity component and its subjective experience with the physical environment. As its name implies, this performance capacity represents the complex interplay among the musculoskeletal, neurological, perceptual, and cognitive abilities required to perform an occupation or enact a behavior. Interaction with the environment occurs through this component. The individual perceives challenges and opportunities in the environment through the perceptual system and processes this information in the brain. According to the meaning ascribed to the perception, the brain plans an action, which is carried to the muscles, joints, and bones of the limbs that perform the action. Whereas an occupation's meaning is ascribed by volition and the social context is determined by habituation, the related actions are enabled though the person's performance capacity. George and Pam like to play bridge (volition subsystem) and do so every Saturday night (habituation subsystem). During the bridge game, George and Pam keep in mind the rules and play accordingly. They sit with others around a table and maintain a grasp on the cards (performance subsystem). The complex interplay between mind, brain, and body inherent in the performance of any occupation occurs through specific skills, including motor skills, process skills, and communication–interaction skills (Table 7.6). Performance capacity, however, entails more than simply possessing intact body structures and functions upon which the actions of occupation are built. The person's subjective experience, or sense of being oneself in one's own body, significantly shapes which occupations are engaged in and the quality of such engagement. Performance capacity involves knowing things, knowing how to do things, and then, finally, actually doing things. The MOHO

TABLE 7.6

Performance Skills

Motor domains and skills	Posture	Stabilizes
		Aligns
		Positions
	Mobility	Walks
		Reaches
		Bends
	Coordination	Coordinates body parts
		Manipulates
		Uses fluent movements
	Strength and effort	Moves objects
		Transports objects
		Lifts objects
		Calibrates force, speed, and movement
	Energy	Endures
		Paces work
Communication and interaction domains and skills	Physicality	Gestures
		Gazes
		Approximates body appropriately
		Postures
		Contacts
	Language	Articulates
		Speaks
		Focuses speech
		Manages
		Modulates
	Relations	Engages
		Relates
		Respects
		Collaborates
	Information exchange	Asks
		Expresses
		Shares
		Asserts
Process domains and skills	Energy	Paces
		Attends
	Knowledge	Chooses tools and materials
		Uses tools and materials appropriately
		Handles tools and materials appropriately
		Heeds directions
		Inquires for directions
	Temporal organization	Initiates
		Continues
		Sequences
		Terminates

Continued

TABLE 7.6

Performance Skills—cont'd		
	Organization	Searches and locates
		Gathers
		Organizes
		Restores
		Navigates
	Adaptation	Notices and responds
		Accommodates
		Adjusts
		Benefits
Social interaction domains and skills	Acknowledging	
		Turns body or face toward others
		Looks at partner
		Confirms understanding
		Touches others appropriately
	Sending	Greets
		Answers
		Questions
		Complies
		Encourages
		Extends
		Clarifies
		Sets limits
		Thanks
	Timing	Times response
		Speaks fluently
		Takes turns
		Times duration
		Completes
	Coordinating	Approaches
		Places self at appropriate distance
		Assumes position
		Matches language
		Disclosure
		Expresses emotion

viewpoint is the bodily experience of doing is intricately intertwined with the embodied mind.[6]

A strength of the MOHO is the holistic view that it provides of dysfunction. Traditional health practice often focuses on one or two particular traits of a dysfunction rather than on all of the contributing factors. All the effects of dysfunction on an individual's life are rarely fully explored.[6] Lack of understanding of the whole situation may be particularly detrimental to the older adult. For example, Calvin is a 78-year-old man recently admitted to the hospital after falling and fracturing his left femur. On admission, an x-ray examination was done, Calvin was taken to surgery, and an open reduction of the fracture was performed. A cast was put on Calvin's leg, and he was referred to physical and occupational therapy (OT) for a brief rehabilitation course. The physical therapist focused rehabilitation on getting in and out of bed and walking with the reduced weight-bearing guidelines recommended by the physician. The OT evaluated Calvin and identified difficulties in dressing and toileting because of the cast and weight-bearing precautions. The OT asked the OTA to train Calvin to dress and toilet with adaptive equipment, to which Calvin easily complied. Calvin was discharged to return home in 2 days, at which time the OT and OTA team documented that Calvin was independent in dressing and toileting with necessary equipment and was aware of home modifications needed to avoid further falls. Unfortunately, nobody on the health team carefully investigated the reason that Calvin fell. Although he can care for himself, he finds living alone unbearably lonely. In addition, three of Calvin's lifelong friends died in the past year. Thus, Calvin has a deep sense of hopelessness. He occasionally tries to alleviate his feelings of loneliness and despair by drinking alcohol. He fell after one of these drinking episodes. When the admitting health worker at the hospital asked him if he consumed alcohol, Calvin responded truthfully that he did so only occasionally. During his hospital stay, Calvin appeared bright and friendly because he received much desired social contact. A more systematic evaluation of Calvin's life would have revealed a deeper problem related to his volition and habituation subsystems. Instead, the OT and OTA team focused on the obvious performance subsystem problem, which was only a symptom of a more complex issue. The OT and OTA team's care also should have addressed Calvin's feelings of hopelessness (volition) and the reduced number of roles he has to help himself organize his days (habituation). Furthermore, the OT and OTA team should have helped Calvin explore community resources.

According to the MOHO, any traditional occupational therapy tool is valid for assessment and intervention. Not one single assessment or intervention tool can completely address the complexity of the individual. Some suggested evaluation tools include the Assessment of Communication and Interaction Skills,[23] the Assessment of Motor and Process Skills,[24] the Assessment of Occupational Functioning,[25] the Occupational Case Analysis Interview and Rating Scale,[26] and the Occupational Performance History Interview.[27] Interest and role checklists, activity configurations, manual muscle tests, range-of-motion tests, and cognitive tests are among the many tools that may be used to evaluate each subsystem. Ultimately, data should be gathered regarding all subsystems of the individual's internal and external environments. Once problems are identified, intervention is prioritized according to all subsystems that are interdependent. In Calvin's case, if the volition and habituation issues had been identified, occupational therapy intervention could have focused on helping Calvin find other meaningful activities and resources for continued social contact, in addition to addressing his dressing and toileting needs.

Alejandro: The Model in Use

Because Alejandro is unable to speak, an observational assessment tool should be used to describe a baseline of occupational functioning. An Assessment of Motor and Process Skills[24] can help us see that although Alejandro is unable to speak, he is able to perform fairly complicated motor tasks. As part of the Assessment of Motor and Process Skills, Alejandro was asked to make a fruit salad. Alejandro positioned his body appropriately for the task, stabilized all objects, including the fruit and knife, maintained a secure grasp on the objects, chose the right tools, sequenced the task correctly, and cleaned the workspace without being asked to do so. Alejandro's actions demonstrated that he continued to consider his role as cook to be very important and that he was motivated to remain active. When tasting the fruit salad, there was no coughing, and it became apparent that part of his problem may have been that his family was feeding him while he was in bed. By making the fruit salad, Alejandro demonstrated to his family that he was not an invalid and that he was motivated to be upright and active. This observation allowed the family to step back and encourage him to increase his level of activity rather than overprotect him as they had been doing. In 2 days, Alejandro's fever was gone and he was developing a system to communicate with his family members through gestures and pictures.

Kawa Model

The models of practice covered thus far in this chapter contributed to the historical development of occupational therapy practice and provide a structure in which occupational therapy defines their scope of practice while providing a foundation to deduce and make sense of the client's narrative. Occupational therapy theory development in modern times has been limited to Western perspectives and focused on the updates to established models of practice with the development of the Occupation Therapy Practice Framework. These models apply concepts and principles collectively across all clients. The Kawa model is a modern-day model that conceives the client's narrative as a whole with a focus on discussion with the client. It was originally published in 2006 by Michael Iwama, an international OT.[28] He developed the model within the Japanese context and culture to provide a client with the ability to name the concepts and principles that become the focus of occupational therapy intervention. Western occupational therapy practitioners that understand the collectivist culture from which the Kawa model has stemmed, will better appreciate the significance of the elements of the model of practice as "culturally relevant occupational therapy."[9]

The Kawa (meaning river in Japanese) model utilizes the metaphor of a river and its elements to represent a client's life flow. Each element of the river (water, river floor and walls, rocks, driftwood, and the spaces around the elements) is a representation of the client's life experiences as social beings within the collective society and the value of their occupations within the natural and spiritual context (Fig. 7.4). The elements provide insight into the client's, the family's, and/or the caregiver's interpretation of what may interrupt the collective's life flow. Occupational therapy intervention focuses on the client's performance, adapting social expectations, and/or adapting the environment in order to remove barriers and enable participation. The ultimate goal is for life to flow freely.[8]

During an occupational therapy intervention, the occupational therapy practitioner discusses with the client a drawing of their river. Either the occupational therapy practitioner, the client, or a caregiver can draw the river. The drawing guides discussion throughout occupational therapy intervention to address what can be changed in order to balance the elements of the river in promotion of life flow. It is important to note that the metaphor of a river was used because it fit the Japanese culture. A metaphor that is culturally relevant to the occupational therapy practitioner and client can be used as an alternative.[7,9] For the purpose of understanding the Kawa model, it will be presented in its original format.

The river in its broadness, curves, and depth holds the water. The beginning of the water flow is birth; where the river meets the sea is death. The water flow is the indicator for the client's life flow and health. A cross-section of the river represents different aspects in a client's time in life and the effects on life flow. The water flow and its relationship with its surroundings allows the occupational therapy practitioner to view the snapshot of the client holistically in relationship to the collective culture (Fig. 7.4). The client assigns the shape and the size to the elements that are drawn into the river and assigns them meaning.[7,9]

The river floor and walls represent the client's physical and social environments. The depth of the river and the shape of the walls are not of primary concern. Of concern, is the ability of the river floor and walls to allow life flow even when obstacles exist. Occupational therapy practitioners can determine ways for the client to improve their interactions within their contexts. Changes in life circumstances such as those that affect body structures and functions are represented by rocks. The size and the placement of the rock indicates the amount of water flow that is blocked in relation to the river's floor and walls. Occupational therapy practitioners discuss with the client whether or not the rocks are impeding with life flow. Driftwood in the river represents personal attributes and

resources (internal or external) that have a positive or negative affect on life flow. Examples of personal attributes and resources are values, personality, living situation, assets, skills, and relationships. Driftwood is fluid and not as stable as the rocks in the river. It can get stuck at times or flow with the water to help create channels increasing life flow. The channels represent the spaces between the objects obstructing water flow. Life flow is free to continue through the spaces and provides the "promise of occupational therapy."[7] Occupational therapy understands where life is flowing and maximizes this strength to increase life flow by guiding the client to reduce the size and shape of the obstacles, shaping the environment surrounding the client, and maximizing existing assets and resources.[9]

The Kawa model is utilized across the lifespan and has application to Amit, Elizabeth, Emilia, and Alejandro. For the older adult, the Kawa model allows for discussion of their past and present and their perspectives and descriptions of their circumstances. Based on the discussion, the OT and OTA team provide interventions to make the changes in the river to increase life flow.

Amit draws his river walls narrow and the river floor shallow. He explains he is feeling as if his environment is closing in on him. He feels helpless in the rehabilitation center. Being in that context, limits his ability to be with his wife and establish a safe place for her. Amit is feeling overwhelmed by his limited time left with his wife and the situation allows for his rocks and driftwood to block his life flow. The occupational therapy practitioner can explore ways for Amit to assist in his wife's care while not being in the same environment. Intervention may focus

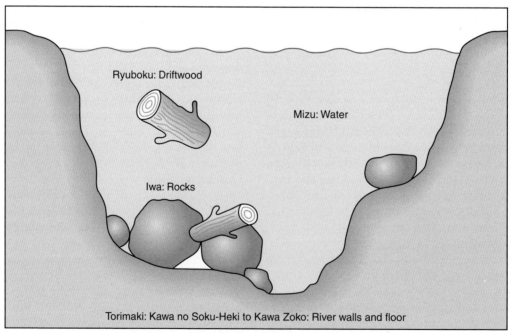

FIG. 7.4 Kawa model. (*Iwama, M. K. (2006). The Kawa model: Culturally relevant occupational therapy. Elsevier Health Sciences.*)

on the inhibitory effect of the river walls and floor to increase life flow.

Elizabeth's completed drawing of her river is evident of her frustration with her current level of functioning with ADLs and mobility. Her rocks are very large and are piled up on the floor of her river. She states she does not have any hope of participating in family events. Her OT begins working with her on increasing her energy and strength to prep herself and participate in social activities at the long-term care facility. Elizabeth's increase in independence in ADLs and satisfaction with interactions with other residents gradually forces the rocks to move and increase life flow.

The occupational therapy practitioner completes Emilia's drawing with her and her husband. During the discussion, the husband adds a piece of driftwood to Emilia's river. The driftwood is explained to be Emilia's inability to socialize with others at the adult day center. Her husband states her personality is such to not trust large groups of people. Emilia states she likes to sit alone and look at magazines at home and does not want to be at the adult day center. The occupational therapy practitioner works with Emilia and her husband to take magazines to the adult day center with her and identify one person at the center to share her magazines. The ability to participate in a familiar activity and begin social interaction allows the driftwood to continue to flow down the river supporting life flow.

Although Alejandro is experiencing multiple functional changes, the occupational therapy practitioner can construct a river with him and focus on the positive aspects of his current life flow. There are multiple spaces between his rocks and driftwood in which the water can flow. His family is present at the hospital daily. When one of his relatives attends treatment, Alejandro engages with the therapist and can follow their commands in his native language. The interaction increases his energy and the water flowing through the spaces start to power through the rocks to make progress in increasing life flow.

CONCLUSION

Building on the use of occupation as a common thread for any occupational therapy intervention, the *OTPF-4* or each of the models of practice provides a unique way to organize and think about information regarding the individual's function. In addition, each model guides the selection of intervention strategies appropriate for the specific needs of the individual. Finally, the use of models of practice assists the OTA in looking beyond the obvious functional deficits, thereby ensuring a more holistic approach to care of complexities of an older adult's life.

This chapter has highlighted only the *OTPF-4* and a few models available to help occupational therapy practitioners understand the person, environment and occupational factors, what should be assessed, and principles

underlying interventions that contribute to the occupational performance of people, groups, and populations we serve. Other models, such as the Canadian Model of Occupational Performance and Engagement[28] and the Person–Environment–Occupation–Performance Model,[29] among others, offer more nuanced insights into occupation, contextual demands, and opportunities, and, therefore, of the complex process of intervention and renewing occupational participation. Readers are encouraged to continually broaden their theoretical repertoire as they gain experience and seek to make unique contributions to healthcare, management, education, science, or policy.

CASE STUDY

Mary is 91 years old and lives with her husband, Hugh, age 90. They recently moved from her home of more than 40 years to a 900-square-foot independent living apartment. The complex also has an assisted living building and a skilled nursing facility (SNF). Mary states, "At some point we might need another level of assistance; neither one of us will be here much longer." Before the move, Mary was ambivalent about leaving familiar surroundings; however, Hugh was motivated and excited to move to a smaller space. Mary had a beautiful garden which she enjoyed caring for, was active in neighborhood parties, attended all family events, and enjoyed going to the symphony, theater, and out to dinner. Mary has also enjoyed travel and has been to many countries; however, in the past few years, travel has become more difficult.

Before her marriage to Hugh, Mary was married to her first husband for more than 50 years, and she was devastated when he died from complications of a stroke. However, with time she resumed her active lifestyle and, at age 84, remarried. Mary has had macular degeneration for more than 10 years, and she is part of study where she gets weekly shots in her eyes. The shots seem to have slowed the progression of the disease; however, she does have visual deficits. She is able to complete all ADLs independently; however, IADLs such as cooking and cleaning were becoming problematic. She gave up driving when she remarried but had only been driving during the day and only to familiar places. Before the move, Mary asked her two children, in-laws, grandchildren, and nieces to pick out an item or two they would like. She enjoyed watching this process and loved to hear the memories associated with each item chosen as a remembrance. Mary is the last living member of her family, which consisted of two brothers and a sister. She was close to all of them, and each death affected her deeply. Upon the death of her last sibling she remarked, "They are all gone now; I am ready to go."

Mary's house sold in a short time, causing anxiety and mild depression; "I'm not sure about this." Before moving day, she was able to choose items that would go to the new "home," and items not taken were put in an estate sale. Moving day was managed by her family. Before moving day, Mary, her daughter, and a niece went through the house and packed items that were to be moved, both personal and household. Hugh on the other had did nothing to prepare for the move and asked that his things not be moved by anyone: "I will take care of them." He had yet to pack anything, even though he was the one who had encouraged the move. His closet still held all his clothes, grooming and hygiene items were still on the bathroom shelves, and his desk was piled with papers, bills, and other miscellaneous items. The day of the estate sale, Mary was tearful and stated, "All those people in my house going through my things? What a sad day this is. How did it come to this?"

On the surface, Mary can recognize the need for someone to cook, clean, and take care of outside maintenance, yet she continues to have days of sadness and tears. Hugh has adapted to the new environment without any difficulty.

■ CASE STUDY QUESTIONS

1 What model of practice best fits Mary's change in lifestyle? Explain your answer and provide a specific example.
2 How can the OTA address Hugh's change in lifestyle based on the *OTPF-4*? Explain your answer and provide a specific example.
3 Refer to Chapter 2. What theory of aging would apply to Mary? What theory would apply to Hugh? Did you choose the same theory for both? Why or why not? What factors about each person helped you decide on a particular theory? Are there other theories you can research not addressed in Chapter 2 that would coincide with the aging factors Mary and Hugh are currently experiencing?
4 What interventions would you provide for Mary and Hugh during their transition to assisted living?

■ CHAPTER REVIEW QUESTIONS

1 Explain the meaning of occupation and why this concept should be at the core of occupational therapy intervention.
2 Describe at least two ways in which a model of practice can help the OTA work with older adults.
3 Explain why it is important to consider context in an older adult's occupational performance.
4 Considering Llorens's Developmental Model, explain the social interaction needs that an older adult is likely to have when placed in a long-term care facility.
5 You have planned a task group for psychiatric clients during which you plan to carve pumpkins for Halloween. Using the Allen's CDM, describe how you would modify the activity if the members of the group are functioning at a cognitive level 4.
6 Using the language of the MOHO, explain how you would prioritize intervention for a Native American elder who was admitted to the hospital after a car accident in which his wife and adult son died. He has severe fractures in all extremities, and there is the possibility of a mild head trauma. When you approach this older adult, he refuses to speak and remains staring out the window.
7 In viewing your client's, who is Hispanic, Kawa model river drawing, you note that there are multiple large rocks blocking the water flow. What approaches to intervention would best allow the client to improve cultural relevant occupations within their context to increase their life flow?

REFERENCES

1. American Occupational Therapy Association. Occupational therapy practice framework: domain and process. 4th ed. *Am J Occup Ther*. 2020;74:1-87. Available at: https://doi.org/10.5014/ajot.2020.74S2001.
2. Llorens L. *Application of a Developmental Theory for Health and Rehabilitation*. Rockville, MD: American Occupational Therapy Association; 1976.
3. Allen C. *Occupational Therapy for Psychiatric Diseases: Measurement and Management of Cognitive Disabilities*. Boston: Little Brown; 1985.
4. Allen C, Earhart C, Blue T. *Occupational Therapy Treatment Goals for the Physically and Cognitively Disabled*. Rockville, MD: American Occupational Therapy Association; 1992.
5. Allen C, Earhart C, Blue T. *Understanding Cognitive Performance Modes*. Ormond Beach, FL: Allen Conferences; 1995.
6. Taylor RR. *Kielhofner's Model of Human Occupation: Theory and Application*. 5th ed. Philadelphia, PA: Lippincott Williams & Wilkins; 2017.
7. Iwama M. *The Kawa Model: Culturally Relevant Occupational Therapy*. Edinburgh, UK: Churchill Livingstone-Elsevier Press; 2006.
8. Cole MB, Tufano R. *Applied Theories in Occupational Therapy: A Practical Approach*. 2nd ed. Thorofare, NJ: Slack; 2020.
9. Turpin MJ, Iwama MK. *Using Occupational Therapy Models in Practice E-Book: A Fieldguide*. New York: Elsevier Health Sciences; 2011.
10. American Occupational Therapy Association. The philosophical base of occupational therapy. *Am J Occup Ther*. 2017;7112410045. Available at: https://doi.org/10.5014/ajot.2017.716S06.
11. American Occupational Therapy Association. Position paper: purposeful activity. *Am J Occup Ther*. 1993;47:1081.
12. American Occupational Therapy Association. Uniform terminology for occupational therapy. *Am J Occup Ther*. 1994;48:1047.
13. Trombly C. Occupation: purposefulness and meaningfulness as therapeutic mechanisms. Eleanor Clarke Slagle lecture. *Am J Occup Ther*. 1995;49(10):960-972.
14. Ma H, Trombly C. Effects of task complexity on reaction time and movement kinematics in elderly people. *Am J Occup Ther*. 2004;58(2):150-158.
15. Ayers AJ. *Sensory Integration and Praxis Test*. Los Angeles, CA: Western Psychological Services; 1991.
16. Atwal A, McIntyre A. *Occupational Therapy with Older People*. 2nd ed. Hoboken, NJ: Wiley-Blackwell; 2013.
17. World Federation of Occupational Therapists. *About Occupational Therapy*. 2012a. Available at: https://www.wfot.org/about/about-occupational-therapy.
18. Katz N. *Routine Task Inventory: Expanded (RTI-E) Manual, Prepared, and Elaborated on the basis of C. K. Allen*. 2006. Unpublished manuscript Available at: http://www.allen-cognitive-network.org/pdf_files/RTIManual2006.pdf.
19. Pollard D, Olin DW. *Allen's Cognitive Levels: Meeting the Challenges of Client-Focused Services*. Monona, WI: SELECTone Rehab; 2005.
20. Burns T, Mortimer JA, Merchak P. Cognitive performance test: a new approach to functional assessment in Alzheimer's disease. *J Geriatr Psychiatry Neurol*. 1994;7(1):46-54.
21. Reilly M. Occupational therapy can be one of the great ideas of 20th century medicine. *Am J Occup Ther*. 1962;16:1-9.
22. Kielhofner G, Burke JP. A model of human occupation, part 1. Conceptual framework and content. *Am J Occup Ther*. 1980;34(9):572-581. https://doi.org/10.5014/ajot.34.9.572.
23. Salamy M, Simon S, Kielhofner G. *The Assessment of Communication and Interaction Skills* (research version). Chicago: University of Illinois; 1993.
24. Fisher G. *Assessment of Motor and Process Skills*. 6th ed. Ft. Collins, CO: Three Star Press; 2003.

25. Watts J, Newman S. The assessment of occupational functioning. In: Hempill-Pearson B, ed. Assessments in Occupational Therapy in Mental Health. 2nd ed. Thorofare, NJ: Slack; 2007.

26. Kalplan K, Kielhofner G. *The Occupational Case Analysis and Interview and Rating Scale*. Thorofare, NJ: Slack; 1989.

27. Kielhofner G, Mallinson T, Crawford C, et al. *A User's Guide to the Occupational Performance History Interview II (OPHI-II)* (version 2.0). Chicago: Model of Human Occupation Clearinghouse, Department of Occupational Therapy, College of Applied Health Sciences, University of Illinois at Chicago; 1997.

28. Townsend E, Polatajko H. *Enabling Occupation II: Advancing an Occupational Therapy Vision for Health, Well-Being & Justice Through Occupation*. Ottawa, ON: CAOT ACE; 2007.

29. Christiansen C, Baum C, Bass J, eds. *Occupational Therapy: Performance, Participation and Well-Being*. 4th ed. Thorofare, NJ: Slack; 2015.

Opportunities for Best Practice in Various Settings

SUE BYERS-CONNON, RENÉ PADILLA, AND AMY L. SHAFFER

(PREVIOUS CONTRIBUTIONS FROM STEVE PARK)

KEY TERMS

adult day care, adult foster home, assisted living, client-centered practice, continued competency, emerging practice, geropsychiatric unit, home health, hospice, inpatient rehabilitation, OTA/OT partnership, *Occupational Therapy Practice Framework*, service competency, skilled nursing facility

CHAPTER OBJECTIVES

1. Illustrate occupational therapy assistant (OTA) practice in traditional and emerging practice settings.
2. Become familiar with the *Occupational Therapy Practice Framework*, fourth edition, and the OTA's role during occupational therapy service delivery.
3. Understand the need for service competency for OTAs and continued competency for occupational therapy practitioners: OTA and occupational therapist (OT).
4. Appreciate the OTA/OT interprofessional relationship.
5. Value the importance of a client-centered practice.

Achieving health, well-being, and participation in life through engagement in occupation is the overarching statement that describes the domain and process of occupational therapy in its fullest sense (p. S4).[1]

Marta works with older adults in a geropsychiatric unit, assisting older adults and families to manage daily life activities on the ward and at home. Arianna works with older adults in an adult foster home, helping older adults engage in leisure and social activities throughout their week. Rachel works in an inpatient rehabilitation unit, helping older adults to regain their competence in basic activities of daily living (ADLs). Jean works as a resident services coordinator at an assisted living facility, overseeing the delivery of services. Drew works with older adults in a skilled nursing facility (SNF), facilitating their ability to participate in basic and instrumental activities of daily living (IADLs) and regain former roles. Amanda works on-call for SNFs and is exploring the possibility of including occupational therapy services at the independently owned hospice where she volunteers. Manisha works in home health, helping older adults engage in a routine of needed and desired daily life activities within their homes. Carlos works at an adult day care center, assisting older adults as they engage in a routine of productive, leisure activities and achieve life satisfaction. Margo works for her city's mayor as part of the council on fitness and well-being, specifically on wellness

initiatives for older adults in the community. Jamie works at a local outpatient facility delivering occupational therapy services virtually using telehealth.

These OTAs attended a reunion for graduates from the Occupational Therapy Assistant program at Blue Lake Community College, established 20 years ago. Of the 150 OTAs in attendance, the majority work with older adults in one capacity or another, reflecting the US national trends of 68% of OTAs working with rehabilitation/disability/productive aging populations and 42.8% working in SNFs.[2] Some OTAs work in more traditional settings, such as a SNF or geropsychiatric unit; others work in emerging practice settings, such as adult foster homes and health and wellness. Despite working in different settings, the common thread is that the OTAs are assisting older adults to engage in daily activities and meaningful occupations. Although the settings differ, the focus and process of delivering OT services are similar.

This chapter addresses the role of OTAs, emphasizing the similar focus and process of occupational therapy service delivery with older adults across different practice settings, using the *Occupational Therapy Practice Framework: Domain and Process*, fourth edition (hereafter known as the OTPF-4)[1] as a guide. Other concepts presented are the importance of the OTA/OT partnership, service competency, continued competency, and practice issues during occupational therapy service delivery. A series of vignettes follow that describe OTAs' work with older adults in specific settings and illustrate best practices for OTAs, that is, when occupational therapy practitioners deliver services "based on knowledge and evidence that reflect the most current and innovative ideas available."[3]

OCCUPATIONAL THERAPY PRACTITIONERS: AN INTERPROFESSIONAL COLLABORATION

To support older adults to achieve health, well-being, and life satisfaction through participation in a meaningful occupation, the OTA/OT team provides valuable occupational therapy services. Even though OTs are ultimately responsible for occupational therapy service delivery and for supervising OTAs, the delivery of occupational therapy services occurs collaboratively between the two partners. According to the American Occupational Therapy Association (AOTA), supervision is viewed as "a cooperative process in which two or more people participate in a joint effort to establish, maintain, and/or elevate competence and performance." This supervisory relationship is necessary to ensure the safe and effective delivery of occupational therapy services and to promote the professional development of the OTA. Moreover, occupational therapy service provision is done in accordance with the Occupational Therapy Code of Ethics,[5] continuing competency and professional development guidelines, relevant workplace policies, and state laws and regulations.[6]

Together, the OTA/OT partners should decide the type of contact (direct or indirect) and frequency of supervision and then develop and document a supervisory plan that details what type of supervision is needed, what areas should be addressed, and how often to meet. For example, an OTA/OT team works in an SNF and meets face-to-face (direct contact) once a week for an hour to review and discuss their clients' concerns and status. In addition, they discuss specific ways to foster the OTA's professional expertise, such as developing advanced therapeutic skills when working with older adults experiencing complex medical problems and better ways to incorporate the learning–teaching process when working with an older adult's family members, significant others, and caregivers. In other settings, such as home health, the OTA and OT meet face to face several times a month for an hour; however, during the week, they keep in frequent contact through telephone calls and email messages (indirect contact). Although these contacts focus primarily on service delivery for clients, they also discuss areas for professional development. The frequency, methods, and focus of supervision vary according to the skills of the OTA and OT, the needs and complexity of clients, the service setting's needs and requirements, and state regulatory requirements.

To establish an interprofessional relationship and deliver quality services, the OTA and OT need to value their common beliefs and skills and honor their different contributions during service delivery.[7] A respectful relationship occurs when partners communicate openly, trust each other, share each other's knowledge, and are willing to learn from each other.[8] Sue, an OTA, worked in a rehabilitation unit for 3 years when Steve, an OT and recent graduate, joined the team. Steve appreciated Sue's expertise in identifying, planning, and adapting therapeutic activities relative to older adults' specific interests and needs, particularly leisure, household, and community activities. Sue appreciated the way Steve fostered her understanding of older adults' specific emotional, cognitive, and physical conditions and how to apply this knowledge during evaluation and intervention. Sue taught Steve new and different ways of engaging clients in activities while Steve modeled a client-centered approach when interacting with older adults. Steve trusted Sue to carry out interventions. Particularly those focusing on adaptation, share her thoughts and professional opinion, and Sue felt comfortable asking Steve for additional supervision when needed. Sue and Steve were respectful of each other's strengths without their partnership being a hierarchical relationship. Together, they were better able to determine the older adults' needed outcomes and design interventions that reached those desired goals as the end result of the occupational therapy process.

Establishing a strong collaborative OTA/OT partnership is an ongoing process that requires active participation by the OTA and OT to identify the partnership's strengths and areas of improvement.[8] To assist with the process, OTAs and OTs should identify each other's competencies, as well as the common knowledge and skills they share. This requires a comprehensive understanding of the roles and responsibilities of OTAs and OTs during the evaluation, intervention, and outcomes process of service delivery. To understand these roles and responsibilities, the fourth (and most recent) edition of the OTPF and its relation to the OTA/OT team process is presented in the following section.

OCCUPATIONAL THERAPY PRACTICE FRAMEWORK

In 2002, AOTA introduced the *Occupational Therapy Practice Framework: Domain and Process*, a document designed to assist OTs and OTAs to more clearly affirm and articulate occupational therapy's unique focus on occupation and daily life activities and to illustrate an intervention process that facilitates clients' engagement in occupation to support their participation in life.[1] Because the *Framework* is an official AOTA document, it is reviewed every 5 years; consequently, a second edition was published in 2008, a third edition in 2014, and the fourth edition in 2020.[1] Following is a brief overview of the two major areas from the latest edition—(1) Domain of Occupational Therapy and (2) Process of Occupational Therapy—that OTAs and OTs should be familiar with when working with older adults. A more general overview is provided in Chapter 7, but because the following sections focus on only highlights from the OTPF-4, occupational therapy practitioners are encouraged to obtain the most recent edition for use in practice.

DOMAIN OF OCCUPATIONAL THERAPY

Occupational therapy practitioners assist clients (persons, groups, and populations) to engage in everyday activities or occupations that they want and need to do in a manner that supports health and participation.[1] "Occupational therapy practitioners recognize the importance and impact of the mind-body-spirit connection on engagement and participation in daily life" (p. 6–7).[1] Achieving health, well-being, and participation in life through engagement in occupation is the overarching statement that describes the domain and process of occupational therapy in its fullest sense. "Occupations are central to a client's health, identity and sense of competence and have particular meaning and value to that client" (p. 7).[1]

In occupational therapy practice, the terms occupation and activity often are used interchangeably, but in the OTPF-4, the term occupation encompasses activity, making a distinction between the two terms. "the term occupation denotes personalized and meaningful engagement in daily life events by a specific client" (p. 7).[1] The term "occupation," then, refers to the daily life activities that have purpose and personal meaning, while an "activity" denotes a form of action that is objective and not related to a specific client's engagement or context (Schell et al., 2019) and, therefore, can be selected and designed to enhance occupational engagement by supporting the development of performance skills and performance patterns (p. 20).[1] In other words, activities are components of occupation that in isolation may not be particularly meaningful but enable occupation. For example, an older adult enjoys growing flowers in his garden, cutting the flowers, then arranging and gifting them to friends and family members. He feels pride in his skill as a gardener and derives pride from the pleasure the flower arrangements bring to others. Another older adult, however, may not place the same value on the activities of gardening and arranging flowers. In fact, some older adults may view gardening outdoors as a chore that requires getting dirty, bug bitten, and hot. If so, then growing flowers would be considered merely an activity, devoid of the meaning that would make it a personal, meaningful occupation.

Although the distinction between activity and occupation is not always clear, it can be helpful for occupational therapy practitioners to consider the distinction between these concepts when working with older adults. If only an older adult's occupations are considered, there may be important activities in the older adult's life that are not adequately addressed during intervention. For example, when using the toilet, it may be important for an older adult to assist to the best of his or her ability to reduce the physical and emotional stress on the caregiver. If an occupational therapy practitioner does not address toileting because the older adult does not think it is important to become as independent as possible, then both the older adult and the caregiver are at risk for physical injury and emotional distress. However, if an occupational therapy practitioner focuses solely on an older adult's performance in activities and ignores the older adult's engagement in meaningful occupation, an important contribution to the older adult's health, well-being, and life satisfaction may be ignored. For example, overemphasizing therapy on increasing an older adult's independence in dressing when he or she does not find much personal meaning in this objective may damage the therapeutic relationship. It may also cause the occupational therapy practitioner to miss an opportunity to enhance the older adult's health, well-being, and life satisfaction through assisting the older adult to engage in meaningful occupation. Enhancing the older adult's engagement in occupation that has meaning to him or her, such as tending to tomato plants, walking the dog around the block twice a day, or washing the dishes after a meal his or her spouse has prepared, may be of greater benefit than achieving "independence" in dressing. The important aspect is that all activities and occupations addressed during occupational therapy intervention consider the contexts in which the older adult lives, loves, works, and plays.

With a primary focus on a client's engagement in occupation, the OTPF-4 outlines five major aspects that constitute the primary domain of occupational therapy (Table 8.1). No one element is considered more important than another. Occupational therapy practitioners need to consider all domain elements and how they affect

TABLE 8.1

Domain of Occupational Therapy	
Occupations	Activities of daily living (ADLs)
	Instrumental activities of daily living (IADLs)
	Health management
	Rest and sleep
	Education
	Work
	Play
	Leisure
	Social participation
Contexts	Environmental factors
	Personal factors
Performance patterns	Habits
	Routines
	Roles
	Rituals
Performance skills	Motor skills
	Process skills
	Social interaction skills
Client factors	Values, beliefs, and spiritual influence
	Body functions
	Body structures

Based on data from American Occupational Therapy Association. American Occupational Therapy Association. Occupational therapy practice framework: Domain and process, 4th ed. Am J Occup Ther. 2020;74(Suppl. 2):1-85. doi: 10.5014/ajot.2020.74S2001.

occupational identity, health, well-being, and participation in life.[1]

The first aspect, *occupation*, identifies the primary categories of occupation that occupational therapy practitioners consider when working with persons, groups, or populations.[1] Occupations are defined by the World Federation of Occupational Therapy as the "things people need to, want to, and are expected to do."[9] These categories represent the primary focus of occupational therapy: a client's engagement in ADLs, IADLs, health management, rest and sleep, education, work, play, leisure, and social participation.[1] Depending on the specific setting in which an OTA works, some occupations may be emphasized more than others. For example, after an acute care hospitalization for pneumonia, it is important for older adults to be able to manage their ADLs when they return home. Although managing ADLs may be a major area of concern for discharge, the OTPF-4 prompts occupational therapy practitioners to also address other potential areas, such as leisure and social participation, which may be equally important to an older adult after discharge.

The second aspect, *contexts*, refers to the varied conditions and surroundings under which people engage in occupation. Engaging in occupation is influenced by the environmental and personal factors unique to the individual client.[1] This could be a person, group, or population. For example, a cultural norm that a family values and follows may forbid female individuals from providing personal, intimate care for male older adults, such as bathing, toileting, or dressing.

The third aspect, *performance patterns*, reflects the combination of habits, routines, rituals, and roles used while engaging in occupations.[1] These performance patterns may support the performance of occupations or hinder the performance of occupations. An important factor for clients is the ability to engage in a series of activities over time that sustain engagement in occupation. For example, an OTA working with an older adult experiencing mild memory loss might assist the older adult to develop a consistent routine to safely prepare toast and coffee each morning.

The fourth aspect, *performance skills*, is composed of goal-directed actions or small units of engagement in daily life[1] and reflects the client's demonstrated abilities (motor skills, process skills, and social interaction skills). A unique skill that occupational therapy practitioners possess is the ability to analyze and grade activities so that their demands match the client's abilities.[10] Each activity "presents" specific demands; some activities require a large outdoor physical environment, such as a lawn to play croquet, whereas other activities require a relatively quiet indoor environment that promotes conversation, such as a living room where coffee and pastries can be served for church members. Furthermore, each activity will demand more or less of a particular body function or body structure; some activities require more fine motor coordination, such as needlepoint, whereas others require greater strength, such as vacuuming. Occupational therapy practitioners use their observation skills to identify those abilities that are effective or ineffective when a person is engaging in occupation. For example, an OTA and an older adult are in a pharmacy where the OTA is primarily interested in the older adult's social interaction skills while picking up a prescription. Throughout the process, the OTA observes the older adult's ability to project his voice to the pharmacist behind the counter and effectively ask questions about a medication's side effects.

The fifth (and final) aspect, *client factors*, represents the underlying characteristics and capacities (i.e., values, beliefs, and spirituality; body functions; and body structures) specific to each client and that influence a client's performance in occupation.[1] Client factors are affected by one's life stages and one's life experiences; and may also be affected by illness, disease, disability, or occupational deprivation.[1]

PROCESS OF OCCUPATIONAL THERAPY: EVALUATION, INTERVENTION, AND OUTCOME

Occupational therapy practitioners view occupation as both the means and end of occupational therapy intervention.[1] With this in mind, service delivery begins with an evaluation of a client's occupational needs, problems, and concerns; continues with an intervention process that emphasizes the therapeutic use of occupations; and ends with a review of outcomes to identify whether the client's occupational needs, problems, and concerns were resolved.[1] The OTPF-4 contains three major elements that represent the process of delivering OT services.

The first element, *evaluation*, represents the first stage and focuses on understanding what the client wants and needs to do with respect to engaging in occupation and identifying the features that support or hinder the client's engagement in occupation.[1] To do so, occupational therapy practitioners must first develop an occupational profile or, in other words, gain a sense of the client's occupational history and experiences, past engagement, personal goals, and so on. After developing the client's occupational profile, the OT analyzes the client's actual occupational performance considering all pertinent aspects identified in the OTPF-4 as the domain of occupational therapy—occupations, client factors, performance patterns, performance skills, and client factors—and how they influence the client's concerns about engagement in occupation and performance of activities.

The evaluation process consists of three steps: (1) creating an occupational profile, (2) conducting an analysis of occupational performance, and (3) synthesizing the evaluation process.[1] Using a client-centered approach, occupational therapy practitioners gather information to create an occupational profile that clarifies what is important and meaningful to a client, focusing on the client's occupational history and experiences, patterns of daily living, interests, values, and needs.[1] The process to create a client's occupational profile will vary, depending on the client and the setting, but the focus remains the same: What are the client's current priorities and problems relative to engaging in occupation? Information from the occupational profile guides the next stage in the evaluation process: analysis of occupational performance. This involves observing clients as they engage in activities and occupations. It requires understanding of the complex and dynamic interaction of the clients' performance patterns and skills, the contexts in which occupation needs to occur, activity demands, and client factors. To analyze a client's performance, specific activities (and the contexts and environments in which they occur) are identified, and the client is observed performing the activities. During this process, the occupational therapy practitioner notes the effectiveness of the client's performance patterns and performance skills. To synthesize the evaluation process, using other information gathered during the evaluation, the occupational therapy practitioner then interprets the data to identify what supports and/or hinders the client's engagement in occupation. OTs are ultimately responsible for initiating and completing the evaluation. OTAs, supervised by an OT, assist during the evaluation process according to their skill level (Table 8.2).[1]

The second element, *intervention*, consists of three steps: (1) developing the plan, (2) intervention implementation, and (3) intervention review.[1] Although OTs are ultimately responsible for developing the intervention plan, OTAs may contribute during the plan's development.[1]

The intervention plan, developed in collaboration with clients (and other professionals), focuses on occupational therapy approaches to create, promote, establish, restore, maintain, or modify clients' engagement in occupation or prevent future problems engaging in occupation. An essential element of the intervention plan is the collaboration between clients and occupational therapy practitioners to identify and set goals for intervention that focus on specific aspects of a client's occupational performance and engagement that could improve or be maintained over the course of intervention.

Interventions are then implemented to address the client factors, activity demands, performance patterns, performance skills, and contexts that hinder the client's engagement in desired activities and occupations.[1] Again, intervention is a collaborative process between clients and occupational therapy practitioners and focuses on facilitating a change in the occupations, contexts, performance patterns, performance skills, and client factors that directly result in improved or maintained engagement in occupation. Throughout intervention implementation, the process is monitored for its effectiveness and progress toward the identified goals and is modified accordingly. OTAs are most active in their role as occupational therapy practitioners when implementing interventions to promote engagement in occupation.[7]

The final element, *outcomes*, focuses on identifying the success of the intervention.[1] Did the intervention foster an improvement with a client's engagement in occupation? Were future problems with a client's engagement prevented? Methods to evaluate outcomes should be used during the evaluation process and throughout intervention

TABLE 8.2

Occupational Therapy Assistant/Occupational Therapist Responsibilities During the Process of Occupational Therapy Service Delivery

	OTA	Framework	OT
Evaluation	Contributes to evaluation process Shares information with OT Administers specific assessments after establishing service competency	Occupational profile Analysis of occupational performance	Responsible for evaluation process, coordinating with OTA Initiates and completes the evaluation Interprets data with input from OTA
Intervention	Provides input to intervention plan	Intervention plan	Responsible for developing intervention plan collaboratively with clients, OTA, and other professionals
	Provides intervention appropriate to demonstrated competency	Intervention implementation	Responsible for intervention, coordinating with OTA
	Provides information to assist with intervention review	Intervention review	Responsible for intervention review and documentation, coordinating with OTA
Outcomes	Provides information to OT related to outcome achievement	Evaluation of outcomes	Responsible for evaluation of outcomes, coordinating with OTA

Based on American Occupational Therapy Association. Guidelines for supervision, roles, and responsibilities during the delivery of occupational therapy services. Am J Occup Ther. 2020;74:7413410020. doi:10.5014/ajot.2020.74S3004.

to identify what progress, if any, a client is making toward the goals and priorities identified at the beginning of occupational therapy intervention. As with evaluation and intervention, OTAs and OTs work collaboratively to monitor intervention outcomes.

OCCUPATIONAL THERAPY ASSISTANT/ OCCUPATIONAL THERAPIST COMPETENCIES WITH EVALUATION, INTERVENTION, AND OUTCOME PROCESS

Continuing competence is a process by which occupational therapy practitioners "develop and maintain the knowledge, performance skills, interpersonal abilities, critical reasoning, and ethical reasoning skills necessary to perform current and future roles and responsibilities within the profession."[10] Demonstration of continuing competency is a requirement of most regulatory boards, employers, and accrediting bodies. The AOTA[10] serves to ensure that occupational therapy practitioners are providing services based on current knowledge and skills. Establishing continuing competency is ongoing and may involve various methods, such as (1) professional service (e.g., volunteering, peer review, and mentoring), (2) completing workshops/courses/independent learning (e.g., attending seminars, lectures, and conferences; reading peer-reviewed journals and textbooks), (3) presenting (e.g., presenting at state, national, and international conferences; serving as adjunct faculty), (4) fieldwork supervision (e.g., Level I or II), and (5) publishing (e.g., journal articles and book chapters).[11] For example, Rachel attended a workshop specifically for OTAs that focused on incorporating a neurodevelopmental approach when providing occupational therapy services for older adults with CVA diagnoses. After returning to the rehabilitation center, she directly applied the knowledge and skills from the workshop with older adults who had experienced a stroke (see Chapter 19). One older adult, Elmer, liked to restore vintage cars. Rachel asked his wife to bring one of their cars to the rehabilitation center. While Elmer polished the car, Rachel worked with him and his wife so that Elmer could learn how to incorporate more normal movement patterns (performance skills) and inhibit muscle tone (client factors).

Establishing competence to practice begins after graduating from an accredited OTA program, successfully completing fieldwork, and passing a nationally recognized entry-level examination for OT assistants.[12] In the United States, OTAs are initially certified by the National Board for Certification in Occupational Therapy (NBCOT).[12] Initial certification permits the use of the COTA credential for 3 years. After the initial certification period, a COTA must recertify, in order to continue using the COTA credential. Recertification also requires the completion of professional development units, indicating continuing competency.[12] Though it is not required, it is strongly encouraged that OTAs maintain their NBCOT certification as it indicates that the OTA has maintained a national standard for professionalism and professional development.[12] Individual state licensure boards and employers may have their own requirements related to maintaining NBCOT certifications beyond the initial certification period. OTAs should ensure their familiarity with expectations of their employment arrangement.

A unique feature within the OTA/OT partnership is the establishment of service competency for the OTA. Establishing service competency is the process by which an OTA collaborates with an OT to demonstrate and document that the OTA's reasoning, judgment, and performance are satisfactory for specific evaluation and intervention methods.[4,7] For example, to establish service competency, an OT may observe an OTA administer the Canadian Occupational Performance Measure (COPM)[13] several times with different older adults. If the OTA consistently administers the COPM according to the manual's instructions, and the OT concurs that the results are accurate with each administration, then the OTA has demonstrated service competency to perform this specific assessment. After demonstrating competence, the OTA may independently administer the assessment and share the results with the OT, although the OTA may not interpret the results.[7] In essence, with the establishment of service competency, less direct supervision is required. Documentation of service competency is recommended and is required by many state regulatory agencies.[4]

When reentering the workforce or changing practice areas, the demonstration of continued competency is important and likely a statutory requirement.[4] For example, Drew had worked in a school setting for 1 year. He always had an interest in working with older adults and accepted a job offer from a SNF. Before he began work, he attended a workshop to become familiar with Medicare guidelines and the prospective payment system (see Chapter 6). He also attended study groups with three other OTAs who worked in SNFs, where they focused on specific skills, such as transfer techniques, use of adaptive equipment, and application of hip precautions during ADLs. By engaging in these educational activities, Drew was actively demonstrating continuing competency relevant to his new area of practice and meeting state regulatory requirements.

BEST PRACTICE FOR INFECTION CONTROL

Infectious materials can be present anywhere—in hospitals, SNFs, ALFs (assisted living facilities), but also in stores in which we shop, workplaces we visit, or the homes of ourselves or others. Using proper infection control methods prevents or stops the spread of infections.[14] It is of utmost importance that OTAs use universal precautions when delivering care to others. Universal precautions begin with proper hand hygiene, before, during, and after providing care. It also includes ensuring one covers their cough or sneeze to prevent microbes from spreading through the air, and ensuring that all items used in the delivery of care are either single-use items or cleaned with appropriate cleansers/techniques between uses.[14]

Inpatient Medical Facilities

Universal precautions should be used in each patient encounter. In an inpatient medical setting, this means performing hand hygiene (soap/water wash or alcohol-based cleanser) followed by donning disposable gloves before touching the patient or anything in the patient's room.[14] Upon exiting, the OTA would doff the gloves and again clean their hands before beginning the next task. The OTA may also encounter patient on various forms of isolation precautions (contact, airborne, droplet, etc.). The type of isolation encountered determines the additional steps that OTA must take to ensure both their own safety and the safety of the patient being treated. These additional precautions include adding additional personal protective equipment (PPE) such as gowns, gloves, booties, hair covering, goggles, face shields, and various types of face masks. It may also include the order in which PPE is donned and doffed as well as any activities or equipment that are further regulated due to the isolation. Signs should be posted outside the isolation areas with instructions regarding the type of isolation as well as the required PPE in use to enter the isolation area. If an OTA is unsure how to properly follow isolation precautions and/or use the PPE, they should seek further instruction from the Infection Control Coordinator at their facility before entering the isolation area.

Home-Based Care

An OTA should expect to use universal precautions whenever they are treating a client in the home.[14] This again includes hand hygiene regimens and glove use. An added burden when providing OT services in a home is the additional universal precaution of providing a barrier between the items you bring into the home and the surface(s) in the home—including one's shoes. OTAs working in home health are expected to provide their own hand hygiene supplies, disposable gloves, and shoe covers, as well as disposable barrier sheets to place on surfaces prior to setting bags, computers, or equipment down in a patient's home. All equipment brought into the patient's home must also be sanitized upon leaving the patient's home and before it can be used again.

OTAs also should expect to provide education on standard precautions to any caregivers present in the home caring for the patient. It is not uncommon for patients to be discharged from inpatient settings to home while still needing to follow isolation precautions. The OTA must know the precautions required to enter the home and should think critically about any materials brought into the home; all items in a medical bag would then have been considered to be exposed to the microbes being isolated. OTAs seeing patients on home isolation may also need to educate the patient and in-home caregivers regarding how to best provide care and adhere to isolation precautions for the safety of all involved parties. This may include developing a hand hygiene regimen, designating specific restrooms, and incorporating enhanced cleaning procedures that are uncommon to people living in a home together as a family unit. The Center for Disease Control and Prevention is a great resource for infection control basics. The CDC website includes a variety of training handouts and videos that can be used across all skill levels.[14]

ISSUES RELATED TO CERTIFIED OCCUPATIONAL THERAPY ASSISTANT PRACTICE

Overuse and underuse of OTAs in the workplace may occur. OTAs may be underused when employers, as well as supervising OTs, do not understand an OTA's degree of skill and knowledge. Restricting an OTA to tasks below his or her skill level, such as those performed by a restorative aide, does not allow OTAs to work to their greatest potential. Tasks such as transporting and scheduling patients, keeping inventory of bath equipment, and assisting patients to eat meals do not reflect the greater knowledge and skills that OTAs acquire during their education. OTAs are underused when they are not permitted to fully contribute when delivering occupational therapy services. OTAs are qualified to provide safe and effective occupational therapy services under the supervision of and in partnership with an OT, including conducting assessments and reporting observations; selecting, implementing, and modifying therapeutic interventions; and contributing to the transition/discharge process.[10]

Overuse may occur when OTAs are asked to contribute beyond the scope of their competency and qualifications. Accepting referrals, conducting initial occupational therapy evaluations, and interpreting data are examples of tasks that OTs are normally required to complete.[10] In some instances, overuse may occur when OTAs are encouraged to take on tasks beyond the legal and ethical scope of practice. For example, an OT may say, "I don't have time to see the client. Why don't you start the initial evaluation?" In other instances, OTAs may be asked to perform these tasks when there is inadequate supervision or there are not enough practitioners to provide occupational therapy services. For example, the facility administrator may ask the OTA to complete the discharge summaries because he or she wants to employ an OT only 4 hours a week. In these cases, the OTA must advocate for proper use of OTAs and discuss the issues with the OT and others who need to understand the legal, ethical, and professional responsibilities of an OTA/OT partnership.

OCCUPATIONAL THERAPY ASSISTANTS WORKING WITH OLDER ADULTS IN VARIOUS SETTINGS

During the class reunion, Chris, the OTA Instructor for the Adulthood and Aging course, invited graduates to share their work experiences with the OTA students during a series of class presentations. She was particularly interested in graduates who worked in traditional and emerging practice settings. A synopsis of each of the presentations is presented and integrates concepts from the OTPF-4.[1]

Geropsychiatric Unit

Marta has worked at a 15-bed geropsychiatric unit in a small urban town for 7 years where she enjoys working with older adults admitted with varied psychiatric diagnoses such as dementia, bipolar disorder, and schizophrenia. Although most older adults are admitted directly from their homes, typically for behaviors with which their family members can no longer cope, such as aggression and confusion, Marta does not let these behaviors become the focus of her practice. Instead, she views each older adult as a unique occupational being, focusing on those daily life activities and occupations of priority and concern to the older adult and their family members. Marta recently worked with one older adult, José, a 62-year-old former migrant farm worker, born and raised in Mexico, who was admitted to the unit with suspected early-onset dementia. After she and Noel, the OT with whom she collaborates, discussed the information from José's occupational profile, they realized that José no longer walked to and visited with friends within the local LatinX community, one of his most meaningful occupations. José's family had become increasingly concerned about his memory loss and confusion and was afraid to let him leave the house for fear he would become lost or have an accident. Furthermore, they wanted to preserve José's dignity and did not want his friends and acquaintances to know about his increasing confusion and memory loss. Although José was admitted to the unit for suspected early-onset dementia, Marta viewed José as an occupational being who was experiencing the loss of meaningful occupations rather than as a confused man who was becoming a burden to his family.

With Marta's 9 years of experience as an OTA, the staff relies on her judgment to identify those daily activities and occupations in which older adult patients can successfully engage and which aspects of their daily routine present additional challenges and require support and assistance. Marta said that the older adults "often look okay and say that they don't have any problems, but the reality is they can get into trouble carrying out simple daily life tasks, if they chose to do them at all." To restore and maintain more successful engagement in routine activities, Marta relies on her skill to analyze an older adult's performance of activities and occupations, identifying those factors that support or hinder the older adult's successful engagement. Although Noel, the OT, works with the older adults during the morning, Marta works from 2:30 p.m. to 8:00 p.m. during the week, providing her with opportunities to observe older adults during their early evening routine of eating dinner, undressing, bathing, toileting, and preparing for bed because performance patterns are important to support successful engagement in activities.[15] Marta works closely with families and staff to establish consistent routines and habits for older adults on the ward, focusing on creating a physical and social environment that promotes success and decreases confusion. With José, she and Noel worked closely with his family so they could create a routine of activities and meaningful occupations when he returned home to help reduce José's confusion and his verbal outbursts.

Because Marta begins her workday at 2:30 p.m. and Noel ends his at 4:30 p.m., they have little scheduled time for consultation and supervision. Both agree, though, that this time is essential, not only to meet state regulatory requirements but also to ensure that patients receive quality occupational therapy intervention. After her meeting with Noel, Marta leads group activities at 3:30 in the afternoon. Depending on the needs of the group of older adults at any one time, Marta will lead groups that focus on life skills, such as crafts and cooking groups. Because of the older adults' short stay on the unit, often less than 2 weeks, Marta finds that engaging them in activities that are familiar and not too challenging helps them to make sense of their daily life in the unit. Marta particularly enjoys leading the reminiscence group activity where she engages older adults with the use of familiar scents, pictures, and objects, encouraging them to interact and share their personal stories. The gardening group activity is particularly enjoyable because Marta can adjust the challenge of the activity to each older adult's capability. For those older adults who experience difficulty potting a plant on their own, Marta decreases the activity demands, such as asking an older adult to help scoop dirt out of the bag or hold a pot while someone else scoops in the dirt. For others, merely sitting at the table and smelling the flowers is enough of a challenge. Those older adults who are more able can choose what they would like to plant and carry out the process more independently, often sharing their own gardening expertise with Marta and other older adults. No matter what capacity an older adult may possess, Marta always ensures that all older adults have a potted plant at the end of the group activity that they can give to a family member or friend during evening visits.

After leading groups in the afternoon and completing her notes on each older adult's participation, Marta works with the unit staff during the evening dinner hour, observing each older adult's ability to eat meals. Because Marta successfully achieved the AOTA Specialty Certification in Feeding, Eating, and Swallowing,[16] and she and Noel have agreed she has achieved service competency to manage eating and feeding problems with older adults on the unit, Marta is responsible for identifying successful strategies to encourage older adults to eat their meals and conveys those strategies to staff members for all meals and snacks. As needed, she will suggest and monitor the use of adaptive equipment. Although it can be challenging at times, Marta also works to create a pleasant and supportive environment during the dinner hour in which older adults can successfully interact with family members when they choose to visit.

Because Marta works a later shift, she is responsible for meeting with family members and educating them not only about their older adult's diagnosis but also about what level of care is currently required. She is particularly adept at identifying what aspects of activities each older adult can do on his or her own and what aspects with which he or she requires assistance. Occasionally, family members may want to protect and help the older adult too much, therefore, Marta works with them to preserve the older adult's independence and dignity while teaching family members to provide the right amount of support.

Although Marta relies primarily on informal observation to gather important information about the older adults, she occasionally administers the Allen Cognitive Level screening tool[17] for which she has established service competency. Although Noel interprets the results, together they share the information with other team members. This information is useful because it provides insight into an older adult's cognitive abilities and his or her capacities in specific tasks or groups. Most of the time, though, Marta relies on her activity analysis skills to analyze an older adult's performance of activities during groups and their evening routine. These informal observations provide her with the valuable information that she needs to help the older adults and their family members plan to return to their own homes.

Inpatient Rehabilitation

After graduating from Blue Lake Community College 5 years ago, Rachel moved to a large metropolitan city and began full-time work at an inpatient rehabilitation facility. She and Beth, the OT with whom she works, share a caseload of 12 patients, the majority of whom are older adults who have experienced a cerebrovascular accident (CVA). Rachel, who does not consider herself a "morning" person, nonetheless arrives at work Monday through Friday at 7:30 a.m. She starts her day working with patients in their rooms, assisting them to achieve greater independence and satisfaction with their morning ADLs, such as eating, grooming, dressing, toileting, and bathing (Fig. 8.1). One of her favorite older adults was Glen, with whom she worked after he experienced a CVA. When Rachel was assisting Glen in the mornings to get ready for the day, Glen would become frustrated because he could never find his hearing aid. One day it would be in the drawer under his clothes and the next it would be under the bed sheets. Rachel communicated with the evening nursing staff to ensure that Glen always put his hearing aid in the top right drawer before he went to bed. Although this seemed like such a small thing to do, Glen was much happier each morning because he could easily locate his hearing aid. Rachel works to establish routines for older adults on the ward, recognizing that establishing performance patterns is particularly

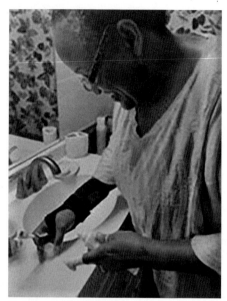

FIG. 8.1 Occupational therapy assistants work with those personal activities of importance to the older adult. *(Courtesy Mia Marrow)*

important for older adults when they are away from their usual home environment.

During the initial OT evaluation conducted by Beth, the OTR, Glen raised a concern that he did not want to be a burden on his wife when he returned home. During Glen's short 12-day admission, Rachel worked diligently to ensure that Glen's wife would be comfortable and safe assisting Glen at home. Thus, although independence with toileting, dressing, and bathing was not the ultimate goal, during Glen's morning routine, Rachel and Beth focused on developing Glen's performance skills so it would be easier for both Glen and his wife when Glen returned home. Although Glen was not pulling up his pants on his own by discharge, Rachel worked out a system whereby Glen was able to stand upright on his own and safely stabilize himself on a solid counter while his wife pulled up and fastened his pants for him.

After morning ADLs and during the remainder of the day, Rachel and Beth work together to help the older adults reach their goals, collaborating to share the responsibility for gathering initial evaluation information, implementing intervention, and evaluating outcomes. During her level II fieldwork, Rachel had observed her supervisor administer the COPM,[13] although Rachel had never done it herself. Because the COPM is an open-ended interview requiring the OT practitioner to solicit the occupational performance issues of concern to the client, Rachel and Beth developed a plan for Rachel to become comfortable and achieve service competency to administer the COPM and other standardized assessments.

When Rachel interviewed Glen using the COPM,[13] Glen identified that he still wanted to be able to take care of his 5-year-old grandson Braden because Glen and his wife provide child care 3 days a week. Because this was a priority for Glen, the afternoon occupational therapy sessions were devoted to help Glen develop the performance skills needed for Glen to play catch and read story books with Braden. Rachel worked with Glen to develop the specific motor skills necessary to play catch, such as bending and reaching for a ball on the ground and grasping and lifting the ball with his affected arm and hand. Rachel also worked with Glen on skills necessary to read story books, such as manipulating the pages and coordinating his affected arm with his other arm to hold the book. On the basis of the occupational profile completed during the initial evaluation, Rachel knew that Glen enjoyed challenging physical activities because he considered himself a sportsman. She particularly enjoyed working with Glen to identify various physical activities, both within the Occupational Therapy department and outside of the hospital, which would further develop his motor skills to help him reach his personal goals. Rachel was able to draw on Glen's strengths, specifically his relatively good communication, social, and cognitive skills, to help Glen improve his ability to perform daily life activities.

An important aspect of Rachel's work, although not her favorite, is documentation. To demonstrate the need for occupational therapy intervention, Rachel and Beth have worked together to develop their documentation skills. They have attended conference workshops and met with local insurance representatives to explain the focus of occupational therapy and to understand the insurance representative's point of view. Rachel and Beth share responsibility to write progress notes for their caseload. Although the OT is ultimately responsible for documenting outcomes,[15] Rachel contributes to the process, sharing her understanding of what has occurred during intervention. Because Beth and Rachel agree it is important that clients also express their views regarding their progress, Rachel often re-administers the COPM[13] before discharge. Although Glen did not make much progress with his morning ADLs in terms of physical independence, the use of the COPM revealed that he was more satisfied with his performance because he believed that he was no longer as much of a burden to his wife. Although he did not believe he was entirely able to take care of his grandson, he felt he was far better than when admitted to the rehabilitation unit. By using a standardized assessment such as the COPM, Rachel and Beth have more credible evidence to document an older adult's progress and communicate the outcomes and benefit of occupational therapy services to help older adults achieve their personal goals.

Adult Foster Home

After graduating 2 years ago, Arianna reflected about what aspects of occupational therapy practice she liked. She decided she liked working with older adults and particularly enjoyed group activities. Because she had the opportunity during her professional education to explore settings that were not based on a medical model, Arianna also recognized that she preferred more nontraditional settings. During her course on adulthood and aging, she spent time at a local senior center where she helped with an exercise program for people with arthritis. Through this experience, she became a certified instructor in exercise and aquatics, which qualified her to teach exercise classes and swim classes.[18] Moreover, a portion of her fieldwork was spent at an assisted living center where she spent time running groups with the activity director. She was able to incorporate the skills and knowledge she learned in her OTA classes, such as designing and organizing groups, leadership strategies, group dynamics, and stages of group process, as well as meeting the individual needs of the group participants.

Arianna noticed an adult foster home in her neighborhood and approached the owners, Elizabeth and Danny, about providing group activities for the older adults. Arianna knew, per state regulations where she lived, that adult foster homes are required to provide 6 hours of activities a week for each resident, not including television and movies. Because the state requires the activities to be of interest and meet each older adult's abilities, her OTA skills to identify, adapt, and implement appropriate activities for older adults were exactly what the owners needed. Arianna talked about her experience working with older adults and her abilities to develop and lead group activities. She explained to the owners that, although she was an OTA, the services she would provide would not be considered occupational therapy. She would use expertise that did not require OT supervision, such as making sure that older adults were seated securely with their feet flat on the floor and using activities that incorporated full range of motion. Elizabeth and Danny were interested because they had been trying to provide activities without any outside help. After clarifying her intent with the state licensing board, Arianna began working, providing[2] half days of activity programming and consultation per week.

Most of the seven older adults at the adult foster home were ambulatory; only one older adult used a wheelchair. Anthony and Florence were legally blind, Maria had a severe hearing loss, Alfred used oxygen 24 hours a day for his chronic obstructive pulmonary disease, Herbert had Parkinson's disease, and Leona and Alfonso had mild dementia. Arianna met with each older adult individually to get to know them and identify their interests. She used her OTA skills to develop a profile that noted each older adult's interests and dislikes, as well as information related to medical needs, such as dietary restrictions, allergies, and "do not resuscitate" status. She also developed a form to document the type of group activity, the length of time each older adult participated, the degree of participation, how each older adult responded during the activity, and whether he or she declined to participate that day. This form was left at the adult foster home at the end of the month for the owners and served the purpose of documenting participation, as well as a time sheet for her hours worked. The owners employed other people, so a payroll tax system was already in place. Because Arianna's husband's employer provided health insurance coverage for spouses, she was fortunate in not having to worry about health insurance benefits.

To provide a solid basis when designing group activities, Arianna organized and implemented a variety of activities, following Howe and Schwartzberg's[19] guidelines for group process. Arianna began each group with small talk, encouraging each resident to discuss current events. Arianna would then incorporate warm-up activities to encourage movement, such as telling a story with the older adults acting out the movements. Activities such as marching in a parade or playing balloon volleyball were popular with the older adults. Then the main activities would follow, focusing on those activities of interest to the older adults, such as preparing the salad for the evening meal, planting herbs in pots, making place mats for holiday meals, and learning new card games. Each group activity closed by asking the older adults to help plan future activities.

As with well-designed groups, the older adults would often direct the activities themselves. For example, while making strawberry shortcake, Leona began reminiscing about growing up in an area where there were many berry farms. She lamented that a community college and housing development now occupy the former berry fields. Others joined in and talked about how they had to pick berries to earn money to buy their school clothes. Despite her memory loss, Leona shared her mother's favorite jam recipe and asked if the group could make the jam at the next meeting. During another activity, Florence shared how she used to enjoy playing bingo but is currently not able to get out to games and cannot see the cards well enough to play. Arianna took note and another activity was designed where the older adults made bingo cards with large black numbers so that everyone could see and participate. Arianna also purchased poker chips to cover the numbers because Herbert had trouble picking up small disks. The older adults' favorite activities, though, were ones that included cooking or baking. They took pride in preparing meals and inviting family members. Even Alfred, who "never cooked a meal in his life," participated and took pride in telling his daughter that he made the cornbread by himself (even though he did require some help). During the majority of the time, Arianna planned activities for all residents to participate. She also made sure that, when an older adult did not want to participate in group activities, she would offer alternative solitary activities.

Not all of the activities were confined to the foster home. The owners had a van and would occasionally take the older adults to eat at local restaurants because they enjoyed getting out and eating their favorite foods. On those occasions when Arianna accompanied them, she sat close to Florence and Anthony, both legally blind, and

suggested that they orient the food on their plate like a clock. Elizabeth took note and followed through with this suggestion at home with the older adults. She reported that both Florence and Anthony were much happier with not needing someone to hover over them during meals. Arianna also suggested a weighted cup for Herbert and provided the phone number of a local vendor. As Arianna became more familiar with the residents, she suggested other community outings such as a trip to a lilac garden, a drive to see Christmas lights, a picnic in the park, and attending local music events at the senior center.

After working at the foster home for 3 months, Arianna expanded her services to other local adult foster homes. The owners were happy with her services and passed along Arianna's business card to other adult foster home owners. Arianna now provides group activities to five foster homes and hopes to find another OTA who is interested in this work, to expand the business. Moreover, with senior centers becoming an emerging practice setting for OT practitioners,[20] Arianna is considering approaching the local senior centers to discuss the development of educational programs. She wants to again contact her state licensing board, however, to understand the parameters under which she can provide health promotion services while also licensed as an OTA.

Skilled Nursing Facility

After graduating 1 year ago, Drew moved to a rural city of 30,000 people and now works full time at a SNF. At the reunion, he shared that, although he is frustrated at times with the facility rules and insurance regulations, he enjoys working with family members to help older adults return home as soon as possible. He shared, "It's tough working toward discharge right away, but then you realize most people's priorities are to get home as soon as they can." Drew primarily sees older adults with CVA, as well as those with hip fractures and recent surgeries. Many have secondary health conditions, such as high blood pressure, diabetes, or pneumonia.

Drew particularly enjoys working with older adults and their families to figure out the best way to manage ADLs at home, including the need for adaptive equipment; thus, the primary intervention approaches he uses with older adults are restore and modify. One of the most problematic issues for older adults leaving the SNF is toileting and bathing at home. Drew particularly prides himself on his ability to analyze each older adult's performance. When observing an older adult on the ward, Drew recognizes that the older adult's home environment may be very different from the accessible and well-equipped rooms at the SNF. For example, he recently worked with Clarence, an older adult who was admitted with a severe case of pneumonia and long-standing arthritis. Clarence and his partner were concerned about Clarence still being able to get in and out of his bathtub and soak in the warm water to relieve his arthritic pain.

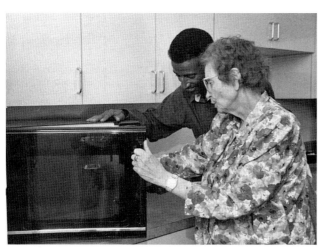

FIG. 8.2 Instrumental activities of daily living are often important for older adults for when they return home.

As best he could in the training bathroom, Drew re-created the layout of Clarence's bathroom at home. He then observed Clarence's partner assisting Clarence to get in and out of the tub. After they tried out different methods, Drew identified the safest and least painful transfer method, which they practiced until Clarence and his partner felt confident. Drew also identified which specific equipment would best meet their needs at home. This was particularly important because many older adults may not start home health immediately after discharge from the SNF, and all necessary equipment needs to be in place before their departure.

Although a main focus of the SNF is promoting independence with ADLs, Drew also addresses other roles that are important to the older adult (Fig. 8.2). Because Clarence was a retired veterinary technician, he was also concerned that he could not take care of his many birds at home. Drew worked with Clarence and his partner to figure how Clarence could safely stand and easily reach while feeding and watering the birds and cleaning the cages. Drew also arranged with the staff for Clarence to play with the resident dog and cat as often as possible when he was not scheduled for therapy. Because Clarence also sang in the church choir, Drew worked with Clarence and his partner to develop a plan so that Clarence could conserve enough energy to attend church twice a week.

In addition to his direct work with the older adults, Drew has additional responsibilities. He participates in the weekly team meetings, sharing the reporting responsibilities with Sheryl, the OT. Drew and Sheryl collaborate to leave clear instructions for Brooke, the OTA who works weekends. Drew also spends part of his time working with restorative aides, ensuring that they can follow through with intervention plans. Drew and Sheryl agree that he would assume the primary responsibility to be aware of current regulatory and reimbursement issues related to SNF (see Chapter 6) and share the information with Sheryl and Brooke.

Assisted Living Facility

Jean has been an OTA for 17 years. After graduating, she took a job at a local rehabilitation hospital and worked mainly with adults experiencing neurological disorders. She enjoyed the work, but, because of budgetary problems, her position was eliminated. She then worked at a large long-term care facility where her level of responsibilities increased over time. Having established service competency with the occupational therapy evaluation and intervention methods used at the facility, she worked fairly autonomously with occasional OT supervision. Four years ago, Jean returned to school on a part-time basis to complete her bachelor's degree in health care administration. As Jean was learning management skills, she decided to apply for a position as the director of the rehab department. Given her competency as an OTA and her current interest and skills in management, she was offered the position. Jean was now responsible for running the department, including scheduling therapy, coordinating the training and supervision of the employees, and maintaining communication between Rehab Services and the other services offered at the facility.

After graduation and the completion of her business degree, she began to seriously consider her future. She enjoyed the management skills that she had learned and developed over the past few years as the Rehab Director. She was not sure that remaining in her current position would allow her to grow further so she began looking at other possibilities. First, Jean compiled a list of her abilities that she could bring to the job. She tried to be as realistic as possible and asked for assistance from her husband, parents, and friends who knew her professionally. She felt that she had good supervisory, interpersonal, verbal, and written communication skills. Finally, she was familiar with health care and rehabilitation in particular. However, her challenges were that she had limited experience in marketing, operations management beyond the rehab department, and budgeting.

At first, Jean looked for jobs related to occupational therapy, rehabilitation, and health care delivery and was discouraged by what she had found. Then, she expanded her search after talking with her neighbor, whose mother was living in an assisted living facility (ALF). Jean searched the internet for information about ALFs and found the website for a corporation that operated a number of facilities in her area. She learned that there were three categories of positions: activities coordinator, executive administrator, and resident services coordinator.

Jean downloaded the three job descriptions and compared them to her list of abilities. The first job description that Jean reviewed was for activities coordinator (Table 8.3). Jean believed that this job was not challenging enough. Moreover, according to state regulations, if a

TABLE 8.3

Activities Coordinator Job Description

Job position	Activities coordinator
Primary purpose	This person is responsible for the development and coordination of individual activity programming for each resident. Responsibilities include planning and coordinating appropriate resident activities, day-to-day operations, supervising staff, and ensuring program quality.
Qualifications/skills needed	Prefer an individual with a minimum of 2 years geriatric experience. Experience working with people with Alzheimer's disease/dementia is essential. Experience in staffing and managing the day-to-day operations is preferred. Must demonstrate good interpersonal skills and excellent written and verbal communication. Reports to resident services coordinator.

TABLE 8.4

Executive Administrator Job Description

Job position	Executive administrator
Primary purpose	This person is responsible for the creation of resident-focused work teams that support the philosophy of partnering with families. Responsibilities include staffing, training, program implementation, budgeting, sales, marketing, and community relations.
Qualifications/skills needed	Prior experience managing senior resident services is required along with a bachelor's degree. Experience in marketing, operations management, and budgeting is essential. Strong leadership skills, including organization and interpersonal skills, are a must. Excellent verbal and written communication skills required, as well as computer experience. Occasional travel required.

TABLE 8.5

Resident Services Coordinator Job Description

Job position	Resident services coordinator
Primary purpose	This person is responsible for overseeing the delivery of resident services and supervising the resident assistant staff. As a member of the management team, responsibilities include supervising unit teams, staff development, and monitoring quality of resident service and staff recruitment. Reports to executive administrator.
Qualifications/skills needed	Person should possess a bachelor's degree in a health-related field. Five years of experience in senior resident services, including staff supervision, is required. Excellent organizational and interpersonal skills are a must. Strong verbal and written communication skills are essential. Computer proficiency is strongly preferred.

perception existed that she was providing direct occupational therapy services, she would require OT supervision. She also felt that the activities coordinator position was not the type of job that interested her enough to leave her current position at the long-term care facility.

The next position that she reviewed was for executive administrator (Table 8.4). Jean compared the job expectations with her abilities and realized that she was lacking in several categories. Although she had experience managing a small department, she lacked the marketing, budgeting, and operational management background required for this position.

The final job description Jean reviewed was for resident services coordinator (Table 8.5). Jean studied the job description and compared it with her list of abilities. Because she believed that this was the right position, Jean contacted the assisted living corporation and requested an application. She applied and was contacted for an interview. Before the interview, Jean wanted to clarify that the services she would provide in the resident services coordinator position were not those of an OTA requiring OT supervision. She contacted her state's Occupational Therapy Licensure Board and asked them to review the job description. On careful review, the Board determined the following: (1) Her status as an OTA in this position did not violate state laws and regulations; (2) although the position oversaw the coordination of programs, including occupational therapy, it did not require Jean to perform hands-on intervention; and (3) Jean could use her OTA initials after her name as long as it was understood that she could not provide any occupational therapy services without the supervision of an OT.

Meanwhile, Jean prepared for the interview by identifying the major points she wanted to emphasize. First, she wanted to stress her belief in the importance of addressing the older adults' needs, including physical, social, emotional, cognitive, and spiritual needs, and how this belief would guide staff recruitment and development, both of which were part of the position description. Second, she wanted to demonstrate how she would coordinate the services in a manner that supported the corporation's philosophy of partnering with families. Third, she wanted to show that her background as an OTA brought a unique perspective on quality of life for older adults. She located information that identified that life satisfaction is multifaceted[21] for older adults and that the manner in which older adults occupy their time contributes to their health, well-being, and quality of life.[21,22]

During the interview, Jean did well and was offered the position. Since then, she has been working with the new executive administrator, assisting with recruitment and development of the resident service teams. One of the first tasks she undertook was to develop a screening tool to identify the physical, social, emotional, cognitive, and spiritual needs of the residents. Her goal was to match the services with the identified needs and eventually demonstrate how the residents' overall needs were being met.

Home Health Agency

Manisha recently changed jobs after working 9 years in an acute care hospital, when she obtained a job at a home health agency within a major metropolitan city. Because Manisha used only public transportation before getting the new job, she needed to purchase her first car, one that was spacious enough to carry needed equipment and supplies. Furthermore, Manisha needed to brush up on her navigation skills because her new supervisor emphasized that she would be traveling extensively, often up to 80 miles a day. The agency she now worked for had recently converted to a computer-based documentation system, so Manisha signed up for a computer course at a local community college. An important issue emphasized during her interview was client confidentiality. Although Manisha was aware of this issue from her work in acute care, Manisha would be visiting many older adults during the day, carrying the required documentation from house to house, and would need to take extra care to ensure that that information was kept confidential during her visits.

During her first few weeks on the job, she traveled with different team members, including nurses, physical therapists and physical therapist assistants, social workers, nutritionists, and home health aides. During these visits, Manisha was surprised by how different things were in the older adults' home environment than what she imagined when she worked in acute care. Sometimes, solutions that

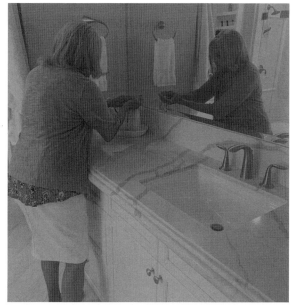

FIG. 8.3 An older adult's home provides many opportunities to problem solve and work on practical skills. *(Courtesy Fitz Johnson)*

were proposed in the hospital (similar to those proposed by Manisha when she worked there) turned out to be impractical, or the older adults just did not want to use them. Recognizing this, Manisha was excited to be working with older adults in their own homes where she could assist them to achieve their goals within their familiar home environment, focusing on practical solutions in context (Fig. 8.3). Manisha looked forward to working with older adults and their caregivers to achieve their goals, such as getting out in the back garden on their own, emptying the trash, getting the mail, operating the radio, or using the telephone to reorder prescription medications.

One older adult, Irene, had lived by herself in a one-room apartment and was getting along fairly well despite her legal blindness. Irene recently broke her foot while getting off a high stool in her kitchen. After receiving the doctor's referral, Antonio, the OT with whom Manisha worked, completed the initial evaluation. Antonio shared the initial evaluation results and developed the intervention plan with Manisha, stressing that her input was important to monitor the effectiveness of the plan. Manisha then assumed primary responsibility for implementing the intervention plan and monitoring the achievement of outcomes. Although Manisha would be on her own visiting Irene over the next month, Manisha would consult as needed with Antonio when they were both in the office in the morning. Furthermore, she frequently communicated with him, as well as with Irene's social worker and physical therapist, through cell phone calls throughout the month.

One of Irene's first priorities was to prepare her own meals rather than rely on the Meals on Wheels initially organized by the social worker. Although it was important to Irene that she prepare her own meals, she did not want to spend a lot of time doing so. After Manisha's first visit, Irene searched for recipes that would be easy to prepare, nutritious, and Manisha arranged for her neighbor to purchase the necessary ingredients. During the next visit, Manisha and Irene problem-solved how to safely prepare simple meals that would not compromise her fractured foot, such as safely using a low chair and safely maneuvering within the kitchen. To make it easier to transport items, Manisha also arranged for Irene to purchase a basket for her walker and to practice safely carrying her recycling items and trash down the hallway.

Because Irene was a volunteer at the blind commission, it was important for her to be able to use public transportation as soon as possible to return to her monthly meetings. Although Irene's home visits would end as soon as she became more mobile, she and Manisha problem-solved how best to manage her walker while using the bus. They practiced skills such as managing doors, stepping up and down different levels while using the walker, and folding up her walker once she was seated. Another priority of Irene's was to plan and be able to execute an emergency exit from her third-floor apartment. She and Manisha developed a plan with Irene's neighbors to deal with different types of emergencies. For some situations, a buddy system would be used; for other situations, Irene could make the necessary arrangements through a telephone call.

Because Irene's broken foot presented additional challenges to safely maneuver within her apartment, Manisha and Irene worked together to rearrange her living and dining room to make it easier and safer for her to listen to the radio and audio books, as well as use her computer. Although Manisha works most of the time with individual older adults, such as Irene, on occasion she is called in to an adult foster home to recommend environmental modifications. For example, she has recommended suitable bath and toilet equipment and more appropriate furniture arrangement to prevent falls. Manisha understands the significant meaning that home has for many older adults,[21] and so when recommending environment modifications, she always considers the older adults' viewpoints.

Manisha enjoys working in home health because it provides a lot of variety. She visits four to five people a day, the majority of whom are older adults. Because she visits older adults in their own homes, Manisha is particularly sensitive to the fact that she is a guest, respecting the older adults' privacy and following their lead to establish intervention priorities. This includes collaborating with older adults and their families/caregivers when determining the best approach to achieve their priorities safely (see Chapter 11). Because Manisha is skilled with body mechanics and safety concerns/issues, she is responsible for home health aide staff training, providing them with information and skills to safely assist older adults (e.g., while toileting, dressing, and bathing).

One of the most important skills that Manisha brings to this particular job is that of observation. Because she has been the primary practitioner working with the older adult, Manisha must provide accurate information to the OT. Often, detailed information is required per regulatory and facility guidelines.[4] In Irene's case, to complete the discharge summary, Manisha needed to provide information to Antonio, not only about Irene's ADL status but also about factors such as Irene's ability to accurately express herself, whether any sanitation hazards were present in the home, which social supports she consistently relied on, and whether she was capable of making safe decisions.

Free Standing Hospice

When Amanda graduated from Blue Lake Community College 14 years ago, her children were toddlers. To balance her work and family life, she chose to work on-call 2–3 days a week at various local SNFs, which she continues to do. For the past 10 years, she has volunteered at Riverview House, an independently owned hospice that provides end-of-life care for individuals who cannot receive services at home. Amanda appreciates the approach at Riverview House where staff and volunteers focus on enhancing a person's quality of life, paying equal attention to the spiritual, emotional, and physical aspects of life. The pace at Riverview House is unhurried with an emphasis on quality time until death. Amanda finds great personal reward in her volunteer work.

Almost 2 years ago, Amanda faced the prospective of death in her own family. Her favorite aunt, Paula, was diagnosed with ovarian cancer and expressed a wish to stay at home. Amanda decided that she could help fulfill her aunt's wish. Her volunteer experience at Riverview House, as well as her OTA experience working in SNFs, provided her with the capacity to feel comfortable with terminally ill individuals and the ability to cope with loss. Moreover, having attended an in-service at Riverview Hospice that emphasized strategies to prevent burnout in hospice personnel,[23] Amanda knew that it was important to maintain her physical well-being, engage in hobbies and interests, take time away from her caregiving, talk with others, and engage in meaningful activities. Amanda arranged for her daughter and niece to provide respite care several times a week so she could spend time with her partner and friends and go to the gym. She and her partner also spent time each week engaged in contemplative activities, walking the labyrinth at a nearby Buddhist retreat and meditating at the local church.

Although Amanda previously experienced the challenges and responsibilities of caring for dying persons, she soon found herself physically and emotionally drained. She was distraught as her aunt experienced a loss of control, diminished ability to engage in her favored daily activities, in addition to physical and emotional pain. As her aunt's condition worsened, home care hospice services were formally instituted. Although a substantial commitment, Amanda decided she wanted to continue as her aunt's primary, live-in caregiver, a usual requirement for home-based hospice services. She also decided to attend a caregivers' support group at the local hospital to help cope with such a challenging, emotional endeavor. Aunt Paula lived long enough to attend the college graduation of her great-grandson and died at home with family by her side.

After her aunt died, Amanda spent time recuperating, re-engaging in projects she had put on hold during the 8 months she cared for her aunt and taking a month-long vacation with a close friend. When she returned, she contacted the director at Riverview Hospice to initiate discussions about the potential inclusion of occupational therapy services. Because the director was familiar with Amanda's volunteer work, she was happy to meet and discuss her ideas. Amanda shared how the philosophy and approach of hospice were very compatible with those of occupational therapy.[24] She then shared her vision of how occupational therapy services might further enhance hospice care.

Amanda emphasized the skills that occupational therapy practitioners possess to facilitate participation in daily activities that people find meaningful, such as cooking simple meals, engaging in art projects, and writing in journals. Amanda then shared one of her volunteer experiences. She was with Joe, an older adult who previously enjoyed fishing and camping and who was complaining that there was nothing he could do now. Amanda gently suggested that Joe might consider barbecuing a trout for the staff at Riverview House; he agreed and contacted his wife to bring in his secret spices to prepare the trout. Meanwhile, Amanda planned with staff to make it easier for Joe to safely use the backyard barbecue. Connecting to his love of fishing and camping through the simple preparation of a barbecued trout provided Joe with a sense of self and connected his current self to his past life.

Amanda went on to explain that occupational therapy practitioners work with individuals throughout the life span, with death and dying being one phase among many. Amanda discussed her experience with Vivian, a lively woman with a sense of humor and quick wit. Vivian enjoyed being with others, especially her family. When she was diagnosed with terminal breast cancer, she decided to move from another state to be near her family of four generations. She would live at Riverview Hospice until her death, where her care could be provided without being a burden to her family, a point she was emphatic about. Vivian was thrilled to be near her 3-year-old great-grandson with whom she shared a special bond (Fig. 8.4). She looked forward to his daily visits but soon found herself exhausted and in pain by the time he usually arrived in midafternoon. Amanda suggested whether it might be possible for Vivian's family to arrange for her great-grandson to arrive during lunch, where they could eat together and cuddle afterward during a nap. Moreover, Amanda suggested that Vivian listen to some relaxation tapes just

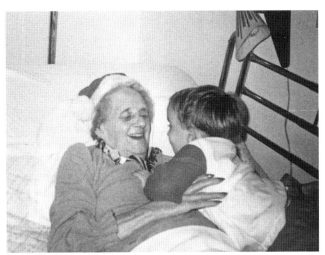

FIG. 8.4 A special bond existed between Vivian and her 3-year-old great-grandson.*(Courtesy Sue Byers-Connon)*

before lunch to help alleviate her pain before her great-grandson arrived. Amanda explained that it was important to not only schedule rest periods but also to consider when to schedule valued activities throughout the day.

Amanda went on to explain that occupational therapy practitioners are committed to facilitating the process of enhancing the quality of life of individuals and that they have particular expertise to modify a person's performance so that he or she can engage in desired activities. She shared the story of Cora, who was experiencing end-stage congestive heart failure and neuropathy in her fingers, making it difficult for her to hold eating utensils. Amanda knew that changing the silverware would make it easier for Cora to eat, but she also understood the enjoyment that eating meals with others can bring. The next week she brought in some silverware with sticky handgrips (which still looked normal) and asked if she could join Cora for lunch in her room. She showed the silverware to Cora and asked if she would like to give them a go. Cora agreed and found eating a bit easier; however, she still chose to eat in her room. A few weeks later, Amanda gently asked if Cora would join her in the dining room for lunch. Cora agreed, and when lunch was over, asked if Amanda would come back next week when Amanda returned the following week, she discovered that Cora had been eating her meals in the dining room. Because Amanda gradually modified Cora's engagement, Cora was able to enjoy her meals, socializing with other residents and family members in the dining room.

The director was impressed with Amanda's understanding of the compatibility of occupational therapy with the practice of hospice and realized that other professional practitioners exist who bring important skills that support the hospice philosophy. Amanda and the director agreed to continue meeting and discuss the possibility of instituting formal occupational therapy services at Riverview House, including the need for an OT/OTA partnership to fully realize the potential of occupational therapy services with older adults at the end of life.

Adult Day Care

Carlos, who graduated 4 years ago, works at an adult day care center in an urban setting. This particular setting has a continuum of care that also includes assisted living, independent apartment living, and adult foster homes. The older adults attend day care 5 days a week from 9:00 a.m. until 3:00 p.m., receiving lunch, health services, and activities in which to participate. Carlos has a dual role at the adult day care center. His primary role is as an activities director, in that he identifies and plans individual and group activities for the day care participants throughout the week. In his other role, he works with Sydney, an OT, in providing occupational therapy services for all clients along the care continuum.

To determine whether an older adult requires individual occupational therapy intervention, Sydney begins the initial evaluation with an occupational profile, identifying what is currently important and meaningful in regard to the older adult's occupational needs. Mr. Kirov, a new day care attendee, had recently fractured his humerus and was having difficulty performing activities with only one arm and hand; consequently, Sydney conducted an initial evaluation. As a result, a specific occupational therapy treatment plan was initiated to address his problems with performing activities. To identify which group and individual activities would be appropriate for each older adult attending the day care center, Carlos (in his role as the activities director) meets with each older adult (and the family, when possible). Carlos also met with Mr. Kirov, who identified that he enjoyed using his hands to make things and that he liked to talk with people. Carlos recommended that he participate in the crafts and other activities that included discussion, such as current events and reminiscence. Note: In his role as the Activities Director, Carlos does not provide occupational therapy services.

Carlos starts off his day by attending a team meeting. At the center where Carlos works, the bus drivers, the chaplain, the custodial staff representative, and home health aides attend team meetings, as do the more typical team members such as nurses, social workers, physicians, physical therapy and occupational therapy practitioners. Everyone contributes during the team meetings. Recently, the bus driver reported that Mrs. Chang experiences shortness of breath while getting on the bus, and a home health aide shared the progress that Millie has made with feeding her cat by herself. After the team meeting, Carlos divides his time—he provides one-on-one occupational therapy intervention under the supervision of Sydney and designs and implements group and individual activities for the day care attendees. Because social participation is integral to an older adult's health and well-being,[25,26] Carlos uses his OTA background to plan and implement groups to ensure that the older adults engage in culturally rich and sensitive social activities that they enjoy and find meaningful. One of the most popular groups is the Helping Hands group. The theme of this group is to provide the older adults with a sense of contribution to the community. In the past, they have put together gift baskets for migrant workers, solicited grooming and hygiene products for military personnel, read to preschool children, and stuffed envelopes for a local school board election. Carlos enjoys working with the Helping Hands group because he knows that older adults enjoy engaging in altruistic activities in which they help other people.[27] Other groups that Carlos plans and implements weekly and monthly are gardening, music, reminiscence, movement, and crafts. In addition, Carlos makes an extra effort to contact family members to discuss options for activities at home in which the older adults can successfully engage and enjoy.

During one-on-one occupational therapy interventions, Carlos addresses specific concerns with performance of daily living activities and occupations. Recently, Carlos worked with Mrs. Chang after she began experiencing increased breathlessness caused by her chronic bronchitis. Mrs. Chang's family reported that, during the weekends, she wanted to help her daughter and son-in-law with household chores and would push herself too far and become breathless. Because Mrs. Chang valued her role as a family member, Carlos worked with her and her family to identify which activities she considered important and which activities her family felt comfortable allowing her to do. Carlos then worked with Mrs. Chang and her family to develop a routine, incorporating energy conservation techniques that would allow her to complete activities without becoming breathless and tired.[28] Within a month, Mrs. Chang's family reported that she was helping with household chores without getting tired and breathless. More importantly, she was extremely happy to be able to make a valuable contribution to the family and felt that her health, well-being, and life satisfaction were better than before. Because health promotion is a primary focus of the organization, Carlos also works with other team members to deliver a falls prevention program during which older adults meet in small groups for 7 weeks.[29] Carlos is particularly proud that he is the team member responsible for the follow-up home visit to oversee the implementation of safety strategies by the group participants in their home environment. In doing so, Carlos can see firsthand the important role that OTAs can play to promote health for older adults.

Community Wellness

Margo, who graduated 6 years ago, works as a consultant in health promotion activities for her city's mayor's office. As part of the city's council on fitness and well-being, Margo is especially concerned with wellness initiatives for older adults in the community. She uses her knowledge on aging to assist in planning for the development of accessible communities and supporting programs that can contribute to continued occupational engagement of older adults well into their senior years. For example, she helped develop a citywide wellness festival that featured adventure, leisure, and post-retirement volunteer opportunities for active seniors. Additionally, she participated in a task force to promote physical activity in the city and made sure that bicycle lanes were brightly marked and routes were identified that could circumvent major hills so that older adults could use them safely, without undue fatigue. She then advocated for public bicycle check-out stands that provided coupons for reduced cost on bicycle helmets and other protective gear. Finally, she helped establish an annual, multigenerational bicycle ride across the city.

Telehealth

Jamie is an OTA with 8 years of experience and is working in an outpatient setting in a rural area. The OT and Jamie treat clients who live over 100 miles away from the nearest medical clinic. Since it is often difficult for clients in this rural area to access services such as occupational therapy, the outpatient clinic in which Jamie works has developed a telehealth practice. In its most basic form, telehealth is described as using technology to provide medical services.[30] Providing occupational therapy to clients using a telehealth platform provides many benefits to both client and provider. Firstly, telehealth removes travel time as a barrier for both client and therapy practitioner. Secondly, conducting a virtual telehealth visit in a client's home allows for Jamie to both see the client's personal environment and to tailor interventions to fit the client's specific needs. Third, telehealth reduces interactions between provider and client which also eases potential exposures to airborne or surface transmittable microbes. This is especially helpful when clients have compromised immune systems. Lastly, telehealth services allow Jamie to provide therapy clients with digital home exercise programs, patient education information, and even short video clips demonstrating exercises and techniques to facilitate carryover and use of the information.

The telehealth model has several barriers to its use as well. Telehealth relies on the use of technology platforms, technological devices, and internet transmission signals. All of these items have multiple versions and providers. Terrain and location both affect the internet signal available in an area. Further, telehealth requires that OTAs possess some technology skills and be able to troubleshoot common problems quickly and independently. They must also be able to troubleshoot the potential problems their clients may encounter as well. The telehealth model may not be appropriate for all clients referred for occupational therapy services. Persons without the appropriate level of digital skills knowledge may not benefit from treatment delivered in this way. Further, many occupational therapy interventions require direct patient access for assessment

and treatment (edema management, transfer training, MMT, and goniometry just to name a few). Finally, OTAs need to know the regulations in their state that govern telehealth services.

CONCLUSION

Over the next three to four decades, the population of older adults will increase significantly, the number of older adults with disabilities living in the community will expand sharply, and the percentage of older adults (particularly those over age 85 years) residing in SNFs will rise dramatically.[31] Such trends suggest that OTAs will continue to work with older adults in both traditional and emerging practice settings, focusing on daily life activities that are meaningful to older adults (Fig. 8.5). In doing so, OTAs will continue to provide a valuable contribution during the delivery of occupational therapy services.

After the series of presentations at Blue Lake Community College, the OTA students were excited and enthusiastic about the variety of opportunities waiting for them after graduation. Their instructor, Chris, emphasized that their unique OTA skills and knowledge prepared them to work with older adults in traditional settings such as SNFs, rehabilitation centers, geropsychiatric units, and home health. She went on to say that the job opportunities did not stop there. As Arianna and Jean demonstrated, they used their OTA background to create new job opportunities in emerging practice areas. Chris concluded that Carlos, who worked in adult day care, was a good example of an OTA who works in collaboration with an OT to provide occupational therapy services but also can use his OTA background to assist older adults in engaging in meaningful activities that do not require the direct

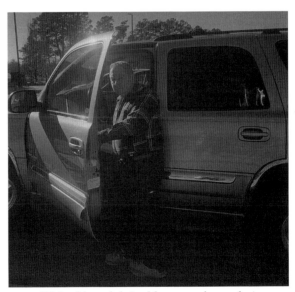

FIG. 8.5 This older adult is able to employ techniques learned in an occupational therapy session to independently transfer into and out of the vehicle. *(Courtesy Amanda Caldwell)*

supervision of an OT. In all cases, whether in typical or emerging practice settings, the Blue Lake Community College graduates were engaged in opportunities that brought satisfaction to themselves and quality services for older adults.

■ CHAPTER REVIEW QUESTIONS

1 Discuss service competency and continued competency for OTAs and ways to establish each.

2 An OTA and OT work together in a rehabilitation setting and have different ideas regarding intervention for older adults. Suggest three ways that they can learn from each other and form a collaborative partnership.

3 An OTA who is a new graduate, and an OT who recently moved from another state, are working to develop a supervision plan. Locate three resources to assist them in developing this plan, and explain what information they would seek from each resource.

4 Identify three activities that you consider meaningful (an occupation) and identify three that you consider merely an activity. Explain the differences.

5 Explain why it is important to focus on both occupations and activities to enhance an older adult's health, well-being, and life satisfaction.

6 Why should OTAs consider the caregiver/significant other/spouse/familywhen collaborating to develop an intervention plan for an older adult?

7 Three OTAs have been hired to work in an SNF. One is a new graduate, one has 5 years of experience working in a rehabilitation setting, and one previously worked in an outpatient adolescent psychiatric unit. Develop a continued competency plan for each OTA.

8 Identify three different potential emerging practice settings in which OTAs might consider working. List five skills for each setting that OTAs receive during their education that would be helpful to secure a position in that specific setting.

9 What previous experience should an OTA have before considering hospice work?

10 What knowledge could OTAs bring to community wellness programs to support continued occupational engagement of well older adults?

REFERENCES

1. American Occupational Therapy Association. Occupational therapy practice framework: domain and process. 4th ed. *Am J Occup Ther.* 2020;74(suppl 2):1-85. doi:10.5014/ajot.2020.74S2001.

2. National Board for Certification in Occupational Therapy. *Executive Summary for the Practice Analysis Study: Certified Occupational Therapy Assistant, COTA.* Gaithersburg, MD: Author; 2018.

3. Leland N, Elliot S, Johnson K. *Occupational Therapy Practice Guidelines for Productive Aging for Community-Dwelling Older Adults.* Bethesda, MD: Author; 2012.

4. American Occupational Therapy Association. Guidelines for supervision, roles, and responsibilities during the delivery of occupational therapy services. *Am J Occup Ther.* 2020;74: 7413410020. doi:10.5014/ajot.2020.74S3004.

5. American Occupational Therapy Association. AOTA 2020 occupational therapy code of ethics. *Am J Occup Ther.* 2020; 74:7413410005. doi:10.5014/ajot.2020.74S3006.

6. American Occupational Therapy Association. Scope of practice. *Am J Occup Ther.* 2014;68:S34-S40. doi:10.5014/ajot.2014.686S04.

7. Schell B, Gillen G, Coppola S. Contemporary occupational therapy practice. In: Schell B, Gillen G, eds. *Willard and Spackman's Occupational Therapy.* 13th ed. Philadelphia: Wolters Kluwer; 2019:56-70.

8. Turnosa N, Lach H, Orr L, et al. Intradisciplinary and interdisciplinary processes in gerontological care. In: Barney K, Perkinson M, eds. *Occupational Therapy with Aging Adults: Promoting Quality of Life Through Collaborative Practice.* St Louis, MO: Elsevier; 2016.

9. World Federation of Occupational Therapists. *About Occupational Therapy.* 2012. Available at: https://www.wfot.org/about/about-occupational-therapy.

10. American Occupational Therapy Association. Standards for continuing competence. *Am J Occup Ther.* 2015;69:6913410055p1-6913410055p3. doi:10.5014/ajot.2015.696S16.

11. National Board for Certification in Occupational Therapy. *Certification Renewal Handbook.* Gaithersburg, MD: Author; 2016.

12. National Board for Certification in Occupational Therapy. *Occupational Therapist Registered OTR® Certified Occupational Therapy Assistant COTA® Certificant Renewal Handbook.* 2021. Available at: https://www.nbcot.org/-/media/NBCOT/PDFs/Renewal_Handbook.ashx?la=en&hash=51470DC8F06EE7305E13D8C88704D212048F870A.

13. Law M, Baptiste S, Carswell A, et al. *Canadian Occupational Performance Measure.* 2021. Available at: http://www.thecopm.ca/about/.

14. Center for Disease Control and Prevention. *Infection Control. Training and Education Resources* (2020). Available at: https://www.cdc.gov/infectioncontrol/training?Sort=CE%20Expiration%20Date%3A%3Adesc.

15. Patnaude ME. Effectiveness of occupational therapy services. In: Patnaude ME, ed. *Early's Physical Dysfunction Practice Skills for the Occupational Therapy Assistant.* St Louis, MO: Elsevier; 2022:61-78.

16. American Occupational Therapy Association. *AOTA's Advanced Certification Program.* 2021. Available at: https://www.aota.org/Education-Careers/Advance-Career/Board-Specialty-Certifications-Exam.aspx.

17. Allen CK, Austin SL, David SK, et al. *Allen Cognitive Level Screen-5 (ACLS-5) and Large Allen Cognitive Level Screen-5 (LACLS-5).* Camarillo, CA: ACLS and LACLS Committee; 2007.

18. Arthritis Foundation. *Health & Wellness: Healthy Living.* n.d. Available at: https://www.arthritis.org/health-wellness/detail?content=healthyliving.

19. Howe MC, Schwartzberg SL. *A Functional Approach to Group Work in Occupational Therapy.* Philadelphia: Lippincott Williams & Wilkins; 2001.

20. American Occupational Therapy Association. *Occupational Therapy's Role in Senior Centers.* Bethesda, MD: American Occupational Therapy Association; 2016.

21. Pega F, Kvixhinadze G, Blakeley T, et al. Home safety assessment and modification reduces injurious falls in community-dwelling older adults: cost utility and equity analysis. *Inj Prev.* 2016;24(6):420-426. doi:10.1136/injuryprev-2016-041999.

22. van Leeuwen KM, van Loon MS, van Nes FA, et al. "What does quality of life mean to older adults? A thematic synthesis." *PloS One.* 2019;14(3):e0213263. doi:10.1371/journal.pone.0213263.

23. Dijxhoorn AQ, Brom L, van der Linden YM, Leget C, Raijmakers NJ. Prevalence of burnout in healthcare professionals providing

palliative care and the effect of interventions to reduce symptoms: a systematic literature review. *Palliat Med.* 2021;35(1):6-26. Available at: https://doi.org/10.1177/0269216320956825.

24. Sleight A, Stein L. Toward a broader role for occupational therapy in supportive oncology care. *Am J Occup Ther.* 2016;70: 7004360030p1-7004360030p8. doi:10.5014/ajot.2016.018101.

25. Cushing D, van Vliet W. Intergenerational communities as healthy places for meaningful engagement and interaction. In: Punch S, Vanderbeck R, Skelton T, et al., eds. Families, Intergenerationality, and Peer Group Relations. Singapore: Springer Science+Business Media; 2016:1-27.

26. McDonald K, Coles M. Conditional independence: development of a grounded theory to enable productive aging. *Am J Occup Ther.* 2016;70:7011515250p1. doi:10.5014/ajot.2016.70S1-PO1100.

27. Martins ELM, Salamene LC, Lucchetti ALG, Lucchetti G. The association of mental health with positive behaviours, attitudes and virtues in community-dwelling older adults: results of a population-based study. *Int J Soc Psychiatry.* 2021;20764021999690. Available at: https://doi.org/10.1177/0020764021999690.

28. American Occupational Therapy Association. *The Role of Occupational Therapy in Chronic Disease Management.* 2015. Available at: http://www.aota.org/~/media/Corporate/Files/AboutOT/Professionals/WhatIsOT/HW/Facts/FactSheet_ChronicDiseaseManagement.pdf.

29. Hu Y, Vance K, Strak S. Elements of effective fall prevention programs: perspectives from medically underserved older adult. *Am J Occup Ther.* 2016;70:7011515247p1. doi:10.5014/ajot.2016.70S1-PO1064.

30. Health Resources and Services Administration. *What is Telehealth?* 2021. Available at: https://telehealth.hhs.gov/patients/understanding-telehealth/?gclid=Cj0KCQiAvP6ABhCjARIsAH37rbSjaPoU4Hv5fMVFU6LQrKsirnfMM99mD5MdcVsaWD0NZ5Q8MCAsTCU-aArpTEALw_wcB.

31. Administration on Aging. *Aging into the 21st Century.* 2014. Available at: https://aoa.acl.gov/Aging_Statistics/future_growth/aging21/preface.aspx.

chapter 9

Cultural Diversity of the Aging Population

RENÉ PADILLA AND AMY L. SHAFFER

KEY TERMS

abstractive, ageism, associative, cognitive style, collectivism, culture, cultural competence, cultural context, cultural norms, cultural pluralism, ethnicity, ethnocentricity, individualism, LGBTQ+, minority, prejudice

CHAPTER OBJECTIVES

1. Explain the meaning of diversity and related terms.
2. Explore personal experiences, beliefs, values, and attitudes regarding diversity.
3. Discuss the need to accept the uniqueness of each individual and the importance of being sensitive to

issues of diversity in the practice of occupational therapy with older adults.
4. Present strategies to facilitate cultural competency in interactions with older adults of diverse backgrounds.

Today is Mia's first day at her first job as an occupational therapy assistant (OTA). She was hired to work as a member of the rehabilitation team in a small nursing home in the town where she grew up. Mia is excited because this job will permit her to stay close to her family and work with older adults. When she arrives at the nursing home, she and the occupational therapist (OT) discuss the older adults who are participating in the rehabilitation program. Mia is told about Mr. Chu, a Chinese gentleman who experienced a stroke and often refuses to get out of bed; and Mrs. Pardo, a Filipino woman who is constantly surrounded by family and consequently cannot get anything accomplished. The OT also tells Mia about Mr. Cooper, an older adult man dying of acquired immunodeficiency disorder (AIDS); Mrs. Blanche, a retired university professor who is a quadriplegic; and Mr. Perez, who was a migrant farm worker until the accidental amputation of his left arm 4 weeks previously. Mia notes the distinct qualities of each of these older adults.

OVERVIEW OF CULTURAL DIVERSITY

The cultural diversity of clients adds an exciting and challenging element to the practice of occupational therapy. Each client comes from a cultural context with a unique blend of values and beliefs. This uniqueness affects all aspects of the client's life, including the domains of occupation. The ways in which a person chooses to do a task, interact with family members, move about in a

community, look to the future, and view health are in many ways, the result of past experiences and the expectations of the people with whom that person comes in contact. OTAs have an important role in supporting older adults' health and participation in life through engagement in occupation.[1] Consequently, OTAs have to manage opportunities and many issues that arise from interactions with persons unlike themselves in terms of race, sex, age, ethnicity, physical ability, sexual orientation, family composition, place of birth, religion, level of education, and work experience (including retirement status) or professional status, among other factors.[2,3]

Culture, ethnocentrism, assimilation, and diversity are discussed to provide a framework for working with older adults in a sensitive manner. This chapter includes general guidelines for assessment and intervention. The challenge for OTAs is to contribute to the creation of a therapeutic environment in which diversity and difference are valued and in which older adults can work to reach their goals.

WHAT IS CULTURE?

The United Nations Education, Scientific and Cultural Organization (UNECO) defines culture as "the set of distinctive spiritual, material, intellectual and emotional features of society or a social group … [which] encompasses, in addition to art and literature, lifestyles, ways of living together, value systems, traditions and beliefs."[4] The World Health Organization (WHO) has also adopted this definition. The concept of culture has long been considered important in the practice of occupational therapy, because one's culture has an impact on their daily life. As such, culture is woven throughout the domains of the OTPF-4.[1] In fact, when analyzing an activity, culture, in various forms, can both facilitate occupational performance and inhibit it. Due to the importance of culture in the domains of occupational therapy, the accreditation standards, and educational programs for the Occupational Therapy Assistant,[5] the Code of Ethics,[6] and the *Occupational Therapy Practice Framework: Domain and Process*[1] all support the consideration of culture in intervention. Culture has been a constantly evolving term and has not been clearly defined or described in occupational therapy professional literature, nor been consistently considered in the assessment and intervention process.[7,8] Part of the reason for this lapse may be the breadth of complex concepts encompassed by this one term. The *OTPF-4*[1] identifies culture among the contexts that influence performance patterns (observable behaviors of occupations used to establish lifestyle and occupational balance). Culture is listed with physical, social, personal, and temporal factors that influence occupation within particular contexts and environments. Culture may be seen as a factor that will: change how a client views success, shape expected roles and behaviors, and outline activity demands.[1] Kielhofner,[9] also offered a broad perspective when he defined culture as the beliefs and perceptions, values and norms, and customs and behaviors shared by a group or society and are passed from one generation to the next through both formal and informal education.

This broad and consequently vague definition of culture is not unique to the occupational therapy profession. Entire books in other fields are devoted to describing culture, and authors have been unable to agree on a single definition. Most include concepts relating to observable patterns of behavior and rules that govern that behavior. They also emphasize the conscious and subconscious nature of culture in the way it is dynamically shared among people. Some of the commonalties in those definitions, including that culture is learned, shared with others, and used to influence daily life, may be used as a basis for an understanding of culture.[7,8]

Culture is learned or acquired through socialization. Culture is not carried in a person's genetic makeup; rather, it is learned over the course of a lifetime. Obviously, then, the context and environment in which each person lives are central to his or her culture. A person's environment may demand or offer opportunities for some types of behaviors and restrict opportunities for other types. For example, individuals in the United States are offered the opportunity to choose the color of their clothing, but generally wearing dresses is culturally restricted to females. In the United States, persons are generally expected to drive on the right side of the street, pay taxes, and arrive at work according to schedule. Through interaction with the environment, individuals learn a variety of values and beliefs and eventually internalize them. Internalized values direct the interactions among people and with the environment. As a result, people assume that others have internalized the same values and beliefs and consequently behave in the same ways.[10,11] However, culture is the result of each person's unique experiences with his or her environment and thus is an ongoing learning process.

Another commonality in the various definitions of culture is that, because it is learned from others, it is also shared. What is shared as culture, however, is very dynamic. Because culture is learned throughout one's lifetime, each person learns it at different points. On the basis of each person's status in learning culture, the person expects something from others and contributes to others' cultural education. In this way, each person learns and teaches something about culture that is unique. Over time, shared beliefs and values change. These changes in cultural beliefs and values may not be easily observed because the actual behaviors that express them seem to remain the same. However, over time, a periodic recommitment to the dynamic transmittal of beliefs and values has occurred.[12] For example, the attire of women in some regions of the Arabian Peninsula has changed very little in the past 200 years. Originally, the black gowns, robes, and veils were probably intended to guard the woman's modesty. Many women who wear these garments today, in addition to guarding modesty, do so as a symbol of resistance to westernization, a concern that was probably not common 200 years ago.[13,14]

Finally, culture is often subconscious.[15,16] Because learning of culture occurs formally and informally, a person is not usually aware, particularly at a young age, of learning it. Instead, the person simply complies with the demands and restrictions of behavior set in particular environments and chooses behaviors from among those that are allowed. For example, when a child is not permitted to touch a frog found by a pond during a family outing, that child is being formally taught that frogs are dirty and therefore should not be touched, a value the child might internalize and then generalize to other animals. This value is informally reinforced when the child sees other people wince and make gestures of repulsion when they see certain types of animals. When the child sees a younger sibling attempting to touch a frog, the child might tell the sibling not to do so because touching it is "bad." In effect, the child internalized a value received from the culture of his or her family and passed it on to a sibling with the slight reinterpretation that it is bad to do the particular behavior. In a similar way, all persons continue to learn culture from each physical and social environment in which they participate. When older adults enter a nursing home for a short-term or long-term stay, for example, some of the facility's rules of behavior are formally explained, whereas others are implied, including meal times (and consequently when older adults must eat), visiting hours (and consequently when older adults must and must not socialize), visiting room regulations (and consequently where and how older adults may socialize), and "lights out" time (and consequently when older adults must sleep). Older adults also informally learn an entirely different set of rules. As they experience the daily routine in the nursing home, they also learn whether it is acceptable to question the professionals who work there, to decline participation in scheduled group activities, and even to express their thoughts, feelings, desires, and concerns. Staff members have likely not formally stated, "You are not permitted to state your feelings here." However, staff members may communicate this value informally if they cut off conversation when an older adult begins to explain feelings or simply never take time to invite an expression of the older adult's feelings. In this way, values and beliefs become sets of unspoken, implicit, and underlying assumptions that guide interactions with others and the environment.[17]

Culture is a set of beliefs and values that a particular group of people share and re-create constantly through interaction with each other and their environments. These beliefs and values may be conscious or unconscious, and they direct the opportunities, demands, and behavior restrictions that exist for members of a particular group. Essentially, every belief and value that humans acquire as members of society can be included in their culture, thus explaining the broadness of the concept of culture. Therefore, the beliefs and values on which we form our own understanding of older adults' behaviors and the rules for these behaviors have also been socially constructed and form part of our own culture.

Each person has a culture, and is part of a larger culture as well. Families have unique and individual cultures based on roles, rituals, and routines. Those cultures are often based on or inclusive of larger societal, religious, or national cultural norms. Cultural norms are expectations or rules that guide the behaviors of the membership.[18] Learning about and understanding cultural norms and cultural values that are important to the culture of an older adult will facilitate not only developing a therapeutic relationship, but it will also assist the OTA with task analysis and intervention planning skills required to enable success with an older adult client. Developing skills of cultural competence, or the "integration and transformation of knowledge" about individuals and groups of people into specific standards, policies, practices, and attitudes used in appropriate cultural settings to increase the quality of services; thereby producing better outcomes[19] is an imperative skill that should not be overlooked by the OTA. As society continues to expand, so too, do the cultural considerations required for optimal care of older adult client.

LEVELS OF CULTURE

Various levels of culture exist at which values and beliefs are shared. Many authors[20-22] have proposed that a multidimensional view of culture be adopted. In this view, culture can be defined in terms of the individual, the family, the community, and the region. At the individual level are the relational, one-to-one interactions through which people learn and express their unique representations of culture. Examples of the individual level of culture are each person's use of humor, definition of personal space, coping style, and role choices. Included at the level of the family are beliefs and values that are shared within a primary social group—the group in which most of the person's early socialization takes place. The family level of culture includes issues such as gender roles, family composition, and style of worship. Each family can be seen as a variation of the culture shared at the level of a community or neighborhood, in which economic factors, ethnicity, housing, and other factors may be considered. Communities may be seen as variations in the culture shared with a larger region, such as language, geography, and industry. Erez and Gati[20] noted that variation exists at each level and within each group.

Adopting a more relational framework helps overcome some of the difficulties inherent in viewing culture as synonymous with ethnicity. Ethnicity is the part of a person's identity derived from membership in a racial, religious, national, or linguistic group.[23] The viewing of culture as synonymous with ethnicity relies on generalizations about the people who belong to a particular group and can lead to mistaken assumptions about an individual's personality and beliefs. For example, the assumption that all persons of Hispanic ethnicity have brown skin and black hair is not true, because Hispanics of all racial backgrounds exist. Equally, people cannot assume that all white individuals are educated, that all Jewish people observe kosher practices, or that everyone who speaks English attaches the same meaning to the word *gay*.

Equating ethnicity with culture can lead to many misinterpretations.[24] In addition, this practice is often used to justify superiority of one group over another. The term *ethnocentricity* describes the belief held by members of a particular ethnic group that their expression of beliefs and values is superior to that of others, and consequently that all other groups should aspire to adopt their beliefs and values. In extreme cases of ethnocentricity, a particular ethnic group has attempted to destroy other ethnic groups, as in Germany during World War II when Jewish people were targeted, Bosnia in 1992 when it declared independence from Yugoslavia and Bosnian Muslims were targeted, and Sudan in the early 2000s when Darfuri men, women, and children were targeted. Ethnocentrism can be, and often is, an underlying, subconscious belief that powerfully guides a person's behavior. An unexamined ethnocentric attitude may lead OTAs to place particular emphasis on certain areas of rehabilitation and disregard others that older adults may consider essential for their recovery. Occupational therapy itself can be viewed as a subculture with beliefs and values that guide practitioners toward independence, productivity, leisure, purposeful activity, and individuality. This bias may sometimes lead practitioners to ignore the client's wishes and impose their own values in the belief that they are more important and worthwhile.

THE ISSUE OF DIVERSITY

The variety of clients whom Mia, the OTA, introduced at the beginning of this chapter, will work with underscores a well-known fact about the United States: It is a country of immigrants, a conglomeration of diverse peoples. How is it possible that all of these groups live together? The metaphor of the "melting pot" has been used to describe the way in which distinct cultural groups in the United States "melt down" and how differences between groups that were once separate entities disappear. This process is the result of the continuous exposure of groups to one another.[25] Kimbro[26] described a process of conformity in which an individual or a cultural group forsakes values, beliefs, and customs to eliminate differences with another culture. In the United States, conformity may be demonstrated by people who Americanize their names, speak only English, abandon religious practices or social rituals, shed their ethnic dress, attend night school, and work hard to take part in the "American dream." Both conformity and the melting pot metaphor imply that new ethnic groups entering the United States will be judged by the degree to which their differences with the values and beliefs of the established American culture disappear. Some people accept the pressure to abandon their cultural identity as an inevitable or even desirable fact of life, whereas others avoid it at all costs.[25] This expectation can easily create bias, prejudice, and discrimination toward many individuals. The term *minority* is an outgrowth of these views and is used to designate not only smaller groups but also groups that have less power and representation within an established culture despite their size.

The realization that some differences such as age, race, sex, and sexual orientation can never be eliminated, even with effort and education, has led many people to discern that they should also value the characteristics that make them unique, such as their cultural heritage and their religious practices. Cultural pluralism is a value system that recognizes this desire and focuses not on assimilation but on accepting and celebrating the differences that exist among people.[7] Those who value cultural pluralism believe that these differences add richness to a society rather than detract from it.

Valuing Diversity

People in the United States are clearly diverse. Diversity is demonstrated through race, sex, age, ethnicity, sexual orientation, family composition, place of birth, religion, and level of education. In addition, people also differ from each other in physical ability or disability, intelligence, socioeconomic class, physical beauty, and personality type. In essence, any dimension of life can create identity

groups or cohorts that may or may not be visible. Most people find that several of these dimensions have particular meaning for them.[27]

Ironically, diversity becomes an inclusive concept when we view it as that which makes us different from each other. This view of diversity embraces everyone because each person is in some way different from everyone else. At the same time, however, each person in some way is also similar to someone else. This viewpoint provides a framework for approaching the diversity that one encounters when working with older adults; OTAs can recognize the ways in which they are both different from and similar to older adults. These differences and similarities can be used during therapy to enrich the older adult's life. A welcome side effect of this approach is that the OTA's life is often enriched as well.

DIVERSITY OF THE AGED POPULATION

A summary of statistical reports on the older adult population is presented in Chapter 1. Each of these reports is an example of diversity. While each generational cohort has specific criteria that defines it, there is diversity of the older adult population within the generational cohort as well. The following facts should also be considered when considering diversity among the rapidly growing older adult population.

Minority Populations

Persons older than age 65 years represent 16.5% of the US population, or about 43 million people.[28] In 2018, 23% of older adults belonged to minority populations, 9% were African Americans, and persons of Hispanic origin (who may be of any race) represented 8% of the older population. About 5.1% were Asian or Pacific Islander, and less than 1% were American Indian or Native Alaskan. In addition, 0.8% of persons age 65 and older identified themselves as being of two or more races. The overall number of minority older adults is expected to grow to 34% by 2040.[28] A growth of 81% is expected in the white non-Hispanic older adult population in that same period. The growth among Hispanic older adults is projected to be the largest (175%), followed by Asian and Pacific Islander older adults (113%), American Indian, Eskimo, and Aleut older adults (75%) and African American older adults (88%).[29] A breakdown of the US racial and ethnic population is provided in Fig. 9.1. Notably, these figures represent the numbers of older adults who belong to broad categories only, not cultural distinctiveness. Each of the categories listed may include numerous subcultures. These numbers are used here simply to emphasize that the population served by occupational therapy practitioner will increasingly include older adults from diverse backgrounds.

LGBTQ+

In addition to cultural factors rooted in one's ethnic or racial identity, OTAs should be aware of the cultural factors related to one's sexual and gender identity. There

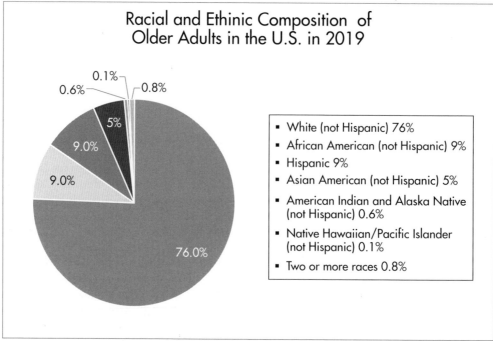

FIG. 9.1   Breakdown of older adult population by race and ethnic origin. *(Data from Profile of Older Americans: 2020 Data Release. United States Administration on Aging, and American Association of Retired Persons. A profile of older Americans. [Washington, DC: U.S. Dept. of Health and Human Services, Administration on Aging] 2021.)*

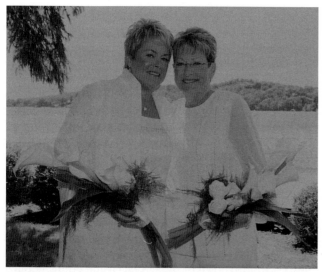

FIG. 9.2   A same sex couple shares their wedding day with family and friends.

is no official US Census data reporting Lesbian, Gay, Bisexual, Transgender, Queer, or Questioning (LGBTQ+) older adults who reside in the United States; however, data from The Williams Institute reports 7% of the LGBTQ+ community population encompasses older adults over age 65 (Fig. 9.2).[30] The same report indicates 21% of the total US population was over age 65 at the time of their research.[30] A separate study indicated there were over 2.4 million LGBTQ+ adults over the age of

50 in the United States. It is estimated that this number will grow to over 5 million by 2030.[31] The Williams Institute further reported that the LGBTQ+ population nationwide of all ages was 4.5% or 13,042,000 (age 13+). Population density for persons in the LGBTQ+ community vary with the largest numbers seen in the Northeastern states as well as states on the West coast.[30] Members of the LGBTQ+ community are reported to be a marginalized group when it comes to seeking and obtaining health care services. It is important that OTAs use gender neutral terminology such as partner, significant other, they, or them when the gender identity of an older adult and/or their partner is not known. OTAs should also feel comfortable asking an older adult client their preferred pronouns upon first meeting.

Religion

The United States is one of the most diverse countries in the world in terms of religious affiliation. Approximately 70% of people in the United States claim to have a definite religious preference.[32] The trend toward increased religious diversity is fueled both by conversion and immigration. Since 1957, the Christian population (i.e., Catholics and Protestants) in the United States has decreased from 92% to 70.6% of the total population, whereas the number of practitioners of other religions, including Buddhism, Hinduism, and Islam, have increased from 1% to 5.9%. Information on the distribution of faiths of the general US population is provided in Fig. 9.3.

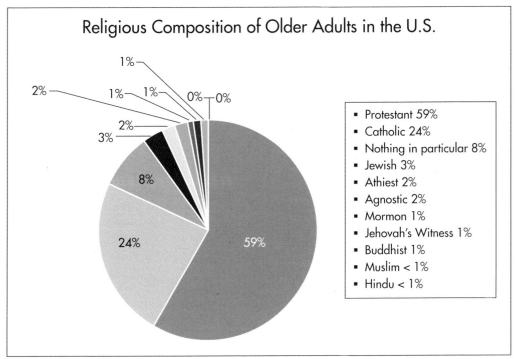

FIG. 9.3 Religious composition of adults ages 65 and older in the United States. *(From Pew Religious Landscape Study. Washington, DC: Pew Research Center; 2015.)*

Socioeconomic Status

In 2019, the overall poverty rate in the United States was 10.5%.[33] This rate is the lowest poverty rate observed by the US Census since it began tracking this data in 1959, and the rate of poverty decreased across all age and all racial/ethnic groups reported.[33] The poverty rate for people age 65 and older was 8.9% in 2019.[33] Despite the percentage of older adults living below the poverty level dropping, the number of people composing that percentage is increasing, as members of the Baby-Boomer generation continue to age.[34] In 2017, the number of older adults living in poverty was 4.7 million people. When reviewing racial/ethnic backgrounds, the poverty rates for non-Hispanic white older adults was reported to be the lowest in groups studied at 5.8% for men and 8.0% for women. Conversely, the poverty rates for older adults identifying as black or African American was the highest in the age cohort at 16.1% for men and 21.5% for women. The oldest older adults (those over age 80) have the highest overall rates of poverty at 11.6%. Women over age 80 living alone experienced the highest poverty rate of this group at 18.6%.[34]

SENSITIVITY TO CULTURE AND DIVERSITY IN INTERVENTION

To be culturally sensitive, people must acknowledge their own prejudices and biases. OTAs should realize that prejudices are learned behaviors that can be unlearned through increased contact with and understanding of people of diverse cultural groups. Furthermore, communication always takes place between individuals not cultures. Research on cultural competence suggests that, in the clinical encounter, the cultures of both the client and the clinician play important roles in successful outcomes.[35] Cultural differences probably account for most misunderstandings and miscommunications between clients and clinicians.[35] Clinicians must learn to work within the client's culture rather than demand that the client, who may be going through a difficult or vulnerable phase, adapt to the clinician's or the organization's culture.[35] Ofahengaue, Giunta, and Simpson[3] as well as numerous other experts have posited that, in addition to the cultures of the client and the clinician, the culture of the institution in which the interaction takes place in many ways directs the interaction between the client and clinician. In health care, institutional culture has strongly valued the biomedical approach to intervention, which places the control of health care with the physician rather than with the client. In addition, the US medical system has placed little emphasis on the development of specific programs to address the needs of older adults from culturally diverse groups.

Culture and diversity are extremely broad and complex concepts. Attempts to make generalizations about various groups would be useless because OTAs are certain to come across older adults who do not fit into the expected behavior. Few persons are perfect representations of their culture. Generalizations may also limit the OTA's ability to see each client as a unique individual. Consequently, OTAs should be cognizant of general issues about culture that should be assessed and remembered at every step of the occupational therapy process. OTAs must realize that cultural sensitivity is an ongoing process.[23] In addition, OTAs should not assume that, by following the guidelines presented in the following sections, they have done everything necessary to provide culturally appropriate occupational therapy services. The OTA's responsibility is to develop ongoing cultural competence strategies that allow the client to maintain personal integrity and be treated with respect as an individual.

The two most important strategies OTAs can use are asking questions and observing behavior carefully. The values and beliefs that encompass culture direct older adults in their particular ways of performing activities of daily living (ADL) functions and work and leisure occupations. Consequently, OTAs must be oriented toward each older adult's culture to provide relevant and meaningful intervention. Cultural orientation should include an understanding of the following: (1) the cognitive style of the older adult, (2) what he or she accepts as evidence, (3) the value system that forms the basis of the older adult's behavior, and (4) the final area of understanding has to do with communication style.[23] If an older adult is unable to directly answer questions regarding these areas, OTAs should attempt to obtain this information from the older adult's family or friends. If this is not an option, the OTA should obtain information about the older adult's culture from other sources, such as a coworker who is of the same national origin as the older adult or from library materials. However, OTAs should remember that the more removed the information source is from the older adult, the less likely that the information will apply to that particular older adult.

Let us return briefly to Mia, the OTA starting a new job, who was introduced at the beginning of the chapter. One of the older adults with whom Mia would be working was Mr. Chu, a Chinese gentleman who refused to get out of bed. The OT informed Mia that soon after Mr. Chu's admission, several of the older adults who had Alzheimer's disease and were disoriented had become agitated in Mr. Chu's presence because they associated him with World War II experiences. The nursing home staff did not want Mr. Chu to be offended by this behavior, so they moved him to a private room. When Mia entered Mr. Chu's room, she said, "Hello! I'm from occupational therapy, and I'm here to help you get out of bed and do your ADLs." As anticipated, he signaled his refusal to cooperate by turning his head and closing his eyes. He remained silent whenever Mia spoke to him. When she attempted to put her hand behind his shoulder to help him sit up, he grabbed her wrist and pushed her arm away. Mia was perplexed. She called Jon, an OT of Japanese descent whom she had met at an orientation session a week earlier, and asked him to provide any insight into Mr. Chu's behavior. Jon told Mia that, in

general, Asians are very circumspect, preferring to be with members of their own group, and that Mr. Chu was probably reacting to Mia not being Asian. Jon suggested that a family member be called in to enlist Mr. Chu's cooperation. Mia contacted Mr. Chu's son, Edwin, who met her later that afternoon at Mr. Chu's bedside. After some discussion with his father, Edwin informed Mia that Mr. Chu refused to get out of bed because he believed he had been placed in a private room to isolate him because he was Chinese. He viewed being informed about occupational therapy intervention plans as further evidence that he was being treated differently. Mia explained the staff's concern that Mr. Chu would be offended by the comments and behavior of the other older adults. Mr. Chu said he understood that such behavior was part of an illness. Mia facilitated Mr. Chu's move to a room with three other older adults, and he began to participate daily in the occupational therapy plan of care. Mia was careful to ask Mr. Chu what he wanted to accomplish in each session. Jon's report about Asians wanting to be with members of their own group was only partially true. Mr. Chu wished to be with other older adults, not specifically other Chinese people. Mia was only able to discover this with the help of someone very familiar with Mr. Chu.

Cognitive Style

OTAs need to understand how older adults organize information. This process does not refer to an assessment of cognitive functions that indicate the presence or absence of brain dysfunction.[36,37] Rather, cognitive style refers to the types of information a person ignores and accepts in everyday life. Because cognitive style is the result of habits, it tends to be automatic or subconscious. Studies of cognitive style suggest that people vary along a continuum of open-mindedness or closed-mindedness, and that cultural patterns are reflected in these styles.[38] Depending on the situation, people may vary along this continuum, and no one is likely to always operate from one of the poles. Open-minded persons seek out additional information before making decisions and tend to admit that they do not have all of the answers and need to learn more before reaching proper conclusions. Open-minded persons usually ask many questions, want to hear about alternatives, and often ask OTAs to make personal recommendations regarding alternatives. Closed-minded individuals, however, see only a narrow range of data and ignore additional information. These persons usually take this approach because they function under strict sets of rules about behavior. For example, a devout Hindu older adult would likely be appalled at being served beef at a meal and would not be willing to consider the potential nutritional benefits of the meal. Similarly, the dietitian who offers this meal to a Hindu older adult may do so on the basis of a closed-minded cognitive style, assuming that beef is the ideal and only source of the particular nutrients the older adult needs. Both persons are functioning under rules of behavior, with the Hindu older adult's rules dictated by religious practice and the dietitian's rules dictated by professional training. Other examples of a closed-minded cognitive style include the female older adult who refuses to work with a male OTA during dressing training because she believes it is not proper, and the explosive retired executive who bellows that he does not wish to walk with a cane despite safety concerns. Both of these people have attended to only part of the data available—that is, the data contrary to the rules of behavior under which they function. Their cognitive styles have limited their abilities to consider the benefits of the alternatives. Studies show that most cultures produce closed-minded citizens.[38]

Another aspect of cognitive style is the way in which people process information, which can be divided into associative and abstractive processing styles. As with open-mindedness and closed-mindedness, people may vary along this continuum, and no one is likely to always operate from one of the styles. People who think associatively filter new data through the screen of personal experience; that is, these people tend to understand new information in terms of similar past experiences only. Conversely, abstractive thinkers deal with new information through imagination or by considering hypothetical situations. An example of an associative thinker is an older adult who has had a stroke and wants the OTA to provide him with a set of weights because using weights was how he increased upper extremity strength when he was younger. An example of an abstractive thinker is an older adult woman who asks the OTA to write down the principles of joint protection and is able to apply that information to all situations in which she may find herself. When approaching an associative thinker with a new task, OTAs should point out the ways in which it is similar to other tasks that the older adult has accomplished. Often, older adults who are associative thinkers need one or more demonstrations of the task and do best with small incremental increases in task complexity. Alternately, when approaching an abstractive thinker with a new task, OTAs should emphasize the desired outcome and permit the older adult to think of ways in which to reach the goal. For example, when teaching an older adult who thinks associatively to transfer to the toilet, OTAs should point out the ways in which this transfer is similar to the transfer of getting to the wheelchair from the bed. When teaching the older adult who thinks abstractly to transfer to the toilet, OTAs should point out that the goal is to maintain alignment when standing, pivot on both legs, and sit by bending the knees.

What Is Accepted as Truth?

When OTAs engage people in therapy, they assume the individuals will act in their own best interest. On the basis of this assumption, OTAs can ask the question: How do clients decide if it is in their best interest to learn the task presented to them? Or, in a broader sense, what is the truth? People from different cultures arrive at truth in different ways. These methods of arriving at truth can be separated into faith, fact, and feeling. The process of evaluating truth tends to be more conscious, in contrast to the automatic cognitive style discussed previously. Furthermore, most people use combinations of methods, but for reasons of clarity, these methods are explained separately in the chapter.

The person who acts on the basis of faith uses a belief system such as that derived from a religion or political ideology to determine what is good or bad. For example, many people believe in self-sufficiency and may decline to use a wheelchair or other adaptive equipment that would clearly help them reduce fatigue. Their belief in self-sufficiency operates independently of the fact that they are too fatigued to stay awake for more than an hour. Other examples of people who act on the basis of faith include the older adult who refuses a blood transfusion because it is explicitly prohibited by his or her religion, and the older adult who calls on a priest, rabbi, pastor, or other spiritual advisor before making a decision about care. Before occupational therapy intervention is initiated, OTAs should always ask whether the older adult wishes to observe any particular rules and should consider the older adult's response when selecting therapeutic occupations.

Obviously, people who act on the basis of fact want to see evidence to support the OTA's recommendation or prioritization of a certain intervention. These people often want to know the benefits that a certain intervention has proven to give in the past. To make plans for their future, these people often wish to know the length and cost of required occupational therapy services. People who act on the basis of fact may stop participating in a particular activity if they do not see the exact results that they anticipated. OTAs may find it helpful to have these older adults participate in some form of group intervention that allows them to directly observe results of occupational therapy intervention with other older adults. In addition, written information about their conditions and about resources can be useful for these older adults.

The most common group is people who arrive at truth on the basis of feelings.[38] Such people are those who "go with their gut instincts." When faced with a difficult decision, they often choose the option that "feels right" over the one that seems most logical if the more logical option makes them too uncomfortable. People who function on the basis of feelings often need to establish a comfortable rapport with the OTA before committing themselves wholeheartedly to working with the OTA. Building a relationship with these individuals may take a long time. However, once the relationship is established, it is very strong. People who function on the basis of feeling will probably want the OTA to continue treating them after they are discharged from a facility if further services are needed; they place less importance on cost considerations than on continuing the relationship. As with any client, OTAs should consistently and periodically ask older adults how they are feeling about their situations and permit them time to process these feelings as needed.

Value Systems

Each culture has a system for separating right from wrong or good from evil. A person's cognitive style and the way in which the person evaluates truth provide general clues about the values of that person's culture. However, more specific value systems exist that form the basis for behavior. Datesman[39] identified six values and assumptions that characterize dominant American culture, including the importance of individualism and privacy, the belief in the equality of all people, and competition within interpersonal interactions. In addition, Datesman[39] described self-reliance, material wealth, and hard work as salient American values. In the chapter, the locus of decision making, sources of anxiety reduction, issues of equality and inequality, and use of time are discussed. Numerous other value systems also direct behavior, but these four systems are discussed here because they are more related than other systems to the concerns of OT.

Locus of Decision Making

Locus of decision making is related to the extent to which a culture prizes individualism as opposed to collectivism. Individualism refers to the degree to which a person considers only himself or herself when making a decision. Collectivism refers to the degree to which a person must abide with the consensus of the collective group. Pure individualism and collectivism are rare. In most countries, people consider others when making a decision, but they are not bound by the desires of the group. Returning to the concept of levels of culture discussed previously in the chapter may be helpful in understanding individualism versus collectivism. Locus of decision making may be considered as a series of concentric circles (Fig. 9.4). In the center is the smallest circle: the individual. At this level, the individual considers mainly himself or herself when making a decision. The next circle represents a slightly larger group: usually the family. Many cultures expect the individual to consider what is best for the family when making a decision. The next circle represents a larger group: the community. This community could be an ethnic group, a religion, or even the individual's country. Some cultures expect people to consider the best interests of the entire, expansive group.

Examples of the ways that people use these different levels of consideration when making a decision are easy to find in occupational therapy practice. An individualistic older adult is one who makes decisions about when and how he will be discharged home without consulting his or

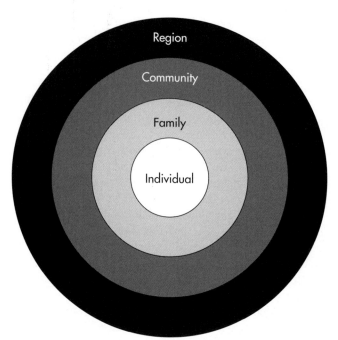

FIG. 9.4 Levels of culture.

her spouse or family. These older adults might believe that their spouse or family has a responsibility to care for them—a value that may not necessarily be shared. Another older adult who considers his or her family when making a decision may refuse to be discharged home out of consideration to his or her grown children because they would have to adjust their lifestyles to accommodate the older adult's needs. Another older adult may decide to attempt to continue living independently to defy society's stereotype of dependence of older adults.

Another way of thinking about individualism versus collectivism is to consider the degree of privacy a person seeks. Older adults from cultures that highly value privacy may be quite perplexed by the number of health care professionals who seem to know about their issues. Conversely, older adults from other cultures who do not have rigid standards of privacy may feel isolated if they are not permitted to have constant contact with family or friends. The occupational therapy culture values independence, privacy, and individualism, but these values may be in conflict with an older adult's needs if not carefully considered. One of the paradoxes of medical care in the United States is that, at the same time that we defend privacy rights in documentation, we assume that the individual will be completely comfortable undressing or toileting in our presence, and we do not give thought to the possibility that the older adult may feel embarrassed by these experiences.

Sources of Anxiety Reduction

Every human being is subject to stress. How do individuals handle stress and reduce anxiety? Most people turn to four basic sources of security and stability: interpersonal relationships, religion, technology, and the law.[38,40-42]

A person who must make a decision about an important health-related issue or adapt to a traumatic event is under stress. OTAs will find it helpful to know where or to whom older adults turn for help and advice. If an older adult is going to ask his or her spouse or family for advice, the OTA should include that spouse or family in therapy from the beginning of intervention so that they clearly understand the issues involved.

Older adults who rely on religion as a source of anxiety reduction often need OTAs to help them obtain special considerations regarding religious practices. Understanding every nuance in the older adult's religion is not as important as acknowledging the importance and appreciating the comfort that the older adult finds in religious observances.

Reliance on technology as a source of anxiety reduction can be manifested when older adults seek yet another medical test to confirm or refute a diagnosis. These clients may rely on medication as the solution to their problems or may collect a myriad of adaptive equipment or "gadgets." Occupational therapy practitioners often have a bias toward relieving anxiety by prescribing the use of adaptive equipment without considering fully the extent to which the older adult truly needs it.

Issues of Equality/Inequality

An important characteristic of all cultures is the division of power. Who controls the financial resources and who controls decision making within the family? A sacred tenet in the United States is that "All men are created equal." Despite this tenet, prejudice against many groups still exists. All cultures have disadvantaged groups. Unequal status may be defined by economic situation, race, age, sex, or other factors. Members of socially and economically advantaged classes may project a sense of entitlement to health care services and may treat OTAs and other health care workers as servants. Conversely, members of a poverty-stricken underclass may eye OTAs with suspicion or defer to any recommendation out of fear of retaliation through withdrawal of needed services.

OTAs also should analyze issues of male and female equality. Female OTAs, in particular, may find it useful to know the way women are regarded in the older adult's culture. In most cultures, men are more likely to be obeyed and trusted when they occupy positions of authority, but the same is not always true for women. There may also be a generational effect on perceptions of authority and leadership in terms of effectiveness.[43,44] OTAs must understand who will be best suited to act as a caregiver on the basis of the older adult's cultural values regarding gender roles as well as age of the OTA. An OTA who is of the opposite sex of the older adult may decide to initiate occupational therapy intervention around issues less likely to bring up conflicts regarding privacy or authority until more rapport is built and the older adult is able to appreciate the OTA's genuine concern for their welfare.

Another factor to be considered is the status awarded to people because of age. Ageism refers to the belief that one age group is superior to another. Often, the younger generation is more valued. The physical appearance of age is frequently avoided through the use of cosmetics to conceal and surgery to reverse manifestations of age. Some people attempt to delay the natural developmental process through adopting healthier lifestyles of exercise, diet, rest, and so on. The avoidance of the appearance of age can contribute to the undervaluing of older adults. Stereotypical descriptors such as "senile," "dependent," or "diseased" are used to describe the aging population as needy people. Because of these views of age, it can be easy for the OTA to assume a position of power over older adults and place them in a position of inferiority and need of services to justify the existence of the profession.[45] McKnight[46] described how "ageism" has resulted in the view that age is a problem to be avoided. He argued that our assumptions and stereotypical myths surrounding the results of normal development contribute to ageism. These stereotypes of older adults cast them as "less" in terms of sight, hearing, memory, mobility, health, learners, and even productive members of society. In contrast, McKnight described how his mother-in-law, whom he refers to as "Old Grandma," views "old":

> ... *finally knowing what is important ... when you are, rather than when you are becoming ... knowing about pain rather than fearing it ... being able to gain more pleasure from memory than prospect ... when doctors become impotent and powerless ... when satisfaction depends less and less on consumption ... using the strength that a good life has stored for you ... enjoying deference ... worrying about irrelevance (p. 27).*[46]

OTAs must be prepared to overcome and critically reflect on their own bias related to growing old to provide culturally sensitive care to the older adults they serve.

Occupational Justice

Wilcock and Townsend define the term occupational justice as "the right of every individual to be able to meet basic needs and to have equal opportunities and life chances to reach toward her or his potential but specific to the individual's engagement in diverse and meaningful occupation."[47] In other words, a person has the right to have access to occupations that they find meaningful and valuable (Fig. 9.5). As such, life experiences vary and each person has differing occupational needs. These needs should be acknowledged and honored.[48] In the US society, however, access to occupations that are meaningful and valuable is not distributed equitably. Disparities in equity and inclusion, and therefore occupational justice, exist either explicitly or implicitly due to various factors. Health disparities such as health care access and quality, economic stability, water quality, food deserts (areas with no access to fresh fruit/vegetables) are systemic issues facing many older adults around the United States.[49] Additionally,

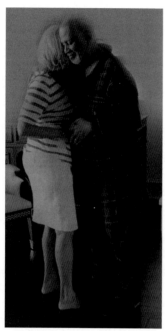

FIG. 9.5 An older adult couple shares an intimate moment dancing together. *(Courtesy Fitz Johnson.)*

marginalized groups, which include older adults, have greater difficulties accessing meaningful occupations. Older adults who also identify as members of other marginalized groups (Immigrants, People with disabilities, People of Color, LGBTQ+) tend to have even larger difficulty with occupational justice due to being members of groups systemically excluded from mainstream American culture.[50] The OTA should be aware of these disparities as well as community resources that may be available to the older adult to assist with accessing meaningful occupations.

Use of Time

Time is consciously and unconsciously formulated and used in each culture. Time is often treated as a language, a way of handling priorities, and a way of revealing how people feel about one another. Cultures can be divided into those who prefer a monochronic use of time and those who prefer a polychronic use of time.[51,52]

Older adults from monochronic cultures will probably prefer to organize their lives with a "one thing at a time" and "time is money" mentality. For these older adults, adherence to schedules is highly important. They are likely to be offended if they are kept waiting for an appointment or if they perceive that the OTA is attending to too many issues at once. People from a monochronic culture prefer having the OTA's undivided attention and expect time to be used efficiently. These people are not necessarily unfriendly but prefer social "chit-chat" to be kept to a minimum if they are paying for a particular technical service. In contrast, older adults from a polychronic culture organize their lives around social relationships. For them, the time spent with someone is

directly correlated to their personal value. Often, these older adults feel rushed by schedules. They may be late for an appointment because they encountered an acquaintance whom they did not want to offend by rushing off to a therapy appointment. With these older adults, OTAs may find that sessions are most effective when a lot of conversation takes place. People from polychronic cultures may also wish to know many details about the OTA's life as a way of showing that they value the professional. When older adults of a polychronic culture arrive late for an appointment, they may be offended if the OTA refuses to squeeze them into the schedule.

Communication Style

The meaning people give to the information they obtain through interaction with others largely depends on the way that information is transmitted. Cultures differ in the amount of information that is transmitted through verbal and nonverbal language. Cultures also differ in regard to the amount of information that is transmitted through the context of the situation.[53] Context includes the relationship to the individual with whom one is communicating. For example, after living together for more than 50 years, an older adult couple does not always have to spell things out for each person to know the other's feelings. Each partner may know the other's feelings simply by the way that the other person moves and the tone of his or her voice. Their shared experiences over 50 years have given them high context; therefore, meaning is not lost when words are not spoken.

Hall[51] noted that high-context cultures rely less on verbal communication than on understanding through shared experience and history. In high-context cultures, fewer words are spoken and more emphasis is placed on nonverbal cues and messages. High-context cultures tend to be formal, reliant on hierarchy, and rooted in the past; thus, they change more slowly and tend to provide more stability for their members.[44,54] When words are used in high-context cultures, communication is more indirect. People in these cultures usually express themselves through stories that imply their opinions.[44,53]

In contrast, persons from low-context cultures typically focus on precise, direct, and logical verbal communication. These persons may not process the gestures, environmental clues, and unarticulated moods central to communication in high-context cultures. Low-context cultures may be more responsive to and comfortable with change but often lack a sense of continuity and connection with the past.[45]

Misunderstanding may easily arise when OTAs and older adults, family members, or caregivers use a different level of context in their communication. Persons from high-context cultures may consider detailed verbal instructions insensitive and mechanistic; they may feel they are being "talked down to." Persons from low-context cultures may be uncomfortable with long pauses and may also feel impatient with indirect communication such as storytelling. It is the responsibility of the OTA to become aware of the style of communication of the older adult, family member, or caregiver and adapt to that style. OTAs must note that nonverbal communication such as facial expressions, eye contact, and touching may have completely different meanings in different cultures. OTAs can learn these things by listening carefully, observing how the family interacts, and adapting their OT practice style as new discoveries are made about the older adult's culture.

CASE STUDY

Mrs. Pardo is a 70-year-old Filipino woman who was admitted to a skilled nursing facility after an infection developed in her right hip. She had a total hip replacement 3 weeks before being transferred to the skilled nursing facility. Because of the infection, Mrs. Pardo had received little therapy. A week ago, the OT was finally able to complete an occupational therapy evaluation. Melissa, a newly hired OTA, is going to be working with Mrs. Pardo. When discussing the case with Melissa, the OT stated that, although Mrs. Pardo has been trained in getting from a supine position to a sitting position at the edge of the bed and in dressing, her family routinely provides assistance. The OT has not discussed with Mrs. Pardo or her family the need for these activities to be done independently. Part of Melissa's responsibility, according to the OT, is to "convince them to not fuss over her so much."

Melissa reviewed Mrs. Pardo's medical record before meeting her. It appeared that Mrs. Pardo's condition was stable, and the infection was under control. Several professionals had documented that she was quite weak and deconditioned, presumably because of prolonged bed rest. Melissa reviewed the occupational therapy evaluation results and intervention goals, which seemed quite straightforward. The general objective was for Mrs. Pardo to become independent in ADL functions and transfers while observing specific hip precautions for at least 6 more weeks. These precautions included touch-toe weight bearing on the right leg, as well as avoiding right leg internal rotation and right hip flexion greater than 60 degrees. Melissa also noted that Mrs. Pardo was a widow who lived with one of her five adult daughters.

One of Mrs. Pardo's daughters and two of her adolescent grandchildren were present when Melissa met Mrs. Pardo. When Melissa introduced herself, Mrs. Pardo smiled and introduced her relatives. She also told Melissa she reminded her of someone she had met years ago while working as a sales representative for an American firm. Once Mrs. Pardo found out where Melissa was from, she asked if Melissa knew the relatives of an acquaintance of hers, who was from Melissa's town. Finally, Melissa stated she was there to work on transfers and dressing. Because Melissa wanted to see how Mrs. Pardo performed these activities independently, she asked the relatives to leave the room for a few minutes. Once they left, Melissa sensed a change in Mrs. Pardo. Although she followed all of Melissa's directions quickly, she seemed to be avoiding eye contact. When Melissa asked her if everything was all right, Mrs. Pardo responded affirmatively. Melissa observed that Mrs. Pardo required minimal assistance to get out of the hospital bed, sit in a commode chair, and dress herself with a gown while observing all hip precautions. Noting that Mrs. Pardo appeared fatigued, Melissa said she would return at 3:00 p.m. to work on Mrs. Pardo's self-bathing ability. Melissa asked whether Mrs. Pardo was aware of any scheduling conflicts, to which Mrs. Pardo responded,

"No." When Melissa left the room, she asked Mrs. Pardo's daughter if she would be available to observe the bath that afternoon. The daughter said she would be there without fail.

Later that afternoon, Melissa entered Mrs. Pardo's room at the same moment that a different daughter was helping Mrs. Pardo get into bed. Alarmed that hip precautions were not being followed, Melissa immediately asked the daughter to let her take over and demonstrate the appropriate method of transferring to the bed. The daughter angrily stated that Mrs. Pardo was too tired for therapy and proceeded to complete the task without Melissa's assistance. Melissa was taken aback and told Mrs. Pardo she would return in the morning for the bath.

That evening, Melissa could not stop thinking about the afternoon's events. She was aware that she had somehow offended Mrs. Pardo's daughter, and she wondered why Mrs. Pardo had gone back to bed knowing that Melissa would be coming to work with her at 3:00 p.m. Melissa decided to carefully analyze what had happened. She remembered how friendly and talkative Mrs. Pardo had been at the beginning of the session, which was perhaps a sign that she valued relationships highly and wanted Melissa to know she was appreciated. Then Melissa thought about the change in Mrs. Pardo when her family left and wondered if she had felt alone without family to support her. Why had Mrs. Pardo said that everything was all right but then avoided eye contact? Was this her way of letting Melissa know that she did not want to do the task without directly opposing the plan for the session? Melissa thought about the tasks they had accomplished and wondered whether Mrs. Pardo had ever before been required to get out of a hospital bed, sit on a commode in front of another person, and dress in a hospital gown? Did these tasks have anything to do with her real life? Finally, Melissa remembered how she had entered the room while Mrs. Pardo's daughter was helping her get into bed. Melissa realized that she had blurted out orders without even introducing herself. Had she caused the daughter to feel embarrassed and incompetent? Was the daughter's anger a way of regaining control?

After evaluating the situation, Melissa concluded that Mrs. Pardo probably could not relate to the artificial ADL tasks presented to her. She also suspected that Mrs. Pardo relied on family members for support in making decisions and reducing anxiety. Mrs. Pardo also seemed to value the feelings of other people and avoided direct confrontation. The daughter might have been angry because Melissa confronted her directly. Melissa decided that the next day she would approach the intervention session with Mrs. Pardo differently. First, she would schedule the session when a family member could be present. She also planned to spend some time simply conversing with Mrs. Pardo and her family members, and she planned to spend more time chit-chatting during the session. Melissa decided to take Mrs. Pardo to the simulated apartment in the rehabilitation department, where they could work in a more realistic home setting with a real bed and chair, and Mrs. Pardo could also work on dressing with her own clothes.

The next day, Melissa carried out her plan with great success. Melissa had realized that Mrs. Pardo was an associative thinker who needed new tasks to be associated with more familiar routines. Melissa had also realized that Mrs. Pardo valued family ties and social relationships greatly and consequently would not risk offending others with a direct refusal. In addition, Melissa realized that Mrs. Pardo relied on family as a source of anxiety reduction. Finally, Melissa had recognized that Mrs. Pardo was from a polychronic culture that valued a more social than prescriptive approach to rehabilitation.

CONCLUSION

Descriptions of particular cultural values or beliefs about aging have not been detailed in the chapter because such generalizations are inherently bound to foster assumptions and create stereotypes.[55] Even if stereotypes are positive, they may discourage practitioners from discovering the unique personality and aspirations of a client because they become shortcuts to communication. For example, sociologists have said that Hispanic families are a close-knit group and the most important social unit.[56] The term *familia* usually goes beyond the nuclear family and includes not only parents and children but also extended family. Individuals within a family have a moral responsibility to aid other members of the family who experience financial problems, unemployment, poor health conditions, and other life issues. If the OTA assumes this to be true about an older adult Hispanic patient, she may jump to the conclusion that family training needs to begin immediately and may not inquire whether the older adult would prefer to be completely independent and live alone. The same value that may lead family members to take care of a grandparent may be leading the older adult to avoid becoming a burden for others. Likewise, the assumption that a Japanese older adult may prefer a highly structured and predictable daily routine, a Japanese cultural feature described by some scholars,[57] may lead the OTA to not offer opportunities for spontaneous activities. Finally, the assumption that an older adult refugee from Sudan would prefer to let her husband make decisions about her care, as is customary in some Muslim cultures,[13] may lead the OTA to ignore that this particular couple customarily shared decision making and were mutually supportive. Although it is advisable that the OTA be informed about the many features of cultures around the world, such knowledge should always be considered tentative and not a replacement for asking questions and letting the older adult guide the selection of goals and interventions in the therapeutic process.

The chapter provides a framework that OTAs can use to approach older adults from diverse backgrounds. Concepts of culture and diversity have been discussed, with special attention given to the ways that these differences can contribute to the older adult's ability to obtain meaning in therapy. Emphasis also was placed on the fact that both culture and diversity are very broad and complex terms. Consequently, a cultural model was presented to aid OTAs in designing individualized occupational therapy services for each older adult. OTAs may use this information as a guide for culturally sensitive practice and remain open to new experiences that they encounter with each older adult. Before attempting to treat older adults from other backgrounds, OTAs must become aware of and analyze their own prejudices and biases about the dimensions of life that create diversity (Box 9.1). Such inner reflection should

BOX 9.1

Attitude Self-Analysis

- Do I believe it is important to consider culture when treating older adults?
- Am I willing to lower my defenses and take risks?
- Am I willing to practice behaviors that may feel unfamiliar and uncomfortable to benefit the older adult with whom I am working?
- Am I willing to set aside some of my own cherished beliefs to make room for others whose values are unknown?
- Am I willing to change the ways I think and behave?
- Am I sufficiently familiar with my own heritage, including place of family origin, time of, and reasons for immigration, and language(s) spoken?
- What values, beliefs, and customs are identified with my own cultural heritage?
- In what ways do my beliefs, values, and customs interfere with my ability to understand those of others?
- Do I view older adults as a resource in understanding their cultural beliefs, family dynamics, and views of health?
- Do I encourage older adults to use resources from within their cultures that they see as important?

always accompany the exploration of the client's values, beliefs, and preferences (Box 9.2).

CHAPTER REVIEW QUESTIONS

1 Explain why it is difficult to define the term *culture*.
2 Give examples of ways in which you have learned and shared a particular value.
3 Give examples of values and beliefs that connect individuals with the various other levels of culture, including family, community, and country.
4 Explain how cultural competence can affect occupational therapy intervention with older adults.
5 Describe your own cognitive style and explain how you base your actions on faith, fact, or feelings. Also, describe how you arrive at decisions about your own health behaviors and what you rely on to reduce anxiety in difficult times.
6 Describe at least three ways in which issues of equality and inequality may affect occupational therapy intervention with older adults.
7 Explain ways in which you tend to behave on a monochronic or polychronic basis. Describe how this tendency may interfere with your ability to provide intervention to older adults.
8 Describe at least three other strategies that Melissa could use with Mrs. Pardo that would take into consideration Mrs. Pardo's cultural context.

BOX 9.2

Exploring the Older Adult's Values, Beliefs, and Preferences

Observation

- If possible, before beginning intervention with an older adult, take some time to observe him or her from afar. How does the older adult interact with others? How do family members and friends interact with the older adult? To what degree is the communication direct? How frequent does eye contact appear to be? While the OTA should not simply mimic the older adult's gestures, they should serve as cues to potentially preferred forms of interaction.
- Are there particular objects the older adult has brought with them to the hospital? Are there any objects that seem to be prominently featured in the older adult's home? Note any specific items and consider them of value, even though you may not at first understand why the older adult chose them. Seek to integrate these items into therapy sessions.

Interaction

- Always approach the older adult respectfully with a greeting. Ask the older adult how he or she would prefer to be greeted and/or addressed. Note that even if an older adult encourages you to use their first name that you do not immediately take other freedoms.
- Ask the older adult how they understand the reasons for therapy. Ask questions to obtain the older adult's explanatory health model:
  - What happened that you now were referred to therapy?
  - What do you think you/your body needs in order to heal?
  - What have you already tried to help yourself recover?
- Always ask the older adult whether they would prefer to have someone present during therapy sessions. Note that an older adult may not feel comfortable answering

truthfully if relatives and/or friends are in the room, so ask the question when the older adult's privacy can be protected.

- Always ask the older adult whether a planned activity is acceptable before initiating it. Explain the goals and inquire whether there are preferred activities that are more meaningful/useful to the older adult in their everyday life.
- Build trust slowly. Encourage the older adult to tell you their life story in increments while working on a therapeutic activity. Follow the older adult's lead; if they prefer to focus quietly on the task, do not insist on having a conversation.
- Share your personal story sparingly and only when or if the older adult asks you to. Remember that the relationship should be centered on the older adult, and your story should build trust not simply make idle conversation.
- Be careful with the frequency with which you ask questions. Permit the older adult to answer fully, and pause before asking another question. Assess the level of comfort with answering questions and adjust accordingly.
- Express interest and openness about the ethnic and cultural heritage of the older adult, and assess the level of comfort they have in speaking about it. Ask the older adult to help you better understand their heritage. Be very careful that your gestures do not inadvertently communicate disgust. Remember that the older adult is relaying information that for them is familiar and often a source of identity. Be culturally humble and communicate your desire to learn from the older adult.
- Paraphrase what the older adult tells you, particularly if related to decisions about their care. This will permit you to check your understanding and assure the older adult that you care.

For additional video content, please visit Elsevier eBooks+ (eBooks.Health.Elsevier.com)

REFERENCES

1. American Occupational Therapy Association. Occupational therapy practice framework: domain and process, 4th ed. *Am J Occup Ther.* 2020;74(suppl 2):1-96. Available at: https://doi.org/10.5014/ajot/2020/74S2001.
2. Healey J. *Diversity and Society: Race, Ethnicity, and Gender.* Los Angeles, CA: SAGE Publications, Inc; 2013.
3. Ofahengaue Vakalahi H, Giunta N, Simpson G, eds. *The Collective Spirit of Aging Across Culture.* New York, NY: Springer; 2014.
4. United Nations Education, Scientific and Cultural Organization (UNESCO). *UNESCO Universal Declaration on Cultural Diversity.* 2001. Available at: http://portal.unesco.org/en/ev.php-URL_ID=13179&URL_DO=DO_TOPIC&URL_SECTION=201.html.
5. Accreditation Council for Occupational Therapy Education. *Standards and Interpretive Guide: Accreditation Standards for an Associate-Degree-Level Educational Program for the Occupational*

Therapy Assistant. 2018. Available at: https://acoteonline.org/wp-content/uploads/2020/10/2018-ACOTE-Standards.pdf.
6. American Occupational Therapy Association. Occupational therapy code of ethics. *Am J Occup Ther.* 2020;74:7413410005p1-7413410005p13.
7. Black R, Wells S. *Culture and Occupation: A Model of Empowerment in Occupational Therapy.* Bethesda, MD: AOTA Press; 2007.
8. American Occupational Therapy Association. *Advisory Opinion for the Ethics Commission: Cultural Competence and Ethical Practice.* 2018. Available at: https://www.aota.org/~/media/Corporate/Files/Practice/Ethics/Advisory/Cultural-Competency.pdf.
9. Kielhofner G. *A Model of Human Occupation: Theory and Application.* 5th ed. Baltimore: Lippincott Williams & Wilkins; 2017.
10. Peters-Golden H. *Culture Sketches: Case Studies in Anthropology.* 6th ed. New York: McGraw-Hill; 2011.
11. Edberg M. *Essentials of Health, Culture, and Diversity: Understanding People, Reducing Disparities.* Burlington, MA: Jones & Bartlett; 2013.
12. Baumesiter R. *The Cultural Animal: Human Nature, Meaning, and Social Life.* New York: Oxford University Press; 2005.
13. Gregg G. *Culture and Identity in a Muslim Society.* Oxford, England: Oxford University Press; 2008.

14. Ross HC. *The Art of Arabian Costume: A Saudi Arabian Profile*. San Francisco, CA: Players Press; 1993.

15. Arnett J. *Human Development: A Cultural Approach*. 3rd ed. Boston, MA: Pearson; 2019.

16. Haviland W, Prims H, McBride B, et al. *Cultural Anthropology: The Human Challenge*. 15th ed. Belmont, CA: Wadsworth Publishing; 2017.

17. Kim G, Chiriboga D, Jang Y. Cultural equivalence in depressive symptoms in older white, black, and Mexican-American adults. *J Am Geriatr Soc*. 2009;57(5):790-796.

18. Goyal N, Adams M, Cyr TG, Maass A, Miller JG. Norm-based spontaneous categorization: cultural norms shape meaning and memory. *J Pers Soc Psychol*. 2020;118(3):436-456. Available at: https://doi.org/10.1037/pspi0000188.

19. Centers for Disease Control and Prevention. *Health Communications: Cultural Competence in Health and Human Services*. 2021. Available at: https://npin.cdc.gov/pages/cultural-competence.

20. Erez M, Gati E. A dynamic, multi-level model of culture: from the micro level of the individual to the macro level of a global culture. *Appl Psychol Int Rev*. 2004;53(4):583-598.

21. Eakman A. Person factors: meaning, sensemaking, and spirituality. In: Christiansen C, Baum C, Bass J, eds. Occupational Therapy: Performance, Participation and Well-Being. 4th ed. Thorofare, NJ: Slack; 2015:313-331.

22. Van de Vijver FJ, Van Hemert DA, Poortinga YH. *Multilevel Analysis of Individuals and Cultures*. New York: Psychology Press; 2015.

23. Padilla R. Environment factors: culture. In: Christiansen C, Baum C, Bass J, eds. Occupational Therapy: Performance, Participation and Well-Being. 4th ed. Thorofare, NJ: Slack; 2015:335-358.

24. Alegria M, Pescosolido BA, Williams S, Canino G. Culture, race/ethnicity and disparities: fleshing out the socio-cultural framework for health services disparities. In: Handbook of the Sociology of Health, Illness, and Healing. New York, NY: Springer; 2011:363-382.

25. Bucher R. *Diversity Consciousness: Opening Our Minds to People, Cultures, and Opportunities*. 4th ed. Englewood Cliffs, NJ: Prentice Hall; 2014.

26. Kimbro R. Acculturation in context: gender, age at migration, neighborhood ethnicity, and health behaviors. *Soc Sci Q*. 2009; 90(5):1145-1166.

27. Johnson A. *Privilege, Power, and Difference*. 3rd ed. New York: McGraw-Hill; 2017.

28. United States Census Bureau. *American Community Survey: 2019 Data Release*. 2019. Available at: https://www.census.gov/programs-surveys/acs/news/data-releases.html.

29. Administration on Aging. *A Profile of Older Americans: 2018*. Washington, DC: U.S. Department of Health and Human Services; 2019.

30. The Williams Institute, UCLA School of Law. *LGBT Demographic Data Interactive*. 2019. Available at: https://williamsinstitute.law.ucla.edu/visualization/lgbt-stats/?topic=LGBT#about-the-data.

31. Choi SK, Meyer IH. *LGBT Aging: A review of Research Findings, Needs, and Policy Implications*. National Resource Center on LGBT Aging; 2016. Available at: https://www.lgbtagingcenter.org/resources/resource.cfm?r=825.

32. Pew Forum on Religion and Public Life. *America's Changing Religious Landscape*. Washington, DC: Pew Research Center; 2015. Available at: https://www.pewresearch.org/religion/2015/05/12/americas-changing-religious-landscape/.

33. Semega J, Kollar M, Shrider EA, Creamer J. *Income and Poverty in the United States: 2019 Report Number P60-270*. United States Census Bureau; September 15, 2020. Available at: https://www.census.gov/library/publications/2020/demo/p60-270.html.

34. Li Z, Dalaker J. *Poverty Among Americans Aged 65 and Older. Report R45791*. Congressional Research Service; July 1, 2019. Available at: https://fas.org/sgp/crs/misc/R45791.pdf.

35. Cuevas AG, O'Brien K, Saha S. What is the key to culturally competent care: reducing bias or cultural tailoring? *Psychol Health*. 2017;32(4):493-507.

36. Allen C. *Occupational Therapy for Psychiatric Diseases: Measurement and Management of Cognitive Disabilities*. Boston: Little Brown; 1985.

37. Allen C, Earhart C, Blue T. *Occupational Therapy Goals for the Physically and Cognitively Disabled*. Rockville, MD: American Occupational Therapy Association; 1992.

38. Hofstede G, Hofstede G. Part 1: The concept of culture. In: Hofstede G, Hofstede G, Minkov M, eds. *Cultures and Organizations: Software of the Mind*. 3rd ed. New York: McGraw-Hill; 2010:24.

39. Datesman M, Crandall J. Chapter 2: Traditional American values and beliefs. In: Datesman M, Crandall J, Keamy EN, eds. *American Ways: An Introduction to American Culture*. 4th ed. New York, NY: Pearson; 2014.

40. Hall E. *Beyond Culture*. New York: Anchor; 1981.

41. Harris M. *Theories of Culture in Postmodern Times*. Pueblo, CO: AltaMira Press; 1998.

42. Gesteland R. *Cross-Cultural Business Behavior: A Guide for Global Management*. 5th ed. Copenhagen, Denmark: Copenhagen Business School Press; 2012.

43. Johnson N. Leadership through policy development: Collaboration, equity, empowerment, and multiculturalism. In: Chin J., Lott B., Rice J., et al., eds. *Women and Leadership: Transforming Visions and Diverse Voices*. Malden Boston: Blackwell; 2007:141-156.

44. Bonvillain N. *Language, Culture, and Communication: The Meaning of Messages*. 8th ed. Lanham, Maryland: Rowman & Littlefield; 2019.

45. Hasselkus BR. *The Meaning of Everyday Occupation*. 3rd ed. Thorofare, NJ: Slack; 2021.

46. McKnight J. *The Careless Society: Community and Its Counterfeits*. New York: Basic; 1995.

47. Wilcock AA, Townsend EA. Occupational justice. In: Crepeau EB, Cohn ES, BoytSchell BA, eds. Willard & Spackman's Occupational Therapy. 11th ed. Baltimore: Lippincott Williams & Wilkins; 2009:192-199.

48. Canadian Association of Occupational Therapists. *Occupational Justice: New Concept or Historical Foundation of Occupational Therapy?* (Slide 8) n.d. Available at: https://caot.in1touch.org/document/3763/f26.pdf.

49. US Department of Health and Human Services Office of Disease Prevention and Health Promotion. *Healthy People 2030: Social Determinants of Health*. n.d. Available at: https://health.gov/healthypeople/objectives-and-data/browse-objectives#social-determinants-of-health.

50. Sevelius JM, Gutierrez-Mock L, Zamudio-Haas S, et al. Research with Marginalized Communities: challenges to continuity during the COVID-19 pandemic. *AIDS Behav*. 2020;24(7):2009-2012. doi:10.1007/s10461-020-02920-3.

51. Hall E. *The Dance of Life: The Other Dimensions of Time*. New York: Anchor; 1984.

52. Wittmann M. *Felt Time: The Psychology of How We Perceive Time*. Cambridge, MA: Massachusetts Institute of Technology; 2016.

53. Deachslin J, Gilbert M, Malone B. *Diversity and Cultural Competence in Health Care: A Systems Approach*. San Francisco, CA: Jossey-Bass; 2013.

54. Luquis R. Health education theoretical models and multicultural populations. In: Pérez M, Luquis R, eds. Cultural Competence in Health Education and Health Promotion. 2nd ed. San Francisco: Jossey-Bass; 2014:145-170.

55. Cruikshank M. *Learning to Be Old: Gender, Culture and Aging*. 3rd ed. Lanham, MD: Rowan & Littlefield; 2013.

56. De Meante B. *Why Mexicans Think & Behave the Way They Do!: The Cultural Factors that Created the Character & Personality of the Mexican People*. Blaine, WA: Phoenix; 2009.

57. Meng Y, Rahman T, Pickett M, et al. *Health and Health Behaviors of Japanese Americans in California: A Sign of Things to Come for Aging Americans?* Los Angeles, CA: UCLA Center for Health Policy Research; 2015.

10

Ethical Aspects in the Work With Older Adults

BRENDA KORNBLIT KENNELL AND LEA C. BRANDT

(PREVIOUS CONTRIBUTIONS FROM KATE BROWN AND CAROL SCHWOPE)

KEY TERMS

advance directives, American Occupational Therapy Association (AOTA) Ethics Commission (EC), autonomy, benefits, burdens, creative documentation, confidentiality, distributive justice, elder abuse, ethical dilemma, ethical distress, ethics committee, HIPAA, informed consent, least restrictive environment, National Board for Certification in Occupational Therapy (NBCOT), stakeholders, State Regulatory Board (SRB)

CHAPTER OBJECTIVES

1. Discuss steps for ethical considerations.
2. Describe the language of ethics.
3. Differentiate between ethical and legal standards of practice.
4. Refine and explain personal and professional ethical commitments.

Sara, Miya, Jaime, and Deon are four friends who graduated from the same occupational therapy assistant (OTA) program a few years ago. They have gathered to discuss ethical conflicts they each experienced where they work. Sara works in a skilled nursing facility, Miya works for a home health agency, Jaime works on the geropsychiatric unit at the hospital, and Deon is employed at an outpatient clinic.

In this chapter, the four previously mentioned OTAs discuss a variety of ethical questions arising from the complexities of their job demands. These discussions include a series of steps for ethical consideration that students and clinicians can use in responding to ethical challenges in their practices. In addition to applying components of the Occupational Therapy Code of Ethics,[1] other ethics commentaries that guide professional practice are introduced in this chapter. The author hopes that OTAs will take the opportunity to refine and explain the ethical commitments that shape their practice when working with older adults. OTAs should understand that being confronted with ethical conflict is inevitable in all areas of occupational therapy practice. Therefore, in addition to one's ongoing cultivation of clinical reasoning skills, it is equally important to develop skills related to ethical decision-making.

AN OVERVIEW: ETHICS AND CARE OF OLDER ADULTS

Before we can really talk about ethics with older adults, we need to know what ethics means and how it relates to the practice of occupational therapy. Although ethics principles were first introduced by the ancient Greek philosophers, modern health care ethics really began with Beauchamp and Childress in 1985 in their book *Principles of Medical Ethics*.[2] Their principles of respect for autonomy, beneficence, nonmaleficence, and justice have been joined by other principles such as veracity and fidelity. Simply put, beneficence means "doing good" and caring for the well-being of others, such as our clients. This can mean ensuring that clients receive appropriate services, using appropriate tools, and delegating services to the appropriate person. Nonmaleficence means to "do no harm"; in other words, to refrain from illegal, inappropriate, or harmful behaviors. This includes things like not stealing from clients, not engaging in sexual relations with clients, or not working when impaired. Autonomy means "personal choice" which is exhibited by allowing people to make informed decisions about their own health care, including refusing services. Justice means "doing the right thing" such as following appropriate rules, regulations, and laws. Veracity means truthfulness, such as ensuring that all billing, documentation, marketing, and promotion is honest and accurate. Fidelity relates to keeping commitments. This includes stewardship of employer resources and showing respect for colleagues. Other ethical and moral concerns such as social justice and confidentiality are addressed by various principles, such as beneficence, autonomy, justice, and fidelity. Some of these principles are reflected in the Core Values of American Occupational Therapy Association (AOTA)—altruism, equality, freedom, justice, dignity, truth, and prudence.[3]

Although the principles themselves have not changed much in the ensuing years, the world of health care has changed dramatically, requiring a closer look at ethical principles and ethical behavior. This includes the many advances in diagnosing and treating various health conditions, longer life expectancy, and technology. Although new technology and treatments exist, there is increasing disparity of health care access among different racial, ethnic, and socioeconomic populations.[4] Changes in the reimbursement systems in health care also set the stage for ethical challenges regarding the quantity, location, and duration of health care and therapy services. More information is available to the public via the internet, but lack of health literacy and disagreements among clients, families, and health professionals may cause barriers to both making informed decisions and accessing appropriate and sufficient health care.[5]

In the United States, most older adults have some form of Medicare and supplemental policies as their main form of health insurance. Medicare is a federal program funded through payroll taxes. Some older adults also have Medicaid which is a joint federal and state program available for people with limited income and resources. The federal government is the "single largest payer for healthcare in the United States."[6] The Centers for Medicare and Medicaid (CMS) which oversee these programs play a role in determining which treatments and technology should be covered, and what is appropriate reimbursement for various services.[6] Many insurers follow what CMS does, so when CMS puts out rules regarding limitations on treatment or reimbursement for treatment provided by occupational and physical therapy assistants or students, medical facilities and other insurers often enact the same policies.

With mounting concerns related to excessive expenditures and lack of correlation between cost and health outcomes, OT practice is especially influenced by pressures to do more with fewer resources. In some ways, these pressures have contributed positively to OT practice. Increased attention to the way health care dollars are spent has made OT practitioners focus more carefully on which interventions to use and the rationale for using them. More attention is being paid to the "distinct value" of occupational therapy and distinguishing our profession from others. Returning to our roots and providing occupation-based services instead of exercises is a way to demonstrate that OT is not an extension of PT. Providing interventions

and billing CPT codes for "self-care" and "therapeutic activities" can help avoid the presumption that services were duplicated by two disciplines both billing for "therapeutic exercises."[7] Understanding the rationale for use is very important when using physical agent modalities (PAMs). Studies and anecdotal evidence have shown widespread use of PAMs in skilled nursing facilities, yet clinicians do not always understand why they are being used, if they are necessary, or if they are effective.[8] An ethical concern may arise when being asked to use PAMs on older adult clients who do not need them, or being asked to use a modality for which the OTA is not competent. Unnecessary or inappropriate treatment can result in harm to a client and is not consistent with the AOTA position that PAMs are to be used "preparatory to occupation" or "concurrent to therapeutic occupation or purposeful activities."[9] Using PAMs when not competent also contradicts the AOTA position that "occupational therapy practitioners possess the foundational knowledge of basic sciences, understanding of relevant theory and evidence, and clinical reasoning to recommend and safely apply PAMs…"[9]

Cost-control strategies can also create ethical challenges for practitioners. Traditionally, health care professionals have provided clinical services based on the occupational needs of clients. Increasingly, however, financial constraints impede practitioners' ability to uphold this commitment. For instance, third-party payers often dictate the number of paid visits a patient may receive for a particular condition, and the number is not always reflective of clinical need. If a practitioner recommends more visits than allocated, clients may be required to pay some or all of the additional amount out of pocket, which may result in an insurmountable financial burden. Other ethically problematic cost-driven practices include "creative documentation" for reimbursement and accepting referrals for marginally necessary or needless interventions. "Creative documentation" refers to the practice of exaggerating a problem, altering a diagnosis, or implying a better prognosis so that more client visits can be approved. When actual fraud exists, such practices are also subject to legal inquiry and penalty.

Like other health professions, OT is also affected by evolving health care technologies. Although some technologies such as improved joint replacement componentry have enhanced clinical outcomes, other technologies capable of sustaining life sometimes pose complex questions that clients, practitioners, and society are ill prepared to answer. For example, continuing to provide artificial nutrition and hydration to a person in a persistent vegetative state elicits complex ethical questions. As stated previously, autonomy means allowing people to make their own health care choices, yet sometimes a person's wishes are not known. Additional ethical issues arise when family members disagree with one another on what care to permit, and they may try to involve occupational therapy practitioners into their arguments.

Other questions concern the ethics involved in equitable access to health care services for all persons. Artiga, Orgera, and Pham remind us that health care disparities "are commonly viewed through the lens of race and ethnicity, but they occur across a broad range of dimensions … [including] socioeconomic status, age, geography, language, gender, disability status, citizenship status, and sexual identity and orientation."[4] The coronavirus pandemic of 2020–2021 has shown us that even when new technology like telehealth and virtual visits exist, people with limited or inconsistent internet access or poor English proficiency may not be able to utilize them. Having to share computer bandwidth with family members who are working or attending school from home, may make it impossible for an older adult to seek virtual health care during the hours it is offered.

Frequently, cost controls can translate into fewer staff for more clients. During temporary or chronic staffing shortages, how is it determined which clients receive services? The ethical principle of distributive justice says that resources should be shared "fairly," but what does that mean? The principle of utility says that "the most ethical choice is the one that will produce the greatest good for the greatest number."[10] But what does that mean? If there is only one OTA who can treat for 6 hours, should she treat 10 clients with mild-moderate deficits or 4 clients with significant deficits? There is not a definitive answer to this question. Ethical practitioners should consider the needs of each client before making such decisions.

When these staffing changes contribute to inadequate supervision, OTAs can be placed in ethically questionable positions in terms of their professional standards of practice. This can include being asked to conduct initial evaluations, provide treatment to clients who have not yet been evaluated, use modalities or equipment for which the OTA is not adequately trained or competent, or work at a level of client acuity for which the OTA is not skilled or safe. OTAs need to be familiar with ethical principles and professional regulations to protect themselves and their clients from these situations.

In addition to the clinical and financial environment of practice, special ethical concerns arise for OTAs who work with older adults. Older adults have a wide range of health care needs, and their occupational goals are diverse. All clients require personalized intervention plans, and the practitioner working with older adults may need to develop particular ethical sensitivities given the resources, practice environment restrictions, and client context.

Consider the example of how clinical decisions are made in the health care setting. Generally, in the United States, most people believe that adults should be the primary decision makers about their own health care because respecting client autonomy is important. In the health care setting, respect for autonomy refers to the idea that

adults have the right to be involved in determining their plan of care and relevant intervention decisions.

In other cultures, however, someone else may be the primary decision maker, or control the flow of information. For example, in Mexico, a father may be responsible for making most decisions, but the mother must be involved as it will be her role to follow through with care plans. In some cultures it will be the elder family members who lead the decision-making. Within certain cultural contexts, family members are informed about the seriousness of an illness and may withhold that information in order to alleviate the stress on the sick person.[11] To ensure that clients and their family members have the information they need to make decisions that lead to good clinical outcomes, practitioners must understand their role as clinical advisors and communicate effectively regarding the benefits and burdens of potential interventions. Informed consent serves as a legal requirement associated with the ethical principle of respect for autonomy. True informed consent hinges on appropriately applying this principle as well as practitioners' ability to effectively communicate potential outcomes.

If practitioners only focus on the signing of an informed consent document, they may be upholding a legal standard, but they are not adhering to the ethical intent associated with respect for autonomy. To support clients' autonomous choice, health care providers must also engage in shared decision-making processes that assist clients in understanding the procedure to which they are consenting or declining. Shared decision-making is predicated on the idea that both the clients and clinicians play essential roles; clients know their values and preferences and the practitioners have clinical knowledge.[12] The higher the risk of harm, the more thorough the consent process should be. The process is more than relaying risks and benefits. In addition, practitioners and clients should engage in dialogue regarding the best decision based on the clients' personal values. Once clients have the necessary information, respect for autonomy necessitates that they be allowed to accept or refuse interventions. Further, respect for autonomy does not include offering interventions that are not clinically indicated. Instead, when clients demand interventions not supported by evidence-based practice, it is the practitioners' ethical responsibility to explain why the interventions cannot be provided and discuss how the burdens outweigh the benefits of the interventions.

Of course the ability to weigh the pros and cons of treatment options is dependent upon understanding the situation and the options. Even without issues such as limited English proficiency, functional illiteracy, and vision and hearing impairment, older adults vary in their capacities for independent function and thought, and thus their capacities for autonomous decision-making. Some older adults are no longer able to make decisions on their own behalf. Often, the extent of this inability and its

BOX 10.1

The Scott Four-Step Process for Ethical Decision[13]
1. Gather the facts, and specify the dilemma
2. Analyze possible courses of action
3. Select and implement a course of action
4. Evaluate the results of the action

consequences for decision-making are unclear. This state of fluctuating ability for decision-making is often referred to as diminished capacity. A decline in physical independence is not always accompanied by mental dependency, and OTAs must keep in mind that older adults who have lost most of their physical independence may still retain the ability to make independent decisions.

In addition, older adults may retain the ability to make decisions in some situations and not in others. Decision-making capacity is situation-dependent and should therefore constantly be reassessed in practice. Caregivers need to appreciate that an older adult's capacity for independent decision-making may fluctuate because of his or her physical or mental conditions. For instance, older adults with Alzheimer's disease, Parkinson's disease, or stroke may be more fully alert at certain times of the day than at other times. Older adults also vary in their capacities to respond to different kinds of decision-making tasks. In a nursing home, for example, a resident who may have the mental capacity to decide what to eat may not have the ability to independently weigh and balance the risks and benefits of medical procedures. Conversely, just because a resident may not have the capacity to independently make medical decisions, his or her right to make daily decisions regarding routine or activities of daily living should not be usurped. The task, the circumstance, and the older adults' mental and emotional state determine their decision-making capacities.

Client decision-making is only one area of ethical concern for OTAs. Through an exploration of the situations presented by the four OTAs, Deon, Miya, Jaime, and Sara, the chapter presents a number of other issues. The chapter is organized around the Scott four-step process for ethical decision-making[13] (Box 10.1). Each step is illustrated with specific cases experienced by the four friends.

STEP 1: GATHER THE FACTS, AND SPECIFY THE DILEMMA

The first step in approaching an ethical problem is to figure out what is going on. This may seem obvious at first, but actually the situation can be quite complicated, and, OTAs must consider a number of factors before taking action. Often, practitioners see problems only as clinical in nature and do not initially ask about or understand the underlying ethical concerns. Like other health care providers, if OTAs do not ask ethical questions, they may arrive at decisions that can be clinically implemented but are ethically problematic.

What Kind of Ethical Situation Is It?

OTAs may find it helpful to start by figuring out the kind of issue they are facing. Clinical ethicists often refer to ethical dilemmas and moral or ethical distress.[14] An ethical dilemma refers to a situation in which there are two or more options for action; but each option compromises some ethical principle. Moral distress occurs when the OTA knows what is the "right" course of action to take but feels constrained to act in accordance with what is believed to be commonly done or is pressured not to take action. Often, the constraint is imposed by someone who has more institutional authority than the OTA. This can become an ethical issue; for example, failing to report a colleague who is practicing while impaired or falsifying billing logs violates the ethical principles of veracity, nonmaleficence, and justice. In other situations though, it could be a matter of misunderstanding between two or more parties, such as when the OTA is addressing medication management with a client but was unaware that the family had taken over that task due to the older adult's declining cognitive status. A situation can also be a personnel issue such as when there is insufficient staff, which can lead to a potential legal issue when the OTA is asked to work outside her scope of practice and licensure law (Box 10.2).

Who Is Involved?

When approaching an ethical problem, one must determine the "stakeholders" or who is involved. Of course this includes the OTA and the client, but who else has a stake in the ethical situation? Stakeholders can include family members, caregivers, health care practitioners, the facility, and the payer source. OTAs must also consider stakeholders' beliefs, values, and biases to anticipate areas of agreement and disagreement about the proposed course of action. The family often needs to be involved in medical decision-making, but involvement may result in an ethical dilemma for the OTA.

For example, Miya is working with a home care client named Mr. Romero. The Romero family asks Miya for help in pursuing long-term care placement for their father who has begun to wander from his home and has gotten lost several times. Miya knows that Mr. Romero values his independence and will resist the move to a facility; however, Miya recognizes that he might endanger himself. Miya must first consider Mr. Romero's decision-making capacity. Does the fact that he wanders indicate that he lacks capacity? Does Mr. Romero have the right to stay in his home even if Miya and his family believe it is a poor or unsafe choice? Respecting the client's choice is difficult when one does not agree with that choice or the decision

BOX 10.2

Examples of Ethical Problems

Ethical dilemma

Jaime works at a geropsychiatric unit in a hospital. He has just learned that his client is to be discharged the following day. Jaime knows he lives alone and will most likely not be able to regulate his medications appropriately. Jaime voices his concerns, but the supervisor says that the man's insurance coverage has run out, so they have no choice but to discharge him. Jaime wonders if he can check on him daily by phone after he discharges?

- Is it ethically wrong to discharge this client? Why or why not?
- Is it ethically wrong not to advocate for the client to remain in the hospital when he has no insurance? Why or why not?
- Is it ethical for Jaime to call the client daily after he is discharged? Why or why not?

Ethical/moral distress

In the past, Sara, an OTA, treated Mr. Walker, who is 96 years old with advanced prostate cancer and Parkinson's disease. He had no energy and rarely got out of bed. The last time she saw him, he said "I just want to relax and enjoy watching television until I die, which I hope is soon." Mr. Walker has new orders to be followed by occupational therapy. Sara approaches the OT who is the Rehab Director and suggests that they do not put Mr. Walker back on the caseload, since he is in a lot of pain, is not motivated, and shows no potential to improve his functional skills. The OT tells Sara to "get with the program, or we can use the other OTA for more hours instead of you."

- Why is this an issue of ethical or moral distress?
- What is the barrier to Sara refusing to treat Mr. Walker?
- What would you do if you were Sara?

Ethical dilemma and ethical distress: distributive justice

The other OTA, Ben, in the outpatient clinic where Deon works, goes on an unexpected leave of absence, leaving the department short-staffed for several weeks.

There are four of Ben's clients that need to be seen:

- A 66-year-old woman with Medicare, recovering from a wrist fracture
- A 68-year-old man with Medicare, who has lateral epicondylitis
- A 62-year-old man with Medicaid, with dense hemiplegia, visual perceptual deficits, and cognitive impairments following a CVA
- A 64-year-old woman with no insurance, recently diagnosed with Myasthenia Gravis

Deon has five open slots in his schedule. The clinic manager schedules both older adults with Medicare for twice weekly and the man with Medicaid who has a CVA for one time weekly. The clinical manager says that the uninsured woman with myasthenia gravis will have to wait until the other OTA returns. Deon questions the allotment of appointments, noting that the less involved orthopedic clients are getting more appointments than the more involved neurological clients. The manager tells Deon it is because they can overlap the orthopedic clients for intervention and also add modalities. Therefore, they can bill more units with the two patients on Medicare, which minimizes the loss of revenue while the other OTA is out. Deon offers to work overtime for a few weeks to enable all the clients to be seen, but the manager says the budget is tight and it is too much paperwork to get overtime authorization. The manager also says that when Ben returns, the clinic may cut one OTA position. Deon is concerned because Ben has been there 5 years, and Deon has been there for only 1 year.

- What are the ethical principles and standards of conduct being violated here?
- Why is this an issue of ethical or moral distress for Deon?
- How is this an example of the principle of distributive justice? In what other scenarios might distributive justice be an issue in the clinic?
- What would you do if you were Deon?

---

could result in harm. However, older adults often make decisions that therapy practitioners must respect without agreeing to the choice. Is this an instance when the practitioner should respect the wishes of the client? At what point should decision-making capacity be questioned? Does the client's family have the right to make decisions for their loved one? What if one son wants to move Mr. Romero to a long-term care setting, but another son wants their father to remain in the family home with assistance? What are the family basing their decisions on—financial concerns, Mr. Romero's safety, or Mr. Romero's happiness? In this situation, what other values, besides Mr. Romero's autonomous choice, should Miya consider? Who else should be involved in addition to Miya, the family, and Mr. Romero?

STEP 2: ANALYZE POSSIBLE COURSES OF ACTION

To determine what action to take, one must first consider core values, ethical principles, professional standards; federal, state, and local laws and regulations; institutional policies and procedures, and reimbursement requirements. Evaluating the facts of the ethical situation in the context of these factors can help the OTA analyze the options and select the appropriate course of action.

Which Laws and Institutional Rules Apply?

There are distinct differences between the law and ethics. While ethical and moral principles attempt to guide our behavior toward what is "right" versus "wrong," legal statues guide our behavior in terms of what is legally permitted and what is illegal. An action can be legal but morally "wrong" to someone based on that person's beliefs and values, such as abortion or the death penalty. Violating an ethical or moral principle may result in personal distress, stigma in a social or cultural circle, public censure, or professional embarrassment. Illegal action, however, can result in monetary fines or even prison time. Both types of action can affect an OTA's ability to work in the field, as licensure laws and practice acts often dictate adherence to the AOTA Code of Ethics. Penalties can be as mild as a letter of reprimand or as severe as loss of certification and licensure.

Sometimes, laws and institutional rules help clarify the role of OTAs with a given ethical problem. Some laws are federal, meaning that they apply in every state, but other laws apply only within a particular state's jurisdiction, such as each state's Occupational Therapy Practice Act. Many health care facilities and institutions have legal counsel who can answer questions about specific laws and regulatory requirements. Generally, institutions have established guidelines and rules that specify the expectations for staff, clients, and administrators. OTAs are responsible for knowing which laws and policies apply to their practice and, according to the Occupational Therapy Code of Ethics, are expected to "comply with current federal and state law, state scope of practice guidelines, and AOTA policies and Official Documents that apply to the profession of occupational therapy" and "Abide by policies, procedures, and protocols when serving or acting on behalf of a professional organization or employer...."[1]

The influence of law in guiding ethical practice is illustrated in a case regarding the use of restraints that Jaime was asked to help resolve at the hospital where he works. Jaime's client Mrs. Taylor is a 68-year-old woman who was admitted to geropsychiatric unit because of agitation and uncontrollable behavior. Her charted diagnosis read, "Axis I schizoaffective bipolar type, axis III hypertension, degenerative joint disease, chronic obstructive pulmonary disease, chronic constipation, head trauma (grade 9; no further details)." Staff members have expressed that they do not particularly like Mrs. Taylor; they often construe her behavior as violent. She calls other clients and staff derogatory names; she also tells lies about them and accuses them of mistreating her. At times, she claims she is unable to walk and demands use of a wheelchair. She often stages a fall by throwing herself from the wheelchair onto the floor. The staff recommends that she be restrained in a chair for her own safety.

When Jaime brought this case to his friends for discussion, Sara pointed out that, given Mrs. Taylor's age, her case was most likely covered by Medicare. She goes on to state that she thinks this means that, legally, like the staff in her nursing home, the staff in the psychiatric hospital should follow the guidelines for restraints defined by the Omnibus Budget Reconciliation Act (OBRA) of 1987. Sara explained that this federal legislation requires health care providers to ensure client safety in the least restrictive environment. Jaime voiced his suspicion that maybe the restraints were being used as punishment, not client safety, but was not sure whether OBRA applied to psychiatric facilities. Deon then posed the following question, "Regardless of the legal implications, shouldn't we strive for what is most ethical?" The others agreed that striving for the least restrictive environment is certainly ethically indicated, but it also would not hurt to understand how OBRA applies to psychiatric facilities. The four friends began thinking of ways that occupational therapy could help in designing the least restrictive environment for this older adult and whom to contact regarding OBRA guidelines. "After all," said Miya, "even unpleasant people deserve the right to make choices and have some liberty, as long as they are not hurting others." While this case demonstrates how the law and ethics may support a single course of action, it also shows that there is a distinct difference between applying ethical standards and the law. When in doubt, it is best to ethically reason through options in line with the standard of care set by the profession. OT practitioners should always strive to provide ethical care, which is often a higher standard than what is legally required. Deon, Miya, Jaime, and Sara question whether there are situations when there would be a conflict between what is legally required and what is ethically indicated.

Many regulations and health care laws were developed with the intent to protect patients' privacy and support their right to self-determination. In particular, laws related to confidentiality and advance directives were adopted in response to cases where the rights of patients were violated. These legal aspects of care delivery are especially complex when working with older adults.

According to Pozgar (2020), an estimated 70% of the 1,600,000 Americans who die each year in hospital and nursing homes, die after a decision was made to forgo life-sustaining treatment. These decisions are based on the individual's beliefs and values but must comply with applicable laws and policies.[15] After court cases on behalf of the families of Karen Anne Quinlan and Nancy Cruzan in 1976 and 1990, respectively; in 1990, the Patient Self-Determination Act was enacted to promote patient understanding of decision-making rights, including the right to create an advance directive.

"Advance directive" is a general term used to apply to documents such as living wills, medical directives, and durable powers of attorney (DPOA) that allow a person to state in advance what kinds of medical care or procedures he or she considers acceptable and unacceptable, in advance of losing decision-making capacity and/or the ability to communicate. The person can appoint a "surrogate decision maker" often called a "healthcare power of attorney" to make those decisions on his or her behalf. This includes decisions about both lifesaving measures like CPR, mechanical ventilation, antibiotics, and feeding tubes; as well as comfort measures such as hydration and pain medication. Appointing a DPOA allows adults to identify the person who can best convey their wishes when they are no longer able to speak for themselves.

Although legislation supporting advance directive documents has been in effect for several decades, there may be barriers when attempting to follow a written advance directive in clinical practice. This is because people often create these documents in response to a legal standard and do not engage in conversations with potential health care decision makers regarding their intent, or do not change the documents when family situations change, for example, financial changes or adult children moving away.

Sara's client Mrs. Sanchez has been working on increasing independence after a fall resulting in a broken hip. Since her initial treatment session, it was clear that Mrs. Sanchez was very close to her daughter Irina, who lives only 8 miles from her mother. Irina is readily available for OT treatment sessions and, when called in for family training, she is supportive of the interventions provided. Mrs. Sanchez' eldest daughter Janice lives on the other side of the country. Although Mrs. Sanchez speaks in high regard of her daughter Janice, it appears that their communication is limited to monthly phone calls secondary to geographical distance. Mrs. Sanchez is proud of Janice's skills as a massage therapist and believes that Janice really understands the human body. A few days after Mrs. Sanchez is admitted to the facility, Janice flies in for a visit to check on her mother and tells Sara that "OT is a bunch of hooey; Mom just needs to be discharged to Irina's house so the family can take care of her. I hold Mom's durable power of attorney and therefore it is my decision to have Mom discharged from OT and this facility. I will relay that decision at the team meeting on Monday." Mrs. Sanchez responds by shaking her head and states, "Janice, I made you the DPOA because you have a health care background, but your sister Irina is the one who should make the decision. She knows more about me and what I can do and what I want."

Sara relays to her friends that she was so uncomfortable she left the room and plans to follow up with the team on Monday. Deon asks his colleagues, "If Mrs. Sanchez is getting better with therapy, can her DPOA make a decision which may be harmful?" Miya replies, "As long as Mrs. Sanchez still has decision-making capacity, I don't think Janice has the authority to make any decisions." Sara responds, "I believe that Mrs. Sanchez has decision-making capacity, but I am most concerned because, if Mrs. Sanchez loses her capacity in the future, Janice will have the legal authority to make decisions, and it doesn't seem like she would be the best surrogate decision maker." Jaime then asks Sara what she is going to do. Sara responds, "I don't feel comfortable addressing all the legal questions involved in this case, but I am definitely going to talk to the social worker and administrators first thing Monday morning before the team meeting about what to

do. While I might not be the best person as an OTA to talk to Mrs. Sanchez about her rights and how the DPOA process works, it is my ethical obligation to address conditions that may prevent her from getting the best care possible, especially the benefit of ongoing OT services."

As is depicted in the scenario, legal decisions do not always appear to be in alignment with the best interests or values of the client. When there are perceived conflicts of interest, it is ethically supported to ask questions. In some cases, this may mean questioning the legal authority of surrogates or documents. Although asking the question may delay the process, it also promotes due diligence to optimize congruency between client wishes and clinical decisions.

Best interest with regard to elderly clients who have at some point held decision-making capacity would be to apply standards of substituted judgment. This is generally the case when working with older adults who have recently lost decision-making capacity or appear to show diminished capacity. Regardless of whether there is an advance directive, providers should work to uphold a substituted judgment standard when attempting to implement decisions for their clients who have lost decision-making capacity. This standard would include involving the client as much as possible in cases of diminished capacity, and discussions with the family regarding previous conversations they may have had with the client and/or reflecting on how the client lived his/her life to determine what he or she would want. Dialogue with the family would also give the health care team insight as to the family's motivations. Hopefully, through dialogue with other team members, the older adult, and/or the family, the conflict can be reconciled. If the intent of conversation is to identify the best course of treatment for an older adult, then practitioners are ethically supported in bringing in stakeholders who can assist in defining the best plan of care. Although confidentiality must be respected, it should not serve as a barrier to caring for older adults.

Laws related to confidentiality, specifically the Health Insurance Portability and Accountability Act (HIPAA), are sometimes cited by practitioners as a barrier to communication. HIPAA was enacted in 1996 with the intent to protect the privacy, confidentiality, and security of patient information.[15] In fact, HIPAA has greatly improved processes related to maintaining confidentiality. Those communication barriers cited as a product of HIPAA can often be resolved if the provider clarifies processes and is truly working to address the needs of the client. According to HIPAA, protected health information (PHI) can be shared as long as the information is needed to effectively treat the patient. Remaining client-centered in making treatment decisions is ethically indicated. By focusing on what is the right thing to do for a client, while understanding the parameters of the law, OT practitioners can engage in best practices with the least amount of legal jeopardy.

In their discussion, Deon shared an experience from fieldwork II at a local hospital where one of the OTs tried to read the medical record of a local politician who was not on her caseload. Luckily after being reminded of the ethical and legal ramifications of a HIPAA violation and the potential consequences to the hospital and to her career, the OT made no further attempts at accessing that person's PHI. However, when the politician was discharged and referred to home health, the therapy staff there were initially denied access to the person' s hospital records. The clinicians worked with the hospital and home health agency's legal counsels to show that they had the right to view these records in order to best serve their client. Deon went on to say that, in his experience, doing the right thing for client is usually not in conflict with the law, and doing the right thing can offer the best legal protection when working in a litigious society.

What Guidance Does the Occupational Therapy Code of Ethics Provide?

The AOTA first published the "Principles of Ethics" in 1977, and now requires that the Code of Ethics is reviewed at least every 5 years by the AOTA Ethics Commission. The purpose of the AOTA Code of Ethics (hereinafter referred to as the Code) is to "address the most prevalent ethical concerns of the occupational therapy profession. It sets forth Core Values and outlines Standards of Conduct the public can expect from those in the profession."[1]

Although most OT practitioners want to "do the right thing," it is sometimes hard to understand what exactly that means. People do not remember what the ethics principles mean and not everyone agrees which principles apply to different situations or behaviors. To make it easier for OT practitioners to know what behavior is expected of them, the AOTA Ethics Commission reorganized the Code of Ethics (2020) from ethical principles to Standards of Conduct. Although these standards are all based on ethical principles, they are now organized into seven professional behavior categories which outline specific behaviors:

- Professional Integrity, Responsibility, and Accountability relates to maintaining awareness and complying with relevant laws, AOTA policies, and employer policies.
- Therapeutic Relationships relates to developing therapeutic relationships to promote well-being in all clientele regardless of any status or attributes.
- Documentation, Reimbursement, and Financial Matters relates to maintaining complete, accurate, and timely records.
- Service Delivery relates to striving to deliver quality, occupation-based, client-centered, culturally sensitive, evidence-based intervention.
- Professional Competence Education, Supervision, and Training relates to maintaining appropriate credentials, licenses, certification, and professional competence.
- Communication relates to upholding confidentiality, informed consent, autonomy, and accuracy in all communication.
- Professional Civility relates to conducting oneself in a culturally sensitive and civil manner are all times.[1]

The reorganization was done in an effort to make the Code of Ethics more inclusive, enforceable, and accessible to practitioners and consumers; and therefore easier to determine the right course of action.[15,16] Not only is the Occupational Therapy Code of Ethics a guide for behavior, but it is also a regulatory code in that guidelines for conduct are stated and sanctions are provided for failure to comply with the code. These sanctions are stated in the Enforcement Procedures for the Code of Ethics.[17] Often, State Regulatory Boards refer to the AOTA Code of Ethics when considering issues related to licensure. Even with the reorganization, OT practitioners sometimes need additional resources to help guide them to understanding and applying ethical reasoning. The Ethics Commission offers other ethics resources in addition to publishing resource books. These include multiple Ethics Advisory Opinions (AOs) which have been developed and are available only to members on the AOTA website.[18] These documents review common ethical issues in practice, with content focused on the systematic processes used when applying the Code of Ethics to various cases and vignettes. The Advisories are consistently reviewed and updated according to the needs of the profession or to current events and technology changes, such as the coronavirus pandemic and the increase in teletherapy. Review of the AOs can assist practitioners in developing ethical reasoning skills in response to common dilemmas.

What Are My Options?

OT practitioners need to be aware of the range of ethical options available to them before deciding what action should be taken in a given case. It is important to note that not all options can be ethically, legally, or in some cases logistically supported. OT practitioners should not offer options to colleagues, older adults, and/or families that are illegal and/or ethically problematic. When OTAs and supervising occupational therapists (OTs) do not agree, OTAs can also find themselves in a compromised position. Identifying reasonable options requires OTAs to understand the constraints and resources available to them in their particular practice setting and role. Deon, Miya, Jaime, and Sara agree that one of the most difficult ethical dilemmas they all experienced was when their ideas regarding the right course of action for a client ran contrary to the supervising OT's recommendations. Jaime lets the others know that one of the AOs available on the AOTA's website[18] is dedicated to ethical issues related to OT and OTA partnerships. Jaime states, "I found reviewing these opinions to be very helpful. The cases are very realistic and they helped me to see how the Code of Ethics could be used to identify what options exist and

STEP 3: SELECT AND IMPLEMENT A COURSE OF ACTION

Reflection: What do I think should happen?

After OTAs are aware of all of the facts and reflect on the options in a given case, they must choose a course of action and be able to explain their position. Each person should find personal methods of reflection that best fit his or her reasoning style in order to determine what actions seem most wrong or right. This process may begin as a gut feeling that persists, and it is important to be sensitive to such feelings. Ethical reflection involves careful consideration of one's feelings and values, cultural beliefs and biases, a rational estimate of benefits and burdens, scope of practice and legally defined roles, and a sense of professional duty. This reflection is most effective when the OTA has engaged in dialogue with the client and/or family to factor in their wishes, values, and motivations. Sometimes emotional and even physical distance may be necessary as OTAs reflect on their ethical commitments and reasoning. If a situation is urgent, rapid reflection is necessary. Otherwise the OTA should take time for serious consideration of preferences, motivations, and potential consequences when choosing a course of action.

Finding a balance between genuine caring for clients and realistic boundaries for professional involvement is a lifelong goal for all health care professionals that requires ongoing ethical introspection. This means examining one's empathetic relationships with clients. In long-term care environments and personal settings such as home health, professionals may find it hard to maintain professional distance. Conversely, older adults must be protected from a health professional's overinvolvement, as in the extreme case of sexual liaisons, and from a health professional's subjective biases, as in the case of bias or discrimination. The four OTA friends shared some thoughts about this.

Jaime reported trying to find excuses not to treat one of his clients, who was charged with physically and sexually abusing his wife and grandchildren. Sara told her friends that she was spending extra time with a client who reminded her of her recently deceased grandmother, with whom she had been very close. Miya recalled postponing family education with an older adult's spouse when she realized they were a same-gender couple. Deon shared terminating a treatment session early when an older adult outpatient said things that were culturally insensitive and hurtful, even though she had not intended that. Reflecting on their feelings helped the four OTAs to recognize that their biases were interfering with their ability to provide the best treatment for certain clients, or that they were developing inappropriate relationship with others. Jaime spoke to his supervisor and was able to switch clients with another OTA on staff. Deon told the outpatient that her words were offensive and she apologized and did not do it again. Miya and Sara reconsidered the amount of time they were or were not spending with their clients, and made the necessary adjustments.

Support: With Whom Can I Talk for Support?

Some health professionals find it useful to talk through a problem with a trusted advisor. In addition to the supervising OT, the OTA may choose other colleagues from the team, or from other disciplines. Two weeks ago, Sara was placed in a difficult position with one of her favorite residents at the SNF, Mrs. Henry. Three months earlier, Mrs. Henry had come to the facility after experiencing a stroke. Despite Sara's best efforts to help Mrs. Henry regain endurance and sitting balance, Sara's supervising OT concluded that Mrs. Henry was not likely to improve any further and recommended discontinuing her therapy. However, Mrs. Henry's family asked Sara to continue the interventions. They could tell how much their mother enjoyed the attention. They were worried that without OT, Mrs. Henry would lose hope and her health would deteriorate further. Sara explained that without demonstrable improvement, Medicare was not likely to reimburse the facility for additional therapy. In response, the family appealed to Sara's sense of loyalty to their mother, asking her to be creative about how she documented the effect of the therapy. Sara faced an ethical dilemma between loyalty to someone she cared for and the obligation to truthfully document OT intervention. She decided to talk to the social worker at the SNF. Sara shared how much she enjoyed working with Mrs. Henry, but that she did not appreciate being pressured by the family to do something that was unethical and illegal. Sara shared that she hated that the decision to discontinue Mrs. Henry's OT services was based on reimbursement. She acknowledged that Mrs. Henry seemed to enjoy her company but had not really made any more progress in OT. Sara wished that the family understood that she would continue to work with Mrs. Henry if she could. While talking, Sara and the social worker came up with the idea that Sara could stop in and check on Mrs. Henry daily, and if she noticed a change she could recommend that the OT reassess the need for OT services. Sara also planned to meet with the family for education that week, to show them exercises and activities they could do with Mrs. Henry. Trying to explain her thoughts to the social worker helped Sara clarify what she was thinking, and be able to create a satisfactory plan of action.

Another alternative is to talk to a trusted group. Such a group can be informal, like the group of OTAs highlighted in the chapter, or more formal, such as a rehab team or an institutional ethics committee. Typically, ethics committees are composed of a multidisciplinary group of health care professionals, including physicians, a bioethicist, administrators, legal counsel, and a community representative. Just as with an informal group of peers, these committees may be helpful in considering the options for addressing a particular ethical dilemma or reviewing the ethics of decisions that have already been made. In most instances, these committees provide a recommendation for resolution, and it is up to the health care team to decide how they wish to move forward based on that recommendation.

When choosing to talk over an ethics problem with someone else, OTAs must respect the confidentiality of those involved. OTAs should make every effort to see that information about clients, colleagues, or institutions is shared in a way that does not reveal anyone's identity unless required to effectively provide intervention for that client. The client's name should not be used with persons not involved directly with the client's care. Similar discretion needs to be taken when the actions of an institution or a peer is discussed.

Ethical decisions can affect other stakeholders than the OTA and the client, including family members, team members, and the facility or institution. Before making decisions, OTAs should solicit the support of others who will be affected by the issue. Sometimes the OTA can receive institutional support from the organization's administration, medical staff, or the ethics committee. There may be more attention given and decision-making authority granted to others who are more involved than the OTA; or who are considered to have more authority, status, expertise, or knowledge relevant to the issue. This decision-making authority does not translate into moral authority, and OTAs should also recognize that they have a professional duty to facilitate dialogue and raise awareness of a potential ethical conflict.

Since OTAs may have limited influence, they must express their position and the reasons that support the position so that others have the benefit of these insights. Also, by expressing their positions, OTAs can sometimes avoid the experience of ethical distress, when asked to participate in an intervention that conflicts with their ethical views. The more rational the OTAs' arguments in support of their position, the more persuasive OTAs will be in defending their objections, even if the course of events cannot be changed. Communication has been identified as a primary strategy in reducing negative outcomes associated with ethical distress. In addition to bringing important information to the table for discussion, OTAs may also acquire information that supports a decision to which they were initially opposed.

In cases in which OTAs are asked to do something that is ethically questionable, they have the responsibility to involve those with supervisory jurisdiction over them. OTAs should document such communications, especially if there are legal ramifications or if job security is at risk. Following is an example of this kind of dilemma.

In the last year since his outpatient clinic changed management, Deon has observed that he is increasingly asked to do interventions that OTRs previously did. Most of the time, Deon appreciates the opportunity for increased responsibility and feels comfortable doing what is asked of him. However, recently he was asked by the referring physician to work with an older adult who needed ultrasound for her elbow. After he explained the situation, Deon and his friends discussed the issue.

"Absolutely not! You haven't had any training for this modality, and you might burn the client or something," said Miya.

"It's not only unfair that they asked you to do this, isn't it illegal? I know you work across the state line in your facility, but I know in my state, we have to be certified in physical agent modalities as does the supervising OT. You need to find out what your state practice act says! They are just trying to save money by asking you to do this instead of asking an OT," added Sara.

"That may well be," replied Deon, "but I still have to deal with it one way or another."

"So what are you going to do?" asked Jaime.

"Well, I like my job and I don't think this is worth quitting over, at least not without first communicating my distress and the legal implications to my supervisor. Like you, Sara, I worry that I might hurt someone inadvertently, and this goes against my sense of professional duty to do no harm. Also in this case, the legal liability is key, I could lose my license, as could my supervising OT. It is not that I am opposed to learning this new skill set, I just wouldn't be able to offer these interventions until I have had the required continuing education. I think that once I communicate this conflict to my supervisor and talk about how this could negatively impact staffing in the long run, she will support me and may even support me in acquiring physical agent modality certification. After all, if the clinic loses both me and the supervising OT because we did not comply with our practice act or AOTA standards of practice, the clinic will be in worse shape."

"We're behind you on this one, buddy. The other OT practitioners at the clinic will be, too. I bet if you emailed the AOTA EC, their staff liaison would back you up," suggested Miya.

"But whatever you do, I think you better carefully document everything that is said and done so there is a clear record of your reasons for refusing and your efforts to negotiate a change in your assignment," cautioned Sara.

STEP 4: EVALUATE THE RESULTS OF THE ACTION: WHAT WILL I DO?

No matter how much thought and reasoning goes into a decision, sometimes it does not turn out to be the right course of action. This includes taking no action. Inaction is actually an action since the person has information and chooses not to act. If the previous steps have been considered in good conscience and the clinical benefits have been prioritized, OTAs usually have an ethical basis for action. OTAs may retain a sense of uncertainty, but at least they will have the comfort of knowing that they have given deep thought to their position to articulate the basis for their action. Generally speaking, OTAs will most likely not have to act alone because of the input received from others. In addition, OTAs must realize that because they are working under the supervision of an OT, their action or inaction will affect both treating OT practitioners. Conversely, even though OTAs work closely with the OT, there is still a level of ethical accountability for one's personal action or inaction.

In the best case scenario, the evaluation results in a sense of well-being, knowing that one did "the right thing." This can help the OTA in future situations, and the OTA can help colleagues faced with similar issues. When the post-action evaluation yields negative results, there is still the opportunity for learning and preventing future problems. Consider what happened when one of Miya's colleagues in the home health agency gave a positive performance appraisal to an OTA who had two incident reports related to older adults falling during her treatment when she was not paying attention to them, and a complaint by a family whose father fell when the OTA left him alone to go get a towel after his shower. The OTA left and took a job at another facility. Her competence had not improved and a client fell and broke a hip when the OTA did not assist her properly during a transfer. When the family found out that similar events had occurred previously with the OTA, they filed a lawsuit and Miya's colleague was subpoenaed in the civil court hearing. Administration met with all therapy and nursing staff and reinforced the need for honest reporting on all competency and performance evaluations for staff and students.

It can be difficult to admit when one is wrong, but often the consequences of not reporting mistakes are much worse. Jaime decides to tell Deon, Miya, and Sara about a recent event that happened at his hospital involving a colleague.

"Well, I wasn't going to bring this up today as I don't want you guys to think poorly about where I work, but we recently had a really terrible situation occur, and I feel kind of conflicted about the outcome. I mean, I know I have probably made a similar mistake and yet, one of my friends was recently terminated by the hospital because she didn't follow policy and a patient died."

"What, you're kidding! Somebody died in an OT session?" Sara exclaimed.

Jaime replied, "Well, not exactly during the session, but this colleague was working with a patient who was unsteady from all of the medications she was taking and of course, older adults often react differently to meds than younger clients. Anyway, the patient lost her balance while working on lower body dressing and bumped her head on the nightstand. The OTA was very apologetic, sat her down, and ran to get the supervising OT. She asked the OT if they should go get a nurse or the doctor, but the

patient seemed fine and her family was arriving for a visit. They decided that she was OK and just told her family to call the nurse if she started feeling sick to her stomach or dizzy. Unfortunately, the patient went to sleep, suffered an intracranial hemorrhage and subsequently died later that evening. Both the OTA and the OT lost their jobs for not following hospital policy, were involved in a civil lawsuit, were given a 2-year probation by the state licensing board, and received a public censure by the AOTA EC."

"Wow, I don't even know what our policy is for reporting a fall in the home health setting. This is something I obviously need to find out," Miya stated with chagrin.

Jaime confided, "It is sad that this had to occur for me to understand how I can actually demonstrate unethical behavior in failing to act. I always assumed if you have good intentions, that is enough. It seems like a really harsh outcome for a seemingly small mistake. If only they had reported the fall to the nurse or doctor."

While frequent, errors in health care practice can be difficult to report because they often result in embarrassment and shame, which create a barrier for disclosure. As with other health care professions, what matters most is how OT practitioners take responsibility and learn from their mistakes. Disclosure is an important first step to foster learning from errors; and it often leads to positive outcomes for clients, OT providers, and future practice.[19]

Although self-disclosure is difficult, reporting the unethical behavior of a client's family, a professional colleague, or an institution is one of the most difficult actions to take. Nevertheless, if unethical conduct has been observed, OTAs have an ethical obligation to report the behavior to the authorities. In some states, this obligation is underscored by law. Thus, if OTAs know of a wrongdoing and do not report it, the law also considers them guilty.

An example of a legal reason to report is with elder abuse. In addition to the ethical obligation to limit harm to older adults under their care, there are legal requirements obligating OTAs and other health care professionals to report elder abuse to the proper authorities. Almost all states have mandatory reporting laws that apply to OT practice. While laws have been enacted beginning with the inception of the Older Americans Act of 1965, elder abuse is consistently underreported. Elder abuse can range from financial exploitation to violence and be inflicted by a family member, a care provider, or even an institution. It is an OTA's ethical responsibility to protect vulnerable populations, which includes reporting abusive situations involving older adults.

Reporting another's unethical behavior is sometimes referred to as whistle-blowing. Especially when the OTA's job may be threatened, it can take courage to follow through with such a report. If possible, OTAs should work with the support of others, especially those in a supervisory position. Obviously, this is difficult when a supervisor is the person engaging in the unethical behavior. Regardless of the circumstance, OTAs should make sure to document their actions so that their systematic efforts to address the problem are well established, especially if the OTA is in a less powerful position than the person being reported. Sometimes in a twist of logic, the whistle-blower becomes a scapegoat or is blamed for another's unethical behavior. If OTAs have kept good records of their attempts to correct or resolve the situation, they will be more easily cleared of such an accusation.

Often coworkers will also have observed unethical behavior and may feel similarly vulnerable. OTAs can sometimes increase the effectiveness of their responses if they work with others. When sharing information with others to gain support for their actions, OTAs must respect the confidentiality of persons and institutions by providing information fairly and appropriately. If warranted, the authorities will dispense an appropriate punishment for wrongdoing after an investigation.

Who are the relevant authorities? This may differ depending on the entity being reported. In the case of elder abuse, each state has a protective services agency and referral to agencies is available from the national Eldercare Locator, a public service of the US Administration on Aging. Many states also have online directories that list local reporting numbers. It is important to work with managers and administrators when making reports to ensure that organizational policies are followed in the reporting process.

When reporting other health care professionals, the profession's State Regulatory Board (SRB) should be contacted. In many cases, the state boards which were created by state legislatures have the power to intervene if they determine the public to be at risk because of a practitioner's incompetence, lack of qualifications, or unlawful behavior. State boards can publicly reprimand a practitioner or, if warranted, suspend or revoke the person's license to practice in that state.

In addition to the SRB, there are two other major bodies with jurisdiction over professional behavior. The AOTA EC has prepared a detailed discussion of where to go to seek guidance about reporting unethical conduct. OT practitioners may call or write the AOTA EC, as can other health care providers and the public. After discussing the possible violation of the Ethics Standards, OTAs can decide whether to file a formal complaint with the EC. The EC is responsible for writing the profession's Ethics Standards and for imposing sanctions on AOTA members who do not comply. Depending on the seriousness of the unethical behavior, the EC will suggest public censure, temporary suspension of AOTA membership, or revocation or permanent loss of AOTA membership.[17]

The National Board for Certification in Occupational Therapy (NBCOT) is responsible for certifying OTRs and OTAs. Depending on the significance of the unethical behavior that is reported, and after a thorough and confidential investigation, the NBCOT may also act against the practitioner in question. The most severe punishment available through the NBCOT is permanent denial or revocation of certification, which means the practitioner can no longer use the credentials OTR or COTA. This can also affect their ability to be licensed, depending on their state. (The NBCOT maintains a webpage with up-to-date information.)

Finally, OTAs should gather copies of their state's licensure laws, the AOTA Code of Ethics,[1] AOs,[18] and other documents from the AOTA that can help clarify ethical issues. Documents such as the Standards of Practice for Occupational Therapy[20] and Guidelines for Supervision, Roles, and Responsibilities during the Delivery of Occupational Therapy Services[21] also can give OTAs a basis for their ethical arguments.

CONCLUSION

Working with older adults carries special rewards and responsibilities. Clinical and ethical competency is necessary to maximize quality outcomes in practice as well as contribute to the dignity and respect of OT clients. OTAs bring comfort to their clients through skillful intervention and by acting as the client's advocate in ensuring ethical care. A healing bond of trust is reinforced each time clients witness OTAs responding with a sense of ethical commitment in the fulfillment of their clients' needs.

The chapter reviewed ethical challenges in older adult care settings and presented a step-by-step method for responding in a conscientious, informed manner. In addition to the steps involved in the ethical reasoning process, the chapter provided the reader with several tips to assist in ensuring thoughtful ethical reflection and application (Box 10.3). The OTA has an ethical duty to ensure that the older adult's voice is heard, as are the voices of those who may be speaking for the client. This is especially important in OT practice with older adults who may at times present with diminished decision-making capacity but who have throughout their lives demonstrated a pattern of independent judgment, indicative of who they are as autonomous persons. While it is important to understand the legal parameters for ethical decision-making, OTAs must ensure that ethical

BOX 10.3

Tips for Ethical Decision-Making

- Ensure that involved parties have their voices heard.
- Ethical dilemmas cannot be collapsed into legal questions.
- Clinical reasoning must accompany ethical analysis.
- Expertise in the clinical health care arena should not be generalized to ethics.
- Disclose and be aware of your own moral values and bias.

reasoning prevails in ensuring professionalism in practice. Ethical dilemmas cannot be collapsed into legal questions. So too, it is important to understand the relationship between good ethical decisions and strong clinical practice. Many ethical dilemmas at the bedside are informed by clinical indicators. The OTA's ethical responsibility includes ensuring that intervention is consistent with what is clinically indicated. OTAs may face situations affected by power differentials within the health care team. Yet OTAs must remember that authority in the clinical arena does not always translate to decision-making authority, and one should not generalize expertise in the clinical health care arena to ethics. Finally, it is imperative that OTAs recognize the influence that personal beliefs may have on practice. Therefore, acknowledgment of bias is ethically required. Health care professionals, including OTAs, need reminders that ethics is about how we should act in consideration of others, not necessarily how we feel or what we believe. The author hopes that readers will follow the strategies described when responding to events in their practices to ensure ethical outcomes for their clients.

 CHAPTER REVIEW QUESTIONS

1 What parameters may ethically limit the autonomous choices of clients?
2 How should decision-making capacity be assessed when working with older adults?
3 How do ethical dilemmas and ethical distress differ?
4 How do ethical and legal standards of practice differ?
5 Explain how cost-control strategies may create ethical challenges for practitioners.
6 What are some practical limitations associated with the Occupational Therapy Code of Ethics?

REFERENCES

1. American Occupational Therapy Association. (AOTA). AOTA 2020 occupational therapy code of ethics. *Am J Occup Ther.* 2020;74(suppl 3):7413410005. Available at: https://doi.org/10.5014/ajot.2020.74S3006.
2. The Ethics Centre. *Big thinkers: Thomas Beauchamp & James Childress.* 2017. Available at: https://ethics.org.au/big-thinkers-thomas-beauchamp-james-childress/.
3. Kanny E. Core values and attitudes of occupational therapy practice. *Am J Occup Ther.* 1993 (updated 2020);47(12):1085-1086. Available at: https://doi.org/10.5014/ajot.47.12.1085.
4. Artiga S, Orgera K, Pham O. *Disparities in Health and Health Care: Five Key Questions and Answers.* Kaiser Family Foundation; 2020. Available at: https://www.kff.org/racial-equity-and-health-policy/issue-brief/disparities-in-health-and-health-care-five-key-questions-and-answers/.
5. Brach C. *Making Informed Consent an Informed Choice: Health Affairs Blog.* 2019. Available at: https://www.healthaffairs.org/do/10.1377/hblog20190403.965852/full/.
6. Troy, Tevi D. *How the Government as a Payer Shapes the Health Care Marketplace.* American Health Policy Institute; 2015. Available at: https://benefitslink.com/news/index.cgi/view/20151203-125461.
7. AOTA. *2021 Selected Occupational Therapy CPT Codes.* 2021. Available at: https://www.aota.org/-/media/Corporate/Files/Secure/Advocacy/Federal/Coding/2021-Selected-Occupational-Therapy-CPT-Codes.pdf.
8. Faucett G, Keeley E. *Current Practices, Protocols, and Rationales of Diathermy Use by Occupational Therapists in Skilled Nursing Facilities* (Unpublished doctoral dissertation). Tacoma, Washington: University of Puget Sound; 2013.
9. AOTA. *Position Paper on Physical Agents and Mechanical Modalities.* 2018. Available at: https://www.aota.org/-/media/Corporate/Files/Secure/Practice/OfficialDocs/Position/PAM-Interim-20181112.pdf.
10. Ethics Unwrapped. *McCombs School of Business.* University of Texas at Austin. Available at: https://ethicsunwrapped.utexas.edu/glossary/utilitarianism.
11. ISI Language Solutions. *Cultural Considerations: Family Decision Making in Health Care.* Available at: https://isilanguagesolutions.com/2019/06/12/family-decision-making-in-health-care/.
12. Lo B. *Resolving Ethical Dilemmas: A Guide for Clinicians.* 5th ed. Philadelphia: Wolters Kluwer; 2013.
13. Scott JB, Reitz SM. Practical applications for the occupational therapy code of Ethics. In: Practical *Applications for the Occupational Therapy Code of Ethics.* Bethesda, MD: AOTA Press/The American Occupational Therapy Association; 2017:42-45.
14. Purtilo R, Doherty R. *Ethical Dimensions in the Health Professions.* 5th ed. Philadelphia: WB Saunders; 2011.
15. Pozgar GD. Legal and ethical issues for health professionals. In: *Legal and Ethical Issues for Health Professionals.* 5th ed. Burlington, MA: Jones & Bartlett Learning; 2020:98-127.
16. Bennett L, Howard B, Kennell B, Erler K. *AOTA Annual Conference (April 2021): Occupational Therapy Code of Ethics 2020: Revisions to meet the needs of stakeholders in today's evolving landscape of practice.* 2021.
17. AOTA. Enforcement procedures for the occupational therapy code of ethics. *Am J Occup Ther.* 2015;69:6913410012p1-6913410012p13.
18. *American Occupational Therapy Advisory Opinions.* n.d. Available at: http://www.aota.org/Practice/Ethics/Advisory.aspx.
19. Mu K, Lohman H, Scheirton L, et al. Improving client safety: strategies to prevent and reduce practice errors in occupational therapy. *Am J Occup Ther.* 2011;65:e69-e76.
20. American Occupational Therapy Association. Standards of practice for occupational therapy. *Am J Occup Ther.* 2015;69:S3. Available at: https://ajot.aota.org/article.aspx?articleid=2477354.
21. AOTA. Guidelines for supervision, roles and responsibilities during the delivery of occupational therapy services. *Am J Occup Ther.* 2020;74(suppl 3):1–6.

11

Working With Families and Caregivers of Older Adults

BARBARA JO RODRIGUES AND PATRICIA J. WATFORD

(WITH PREVIOUS CONTRIBUTIONS FROM SUE BYERS-CONNON, ADA BOONE HOERL, AND RENÉ PADILLA)

KEY TERMS

abuse, caregivers, community, education, family, social support system,
neglect, resources, role changes, stress

CHAPTER OBJECTIVES

1. Define the role of the occupational therapy assistant (OTA) in family and caregiver training.
2. Understand role changes within family systems at the onset of debilitating conditions in older adults.
3. Discuss communication strategies that maximize comprehension during older adult, family, and caregiver education.
4. Identify stressors that affect quality of care, ability to cope, and emotional responses in the older adult-caregiver relationship.
5. Identify techniques to minimize caregiver stress.
6. Define and identify signs of older adult abuse and neglect, and discuss reporting requirements.

Janice woke up early and began her day. She was exhausted, not having had a full night's sleep for more than 3 months since her mother, Lillian, moved in with them. After having a stroke, Lillian had been at a nursing home for rehabilitation and was no longer safe to live on her own. Lillian became very depressed when she was told she could not return home tearfully pleading with Janice, "Please don't put me away at an old folk's home; I couldn't bear it." Janice felt quite distressed. As the working mother of three children, she was overwhelmed thinking of how she would be able to add her mother to her already very busy schedule. Janice consulted with her family and they all agreed to help out and bring Lillian home to live with them. "We can set her up in the dining room. I can make some temporary walls," offered Janice's husband, Mike. A case manager helped Janice get in contact with an agency that provided a caregiver for part of the day while Janice was at work. Physical and occupational therapies were scheduled after a home evaluation. Janice was relieved—it seemed everything was going to work out.

The phone rang while Janice was getting ready to leave for work. "I am sorry, I'm not going to be able to come today—my child is sick," said the home health worker who was scheduled to be with Lillian that day. The agency did not have a replacement. Janice turned to Mike and said, "I guess I'll call work and let them, know I can't come in." Throughout the day she spent with her mother,

Janice noticed Lillian seemed to be confused, forgetting family members' names and thinking she needed to leave to go home to her own house. Later that night, as Janice was getting ready for bed, she heard a crashing sound in the other room. She ran to the dining room and found Lillian sitting on the floor by the bed. Janice called for Mike's help and together they were able to get Lillian into the car and to the emergency room for evaluation.

At the hospital, it was determined that Lillian had experienced another small stroke. Once again, Lillian was transferred to a nursing home so she could receive intensive rehabilitation for a few days. Confusion was much more noticeable when Lillian returned home. She often could not find her way around the house and seemed unable to complete small tasks without constant verbal direction.

Janice was very worried, but the doctor assured her there was not much else that could be done for Lillian except to structure her environment so that Lillian could have some routines and so her safety could be maximized. Another home evaluation was done, and an occupational therapist (OT) and occupational therapy assistant (OTA) team worked with the family to remove tripping hazards and set up Lillian's room, so she could find everything she needed in plain sight. At this point, it was clear Lillian could not be left alone in the house for any period of time, so Janice or Mike had to be home each evening, which meant that only one parent could be present at their children's frequent events. Janice felt it necessary to resign as president of the high school's booster club, as well as take a break from her book club and other regular activities so she could stay at home with her mother.

As the weeks went by, Lillian fell twice more in the middle of the night when she tried to get up to use the bathroom. It seemed to Janice and Mike that Lillian was getting more and more confused as each day passed. Janice began setting her alarm at 2:00 a.m. to help her mother to the bathroom and get her back to bed. Janice would then try to sleep for a couple of hours before it was time to get up and get the family ready for the day. Janice began wondering how they would handle their upcoming annual family vacation in a couple of weeks. She felt guilty that she wanted a break.

More than 50 million people provide care for a chronically ill, disabled, or aged family member or friend in the United States in 2020.[1] The term *caregiver* refers to anyone who provides assistance to someone else who is in some degree incapacitated and needs help. *Informal caregiver* and *family caregiver* are terms that refer to unpaid individuals such as family members, friends, and neighbors who provide care. These individuals can be primary or secondary caregivers, full time or part time, and can live with the person being cared for or live separately. Formal caregivers are volunteers or paid care providers associated with a service system.[1]

Families are the major provider of long-term care, but research has shown that caregiving exacts a heavy emotional, physical, and financial toll.[2] Many caregivers who work and provide care experience conflicts between these responsibilities. Nineteen percent of caregivers are assisting two individuals, whereas 5% are caring for three or more.[1] More than half of all caregivers are age 50 and older, making them more vulnerable to a decline in their own health, and one-third describe their own health as fair to poor.[1]

To provide optimal care, OTAs must consider the many factors that influence an older adult's occupational performance. When planning intervention, the OT/OTA team should not only consider client factors and performance skills but also the contexts and environments that may affect the older adult's occupational performance potential.[3] Social support systems such as spouse and family can significantly affect the outcome of occupational therapy intervention.[4] It is important that OTAs interact with older adults and their social support systems, especially the family, and treat older adults and their families as units of care.

ROLES FOR OCCUPATIONAL THERAPY ASSISTANTS

For OTAs to define their roles in facilitating family interaction, they must first understand the family caregiver's role. Family members are not necessarily inherently skilled at caregiving. Frequently, this role is unfamiliar and possibly unwanted. Caregivers must do more than simply keep older adults safe and clean and ensure that their daily physical needs are met. They must also help older adults maintain socialization and a sense of dignity. These tasks can be overwhelming for a family member who has little or no experience with debilitating and chronic illness. Ensuring that caregivers and older adults work together effectively is crucial.[5] OTAs should act as facilitators, educators, and provide resources.

Development of older adults' and caregivers' skills is achieved through selected activities with graded successes facilitated by OTAs. Activities that include family members and caregivers should be introduced as early as possible in the occupational therapy program to minimize dependence on OTAs. Facilitating interdependence between older adults, their families, and caregivers will ease the transition from one level of care to the next.

Effective older adult, family, and caregiver education is a central component of care.[6] Knowledge is empowering and encourages older adults, family members, and caregivers to be responsible. Activities selected during the early stages of intervention need not be complex. They may include ideas for problem solving, technical skills, support, home modification, community referral, and assistive technology.[7,8] It is important that the relationships between older adults, family members, and caregivers not focus solely on the older adult's functional limitations but on remaining skills, interests, and goals. Helping family members accept functional changes as part of a normal process rather than as a catastrophic decline can encourage preservation of relationships.[9,10] More training can follow as discharge planning progresses and the role of the caregiver becomes more clearly defined.[11]

Older adult, family, and caregiver education is often required for all areas of occupation as described in the *Occupational Therapy Practice Framework (4th edition)* (see Chapter 7).[3] It is most effective to continually help older adults, family members, and caregivers to consider occupational therapy intervention strategies focused on performance skills (such as sensory, motor, cognitive, or communication skills) in the context of meaningful occupations. Changes needed in the older adults' or family routines and habits are more easily accomplished when they are consistent with their values, beliefs, and spirituality. Therefore, it is essential for the OT/OTA team to have a good grasp of the older adult's current preferences, past occupational participation, and future goals. OTAs may help older adults, family members, and caregivers understand the physician's diagnosis and prognosis of the medical condition and its functional implications. Insight regarding the specific physical, cognitive, and psychosocial impairments will aid caregivers in providing safe and appropriate assistance. Sometimes, understanding the reasons for doing a certain task is more important than demonstrating proficiency in its performance.[12] For example, understanding principles of joint protection that

BOX 11.1

Considerations for Effective Communication

- Initially, make frequent, brief contacts to develop the relationship. This will familiarize the older adult, family members, and caregivers with OTAs and their purpose.
- Manage the environment in which communication occurs. Minimize distractions and interruptions.
- Use responsive listening techniques. Maintain good eye contact, intermittently acknowledge statements made, and use body language that allows all parties to listen and respond. Be an active listener.
- Use common terminology that nonmedical individuals understand. If a common term is available, use it. For example, use shoulder blade for scapula. Otherwise, define and explain concepts in simple terms.
- Always respect client confidentiality. If able, secure permission from clients before discussing details with others.
- Use open-ended questions to encourage self-expression. Be comfortable with brief silences.
- Organize your ideas and avoid skipping between subjects. Focus on one topic at a time, and clarify what you do not understand.
- Provide education that will enable older adults and their families to make informed choices. Do not offer advice or your personal opinion. Always acknowledge the right of choice.
- Communicate with respect and warmth. Be supportive. Respond to feedback when given.
- Do not promise if you cannot deliver.

---

can be applied to every situation is more important for caregivers than correctly supervising the older adult's use of radial wrist deviation to open a door each and every time. To maximize the effectiveness of the education, OTAs need to develop communication strategies (Box 11.1).

OTAs also act as resources for older adults, family members, and caregivers. Depending on facility role delineation, OTAs may provide information about community and support services, as well as medical equipment vendors, paid caregivers, and respite programs. In collaboration with OTs, OTAs may also serve as liaisons with other services.

OTAs can learn much about older adults', family members', and caregivers' values, desires, and insights through frequent and close interaction. Older adults may be unable to express themselves for many reasons. Some limitations may be preexisting, whereas others, such as aphasia, may result from illness. OTAs may act as advocates for older adults, helping meet needs that might otherwise go unacknowledged. OTAs may also act as advocates for family members and caregivers. Like older adults, families and caregivers may have needs that become evident only after close and frequent interaction. Because each individual's

ability to provide caregiving differs, the OT/OTA team must consider everyone's abilities when planning for facility discharge and family training.

All members of the treatment team, including OTAs, must educate older adults, family members, and caregivers about the team's treatment recommendations. Recommendations may include plans for discharge, supervision, follow-up treatment, and home/community programs, all of which must be clearly documented. When older adults, families, and caregivers choose not to follow the team's recommendation, it is crucial to document all responses and actions to serve as a legal record if anyone is harmed. The more often older adults, family members, and caregivers are included in the formulation of plans, the more likely they are to comply with home programs and other discharge recommendations.[11]

ROLE CHANGES IN THE FAMILY

Greater therapeutic outcomes are achieved when intervention does not focus solely on older adults but also includes families and caregivers.[2] This is especially important when family lifestyle changes are required because of older adults' functional declines.[13] Ideally, older adults will consult family members when caregiving needs become evident. However, many variables affect a family system's abilities to meet the older adult's needs. Some of these variables may include the treatment setting itself, cognitive deficits, psychological issues, and the prior quality of family relationships, cultural and social influences, geographic distance, scheduling conflicts, financial resources, and advanced directives. OTAs must take all of these factors into consideration during collaborative planning.[11,14]

OTAs must consider role changes that occur for both older adults and family during the course of an illness. Occupational therapy should be designed around older adults' and family members' skill levels. From that foundation, OTAs can facilitate adjustment to disability. With the onset of illness or disability, older adults may feel a loss of independence, which can mean a major change in their sense of control and their role within the family.[15]

Role changes also occur within the family unit during an older adult's illnesses.[16] Spouses may feel a deep sense of loss of a partner and may resent being solely responsible for previously shared tasks. In addition to a sense of loss, children must deal with the role reversal of being a parent to their own parent. Older adults' disabilities and needs for caregiving may come at a time in children's lives when, for the first time, they find themselves free of family responsibilities and are planning for their own retirement. Family members are usually unprepared for the sudden changes that may occur with acute illnesses.[17]

Roles within the family unit tend to be adjusted and adapted to gradually when older adults have chronic or degenerative diseases. However, as the functional impairments accumulate into a major disability with significant activity limitations, modifications in roles are required.[18,19]

Not knowing the length of the illness is often a source of added frustration. In addition, chronic conditions may involve long-term adaptations that demand a greater degree of self-care and responsibility on the part of older adults and caregivers.[20]

Caregiver Stresses

An entire generation is moving into the caregiving role for their aging parents.[13] These caregivers are changing their lives to assist their parents through the illness process. In addition to grieving for their parent, these caregivers may also be experiencing a loss of their own independence, privacy, financial security, safety, and comfort within their own homes. These losses may leave caregivers ultimately feeling guilty about their inadequacies or angry toward the debilitated older adult.[15]

Life changes for caregivers and their families. Changes may be gradual, beginning with the older adult experiencing mild confusion and only requiring assistance with finances. Change also may be sudden and immediate, such as when the older adult survives a stroke and needs total physical care. The care required may be temporary, or it may be permanent with no hope for rehabilitation. No matter what the situation, this change of life is stressful for everyone involved.[2,17]

Advice from physicians, nurses, and therapists and attempts at self-education about an unfamiliar illness also can add stress. The need to learn the language of health care workers can be stressful, especially for caregivers for whom English is a second language or caregivers who are functionally illiterate.

Stress also may be increased by family members who offer suggestions for caring for older adults. When decisions are made by several relatives but one family member or caregiver is responsible for following through with the group's decisions, the caregiver can easily become overwhelmed and feel resentful.

Older adults who need caregiving may require various levels of assistance, and their conditions may change frequently. At times, little assistance may be needed, but there may be long periods when much more assistance is required (Fig. 11.1). Other family members may not understand the fluctuating assistance levels, and their perceptions of the work required to maintain the older adult at home may not be accurate.[21]

Family members may not understand their own emotions or those of the primary caregiver and may deny feelings of guilt, frustration, anger, or grief. They also may be in denial about the level of care required and may not be ready to assist. Family members who are unable to understand their own emotions or the illness and needs of the older adult may become angry with the caregiver for not allowing the older adult more independence.[16] They may be resentful and suspicious of the caregiver's motives or intentions, which can devastate caregivers and reduce the level of care they are willing to provide.

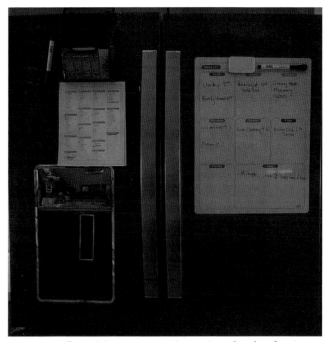

FIG. 11.1 Caregiving may require various levels of assistance. In this home, the older adult's caregiver provides a memory aid on the refrigerator door as a visual reminder of weekly activities and errands. *(Courtesy Amy Schaffer.)*

The demands and constraints of caregiving can become overwhelming. Between 40% and 70% of caregivers exhibit symptoms of depression, with 25%–50% of those meeting the diagnostic criteria for clinical depression.[22] Caregivers may feel isolated and believe that they must be the sole providers of care. Caregivers who are stressed are often affected in their work and social life.[22] They may also think they have no time for friends or support systems. Responsibilities can quickly become burdens, and caregivers may feel that they are not providing the needed assistance and are failing in their responsibilities to the older adult.[23] Caregivers may refuse assistance from others because they feel the home is not clean enough for others to visit, or they believe they are the only ones who can properly care for the older adult. Caregivers may forget that the level of care they now provide is the result of months of practice and learning through trial and error. OTAs must become adept at identifying signs of caregiver stress to ensure that the older adult's needs are being met (Box 11.2).

Family Resources

OTAs should continually assess the family's needs and resources and offer the best referrals possible, keeping in mind that family members may feel isolated and disconnected or may be reluctant to ask for assistance. It may first be necessary to assist family members in identifying their needs and willingness to accept assistance. The suggestion that they read a book about caregivers or attend a caregiver support group may be met with resistance.

BOX 11.2

Signs of Caregiver Stress

Too much stress can be damaging to both the caregiver and the older adult. The following stress indicators experienced frequently or simultaneously can lead to more serious health problems.

- The caregiver may deny the disease and its effect on the person who has been diagnosed: "I know Mom's going to get better."
- The caregiver may express anger that no effective treatments or cures currently exist for chronic conditions such as Alzheimer's disease and that people do not understand what is going on: "If he asks me that question one more time, I'll scream."
- The caregiver may withdraw socially from friends and activities that once brought pleasure: "I don't care about getting together with the neighbors anymore."
- The caregiver may express anxiety about facing another day and what the future holds: "What happens when he needs more care than I can provide?"
- The caregiver may experience depression, which eventually breaks the spirit and affects coping ability: "I don't care anymore."
- The caregiver may be exhausted, which makes it nearly impossible to complete necessary tasks: "I'm too tired for this."
- The caregiver may experience sleeplessness caused by worrying: "What if she wanders out of the house or falls and hurts herself?"
- The caregiver may express irritability, which may lead to moodiness and trigger negative responses and reactions: "Leave me alone!"
- Lack of concentration on the part of the caregiver makes it difficult to perform familiar tasks: "I was so busy, I forgot we had an appointment."
- The caregiver experiences mental and physical health problems: "I can't remember the last time I felt good."

Adapted from *Ten Signs of Caregiver Stress.* The Alzheimer's Caregiver. Alzheimer's Research & Research Foundation; 2020.

However, OTAs must provide support and guidance while family members go through the process of realizing their own needs. When family members are ready to ask for assistance, OTAs must be ready with reliable resources and referrals. Successful experiences encourage families to use available community resources. OTAs must help family members and caregivers understand that caring for themselves and accepting help will ultimately help them care for the older adult. Caring for themselves and accepting help may also make it possible to offer care at home for a longer period (Box 11.3; Fig. 11.2).

Many community and national resources are available for families and caregivers. Support groups, publications, videos, and resources can be found in virtually every large community. In rural areas, organizations may be contacted by phone, in writing, or through computer technology.

RECOGNIZING SIGNS AND REPORTING OLDER ADULT ABUSE OR NEGLECT

Unfortunately, abuse and neglect of older adults do occur.[24] Approximately 1 in 10 persons, age 60 and over have been injured, exploited, or otherwise mistreated by someone on whom they depended for care or protection. Due to the growing older adult population, there are approximately 5 million victims of older adult abuse annually.[25] All professionals working with older adults must be informed of their responsibilities and prepare themselves to act on the older adult's behalf if suspicion of abuse or neglect arises. Older adult abuse is vastly underreported, with only 1 in 23.5 cases reported to any agency.[26] Federal definitions of older adult abuse have been included in the Older Americans Act since 1987. Each state also has its own definition of older adult abuse through legislation on adult protective services. OTAs should contact their state's ombudsman or Adult Protective Services Office for more detailed and specific guidelines. Only general definitions and guidelines are presented in this chapter. Older adults have a right to direct their own care, refuse care, and receive protection from being taken advantage of or hurt by others.

The National Center on Elder Abuse (NCEA) of the US Administration on Aging has identified and defined seven types of older adult abuse.[27] Physical abuse is non-accidental use of physical force that results in bodily injury, pain, or impairment. It may include acts of violence such as striking, shoving, shaking, slapping, kicking, pinching, and burning. Inappropriate use of drugs and physical restraints, force-feeding, and physical punishment of any kind also are considered physical abuse. Sexual abuse is nonconsensual sexual contact of any kind with an older adult. It includes unwanted touching, all types of sexual assault or battery, coerced nudity, and sexually explicit photographing. Emotional or psychological abuse is willful infliction of mental or emotional anguish by threat, humiliation, or other verbal or nonverbal abusive conduct. It may include actions such as verbal assaults, insults, threats, intimidation, humiliation, and harassment. The NCEA also includes treatment of older adults like infants and isolating them from family and friends or from their regular activities as emotional/psychological abuse. Neglect is the willful or nonwillful failure by caregivers to fulfill their obligations or duties as caretakers. Abandonment is the desertion of older adults by the people who have assumed responsibility for providing care for them. Financial or material exploitation is an unauthorized use of an older adult's funds, property, or resources. This may include such actions as cashing an older adult's checks without permission, forging an older adult's signature, misusing or stealing an older person's money or possessions, coercing or deceiving an older adult into signing any document, and the improper use of

BOX 11.3

Ways to Cope With Caregiver Stress

- Participate in joyful activities
  - Do things that make you happy such as exercise, hobbies, relaxing, gardening, music, reading, watching movies, shopping, playing games or cards, visiting family, spending time with pets or animals.
- Use positive self-talk
  - Remind yourself each day how special you are, the good things in your life, and the positive things that happen each day, no matter how small. Challenge and replace negative thoughts with positive dialogue about yourself and how you are doing.
- Identify the benefits of caregiving
  - Research has shown that caregivers who focus on the positive aspects of caregiving have less stress. Take some time each day to think about ways that caregiving has improved your life and the life of your care recipient. Some benefits of caregiving include: giving purpose to life, developing character and personal growth, improving self-esteem, creating satisfaction over a job well done, making you feel appreciated, and giving you comfort that you have helped someone.
- Get regular exercise
  - Exercise in any form helps the mind and body better deal with stress and improves energy and mood. Start slow and gradually build up the intensity and duration of your exercise. Invite a friend to make exercise a social event. Consult with a physician before starting a new fitness program.
- Attend to your own health
  - Eating nutritional food makes you feel better and gives you more energy.
  - Getting enough sleep is critical for mental and physical health.
  - Seeking regular medical care for yourself. If you do not take care of yourself, how can you take care of anyone else?

- Use informal and formal social support systems
  - Informal social supports include: family, friends, neighbors, clubs and organizations, church members, volunteers. They may be able to help with housework, cooking or sharing meals, running errands, shopping, visiting, or daily care of your care recipient.
  - Formal supports include: caregiving and skills training programs, professional counseling, respite care, support groups, and religious or faith-based programs.
- Be organized
  - Set priorities by making a daily list of the thing that need to be done in order.
  - Use a planner to keep track of priorities, activities, appointments, and phone numbers.
  - Organize your environment and reduce clutter to reduce frustrations and making accomplishing tasks easier.
- Maintain a caregiver journal
  - Some caregivers find meaning in their experiences by writing down their experiences. Write down at least one positive accomplishment each day. Journaling is also a good way to keep track of your stress level. Write down the stressors, how stressful they are, how you tried to solve the stressor, and how you coped with it.
- Seek professional help
  - If your symptoms of stress are chronic, unbearable, or overwhelming, or you have symptoms of depression, consult a health care professional, counselor, or therapist. Make taking care of yourself a priority.
- Use relaxation techniques
  - Deep breathing
  - Progressive muscle relaxation
  - Visualization or guided imagery
  - Meditation
  - Yoga
  - Massage
  - Aromatherapy
  - Music therapy

Adapted from *Caregiver Stress: Coping Strategies*. The Alzheimer's Caregiver. Alzheimer's Research & Research Foundation; 2020.

conservatorship, guardianship, or power of attorney. Finally, self-abuse and neglect are behaviors of older adults directed at themselves that threaten their own health or safety, such as refusing to eat or drink, or providing adequate clothing, shelter, personal hygiene, or medications.

Abuse may occur in the home or community setting, as well as in residential care, skilled nursing facilities (SNFs), or day health programs. In an effort to protect older adults, every health care provider must be aware of signs and indicators of abuse. Indicators of abuse have been outlined in many documents available through agencies on aging (Table 11.1).[28]

Many states have enacted mandatory reporting laws that require professionals who regularly work with older adults, including health workers such as OTAs, law enforcement personnel, and human service personnel, to report suspected abuse. State and local agencies designated to receive and investigate reports and provide referral services to victims, families, and older adults at risk for abuse include the Adult Protective Services Agency, long-term care ombudsman programs, law enforcement or local social service agencies, area agencies on aging, aging service providers, and aging advocacy groups. If older adult abuse is suspected, these agencies can assist OTAs.

OTAs must report physical abuse if they witness an incident that reasonably appears to be physical abuse; find a physical injury of a suspicious nature, location, or repetition; or listen to an incident related by an older adult or

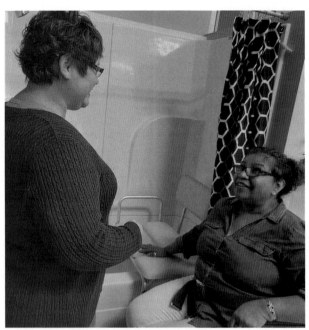

FIG. 11.2 Discharge planning and equipment training can help older adults and caregivers feel more comfortable with changes. *(Courtesy Amy Schaffer.)*

dependent adult. An immediate telephone call followed by a written report is often required. The report should include identifying information about the person filing the report, the victim, and the caregiver. In addition, the incident and condition of the victim and any other information leading the reporter to suspect abuse must be included. Although many facilities have designated personnel to carry out reporting, it is each individual's duty to report suspected abuse. Failure to report is a legally punishable misdemeanor in states with mandatory reporting laws. Further, OTAs have an ethical responsibility to demonstrate a concern for the safety and well-being of the recipients of their services[29] and failure to do so may result in disciplinary action by a professional organization of which the OTA is a member.[30]

The OTA's responsibility does not end with reporting an incident of abuse. Connecting the older adult and/or the family with community resources to help cope with trauma and address conflicts is important.[31] Referrals should be done in a way that is acceptable to the older adult. Many churches, community centers, and organizations such as the Area Agency on Aging can assist in locating resources to support older adults to continue living safely in their communities.

TABLE 11.1

Signs and Symptoms of Abuse	
Type of abuse	**Signs and symptoms**
Physical	Bruises, welts, lacerations Bone fractures Open wounds, cuts, punctures, untreated injuries in various stages of healing Sprains, dislocations, and internal injuries/bleeding Broken eyeglasses Laboratory findings of medication overdose or underutilization of prescribed drugs Older adult's report of being hit or mistreated Older adult's sudden change in behavior Caregiver's refusal to allow visitors to see an older adult alone
Sexual	Bruises around the breasts or genital area Unexplained venereal disease or genital infections Unexplained vaginal or anal bleeding Torn, stained, or bloody underclothing Older adult's report of being sexually assaulted or raped
Emotional/ psychological	Being emotionally upset or agitated Being extremely withdrawn and noncommunicative or nonresponsive Unusual behavior usually attributed to dementia (e.g., sucking, biting, rocking) Older adult's report of being verbally or emotionally mistreated
Neglect	Dehydration, malnutrition, untreated bed sores, and poor personal hygiene Unattended or untreated health problems Hazardous or unsafe living condition/arrangements (e.g., improper wiring, no heat, or no running water) Unsanitary and unclean living conditions (e.g., dirt, fleas, lice on person, soiled bedding, fecal/urine smell, inadequate clothing) Older adult's report of being mistreated
Abandonment	Desertion of an older adult at a hospital, a nursing facility, or other similar institution Desertion of an older adult at a shopping center or other public location Older adult's own report of being abandoned

TABLE 11.1

Signs and Symptoms of Abuse—cont'd

Type of abuse	Signs and symptoms
Financial/ material exploitation	Sudden changes in bank account or banking practice; unexplained withdrawal of large sums of money by a person accompanying the older adult
	Inclusion of additional names on an older adult's bank signature card
	Unauthorized withdrawal of the older adult's funds using the older adult's ATM card
	Abrupt changes in a will or other financial documents
	Unexplained disappearance of funds or valuable possessions
	Substandard care being provided or bills unpaid despite the availability of adequate financial resources
	Discovery of an older adult's signature being forged for financial transactions or for the titles of his or her possessions
	Sudden appearance of previously uninvolved relatives claiming their rights to an older adult's affairs and possessions
	Unexplained sudden transfer of assets to a family member or someone outside of the family
	Provision of services that are not necessary
	Older adult's report of financial exploitation
Self-neglect	Dehydration, malnutrition, untreated or improperly attended medical conditions, and poor personal hygiene
	Hazardous or unsafe living conditions/arrangements (e.g., improper wiring, no indoor plumbing, no heat, no running water)
	Unsanitary or unclean living quarters (e.g., animal/insect infestation, no functioning toilet, fecal/urine smell)
	Inappropriate and/or inadequate clothing, lack of necessary medical aids (e.g., eyeglasses, hearing aids, dentures)
	Grossly inadequate housing or homelessness

Adapted from National Center Elder Abuse. *Types of Abuse.* U.S. Department of Health and Human Services, Administration for Community Living; 2021.

CASE STUDY

After the last fall, Janice called Lillian's physician and received another referral for home health OT services. Paul, the OT, called Janice to set up the initial visit and made arrangements for Diana, a recently hired OTA, to join him during the evaluation because she would be picking up the case if they determined services were needed. On the designated date, Paul and Diana arrived at the home, Janice invited them into the house. They all sat in the living room with Lillian and began the initial interview. "Lillian, please tell us how it came about that a call for occupational therapy services was made? What has been going on?" asked Paul. Lillian responded, "I do not know. I have been doing fine—I can handle everything I need to do." Janice reminded Lillian, "Don't forget you fell a few times, Mom." Lillian at first seemed confused, but then offered, "Oh, yes, I fell getting out of bed because someone had left things on the floor and I tripped. But that was just an accident. It's not going to happen again." Paul asked Lillian to describe her typical day, which she did in large strokes. "I get up and try to help with breakfast before the kids leave. Then I take a shower and get dressed and then watch my morning TV shows. Sometimes I go to visit friends. Then I cook lunch and start with cleaning the house. My daughter is too busy, you know, and she brought me to live here so I could help her. They are all so busy all the time." Paul and Diana noticed that Janice who was sitting behind Lillian, shook her head several times as Lillian described her routines. Diana asked, "Have you needed any help to shower and get dressed?" Lillian shook her head and answered, "Well, I don't really need help, but my daughter has a person stay with me during the day to keep me company, so I let her help me sometimes."

Lillian began telling Paul and Diana about her life before her first stroke. Up to that point, she had been living alone and was very active in her church. She never missed one of her grandchildren's games. She drove a car up to about a month before the stroke. She gave up driving because she felt her eyesight was becoming problematic. She enjoyed cooking, sewing, and gardening. Since the stroke, she had not been outside of the house except for medical appointments, and just recently, she attempted to do some sewing once her work was brought from her own home.

Paul asked Janice if they could talk as Lillian demonstrated how she got dressed, accessed the bathroom, and prepared a simple snack. Janice stated, "I hired someone to help Mom. She doesn't need to do these things for herself anymore. We just need her to walk better so she doesn't fall. That is what worries me the most. She can't be alone because she will fall." Paul and Diana asked Lillian to show them where she slept, and once there asked her to demonstrate how she got in and out of bed. Lillian agreed to do so, but when she began sitting up from the bed, Janice jumped in and provided assistance. Paul encouraged Janice to let Lillian demonstrate her abilities and, with some struggling, finally she was able to get herself to sitting on the edge of the bed. A similar pattern of Paul asking Lillian to demonstrate a skill and Janice jumping in to assist her was evident when Lillian dressed and accessed the bathroom.

When the group was on the way to the kitchen, Janice again noted, "We don't let mother do much cooking. She gets confused, and it ends up being more work for me in the end." When Janice was distracted, Paul took Diana aside and asked her to observe Lillian make a peanut butter and jelly sandwich while he took Janice to the living room to talk to her. In the living room, Paul asked Janice how she was dealing with Lillian's functional changes. Janice tearfully confessed, "I am exhausted. I am so worried she will hurt herself; she just can't be left alone. We can't afford to pay for an attendant all the time, and I keep missing work. I don't sleep because she needs to get up at night to go to the bathroom, and she is so hard-headed—she just will not use the commode by the bed. She only lets me or the home health worker help her with dressing or her bath. I don't want to put her in a skilled nursing facility, but I don't know if I can keep her either!"

In the kitchen, Diana observed Lillian walk to the refrigerator, open the door, and stare into space. Diana asked what steps she needed to follow to make the sandwich and Lillian seemed confused. "Get what you need for a peanut butter and jelly sandwich," Diana encouraged. Still, Lillian appeared confused, so Diana instructed her to find each of the needed materials one by one. Once everything was assembled on the counter in front of her, Lillian was able to assemble a sandwich without any other problems. Diana asked her what she usually cooked, and Lillian answered, "Nothing anymore. Barbie doesn't let me do anything anymore."

▓ CASE STUDY QUESTIONS

1 What are the major issues going on with Lillian and her family?
2 What communication strategies could the treatment team use to integrate the different viewpoints of Lillian and her family?
3 What intervention strategies should the team implement to meet Lillian's needs as well as those of the family?

▌ CHAPTER REVIEW QUESTIONS

1 While working at a skilled nursing facility, you approach a new older adult resident who says, "My husband just left me here all alone. Oh, please help me, I want to go home." How should you respond?
2 You work in a rehabilitation unit. You recommend a tub transfer bench for an older adult with hemiplegia. Medicare will not cover the expense of this bench.

The family says, "We'll just rig something up when we get home." How should you respond?
3 You are working on an Alzheimer's disease special unit. An older adult comes up to you, grabs your arm, and says, "Momma, where have you been? I've been so afraid." As the older adult continues to cling to your arm, you notice the older adult's family members are watching. The older adult's behavior escalates whenever a family member approaches. How should you respond?
4 The grown daughter of an older adult approaches you and states, "My father has been an alcoholic all my life. He has been so mean to my mother. His being in the hospital is the first peace she's had in years. Please don't let my father come home." How should you respond?
5 You have worked closely with an older adult for 2 weeks. After a week-long vacation, you return to learn that the older adult has refused treatment most of the week you were absent. The older adult had stated, "I don't want anyone new! My family doesn't know how to help me." What steps should you have taken to minimize the older adult's dependence on you?
6 On admission of their 87-year-old widowed father to an acute-care hospital, three adult children state that it is their desire to take him home and share the caregiving responsibilities when he is ready for discharge. During the 3-week hospitalization, staff members have seen the children visit only once. They also have not returned repeated phone calls by the social worker. What input should the OTA give to the treatment team in preparation for discharge?

EVIDENCE NUGGETS: EFFECTIVENESS OF INTERVENTIONS FOR CAREGIVERS

1. Abrahams, R., Liu, K., Bissett, M., Fahey, P., Cheung, K., Bye, R., Chaudhary, K., & Chu, L. W. Effectiveness of interventions for co-residing family caregivers of people with dementia: Systematic review and meta-analysis. Australian Occupational Therapy Journal. 2018;65(3), 208–224. doi: 10.1111/1440-1630.12464.
   • Multi-component interventions had a significant positive pooled effect on burden, depression, health and social support for family caregivers of people with dementia.
   • Counseling, support groups, education, stress and mood management, or telephone support are effective intervention strategies for caregivers of people with dementia.
2. Deeken, F., Rezo, A., Hinz, M., Discher, R., & Rapp, M. A. Evaluation of technology-based interventions for informal caregivers of patients with dementia–a meta-analysis of randomized controlled trials. The American Journal of Geriatric Psychiatry: Official Journal of the American Association for Geriatric Psychiatry. 2019; 27(4), 426–445. doi:/10.1016/j.jagp.2018.12.003.

   • There is a small but significant effect for the effectiveness of technology-based interventions for caregivers of people with dementia.
   • A significant effect was found on caregiver depression and burden for caregivers receiving a technology-based intervention comprised of telephone, web-based, and DVD/video technologies.
   • The highest effect sizes were for combined interventions and the smallest effect sizes were for computer/web-based interventions.
3. Hopkinson, M. D., Reavell, J., Lane, D. A., & Mallikarjun, P. Cognitive behavioral therapy for depression, anxiety, and stress in caregivers of dementia patients: A systematic review and meta-analysis. The Gerontologist. 2019;59(4), e343–e362. doi:/10.1093/geront/gnx217.
   • Following cognitive behavioral therapy (CBT), depression and stress were significantly reduced in caregivers but anxiety levels were not.
   • Eight CBT sessions or less were equally effective as more than eight sessions at significantly reducing depression and stress.

EVIDENCE NUGGETS: EFFECTIVENESS OF INTERVENTIONS FOR CAREGIVERS—cont'd

- Participant attitudes toward CBT interventions were mostly positive.
4. Terracciano, A., Artese, A., Yeh, J., Edgerton, L., Granville, L., Aschwanden, D., Luchetti, M., Glueckauf, R. L., Stephan, Y., Sutin, A. R., & Katz, P. Effectiveness of powerful tools for caregivers on caregiver burden and on care recipient behavioral and psychological symptoms of dementia: A randomized controlled trial. Journal of the American Medical Directors Association, 2020;21(8), 1121–1127.e1. doi:10.1016/j.jamda.2019.11.011.
  - A psychoeducational intervention, powerful tools for caregivers (PTC) was found to reduce caregiver burden and depressive symptoms and increase self-confidence.
  - PTC did not significantly reduce behavioral and psychological symptoms of dementia in care recipients.

5. Wawrziczny, E., Larochette, C., Papo, D., Constant, E., Ducharme, F., Kergoat, M. J., Pasquier, F., & Antoine, P. A customized intervention for dementia caregivers: A quasi-experimental design. Journal of Aging and Health, 2019;31(7), 1172–1195. doi:10.1177/0898264318770056.
  - An intervention consisting of classical psychoeducational, Acceptance and Commitment Therapy, and couple interventions among caregivers of people with dementia were found to have a stabilizing effect on the caregivers' perceptions of self-esteem, quality of family support, and feelings of distress.
  - Caregiver's feelings of preparedness, self-efficacy, self-related health, and impact on daily routine were positively affected following intervention.

REFERENCES

1. National Alliance for Caregiving & American Association of Retired Persons. *Caregiving in the U.S.* 2020. Available at: https://www.caregiving.org/wp-content/uploads/2021/01/full-report-caregiving-in-the-united-states-01-21.pdf.
2. Schulz R, Beach SR, Czaja SJ, Martire LM, Monin JK. Family caregiving for older adults. *Annu Rev Psychol.* 2020;71:635-659. doi:10.1146/annurev-psych-010419-050754.
3. American Occupational Therapy Association. Occupational therapy practice framework: Domain and process-fourth edition. *Am J Occup Ther.* 2020;74:1-87. Available at: https://doi.org/10.5014/ajot.2020.74S2001.
4. American Occupational Therapy Association. AOTA's statement on family caregivers. *Am J Occup Ther.* 2007;61:710. doi:10.5014/ajot.61.6.710.
5. Longacre ML, Valdmanis VG, Handorf EA, Fang CY. Work impact and emotional stress among informal caregivers for older adults. *J Gerontol B Psychol Sci Soc Sci.* 2017;72(3):522-531. doi:10.1093/geronb/gbw027.
6. Aksoydan E, Aytar A, Blazeviciene A, et al. Is training for informal caregivers and their older persons helpful? A systematic review. *Arch Gerontol Geriatr.* 2019;83:66-74. doi:10.1016/j.archger.2019.02.006.
7. Jiménez Palomares M, González López-Arza MV, Garrido Ardila EM, Rodríguez Domínguez T, Rodríguez Mansilla J. Effects of a cognitive rehabilitation programme on the independence performing activities of daily living of persons with dementia-A pilot randomized controlled trial. *Brain Sci.* 2021;11(3):319. doi:10.3390/brainsci11030319.
8. Ben Mortenson W, Demers L, Fuhrer MJ, et al. Effects of a caregiver-inclusive assistive technology intervention: a randomized controlled trial. *BMC Geriatr.* 2018;18(1):97. doi:10.1186/s12877-018-0783-6.
9. Dahlke S, Steil K, Freund-Heritage R, Colborne M, Labonte S, Wagg A. Older people and their families' perceptions about their experiences with interprofessional teams. *Nurs Open.* 2018;5(2):158-166. doi:10.1002/nop2.123.
10. Slatyer S, Aoun SM, Hill KD, Walsh D, Whitty D, Toye C. Caregivers' experiences of a home support program after the hospital discharge of an older family member: a qualitative analysis. *BMC Health Serv Res.* 2019;19(1):220. doi:10.1186/s12913-019-4042-0.
11. Krieger T, Specht R, Errens B, Hagen U, Dorant E. Caring for family caregivers of geriatric patients: results of a participatory health research project on actual state and needs of hospital-based care professionals. *Int J Environ Res Public Health.* 2020;17(16):5901. doi:10.3390/ijerph17165901.
12. Chan EY, Glass G, Chua KC, Ali N, Lim WS. Relationship between mastery and caregiving competence in protecting against burden, anxiety and depression among caregivers of frail older adults. *J Nutr Health Aging.* 2018;22(10):1238-1245. doi:10.1007/s12603-018-1098-1.
13. AARP and National Alliance for Caregiving. *Caregiving in the United States 2020.* Washington, DC: AARP. May 14, 2020. Available at: https://doi.org/10.26419/ppi.00103.001.
14. Riffin C, Van Ness PH, Wolff JL, Fried T. Family and other unpaid caregivers and older adults with and without dementia and disability. *J Am Geriatr Soc.* 2017;65(8):1821-1828. doi:10.1111/jgs.14910.
15. Lilleheie I, Debesay J, Bye A, Bergland A. The tension between carrying a burden and feeling like a burden: a qualitative study of informal caregivers' and care recipients' experiences after patient discharge from hospital. *Int J Qual Stud Health Well-Being.* 2021;16(1):1855751. doi:10.1080/17482631.2020.1855751.
16. Bangerter LR, Liu Y, Zarit SH. Longitudinal trajectories of subjective care stressors: the role of personal, dyadic, and family resources. *Aging Ment Health.* 2019;23(2):255-262. doi:10.1080/13607863.2017 1402292.
17. Faronbi JO, Faronbi GO, Ayamolowo SJ, Olaogun AA. Caring for the seniors with chronic illness: the lived experience of caregivers of older adults. *Arch Gerontol Geriatr.* 2019;82:8-14. doi:10.1016/j.archger.2019.01.013.
18. Leocadie MC, Morvillers JM, Pautex S, Rothan-Tondeur M. Characteristics of the skills of caregivers of people with dementia: observational study. *BMC Fam Pract.* 2020;21(1):149. doi:10.1186/s12875-020-01218-6.
19. Ploeg J, Northwood M, Duggleby W, et al. Caregivers of older adults with dementia and multiple chronic conditions: exploring their experiences with significant changes. *Dementia.* 2020;19(8):2601-2620. doi:10.1177/1471301219834423.
20. Szlenk-Czyczerska E, Guzek M, Bielska DE, Ławnik A, Polański P, Kurpas D. Needs, aggravation, and degree of burnout in informal caregivers of patients with chronic cardiovascular disease. *Int J Environ Res Public Health.* 2020;17(17):6427. doi:10.3390/ijerph17176427.

21. Del-Pino-Casado R, Frías-Osuna A, Palomino-Moral PA, Ruzafa-Martínez M, Ramos-Morcillo AJ. Social support and subjective burden in caregivers of adults and older adults: a meta-analysis. *PLoS One*. 2018;13(1):e0189874. doi:10.1371/journal.pone.0189874.

22. Anxiety and Depression Association of America (ADAA). *Caregivers*. Available at: https://adaa.org/find-help/by-demographics/caregivers.

23. Alves LCS, Monteiro DQ, Bento SR, Hayashi VD, Pelegrini LNC, Vale FAC. Burnout syndrome in informal caregivers of older adults with dementia: a systematic review. *Dement Neuropsychol*. 2019;13(4):415-421. doi:10.1590/1980-57642018dn13-040008.

24. Johnson MJ, Fertel H. Elder Abuse. In: *StatPearls*. Treasure Island (FL): StatPearls Publishing; 2020.

25. National Center on Elder Abuse. *Prevalence of Mistreatment*. Available at: https://ncea.acl.gov/What-We-Do/Research/Statistics-and-Data.aspx#prevalence.

26. Nursing Home Abuse Center. *Elder Abuse Statistics*. January 16, 2020. Available at: https://www.nursinghomeabusecenter.com/elder-abuse/statistics/.

27. National Center on Elder Abuse. *Types of Abuse*. n.d. Available at: https://ncea.acl.gov/Suspect-Abuse/Abuse-Types.aspx.

28. National Institute on Aging. *Elder Abuse*. n.d. Available at: https://www.nia.nih.gov/health/elder-abuse#signs.

29. American Occupational Therapy Association. Occupational therapy code of ethics. *Am J Occup Ther*. 2020;74:7413410005. Available at: https://doi.org/10.5014/ajot.2020.74S3006.

30. American Occupational Therapy Association. Enforcement procedures for the occupational therapy code of ethics and ethics standards. *Am J Occup Ther*. 2019;68:S3-S15. Available at: https://doi.org/10.5014/ajot.2014.686S02.

31. Du Mont J, Kosa SD, Kia H, Spencer C, Yaffe M, Macdonald S. Development and evaluation of a social inclusion framework for a comprehensive hospital-based elder abuse intervention. *PLoS One*. 2020;15(6):e0234195. doi:10.1371/journal.pone.0234195.

12

Addressing Sexual Activity of Older Adults

HELENE L. LOHMAN AND CHRISTINA-MARIE K. SLEIGHT

(PREVIOUS CONTRIBUTIONS FROM ALEXANDRIA KOBRIN)

KEY TERMS

LGBTQ+, myths, nursing facilities, physiological changes, PLISSIT model, sexual activity, sexually transmitted diseases, values

CHAPTER OBJECTIVES

1. Discuss ways that values can influence attitudes about older adult sexual activity.
2. Identify primary myths about older adult sexual activity.
3. Discuss how older adults who are lesbian, gay, bisexual, transgender, and queer (LGBTQ+) have been ignored by society.
4. Describe normal age-related sexual physiological changes.
5. Describe sexually transmitted diseases and the older adult population.
6. Discuss the treatment team members' roles in addressing older adults' sexual concerns.
7. Discuss ways older adults' sexual activity is commonly addressed in nursing facilities.

8. List the components of the permission, limited information, specific suggestions, and intensive therapy model (PLISSIT), and discuss ways that the certified occupational therapy assistant (COTA) can apply this model.
9. Identify the differences between the PLISSIT and EX-PLISSIT models.
10. Identify strategies for older adult sexual education.
11. List intervention for sexual concerns of older adults who experience strokes, heart disease, arthritis, joint replacements, and diabetes.
12. Intensify how learning this material has increased personal comfort to discuss older adults' sexual concerns.

Emily is an occupational therapy assistant (OTA) employed at a skilled nursing facility (SNF). A large part of her caseload is older adults who have sustained total hip replacements. Intervention approaches are routine, and transfers, safety precautions, and the person's home situation are typically addressed following a total hip repair. One day, a circumstance happens that results in Emily changing her intervention approach. Emily is working with James, an older adult who had sustained a right total hip replacement. After Emily went through the protocol for total hip replacements, she asks him if he has any questions. "Yes," he responds, "my partner and I want to know when we can have sex again." Emily starts to feel a surge of emotions. She feels perplexed because she does not know how to respond. She recalls blushing with embarrassment, stammering through a sentence stating that she would get back with James, and abruptly leaving the room. Later in day, Emily reflects upon the situation. She wonders why she felt so embarrassed and what she could

have done differently. She questions her own comfort and personal beliefs about older adults engaging in sexual activity. After further reflection, Emily decides to take the initiative to learn more about the sexual activity of older adults and to incorporate this knowledge into future interventions.

OTAs that provide thorough intervention first form a holistic view of their patients and develop an understanding of the person's daily life routines. Part of the daily life routines of many older adults may involve sexual functioning. Sexual activity is categorized as an activity of daily living (ADL) function, according to the *Occupational Therapy Practice Framework: Domain and Process*,[1] fourth edition (OTPF-4). It is defined as "engaging in the broad possibilities for sexual expression and experiences with self or others (e.g., hugging, kissing, foreplay, masturbation, oral sex, intercourse)."[1] The OTPF-4 also recognizes the importance of intimate partners in social participation, defining intimate partner relationships as

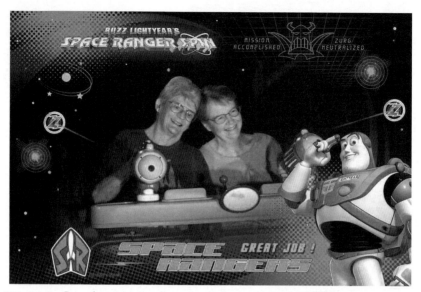

FIG. 12.1   Sexual activity involves touch, hugs, and other forms of expression.

"engaging in activities to initiate and maintain a close relationship, including giving and receiving affection and interacting in desired roles."[1]

Sexual activity is an integral part of an individual's quality of life and is an important aspect for self-concept, self-esteem, and the whole human experience[2] (Fig. 12.1). However, despite sexual activity being so integral to human sexual expression, it may be ignored in clinical intervention for many reasons, including discomfort with one's own sexuality or with an older adult remaining sexually active. Other reasons may include a lack of understanding of normal sexual changes with aging and a lack of knowledge about sexual function with regard to age and disability. Studies have shown some therapists do not address sexual health due to their own beliefs about the influence of older adults' client factors on their sexuality.[3] Therapists may question older adults' age, marital status, and perceived readiness to receive sexual health interventions.[3] These biases continue to place older adults at an occupational injustice* when health care practitioners make judgments on who should and should not receive interventions for sexual health. Addressing older adults' concerns about sexual function should be part of intervention, regardless of therapists' beliefs (Fig. 12.2). This chapter helps OTAs learn about this important, but often ignored area of ADL intervention. Furthermore, the chapter helps clarify myths and misconceptions of older adults and their sexual health.

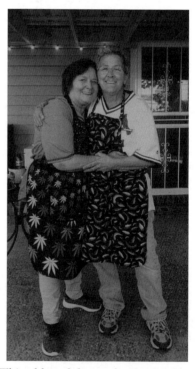

FIG. 12.2   This older adult couple expresses love by shared occupations.

VALUES ABOUT SEXUAL ACTIVITY

Each generation has certain values reflective of society, although such values are not necessarily uniformly held by all members of that generation. All individuals also have their own value systems.[1] The oldest adults coming from The Traditionalists[6] generation (born between 1922 and 1945) may experience internalized sexual stigmas due to

---

*American Occupational Therapy Association's Code of Ethics includes justice as a core value to the occupational therapy profession. Justice is remaining objective and providing occupational therapy services to all persons who require assistance.[4] Occupational justice is the "full inclusion in everyday meaningful occupations for persons, groups, or populations."[4,5]

■ Exercise 12.1: Generational Sexual Attitudes/Values Inventory[a]

Answer the following questions while considering your generation compared to the Baby Boomer generation (born between 1946 and 1964) and/or the Traditionalist generation (born between 1922 and 1945). Fill out "Yes" (*acceptable*) or "No" (*unacceptable*) for each question, then discuss or contemplate your findings. (For more information on generational cohorts, please refer to Chapter 1.)

	Your generation:_____	Baby boomers	Traditionalists
1. It is appropriate to openly discuss sexual needs and concerns.	Yes ___ No ___	Yes ___ No ___	Yes ___ No ___
2. Sexual activity is acceptable in a nonmarriage situation.	Yes ___ No ___	Yes ___ No ___	Yes ___ No ___
3. Sexual activity is appropriate if the purpose is physical pleasure.	Yes ___ No ___	Yes ___ No ___	Yes ___ No ___
4. The main purpose of sexual activity is for procreation.	Yes ___ No ___	Yes ___ No ___	Yes ___ No ___
5. The naked body is very private. Nudity is unacceptable.	Yes ___ No ___	Yes ___ No ___	Yes ___ No ___
6. Women should discuss their sexual needs with their partners.	Yes ___ No ___	Yes ___ No ___	Yes ___ No ___
7. It is appropriate for women to initiate sex.	Yes ___ No ___	Yes ___ No ___	Yes ___ No ___
8. Masturbation is a normal sexual act.	Yes ___ No ___	Yes ___ No ___	Yes ___ No ___
9. Sexual activity between people of the same sex is acceptable.	Yes ___ No ___	Yes ___ No ___	Yes ___ No ___
10. Sexual activity between adults of different generations is unacceptable.	Yes ___ No ___	Yes ___ No ___	Yes ___ No ___

Reflective Comments:

[a]These questions are adapted from a module by Goldstein H & Runyon C. An occupational therapy module to increase sensitivity about geriatric sexuality. *Phys Occup Ther Geriatr.* 1993;11(2):57-75.

lack of education regarding sex and sexuality.[7] For some members of this generation, sexual activity was considered only a necessity for procreation and not a source of enjoyment. These deeply held values can influence the older adult's comfort level when discussing sexual feelings during clinical intervention. However, generational values change, and Baby Boomers are more likely to embrace open-minded and progressive attitudes toward sexual activity than previous generations.[7]

Similar to older adults, health care practitioners may also have explicit (conscious) and implicit (unconscious) biases regarding sexuality formed by their own cultural, religious, and lived experiences. OTAs may feel uncomfortable discussing sexual concerns with older adults because sexual activity may not have been an open topic for some members of their generation as well. These beliefs and discomfort may influence practice with older adults, as OTAs may choose whether to discuss sexual activity. As health care practitioners, OTAs have a responsibility to examine their own biases as this may affect older adults' occupational justice. Sexual activity is a valued occupation for older adults, and occupational justice requires OTAs to help provide "full inclusion in everyday meaningful occupations" including sexual activity.[4,5] This chapter hopes to increase OTAs' self-awareness about possible biases

and increase comfort to address sexuality with older adults. Exercises 12.1 and 12.2 should be completed before further reading to explore values regarding older adults and sexual activity.

MYTHS ABOUT OLDER ADULTS AND SEXUAL FUNCTIONING

The media can provide people with misinformation and myths about older adult sexual functioning. Television, magazines, and online advertisements encourage people to ignore or to cover up the aging process. Greeting cards make fun of aging and suggest that lying about one's age is acceptable. Some media sources encourage myths about sexuality such as "dirty old man syndrome." In addition, myths can be perpetuated by family members, peers, or older adults themselves. With this inundation of misinformation, many people, including older adults, believe myths instead of truths about sexual activity. Exercise 12.3 helps determine personal myths about older adults and sexual activity.

Discussion of Myths

Findings from two surveys by the AARP published in 2010 (n = 1670) and 2017(n = 1002) provide perspective on some of the myths about older adult's sexual activity

■ **Exercise 12.2: Personal Values Assessment**

This exercise helps identify personal values and attitudes. Answer the following questions. On completion of this exercise, any uncomfortable feelings may be handled by using this chapter as an educational tool to help dispel misconceptions and to clarify normal physiological changes resulting from aging. After reading the chapter, the OTA can retake this personal value assessment to determine whether uncomfortable feelings have decreased.

1. Older adults in nursing facilities should not be sexually active.	Agree	Disagree
2. My grandparents (or parents) should not be sexually active.	Agree	Disagree
3. It is acceptable for older adult men to remain sexually active.	Agree	Disagree
4. It is acceptable for older adult women to remain sexually active.	Agree	Disagree
5. It is immoral for older adults to engage in recreational sex.	Agree	Disagree
6. Sexual education is not necessary for older adults.	Agree	Disagree
7. Sexual education is not necessary for nursing facility staff.	Agree	Disagree
8. Nursing facilities should provide large enough beds for couples to sleep together.	Agree	Disagree
9. Nursing facilities should provide privacy for residents who desire sexual activity.	Agree	Disagree
10. Nursing facilities should prohibit older adults residing there from openly identifying themselves as LGBTQ+.	Agree	Disagree

mentioned in Exercise 12.3.[8,9] Both studies examined sexual health for older adults; however, each study had slightly different findings based on the focuses of the studies. The 2010 AARP study surveyed older adults age 45 and older, while the 2017 surveyed older adults age 65 and older.

A key finding in both studies was that more than 50% of older adults considered a satisfying sexual relationship as contributing to their quality of life.[8,9] However, a greater percentage of older adult men respondents than women respondents valued sexual activity as contributing to their quality of life, and more older adult men remain sexually active.[9] Nevertheless, sexual activity was perceived as an integral part of all older adults' lives, not something they avoided.[8,9]

Both studies indicated most older adults, especially the young old (i.e., those 65–75 years of age), have active lives in which sexual activity can and does remain an important component.[8,9] Most likely, if a couple has always been sexually active, they will continue to be so as they grow older. As with any age group, communication is important for a positive sexual relationship. Frailty and disability do not automatically necessitate cause for an older adult to be abstinent. However, findings from both studies suggest having a disability or health condition does contribute to a decrease in sexual activity.[8,9] In addition to having a disability or health condition, other contributing factors leading to a decline in sexual activity included increased stress, health decline of one's partner, and financial instability.[8] The loss of one's partner through death can be a barrier to engagement in sexual activity, especially affecting older adult women.[10] Women outnumber men in the

■ **Exercise 12.3: Myths About Sexual Activity and Older Adults**

For each of the following questions, answer *True (T)* if believed the statement is accurate or *False (F)* if the statement is incorrect or a myth. Refer to discussion in this chapter for clarification of myths.

	True	False
1. Older adults are no longer interested in sexual activity.	____	____
2. Older adults no longer engage in sexual activity.	____	____
3. Older adults engage in a wide variety of sexual activity, including intercourse, masturbation, cuddling, caressing, mutual stimulation, and oral sex.	____	____
4. Older adults in nursing facilities should be segregated according to sex; sexual functioning should be prohibited.	____	____
5. Older adult women are unattractive.	____	____
6. More older adult men remain sexually active than older adult women.	____	____
7. Older adults are too frail to engage in sexual activity.	____	____
8. Inability to maintain an erection (erectile dysfunction) is a natural consequence of aging for all men.	____	____
9. All older adults are heterosexual.	____	____
10. Older adults do not get sexually transmitted diseases.	____	____

Answers to Exercise 12.3 questions: 1. F; 2. F; 3. T; 4. F; 5. F; 6. T; 7. F; 8. F; 9. F; 10. F

These questions are adapted and added from a scale developed by White CB. The aging sexuality knowledge and attitudes scale (ASKAS): A scale for the assessment of attitudes and knowledge regarding sexuality in the aged. *Arch Sex Behav.* 1982;11(6):491-502.

older adult population.[11] Women are less likely to be married in the older cohort than men (69% of men to 47% of women) and the proportion of widows is high in this population (31%).[11]

Furthermore, some older adult women believe the myth that they are unattractive and therefore should remain abstinent from sexual relationships. The 2010 AARP study explored older adults' views on attraction toward sexuality.[8] Findings indicated 51% of males over 65 years old stated that their partners were physically attractive, and 48% of females over 70 found their partner to be attractive.[8] These findings support that many older adults find their partners physically attractive. Thus, this contradicts the myth about unattractiveness associated with older age.

The 2010 AARP study additionally examined older adult's attitudes toward sexuality. Findings were that 22% of individuals over 45 agree that unmarried people should not have sex.[8] Only 8% of individuals over 45 agreed that sex is solely for procreation.[8] The 2010 AARP study verified that older adults valued a variety of sexual activities, including kissing, hugging, caressing, oral sex, anal sex, sexual intercourse, and self-stimulation.[8]

The 2017 AARP study focused on older adult satisfaction with their sex life and discussing sexual health with health care providers.[9] Not only are older adults engaging in sexual activity, more than 73% of older adults age 65 and older reported that they were satisfied with their sex life.[9] Another key finding in this study is that only 17% of older adults reported discussing their sexual health with a health care provider.[9] Of those who spoke with a health care provider, 88% reported being comfortable discussing their sexual health concerns.[9] Although OTAs may feel uneasy addressing sexual health, OTAs should keep in mind most older adults felt comfortable discussing the topic. Additional tools to increase comfort when addressing sexual health will be discussed later in this chapter.

In addition to the AARP studies, findings from literature dispel or add credence to other myths about sexual health and older adults. Literature supports the myth that sexual activity is discouraged in nursing facilities or other institutions.[10] Both older adult men and women may experience pressure from their children to remain abstinent in those settings. Some adult children may find it difficult to think of their parents as having normal sexual desires, especially if the parent resides in a nursing facility.[11] However, residents are not asexual in nursing facilities, as will be discussed later in this chapter.

About the myth regarding erectile dysfunction (ED), most adult men experience occasional impotence or ED with 52% of men between the ages of 40 and 70 experiencing symptoms of ED and up to 70% of men experiencing symptoms by the age of 70.[12] In the 2010 AARP study, 30% of men age 45 years and older admitted to being diagnosed with ED.[8] Furthermore, with normal aging,

older adult men do not have a complete loss of sexual functioning.[10] ED is related to many factors. Psychological reasons can be stress, anxiety, depression, relationship issues, or loss of a partner.[10,12] Lifestyle factors may include little exercise, smoking, excessive alcohol use, and drug use.[12] ED may also be attributed to physical causes such as obesity, cardiovascular disease, hypertension, and diabetes mellitus (DM); men with DM are at quadruple risk for developing ED.[12] Other common causes of ED include stroke, arthritis, multiple sclerosis, dementia, visual or hearing impairments, and urinary problems.[10,12] Side effects of medication and prostate cancer treatments may be linked to ED as well.[10,12] Regardless of the higher incidence of ED as men age, they can continue to have normal sexual activity throughout their lives. Minor physiological changes may have some effect on sexual functioning. For example, a benefit from physiological aging may be delayed ejaculation, which can increase sexual pleasure for the partner.[13]

For older adult men who have ED, medications such as Viagra (sildenafil) and other approved medications,[12] which increases the vascular flow to the genitals, can help. However, caution must be taken with medications because ED is complex, involving physical and psychological factors and they have side effects and interactions.[12] Older adult men with ED should discuss with their physician the benefits and risks involved in medications.[14] Older adult men may also benefit from other compensatory strategies such as a penile injection, vacuum erection device, tension ring, penile support, and penile sleeve to increase vascular flow to the penis and maintain an erection.[15] Older adult men should consult with their physician on an appropriate course of intervention.

OLDER ADULT LESBIAN, GAY, BISEXUAL, TRANSGENDER, AND QUEER+

Society has often ignored older adults with differences in sexual orientation from heterosexuality in older adults. Thus, older adults who are LGBTQ+ are often considered to be an invisible group.[16] However, research estimates there are 1.1 million older adults aged 65 and older who identify as LGBTQ+, and this population will only increase over time.[17] A Gallup poll of more than 340,000 adults found that 8.2% reported being lesbian, gay, bisexual, and transgender (LGBT), with 2.4% of Baby Boomers and 1.4% of Traditionalists self-identifying as LGBT.[18] Researchers speculated that the lower number among older adults may be due to hesitancy to identify as LGBTQ+.[18]

Overall, society has embraced a "heteronormativity" viewpoint or "a general perspective which sees heterosexual experiences as the only, or central view of the world."[19,20] However, the older adult cohort is diverse in terms of income, race, health status, gender identity, and sexual orientation. Similarly, the older adult LGBTQ+

population has a diverse background.[21] There is a great need to research the older adult LGBTQ+ population, especially in occupational therapy literature.[19]

Many older adults who are LGBTQ+ may be uncomfortable sharing about their sexual orientation, having grown up in a time of overt prejudice.[19-21] In fact, homosexuality was defined as a mental illness by the American Psychiatric Association until the early 1970s.[21] In today's society, concern about discrimination remains. In a national survey of LGBTQ+ older adults and other people in their lives (n = 739), respondents expressed concerns about staff discrimination (89%), abuse, and/or neglect (53%). A high percentage of the older adult subjects (43%) reported actual mistreatment such as staff harassment or not being provided basic care.[22] Fear of discrimination may prevent older adults who are LGBTQ+ from seeking out health care support services,[20] especially among the oldest LGBTQ+ persons.[23] An additional survey (N = 2376) comparing LGBT older adults (n = 1857) and non-LGBT older adults (n = 519) reported that more than one-third of LGBT older adults did not disclose their sexual orientation to their health care provider for fear of being judged.[24] These fears of discrimination in the health care setting increases with transgender older adults, with 44% believing their relationships with medical staff would be negatively impacted by their gender identity.[24] In addition, transgender older persons believe their access to health care services will be denied (55%) or limited (65%) as they age.[24] However, in another national survey of LGBTQ+ persons of the Baby Boomer generation (n = 1200), more than half of the respondents expressed confidence that they will be treated with "dignity and respect" by health professionals as they reach the end of their lives.[25]

Working in a long-term care facility, OTAs need to be aware of and sensitive to certain factors that may have an influence on the professional relationship with an older adult who is LGBTQ+. As discussed, some of these older adults have real concerns about safety and mistreatment and may not be open about their sexual orientation.[21,23] Additionally, these older adults may not have biological family members for support but rather a "chosen family." When compared to non-LGBT older people, LGBT older adults were more likely to have smaller support systems and live alone.[24] Therefore, it is more probable that they will need caregiving services.[21,23,25] Some older adults who are LGBTQ+ may fear that their supports will not be allowed to be involved in their care or permitted input with their decisions.[22,23] Older adults may hide their sexuality when they transition into a long-term care facility and possibly label their partner as a close friend.[26] OTAs can demonstrate respect for older adults who are LGBTQ+ by simple actions such as using inclusive gender-neutral language (partner and significant other rather than husband or wife), as well as using the older adult's preferred pronouns (e.g., he/him,

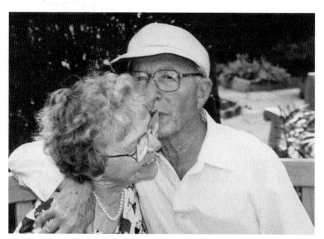

FIG. 12.3 Sexual expression is an important part of a person's life at any age.

she/her, and they/them).[17] Some older adults may prefer to be addressed by a chosen name, which may differ from their legal name. OTAs can also have an attitude of acceptance, help to create an environment of inclusion, and listen to any fears expressed about discrimination.[23] When discussing an older adult's significant other, OTAs should use similar vocabulary as the client. For example, if an older adult uses "roommate" to describe a partner, the OTA should use the term "roommate" when discussing the partner during intervention. If providing any handouts or educational materials, the OTA may also ensure the information is inclusive. For example, when discussing positioning, the OTA should utilize materials that depict a variety of couples, including same-sex couples. If discrimination is found in a long-term care setting, the OTA can suggest that the older adult contact an ombudsman representative or make a formal complaint to the state survey board.[22]

Times are changing because of a Supreme Court decision (*Obergefell v. Hodges*) that allows same-sex couples the right to marry in all 50 states (Fig. 12.3). Therefore, more homosexual couples are recognized as married for determining Social Security benefits or "eligibility for Supplemental Security Income (SSI) payments."[27] Furthermore, because of another Supreme Court ruling (*United States v. Windsor*), Section 3 of the Defense of Marriage Act (DOMA) was deemed unconstitutional, and Medicare can now recognize same-sex marriages for benefits.[28] Advocacy organizations such as the Human Rights Campaign (HRC) and Services and Advocacy for LGBT Elders (SAGE) are improving care for older adults who are LGBTQ+. The HRC works on discrimination in health care facilities through research about policies and promoting patient-centered care by education.[29] SAGE is a national organization that works to increase the quality of life for LGBT aging through services, research, promoting inclusion, and advocacy on a national, state, and local level.[30] SAGE also provides numerous resources for older adults and health care staff through The National Resource Center on LGBT Aging.[30]

NORMAL AGE-RELATED PHYSIOLOGICAL CHANGES IN MEN AND WOMEN

With normal aging, physiological changes might affect sexual functioning. Knowledge of these changes may help the OTA counsel the older adult (Box 12.1). Not all of these changes happen to every older adult, and the degree varies among individuals. For women, hormonal changes and medical conditions can cause sexual dysfunctions such as weaker or fewer orgasms.[31,32] Aging may also result in vaginal dryness and thinning of tissue, which can cause pain and irritation during intercourse.[31] Using water-based personal lubricants and extending the amount of time for foreplay are options for overcoming vaginal dryness.[31] Women may also benefit from the use of additional sex devices such as a vibrator to increase sensation needed for orgasm.[33] Men can experience a loss of libido, which can be caused by medical problems, depression, or side effects from medications that potentially can cause ED.[10,12] Though prevalence of female sexual dysfunctions varies widely across studies, the most commonly reported challenges include vulvovaginal atrophy leading to reduced lubrication and painful intercourse, urinary incontinence, and difficulty reaching orgasm.[32] In addition, OTAs should be aware of the concept "use it or lose it." Older adults who remain sexually active may not experience some of these physiological changes or not to the same degree as older adults who do not remain sexually active. Furthermore, these physiological changes are just one aspect of sexual activity as sexuality is complex and involves psychological, spiritual, social, and cultural dimensions of a human being. The ways a person reacts to and perceives these physiological changes ultimately affects sexual functioning. OTAs can apply the knowledge of normal age-related physiological changes to educate older adults. For example, a commercially available lubricant supplement decreases vaginal secretion and helps reduce abrasion from thinning of the vaginal lining. Lubrication may also prevent dyspareunia, or painful intercourse.[13] Kegel exercises (pelvic floor exercises) help preserve vaginal tone in women, can aid in the intervention of ED in men, and can reduce symptoms of incontinence in both genders.[34,35] Refer to Chapter 17 for additional information on instruction of Kegel exercises.

BOX 12.1

Age-Related Physiological Changes and Sexual Responses

Women

1. Decrease in rate and amount of vaginal lubrication may possibly lead to painful intercourse.[31,36,37]
2. Orgasmic phase decrease may occur in older adult women, resulting in lessened orgasmic intensity.[13,31,36,37]
3. Structural changes or atrophy may occur in the labia or uterus, in addition to a reduction in the expansion of the vagina width and length.[13,13,37,38]
4. Thinning of the lining of the vagina can result in irritation and painful intercourse.[13,31,37]
5. Sexual stimulation from the nipples, clitoris, and vulva may decrease with age due to lessened sensation.[38]

Men

1. Erection is slower, less full, and disappears quickly after orgasm. Erection has a longer refractory period.[13,36]
2. Older adult men may experience a decrease in penile rigidity.[13,36]
3. A decreased volume of sperm occurs; although fertility level is diminished, men do not become sterile.[13,37]
4. Decreased penile sensitivity results in increased need for direct penile stimulation over other forms of stimulation such as visual or psychological.[39]
5. Ejaculatory control enhanced.[13,36,39]
6. Ejaculation and orgasm are less strong.[13,39]
7. Decrease in ejaculatory seminal fluid.[39]

SEXUALLY TRANSMITTED DISEASES AMONG THE OLDER ADULT POPULATION

An often-overlooked aspect of sexual activity in the older adult population is the prevalence and prevention of sexually transmitted diseases (STDs). A Centers for Disease Control and Prevention (CDC) study[40] found that 51% of the diagnoses of HIV/AIDS was among people over 50 in the United States. According to the 2010 AARP study, the most common STD involving older adults is vaginitis, which affects 35% of women.[8] In addition, 5% of men and women have been diagnosed with gonorrhea and human papilloma virus.[8] Without the risk of pregnancy, many older adults forgo using safer sex techniques such as condoms.[41] According to the 2010 AARP study, only one in five of actively dating singles over the age of 45 reported using protection.[8] Older adults may be less knowledgeable about STDs and therefore less likely to use protection.[10,42]

Many health care providers are not comfortable asking older adults about their sexual activity. However, if health care providers do not ask, patients are unlikely to share information about their symptoms until they are debilitating.[42] Prevention and education with older adults should be incorporated with intervention. Promoting the use of condoms, STD testing, and other safer sex techniques is important in discussions of sexual activity with older adults. In the community, older adults can receive testing through their physician's office and with the reauthorization of the Older Americans Act in 2020. Title 1 addresses prevention of STDs through evidence-based programming.[43] OTAs working in long-term care facilities can educate older adults on the importance of safer sex techniques as well as the proper use of condoms. OTAs can also collaborate with other health care professionals to facilitate education on safer sex among the older adult population.

ROLE OF INTERVENTION IN SEXUAL EDUCATION

OTAs, occupational therapists (OTs), and older adults should collaborate to address concerns about sexual activity. In addition, OTAs should be aware of other team members' areas of expertise. Sexual dysfunction such as erectile problems, ejaculatory disturbances, anorgasmia (lack of orgasm), and pain during intercourse may be caused by side effects of medication and other physiological reasons.[36] The physician and pharmacist must be notified about these concerns. Sexual dysfunction has a psychological component.[12,36,44] Therefore, the client should be referred for counseling with a social worker or psychologist who has expertise with older adults who have disabilities and sexual dysfunction. In addition to the OT/OTA team, some physical therapists and nurses may educate the client about sexual positioning. Speech language pathologists may assist older adults who have difficulties with communication.

ADDRESSING OLDER ADULT SEXUAL ACTIVITY IN NURSING FACILITY

Trends in public policy and in professional literature suggest a more accepting attitude of sexual activity in nursing facilities (Fig. 12.4). Federal laws regulate privacy and other rights for institutionalized patients, namely the Omnibus Budget Reconciliation Act (OBRA, 1987) or Nursing Home Reform Act passed in 1987.[22,45] Assisted living facilities are regulated by the states so resident protections vary, but many facilities have the same rights.[22] One national survey found that over half of nursing homes in the United States have experienced issues related to sexual activity and masturbation, yet 63.4% of nursing homes do not have policies related to sexual behavior.[11] In general, most facilities that have policies apply them to all residents though some facilities only apply policies once sexual activity is noted, once it is requested, or to residents with cognitive deficits.[11]

In a systematic review of literature regarding perspectives on sexual behavior of residents residing in institutions, findings were that, generally, residents' attitudes were positive except with regard to sexual orientation.[46] Furthermore, residents think about and want to discuss sexual activity. A major finding was that older adults in institutions are not asexual as is sometimes portrayed and that they engage in a variety of sexual practices.[46] However, despite these positive trends, challenges still exist in nursing home facilities. One of these challenges includes availability of privacy.[47] Very few facilities exist that are designed to accommodate private intimate moments, and residents can anticipate interruptions by well-meaning staff members or schedules. Sometimes, schedules are too standardized to allow for private activities.[47] Even with private rooms, residents may feel inhibited by the close proximity of staff members or other residents.[31]

Another challenge is dealing with sexual behavior of residents who have cognitive impairment, such as dementia. Sexual interest does not disappear with onset of dementia. For example, in the first stage of Alzheimer's disease, a person may experience heightened sexual desire.[48] Sometimes a person with dementia may display inappropriate sexual behavior (e.g., masturbating in public). When such behavior occurs, the interprofessional team should carefully assess the situation to determine the reason for the behavior and the best way to manage it.[49] They should also keep in mind that residents do have rights to express their sexuality as long as both older adults have the mental capacity to participate.[11,50] Inappropriate sexual behavior can sometimes occur because of boredom or loneliness[31] and, in that case, OTAs can provide suggestions for meaningful activities to keep the person involved. It is important to consider the decision-making capacity of residents with dementia and their understanding of sexual activity. Residents with poor understanding should be protected from sexual exploitation.[31,51]

In addition, staff members may have misconceptions and negative attitudes about sexual activity and aging, which can pose a barrier to sexual fulfillment for long-term care residents.[31,47] Staff may express their disapproval in many ways. One subtle way is by joking about sexual activity, which may serve as a means to make older adults conform to the expectation of asexuality in some nursing facilities.

In some institutional settings, envisioning older adults being interested in sex is difficult, and the older adults themselves may be intolerant of peer engagement in sexual behavior.[46,47] Generational beliefs, societal expectations, personal beliefs, and/or religious beliefs may

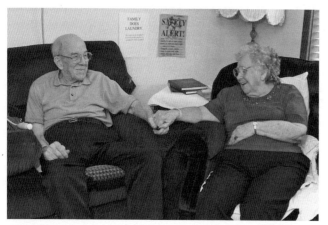

FIG. 12.4 Sharing a room in a long-term care facility, these older adults are able to enjoy the companionship of their lifelong spouse.

influence these attitudes.[46,47] OTAs participating in program planning can suggest dances and other social events that encourage romance and human touch. In addition, OTAs should always be aware of respecting client privacy. Shutting a curtain between beds or going to another room for intervention with personal ADL functions helps preserve privacy rights. Older adults should reside in a supportive environment that encourages sexual expression and involvement in sexual activity when appropriate. Nursing homes should set up policies to allow sexual behavior, and residents should have input with setting up nursing home standards.[46,51]

Finally, education can help dispel myths and misconceptions about sexual activity and older adults in nursing facilities.[52] OTAs and other members of the interprofessional team who have positive attitudes and are educated about sexual activity and older adults can help dispel the ageist attitudes sometimes held by some nursing home staff, family members, or the older adults themselves.

EDUCATING AND COUNSELING THE OLDER ADULT CLIENT

The Permission, Limited Information, Specific Suggestions, and Intensive Therapy Model

Intervention models may help provide sexual education to older adults. The permission, limited information, specific suggestions, and intensive therapy (PLISSIT) model developed by Annon[53,54] is a useful format for presenting sexual education information (Box 12.2).

OTAs can use the first, second, and third stages of the PLISSIT model during intervention. The older adult must be assured of confidentiality throughout the educational process. In the first stage of the PLISSIT model—*permission*—the OTA applies therapeutic listening skills. The verbal and nonverbal body language of the OTA must demonstrate comfort with the topic. OTAs can ask questions using clear and direct language in a nonthreatening manner to build rapport which has been shown to encourage communication about sexual functioning.[55] In addition, the OTA can convey that sexual activity is a normal part of every human's needs throughout a lifetime. Older adults who are interested in discussing sexual activity may have general questions about normal sexual changes with aging or common myths. The spouse or partner should be encouraged to join the discussion.

In the second stage of the PLISSIT model, the OTA can apply *limited information* by relating knowledge of sexual activity gleaned from this chapter and other relevant sources. The OTA may also educate older adults in this stage by using general resources and handouts. This education provides the older adult an opportunity to review the information privately before progressing to specific suggestions. The OTA can provide *specific*

BOX 12.2

The PLISSIT Model

P = Permission.
- This stage involves listening in a nonjudgmental, knowledgeable, and relaxed manner as the client discusses sexual concerns. General questions can be asked in an intake or screening evaluation (e.g., "Do you have any concerns about the effects of your condition on sexual function?").

LI = Limited information.
- At this stage, older adults can be educated about normal physiological changes with aging, myths and stereotypes about the older adult population, and sexual activity and psychosocial factors that may inhibit or stress the older adult.
- Clinicians may provide resources and general handouts for further patient education.

SS = Specific suggestions.
- At this stage, OTAs may make appropriate suggestions for improved sexual functioning. Older adults also may need to be referred to specialists such as social workers, psychologists, and physical or occupational therapists.

IT = Intensive therapy.
- This stage of counseling involves the expertise of a skilled social worker, psychologist, or psychiatrist.

Adapted from Annon JS. *The Behavioral Treatment of Sexual Problems: Brief Therapy* [brochure]. Honolulu, HI: Kapiolani Health Services; 1974; Annon JS. *The Behavioral Treatment of Sexual Problems: Brief Therapy.* New York: Harper & Row; 1976.

suggestions in the third stage. Many suggestions to help older adults who have disabling conditions and their partners maintain sexual function are discussed in this chapter. The OTA should refer the older adult who needs psychological support at any point of the education process to the appropriate counselor. The fourth stage of the model—*intensive therapy*—involves the skills of a trained counselor and is especially important for those older adults experiencing sexual dysfunction.

The Ex-PLISSIT[56] framework expands on Annon's PLISSIT[54] model by requiring practitioners to receive extended permission from their patients. Prior to proceeding with each stage, the practitioner must ask the patient if they are comfortable moving forward with the steps of the PLISSIT model. Health care practitioners also extend permission to the patients to discuss concerns or questions they may have at any time during the intervention process.[56] Extended permission ensures open communication and increases both the patient's and the health care practitioner's comfort level while addressing sexual activity.

Role of the Certified Occupational Therapy Assistant in Sexual Education

To provide older adults with adequate sex education, OTAs must have a general knowledge about medical conditions, awareness of psychological issues, and an understanding of the importance of good communication. Knowledge of the effects of a disease or disabling condition on sexual performance is necessary. OTAs must remember that the manifestations of a disease or condition differs with each older adult. Older adults' ability to adapt to life changes and their coping skills often affect their sexual functioning. Refer to Box 12.3 for some general education suggestions for all conditions.

Safety Considerations With Sexual Activity

Due to multiple factors, safety should be addressed when providing interventions for sexual health. This section provides an overview of different safety suggestions when educating older adults.

- Older adults who sustained strokes may have motor, sensory, and psychological dysfunctions. Sensory and motor dysfunctions should be considered with suggestions for positioning with sexual activity.
- With a cardiac condition, encourage older adults to consult with their physicians before returning to sexual activity. OTAs should educate older adults on the precautions for sexual activity after a cardiac condition: chest pain, shortness of breath, irregular heart rate, dizziness, fatigue the next day, insomnia, or heart palpitations lasting longer than 15 minutes after sex.[57-59] Older adults experiencing these symptoms should seek immediate medical assistance.

BOX 12.3

General Education Suggestions
1. Encourage older adults to maintain good communication with their partners in all aspects of their lives, not just about sexual activity.[13]
2. Encourage older adults to experiment with different sexual positions for increased comfort and pleasure.[13]
3. Provide instruction on energy conservation techniques. Suggest resting before sexual activity.[2,13]
4. Encourage older adults with decreased energy or with a medical condition that prevents participating in intercourse to explore other forms of sexual expression such as hugging, kissing, caressing, masturbation, and oral sex.[13,43]
5. Reassure older adults that once they are medically stable and their physician has assessed them, they can resume sexual activity.[45,58]
6. Talk with older adults about any fears they may have about resuming sexual functioning after sustaining a condition.[43]

- Arthritis can cause pain, fatigue, and joint inflammation during sexual activity. Older adults should be instructed on sexual positions that reduce the risk of these debilitating factors.
- Safety concerns with sexual activity and other activities are necessary for older adults to follow after total hip replacements. Review with older adults who have a posterolateral surgical approach that, with any sexual or life activity, they should not flex the affected hip more than 90 degrees, and the affected hip should not be adducted or internally rotated.[60,61] Evidence suggests that the safest position for sexual activity is supine or missionary position for the person with the total hip replacement.[62] Precautions vary according to surgical approach (anterolateral or posterolateral), and OTAs should consult with the physician for any guidance.
- OTAs need to recognize when to refer older adults with sexual concerns who would benefit from additional services, such as psychological support, to appropriate professionals (Box 12.4 overviews some intervention ideas for working with older adults).

EFFECTS OF HEALTH CONDITIONS ON OLDER ADULT SEXUAL ACTIVITY

Cerebrovascular Accident

OTAs commonly work with older adults who have sustained cerebrovascular accidents (CVAs) or strokes. Approaching sexual concerns after a stroke in intervention is often ignored.[63,64] Addressing sexual activity should be one of many aspects of a thorough evaluation and intervention. Just as the outcomes after a stroke are complex and different for each person, so are the effects of a stroke on sexual activity. It is not unusual for someone after a stroke to experience a decreased desire and satisfaction with sexual activity.[63,64] Changes after a CVA have been linked to a person's attitude about sexual activity and to fears about having ED, experiencing rejection, or having another stroke.[65,66] Changes in one's body image and one's coping skills can be psychological manifestations.[65,66] Being aphasic, having functional changes, displaying difficulties with endurance, feeling fatigued, and taking certain medications that have side effects on sexual performance can influence sexual activity.[63,64,66] Many of these changes may indicate a need for intervention to address sexual activity, and OTAs can play a strong role because of their background in working with people who have had CVAs. However, in considering any intervention, OTAs should keep in mind the concept that sexual dysfunctions after a CVA are likely multifactorial.[63,64,66] Therefore, use of clinical reasoning skills and an interprofessional team-based approach is important.

OTAs should observe for motor abnormalities and other symptoms that can affect sexual function, including hemiplegia, perceptual, cognitive, and visual spatial disturbances. Sensory deficits, speech problems, and emotional

BOX 12.4

Intervention Gems and Older Adult Sexual Activity

- Sexual activity is an ADL listed in the *Occupational Therapy Practice Framework: Domain and Process*, fourth edition.[1] It is a normal part of aging and should be incorporated into intervention if older adults desire.
- Generational values, as well as individual values, influence attitudes and beliefs about sexual activity.
- The current oldest generation of older adults, the Traditionalists, grew up in a time when sexual activity was not openly discussed. The Baby Boomer generation may discuss sexual activity more openly in intervention sessions.
- OTAs should develop rapport with older adults before discussing sexual activity and address sexual activity based on the PLISSIT model.
- OTAs must be comfortable discussing sexual activity with intervention. Possible areas to address include sexual positioning, adaptive equipment, energy conservation strategies, sensory adaptations, compensatory strategies, and sexual education about safe sex practices.
- OTAs should be sensitive to the older adults' sexual orientation, gender preference, and psychological aspects of sexual activity.
- OTAs can also collaborate with the interprofessional treatment team as well as educate staff on the importance of incorporating sexual activity within the older adult's intervention plan. The physician on the interprofessional team should guide older adults with

conditions (e.g., stroke, cardiac, arthritis, and joint replacement) about resuming sexual activity.
- A stroke can have motor, sensory, and psychological manifestations that may affect an older adult's ability to participate in sexual activity, as well as other underlying conditions. Common compensatory techniques for sexual intercourse include lying on the affected side so the unaffected arm is free, using pillows under the affected side, encouraging touch for individuals with aphasia, and a nondistracting environment for individuals with cognitive impairments.
- Older adults with cardiac conditions may have a fear of sustaining a recurrent MI during sexual activity. OTAs can instruct older adults on the use of relaxation techniques and energy conservation for sexual activity.
- Pain, fatigue, joint inflammation, and anxiety can hinder sexual activity with older adults who have arthritis. OTAs can instruct older adults with arthritis to use energy conservation techniques and rest to decrease pain during sexual activity. Heat pads or warm baths can be effective preparatory methods to decrease pain.
- Older adults with hip replacements should be instructed to abide by hip precautions during sexual activity.
- Older adults with knee replacements often prefer a side-lying position for comfort. Pillows can also be used with older adults with knee replacements to maintain comfort and for safety.

---

manifestations are additional symptoms. For example, if older adults have unilateral neglect, they may ignore one side of the body during sexual performance. Motor disturbances such as muscle weakness, decreased range of motion (ROM), and problems with balance, coordination, or endurance can make sexual performance difficult.[63,66] Sensory deficits[66] as well as pain[63] can affect sexual performance. Expressive aphasia may result in difficulty stating sexual needs. If older adults are depressed, they may have no interest in sex. Anxiety may cause sexual performance problems such as ED in males and decreased lubrication leading to painful intercourse in females.[64,66] Other underlying conditions may also affect performance such as impaired bladder function, diabetes, hypertension, or even heart disease.[64,66] Thus, OTAs need to consider the entire medical picture when addressing sexual function. (See Chapter 19 for a detailed discussion about CVA and Chapter 22 for a discussion of cardiovascular conditions.)

After identifying the symptoms that affect sexual performance, the OT and the OTA should collaborate with the older adult to develop specific intervention suggestions. For example, clients with hemiplegia are sometimes advised to lie on the affected side so that the unaffected arm is free to caress the partner[66] or to find a comfortable

position.[13,66] Adaptations such as applying pillows under the affected side and use of a vibrator can help with motor manifestations.[66] Clients who experience spasticity after stroke may benefit from taking a warm bath before sexual activity to relax muscles.[67] Alternative communication cues, such as hand signals or sounds, are useful for those with aphasia. Cues can assist with communicating enjoyable sensations, painful sensations, or directions.[67] Partners of older adults with visual field deficits should be encouraged to approach from the impaired side and use touch on both sides. Minimizing environmental distractions during sexual activity may help older adults with cognitive deficits involving concentration.[66,68] Clients with changes in sensation should consider using body mapping at home. Body mapping consists of touching the affected partner slowly and gently to identify areas of hyposensitivity, hypersensitivity, and areas that are most sexually charged.[67]

Beyond the physical effects of a CVA, some older adults may experience low self-esteem and depression. These symptoms can affect sexual desire and performance.[65,66] In addition, older adults who are in some way dependent on a partner may feel ambivalent about resuming a sexual relationship because of role changes.[65] Older adults with CVA may benefit from counseling services to help address the psychological effects following the injury.

Heart Disease

Heart disease is one of the most common chronic ailments affecting the older adult population.[69] Older adults can have acute cardiac conditions, such as myocardial infarctions (MI), or chronic cardiac conditions, such as hypertension. With either type of cardiac condition, the possible effect on sexual activity must not be ignored. Older adults should consult their physician for recommendations about sexual activity and cardiac conditions. DeBusk and colleagues[70] developed a classification system to use as a guideline for physician's recommendations to manage sexual activity in patients with cardiac disease. With this classification system, patients are grouped into low, medium, or high cardiac risk. Patients with low risk, such as having controlled hypertension or mild stable angina, are recommended to safely resume sex. Patients with moderate risk, such as sustaining a recent MI or displaying moderate angina, require further cardiac evaluation. Patients in the high-risk category, such as having unstable angina or hypertension, are recommended to be stabilized before reassuming sexual activity. A scientific statement from the American Heart Association established guidelines for sexual activity for different conditions such as coronary artery disease, heart failure, valvular heart disease, arrhythmias, and pacemakers.[58]

Once stabilized, and with physician permission, some older adults with cardiac conditions may be instructed to resume sexual activity in a gradual manner.[71] For older adults who gradually reassume sexual activity, especially when experiencing heart symptoms or an exacerbation of heart failure, alternative forms of sexual activity other than intercourse may be suggested.[57,71] However, before reassuming sexual activity, older adults should be instructed by the medical team about precautions and when to notify their physician, or older adults may be directly instructed by their physicians about precautions for specific conditions.

Examples of precautions with cardiac conditions for sexual activity are chest pain, shortness of breath, insomnia, dizziness, and fast or irregular heart rate. Other precautions that should be monitored following sexual activity include excessive fatigue, continuous increase in blood pressure, or heart palpitations lasting longer than 15 minutes.[57-59] The interprofessional team should also be aware of the positive effects of medications in helping to maintain sexual function[57,72] and negative side effects of certain medications that can influence libido or result in sexual dysfunction.[57,72]

Sustaining a cardiac condition can affect a person psychologically, resulting in fears about resuming sexual activity. The resumption of sexual activity after a heart attack is believed by some people to cause future cardiac incidents and even death.[73] Findings from a study (n = 1774)

published in the *Journal of the American Medical Association* (*JAMA*) help clarify anecdotal information.[59] Sexual activity was found to contribute to MIs in a small number of the subjects (0.9%), and regular exercise was related to a decreased risk.[74] The physical demands of sexual activity are equal to mild to moderate exercise ("heart rate rarely increases to greater than 130 beats per minute and systolic blood pressure is rarely greater than 170 mm Hg").[70] For example, sexual intercourse requires no more metabolic energy than walking 1 mile on an even surface.[75] However, a caution to take with some research findings on physical demands of sexual activity is that many studies assessed young to middle age healthy men and may not apply to older adults.[58]

Relaxation is important because fears and anxieties are common after cardiac incidents, especially about resuming sexual relationships.[73] In addition, it is not uncommon to be depressed[76] or to be anxious, which can lead to sexual dysfunction.[76,77] Sexual dysfunctions such as ED[78] also can result from physical reasons such as hypertension leading to arteriosclerosis (hardening of the arteries).[12] Encouraging sexual activity in a familiar environment,[78] using positions that require less energy expenditure, and suggesting relaxation with sexual activity are helpful suggestions.[79] OTAs can teach older adults stress reduction techniques. Energy conservation strategies also may be helpful for those who are gradually building up their endurance. It is also beneficial to wait 1–3 hours after meals to allow the heart to pump blood to assist with the digestive process and to have sex in a cool room.[78] Per the PLISSIT model,[53,54] OTAs may need to refer the older adult to an expert to address any sexual dysfunction. (See Chapter 22 for a more detailed discussion about cardiac conditions and older adults.)

Arthritis

Arthritis is another common chronic condition among older adults.[69] All types of arthritis, including osteoarthritis and rheumatoid arthritis, can influence sexual function with physical and psychological effects. Physical concerns can be pain, functional limitations, fatigue, medication side effects, with some types of arthritis. Psychological issues include, but are not limited to, depression and anxiety which can increase fatigue as well.[61]

Older adults with joint inflammation and pain may be particularly prone to sexual performance problems. A common intervention goal for people with rheumatoid arthritis is to maintain or increase functional abilities in all areas of life,[61,80] including sexual activity. OTAs can make specific suggestions to help older adults reduce joint pain and discomfort and preserve energy. Exercises to increase and maintain muscle strength affect the motor aspect of sexual performance. Older adults should be encouraged to take a warm shower or tub bath before sexual activity to help decrease pain and improve ROM.[81] Older adults and their partners also may experiment with various sexual positions that decrease joint pressure. Rest and energy conservation techniques may help make sexual performance less fatiguing. Finding the best time of day for sexual activity when the older adult is less fatigued and following a daily schedule based on conserving energy help sexual performance.[60,80,81]

Joint Replacements

Older adults with a history of arthritis commonly sustain joint replacements. Older adults after total hip replacements are counseled to follow certain precautions in all areas of their lives, including sexual activity. For an older adult who has had a total hip replacement (posterolateral approach), it is important to review that, with any sexual or life activity, the older adult should not flex the affected hip more than 90 degrees,[60,82] and that the affected hip should not be adducted or internally rotated.[82] Similarly, the older adult should avoid adduction with an anterolateral surgical approach in addition to avoiding external rotation and extension.[82] OTAs should consult with the older adult's physician for any clarification on precautions. After the customary healing period of approximately 6 weeks and with physician approval, these older adults can resume sexual activity as long as they follow precautions.

For intercourse, it is preferable with either sex that the older adult with the total hip replacement be positioned supine or in missionary position (on back) with hips abducted (apart), knees in extension (straight), and legs in neutral (toes pointed up),[62] and not in external rotation (toes pointed out).[60] Intercourse in a side-lying position for the involved older adult woman is accomplished by lying on her unaffected side with a minimum of two pillows between her legs to keep them abducted. The involved man using a side-lying position should also lie on his unaffected side and use his partner's legs to reinforce his affected leg.[60] Thus, the man's affected leg is on top of his partner's leg during sexual intercourse. The older adult man's partner should have a minimum of two pillows between their legs for support and to help their partner follow precautions.[60] Other suggestions are pillows between the knees to help maintain the hip joints in abduction[82] and pillows under the knees while in a supine position to prevent extreme external rotation.[82]

After a total knee replacement, older adults should be instructed to find the most comfortable position for intercourse. When the involved person is in a supine position, pillows can be placed under the knee, and the person can bend the knee within a comfortable range.[60] A side-lying position is often most comfortable after surgery, and pillow support under the knee is beneficial.[82]

Diabetes

According to the CDC, 26.8% of older adults have diabetes.[83] Older adults with diabetes may have physiological symptoms that impact sexual activity. These effects can include neuropathy, decreased circulation, decreased arousal, difficulties with vaginal health, and decreased sensation associated with increased glucose levels.[84] With diabetes, older men might experience ED, decreased libido, and retrograde ejaculation.[84] Older adult women may have less lubrication, difficulty orgasming, decreased libido, and an increased risk of yeast infections.[84] The OTA should recommend the older adult be instructed to see a physician for continual yeast infections. OTAs should also utilize general suggestions for positioning, Kegel exercises, and interventions for ED mentioned earlier in the chapter.

TECH TALK: FOCUS ON SEXUAL WELLNESS

NAME	PURPOSE	APPROX. COST	WHERE TO BUY
Sexuality and Intimacy in OT	Website designed to fill the gap in sexuality-related education and guidance for occupational therapy professionals through continuing education.	$0 to ~$75.00 per course	sexintima-cyot.com
Coral	App designed using evidence and research to support individuals/couples intimacy and sexual occupations.	$0 to ~ $60/yr.	Google Play IOS App Store Getcoral. app
Sportsheets	Website that includes guides for those with physical limitations (arthritis, ED, hip replacement, etc.) and carries sexual wellness products.	Varies by item	Sportsheets. com

CASE STUDY 1

Rita and "Mac" are friends and both have dementia. They reside in a Memory Care Unit at an assisted living facility. They enjoy each other's company and spend most of the day together. They start their day with morning coffee, eat their meals, and partake in social activities. They especially enjoy dances, where they can be observed embracing each other. They hold hands, sit next to each other cuddling, and are frequently observed kissing and hugging. The other residents enjoy seeing the couple embracing, as it appears to bring back memories. This couple sometimes can be seen sitting quietly holding hands and staring off into space. There is a calmness that comes over them when they are together as well as decreased agitation.

Initially, the staff were uncertain on how to react, making jokes and inappropriate comments about Rita and Mac's relationship. They consider their relationship likely to dissipate. As time passes, the staff recognizes and accepts the relationship, as it brings both residents a sense of calmness.

Rita is a widow, who has two adult daughters and one adult son who live nearby. Mac has been married to Donna for over 50 years, and they have one adult son, Mike. Donna and Mike visit Mac frequently at the facility. Initially, Donna is comfortable with her husband, Mac, and Rita spending time together as she notes his decrease in agitation. However, Mac does not recognize Donna when she visits. Disagreeing with his mom, Mike thinks the staff should keep Rita and Mac apart. He expresses concerns for his mother about this relationship mainly based on his own religious beliefs. Mike also is encouraging his mother to move his father to another facility. Although Rita's family is embarrassed about their mother's relationship, they clearly see the difference in her behavior when she is in Mac's company.

Recently, the staff noted that Rita is spending the night in Mac's room. Several times when they try to redirect Rita to her own room, the couple becomes agitated. Some of the staff members insist that Rita return to her room, and others are comfortable with her spending the night with Mac. A family conference is scheduled for each of the older adult's families, and the staff plans to discuss the sleeping arrangement with them.

■ CASE STUDY QUESTIONS

1 What are your personal thoughts about the scenario?
2 Why did the staff initially react by making jokes about Mac and Rita's relationship? Did their response suggest ageism? Explain why or why not.
3 Are Rita and Mac cognitively aware of their relationship?
4 Besides yourself, who else would be appropriate staff members to be at the family conference and why?
5 If the decision is to move Mac to another facility, how would that affect the residents' families and the older adults?
6 How can the OTA educate the staff and family members on the importance of an individual's rights related to sexuality?

CASE STUDY 2

Upon graduating and receiving his license, Ben accepts an OTA position at an assisted living facility. While treating Mary, a 65-year-old patient who has sustained a CVA, Ben asks Mary if she and her partner, Cristina, have any questions about sexual activity following her condition. They both giggle uncomfortably but express they are happy someone on their health care team approached the topic. Mary and Cristina disclose to Ben that sex is an important part of their romantic relationship, and they have questions on positioning and precautions following Mary's condition. Ben answers their questions and provides the couple with resources on safe positioning and body mapping for sensory exploration. Ben's next patient on his caseload is Tommy, an 81-year-old patient, who had also sustained a CVA and is widowed. Ben reviews one-handed dressing techniques and compensatory strategies for IADL participation with Tommy. After leaving Tommy's room, Ben reflects and compares his experiences with both clients. Ben questions himself as to why he initiated the conversation of sexual activity with Mary and not with Tommy.

■ CASE STUDY QUESTIONS

1 Why do you think Ben did not address sexual activity with Tommy?
2 What beliefs may Ben have had toward older adults and sexual activity?
3 What could Ben have done differently to ensure occupational justice for all clients?
4 Do you believe Ben felt comfortable addressing sexuality with his clients? Why or why not?
5 What level(s) of the PLISSIT model did he utilize with his intervention with Mary and Cristina?

■ CHAPTER REVIEW QUESTIONS

1 Discuss common myths related to older adult sexual activity.
2 Discuss the viewpoint held by society about older adults who are LGBTQ+.
3 Describe issues related to STDs and the older adult population.
4 Identify some of the normal age-related physiological changes for women and intervention suggestions.
5 Identify some of the normal age-related physiological changes and intervention suggestions for men.
6 List the members of the interprofessional team and discuss ways that they can work together to address older adults' sexual concerns.
7 Discuss ways that attitudes of health care workers and the older adults themselves in nursing facilities can affect older adult sexual activity.
8 Describe ways OTAs help facilitate older adult sexual expression in a nursing facility setting.
9 List and describe the parts of the PLISSIT model with example of ways OTAs can apply the model in intervention.
10 Identify some advantages of using the EXPLISSIT framework along with the PLISSIT model.
11 Discuss any precautions that OTAs might suggest with sexual expression for someone with a stroke, total hip replacement, and heart condition.

EVIDENCE NUGGETS

1. Bauer, M., Haesler, E., & Fetherstonhaugh, D. Let's talk about sex: older people's views on the recognition of sexuality and sexual health in the health-care setting. Health expectations: An international journal of public participation in health care and health policy. 2016;19(6), 1237–1250. doi.org/10.1111/hex.12418
   - Sexuality is important topic for older adults.
   - Barriers such as embarrassment, dissatisfaction with treatment, negative attitudes, and the appearance of disinterest by health professionals prevent older adults from talking with health care workers about sex.
   - Health care workers should incorporate strategies that are supportive of sexual activity and intimacy with older adults.
2. Hogben, M., Ford, J., Becasen, J. S., & Brown, K. F. A systematic review of sexual health interventions for adults: Narrative evidence. Journal of sex research. 2015;52(4), 444–469. doi.org/10.1080/00224499.2014.973100
   - Face-to-face interventions were more likely to have effects on behaviors and health outcomes, whereas community interventions impacted attitudes and knowledge.
   - Ninety-eight percent of participants reported a positive finding in at least one domain following sexual health interventions.
   - Incorporating principles from existing sexual health definitions in public health efforts may help improve sexual health.
3. Horne, M., Youell, J., Brown, L., Simpson, P., Dickinson, T., & Brown-Wilson, C. A scoping review of education and training resources supporting care home staff in facilitating residents' sexuality, intimacy and relational needs. Age and ageing. 2021; Advance online publication. doi.org/10.1093/ageing/afab022
   - Sexual activity education interventions can improve the care toward older adult's sexuality and intimacy needs.

- The education interventions were focused toward: sexual expression of older people living in residential aged care, sexuality and aging, and expression of sexuality in people with dementia.
4. Lichtenberg P. A. Sexuality and physical intimacy in long-term care. Occupational therapy in health care. 2014;28(1), 42–50. https://doi.org/10.3109/07380577.2013.865858
   - OT practitioners frequently address acts of intimate care during ADL training, which may lead to more opportunities to address intimacy and sexual goals of clients.
   - Occupational therapy interventions addressing sexuality are beneficial to older adults in long-term care.
   - Holistic care must include the OT practitioner's inclusion of sexual needs and concerns of older adults.
5. McGrath, M., & Lynch, E. Occupational therapists' perspectives on addressing sexual concerns of older adults in the context of rehabilitation. Disability and rehabilitation. 2014;36(8), 651–657. doi.org/10.3109/09638288.2013.805823
   - Health care professionals continue to be reluctant to respond to older adult's sexual concerns.
   - Barriers for OT practitioners in discussing sexual concerns with clients included socio-cultural norms related to sexuality, perceived professional competence and confidence with the topic, and prioritization of resources.
   - Education is needed to improve therapist's perceived competence and confidence in addressing sexuality with older adults.

REFERENCES

1. American Occupational Therapy Association. Occupational therapy practice framework: domain and process fourth edition. *Am J Occup Ther.* 2020;74(suppl 2):1-87. doi:10.5014/ajot.2020.74S2001.
2. Tipton-Burton M, Delmonico R, Burton GU. Sexuality and physical dysfunction. In: Pendleton H, Schultz-Krohn W, eds. *Pedretti's Occupational Therapy Practice Skills for Physical Dysfunction.* 8th ed. St Louis: Elsevier; 2018:289-304.
3. Hyland A, McGrath M. Sexuality and occupational therapy in Ireland–a case of ambivalence? *Disabil Rehabil.* 2013;35(1):73-80.
4. American Occupational Therapy Association. AOTA occupational therapy code of ethics. *Am J Occup Ther.* 2020;74(suppl 3):26-47.
5. Scott JB, Reitz SM, Harcum, S. Principle 4: justice. In: Scott JB, Reitz SM, eds. *Practical applications for the Occupational Therapy Code of Ethics.* 2nd ed. Bethesda: AOTA Press; 2015:85-95.
6. Beekman T. Fill in the generation gap. *Strateg Finance.* 2011;93(3):15. doi:10.1109/AINA.2007.72.
7. Syme ML, Cohn TJ. Examining aging sexual stigma attitudes among adults by gender, age, and generational status. *Aging Ment Health.* 2016;20(1):36-45. doi:10.1080/13607863.2015.1012044.
8. Fisher LL. *Sex, Romance, and Relationships: AARP Survey of Midlife and Older Adults.* AARP, Knowledge Management; 2010. Available at: http://assets.aarp.org/rgcenter/general/srr_09.pdf.
9. University of Michigan. *National Poll on Healthy Aging - Let's Talk About Sex.* 2018. Available at: https://deepblue.lib.umich.edu/bitstream/handle/2027.42/143212/NPHA-Sexual-Health-Report_050118_final.pdf?sequence=1&isAllowed=y.
10. Dhingra I, DE Sousa A, Sonavane S. Sexuality in older adults: clinical and psychosocial dilemmas. *J Geriatr Ment Health.* 2016;3(2):131-139. doi:10.4103/2348-9995.195629.
11. Lester P, Kohen I, Stefanacci R, Feuerman M. Sex in nursing homes: a survey of nursing home policies governing resident sexual activity. *J Am Med Dir Assoc.* 2016;17(1):71-74. doi:10.1016/j.jamda.2015.08.013.
12. Mobley D, Khera M, Baurn N. Recent advances in the treatment of erectile dysfunction. *Postgrad Med J.* 2017;93(1105):679-685. doi:10.1136/postgradmedj-2016-134073.
13. Laflin M. Sexuality and the elderly individuals. In: Lewis CB, ed. *Aging: The Health-Care Challenge.* 4th ed. Philadelphia: FA Davis; 2002.
14. Mayo Clinic. *Erectile Dysfunction.* 2020. Available at: https://www.mayoclinic.org/diseases-conditions/erectile-dysfunction/diagnosis-treatment/drc-20355782.
15. Wassersug R, Wibowo E. Non-pharmacological and non-surgical strategies to promote sexual recovery for men with erectile dysfunction. *Transl Androl Urol.* 2017;6(suppl 5):S776-S794. doi:10.21037/tau.2017.04.09.

16. Lof J, Olaison A. 'I don't want to go back into the closet just because I need care': recognition of older LGBTQ adults in relation to future care needs. *Eur J Soc Work*. 2020;23(2):253-264. doi:10.1080/13691457.2018.1534087.

17. Fredriksen-Goldsen KI. The future of LGBT+ aging: a blueprint for action in services, policies, and research. *Generations*. 2016;40(2):6-15.

18. Newport F. *In U.S., Estimate of LGBT Population Rises to 4.5%*. 2018. Available at: https://news.gallup.com/poll/234863/estimate-lgbt-population-rises.aspx.

19. Twinley R. Sexual orientation and occupation: some issues to consider when working with older gay people to meet their occupational needs. *Br J Occup Ther*. 2014;77(4):623-625. doi:10.4276/030802214X14176260335381.

20. Ezhoa I, Savidge L, Bonnett C, et al. Barriers to older adults seeking sexual health advice and treatment: a scoping overview. *Int J Nurs Stud*. 2020;107:103566. doi:10.1016/j.ijnurstu.2020.103566.

21. Kimmel D. Lesbian, gay, bisexual and transgender aging concerns. *Clin Gerontol*. 2014;37:49-63. doi:10.1080/07317115.2014.847310.

22. National Senior Citizens Law Center. *LGBT Older Adults in Long-Term Care Facilities: Stories from the Field*. 2011. Available at: http://www.lgbtagingcenter.org/resources/pdfs/NSCLC_LGBT_report.pdf.

23. Schwinn SV, Dinkel SA. Changing the culture of long-term care: combating heterosexism. *Online J Issues Nurs*. 2015;20(2):7. doi:10.1080/03601277.2012.682953.

24. Espinoza R. *Out and Visible: The Experiences and Attitudes of Lesbian, Gay, Bisexual, and Transgender Older Adults, Ages 45-75*. 2014. Available at: https://www.sageusa.org/wp-content/uploads/2018/05/sageusa-out-visible-lgbt-market-research-full-report.pdf.

25. MetLife Study. *Still Out, Still Aging: The MetLife Study of Lesbian, Gay, Bisexual, and Transgender Baby Boomers*. 2010. Available at: https://www.asaging.org/sites/default/files/files/mmi-still-out-still-aging.pdf.

26. Serafin J, Smith GB, Keltz T. GAPNA Section. Lesbian, gay, bisexual, and transgender (LGBT) elders in nursing homes: it's time to clean out the closet. *Geriatr Nurs (Minneap)*. 2013;34(1):81-83. doi:10.1016/j.gerinurse.2012.12.003.

27. Social Security Administration. *Same-Sex Couples*. 2015. Available at: https://www.ssa.gov/people/same-sexcouples/.

28. CMS.gov. *HHS Announces Important Information for Individuals in Same-Sex Marriages*. 2014. Available at: https://www.cms.gov/newsroom/press-releases/hhs-announces-important-medicare-information-people-same-sex-marriages.

29. Human Rights Campaign. *Human Equality Index 2020*. 2020. Available at: https://hrc-prod-requests.s3-us-west-2.amazonaws.com/resources/HEI-2020-FinalReport.pdf?mtime=20200830220806&focal=none.

30. Sageusa.org. *SAGE Mission and Core Values*. Available at: https://www.sageusa.org/wp-content/uploads/2018/07/sage-mission-and-core-values.pdf.

31. Rheaume C, Mitty E. Sexuality and intimacy in older adults. *Geriatr Nurs (Minneap)*. 2008;29(5):342-349. doi:10.1016/j.gerinurse.2008.08.004.

32. Granville L, Pregler J. Women's sexual health and aging. *J Am Geriatr Soc*. 2018;66(3):595-601. doi:10.1111/jgs.15198.

33. Schwartz P. *Sex Toys for Older Couples*. 2013. Available at: https://www.aarp.org/home-family/sex-intimacy/info-07-2013/couples-guide-to-sex-toys-schwartz.html.

34. Lo CC, Goldman R. *Exercises to Eliminate Erectile Dysfunction*. 2015. Available at: http://www.healthline.com/health/erectile-dysfunction/exercises#Overviewl.

35. United States National Library of Medicine. *Kegel Exercises-Self-Care*. 2016. Available at: https://www.nlm.nih.gov/medlineplus/ency/patientinstructions/000141.htm.

36. Gentili A, Godschalk M. Sexual health & dysfunction. In: Williams BA, Chang A, Ahalt C, et al., eds. Current Diagnosis & Treatment: Geriatrics. 2nd ed. New York: McGraw-Hill Education; 2014:340-346.

37. Zhao PT, Su D, Seftel AD. Geriatric sexuality. In: Guzzo TJ, Drach GW, Wein AJ, eds. *Primer of Geriatric Urology*. New York: Springer; 2013:143-200.

38. Basson R, Wierman ME, van Lankveld J, et al. Summary of the recommendations on sexual dysfunctions in women. *J Sex Med*. 2010;7:314-326. doi:10.1111/j.1743-6109.2009.01617.x.

39. Hillman J. Men's issues in sexuality and aging. In: Hillman J, ed. *Sexuality and Aging: Clinical Perspectives*. Boston: Springer US; 2012:199-227. doi:10.1007/978-1-4614-3399-6_8.

40. Center for Disease Control and Prevention. HIV.gov. Aging with HIV. *Growing older with HIV*.2021. Available at: https://www.hiv.gov/hiv-basics/living-well-withhiv/taking-care-of-yourself/aging-with-hiv

41. Amin I. Social capital and sexual risk-taking behaviors among older adults in the United States. *J Appl Gerontol*. 2016;35(9):982-999. doi:10.1177/0733464814547048.

42. Benjamin Rose Institute on Aging. *Sexually Transmitted Diseases in Older Adults*. 2015. Available at: http://www.benrose.org/Resources/article-stds-older-adults.cfm.

43. *Supporting Older Americans Act of 2020*. 2020. Available at: https://www.congress.gov/116/plaws/publ131/PLAW-116publ131.pdf

44. Zhao PT, Su D, Seftel AD. Geriatric sexuality. In: Guzzo TJ, Drach GW, Wein AJ, eds. *Primer of Geriatric Urology*. New York: Springer; 2013:143-200.

45. *Omnibus Budget Reconciliation Act*. Baltimore: Health Care Financing Administration; 1987.

46. Mahieu L, Gastmans C. Older residents' perspectives on aged sexuality in institutionalized elder care: a systematic literature review. *Int J Nurs Stud*. 2015;52(12):1891-1905. doi:10.1016/j.ijnurstu.2015.07.007.

47. Villar F, Celdrán M, Fabà J, et al. Barriers to sexual expression in residential aged care facilities (RACFs): comparison of staff and resident's views. *J Adv Nurs*. 2014;70(11):2518-2527. doi:10.1111/jan.12398.

48. Tabak N, Shemesh-Kigli R. Sexuality and Alzheimer's disease: can the two go together? *Nurs Forum*. 2006;41(4):158-166. doi:10.1111/j.1744-6198.2006.00054.x.

49. Wilkins JM. More than capacity: alternatives for sexual decision making for individuals with dementia. *Gerontologist*. 2015;55(5):716-723. doi:10.1093/geront/gnv098.

50. Mendes A. Companionship, intimacy and sexual expression in dementia. *NRC*. 2015;17(7):390. doi:10.12968/nrec.2015.17.7.390.

51. Heath H. Older people in care homes: sexuality and intimate relationships. *Nurs Older People*. 2011;23(6):14-20.

52. Katz A. Sexuality in nursing home facilities. *Am J Nurs*. 2013;113(3):53-55. doi:10.3109/07380577.2013.865858.

53. Annon JS. *The Behavioral Treatment of Sexual Problems: Brief Therapy [brochure]*. Honolulu, HI: Kapiolani Health Services; 1974.

54. Annon JS. *The Behavioral Treatment of Sexual Problems: Brief Therapy*. New York: Harper & Row; 1976.

55. Sinkovic M, Towler M. Sexual aging: a systematic review of qualitative research on the sexuality and sexual health of older adults. *Qual Health Res*. 2019;29(9):1239-1254. doi:10.1177/1049732318819834.

56. Davis S, Taylor B. From PLISSIT to ex-PLISSIT. In: Davis S, ed. *Rehabilitation: The Use of Theories and Models in Practice*. Edinburgh: Elsevier; 2006:101-129.

57. Steinke EE, Jaarsma T. Sexual counseling and cardiovascular disease: practical approaches. *Asian J Androl*. 2015;17:32-39. doi:10.4103/1008-682X.135982.

58. Levine GN, Steinke EE, Bakaeen FG, et al. Sexual activity and cardiovascular disease: a scientific statement from the American Heart Association. *Circulation*. 2012;125(8):1058-1072. doi:10.1161/CIR.0b013e3182447787.

59. Cambre S. *The Sensuous Heart: Guidelines for Sex After a Heart Attack or Heart Surgery*. Atlanta: Pritchett & Hull Associates Inc; 2010.

60. Whittington C, Mansour S, Sloan SL. *Sex After Total Joint Replacement: A Guide for You and Your Partner.* Atlanta: Media Partners; 2001.

61. Crites A, Samuel P. Rheumatoid arthritis and osteoarthritis. In: Radomski MV, Latham CAT, eds. *Occupational Therapy for Physical Dysfunction.* 8th ed. Philadelphia: Wolters Kluwer Health/Lippincott Williams & Wilkins; 2021:877-894.

62. McFadden B. Is there a safe coital position after a total hip arthroplasty? *Orthop Nurs.* 2013;32(4):223-226. doi:10.1097/NOR.0b013e31829b0349.

63. Rosenbaum T, Vadas D, Kalichman L. Sexual function in poststroke patients: considerations for rehabilitation. *J Sex Med.* 2014;11(1):15-21. doi:10.1111/jsm.

64. Dusenbury W, Johansen P, Mosack V, et al. Determinants of sexual function and dysfunction in men and women with stroke: a systematic review. *Int J Clin Pract.* 2017;71(7):12969. doi:10.1111/ijcp.12969.

65. Thompson HS, Ryan A. The impact of stroke consequence on spousal relationships from the perspective of the person with a stroke. *J Clin Nurs.* 2009;18:1803-1811. doi:10.1111/j.1365-2702.2008.02694.x.

66. Hattjar B, Gillen G. Sexual function and intimacy. In: Gillen G, Nilsen D, eds. *Stroke Rehabilitation: A Function-Based Approach.* 5th ed. Philadelphia: Elsevier; 2021:262-279.

67. Mioduszewski M. Stroke and sexuality. In: Hattjar B, ed. *Sexuality and Occupational Therapy: Strategies for Persons with Disabilities.* Bethesda, MD: American Occupational Therapy Association, Inc; 2012:163-185.

68. Neistadt ME, Freda M. *Choices: A Guide to Sexual Counseling with Physically Disabled Adults.* Malabar, FL: Robert E. Krieger; 1987.

69. Department of Health and Human Services. *2019 Profile of Older Americans.* 2020. Available at: https://acl.gov/sites/default/files/Aging%20and%20Disability%20in%20America/2019ProfileOlderAmericans508.pdf.

70. DeBusk R, Drory Y, Goldstein I, et al. Management of sexual dysfunction in patients with cardiovascular disease: recommendations of the Princeton Consensus Panel. *Am J Cardiol.* 2000;86(2):175-181. doi:10.1016/j.mayocp.2012.06.01.

71. Steinke EE, Jaarsma T, Barnason SA, et al. Sexual counselling for individuals with cardiovascular disease and their partners: a consensus document from the American Heart Association and the ESC Council on Cardiovascular Nursing and Allied Professions (CCNAP). *Circulation.* 2013;128:2075-2096. doi:10.1161/CIR.0b013e31829c2e53.

72. Steinke EE, Mosack V, Hill TJ. Changes in sexual activity after a cardiac event: the role of medications, comorbidity, and psychosocial factors. *Appl Nurs Res.* 2015;28:244-250. doi:10.1016/j.apnr.2015.04.011.

73. Bispo GS, de Lima Lopes J, de Barros ALBL. Sexuality and chronically ill clients. *J Clin Nurs.* 2013;22:3522-3531. doi:10.1111/jocn.12143.

74. Muller J, Mittleman M, Maclure M, et al. Triggering myocardial infarction by sexual activity. Low absolute risk and prevention by regular physical exertion. Determinants of myocardial infarction onset study investigators. *JAMA.* 1996;275(18):1405-1409.

75. Jackson G. Sexual response in cardiovascular disease. *J Sex Res.* 2009;46(2-3):233-236. doi:10.1136/heart.86.4.387.

76. Jaarsma TT, Fridlund B, Martensson J. Sexual dysfunction in heart failure patients. *Curr Heart Fail Rep.* 2014;11:330-336. doi:10.1007/s11897-014-0202-z.

77. Hoekstra T, Lesman-Leegte I, Luttik ML, et al. Sexual problems in elderly male and female patients with heart failure. *Heart.* 2012;98(22):1647-1652. doi:10.1136/heartjnl-2012-302305.

78. Steinke EE, Jaarsma T, Barnason SA, et al. Sexual counselling for individuals with cardiovascular disease and their partners. *Eur Heart J.* 2013;34(41):3217-3235. doi:10.1093/eurheartj/eht270.

79. Hattjar B. Cardiovascular disease and sexuality. In: Hattjar B, ed. *Sexuality and Occupational Therapy: Strategies for Persons with Disabilities.* Bethesda, MD: American Occupational Therapy Association, Inc; 2012:109-133.

80. Helewa A. Management of persons with rheumatoid arthritis and other inflammatory conditions. In: Walker JM, Helewa A, eds. *Physical Rehabilitation in Arthritis.* 2nd ed. St Louis: WB Saunders; 2004:191-212.

81. Hattjar B. Arthritis. In: Hattjar B, ed. *Sexuality and Occupational Therapy: Strategies for Persons with Disabilities.* Bethesda, MD: The American Occupational Therapy Association, Inc; 2012:11-33.

82. Lawson S, Murphy LF. Orthopedic conditions: hip fractures and hip, knee, and shoulder replacements. In: Pendleton HM, Schultz-Krohn W, eds. *Occupational Therapy: Practice Skills for Physical Dysfunction.* 8th ed. St Louis: Elsevier; 2018:1004-1029.

83. Center for Disease Control and Prevention. *National Diabetes Statistics Report.* 2020. Available at: https://www.cdc.gov/diabetes/pdfs/data/statistics/national-diabetes-statistics-report.pdf.

84. Hattjar B. Diabetes and sexuality. In: Hattjar B, ed. *Sexuality and Occupational Therapy: Strategies for Persons with Disabilities.* Bethesda, MD: American Occupational Therapy Association, Inc; 2012:61-80.

13

Use of Medications by Older Adults

BRENDA M. COPPARD, KELLI L. COOVER, AND MICHELE A. FAULKNER
(PREVIOUS CONTRIBUTIONS FROM BARBARA FLYNN)

KEY TERMS

adverse drug reactions, drug interactions, medication therapy management,
over-the-counter, polypharmacy, self-medication, side effects

CHAPTER OBJECTIVES

1. Identify factors that predispose older adults to adverse drug events and discuss strategies to detect medication problems.
2. Define polypharmacy and identify recommended interventions to diminish drug-related problems of polypharmacy in older adults.
3. Identify classes of medications commonly associated with adverse drug reactions in older adults.
4. Identify and describe skills needed for safe self-medication.
5. Apply the Occupational Therapy Practice Framework: Domain and Process (fourth edition) to analyze self-medication for individuals with various conditions.
6. Explain the ways that adaptive devices compensate for skills needed for safe self-medication.
7. Describe older adult and caregiver education needs regarding self-medication.

Kate is a occupational therapy assistant (OTA) working in a skilled nursing facility 3 days a week. Her time for seeing the residents is dependent on the needs of the facility. One of the residents she follows is Esther, a 79-year-old female with a history of a recent stroke, high blood pressure, depression, and insomnia. Kate has noticed changes in Esther's alertness and behavior, based on the time of day that she is seen for intervention. When Kate follows Esther in the morning, she seems very tired, unfocused, and often complains of dizziness. Kate has found such morning therapy sessions to be less productive toward meeting Esther's intervention goals. When she sees Esther in the afternoon, she seems to be almost a completely different person, exhibiting much more energy and enthusiasm to do intervention tasks. Kate began to question the inconsistency of Esther's behaviors. Could Esther be experiencing poor sleep, resulting in the morning fatigue? But why the dizziness? Is Esther more depressed? If that is the case, why does she seem to be in a much better mood in the afternoon? Kate also questions whether the behavioral differences could be related to the medications that Esther is taking. Kate decides to consult with the treatment team about Esther's inconsistent behavior and her dizziness.

The other health care practitioners on the treatment team are a physical therapist, a nurse, a speech therapist, and a pharmacist. There is much discussion about Esther because other members of the treatment team have noticed her inconsistent behavior too. Some members suggest asking for laboratory work to review laboratory level values. The pharmacist, Juan, looks at Esther's medications and points out a possible correlation between the timing and the dosages of the medications with the behaviors that Esther is exhibiting. He questions whether Esther is experiencing some common side effects from the medications that she is taking and informs the team that he plans to consult about Esther's medication with her physician. The following week when Kate follows Esther for the morning intervention sessions, she is much better focused. Kate learns that, as a result of the team meeting, Esther's medications were readjusted.

OTAs often work with older adults on a daily basis in a variety of treatment settings. Because OTAs spend a considerable amount of time with the older adult population, they are a valuable asset in addressing medication routines. OTAs also may convey vital information regarding medications and side effects to the health care team. When specific medication information is required, advice should be sought from a pharmacist or other medication expert. Common medications and medication-related problems encountered by older adults are discussed in the chapter. Skills for self-medication and intervention programs for older adults and caregivers are also discussed.

FACTORS AFFECTING MEDICATION RISK IN OLDER ADULTS

Older adults consume the majority of prescription and over-the-counter (OTC) medications in the United States. Because of the aging population and individuals are living longer, often with chronic diseases that require medication therapy, it is no surprise that 89% of adults 65 or older report they currently take at least one prescription medication.[1] More than half (54%) of older adults report taking four or more prescription drugs medication.[1] Subsequently, 21% of older adults report that did not take their medicines at some point in a given year because of the cost.[1] When OTCs are included, the number of medications consumed per day often exceeds 10 or more.[2] OTC medications are often used for to address colds, cough, congestion, pain, heartburn, constipation, and diarrhea.[2] It is important to note that natural products (such as health foods, supplements, and vitamins) may also be consumed by this population. Yet, because they are erroneously not considered medications by some, they may not be reported when an older adult is questioned about medication use.

POLYPHARMACY

Polypharmacy (use of multiple medications in a single individual) has been positively associated with increasing age, multiple diseases, and disability. The use of multiple medications has been shown to increase nursing home placement, difficulty with ambulation, admissions to the hospital, and mortality.[3] Several components contribute to the incidence of polypharmacy. Sometimes, the use of many medications is the right thing for patients to control their diseases and ensure a better quality of life. However, there are risks associated with polypharmacy. When a person consumes more drugs, then drug interactions happen with increased frequency. These interactions may include the increase or decrease in effectiveness of one drug. Changes in effectiveness are caused by another or a more pronounced manifestation of an adverse event due to the older adult taking two drugs that have a similar side effect profile. In addition, sometimes new medications are introduced for the specific reason of offsetting a troublesome effect caused by another. Providing new medications may be appropriate, but this scenario often occurs because the problem is not recognized as drug-induced. Risk factors that contribute to polypharmacy include the use of multiple physicians with different specialties who may prescribe similar medications, the use of multiple pharmacies, and the fact that older adults often have multiple conditions requiring medication therapy. An additional risk factor is inappropriate medication reconciliation upon discharge from the hospital. The prevalence of polypharmacy posthospital discharge has been shown to be higher than at the time of admission.[4]

PHYSIOLOGY AND THE AGING PROCESS

Many factors are involved in the increased incidence of medication-related adverse events in older adults. With aging, kidney and liver functions decline. Many medications are excreted by the kidney and metabolized, or degraded, by the liver. Therefore, changes in organ function may frequently lead to drug accumulation in the body. This accumulation may result in toxic levels of drugs. To avoid drug accumulation, it is imperative that consideration be given to modifying doses for older adults.

Although not all of the reasons are well understood, older adults tend to be more sensitive to the effects of certain medications.[5] Body composition (lean tissue to fat ratio) changes as we age. Changes in body composition may result in alterations in how the body distributes a medication, making more or less of the drug available to have an effect. This is true for both the desired effects and for unwanted side effects. The adage "start low, go slow" should generally be used when initiating a new medication therapy for an older adult.

OLDER ADULT MEDICATION USE AND IMPLICATIONS FOR THE OTA

When medical records are available, OTAs should always check the medication section to determine which medications are being used. This information helps OTAs be aware of possible side effects and drug interactions that might be observed with clinical intervention. OTAs should contact the older adults' physicians and pharmacies with any medication-related concerns or questions. (Common drug-related abbreviations and definitions are listed in Table 13.1. Medications commonly used by older adults are listed in Table 13.2. Note that this is not an all-inclusive listing of medications used by older adults or those that may contribute to side effects. Only generic names are listed, and they should be cross-referenced with trade names when necessary.)

Cardiovascular diseases (high blood pressure, congestive heart failure, irregular heart rhythm, chest pain, heart attack, and stroke) are common in older adults.[6] Medications used to treat these diseases may alter a patient's blood pressure and/or heart rate, resulting in dizziness and the potential for falls. One class of medication, the diuretics, may cause excessive urination. As such, it is recommended that nighttime dosing be avoided because of the risk of falls and interruption of rest. OTAs may notice that the client needs frequent breaks during therapy to use the restroom or may be incontinent, indicating that the timing of the medication dose may need to be altered to avoid this. Persons taking one or more of the medication types mentioned previously should be closely monitored during therapy for the emergence of side effects, and consideration should be given to routine monitoring of blood pressure and heart rate by the OTA. In addition, many of these same clients will be using medications to treat high

TABLE 13.1

Common Drug-Related Terminology

Abbreviations	Definitions
PO	By mouth
IM	Intramuscular
IV	Intravenous
Sub Q	Subcutaneous
(Do not use SC or SQ)	
PR	Rectally
SL	Sublingually (under the tongue)
Daily or Q Day	Once a day
(Do not use QD)	
BID	Twice daily
TID	Three times daily
QID	Four times daily
Every other day	Every other day
(Do not use QOD)	
HS	Hour of sleep (Bedtime)
PRN	As needed
AC	Before meals
PC	After meals

cholesterol. Some of these drugs may cause diffuse muscle pain when they are started, with a dose increase, or with the addition of another medication, which may increase blood levels of the former. The OTA can help identify this type of drug-induced musculoskeletal pain and see to it that it is addressed by the appropriate individual. Although usually not serious, in some cases, the consequences of this side effect can be severe and even life-threatening.

Drugs that affect the blood's ability to clot are also frequently used in persons with cardiovascular diseases. The OTA must be aware of clients using one of these agents as the risk of a serious bleed is increased and therapy may have to be adjusted. One sign associated with the use of these medications is easy bruising. This is not necessarily unexpected, but if the OTA believes that the amount of bruising is excessive, referring such clients to have their medication therapy evaluated may be prudent. It is especially important to ensure that these clients do not fall because internal bleeding may result. In addition, the OTA should report balance issues or falls to the prescriber without delay.

Another common complaint of older adults is pain, which can be either chronic (such as arthritis pain) or short term because of an acute injury. The use of OTC pain medications is common when older adults choose to self-treat. These medications include acetaminophen, aspirin, ibuprofen, and naproxen. Commonly observed side effects associated with these agents include gastrointestinal distress (which may be a symptom of a more serious condition such as a stomach ulcer) and increases in blood pressure, because some of these medications can cause fluid retention. With more severe pain, prescription medications are used. Most prescription pain medications (primarily narcotics such as codeine, hydrocodone, oxycodone, and morphine) exert their action in the central nervous system (CNS) and therefore may cause dizziness, drowsiness, and confusion. These symptoms add to the risk of falls and may make successful therapeutic intervention by the OTA a challenge if the client is unable to fully participate because of cognitive impairment. All narcotics have the potential to cause constipation so the OTA should be aware if stimulant laxatives are concurrently prescribed with scheduled narcotic pain medications. Use of these medications may contribute to fecal incontinence.

Many older adults experience a variety of psychosocial, psychiatric, and cognitive disorders. Drugs that may be used to treat such diagnoses include antipsychotics, antidepressants, antianxiety agents, and medications used to slow the progression of cognitive impairment, such as those used in the treatment of Alzheimer's dementia. These medications are all active in the CNS and therefore have the potential to affect sensorium, alertness, and balance.[7,8] Additionally, some of them may have effects on other body systems causing disturbances in sleep and bodily functions (dry eyes, dry mouth, urinary retention, constipation, elevated heart rate, and the inability to perspire). Some of the agents used to treat psychosis also cause extrapyramidal symptoms that may manifest as abnormal movements of the limbs, head, neck, and the tongue.[7] Sometimes, these symptoms can be controlled with another medication or by discontinuing the offending agent. However, other times the benefit of continuing the medication may outweigh the risk associated with developing these symptoms, and the client and OTA may need to find a way to work around them. Furthermore, use of these medications is likely to aid the OTA in working with a client when symptoms of these types of disorders are controlled.

Sleep disturbances are frequently encountered by older adults. Such disturbances include the inability to fall asleep, early morning awakening, and daytime drowsiness. Sleep-inducing medications are often used to help older adults sleep. However, it is important to note that, as people age, sleep patterns change and older adults tend to wake up more frequently during the night. This can contribute to daytime sleepiness. Education of older adults is necessary to help them differentiate between insomnia and the normal aging process as it pertains to sleep. Some sleep agents may cause clients to be drowsy during the morning hours, which may interfere with the therapy process. Proper sleep hygiene (going to bed and getting up at the same time each day, minimizing daytime napping, using the bed for sleep and sex only, and avoidance of caffeine and exercise late in the day) can make a

TABLE 13.2

Disease States, Medications, and Common Side Effects

Disease states	Medications	Common side effects
Cardiovascular (high blood pressure, congestive heart failure, high cholesterol, irregular heart rhythm, chest pain, heart attack, stroke)	ACE inhibitors (e.g., lisinopril, enalapril, captopril, benazepril, ramipril, fosinopril) Angiotensin receptor blockers (ARBs) (e.g., losartan, valsartan, irbesartan, candesartan, olmesartan) Direct renin inhibitors (e.g., aliskiren) Beta blockers (e.g., metoprolol, carvedilol, atenolol, propranolol) Calcium channel blockers (e.g., amlodipine, felodipine, nifedipine, diltiazem, verapamil) Cholesterol medications (e.g., atorvastatin, simvastatin, lovastatin, rosuvastatin, pravastatin, gemfibrozil, fenofibrate, niacin, ezetimibe, evolocumab, alirocumab) Diuretics (e.g., hydrochlorothiazide, triamterene, furosemide, bumetanide, chlorthalidone, torsemide, spironolactone) Miscellaneous (e.g., clonidine, doxazosin, prazosin, terazosin, minoxidil)	Low blood pressure, dizziness, joint or muscle pain, low heart rate, irregular heart rate, drowsiness, urinary frequency or incontinence, increased fall risk, fluid in the extremities/swelling, cough, elevated potassium levels in the blood
Blood-thinning agents	Warfarin, clopidogrel, aspirin, ticlopidine, prasugrel, ticagrelor, enoxaparin, heparin, dalteparin, dabigatran, apixaban, rivaroxaban, edoxaban	Bleeding, bruising
Pain medications	Nonsteroidal drugs (e.g., aspirin, ibuprofen, naproxen, celecoxib, meloxicam, diclofenac, ketorolac) Narcotics (e.g., codeine, hydrocodone, oxycodone, morphine, hydromorphone, fentanyl, methadone) Drugs for neuropathic pain (e.g., gabapentin, pregabalin, amitriptyline, sodium valproate, venlafaxine, duloxetine, lidocaine patch, capsaicin topical) Miscellaneous (e.g., acetaminophen, tramadol)	Bleeding, bruising, gastrointestinal pain, swelling of the extremities, dizziness, drowsiness, increased fall risk, confusion, nausea, constipation, hallucinations, weight gain, dry eyes, dry mouth
Psychiatric medications	Antidepressants (e.g., sertraline, fluoxetine, venlafaxine, desvenlafaxine, mirtazapine, bupropion, citalopram, escitalopram, amitriptyline, trazodone, duloxetine, levomilnacipran, vortioxetine) Antipsychotics (e.g., quetiapine, risperidone, haloperidol, olanzapine, aripiprazole, ziprasidone, brexpiprazole, paliperidone, asenapine, iloperidone, lurasidone) Antianxiety agents (e.g., diazepam, alprazolam, lorazepam, buspirone) Drugs for cognitive impairment (e.g., donepezil, rivastigmine, galantamine, memantine)	Drowsiness, dizziness, confusion, seizures, extrapyramidal side effects, nausea, diarrhea, weight loss or gain, insomnia, erectile dysfunction
Sleep disorders	Diazepam, alprazolam, temazepam, lorazepam, trazodone, doxepin, zolpidem, eszopiclone, zaleplon, ramelteon, diphenhydramine	Drowsiness, dizziness, increased fall risk, sleep walking, amnesia, hallucinations
Diabetes	Metformin, glipizide, glyburide, pioglitazone, rosiglitazone, insulin, exenatide, sitagliptin, saxagliptin, linagliptin, liraglutide, semaglutide, canagliflozin, dapagliflozin, empagliflozin	Low blood sugar, dizziness, tremor, sweating, headache, confusion, nausea, weight loss, urinary tract infections
Urge incontinence	Tolterodine, oxybutynin, dicyclomine, solifenacin, darifenacin, fesoterodine, trospium, mirabegron, vibegron	Dry mouth, dry eyes, urinary retention, constipation, elevated heart rate, inability to perspire, elevated blood pressure
Benign prostatic hyperplasia (BPH)	Dutasteride, finasteride, tadalafil, terazosin, alfuzosin, tamsulosin, doxazosin, silodosin	Erective dysfunction, low blood pressure

large difference in the client's ability to fully participate in therapy. If daytime drowsiness is a concern, the OTA may wish to inquire about the use of sleep agents (both prescription and OTC) to determine whether a change needs to be made.

As persons age, the diagnosis of type 2 diabetes becomes more common. Drugs used for the treatment of elevated blood glucose are associated with several side effects that may be observed by the OTA. The most common of these is hypoglycemia, or low-blood glucose. Symptoms associated with hypoglycemia include sweating, dizziness, weakness, tremor, elevated heart rate, and confusion. These symptoms may be more common if the client has not had a normal amount of food before therapy. Additionally, diabetes can cause impaired sensation in the extremities, also known as neuropathy. This can result in numbness or extreme pain and may present a substantial challenge for the OTA. It is important that therapy be tailored for older adults with impaired sensation to ensure that they remain safe during therapy and in their living environment. Medications are available to help with the pain of neuropathy, and the OTA may wish to refer patients if the pain interferes with quality of life. Many of the medications used to treat neuropathic pain are primarily used to treat other disorders (e.g., depression and epilepsy). It is important for the OTA to identify the diagnosis for the use of these medications.

Although not a normal part of aging, urinary incontinence may be frequently encountered in the older adult population.[9] Incontinence presents its own challenges such as those associated with social isolation, the need for frequent toileting, and skin breakdown as a result of excessive exposure to moisture. Medications used to treat one type of incontinence, overactive bladder or "urge" incontinence, can cause a multitude of side effects similar to those mentioned as associated with the psychoactive medications (dry eyes, dry mouth, urinary retention, constipation, elevated heart rate, and the inability to perspire).[10] Males may experience urinary incontinence due to benign prostatic hyperplasia (BPH). This type of incontinence is due to noncancerous enlargement of the prostate gland. Males with this condition have "overflow" incontinence causing incomplete bladder emptying, difficulty initiating urination, interruptions in urinary flow, and urinary frequency. The OTA can assist individuals with this condition by ensuring they have toileted before beginning a therapy session and assisting them in their ability to safely toilet thereby preventing falls and episodes of incontinence.[11]

STRATEGIES FOR MINIMIZING MEDICATION PROBLEMS IN OLDER ADULTS

There are multiple reasons why older adults may be at higher risk for medication problems than younger persons. It is imperative that health care providers ensure that clients can safely manage their medications.

Psychiatric diagnoses, such as dementia and depression, are common in this population and may affect the client's ability to manage drug therapy without assistance. Often, the first indication that there may be a problem in this area is the inability to manage other daily tasks such as keeping good finances or managing basic household responsibilities.

Older adults are often apprehensive when it comes to questioning health care providers, and this may lead to a lack of active participation in their own care. In many cases, a medication regimen can be simplified, but if the health care provider is not asked to do this, it is unlikely to occur. Additionally, if information about medications or their side effects is not readily offered, an older adult might not directly ask about such things, and this may lead to underrecognition of side effects. It is also important that clients understand why they are taking each medication and its intended purpose so that they may self-monitor for problems.

There are many reasons that clients may not adhere to a medication regimen as prescribed. Medication overuse may occur, either by mistake because clients cannot remember whether a medication has already been taken, or because they may believe that "if a little is good, more must be better." On the other hand, nonadherence also occurs for various reasons. Avoidance of side effects may lead a client to skip medication doses. Additionally, if money is a concern, clients may choose to alter their regimen by deliberately taking a medication less often than prescribed. Cutting pills in half and taking partial doses is another common occurrence when saving money is an issue.

Self-treatment of symptoms or side effects with OTC medications may also result in problems. Although OTC medications are available without a prescription, it is incorrect to believe that they are without risks. Drug interactions may occur with medications that have previously been prescribed. It is also incorrect to believe that "natural" products are inherently safe. They too may interact with other drugs and cause side effects that may be more difficult to recognize because of a lack of regulation and standardization.

If the OTA suspects or recognizes that a client is having difficulty managing their medication regime, consideration may be given to referring the client for medication therapy management (MTM) services. MTM is a formal process whereby the patient works with the pharmacist in collaboration with other health care providers to optimize drug therapy and ensure positive therapeutic outcomes.[12]

APPLICATION OF THE OCCUPATIONAL THERAPY PROCESS TO SELF-MEDICATION

Medication routines of clients are often not addressed by occupational therapy.[13] This is evident in the lack of literature on self-medication programs and OT interventions with medication routines. Medication routines are instrumental activities of daily living (IADLs). According to the OTPF-4, medication routines are classified as a health management and maintenance IADL.[14] Thus, assessment of routines and instruction in proper use of medication should be dealt with as part of activities of daily living (ADL) routines.[14] Participation in one's medication routine includes obtaining medication, opening and closing containers, interpreting and following prescribed schedules, administering correct quantities by using prescribed methods, filling and refilling prescriptions in a timely manner, and reporting problems and adverse effects.

CLIENT FACTORS

Values, beliefs, spirituality, body functions, and body structures that reside within the client and may affect performance in medication routines should be analyzed by the occupational therapist (OT) and OTA. This section overviews how each of these client factors can potentially affect one's medication management.

Values, Beliefs, and Spirituality

A variety of factors related to adherence to medication routines has been researched, including people's values, beliefs, and spirituality.[15-17] The self-regulations theory is a patient-centered understanding to such factors that affect adherence.[17-19] The theory suggests that people attempt to understand their illness by developing a representation of their illness, its causes, its effects, the duration of the illness, and whether the illness can be cured or controlled. In this view, it is thought that people are motivated to reduce their health-related risks and will work on eliminating health threats in ways that are congruent with their perceptions.

In addition to forming representations of illness, it is hypothesized that clients also form representations of their treatments.[20] Researchers have demonstrated the link between values and behaviors.[21-23] Decisions about taking medication are likely to be affected by the beliefs about the medicines, the illness, and the treatment providers.[24] Values are often the underpinnings of behaviors. People typically decide what is important for them and then act on such decisions. Although a paucity of literature exists on the influence of spirituality on medication routines, persons diagnosed with terminal illnesses have reported a high level of spirituality (and they have been correlated highly with psychological adaptation and positive health outcomes).[15,25-27]

Bodily Functions

Bodily functions are "physiological functions of body systems (including psychological functions)."[14] Bodily functions affect one's ability to perform and participate in an occupation. Medication routines require extensive performance from multiple bodily functions, including the following:
- Mental functions
- Sensory functions and pain

- Neuromusculoskeletal and movement-related functions
- Cardiovascular, hematological, immunological, and respiratory system function
- Voice and speech function
- Digestive, metabolic, and endocrine system function
- Genitourinary and reproductive functions
- Skin and related structure functions

Mental Functions

Various types of memory are involved with medication regimes as medication adherence involves complex cognitive abilities.[28] "Verbal memory, working memory, processing speed and reasoning"[28] are components. Verbal memory is important for understanding the names of medications, and reasoning is necessary to understand the purposes for medications. Working memory, which includes simultaneous storing and processing of information, is needed to avoid undermedication or overmedication. This frequently occurs when older adults do not remember whether they took a medication. Long-term memory[29] is required for independent self-medication. Older adults need long-term memory to understand which condition is being treated, and long-term memory along with reasoning helps with understanding the purpose for the medication(s) they take. Understanding and remembering the nature of the regimen also is required for self-medication. Older adults use long-term memory to remember where the medication is stored. Various items such as programmable alarms, medication tracker apps on mobile phones, auditory devices that exclaim, "time to take your pill," pill packs, and pill storage boxes can aid self-medication. Home health aides and pharmacists may assist in filling self-medication boxes. A fee may be charged for this service. One advantage of involving a home health aide or pharmacist is that he or she can make sure the older adult is actually taking the medicine, as prescribed, when it is time to refill the storage container.

A great deal of problem-solving is needed to properly self-medicate. Older adults must decide whether to contact the physician when changes in a condition occur. For example, Ken goes to his physician because he wonders whether his frequent headaches indicate that his blood pressure medication is not working or whether he needs a new prescription for his glasses. Problem-solving also is needed to determine when refills need to be obtained and how to safely store medication. Even more complex is the problem-solving needed to determine Medicare prescription plan options.[30] Some pharmacies and health care agencies will provide individualized consults for older adults who need assistance in understanding and choosing such plans.

Older adults must be motivated to comply with their medication regimen. Depression, uncertainty, misunderstanding, financial worries, lack of confidence, side effects, and social or cultural taboos are all factors that may contribute to a lack of motivation. For example, Hazel, a 74-year-old female with a history of heart failure and high blood pressure, sometimes takes her medication tablets once a day instead of three times a day as prescribed. Hazel does this when she feels "better" to save money. In addition, some older adults are embarrassed by the diagnosis of depression, or other emotional disorders, and are reluctant to take prescribed antidepressants or other medicines used to treat psychological problems.

Mental function impairment may affect older adults' ability to manage their medication. The ManageMed Screening (MMS) is a quick assessment tool for interdisciplinary use.[31,32] The MMS was created by occupational therapists to assess medication management of the general adult population. The screen is standardized and consists of 30 questions and performance tasks that screen reading, medication knowledge base, problem solving, short-term and prospective memory, and calculations. The MMS demonstrated it can differentiate between persons who need assistance and those who are independent with medication management.[31] The MMS manual is available online.

Sensory Functions and Pain

Visual perception skills may be required by older adults who take multiple medications. Visual perception skills include color discrimination, depth perception, and figure-ground perception. Visual acuity and perception are required to distinguish between different containers of medication and to read instruction labels. If needed, glasses should be worn when older adults self-medicate. Adaptations may be used to assist older adults who have visual impairments (Fig. 13.1). Magnifying lenses and large type or contrasting print may be helpful. For severe visual impairments, different size, different shape, or multicolor containers can be used for medication storage. Instructions for administration can be tape recorded to relay information that cannot be read. Depth perception skills are needed to obtain pills in a multipartition container. Figure-ground perception also is needed to see white pills in a white pill box. OTAs should suggest that older adults use colored pill containers for white pills.

According to the National Institute on Deafness and other Communication Disorders, there is a relationship between age and hearing loss. For example, 25% of adults who are ages 65–74 years and 50% of adults age 75 years and older have a disabling hearing loss.[33] OTAs should remember this when educating older adults, family members, and caregivers. The ability to hear is important for older adults to understand patient education, medication dosages, and changes. OTAs should provide both verbal and written instructions when educating older adults. For example, José, an OTA, meets with Vladimir, who has difficulty hearing, to review his discharge program. He first checks to make sure Vladimir is wearing his hearing aid and then reviews the information in his client education packet. José speaks slowly and clearly and is sitting directly at eye level with Vladimir. He also frequently asks Vladimir

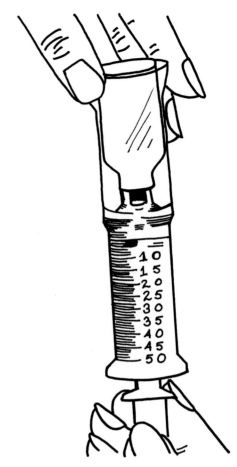

FIG. 13.1   This magnifier device consists of a plastic cylinder in which the medication and syringe fit at each end and permits elders older adults with visual impairments to view amounts easily.

whether he has any questions and encourages him to repeat back to him what he understands (see Chapter 16).

Movement-Related Functions and Neuromusculoskeletal

Usually, a great deal of fine motor coordination, finger dexterity, and some degree of strength are needed to open and close medication containers and use syringes. Prehensile and grasp patterns are required when picking up pills or tablets. Therefore, older adults with conditions such as rheumatoid arthritis or Parkinson's disease may have difficulty opening childproof containers. Nonchildproof tops can be provided by the pharmacist, if requested. If nonsafety caps are dispensed by the pharmacist, it is essential that older adults store their medication out of the reach of children.

Manipulating medication containers requires strength. Occasionally, a medication routine involves crushing pills or splitting them in half. Such assists as pill crushers and pill splitters can help an older adult who has poor hand strength. Older adults should never use a razor blade to cut tablets. Many medications are released over time (known as extended or sustained release) and should not be crushed. A pharmacist is an invaluable resource person to find out whether a tablet can be crushed. Furthermore, sometimes a liquid form of the medication (if available) may be a better choice for an older adult who needs to crush several medicines.

Older adults taking medications need to have a way of getting prescriptions filled on a regular basis. Older adults who do not drive or are wheelchair-bound may need to seek out community resources to obtain rides to medical appointments and the pharmacy. Many pharmacies will deliver medications or mail medications to the person's home. Sometimes these services are free and other times there may be a fee. In addition, some communities have volunteer programs that provide this transportation service at no cost. For example, Leo is unable to drive because of his poor vision, but he is able to renew prescriptions by using a free transportation service provided by his church. Automated systems are available at many pharmacies, which allow people to renew their prescriptions over the phone. Some pharmacies also provide automatic refill reminders and service for maintenance prescription medications.

It is estimated that dysphagia affects more than 30% of patients who have had a stroke, 52%–82% of older adults with Parkinson's disease, 84% of those with Alzheimer's disease, nearly 40% of older adults 65 years and older, and more than 60% of institutionalized older adults.[34,35] Patients and caregivers (n = 477) were surveyed about swallowing medicine. Results of the survey included 68% of persons who reported opening a capsule or crushing a tablet, whereas 64% reported not taking their medication because of difficulty swallowing.[36] Health professionals must facilitate medication routines of patients who cannot properly swallow medications by reviewing regimens, omitting medications that are unnecessary, and determining alternative forms of medications when needed.

Cardiovascular, Hematological, Immunological, and Respiratory System Function

Some medications, including nebulizers and inhalers, require the ability to inhale medication through the mouth or nostrils. Inhalers are used to deliver medication directly to the lungs. A nebulizer is a type of inhaler used to spray a fine mist of medication through the use of a mask. A mouthpiece is often connected to a machine and plastic tubing to deliver the medication to the person. Inspiration must be satisfactory to receive the medication, and in the case of some inhalers, it is necessary to activate the device with a deep, forceful inhalation It is essential to follow the instructions for cleaning nebulizers and inhaler devices to prevent upper and lower respiratory infections.

Voice and Speech Functions

Older adults must be able to communicate their medication regimen with health care providers and caregivers.

Health care providers must reciprocate communication in an effective manner. Demonstration, web-based, verbal, and written formats can be used for communication. Older adults may find it helpful to keep names, phone numbers, and addresses of health care providers and agencies in a regular place so they are available for emergencies. Posting this information on the refrigerator may also be helpful. For example, Greta has been deaf since birth but is able to communicate by using a notebook that contains information regarding her past and present medical condition. She stores this notebook in a drawer in the nightstand by her bed. She also has notified family members where the notebook is located in case of an emergency.

Digestive, Metabolic, and Endocrine Functions in Older Adults

As people age, less saliva is produced, which means the older adult may experience difficulty in chewing and swallowing dry food.[37] Older adults also produce less salivary enzymes, which helps digest starches and fats. Ill-fitting dentures and a decreased ability to taste food may make chewing difficult and eating less pleasurable. Swallowing problems are related to esophageal changes caused by decreased motility and upper sphincter pressures. This can lead to gastroesophageal reflux disease and hiatal hernia. Consequently, these conditions put older adults at risk for dysphagia, aspiration, and pill-induced esophagitis. Stomach motility slows down with age, so gastric emptying is slower. This makes older adults feel full longer.

Older adults experience physiologic changes as they age including delayed gastric emptying, decreased peristalsis, and slowed colonic transit, all of which can effect drug absorption.

Changes in the older adult's metabolism often effects the body's ability to excrete the compounds, which typically occurs in the liver. The liver's metabolism of drugs depends on hepatic blood flow, hepatic enzymes, and the proportion of drug not bound to plasma proteins. Since hepatic blood flow decreases by 40% in older adults, toxicity issues are a concern.[38] Thus, appropriate medication dosage is often adjusted for the older adult's physiologic status and side effect and toxicity profile.[39]

Skin and Related Structure Functions

While some medications are specifically used to treat wounds and infections, certain topical medications must not be applied to skin where integrity has been compromised. These skin areas include places where cuts, sores, abrasions, or open wounds exist, because this may result in unintentional absorption or irritation. When uncertainty exists, consult prescribers or pharmacy personnel. Thus, the skin must be free from wounds, abrasions, and cuts.

ACTIVITY DEMANDS

Medication routines involve activity demands (formerly cited in the *Occupational Therapy Practice Framework*, third

TABLE 13.3

Activity Demands and Examples Related to Medication Routines

Activity demand aspect	Examples related to medication routine
Objects and their properties	Common objects used in medication routines include pill bottles, pill storage boxes, syringes/pens, inhalers, tubes, gloves, and such.
Space demands	Space to complete a medication routine commonly requires appropriate lighting to see what one is doing, ample room to manipulate any equipment or objects used, and proper space for medication storage. Occasionally, medication must be stored in special environments—for example, environments that adhere to recommended temperature ranges and restricted exposure to sunlight.
Social demands	Medication routines require communicating when one may need medication to refill prescriptions or report outcomes or concerns to one's physician(s).
Sequence and timing	Medication routines often require timing of medication. Occasionally, medications must be taken properly throughout the day. For example, sequencing the medication routine involves selecting the container, opening the container, securing the medication tablet, and swallowing the medication.
Required actions and performance skills	Skills used to perform medication routines include opening and closing containers, manipulating any objects needed in medication routines, and such.
Required body functions	Body functions needed in medication routine often include mental, neuromusculoskeletal, and speech functions.
Required body structures	Body structures often needed to perform medication routines include use of hands, eyes, and such.

edition). Table 13.3 offers examples of activity demands typically involved in medication routines.

Performance Skills

Performance skills are "observable, goal directed actions that result in a client's quality of performing occupations."[14] Performance skills include "motor skills, process skills and social interaction skills."[14] Examples of performance skills required during medication routines are presented in Table 13.4.

OCCUPATIONAL THERAPY PROCESS

According to the OTPF-4,[14] evaluation, intervention, and outcomes comprise the process of occupational therapy. Evaluation includes consultation and screening, the occupational profile, analysis of occupational performance, and a synthesis of the evaluation process. Intervention constitutes the plan, implementation, and review. Finally, the outcomes are the determination of success of the desired outcomes, transition, and discontinuation. The following section outlines the process as applied to medication routines.

Consultation and screening with an older adult is completed to determine if further evaluation should be completed. The occupational profile provides an understanding of the client's occupational history and experiences, patterns of daily living, interests, values, and needs. The client's problems and concerns about performing occupations and daily life activities are identified, and the client's priorities are determined.[14] OTAs often assist in gathering information from the client and/or caregiver during the

TABLE 13.4

Examples of Skills Needed for Medication Routines

Skill	Example
Motor and praxis skills	Planning and executing movements to successfully open and close medication containers; maintaining balance while taking medication; adjusting posture, for example, to extend neck when applying eye drops.
Sensory perceptual skills	Sensing that a pill is on your tongue and ready to be swallowed; feeling relief after an antitch cream has been applied to an itchy and irritated area; seeing the volume marks on a syringe.
Cognitive skills	Ability to recognize when one needs a prescription refill; ability to remember taking medication, judging whether the symptoms being addressed are getting better, worse, or staying the same.
Communication and social skills	Ability to communicate with family, caretakers, pharmacists, and physicians about one's medication routine; ability to answer questions posed by health care providers and caretakers about medication routine.

profile. Questions and items to be used as part of the occupational profile related to medication routines include the following:

- Tell me about any medications you take. Do not forget to include prescriptions, OTC medications, supplements, and natural products.
- Tell me about any vitamins or nutritional supplements you use.
- Describe your routine of taking medications.
- Tell me how often you miss taking a dose of your medications. Can you identify any barriers to successfully taking your medications as prescribed?
- Describe any concerns you might have about your medication routine.

Depending on the issues that arise from the occupational profile, the therapist may determine to analyze the person's performance related to the medication routine. Analysis of occupational performance is part of the evaluation process during which the client's assets, problems, or potential problems are more specifically identified. Actual performance can be observed in context to identify what supports and what hinders performance. Performance skills, performance patterns, context or contexts, activity demands, and client factors are all considered; however, only selected aspects may be specifically assessed. "Targeted outcomes" are then identified.[14] For example, a therapist may suspect that the older adult's grip strength is insufficient to open a medication container and thus test grip strength using a dynamometer or asking the person to open his or her medication container(s). Based on the analysis of occupational performance, the therapist is able to plan the intervention.

The intervention consists of a plan of actions and is developed collaboratively with the client. Interventions are based on selected theories, frames of reference, and evidence. Outcomes to be addressed are confirmed.[14] For example, the therapist may use a rehabilitative frame of reference and focus on the person's abilities and compensate for disability. Thus, the therapist may decide that the person's grip strength is not sufficient to open childproof medication containers and has the client practice opening a nonchildproof container. The therapist may provide information on how to request such containers for future prescriptions. This action is the intervention implementation or the ongoing actions taken to influence and support improved client performance. Interventions are directed at targeted outcomes. The client's response is noted and documented.[14] The therapist will then review the implementation plan and the progress toward targeted outcomes.[14] The following section addresses ideas for medication intervention with older adults.

ASSISTIVE AIDS FOR SELF-MEDICATION

Many commercial or homemade aids and services can assist individuals with self-medication.[40] Each aid has advantages and disadvantages.

Commercial Aids

It is important to understand that no modifications to any medication dosage should be undertaken without the advice of a pharmacist to prevent loss of efficacy or risk of compromising patient safety.

Calendars

Calendars are helpful for tracking medication schedules. A pocket calendar or a calendar hung near the place where medication is taken can be used to mark each time medication is taken. At the end of the day, marks are counted to make sure that the medication schedule was followed. The advantage of using calendars is that the medications are stored in their original containers and remain properly labeled. Calendars are also inexpensive and readily available. The disadvantage of using a calendar is that it requires vision, some basic reading, comprehension, and memory skills to mark the calendar each time medications are taken.[40]

Pill storage boxes/storage boxes

For people who take medications on a regular basis, a pill box or pill reminder is a useful item. Pill storage boxes are containers with compartments in which to put medications (Fig. 13.2). Pill boxes are easy to use and can be useful to adhere to one's medication schedule regardless of whether one is at home or traveling. Pill boxes are organized daily, weekly, or monthly. Some have the capacity to organize medications throughout the day (e.g., breakfast, lunch, and dinner and bedtime). Added features such as locks or timers and alarms can be ideal when safety is a concern or when a cognitive reminder is needed. Some boxes are made to look like jewelry boxes. There is certainly one likely to be available to suit one's needs and style.

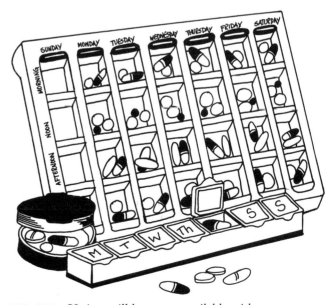

FIG. 13.2 Various pill boxes are available with compartments for single or multiple daily and weekly doses.

Pill boxes require manual dexterity skills to open and close and to manipulate pills. Visual discrimination also is required to identify desired pills. Pill boxes usually do not provide tight storage for medications that require tight containers, such as nitroglycerin. In addition, the pills are no longer in labeled, childproof containers.

There are advantages and disadvantages for using daily and 7-day pill boxes.[40] An advantage of a daily pill box is a better chance of taking all daily doses. Any errors made in setting up this pill box would be experienced for 1 day only. A disadvantage of a daily pill box is that each compartment could contain several unlabeled pills. The older adult would have to identify the medication(s) by physical appearance. This is a serious safety concern if pills are similar in size, shape, or color, especially if the older adult has impaired vision or is easily confused.

Weekly pill boxes store medication for 7 days. The design of some pill boxes allows the separation of multiple daily doses. These boxes often consist of four rows and seven columns. The four rows are marked with times of the day (morning, noon, evening, and bedtime), and the seven columns are marked with the day of the week. The advantage of using a 7-day pill box is that set up is required once a week only. The disadvantage is that set up requires more accuracy.[30] If there is a mistake, it is repeated seven times.

A pill box with an alarm is an option for older adults who must take their medication at specific times. The advantage of this type of pill box is that it alerts older adults of the medication schedule. A disadvantage is that older adults must be able to read, understand, and follow in-depth instructions. These devices often need to be programmed and may require very fine manipulation to set the clock or the alarm. If the device breaks, repairs may be difficult and expensive. Another disadvantage is the risk of not hearing the alarm when it sounds.

Insulin pens

Insulin pens do not eliminate the need to inject oneself, but they make measuring and delivering insulin easier. The pens come in two forms: disposable and reusable. Disposable pens contain a prefilled cartridge and the entire pen is thrown away when empty. Reusable pens allow a person to replace the insulin cartridge when it is empty. Benefits of using insulin pens versus vial and syringe include: 1) accuracy of dosage, 2) easy to read dosing, 3) may facilitate adherence to the therapy routine, 4) easy storage, 5) portable and discrete, 6) less time to administer the insulin.[41]

Pill splitters

Pill splitters are useful devices when a pill must be split for proper dosage or to reduce the pill size for easier swallowing (when appropriate). Pill splitters are often lightweight and use a leverage design to reduce the amount of strength needed to use it. As previously stated, a razor blade should never be used to cut a tablet.

Pill crushers

A pill crusher is a device used to pulverize tablets into a fine powder. Similar to the design of pill splitters, pill crushers use a leverage system so that an abundance of strength is not required. Pill crushers can be beneficial when individuals have difficulty swallowing whole tablets. (Remember that not all tablets can be crushed or split.)

Talking and shaking alarms, watches, mobile phone apps, and prescription bottles

For older adults who experience difficulty remembering to take their medications or what their medication routine is, several devices such as talking or shaking alarms and talking prescription bottles may be beneficial. Talking alarms are devices that are programmed to send a "beep," voice message, or visual cue when it is time to take a medication. Medication tracker apps on a mobile phone can provide reminders to take medication.[42] Shaking alarms can be clipped to the bedding to wake older adults when it is time to take their medication. The device can be put in one's pocket when in public and it will provide a quiet vibration to indicate the medication time. A talking prescription bottle is a device attached to a prescription bottle. A pharmacist or physician records the prescription information into the device. To operate, one pushes a button on the device to play a recorded message about the contents; how many pills to take, when, and what for; and any warnings. The talking prescription bottle is intended for those who have low vision or hearing impairments. It is also beneficial for older adults for whom English is a second language or for older adults who have difficulty reading.

Homemade aids

Medication diary

A medication diary is another aid for tracking medication use (Table 13.5).

OTAs may assist older adults in making a diary, which can be kept in a notebook. This information can then be shared with other health care professionals, as needed.

Storage cups

Storage cups can be made at home by using small plastic or paper cups that are stacked and ordered according to the number of times the medication must be taken throughout the day. The cups should be marked in relation to when medications are taken (e.g., morning, noon, dinner, and bedtime) (Fig. 13.3). After the morning medication is taken, the "morning" cup is moved to the bottom of the stack. This allows the next medication dose to be on the top. This system requires that older adults have good manual dexterity, visual-perceptual, and memory skills. A similar system can be made using egg cartons. For liquid or powder medications, a system can be set up

TABLE 13.5

Contents of a Medication Diary

Section	Information
1: Demographics	Name
	Date
	Address
	Phone number
	Date of birth
	Medication allergies: date of occurrence and type of reaction
	Vaccinations (e.g., COVID-19, shingles, pneumococcal, etc.) (year, date)
	Flu shots (year, date)
2: Health care providers	List names and phone numbers of all health care providers (tape their business cards here).
3: Past medications	List all medical conditions that required treatment with medication over the years.
	List all medical conditions that currently require treatment with medication.
4: Special equipment	List all adaptive or special equipment required (such as a nebulizer, ostomy products, and incontinence products). Include the brand, size, model, and the supplier's name and phone number.
5: Recent medications	Enter the name of new medications used, the date, the reason the medication is being used, the strength of the medication, and how often the medication is taken each day.
	Keep track of any dosage changes, discontinuation, the date, and the reason for the change or discontinuation.
6: Over-the-counter medications	List any over-the-counter medications used for the eyes, ears, skin, and other organs and tissues.
	Enter how often the medications are used.
7: Questions for health care providers	List any questions to ask the doctor or pharmacist.

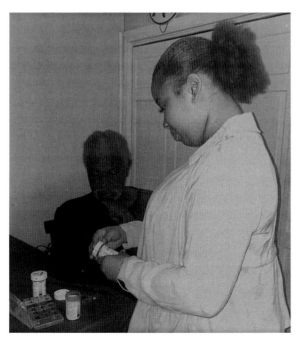

FIG. 13.3 Pill sorting and medication management is an important IADL for this older adult to complete to remain independent in his home. *(Courtesy Alexis Gordon.)*

using small, labeled, airtight containers. Using a home-made system is simple and inexpensive. However, using a homemade system may cause medication to be exposed to improper storage conditions.[40] Also, pills in open view may tempt small children who live in or visit the older adult's home. This risk can be reduced by storing the medication out of view and reach.

SELF-MEDICATION PROGRAM

A formal self-medication program may prevent problems with polypharmacy. The program is designed to (1) use an interdisciplinary team approach, (2) educate older adults about their medications, (3) develop older adults' motor skills for proper administration, (4) offer practice opportunities to older adults, (5) assess older adults for any adaptive devices that may be useful, and (6) evaluate older adults' skills in medication administration before discharge.

The older adults' plan should include interventions to maximize independence with self-medication. Depending on older adults' limitations and deficits, OTAs should engage them in simulated medication tasks. An example of such a task is using small, colored candy pieces to practice color discrimination and fine prehensile patterns. Reading and comprehending general labels can aid in reading medication labels. Opening and closing medication containers should be practiced. In addition, older adults should master any adaptive aids before being discharged from OT.

Relatives, friends, and home care personnel who assist in the delivery of medications often have not been included in discussions of medications.[43] Family and caregivers should be able to name the older adult's medications, describe the purpose of each medication, and describe any precautions associated with each medication. OTAs can refer to Box 13.1 to help educate family and other caregivers. Box 13.2[9] addresses safety issues for OTAs' consideration.

BOX 13.1

Guidelines for Caregivers Who Administer Medications

Older adults most at risk to experience problems with medications are those who are:
- Seeing more than one physician.
- Taking many medications.
- Using more than one pharmacy.

Keep track of the following information on the older adult(s) you are caring for:
- All of the prescription drugs the older adult is taking.
- All of the nonprescription (OTC) drugs the older adult is taking.
- All other medicinal items the older adult uses from a health food store or supermarket.
- When and how much medicine to give.
- What results to expect from the medicine.
- Any physical or mental change in the older adult (report to physician).
- What to do if a dose is missed.

Prescriptions
- The need for the medications should be reevaluated at least every 3–6 months.
- Do not save unused medication for future use without the physician's approval. Take the entire course of any antibiotic that is prescribed.
- Do not share medications with anyone. Closely check expiration dates and dispose of expired medicine.
- If you are not clear about what the directions you are given mean, clarify them with your pharmacist or the prescriber. For instance, look at the following directions:
  - Take as directed.
  - Take before meals.
  - Take as needed.
  - Take four times a day.
  - What does four times a day really mean?
  - Does it mean every 6 hours? Does it mean with meals and at bedtime?
  - Does before meals mean before each meal or on an empty stomach?
  - How often is it safe to take a medication prescribed on an "as needed" basis?

These are the types of questions that a patient or caregiver should ask.

Written directions should always be given, and "take as directed" should not be considered adequate direction.

To reduce the risk for aspiration and swallowing problems, never give tablets or capsules while the elder is lying down. Always give medications with plenty of fluids to reduce stomach upset unless directed otherwise.

Medication storage
- Store medications properly.
- Keep them in a cool, dry place, away from the sunlight unless directed to refrigerate.
- Keep medications away from children.
- Keep the label on the medication container until all medicine is used or destroyed.
- When traveling, take the original medicine container with you in case of an emergency.

Medication disposal
- Do not flush medications down the toilet unless the label or instructions specifically tell you to do so.
- Medications can be disposed of through a drug take-back program in your community.
- Find a drug take-back program by calling your local pharmacy, city or county.
- If a drug take-back program is not available, discard medications as follows:
  - Take the drugs out of their original containers.
  - Mix them with an undesirable substance (kitty litter, used coffee grounds).
  - Seal the mixture in a disposable container and place in the trash.
  - Make sure that personal information and prescription numbers are made illegible, and discard the original medication containers.

Take precautions with the following:
- Chewable tablets: Older adults often do not like chewable tablets because they can interfere with dentures. One option is to have the older adult suck on the tablet to dissolve it. Chewable tablets should not be swallowed whole.
- Crushing tablets or opening capsules: Many pills should not be crushed because they are designed to be long-acting. Other pills should not be crushed because the contents may cause stomach upset or inflammation.

Always check with the pharmacist. Occasionally, a liquid substitute is available.
- Liquid medications: Because liquid medications are difficult to measure accurately, ask the pharmacist for a measuring device to ensure the correct dose.
- Applying ointments: Because medications applied to the older adult's skin will have an effect on your skin, wash

BOX 13.1

Guidelines for Caregivers Who Administer Medications—cont'd

hands after each application. Use gauze or gloves to apply.

- Applying patches: Always remove old patches. Know how often and where to apply the patch on the body. Remove old patches gently because older adults have delicate skin. Notify the pharmacist if the skin becomes irritated or the patch does not stick. Wash hands after the removal and application of the medication patch.
- Giving injections: Practice administration techniques with a nurse or pharmacist.
- Tube feedings: Tube feedings with medication require special instructions. Liquid medications, if available, work best when medicine needs to be given down a feeding tube. Some medications may actually directly interact with the enteral supplement. Contact the pharmacist for instructions on how to properly give the medication.

Discharge plans from the hospital or nursing home
This can be a very confusing time! Medications often change while the older adult is in the hospital. Everyone must know which medications to take and which not to take.

- Know about any generic drugs.
- Tablets or capsules may look different and have a different name, but the medications contain the same ingredient in the same amount.
- Keep an accurate list or bring all of the medications to every doctor appointment.
- Shop at one pharmacy to avoid medication duplication.
- When moving to another area, ask the pharmacist to forward your prescription records to your new pharmacist.
- Monitor the older adult's nutrition, diet, and fluids.
- Monitor the older adult's appetite and notify the physician with any concerns, such as weight gain or loss.
- Be aware of dietary requirements or restrictions.
- Administer medication by offering plenty of liquids, unless otherwise instructed.

BOX 13.2

Safety Gems for OTAs to Consider With Medication Provision for Older Adults

- Critically consider and bring forward concerns about possible common medication side effects for symptoms that the older adult may be exhibiting.
- Be aware of possible medication side effects that may cause symptoms that could lead to safety issues such as falls or cognitive impairment. (Refer to Table 13.2.)
- Share results of assessments (particularly cognitive, communication skills, neuromuscular and movement, and sensory assessment findings) with members of the treatment team to help inform others about the older adult's ability to safely manage and self-administer medications.
- Communicate any medication issues, such as the alteration of medications to save money or difficulty with a particular dosage form (for instance, those that need to be swallowed), with appropriate health care team members.
- Make appropriate adaptations so that older adults can safely take medications.
- Train older adults and care givers in proper infection control prior to the administration of medications

including hand hygiene. An alcohol-based hand gel may be used if hands are not visibly soiled. Rub product into hands covering all surfaces until the alcohol product has dried. If the hands are visibly soiled, they must be washed with soap and water.
- Remove jewelry from the wrist down.
- Lather with warm water and soap for 30 seconds (preferably antibacterial), paying special attention between fingers, creases, breaks in skin, and under nail beds.
- Avoid touching area around sink.
- Rinse hands and dry thoroughly with paper towels.
- Turn facet off with dry paper towel.
- Be careful not touch trash can when disposing of paper towels.
- After hands are cleaned, gloves may be optionally used.
- After administration of medications is complete, remove gloves turning the inside out, being careful not to touch the outside of the gloves and dispose of them without touching the outside of the trash can.

191

TECH TALK: FOCUS ON MEDICATION MANAGEMENT

NAME	PURPOSE	APPROX. COST	WHERE TO BUY
MedaCube	In home automatic pill dispenser designed to dispense up to 90-day supply for up to 16 medications. Includes text, email, and voice notifications.	~$1800	Medacube.com
Medisafe	App designed to provide personalized medication reminders for individual medications along with drug interaction and missed mediation alerts.	$0 to ~$39/yr.	Google Play IOS App Store
MyTherapy	App designed to provide personalized medication reminders, refill reminders and tracks intake, symptoms, other health info such as BP, activity, etc.	$0	Google Play IOS App Store

CASE STUDY

Roman is a 74-year-old widower who lives alone in a ground floor apartment. He was recently discharged from the hospital after receiving treatment for a blood clot in his leg. He wakes up frequently during the night to urinate. Recently, he sustained a fall upon arising from his bed to go to the bathroom. He has had diabetes for 13 years and complains of loss of sensation in both of his feet. He is receiving therapy to regain his strength after his hospitalization.

Disease state	Medication	Dosage
Deep vein thrombosis (blood clot)	Dabigatran	150 mg po bid
Benign prostatic hyperplasia	Tamsulosin	0.4 mg po daily
Diabetes	Metformin	1000 mg po bid
	Glipizide extended release	10 mg po daily
	Aspirin	81 mg po daily
Neuropathy	Amitriptyline	25 mg po HS
Hypertension	Lisinopril	10 mg po daily
	Chlorthalidone	50 mg po HS

■ CASE STUDY QUESTIONS

1 Which medication-related problems might be of concern to the OTA?
2 Could any of Roman's current medical problems be caused by his medications? If so, which medications cause which side effects? (Refer to Table 13.2.)
3 What other factors may place Roman at risk for polypharmacy and medication-related problems?
4 The OTA is concerned about Roman's fall and the risk of bleeding but is unsure whether any medications contributed to the fall. What is a reasonable course of action to address this plausible medication-related concern?
5 What skills for safe self-medication are affected in Roman's case?
6 What assistive devices may help with his medication routine and why?
7 Who should be involved in a self-medication program to help Roman with his medications?

EVIDENCE NUGGETS: EVIDENCE OF EFFECTIVENESS OF INTERVENTIONS TO IMPROVE SAFETY AND COMPLIANCE OF MEDICATION USE

1. Miguel-Cruz A., Bohorquez A. F., & Parra, P. A. A. What does the literature say about using electronic pillboxes for older adults? A systematic literature review. *Disabl Rehabil: Assist Technol.* 2019;14(8), 776-787. Doi:10.1080/17483107 .2018.1508514
   - Electronic pillboxes with multiple reminders such as "voice of a friend" or relative are advisable. This implies the pillboxes adopt a "social role."
   - Electronic pillboxes have a clinically positive impact on adherence.
   - The overall adherence to medication when utilizing an electronic pillbox was 88.8%.
2. El-Saifi N., Moyle W., Jones C., & Tuffaha H. Medication adherence in older patients with dementia: A systematic

literature review. *J Pharm Pract.* 2018;31(3), 322-334. doi:10.1177/0897190017710524
   - Barriers to medication adherence include increasing age, choice of medication, use of concomitant medications, and cost of medications.
   - Telehealth home monitoring and treatment modifications were found to be effective interventions in improving medication adherence for older adults with dementia.
   - Daily reminders to take medication have been found successful in improving compliance of medication use in older adults.
3. Marcum Z. A., Hanlon J. T., & Murray M. D. Improving medication adherence and health outcomes in older adults: An

evidence-based review of randomized controlled trials. *Drugs Aging.* 2017;34(3), 191-201. doi:10.1007/s40266-016-0433-7

- Patient-centered and multidisciplinary interventions have shown to improve medication adherence and health outcomes in older adults.
- Virtual reminders were found to be effective intervention tools to increase medication compliance in older adults.

4. Tarn D. M., Pletcher M. J., Tosqui R., et al. Primary nonadherence to statin medications: Survey of patient perspectives. Prev Med Rep. 2021;22, 101357. doi: 10.1016/jpmedr.2021.101357

- Only 35.8% of participants with primary nonadherence believe that statins are safe medications.
- 56.6% of participants with nonadherence strongly or somewhat agreed that they worried about becoming dependent or addicted to a statin.

- The most important reasons participants gave for nonadherence of statins were worry about side effects, wanting to try diet or exercise first, preferring to take natural remedies or dietary supplements.

5. Spears, J., Erkens, J., Misquitta, C., Cutler, T., & Stebbins, M. A pharmacist-led, patient-centered program incorporating motivational interviewing for behavior change to improve adherence rates and star ratings in a medicare plan. *J Man Care Spec Pharm.* 2020; 26(1), 35–41. https://doi.org/10.18553/jmcp.2020.26.1.35

- Motivational interviewing is an intervention tool that can be used to improve safety and compliance of medication use by older adults.
- Behavior change through didactic learning and coaching interventions resulted in quality improvements of medication use in older adults.

CHAPTER REVIEW QUESTIONS

1 Considering the information in the chapter, explain why the OTA is an important player in the health care team to address medication issues with older adults.

2 What are some reasons for polypharmacy among older adults?

3 What is one side effect of each of the following: diuretics, OTC and prescription pain relievers, antidepressants/antipsychotics, and insulin? (Refer to Table 13.2.)

4 What resources and personnel are available to address the concerns or questions of OTAs regarding medications?

5 Explain skills needed for safe self-medication.

6 What aids are available to older adults with poor vision, memory, or hearing, or lack of transportation?

7 What should be included in a medication diary?

8 What are some essential components to a self-medication program?

9 What information should OTAs provide to educate caregivers?

REFERENCES

1. Kirzinger A, Neuman T, Cubanski J, Brodie M. *Data Note: Prescription Drugs and Older Adults.* 2019. Available at: https://www.kff.org/health-reform/issue-brief/data-note-prescription-drugs-and-older-adults/.
2. Rolita L, Freedman M. Over-the-counter medication use in older adults. *JOGN.* 2008;34(4):8-17.
3. Garfinkel D, Mangin D. Feasibility study of a systematic approach for discontinuation of multiple medications in older adults. *Arch Intern Med.* 2010;170(18):1648-1654. doi:10.1001/archinternmed.2010.355.
4. Nobili A, Licata G, Salerno F, et al. Polypharmacy, length of hospital stay, and in-hospital mortality among elderly patients in internal medicine wards. The REPOSI study. *Eur J Clin Pharmacol.* 2011;67(5):507-519. doi:10.1007/s00228-010-0977-0.
5. Deranged Physiology. *Change in Drug Response in the Elderly.* Available at: https://derangedphysiology.com/main/cicm-primary-exam/required-reading/variability-drug-response/Chapter%20245/changes-drug-response-elderly.
6. Centers for Disease Control and Prevention. *National Center for Health Statistics. Older Persons' Health.* Available at: https://www.cdc.gov/nchs/fastats/older-american-health.htm.
7. Divac N, Prostran M, Jakovcevski I, et al. Second-generation antipsychotics and extrapyramidal adverse effects. *Biomed Res Int.* 2014;2014(65):63-70. doi:10.1155/2014/656370.
8. Do D, Schnittker J. Utilization of medications with cognitive impairment side effects and the implications for older adults' cognitive function. *J Aging Health.* 2020;32(9):1165-1177.
9. Milsom I, Gyhagen M. The prevalence of urinary incontinence. *Climacteric.* 2019;22(3):217-222.
10. Lieberman J. Managing anticholinergic side effects. *Prim Care Companion J Clin Psychiatry.* 2004;6(suppl 2):20-23. doi:10.1111/j.1532-5415.2012.03923.x.
11. Speakman M, Kirby R, Doyle S, et al. Burden of male lower urinary tract symptoms (LUTS) suggestive of benign prostatic hyperplasia (BPH)—focus on the UK. *BJU Int.* 2015;115(4):508-519. doi:10.1111/bju.12745.
12. American Pharmacists Association. *APhA MTM Central: What is Medication Therapy Management?* Available at: https://portal.pharmacist.com/node/29279?is_sso_called=1.
13. Guariglia S, Smallfield S. The role of occupational therapy in medication management in acute care. *Gerontologist.* 2015;38:1-3. doi:10.1093/geront/gns103.
14. American Occupational Therapy Association. Occupational therapy practice framework: domain and process fourth edition. *Am J Occup Ther.* 2020;74(suppl 2):1-87.
15. Badanta-Romero B, de Diego-Cordero R, & Rivilla-Garcia E. Influence of religious and spiritual elements on adherence to pharmacological treatment. *J Relig Health.* 2018;57:1905-1917.
16. Kressin NR, Elway AR, Glickman M, et al. Beyond medication adherence: the role of patients' beliefs and life context in blood pressure control. *Ethn Dis.* 2019;29(4):567-576.

17. West LM, Theuma RB, Cordina M. The "Necessity-concerns framework" as a means of understanding non-adherence by applying polynomial regression three chronic conditions. *Chronic Illn.* 2018;6(4):253-265.

18. Diefenbach MA, Leventhal H. The common-sense model of illness representation: theoretical and practical considerations. *J Soc Distress Homeless.* 1996;5:11-38. doi:10.1007/BF02090456.19.

19. Leventhal H, Benyamini Y, Brownlee S, et al. Illness representations: theoretical foundations. In: Petrie KJ, Weinman JA, eds. *Perceptions of Health and Illness: Current Research and Applications.* Singapore: Harwood Academic; 1997:19-45.

20. Gauchet A, Tarquinio C, Fischer G. Psychosocial predictors of medication adherence among persons living with HIV. *Int J Behav Med.* 2007;14(3):141-150. doi:10.1007/BF03000185.

21. Church RM. Pharmacy practice in the Indian Health Service. *Am J Hosp Pharm.* 1987;44(4):771-775. doi:10.1016/S0003-0465(15)32840-8.

22. Lefley HP. Culture and chronic mental illness. *Hosp Community Psychiatry.* 1990;41(3):277-286. doi:10.1176/ps.41.3.277.

23. Whetstone WR, Reid JC. Health promotion of older adults: perceived barriers. *J Adv Nurs.* 1991;16(11):1343-1349. doi:10.1111/j.1365-2648.1991.tb01563.x.

24. Horne R. Representations of medication and treatment: advances in theory and measurement. In: Petrie KJ, Weinman J, eds. *Perceptions of Health and Illness: Current Research and Applications.* London: Harwood Academic; 1997:155-187.

25. Margolin A, Schuman-Olivier Z, Beitel M, et al. A preliminary study of spiritual self-schema (3-S[+]) therapy for reducing impulsivity of HIV-positive drug users. *J Clin Psychol.* 2007;63(10):979-999. doi:10.1002/jclp.20407.

26. Ironson G, Stuetzle R, Fletcher MA. An increase in religiousness/spirituality occurs after HIV diagnosis and predicts slower disease progression over 4 years in people with HIV. *J Gen Intern Med.* 2006;21(suppl 5):S62-S68. doi:10.1111/j.1525-1497.2006.00648.x.

27. Leach CR, Schoenberry NE. Striving for control: Cognitive, self-care, and faith strategies employed by vulnerable black and white older adults with multiple chronic conditions. *J Cross Cult Gerontol.* 2008;23(4):377-399. doi:10.1007/s10823-008-9086-2.

28. Campbell NL, Boustani MA, Skopelja EN, et al. Medication adherence in older adults with cognitive impairment: a systematic evidence-based review. *Am J Geriatr Pharmacother.* 2012;10(3):165-177.

29. Andiel C, Liu L. Working memory and older adults: implications for occupational therapy. *Am J Occup Ther.* 1995;49:681-686. doi:10.5014/ajot.49.7.681.

30. Aruru MV, Salmon JW. Development of a Medicare beneficiary comprehension test: assessing medicare part D beneficiaries' comprehension of their benefits. *Am Health Drug Benefits.* 2013;6:453-460. doi:10.1053/j.ajkd.2012.10.009.

31. Bolduc JJ, Robnett RH. Usefulness of the ManageMed Screen (MMS) and the Screening for Self-Medication Safety Post Stroke (S5) for assessing medication management capacity for clients post-stroke. *IJAHSP.* 2015;13(2):Article 3.

32. Robnett RH, Dionne C, Jaques R, LaChance A, Mailhot M. The ManageMed Screening: an interdisciplinary tool for quickly assessing medication management skills. *Clin Gerontol.* 2007;30(4):1-23. doi:10.1300/J018v30n04_01.

33. National Institute on Deafness and Other Communication Disorders. *Quick Statistics about Hearing.* n.d. Available at: http://www.nidcd.nih.gov/health/statistics/pages/quick.aspx.

34. Schiele JT, Penner H, Schnneider H, et al. Swallowing tablets and capsules increase the risk of penetration and aspiration in patients with stroke-induced dysphagia. *Dysphagia.* 2015;30:570-582. doi:10.1007/s00455-015-9639-9.

35. McGillicuddy A, Crean AM, Sahm LJ. Older adults with difficulty swallowing oral medicines: a systematic review of the literature. *Eur J Clin Pharmacol.* 2016;72:141-151. doi:10.1007/s00228-015-1979-8.

36. Kelly J, D'Cruz G, Wright D. A qualitative study of the problems surrounding medication administration to patients with dysphagia. *Dysphagia.* 2009;24:49-56. doi:10.1007/s00455-008-9170-3.

37. Molle E. Keep the upper GI tract from going downhill. *Nursing.* 2005;35(10):28-29.

38. Sera L, Uritsky T. Pharmacokinetic and pharmacodynamic changes in older adults and implications for palliative care. *Prog Palliat Care.* 2016;24(5):255-261. doi:10.1080/09699260.2016.1192319.

39. Kucukdagli P, Bahat G, Bay I, et al. The relationship between common geriatric syndromes and potentially inappropriate medication use among older adults. *Aging Clin Exp Res.* 2020;32:681-687. doi:10.1007/s40520-019-01239.

40. Meyer ME. *Coping with Medications.* San Diego, CA: Singular; 1993.

41. Felman A. What are insulin pens and how do we use them? *Medical News Today.* 2019. Available at: https://www.medicalnewstoday.com/articles/316607#:~:text=People%20with%20diabetes%20use%20insulin,a%20pen%20to%20administer%20insulin.

42. Sullivan D. *6 of the Best Reminders for Your Medications.* Healthline; 2020. Available at: https://www.healthline.com/health/best-medication-reminders.

43. Wieder AJ, Wolf-Klein GP. When medications change, tell the caregiver, too. *Geriatrics.* 1994;49:48. doi:10.1093/geronb/gbp033.

14

Considerations of Mobility

STEPHANIE JOHNSON, BRYAN CLEVER, AND SHARON COSPER
(PREVIOUS CONTRIBUTIONS FROM CYNTHIA GOODMAN, LOU JENSEN, MARY ELLEN KEITH, IVELISSE LAZZARINI, HELENE L. LOHMAN, MICHELE LUTHER-KRUG, TRACY MILIUS, CANDICE MULLENDORE, AND SANDRA HATTORI OKADA)

KEY TERMS

alternative transport, community mobility, driving, falls, fall reduction, fall recovery, fall prevention, fall protocols, mobility and seating assessment, OBRA, restraints, pedestrian, restraint reduction, seating components, wheeled mobility devices

CHAPTER OBJECTIVES

1. Discuss the Omnibus Budget Reconciliation Act regulations pertaining to the use of physical restraints.
2. Describe the steps in the establishment of a restraint reduction program.
3. Describe the role of the occupational therapy assistant in restraint reduction.
4. Outline the basic steps in evaluating the fit of a wheelchair.
5. Describe the major precautions to consider when older adults should use wheelchairs.
6. Describe essential considerations when evaluating and fitting a person of larger size with a wheelchair.
7. Identify three reasons that older adults are at a greater risk for falls than the general population.
8. Identify environmental, biological, psychosocial, and functional causes of falls.

9. Describe key considerations during the evaluation process for older adults at risk for falls.
10. Describe recommended and evidence-based interventions to prevent falls.
11. Discuss potential desired outcomes of fall prevention interventions.
12. Discuss the performance components and personal factors that are essential for safe driving.
13. Describe physical, sensory, and cognitive changes that can occur with aging that may affect independent driving.
14. Discuss intervention strategies and modifications that can be used for continued safe driving.
15. Discuss pedestrian safety and aspects related to continued community mobility.
16. Be knowledgeable about alternative transportation and ADA criteria for qualifying for transportation services.

STEPHANIE JOHNSON
(PREVIOUS CONTRIBUTIONS FROM KAI GAIYEN, TRACY MILIUS, CANDICE MULLENDORE, IVELISSE LAZZARINI, AND HELENE L. LOHMAN)

PART 1 Restraint Reduction

The use of physical restraints in health care practice has been common for many years.[1] The American health care system has used physical restraints throughout the continuum of care ranging from hospital emergency rooms, psychiatric units, and med-surgical units to nursing homes and other institutions. However, mounting evidence exists of patient safety risks related to the use of physical restraints.[2,3]

The Omnibus Budget Reconciliation Act of 1987[4] (OBRA) forbids the use of physical restraints for the purposes of discipline or staff convenience in nursing homes. Even with the OBRA law, it took years to decrease the usage of restraints in nursing homes. This decreased usage was accelerated in 2006 when the Centers for Medicare and Medicaid Services (CMS) tightened the regulations regarding the use of restraints by requiring health care workers to undergo more extensive training about the appropriate use of restraints to help ensure patient safety.[5] These CMS regulations were followed by a 2-year campaign in 2008 to reduce the use of restraints

BOX 14.1

Negative Effects of Restraints

PSYCHOSOCIAL	PHYSICAL
Depression	Hazards of immobility
Lethargy	Incontinence
Withdrawal	Constipation
Anxiety	Disturbed spell pattern
Distress	Loss of balance
Fear	Falls
Panic	Pressure ulcers
Anger	Bone demineralization
Agitation	Loss of muscle tone and mass
Increased aggression	Respiratory difficulties
Reduced opportunity for	Pneumonia
social contact	Infection
Threat to identity	Thrombophlebitis
Embarrassment	Dehydration
Humiliation	Impaired circulation
Demoralization	Respiratory problems
Decreased feelings of	Orthostatic hypotension
dignity	Decreased appetite
Decreased sense of	Decreased ability to care for
self-esteem	self
Decreased autonomy	Abrasions
Helplessness	Cuts
Dependence	Bruises
Regression	Decreased functional status
Increased confusion	Loss of freedom
Increased disorientation	Death caused by suffocation or
Increased disorganized	strangulation
behavior	Broken human spirit

in nursing homes because of the high risks of harm.[6] According to data from 2013, the usage of physical restraints in nursing homes decreased to 2.2% compared to 5% in 2007 and 10.4% in 2000.[7,8] Box 14.1 lists some of the negative effects of the use of restraints.

Restraint use within settings, such as acute care and intensive care units, are utilized to restrict clients from interfering with the provision of life-saving treatment or are necessary because less restrictive devices have failed. Researchers within one hospital system reported an estimated 46% of ICUs utilized restraints.[9] Within these settings, a documented medical need and physician's order for restraints must exist, including new orders every 24 hours, as well as client status re-assessment pending the restraint type and client age every 1, 2, or 4 hours.[10]

OMNIBUS BUDGET RECONCILIATION ACT REGULATIONS

OBRA was drafted to protect older adults from abuse and to promote choice and dignity. The ultimate goal of OBRA is that each person reaches his or her highest practical level of well-being. A reduction in the use of restraints is only a small part of this intent. OBRA requires caregivers to develop an individualized plan of care that supports each older adult in the least restrictive environment possible.[5,11,12] Occupational therapy assistants (OTAs) should become familiar with OBRA guidelines regarding restraints.

OBRA defines two types of restraints: chemical and physical. "Physical restraint can be any manual method, such as any physical or mechanical device, that restricts the patient's freedom of movement."[5] Some examples of direct physical restraints with the older adult may include restrictive chairs with full lap trays and small wheels that limit mobility, vests used to secure patients to their chairs or beds, wrist or ankle restraints, or bedrails. Indirect physical restraints can include no response or lack of response to call bells, sitters utilized for monitoring, mobility aids placed out of client's reach, or passive interactions.[13] "Chemical restraints are described as a drug or medication when it is used as a restriction to manage the patient's behavior or restrict the patient's freedom of movement and is not a standard treatment or dosage for the patient's condition."[14] A third type of restraint is seclusion or confinement of the individual to a space. Utilization of the least restrictive form of restraint is recommended, while offering protection to clients, staff, and/or others as needed.[10]

As discussed, through the OBRA guidelines and with other efforts, the improper usage of restraints in the United States has decreased. However, OTAs have an ethical and legal obligation to report older adult abuse, which includes using restraints as punishment for clients or as a convenience to staff. OTAs should also participate in educating others about restraints and may wish to initiate a restraint reduction program in their own facility and offer restraint alternatives.

ESTABLISHING A RESTRAINT REDUCTION PROGRAM

Reducing restraints is a complex matter. OTAs must evaluate and appropriately address ethical considerations, regulatory and professional standards, legal liability concerns, and health care team members' education regarding restraint use. It is also important to identify areas for, and participate in, research concerning physical restraints to assist staff nurses and other members of the health care team with making informed decisions regarding patient care.[15]

Philosophy

The philosophical premises of an educational program aimed at restraint reduction include beliefs about quality of care, commitment to understanding the meaning of behavior, and desire to shift practice from control of behavior to individualized approaches to care. An educational program with members of the interdisciplinary team is vital to assist in implementing restraint reduction programs. Results of testing a restraint education program suggested that altering staff beliefs and increasing knowledge produced a change in restraint practices, at least in the short term.[16]

A fundamental philosophical concept in the care of older adults is the empowerment of both older adults and staff. This empowerment is expressed in collaborative solutions to problems. The ability to contribute to solutions returns dignity to older adults and adds meaning and quality to their lives.[17]

In addition, it is also paramount to teach family members about the potentially harmful effects of restraint use and the regulatory restrictions and oversight on using restraints. Although family members may incorrectly believe that a restraint prevents injury, OTAs or other health care providers play an important role in educating family members on the aspects of patient autonomy and freedom of movement.

Policy

Health care providers' written policies and procedures should be consistent with each of the requirements listed in the regulations. Yearly mandatory training for staff should be provided, and all training and education programs should be documented. Documentation of events of restraint use should meet required regulations.[15] The CMS Federal Register indicates that staff must be trained regarding restraint use and regulations, and all training must be documented.[18]

When a facility makes a philosophical decision to reduce restraint use, education must be incorporated to help change the organizational culture and to provide strategies for the successful removal of restraints.[19]

Education

Practitioners should educate and work toward restraint reduction to not only comply with federal regulations but also to facilitate overall improvement in older adults functioning.[20]

An effective education program includes an experiential component, such as applying a variety of restraints to participants to allow participants to experience the feelings of helplessness and degradation of being restrained. Restraint reduction education should include and affirm participants' life experiences. This will lead to a decreased reliance of restraints and inclusion of all members of the interdisciplinary team, as well as board members, volunteers, and facility employees (i.e., kitchen workers, bookkeepers, administration, chaplains, maintenance workers, etc.) is important.[21,22] Education must also include possible consequences of restraint use. Physical consequences can include, injuries, falls, physical deconditioning, incontinence, malnutrition, dehydration, bone demineralization, and even death. Muscle atrophy, skin tears, pressure ulcers, contractures, cardiac rhythm disturbances, and infection can be other consequences of being restrained.[23] Possible psychosocial and behavioral consequences associated with restraint use may include increased delirium, agitation, frustration, fear, and loneliness. Mistrust in nursing and exacerbated behavior outbursts, such as yelling are also reported in the literature.[24-26]

Steps for Success

A key to eliminating the use of restraints is individualized care, which depends on staff knowing the client as a person.

One strategy for fostering staff-client relationships is the consistent assignment of staff to clients, which may help promote this individualized care. When these staff members are not working, they should have regular replacements. Permanence in staffing fosters relationships between older adults, families, and staff who contribute to feelings of safety and connectedness. Permanent staff are particularly important to older adults with cognitive impairment. Initial success will help staff members feel confident about continuing restraint reduction. Staff members responsible for care planning should try and document various options to avoid the use of restraints (Box 14.2).[23]

All members of the interdisciplinary team, including client and family members, should be included in all stages of the program with consistent open communication. Family members can, for example, describe the older adult's previous routines and preferences. In addition, family involvement that ranges from simply being notified of the restraint reduction to formal family educational programs has proven effective in a reduction program.[19] Kari and Michels assert that nursing assistants (CNAs) have essential knowledge of older adults and that their usual

BOX 14.2

Suggestions to Facilitate a Successful Restraint-Free Environment

- Develop a restraint committee involving all disciplines and departments in the facility.
- Determine the goal for the restraint reduction program. Is it to minimize restraints or completely ban restraints?
- Develop a strategic plan including protocols for specific restraint cases.
- Recruit specialists (geriatric nurse specialist, occupational therapy personnel, etc.) for consultation.
- Determine a protocol for how restraints are ordered by physicians.
- Limit restraint usage to a 24-hour trial. If the restraint usage exceeds that time period, consult with the physician.
- Provide documentation of both alternatives and reasons for restraint usage when requesting physician's orders.
- Implement a gradual process of change when starting the restraint reduction program.
- Start with the easiest cases first and move on to more difficult cases once initial success is achieved.
- Complete ongoing resident assessments. Provide restraint alternatives and interventions based on an individualized resident-specific approach. Include family participation. Learn from others who have successful restraint reduction programs.

From Joanna Briggs Institute. Physical restraint—Part 2: Minimization in acute and residential care facilities. *Best Pract.* 2002;6(4):1-6. Asia: Blackwell Publishing Asia.

lack of influence in decision-making negatively affects the quality of care.[17] CNAs may be the team members who first notice behavioral changes and the need for removal of restraints in older adults.[21] Strumpf and colleagues indicate that respect for the dignity of the CNA's work is vital for any significant reduction in the use of restraints.[16] An interdisciplinary team assessment of the need for restraint is helpful in reducing reliance on restraints.[22,27]

Rader found that the biggest obstacles to eliminating restraints are fears, biases, and unwillingness to change and proposes that caregivers, clients, advocates, and regulators work together to create new interventions on the basis of the older adult's perspectives and wishes.[28] Reducing restraints should be only the beginning of providing safe care in a dignified and less restrictive environment that promotes the older adult's abilities.[29,30]

ROLE OF THE OCCUPATIONAL THERAPY ASSISTANT

In collaboration with an occupational therapist (OT), OTAs may assess the need for restraints, consult with staff about alternatives to restraint, and provide intervention to eliminate restraint use. The type or technique of restraint used must be the least restrictive intervention that will be effective to protect the patient, staff member, or others from harm.[5]

Assessment

Once the need for intervention is documented and an occupational therapy order has been received, the OT/OTA team performs an evaluation. Specific assessments of posture, alignment, balance, strength, and visual acuity are necessary. Assessments of head control, trunk stability, upper extremity support, and the ability to self-propel are added to evaluate seating needs.[31,32] Perceptual and cognitive assessments should be included only as appropriate. Practitioners should not embarrass or agitate cognitively impaired older adults by assessing areas already documented as deficient.

Consultation

The assessment may reveal minimal intervention needs, perhaps consultation only. Patterson and colleagues include the roles of advocate, observer, teacher, information specialist, team problem solver, and identifier of resources and alternatives in their definition of consultant.[33] They also report that the combination of consultation with formal restraint reduction training significantly reduces the use of restraints. OTAs are uniquely qualified to function as consultants in developing alternatives to restraints, especially if they are familiar with restraint reduction principles, OBRA regulations, and the basic principles of positioning. For example, an elbow air splint may be all that is necessary for an older adult who continually scratches at sutures on a healing incision. Although an air splint is restrictive, it allows more movement than wrist restraints, thereby meeting the criterion for "least restrictive environment." Because wound healing is temporary, the air splint is a temporary measure. A protocol for use of the air splint should be provided by the consulting OTA. The care plan should document the reason that the splint is being used, the way it will be used, and the way it will be reassessed by the nursing staff. Communication is a key element, as part of the interdisciplinary team, with the attending physician, nursing staff, client, and caregiver.

OTAs may recommend other environmental, psychosocial, and activity-related alternatives (Table 14.1). The alternatives outlined are not a complete list as options are vast, depending on the OTA's creativity. Each measure considered should provide as much free choice and control as possible for older adults. Eigsti and Vrooman claim that the basic ingredient in reducing restraint use is teaching the staff to understand and believe that alternatives exist.[34]

TABLE 14.1

Alternatives to Restraints	
Environmental objects	**Specific examples of alternatives**
Chairs	Deep seats
	Tilted
	Recliners
	Rockers
	Gliders
	Bean bag
	Adirondack type
	Customized
Beds	Water or concave-type mattress
	Create bed boundaries with swim noodles under sheets or body pillows
	Positioning cushions
	Individual height mattresses, including floor mattresses
	Trapeze for bed mobility

TABLE 14.1

Alternatives to Restraints—cont'd

Environmental objects	Specific examples of alternatives
Monitoring systems	Television monitoring
	Enclosed courtyards
	Alarms
	Exit alarms
	Door buzzers
	Nursery intercom
	Personal alarms for bed or chair
	Wandering alarms at doorways and exits
	Pressure-sensitive pads
	Positional alarms
	Limb bracelet alarms
Signs	Directional
	Stop or Keep Out
	Identifying (elder's name)
Safety adaptations	Nonskid surfaces
	Low bed
	Mattress or sleep mat on floor
	¾ to ½ length bed rails (instead of full length)
	Lowered or no bed rail
	Accessible call lights
	Move furniture and other obstacles from walkways
	Accessible light switches
	Safe walking routes
	Encouraged use of handrail
	Bedside commode or urinal
	Items within reach
	Shoes or nonskid socks worn in bed
Personalized room	Familiar furniture
	Familiar objects to hold
	Meaningful pictures and photographs
Other adaptations	Lighting (easy to turn on switches and access)
	Locked exit doors
	Cloth barrier doorways attached with Velcro
	Activity area at end of corridors
	Bean bags (different sizes)
	Pillows
	Foam
	Nonslip mats
	Firm wheelchair seats
	Air-splints
	"Wrap-around" walkers with seats
Psychosocial alternatives	Specific examples of alternatives
Behavioral strategies	Remotivation
	Reality orientation (if helpful)
	Frequent reminders
	Active listening
	Responding to agenda behavior
Decrease or increase	Interactions
	Visiting
	Sensory stimulation (especially noise such as that from overhead paging, television, radio, among others)
	Identification of antecedent to the unwanted behavior and appropriate measures to address

Continued

TABLE 14.1

Alternatives to Restraints—cont'd	
Environmental objects	**Specific examples of alternatives**
Activities	Companionship
	Encourage resident/staff interactions
	Consistent staff for familiarity
	Decreased sensory stimulation
	Decreased noise
	Structured daily routines
	Self-care
	Permit or encourage wandering and pacing
	Exercise
	Bowling
	Nature walks
	Wheelchair aerobics, dances, ball games
	Ambulation programs
	Toileting every 2 hours
	Nighttime activities
	Volunteer and family assistance
	Buddy system
	Activity kits
	Diversional opportunities
	Relaxation techniques
	Massage
	Therapeutic touch
	Warm bath
	Music specific to elder tastes

ENVIRONMENTAL ADAPTATIONS

There are several strategies that can be used to modify the environment to move toward making it restraint-free, such as equipment, alarms, and signage—both with high and low tech options. For example, using chairs that are personalized for seat height, depth, and level of backing for each resident can reduce the risk and need for restraints, especially in public areas, such as a dining room.[23]

An inexpensive and less restrictive alternative for older adults who are unsteady with functional mobility, but also have cognitive or impulsivity deficits, who rises, might be a personal alarm, alerting staff of their movement. While these do not prevent the older adult from rising, the alarm sounds when the older adult stands, warranting attention from the caregiver. A personal alarm may frighten or agitate the older adult or surrounding residents; therefore, the use of the alarm should be with caution and take into account the environment, older adult, and other residents. Many facilities have discovered that nursery intercoms are an inexpensive and effective way to monitor safe ambulators who wander. Directional signs may help these older adults locate their rooms and deter them from entering someone else's room. An alternative to direction signs are signs with familiar pictures instead of words.

Providing cues to help orient residents who wander may also be helpful. Cues can include memory boxes by a resident's door, personal furnishings that residents will recognize, or large visual signs or pictures for bathrooms and other frequently sought areas.[23] Simple Velcro signs can be placed across doorways that wandering residents should not enter (e.g., exit doors). These signs are generally red or yellow and may read "Stop" (Fig. 14.1). These visual cues help the wandering resident return to another area of the building.

There are a variety beds on the market that will allow a facility to reduce bed rail use (a possible indirect restraint pending utilization) and decrease incidence of falls. For residents at a higher risk for falls, beds can be adjusted from a standard height to 7 inches off the floor, so that if a fall occurs, injury is potentially mitigated. Safety alarms, special mattresses and pillows, and thick rubber bedside mats can also be installed. Placing squeak toys between the sheets and mattress pads reminds residents when they are getting too close to the edge of the bed. When side rails must be used, staff can set foam "swim noodles" between the mattress and side rail to reduce the risk of a resident getting trapped against the rail.[35]

PSYCHOSOCIAL APPROACHES

Qualitative studies and other literature indicate negative experiences of people who have been restrained, including emotional distress, loss of dignity and independence,

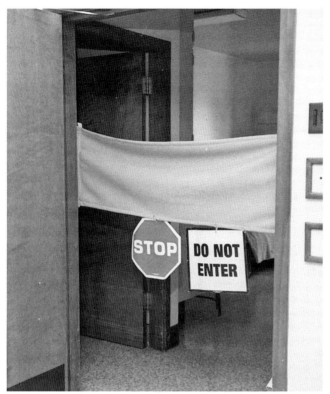

FIG. 14.1 Environmental adaptations should help older adults with cognitive deficits from wandering into other people's rooms without restricting access to hallways.

dehumanization, increased agitation, and depression.[1,23] Clients may experience emotions ranging from frustration and anxiety to anger and terror when restrained. Therefore, psychosocial approaches to reduce restraint use are important.

Wandering or attempts to get up from a chair may be part of an older adult's agenda behavior and may lead to agitation if the older adult is restrained. Evans and colleagues indicate that the keys to responding successfully to agenda behavior are to allow older adults to act on their plans, identify a point at which they may accept a suggestion or guidance, and allow them to keep their dignity throughout an incident.[36] The important difference in the result of this approach compared to others is that allowing the older adult to play out the behavior provides a sense of identity and promotes feelings of belonging, safety, and connectedness. This diminishes the older adult's need to seek those feelings elsewhere and further incidences of wandering are subsequently decreased or eliminated.[37] Brungardt adds that this method works well if the older adult's welfare is considered before the needs or routines of the facility.[20]

ACTIVITY ALTERNATIVES

Activity zones with recreational activities, such as multi-sensory theme boxes, and offering substitute physical activities that interest clients such as dance, exercise, or rocking, may be ways to engage clients in something of interest and reduce the occurrence of wandering. Providing cues to help orient residents who wander may also be helpful. As previously discussed, memory boxes or signage are examples of appropriate cues to focus the client.[23]

Providing meaningful activity alternatives can decrease behavior such as restlessness that has traditionally led to the use of restraints. An activity kit, perhaps in the form of a sewing basket, briefcase, fanny pack, or tackle box, may be helpful. The kit may be assembled by family members who are familiar with the older adult's interests.[28,38] The idea is to provide something familiar, comfortable, and safe that engages the older adult's attention.

INTERVENTION

Although not all referrals require intervention beyond consultation, the assessment may identify a need for ongoing intervention. Examples of intervention to eliminate the need for restraints include the development of self-care techniques, upper body positioning, and seating adaptations. Because restraint use is associated with the inability to perform self-care, older adults and their caregivers should be taught strategies for accomplishing this goal. Determining the routines the older adult followed in the past to maintain a sense of continuity and predictability is particularly important. Because part of the objective is to reduce anxiety and agitation, self-care must be done according to the older adult's agenda and routine rather than those of the OTA or facility.

Older adults with hemiplegia are often provided with half-tray style lapboards to assist with upper body positioning. Because these older adults may need support for their affected upper extremity and/or trunk, as well as may have balance and motor control deficits, this is one of the few cases in which it may be advantageous to begin with the most restrictive device, a full lapboard, and adapt if necessary. If a full lapboard causes agitation or seems too restrictive (perhaps the older adult is unable to use a urinal independently), a swing-away half lap tray may be used. Another solution is a foam wedge or cylindrical bean bag, which can extend the width of the armrest for safe positioning without a lapboard. As with any restrictive device, however, less than perfect positioning may be necessary to accommodate the older adult's choice.

Another specific occupational therapy intervention aimed at reducing the need for restraints is a positioning assessment for older adults who are wheelchair-bound. Ill-fitting wheelchairs contribute to restraint use, which can lead to an abnormal sitting posture and the eventual loss of function.[39] For example, wheelchairs usually found in nursing homes are not designed for independent mobility or long-term sitting. Necessary adaptations for comfort and function include dropping the seat so that older adults can reach the floor with their feet, replacing the sling seat with a firm seat and cushion, and replacing the sling back with a firm back. A narrower chair may help older adults propel themselves more comfortably.[40] Knowledge of the principles of positioning is essential. (Basic alignment principles applicable to any older adult are outlined in Part 2 of this chapter.) Once adaptations have been designed and implemented, the older adult's verbal, behavioral, and postural response must be observed. The system should be reassessed and adapted as necessary until the positioning goals have been met. Documentation should accompany every step of this process, especially if the older adult declines the intervention. With very difficult cases, consultation with a seating expert may be helpful. However, even the nonexpert can make many "low-tech" foam supports or recommendations. More detailed information on wheelchair positioning is included in Part 2 of the chapter.

Relatively inexpensive foam is available in large sizes at the local building or craft store and can easily be cut and shaped with an electric knife. This type of foam works well for the addition of width to an armrest, the fabrication of forearm wedges to elevate edematous upper extremities, or the provision of lightweight lateral trunk support. Egg crate foam is another inexpensive material suitable for limited purposes. Neither of these low-density foams is adequate to support entire body weight while sitting or during episodes of spasticity however. For long-term positioning, manufactured cushions of mixed density foam, gel, or air cushions are more durable and are recommended for both comfort and maintaining skin integrity. The therapeutic role of orthotic devices in achieving proper body position, balance, and alignment and improving overall functional capacity without the potential negative effects of restraint use is recognized by the CMS.[11,12] This recognition does not provide the license to use wedges, reclining chairs, or seat belts as restraints, even for cognitively intact older adults. However, it does allow the legitimate use of positioning devices to increase function, given a demonstrated necessity. Any adaptation should maintain the dignity of older adults and augment their quality of life.

CONSIDERATIONS FOR OTAs IN FACILITIES UTILIZING RESTRAINTS

If working in a facility that utilizes restraints, it is the OTA's responsibility to comply with the facilities policies regarding restraint usage, including but not limited to: proper training and education of how to utilize/apply restraints, inquiring as to reasons for restraints, and receiving authorization to remove restraints prior to any therapy session. It is also vital that posttherapy sessions, the client—if restrained prior to therapy session—is returned to the same restraint usage and nursing notified. As an OTA, documentation of how the client presented, participated in therapy, as well as how they are left when exiting the room is vital. Being a part of the interdisciplinary team, the OTA has the opportunity to discuss with the team progress for client status, which could potentially

lead to a less restrictive state. It is the OTAs responsibility to both document and communicate any progress or changing needs of the client to health care team, including the treating physician and nursing staff.[41,42]

CASE STUDY

Sandra, a 79-year-old woman with the diagnosis of dementia, resides in a long-term care facility. Other medical history includes multiple transient ischemic attacks (TIAs) and skin breakdown on the buttocks area. Sandra requires total assist transfers from the bed to the wheelchair. Her current wheelchair positioning includes a pressure relief cushion and a self-release pelvic belt to prevent sliding forward in the wheelchair. Sandra is able to self-release the pelvic positioning belt; therefore the belt is not considered to be a restraint. However, when she releases it because of agitation or trying to take herself to the bathroom, she tends to slide forward in her chair and is at risk for falls. To prevent this from happening, the nursing staff have requested that the pelvic belt be replaced with one that Sandra is not able to release herself. The new pelvic belt then becomes a restraint. The nursing staff order the OT/OTA team of Logan and Taylor to address this case.

Because Logan and Taylor are aware of restraint reduction guidelines, they provide interventions to promote optimal positioning using the least restrictive methods. They install a manual tilt pack on the wheelchair to reduce sliding forward and remove the pelvic positioning belt. They also install a drop seat to allow Sandra's feet to touch the ground and self-propel throughout the facility. They provide a wedge cushion for optimal positioning. To involve the other members of the health care team, they educate nursing staff on proper positioning devices and techniques.

Finally, they focus on the resident and encourage Sandra to self-propel her wheelchair for increased independence. They talk with staff about engaging Sandra in various activities throughout the day and evening and suggest moving her to various interesting areas during the day (high traffic areas, such as nursing stations or activity room, or near windows to see outside). As a result, Sandra is able to make her needs known when placed near the nursing station and enjoys increased independence with mobility. The pelvic belt is replaced by a recliner back, drop seat, and wedge cushion. These interventions collectively position Sandra correctly and reduce her incidences of sliding forward and fall risk. Most importantly, Sandra does not have a restraint.

■ CASE STUDY QUESTIONS

1 How is addressing Sandra's wheelchair positioning in this study related to restraint reduction?
2 How did Logan and Taylor help maintain Sandra's dignity and quality of life?
3 How did the OT/OTA team work as part of the interdisciplinary team to eliminate Sandra's restraint and improve her functional abilities?

CONCLUSION

OTAs have a responsibility to clearly state their professional opinion and recommendations regarding restraint reduction. Clients must choose whether to act on that advice. True restraint reduction requires an examination of attitudes about the rights of older adults, especially those with cognitive impairment, to make choices and take risks. OTAs must be willing to become advocates for older adults. An understanding of OBRA regulations and positioning principles and the ability to be flexible and creative within an interdisciplinary team permit OTAs to contribute effectively to restraint elimination programs. If OTAs have diligently attempted to increase the function and dignity of the older adults they serve, they will have followed not only the letter of the law but also the intent and spirit.

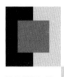

BRYAN CLEVER

(PREVIOUS CONTRIBUTIONS FROM (CANDICE MULLENDORE

AND CYNTHIA GOODMAN)

PART 2 Wheelchair Seating and Positioning: Considerations for Older Adults

According to the 2019 *American Community Survey* performed by the US Census Bureau, an estimated 11.3 million adults over the age of 65 had some form of disability that directly affected their ability to safely ambulate.[43] In 2011, the National Health and Aging Trends Study found that 2.135 million adults in the United States over the age of 65 were using a wheelchair, with the greatest percentage being female.[44] A national study that analyzed wheelchair demographics data from 1990 to 2005 showed a 5% increase among older adult wheelchair users each year.[45] As the Baby Boomer generation continues to age and life expectancy in the United States rises, the number of older adults relying on wheelchairs for mobility is expected to increase.[46] Older adults are more likely to be provided manual wheelchairs than power wheelchairs[47]; however, with advances in technology, standard wheelchairs are being made with higher quality material and with more adjustable features to accommodate individual needs.[48] The use of a wheelchair for mobility in the home, community, or both is important in improving individuals' level of independence and ability to participate in chosen occupations.

Many health care professionals assume that a basic standard wheelchair (Fig. 14.2) is suitable for most adults, regardless of the individual's shape, size, functional abilities, and living situation. This is, in part, due to Medicare's strict rules regarding which older adults are eligible for financial coverage of mobility equipment. Medicare only pays for more complex wheeled mobility devices if a client has specific neurological diagnoses and if a formal evaluation is performed by either a physical therapist (PT) or an OT with an assistive technology professional (ATP) present. The specific neurological diagnosis and in-depth evaluation are not required for Medicare coverage of standard wheelchairs, making them easier to obtain.

Another roadblock to obtaining a custom-fitted wheelchair is the 20% copay for the equipment. This is often difficult for older adults to afford, as they are commonly on a fixed income and may not have secondary insurance to cover the copay. Custom manual wheelchairs can cost $6000+ depending on options and positioning accessories,

and powered mobility can range from $5000–$45,000. A standard wheelchair which costs between $100 and $500 is often the most affordable option.

Since standard wheelchairs are more affordable and are more easily covered by insurance, why are not they the mobility solution for all older adults? The main reasons are that standard wheelchairs are meant to be used for short periods (<2 hours at a time), have minimal opportunities for adjustment, come in limited sizes, and provide little postural support due to the sling upholstery.[49] Placing older adults in standard wheelchairs for extended periods of time can put them at risk of developing complications such as pressure injuries and joint contractures.[50] Unfortunately, many long-term care facilities primarily utilize standard wheelchairs because of their low cost and the ease of operation and storage.

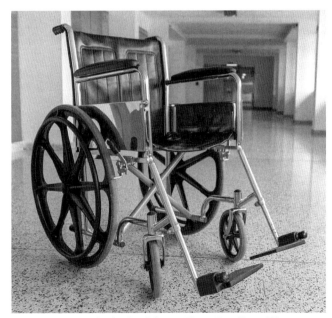

FIG. 14.2 Standard wheelchair. *(From Pendleton H, Schultz-Krohn W. Pedretti's Occupational Therapy – Practice Skills for Physical Dysfunction, 8th edn. Chapter 11. Mobility, Figure 11.6.)*

TABLE 14.2

Physical Changes of Aging	
Thinning, fragile skin	More prone to skin injuries due to pressure and shearing
Decreased body fat and fluids	Provides less protection over bony prominences, also leading to an increased chance of skin injuries
Visual changes	Requires more light to see, especially with glare on glossy surfaces
Cardiovascular changes	Can decrease blood pressure upon standing, leading to a higher risk of falls. Results in longer recovery times following exercise and even daily tasks.
Changes in bladder and kidney function	Increased urinary urgency and frequency and decreased control. Sitting while wet increases the potential for skin breakdown.
Respiratory changes	Results in increased energy expenditure, fatigue, and shortness of breath with activity, increased susceptibility to respiratory infection.
Musculoskeletal changes	Decreased muscle mass leads to increased energy consumption for daily tasks. Decreased bone density and increased osteoporosis increase the risk of severe injury with falls. Decreased range of motion (ROM) affects the ability to perform daily tasks.

AGING

Due to the physical changes that occur to the body as we age (Table 14.2), older adults require a different approach to seating and mobility than younger adults.[51] Aging can lead to postural changes, functional changes, and several different health conditions that can greatly affect older adults' ability to safely perform their activities of daily living (ADLs). Some health conditions frequently seen that impact mobility include cerebral vascular accident (CVA), osteoporosis, orthopedic injuries and trauma, respiratory diseases such as chronic obstructive pulmonary disease (COPD), rheumatoid arthritis (RA), diabetes, Parkinson's disease, and dementia.[51] Within the older adult population, women are more likely to require specialized seating due to longer life spans, increased frailty, and higher instances of mobility disabilities.[52,53] When deciding on a seating and mobility solution, the older adult's primary diagnoses and comorbidities along with the prognoses should be carefully considered.

RISKS OF IMPROPER SEATING

A standard or improperly fitted wheelchair used over an extended period of time can lead to several problems such as poor posture, pain, inhibited mobility, and possibly increased use of restraints.[54] Many of the problems caused by a standard wheelchair are the result of the sling upholstery on the seat. This type of seat is unable to provide adequate postural support over an extended period of time and can lead to posterior pelvic tilt, kyphosis (forward rounding of the spine), and neck flexion.[51] These abnormal postural positions are not only uncomfortable, but they may require the older adult to exert more energy than necessary to accomplish ADL tasks.

Another risk for older adults when placed in an improper seating system is that the person may lean forward in an attempt to stabilize themselves or to participate in functional activities, which places them at risk of falling out of the wheelchair. Also, if a person is of shorter stature and unable to adequately access the handrim of the wheels for propulsion, they may attempt to propel themselves with their feet. Propelling with the feet in a standard wheelchair can cause the pelvis to shift forward which could cause the client to fall from the chair. Frequent falls from wheelchairs can result in restraints being placed in the wheelchair or the older adult being labeled a "fall risk" and removed from any type of mobility device. This could lead to the person spending most of their time in a recliner or bed, increasing the potential for further decline in function and health.

Another negative effect of improper positioning is that older adults with communication deficits, such as dementia or aphasia, may not be able to communicate their discomfort, which may lead to agitation or aggression. Other issues that can arise are skin breakdown, the progression of skeletal and musculoskeletal deformities (scoliosis, joint contractures, etc.), disruptions in swallowing, digestion, altered bowel and bladder performance, decreased respiratory function and visual field. As a result of these conditions, the older adult may experience an increase in physical comorbidities, decreased socialization, and an increased risk of depression.[51]

DECIDING ON A WHEELED MOBILITY DEVICE

The solution for the complex dilemma of seating and positioning is an individualized system placed on a mobility base that is built to suit the person's specific dimensions and functional needs. This requires a formal seating and mobility evaluation. Because an evaluation is required, this does not mean that the OTA is excluded from this process, as the OTA plays an integral role in the interdisciplinary team deciding on the optimal mobility solution.

The Interdisciplinary Team

The team is led by the patient's physician due to Medicare and other insurances requiring a prescription to cover the cost of the mobility system. It is recommended that a physician write the prescription for a device based on a seating and mobility evaluation by a PT or an OT. This allows the therapist(s), ATP, client, caregiver, and family members to come together during the evaluation and determine the best equipment for the older adult.

The ATP, who is required to be present at the time of evaluation, has extensive knowledge in equipment and funding and is an invaluable resource. Occupational therapy practitioners should work with an ATP professional to determine the best system for their client. ATPs work with the seating and mobility issues of patients on a daily basis and have experience with many different diagnoses and devices. The oversight for ATP certification is by the Rehabilitation Engineering and Assistive Technology Society of North America (RESNA) and is available to those who wish to pursue an advanced role in seating and mobility, including OTAs.

The role of the therapy practitioner in the interdisciplinary team is to holistically evaluate the client using an interview and mat assessment. It is within the OTA's scope of practice to perform the mat assessment and present the findings to the supervising OT.[55] The OTA should also provide any additional information about the client such as information about current abilities or equipment options.[55] The OT then interprets the findings of the assessment and can strategize with the OTA and the interdisciplinary team.

During this entire process, the therapy practitioners serve as the older adult's primary advocates, as many clients and family members do not have extensive knowledge of mobility solutions or how to obtain them.

The final and most important members of the interdisciplinary team are the client, their family, and caregivers. Because the client will be the one to use the device on a daily basis to perform occupations and interact with their environment, a comprehensive look at the client and every aspect of their lives should be taken into consideration. The family or caregivers should also be asked to provide input, especially if they will be assisting the client in the use of the device. If the client and/or caregiver is unable to easily and safely operate the mobility device, there is an increased risk of the mobility device being discarded and abandoned.

Wheeled Mobility Bases

For the OTA to be able to recognize a need and bring recommendations to the OT, it is necessary to have a basic knowledge of seating and positioning equipment. For mobility devices, an excellent place to begin that journey of knowledge is with mobility bases. As mentioned earlier, different types of manual and power wheelchairs can provide different levels of customization to address a person's specific needs (Table 14.3).

TABLE 14.3

Wheelchair Types	
Transport chairs (Fig. 14.3)	▪ Made for a caregiver to push ▪ No adjustments ▪ Lightweight ▪ Easy to transport ▪ Temporary use
Standard wheelchairs (Fig. 14.2)	▪ Can be self-propelled ▪ Utilized for multiuser environments—hospitals ▪ Can weigh over 50 pounds ▪ No adjustments of components
Lightweight wheelchairs (Fig. 14.4)	▪ Weigh 30+ pounds ▪ Used for short intervals of time ▪ Limited adjustment of components—leg rest height, armrest height, overall wheelchair height within a couple of inches
Ultralightweight wheelchairs (Fig. 14.5)	▪ Full adjustability of all components ▪ Custom frame dimensions made to fit the user ▪ For full-time, independent users ▪ Less than 30 pounds ▪ Rigid and folding frames ▪ Rigid frames are the lightest
Tilt-in-space wheelchairs (Fig. 14.7)	▪ For dependent users ▪ Very heavy, typically between 40 and 60 pounds depending on the seating system ▪ Used for those unable to perform independent pressure relief
Power-operated vehicles (Scooters) (Fig. 14.8)	▪ Standard seat dimensions ▪ Lightweight and transportable ▪ Short-term use over longer distances and stable terrain ▪ Best used outside the home due to poor turning radius

Continued

TABLE 14.3

Wheelchair Types—cont'd	
Power mobility device (PMD) (Fig. 14.9)	▪ Full-time use—in the home and outside ▪ Some options may accommodate custom seating ▪ Smaller device footprint ▪ More powerful motors ▪ Longer lasting batteries
PMD with complex rehabilitation technology (CRT) (Fig. 14.10)	▪ Full-time users ▪ Able to accommodate all custom seating options ▪ Addition of powered positioning aides—tilt, recline, elevating leg rests, seat elevate, etc. ▪ Able to accommodate alternate drive controls—head array, sip and puff, eye gaze, etc.

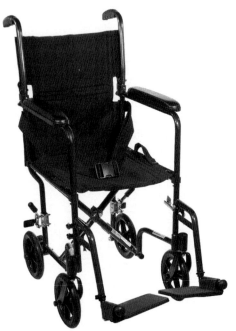

FIG. 14.3 Transport chair. *(Taken from DriveMedical.com. https://www.drivemedical.com/us/en/products/mobility/ wheelchairs/transport-chairs/aluminum-transport-chair/ p/950-1.)*

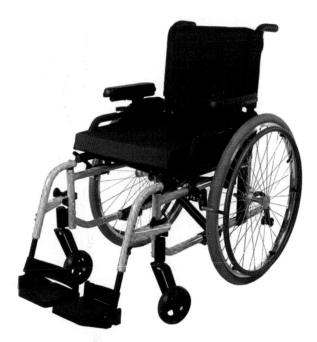

FIG. 14.4 Lightweight wheelchair. *(Taken from karmanhealthcare. com. https://www.karmanhealthcare.com/product/s-ergo-115-ultra- lightweight-wheelchair/.)*

Manual Wheeled Mobility

The simplest type of wheelchair is the transport chair (Fig. 14.3). This type of wheelchair is primarily used for quick transport of a person as they are being pushed.[49] Transport chairs are exceptionally lightweight without the large heavy rear wheels of a standard wheelchair. They can be folded and placed in vehicles easily due to their light weight. The next type of manual wheelchair is the standard wheelchair (Fig. 14.2). This type of wheelchair is typically found in multiuser facilities like hospitals, skilled nursing and rehab facilities, medical offices, etc.[49] Standard wheelchairs are heavy, weighing over 50 pounds, and do not provide any adjustments for individual users. Even though they have larger rear wheels for self-propulsion, the position of the rear wheels

is not optimal for continued independent use and are primarily for temporary use and transport.[56]

Lightweight wheelchairs, the next device in this category, are more suited for self-propulsion; however, they are still not ideal for full-time use (Fig. 14.4). They do offer some adjustability of components like the length of the leg rests, the height of the armrests, and overall seat height. By raising the position of the rear wheels and casters, the seat height becomes lower to better accommodate foot-assisted propulsion of the wheelchair.[56] Ironically, despite the name, lightweight wheelchairs are still considered heavy, weighing over 30 pounds. The weight combined with the fixed horizontal position of the rear wheel makes it inefficient, especially for older adults.[49]

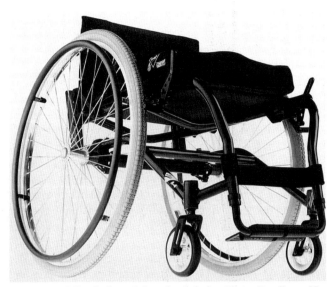

FIG. 14.5   Ultralightweight wheelchair. *(From Pendleton H, Schultz-Krohn W. Pedretti's Occupational Therapy – Practice Skills for Physical Dysfunction, 8th edn. Chapter 11. Mobility, Figure 11.5B.)*

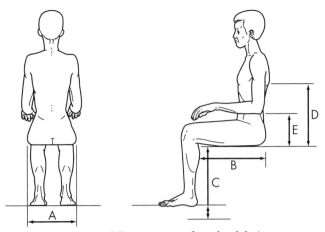

FIG. 14.6   Measurements for wheelchairs.

Ultralightweight manual wheelchairs are the best option for full-time wheelchair users (Fig. 14.5).[49] These types of wheelchairs come in two frame options, rigid and folding. The rigid frame is the most energy-efficient type of frame because it has no moving parts which allows the transfer of the majority of the user's energy straight to the ground in the form of propulsion.[56] Rigid frame chairs are also lighter and require less energy to be exerted by the user during propulsion. The decreased weight and increased efficiency of an ultralight manual wheelchair can often mean the difference between a client being able to participate in mobility related ADLs (MRADLs) for the entire day or needing more assistance as the day progresses due to fatigue. Folding frame ultralightweight manual wheelchairs are easier to transport and store due to the low profile of the frame once it is folded. Both ultralightweight options are fully customizable and adjustable.

Frame Dimensions

Frames for any custom-fitted mobility device are built according to the dimensions agreed upon by the ATP and the occupational therapy practitioner. The seat depth (Fig. 14.6B) provides the needed support and pressure distribution through the buttocks and thighs. To achieve optimal pressure distribution, it is important to have the greatest amount of surface area of the body possible in contact with the support surface (the seat cushion). If the seat depth is too long, it could result in posterior pelvic tilt, increasing the pressure placed at the sacrum and lead to skin breakdown.[56] In addition, the user may slide down in the chair to relieve the pressure on the back of the lower legs causing shearing of the skin. If the seat depth is too short, it will not provide adequate support or pressure

distribution and could result in pressure injuries to the back of the thighs or the buttocks.[56]

A properly fitted seat width (Fig. 14.6A) allows for pelvic support and the best access to the wheels for optimum propulsion.[56] The seat width should fit snug, if the seat is too wide it can allow the pelvis to reposition in the seat creating an unstable posture and can make the wheels less accessible putting an unnecessary strain on the shoulders and wrists during propulsion. Conversely, if the seat is not wide enough, then the wheels could rub against the hip putting the skin at risk for breakdown.

Seat to footrest height (Fig. 14.6C) provides the proper amount of contact for the thighs on the seating surface. If the footrest is set too high, then the user's weight is shifted back to the ischial tuberosity (IT), increasing possibility of skin breakdown. If the footrest is too low, pressure increases at the back of the thigh at the edge of the seating surface.[56] This can lead to the user sliding forward in the chair to relieve pressure and reach the footrest.

The front frame angle and leg rest angle should be set according to the user's knee range of motion (ROM). Ideally, this angle should be as close as possible to 90 degrees to allow the feet to sit slightly under the user. This allows for the smallest possible footprint for the chair and the greatest amount of maneuverability.[56] The further out a person's feet are from the seat, the more likely they are to settle into posterior pelvic tilt.

The front seat height is typically dictated by the length of the lower leg, or the distance required from the seating surface to the footplate.[56] The team must take into consideration not only the user's lower leg length but also the thickness of the cushion to be used, this will reduce the distance based on leg length. Another consideration is the user's access to tables and other surfaces. If the front seat height is set too high, the user may not be able to fit underneath the surface to be able to perform necessary tasks. The height should accommodate for ground clearance of the footplate as well, which is typically at least 2 inches above the ground.[56]

Rear seat height can be used to provide postural support and is important for the vertical placement of the rear wheel.[56] It is not uncommon to have the rear seat height lower than the front to provide pelvic stability to individuals with paraplegia and quadriplegia. This places the pelvis in a neutral position, and possibly some anterior tilt, which compensates for the lack of strength and provides the support needed to maintain an upright posture. If the rear seat height is too low it can cause excess elbow flexion and shoulder abduction to reach the top of the handrim, eventually leading to shoulder injuries.[56] Placing the rear seat height too low compared to the front seat height may affect the user's ability to perform transfers. Conversely, if the rear seat height is too high, the user will have to extend the elbow to reach the handrim resulting in an inefficient push. The ideal position is a height where the user's elbow is flexed between 100 and 120 degrees with their hands placed at the top of the handrim.[57]

The back angle is the relation of the backrest to the ground. The ideal position would be 90 degrees to achieve an upright posture. When dealing with the older adult population, there is an increased incidence of kyphotic postures.[56] This would require a greater back angle to compensate for the excessive spinal curvature and allow for the head to remain in an upright position. Some backrests are available to assist in accommodating a kyphotic posture which reduces the amount of back angle required and lessens the pressure placed on the sacrum in a reclined position. Back height (Fig. 14.6D) is typically determined by the user's amount of trunk control. The less trunk control a user has, the taller the back height will need to be to provide postural support.[57] It is important to note that if the backrest contacts the scapula it will impede the natural movement of the scapula during propulsion. This will decrease the efficiency of the push stroke

and require more strokes and energy to propel the same distance. It is ideal to have the backrest below the bottom of the scapula while still maintaining lumbar support, if the user has adequate trunk control.[57]

Center of gravity (COG) is crucial to the efficiency of the wheelchair. If the rear wheels are placed too far back, the user's weight is distributed too far over the casters making it more difficult to turn and overcome thresholds and uneven terrain. It also causes the user to have to reach behind them to access the wheels which can lead to shoulder strain.[51] If the rear wheels are placed too far forward, it can cause the chair to be unstable and fall over backward when the user is navigating inclines. For each client there is an ideal placement for the rear wheel that balances ease of use with stability.

A manual wheelchair solution for those that are dependent on caregivers for their mobility, transfers, and pressure relief is the tilt-in-space wheelchair (Fig. 14.7). The main objective for this type of manual wheelchair is pressure relief as it allows the caregiver to tilt the person back to offload pressure from the bottom to the back. This typically requires a tilt angle of at least 30 degrees.[58] To allow for the greatest return of blood flow to the tissue, tilt should be used in conjunction with recline; with the greatest angles achieving the greatest amount of return blood flow.[59]

Power Wheeled Mobility

Clients who are not able to physically propel themselves in a manual wheelchair but have sufficient cognitive ability should use power wheelchairs. The most common power devices encountered in the older adult population are Power Operated Vehicles (POV) and scooters (Fig. 14.8).[60] They only come in basic seat styles and sizes, typically either 16"w × 16"d or 18"w × 16" deep. Devices in this

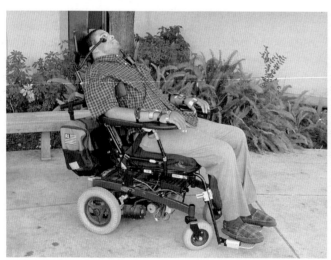
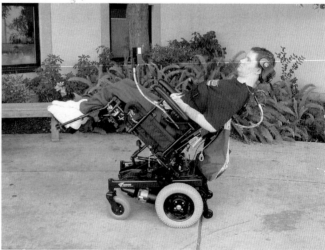

FIG. 14.7 Tilt-in-space wheelchair. *(From Pendleton H, Schultz-Krohn W. Pedretti's Occupational Therapy – Practice Skills for Physical Dysfunction, 8th edn. Chapter 11. Mobility, Figure 11.4C.)*

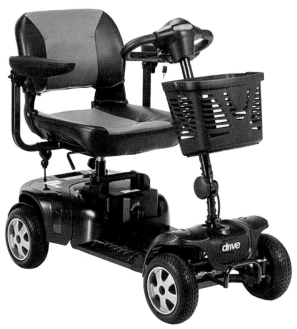

FIG. 14.8 Scooter. *(From Drivemedical.com. https://www. drivemedical.com/us/en/products/mobility/mobility-scooters/compact-travel-scooters/phoenix-hd-4/p/583-1.)*

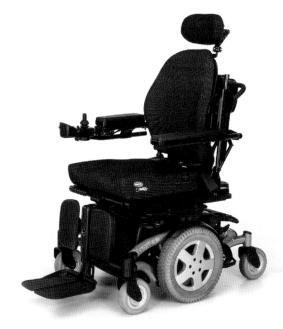

FIG. 14.9 Power mobility device (PMD). *(From Pendleton H, Schultz-Krohn W. Pedretti's Occupational Therapy – Practice Skills for Physical Dysfunction, 8th edn. Chapter 11. Mobility, Figure 11.3B.)*

category are lightweight and can be easily transported by breaking down into smaller parts.[60] Because they are lightweight, they have small batteries, which decreases the distance that they can cover. These devices, like standard wheelchairs, are intended for temporary use.

Power mobility devices (PMD) should be examined for clients that require a power option for full-time use, do not need specialized seating or power seating features, and can perform independent to minimal assist transfers (Fig. 14.9).[60] These power chairs feature larger drive wheels to navigate uneven terrain, more powerful drive motors for durability and speed, increased suspension, and larger batteries for longer use. The seating on these chairs is usually a "captain's seat" style, but some models can accommodate more specialized seating.

For older adults who are full-time users and are dependent on caregivers for most of their ADLs, a PMD with complex rehabilitation technology (CRT) is the best option (Fig. 14.10).[60] Power chairs in this category can accommodate custom seating, alternative drive methods, and power seating functions. Aside from the standard joystick used to operate some POVs and PMDs, CRT power chairs can be operated by different styles of joysticks, head arrays, sip and puff mechanisms, and even eye gaze. Switches can be added to the wheelchair to control specific functions if the user is unable to reach or utilize the traditional controls. Some options can be added to control a user's environment as well, such as using the joystick as a computer mouse or to operate their smartphone, controlling smart home functions, and controlling communication devices. These chairs also offer power seating functions to assist

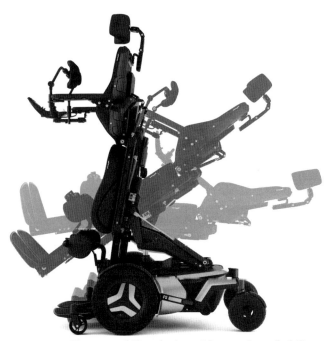

FIG. 14.10 Power mobility device with complex rehabilitation technology (CRT). *(From permobile.com. https://www. permobil.com/en-us/products/power-wheelchairs/permobil-f5-corpus-vs.)*

with positioning and pressure relief.[60] Power elevating leg rests allow the user to adjust the angle of the leg rests to allow for more ground clearance when navigating obstacles. They are also able to achieve a flat lying position for pain relief, rest, caregiver assist with ADLs, and have the ability to raise the feet above heart level to aid in lower extremity edema reduction.[60] The power seat elevator lifts the entire seating surface around 12" so that the user can access objects in higher places, interact at eye level for those who are standing, increase independence with transfers to surfaces with varying heights, and improve the visual field in crowded areas.[60]

ASSESSMENT

The first step in determining the type of wheelchair, seating, and positioning accessories that are needed is to assess the client's strength and skeletal and musculoskeletal abnormalities. Skeletal abnormalities can either be fixed and must be accommodated for, or flexible and can be corrected. Ideally, the physical assessment of the client should take place on a stable surface like a mat table, not in a mobility device.[61] While performing this assessment, the occupational therapy practitioner should use their hands as if they are the support surfaces for each area of the body. This will give the practitioner a feel for how much pressure is required to correct or accommodate a deformity.[61] Too much pressure at a single point will lead to skin breakdown. After the mat evaluation, the OT will interpret the results of the assessment and the OTA and OT can then discuss the best options for the client. Medicare requires that certain areas be addressed during the seating and mobility evaluation. The Houston Methodist Functional Mobility and Wheelchair Assessment was designed to satisfy the Medicare algorithm and is a great guide for obtaining the required information.[62] See Additional Resources below on how to obtain a copy of this assessment.

The Pelvis

The first area of the body to assess when attempting to reduce any postural instability in a seated position is the pelvis.[61] For the pelvis to effectively support a seated person, it should be in a flat, level, and neutral position.[59] The most common misalignment of the pelvis is pelvic tilt, with posterior pelvic tilt being more prevalent than anterior pelvic tilt. Posterior pelvic tilt is often seen in conjunction with kyphosis.[51] If the person presents with a mild posterior tilt, an antithrust cushion can be enough to correct the posture. For more involved cases, the addition of a two-point pelvic belt with pads may be required.[51] If the posterior pelvic tilt is fixed, then accommodations will need to be made, typically by using a cushion to offload and redistribute pressure.[51] If the client presents with flexible or fixed anterior tilt, the use of the two-point belt with pads is suggested. Another solution for anterior pelvic tilt is the use of a tilt-in-space wheelchair that places the client in a position where gravity can assist in pulling the lumbar spine back toward neutral, decreasing the pressure on the spine, and increasing the comfort of the individual.[63]

Another misalignment of the pelvis is right and left pelvis rotation. This is typically a result of a neuromuscular condition that increases muscle tone and twists the body.[61] If the rotation is flexible, it can be corrected by using either a two-point pelvic belt or a four-point pelvic belt depending on the intensity of the rotation.

The final pelvic misalignment is pelvic obliquity. This occurs, typically, in conjunction with scoliosis and presents as either the right or left iliac crest being higher than the opposite side. If the person presents with a flexible obliquity, building up the cushion under the lower IT will help to align the pelvis back to neutral. If the obliquity is fixed, building up the cushion under the higher IT and removing material under the lower IT will help to distribute the pressure evenly across a greater surface area.

The Lower Extremities

After assessing the pelvis, the lower extremities should be examined next, beginning with the hips. This part of the assessment should begin by measuring strength as this can help to narrow down the type of mobility device that may be needed.[61] If a client is able to ambulate short distances and can transfer in and out of the wheelchair independently, they may not require a CRT device. Next, hip ROM and thigh positioning are measured.[61] Increasing the seat to back angle of the chair, or "opening it up," will accommodate a lack of hip flexion preventing the person from sliding forward in the chair. If the person has a lack of hip extension and remains in flexion, a seat wedge which lowers the rear seat height in relation to the front could provide the needed support. If there is tightness toward adduction, but it is flexible, the use of a medial thigh support (or abductor pad) or placing the lower legs in a different position may relive the problem.[61] Adduction tightness is especially common in users of standard wheelchairs with sling seats, placing the person at risk of skin breakdown over the medial condyles and making hygiene tasks difficult. If the tendency is toward abduction, then the use of lateral thigh supports is indicated. Like adduction, abduction could be a result of external hip rotation and could also be addressed by positioning the lower legs differently.[61] This is prevalent with clients who are overweight. Due to additional medial thigh tissue, the hips are forced into abduction and external rotation. Hip abduction left unaddressed poses a safety risk as they are likely to strike their knees on corners, doorways, and protrusive obstacles.

Knee ROM and lower leg positioning should be assessed next. If a client tends to pull the knees into flexion and it cannot be comfortably corrected, then the seat depth may need to be shortened and cushioned with an undercut used to accommodate for the legs being tucked underneath the chair. If the tendency toward knee flexion can be corrected, the use of a calf straps, ankle straps, or shoe holders may be needed. If this is unaddressed, the feet could end up getting caught under the chair which can pull the client out of the chair or possibly cause a fracture. The use of ankle straps or shoe holders can be successful with flexible extension issues as well. Fixed knee flexion may require the use of elevating leg rests to support the lower leg in a comfortable position.

Finally, the ROM and positioning of the feet and ankles need to be assessed.[61] If able to be placed into a neutral position, the foot should be fully supported by the footplate.[61] If the foot and ankle are prone to or fixed in dorsiflexion, an adjustment in the angle of the footplate with the addition of something to block the heel should be enough to accommodate for this. If the tendency is toward plantarflexion, adjusting the angle of the footplates may be enough, or the person may need a padded foot box. A foot box made of iscoelastic foam or gel-infused foam will help to reduce the amount of pressure placed at the point of contact at the base of the foot box and can also be a viable solution to ankle inversion and eversion, depending on flexibility.

The Trunk

Once the pelvis and lower extremities have been considered, the strength and posture of the trunk can be assessed. Trunk strength will determine the type of back rest, the height of the back rest, if lateral trunk supports are needed, and if any additional anterior supports are needed.[61] The lower the strength, the more positioning that individual will require. Clients who have experienced cerebrovascular accidents will sometimes present with hemiplegia that can cause an individual to lean to one side, requiring the use of lateral supports. A deficit in trunk strength, with no evidence of skeletal deformation, can cause someone to fall forward when placed in an upright position. This can be corrected by slight adjustment to the seat-to-back angle, the use of a tilt-in-space wheelchair, or by utilizing shoulder straps or a chest harness.

Spinal deformities must also be considered in determining the amount of trunk support needed. As previously mentioned, the most common spinal abnormality found in the older adult population is kyphosis.[51] If addressing the pelvis is not enough to remedy the problem, the seat-to-back angle should be increased, and the backrest should be examined. There are several options for backrests on the market that can accommodate kyphosis. This is a situation where the ATP's knowledge of the availability of different products can assist in selecting the best solution for the client.

Another spinal deformity, lordosis, the excessive inward curve of the spine, can be more challenging to manage. In mild cases of lordosis, it is recommended to increase the seat to back angle and employ a backrest for increased lumbar support.[64] In more extreme cases, a common solution is to use a tilt-in-space wheelchair to allow gravity to assist in positioning and prevent collapsing of the spine.

Scoliosis, a sideways curvature of the spine, is the final spinal deformity among older adults that is commonly addressed. Correcting and supporting scoliosis requires three points of contact (Fig. 14.11) using two lateral trunk supports and one lateral hip support.[65] The pads of the lateral

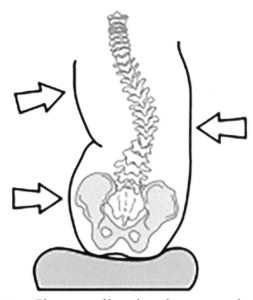

FIG. 14.11 Placement of lateral trunk supports—three points of contact. *(From leckey.com. https://www.leckey.com/products/mygo-seat.)*

trunk supports should be big enough to distribute as much pressure as possible without interfering with function.

The Upper Extremities

Assessment of the upper extremities can be a determining factor between a manual wheelchair and a power wheelchair, and the type needed. For this reason, assessment of the upper extremities should begin with determination of strength.[61] Cervical spinal cord injuries can present with varying degrees of weakness in the distal upper extremity. This can affect the grip on the handrim of a manual wheelchair. If this is the case, protrusions can be added to the handrim to provide something to push against. If an individual does not possess the strength to propel a manual wheelchair, a tilt-in-space manual or power wheelchair should be considered.[60,63] If a client who is using a power chair is unable to maintain placement of the arms on the armrests while in a tilted position, the use of an arm trough or an elbow prop combined with forearm laterals should be considered. ROM should also be assessed at this time. If a client in unable to fully extend the elbow during propulsion, this will decrease the amount of force applied and increase the amount of energy needed.[57] For someone who has limited external rotation, placing the joystick control more midline could allow for independent use of a power wheelchair.

The upper extremities can also assist in supporting the trunk and maintaining an upright posture. If there is edema and developing contractures in a hemiplegic upper extremity resulting from a CVA, the use of elevating hardware on an arm trough with an appropriate hand prop should be considered. If someone has hemiplegia and a subluxed shoulder, and tends to lean toward the affected side, securing the affected arm in an arm trough can reduce pain by keeping the humeral head in contact with the glenoid surface and provide enough pressure to help counteract the tendency to lean. This can also positively affect the position of the head and neck.

The Head and Neck

A neutral neck and head position and neck strength are important to the most basic of human functions such as breathing and swallowing, and the accessible visual field.[66] A kyphotic posture can cause the cervical and craniocervical extensor muscles to fatigue quickly from having to overcome the curve of the spine in order to eat, see, and interact with others.[66] To accommodate for this flexion, a slight tilt to the seating may be enough to overcome gravity and weakness, if the ROM allows. In this position, a standard contoured headrest would be sufficient to support the head. A headrest with adjustable "wings" or lateral supports may be considered if lateral control is compromised. Some type of anterior head support should be considered if extension ROM is restricted, which also decreases the progression of the contracture. Anterior head supports are typically a strap mounted to the headrest that goes around the forehead. This type of support may result in cervical protrusion, further complicating breathing and swallowing. Another option is a cervical collar with a chin prompt that can eliminate the protrusion but may interfere with eating and communication. A cervical collar can also be useful in minimizing the effects of torticollis.

ROLE OF THE OTA AFTER DELIVERY OF MOBILITY DEVICE

After a mobility device has been selected and delivered to the client, the OTA continues their involvement by training the client, family members, and caregivers how to safely use and operate the mobility device.[49] Because the device will be integral to the client's functional movement and participation in ADLs, therapy practitioners will need to provide MRADL training. Safe and proper use of a mobility devices is especially important for older adults with a mobility disability as they are at increased risk of developing a chronic condition related to use of the device. The most prevalent of these is chronic conditions is arthritis, typically in the shoulders.[67]

With adequate training and knowledge, an additional role of the OTA is to make adjustments to all but the most complex seating systems. Most mobility devices and their components require a small number of basic tools in order to make necessary adjustments. By combining this skill with the ability to recognize improper positioning, the OTA can be an invaluable asset to the team, client, and their family, even after delivery of the mobility device.

CONCLUSION

When working with older adults, it is important to keep in mind that every client, even if those with the same diagnosis will present differently and will have their own specific set of circumstances that determine individual goals and the interventions used to achieve those goals. The responsibility of occupational therapy is to help individuals increase their ability to functionally participate in their occupations, thus increasing their quality of life.[49] The responsibility of an OTA is to recognize a client's need and advocate for a proper wheeled mobility device with the appropriate seating and positioning devices. This should be determined by an assessment of their skeletal and musculoskeletal limitations to allow older adults to interact with their environment and participate in their chosen occupations. When the optimal configuration is reached, it can provide comfort, independence, increased function, increased socialization, and a decrease in further medical complications. As the older adult population continues to grow, it is imperative that seating, positioning, and mobility independence remain an important part of occupational therapy interventions.

ADDITIONAL RESOURCES

- Lange ML, Minkel JL. Seating and Wheeled Mobility: A Clinical Resource Guide. Thorofare, NJ: Slack Incorporated; 2018.
- Permobil's resource guides: https://hub.permobil.com/permobil-resources
- To pursue an ATP certificate or to find an ATP in your area visit: https://www.resna.org/
- Houston Methodist Functional Mobility and Wheelchair Assessment: https://www.numotion.com/blog/october-2017/best-practice-houston-methodist-functional-mobili

STEPHANIE JOHNSON
(PREVIOUS CONTRIBUTIONS FROM LOU JENSEN, SANDRA HATTORI OKADA, AND CANDICE MULLENDORE)

PART 3   Fall Prevention

Falls among older adults are a complex and significant health problem that can lead to participation restrictions, activity limitations, altered living situations (e.g., premature nursing home admissions), injury, and even death. A fall is "an unexpected event in which the participant comes to rest on the ground, floor, or lower level."[68] Roughly one out of every four adults age 65 and older experience at least one fall per year with a higher increase in likelihood of falls, if female, over 85 years of age, or of Alaskan Native or American Indian ethnicity.[69] Accidental falls are the leading cause of nonfatal injuries treated in hospital emergency departments in all adult age groups (except 10–24 year olds), and nonfatal falls are the leading cause of hospital admissions in older adults.[70,71] Of those older adults hospitalized for injuries related to a fall, about half are discharged to nursing homes.[72] While falls may not result in injury, approximately 20% of falls result in serious injury, including various fractures and head trauma.[73,74] Approximately 95% of hip fractures are due to falls. Older adults who sustain a hip fracture as a result of a fall have an increased risk of mortality within 1 year of 33% and an overall higher mortality rate than the general population for at least 10 years.[75-77] Unintentional falls are the leading cause of death from injury in those age 65 and older.[78] Falls that do not cause physical injury often cause a fear of falling that results in a decrease in occupational participation and independence, and impairments in client factors such as strength and balance because of a decrease in overall activity level.[79,80] Of those older adults that fall, only roughly half, notify their physician of the fall, with women more often discussing a fall with their physician versus men.[81]

Considering the above discussion, let us look at Jona and her experience with a fall.

Jona is a 74-year-old woman who was recently widowed. Jona is independent in most of her basic ADL but had required her husband to assist her in getting into and out of her bathtub. Since his death, Jona has attempted this task by herself but has had several near-falls. She was accustomed to relying on her husband, Nathan, for many instrumental activities of daily living (IADL) such as housework, yard maintenance, shopping, and driving. Jona has the reputation among her friends as being a wonderful cook, but in recent years, she was finding herself relying on her husband to be her "eyes in the kitchen" as Jona's macular degeneration was progressing, making it increasingly difficult to read the dial on the stove and to see as she prepared meals. After her husband's death, Jona has had increasing difficulty keeping up with her home maintenance. Additionally, she does not want to burden her friends and neighbors for transportation, so she has drastically decreased time spent in activities outside of her home such as medical appointments, church activities, and other social events. This decrease in physical activity coupled with situational depression has left Jona feeling isolated, weak, and fearful of the future.

Recently, Jona was visiting on the phone with her daughter who lives out of state and admitted that she has fallen inside her home twice in the past week. Jona's daughter is quite concerned and encouraged her mother to visit with her physician. Jona is hesitant, stating, "I don't want to tell my doctor I fell! The next thing you know, I'll have to move into a nursing home, and I can't bear to leave my house. If I leave here, I'm afraid my memories of Nathan will quickly fade away. This is my home! I want to stay here."

The effect of a fall on the life of an older adult alone emphasizes the importance of including fall prevention into the care plan of any older adult. However, the financial effect of falls on the health care system and society adds additional justification for addressing this important health problem. In the United States, the total cost of fatal and nonfatal fall-related injuries of older adults is estimated at $50 billion.[82]

On an individual level, costs associated with a fall-produced fracture are $58,120 for the first year and $86,967 for a lifetime.[83] As the older adult population increases in the next 30 years, so will the incidence of falls and the costs associated with them. Therefore, it is important for OTAs to be knowledgeable about the risk factors and causes associated with falls, as well as how the occupational therapy process can be used to effectively reduce falls in older adults.

RISK FACTORS AND CAUSES OF FALLS

Falls are multifactorial in nature and can have a variety of precipitating causes (Box 14.3). Older adults are particularly vulnerable to falls because of the increased prevalence of intrinsic risk factors such as comorbid clinical conditions, multiple medication regiments, cognitive disorders, and age-related physiological changes (e.g., decreased vision and decreased muscle strength).[84-86] More important, a delicate balance exists between intrinsic factors and common environmental hazards; even a small disruption in this dynamic system can lead to a devastating fall. For example, an accidental trip over a new throw rug may cause a fall that could be attributed to the throw rug (i.e., the environment). However, the fall could have been more likely because the older adult had

BOX 14.3

Causes of and Risk Factors for Falls in Elderly Persons	
CAUSE	**RISK FACTOR**
Accident and environment related	Lower extremity weakness
	History of falls
Gait and balance disorders or weakness	Gait deficit
	Balance deficit
Dizziness and vertigo	Use of assistive device
Drop attack	Visual deficit
Confusion	Arthritis
Postural hypotension	Impaired ADL
Visual disorder	Depression
Syncope	Cognitive impairment
	Age >80 years

Data from Rubenstein LZ, Josephson, KR. Falls and their prevention in elderly people: What does the evidence show? *Medi Clin North Am.* 2006;90;807-824.

impaired vision, lower extremity weakness, and balance deficits (i.e., intrinsic risk factors). Falls in the older adult population can occur in a variety of environments, including the home, community, hospital, or nursing home.[87]

Environmental Causes

Accidents related to the environment are the primary cause of falls among older adults, comprising 31% of falls.[87] According to the National Institute on Aging, 6 out of every 10 falls occurs at home.[88] Disease processes associated with aging are often strong determinants for falls, but environmental factors in the home also have an effect.[84,85] About 28% of older adults are aging in place, a 30% increase from previous decades, increasing the need for older adults to be safe in their own home.[1] A poorly kept home or yard may be an environmental sign of age-related changes. As people age, they may lose the endurance, strength, and cognitive ability to structure tasks and deal with their environment. Common environmental hazards in the home include poor lighting or glare, uneven stairs, lack of handrails by stairs, and uneven or unsafe surfaces (frayed rug edges, slippery floors in the shower and tub, polished floors, cracks in cement, high doorsteps, and so on). Other hazards may involve old, unstable, or low furniture (chairs, beds, or toilets); pets; young children; clutter or electric cords in walkways; inaccessible items; and limited space for ADL functions (Fig. 14.12). New, used, or improperly installed equipment and unfamiliar environments may also be hazardous.

According to Carpenter and colleagues, approximately 55% of falls in the older adult population occur outside of the home.[86] Common areas in the community where falls occur include public buildings, streets, sidewalks, transferring to or from transportation, or another person's home. In addition, the greatest proportion of persons with repeated falls occur in the community, specifically on

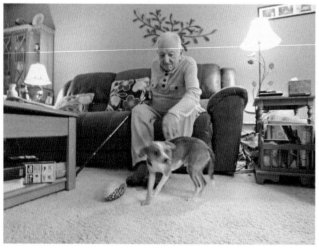

FIG. 14.12 Common potential hazards that may cause falls include rugs and pets that may get under foot.

the street or sidewalk. The most common activities that older adults engage in when they fall include walking on uneven ground, tripping (over curbs, rugs, or objects), and slipping on wet surfaces. Other examples of activities associated with falls include lifting heavy objects, reaching, balancing on items of unstable support (overturned box), or turning quickly. Therefore, the OTA should take into consideration the context and environment, as well as the activity engaged in during a fall when determining a fall prevention plan.[86]

Biological Causes

Sensory

Visual changes associated with aging that may influence falls include decreases in depth perception, peripheral vision, color discrimination, acuity, and accommodation. Approximately, 30% of persons age 65 and older have visual impairments. This number is expected to dramatically increase as the youngest of the Baby Boomer generation reaches 65 by the year of 2029.[89,90] By the year 2050, it is expected that nearly 8 million Americans will have some sort of visual impairment or blindness.[91]

Older adults visual impairment can affect a person's ability to participate in functional mobility in the home and in the community, such as stair or curb navigation, with 75% of all stair accidents occurring while descending and most frequently occurring in the bottom half of the stairs.[32,92] While bifocals or trifocals may assist in visual correction, they require adjustment time for visual use. Stair navigation also requires increased motor coordination, requiring increased head and eye adjustments.

Medical conditions affecting vision include macular degeneration, cataracts, diabetic retinopathy, glaucoma, and stroke.[89,90] These conditions may manifest as scotomas (blind spots), which may impair safety in mobility and make objects in one's walking path not apparent, such as telephone cords, small animals, or even furniture. Decreased visual input caused by disease processes may result in a decrease in postural stability.[93] In turn, this affects an older adult's balance and may contribute to the greater incidence of falls among this population.

A disorder involving spatial organization or figure ground may cause older adults to perceptualize incorrect variances in their environment. For example, an older adult may perceive a change in rug color or flooring as a stair or a glare on the linoleum as spilled liquid. A dark stairway may be perceived as a ramp. Misinterpreting this information may cause a misjudged step and a fall. (Chapter 15 provides more detailed information on age-related changes in vision and recommended adaptations.)

Vestibular disorders that cause dizziness and vertigo may also contribute to falls. One such disorder leading to dizziness is benign paroxysmal positional vertigo (BPPV), which is a mechanical vestibular problem caused by displaced otoconia in the inner ear as a result of trauma or age and is the most common cause of vertigo in persons over the age of 65 years.[94] BPPV can cause severe dizziness and vertigo, especially with changes in position or head movements. An older adult, particularly one who has a history of falls, may be susceptible to this disorder, possibly leading to an increase in falls. BPPV is treatable, however, through vestibular rehabilitation and specific therapeutic techniques, which may decrease the likelihood of falls as a result of this diagnosis.[95]

Neurological/musculoskeletal

Conditions that affect posture and body alignment cause changes in the center of gravity, gait, stride, strength, and joint stability, all of which increase the risk for falls. Age-related changes in postural control include decreased proprioception, slower righting reflexes, decreased muscle tone, and increased postural sway.[93] Changes in gait include decreased height of stepping; also, men tend to have a more flexed posture and wide-based, short-stepped gait, whereas women tend to have a more narrow-based, waddling gait.[96] Medical conditions that affect instability include degenerative joint disease, deconditioning, malnutrition, dehydration, and neurological disorders such as neuropathy, stroke, Parkinson's disease, and dementia.[32,92,94] Older adult women are more susceptible to brittle bones as they age, with a greater incidence of osteoporosis after menopause. In the case of brittle bones, it may be a fractured bone that causes the fall rather than the fall causing the fracture. However, falls in older adults cause 90% of the incidence of hip fractures.[97] Musculoskeletal conditions that contribute to falls in older adults include osteoarthritis, spondylosis, and a general decrease in joint range of motion.[96]

Various conditions can also impact gait in specific ways; for example, a person may drag a foot or lose their balance toward their weaker side (CVA) or present with a shuffling gait (Parkinson's disease). To compensate for changes in gait and decreased balance, older adults may "furniture glide" by holding on to furniture for support while they walk (Fig. 14.13). Older adults may hold on to faucets or towel racks to get into the tub or shower or lean against the shower wall for stability while bathing. Each of these may increase the likelihood of falls. Furniture gliding, holding onto towel racks or faucets are generally not recommended and should be avoided; if utilizing, another option, such as a mobility aid, should be assessed and offered to improve functional stability and balance.

Cardiovascular

Age-related changes include orthostatic hypotension, which affects approximately 30% of the older adult population and are a significant risk factor for falls among older adults.[92,98] Other medical conditions that cause blood pressure changes include hypertension, neuropathy, and diabetes. In addition, these changes can occur as side effects of certain medications. Arrhythmias may cause up to 50% of syncopal episodes (temporary loss in

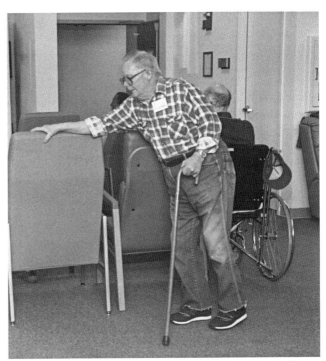

FIG. 14.13   Older adults often "furniture glide" by holding on to furniture to compensate for changes in gait and decreased balance.

consciousness due to a drop in blood pressure) in older adults.[92] Older adults may experience a greater incidence of dizziness or light-headedness, with lower cardiac output, autonomic dysfunction, impaired venous return, and prolonged bed rest. Underlying cardiac disease is the most common cause of syncope that may result in a fall.[84] Together with extrinsic or environmental factors, these biological or intrinsic factors are the primary causes of falls among older adults.[32,87]

Cognitive/Psychosocial Causes

Psychosocial and cognitive risk factors that may influence falls include poor judgment insight, and problem-solving skills; confusion; and inattention resulting from fatigue, depression, and dementia. Other factors may include reactions to psychotropic medications, fear of falling, unfamiliarity with a new environment or caregiver, and a strong drive for independence. Functional mobility requires a balance between strength, coordination, balance, and reaction time. Cognitive risk factors that may influence one's ability to safely navigate include attention, inhibitory control, and executive functioning skills, such as problem solving, judgment, and awareness. Decline in the aforementioned cognitive skills may yield a decline in overall stability, gait speed, and an increase in likelihood of falls, including falls with serious injury.[99,100] Anxiety, fear of falling, and other fall-related psychosocial concerns, such as balance confidence should also be considered for older adults when assessing fall risk, as well as family support, knowledge, concern for a caregiver's fall risk, and family dynamic.[101-102] Older adults and their families may not comply with recommended safety modifications because of cultural or personal preferences, esthetic values, and limited financial or social resources. Consequently, both the caregiver and the client are at greater risk for having a fall.

Depression and psychotropic medications have both been associated with an increased fall risk. Depression increases the risk of falling two-fold, presumably because of an inattention to the environment and a disregard for safety.[87] Metaanalyses concluded that not enough has been done to address fall risk due to depression and psychotropic medications.[103] Recent research demonstrates that gradually reducing the use of psychotropic medications significantly reduces an older adult's risk of falling, providing an additional intervention option for fall reduction in older adults.[104]

Functional Causes

As stated in the 2018 *Profile of Older Americans* report, retrieved from the US Census Bureau, American Community Survey and National Center for Health Statistics, National Health Interview Survey, 35% of older adults (aged 65 years and older) reported some type of disability and 46% of individuals 75 years of age and older, reported difficulty with physical functioning (twice the rate of those aged 45–64 years).[105] The report details that of those aged 65+, 14% reported difficulty living independently, 8% reported difficulty with basic self-care; 22% reported difficulty with ambulation; 9% reported cognitive decline; and 20% reported vision or hearing difficulties.[105]

Functional mobility problems that may lead to falls include difficulty with performing transfers (to or from a lounge chair, bed, toilet, tub or shower, wheelchair, and car), dressing and bathing (especially the lower body), reaching, sitting, standing, and walking unsupported. Other factors may include the lack of assistive devices for ambulation or an inability to use them correctly. Older adults with dementia may forget where they left a cane or walk carrying their walker rather than using it for support. Old, lost, borrowed, or smudged glasses may impair vision. Poorly fitting shoes, loose pants with dragging hems, and flimsy sandals or flip-flops can affect balance. Falls most commonly occur in places where older adults perform most self-care activities: by the bed and in the bathroom.[32]

Knowledge of the most common risk factors and causes of falls in older adults can significantly inform the occupational therapy process, as described in the fourth edition of the *Occupational Therapy Practice Framework: Domain and Process*.[55] OTAs are important team members in all parts of the process and therefore must understand components of a comprehensive fall risk assessment, fall prevention and reduction interventions, and meaningful ways to measure the outcomes of interventions designed to reduce falls in the older adult population.

EVALUATION

Because falls in older adults typically result from a combination of several intrinsic and extrinsic risk factors, multiple precipitating causes, and in a variety of environments, fall prevention strategies, education, and goal setting are vital for the entire health care team. Team members, including the OTA, can collaborate to perform an accurate evaluation of the client and to obtain a detailed fall history before designing an individualized fall prevention program. Stevens and Colleagues reported less than half of older adults who fell discussed the fall with their physician, and less than one-third who discussed the fall also discussed fall prevention techniques with their physicians.[81] Open communication with the health care team or family regarding falls is essential. Older adults may be ashamed to admit that they have fallen or may fear they will be forced to leave their home or lose their independence if they disclose a fall. Conversely, older adults may not consider it important or relevant to report a fall in which no injury was sustained. However, open and honest communication is important to successfully address fall prevention. The OT/OTA team can collaborate to obtain a complete occupational profile that includes fall-related history and must make the establishment of therapeutic rapport a priority to ensure that the information is complete and accurate.

OTAs, in collaboration with OTs, are well equipped to assess older adults fall risk, educate on fall prevention strategies, and provide other resources. In addition to assessing client risk factors related to body structures and functions and performance skills, an interview to obtain an accurate history of falls is necessary. Body functions that need to be assessed can include but are not limited to: mental functions, such as cognition, attention, and memory; sensory function, such as vision, proprioception, sensation, and pain; and neuromuscular functions, such as joint mobility and stability, muscle strength, endurance, and tone, balance, functional ambulation.[55] Careful attention to blood pressure, especially orthostatic hypotension should be noted, recorded, and assessed for as well.[106] When assessing for history of falls, clients should be asked to describe the frequency, timing, and location of their fall(s); the activities they were involved in during their fall(s) and any devices or equipment used; their medical history and symptoms; and medications taken and their side effects.[32,107] Near-fall experiences, where clients lost their balance but were able to stop the fall with an environmental object such as a grab bar, should also be recorded. Such events need to be addressed as they could have been a more serious incident had the environmental object not been present to break the fall.[32] If an older adult reports no history of falling, care should still be taken to identify potential risk factors. When asking about functional status, OTAs should not only ask whether the older adult is able to perform ADL functions but also observe the way these are done. In other words, the OT evaluation process includes obtaining a detailed occupational profile and analyzing occupational performance.[55]

For example, when the OTA asked Jona whether she could get off the toilet by herself, she responded that she was independent with toileting. When the OTA asked her to demonstrate this transfer, Jona hooked her cane on a towel rack to pull herself off of the toilet. The OTA was able to determine a high risk for falling only because the transfer was observed. If the OTA had simply accepted Jona's report of independence, she would not have been able to recommend a raised toilet seat and toilet rails or replacement of the towel racks with sturdy grab bars.

Performance patterns, including habits, routines, and roles should also be assessed during the evaluation process. Inclusion about beliefs about falls, fall understanding and knowledge for the client and caregiver, risk patterns, and home and community access is also needed. If possible, a home assessment would be beneficial to determine safety implications within the natural environment for the client.[106,108]

The extensiveness of the evaluation process and team members involved depends on the planned fall prevention strategy. An interdisciplinary team approach may be the most beneficial method to address fall prevention. For example, occupational therapy practitioners are well suited to address safe performance of daily occupations and the home environment. A referral to physical therapy may be indicated to address weakness, balance and coordination deficits, and overall endurance. A nutritionist or dietitian may be included to determine the adequacy of a client's diet and whether modifications that would improve overall health and strength need to be made. Pharmacists can review medications and potential side effects that may lead to an increased risk of falling. Referrals to any number of medical specialists could be indicated if a client has an underlying medical condition that affects their fall risk. Once the necessary referrals are made and the team has established goals with the client, intervention can begin.

FALL PREVENTION INTERVENTIONS

Rubenstein and Josephson classified current fall prevention interventions for older adults into five broad categories: multidimensional fall risk assessment and risk reduction; exercise-based intervention; environmental assessment and modification; institutional approaches; and multifactorial approaches, including medical management of the older adult.[87] OTAs can be involved, in varying degrees, in each of these interventions.

Several Cochrane systematic reviews of the available evidence for preventing falls in older people have been conducted. One Cochrane review for preventing falls of older adults living in the community considered 159 randomized controlled trials with 79,193 participants.[104] This review targeted exercise-based interventions and multifactorial trials. Findings were a significant reduction of rate and risk of falls with multiple-component

group exercise. Tai chi as an exercise approach showed statistical significance in reducing the risk of falls and was borderline statistically significant in reducing the rate of falls. Furthermore, multifactorial intervention involving individual risk assessments and interventions for fall prevention reduced the rate but not risk for falls. Vitamin D supplements did not decrease falls. Home safety assessments along with home modifications were statistically effective in reducing risks of falls, especially for people with severe visual impairments and for people at increased risk. An exciting finding from this Cochrane review was that home safety interventions appear most effective when completed by occupational therapy practitioners.[104]

Another Cochrane review focused on fall prevention interventions in care facilities and hospitals.[109] It included 60 studies with 60,345 participants in care facilities and 17 studies with 29,972 participants from hospitals. A finding was that multifactorial interventions in hospitals did decrease the fall rate, but the research evidence for risk of falling was not conclusive. In care facilities, findings were that vitamin D reduced falls likely because residents had low levels.[109] Findings were not clear from the 13 studies on the effect of exercise on fall prevention, and some studies even found exercise programs as nonbeneficial. It was surmised that these nonbeneficial exercise programs might have increased the fall risk among frail older adults.[109] However, multifactorial interventions that targeted multiple fall risks were found to be effective in care facilities, but more research is needed. In hospitals, more physiotherapy reduced fall risks on subacute rehabilitation units as well as those targeting multiple risk factors.[109]

The American Geriatric Society (AGS) and the British Geriatric Society (BGS) published clinical practice guidelines for fall prevention with older adults based on levels of evidence from the research for assessment and intervention of older adults living in the community and care facilities.[110] An included rating system built on research findings identifies intervention that helps older adults. For example, areas with high recommendation are "exercise programs that incorporate balance, gait, and strength training for all older adults" and specific to community-dwelling older adults are exercises as part of multifactorial intervention.[110] However, with older adults in care facilities who are frail and at risk for injury, exercise programs were given a rating of fair evidence, with modification of home environments receiving the highest level of recommendation.[110]

OTAs are encouraged to consider these guidelines along with the discussed Cochrane reviews with assessment and intervention. Based on these guidelines, the Centers for Disease Control developed the initiative of STEADI (Stopping Elderly Accidents, Deaths, and Injuries); this initiative aims to standardize health care providers screening process for clients (aged 65+) fall risk, as well as modifiable risk factors and interventions to reduce falls.[111] OTs and OTAs are both vital members of the interdisciplinary team, which can help screen, educate, and then treat clients who are at risk for a fall. Free training is available for the STEADI program via the CDC's STEADI-Older Adult Fall Prevention Web page.[111]

Multidimensional Fall Risk Assessment and Risk Reduction

The goal of the multidimensional approach for fall prevention in the older adult population is to target the multiple risk factors associated with falls to reduce fall risk, most often including some sort of combination of both exercise and education.[112] This approach can be used for both individuals and populations. For example, a multidimensional fall prevention program can be offered to a population of community-dwelling well older adults to educate them on ways to prevent falls (Table 14.4) and to screen older adults to determine their fall risk. Health fairs and community educational programs are two examples of a population-based multidimensional approach for fall prevention. Conversely, an individualized multidimensional fall prevention program may be instituted for an older adult who has a history of falls or is at high risk for falling, targeting: education about roles, habits, and routines that may contribute to falls; improvement of physical abilities; and/or home modifications suggestions.[113] In either case (individual or population based), fall risk assessment precedes intervention and consists of a fall history, general medical and medication history, and an assessment of client factors and performance skills. Elliott and Leland found within a systematic review strong evidence for multicomponent group-based fall prevention interventions (exercise + education); mixed evidence for individually tailored multifactorial (target clients multiple fall risks) fall prevention interventions; moderate evidence for population-based fall prevention interventions; and mixed evidence for single component fall prevention interventions.[112] As a result of the review, the authors recommended within occupational therapy

TABLE 14.4

Checklist for Fall Prevention for Older Adults at Home

Area	Considerations	Possible interventions
Floors	Do you have a clear path to walk around furniture?	Ask someone to move the furniture so your path is clear.
	Are there any throw rugs on the floor?	Remove rugs, or use nonslip backing so the rugs won't slip. If you use a walker, remove rugs from the home because they can catch on the walker and cause a fall.
	Are there objects (e.g., books, shoes, boxes, papers) on the floor?	Pick up things that are on the floor. Always keep objects off of the floor.
	Are there wires or lamp cords on the floor that you must walk over?	Tape electrical cords and wires to the wall to prevent tripping on them. An electrician may need to install another outlet.
Stairs and steps	Are there papers, shoes, or other objects on the stairs?	Remove all objects from the stairs.
	Is there a light over the stairway?	Have an electrician install an overhead light at the top and bottom of the stairs. Make sure you have a light switch at the top and bottom of the stairs, and preferably a switch that glows for nighttime.
	Are the handrails loose or broken? Are they on both sides of the stairs?	Make sure handrails are on both sides of the stairs and as long as the stairs.
Kitchen	Are the most frequently used items on high shelves?	Move frequently used items to lower shelves. (Keep these at waist level.)
	Is your step-stool unsteady?	It is best not to use a step-stool, but if you must, get a sturdy one with a bar to hold on to. Never use a chair as a step-stool.
Bathroom	Is the tub or shower floor slippery?	Place a nonslip rubber mat on the floor of the tub or shower.
	Is there a grab bar in place near the tub or shower for stability when entering?	Have a carpenter install a grab bar inside the tub or next to the shower.
	Is it difficult to get up from the toilet?	Consider a toilet riser or having a grab bar installed near the toilet to help in rising from the toilet.
Bedroom	Is there a light near the bed within easy reach?	Place a lamp close to the bed where it is easy to reach.
	Is the path dark from your bed to the toilet?	Use a night-light to see where you are walking during the night.

TABLE 14.5

Evidence-Based Fall Prevention Programs

Name of program	Time frame	Focus
A Matter of Balance[112]	8 weeks: 2 hour session/week	Multidimensional: Address view of falling, increase activity level, exercise, home modifications
Community Aging in Place-Advancing Better Living for Elders (CAPABLE)[113]	5 month structured program	Client directed; home based: Address increasing mobility, functionality, and aging in place. Services provided by OT, nurse, and hand worker
YMCA Moving Better for Balance[114]	12 weeks	Address: mobility, flexibility, strength, and balance through Tai Chi movements
Stepping On[115]	7 weeks; 2 hour session/week	Address: balance, strength, fall hazard topics, vision, medication management

practice that exercise and education occur within multicomponent or population-based fall prevention, as well as individualized fall risk assessment, education, and home assessment. The authors also recommend education of evidenced-based fall prevention programs, such as those listed in Table 14.5 for students within the field of occupational therapy.[112]

Exercise-Based Intervention

As mentioned previously, exercise-based interventions have been found to effectively reduce falls in older adults, especially older adults who are not considered frail.[104,110,116] General strengthening programs incorporated in the older adult's daily routine can help decrease deconditioning, especially that caused by a sedentary lifestyle. In addition to OT-led exercise programs, OTAs may also refer older adults to physical therapy for general lower extremity strengthening and balance exercises.[93] Community exercise programs, such as dancing, water aerobics, swimming, and walking clubs, are also appropriate recommendations.

Activities that target balance can be incorporated into the occupational therapy treatment plan. A careful balance of activities designed to remediate balance with those that allow compensation needs to be considered. As discussed, tai chi is a form of exercise that has been shown to be effective in reducing falls and improving balance.[104,110,117,118] Tai chi focuses on building strength, balance, flexibility, and coordination. Tai Chi Prime, a 6-week program featuring the basics of tai chi and qi gong, has been shown to improve overall mobility, balance, strength, and cognitive skills among community dwelling older adults.[114] Other evidence-based exercise focused groups, some with multidimensional components, are listed in Table 14.5.

Gradual increases in activity are recommended for people with conditions that affect endurance (such as cardiac conditions and deconditioning). Strategically located sturdy chairs may be useful for older adults who require rest periods when going from one room to another. Sitting while bathing and avoiding long hot baths are also recommended. A commode chair by the bed may save energy. Activities that involve straining and holding one's breath (such as during toileting, strenuous transfers, or exercise) can cause light-headedness and should be avoided. Clients should be educated on breathing techniques when completing exercise or daily activities to help prevent the aforementioned complications.

If a fall does occur, older adults need to be aware of techniques for fall recovery and OTAs can also educate to a lifeline support. OTAs should be proactive and educate clients on a more safe way to fall (if a fall does occur), as well as how to recover following a fall.[119] Practice during therapy sessions of how to recover from a fall is recommended.[120] The older adult should be educated with the following considerations that should be taken following a fall. OTAs can assist in tailoring these steps to meet the individual needs of an older adult during therapy sessions that focus on fall prevention and recovery.

Instruct your older adult (if a fall occurs):

1. Do not panic and lie still for a few minutes following a fall, assessing for any injuries and overall how one feels.
2. Look for a sturdy piece of furniture that is close and log roll to one's side, then stomach slowly, making sure no dizziness occurs.
3. Push up onto hands and knees, again making sure no dizziness occurs.
4. Crawl to the sturdy piece of furniture and place hands on the furniture.
5. Move one foot forward, leaving the other leg and foot bent in contact with the floor.
6. Push up slowly with hands and foot that is forward to sit in the chair.
7. Rest, sitting in the chair, until recovered and stable.
8. Notify your physician and caregiver that a fall occurred.[120]

Environmental Assessment and Modifications

As noted in several reviews of research evidence, adaptation of the home is proven to be highly beneficial.[104,110]

Occupational therapy practitioners play a significant role in home adaptations with their focus on the importance of the environment on occupation and are trained to identify the interaction of the person and environment, assisting to identify barriers or features that hinder or support a client's performance in their home.[121] Home safety checklists can be provided to clients and caregivers as a preventive measure as well, such as the STEADI "Check for Safety" brochure.[122]

The following are examples of modifications or adaptive ways to decrease fall risk in various areas of the home:

Bathroom modifications/adaptations may include:

- A tub or shower bench with armrests and back and a handheld shower hose and soap on a rope.
- Grab bars strategically placed in/outside the tub and/or around the toileting area.
- Adaptive equipment, such as a raised toilet seat.
- Throw rugs should be removed, or nonskid backing should be applied under them (applicable throughout the home).
- Nonskid stripping or rubber mats can be placed on tub or shower floors.
- Sliding glass doors should be removed to allow for wider access into the tub.
- A shower curtain may be hung from a pressure mounted bar to provide privacy, if the glass doors are removed.
- Heat-sensitive safety valves can be installed to prevent scalding.
- If the older adult uses a wheelchair and the door to the bathroom is too narrow, a rolling shower bench or commode chair with wheels may help or removal of the door jamb to allow for a few extra inches in the doorway entrance.
- Placing a commode chair by the bed may eliminate unsafe night transfers to the bathroom toilet.
- A three-in-one commode chair is an inexpensive solution. This type of commode is light and can be used at bedside, over the toilet, or in the tub or shower. Caregivers should remember, however, that emptying the commode bucket and lifting and relocating the commode can be difficult.
- Clients should be discouraged from using soap dispensers, towel racks, and toilet paper holders for support. Hygiene items should be placed within reach.
- Mirrors may be tilted or lowered for better viewing during ADL functions.
- Doors under the sink can be removed to give the older adult more leg room while sitting in front of the sink.

Kitchen modifications/adaptations may include:

- Step stools should be avoided, and frequently used utensils and dishes should be rearranged so they are within safe reach, ideally between knee and shoulder height.
- Use of energy conservation techniques during meal preparation may decrease the risk for falling because of fatigue or orthostatic hypotension.
- Simple meal preparation packages are widely available in grocery stores.
- Use of a microwave can help decrease the amount of time an older adult spends standing at a stove to prepare a meal.

Halls and entry way modifications:

- Caregivers must ensure that stairs are well lit, with no glare, and equipped with railings running along the entire length of the stairwell on both sides.
- Striping of various colors can be used at the edge of each step to distinguish steps from each other.
- Safety grip strips may be placed on each step as well.
- Light switches should be within reach at both the top and bottom of the stairway.
- OTAs should discuss safe ways to change a light bulb with older adults. User-friendly, touch-sensitive, and motion-sensor light switches are also available.
- Transition areas such as doorways, garages, and patios are common sites for falls.

OTAs should also look at the outdoor environment, transition areas, and the indoor environment to help prevent falls.

Interventions to compensate for visual loss include increased lighting with limited glare, improved contrast for steps and furniture, decreased clutter in walkways, and well-maintained flooring. OTAs should anticipate older adults' performance at different times of the day, with varied natural lighting and indoor lighting. Referrals to vision specialists may be appropriate to ensure that older adults are wearing the appropriate eyewear.

Environmental modifications can also include modifications of the objects commonly used during ADLs by the older adult. OTAs should encourage older adults to wear sturdy, comfortable, rubber-soled footwear (e.g., athletic shoes) to help obtain a more secure footing. Some older adults may wear slip-on shoes because tying or fastening shoes is difficult; however, unsteady footwear may increase the likelihood of a fall. Assistive devices such as elastic laces or Velcro closures may help address this difficulty and provide the older adult with more stable footwear to help prevent falls. When dressing, older adults should pull pant legs above their knees before standing. Pants should be pulled down after transferring from the wheelchair to the toilet to avoid tripping.

Approximately, 30% of all falls in older adults occur in the home.[86,104,123] Of those older adults who fell during ADLs, 22% had falls that occurred when they tried to get out of bed or up from a chair.[124] The height of seats (beds, sofas, chairs) can be increased with firm cushions and worn mattresses or cushions should be rotated. Chairs with armrests are recommended to facilitate rising from the chair and chairs with wheels should be avoided. When completing ADL transfers, the brakes of wheelchairs and commodes must be secured before transfers are attempted. Older adults should lean forward in the wheelchair only when both feet are flat on the floor (not on the footrests).

Electronic lift chairs are typically available in furniture stores; however, safety and appropriateness for lift chairs should be assessed before purchasing.

Older adults with a reach of less than 6–7 inches are also limited in their mobility skills and are the most restricted in ADL functions.[96] Limited reach puts older adults at higher risk of falling and may decrease their independence at home. In such cases, individuals should be assessed for home safety and home modifications to compensate for limited reach.[104] Possible home interventions may involve incorporating assistive devices for the completion of tasks.[110] Reachers, long-handled bath sponges or shoe horns, carts, walker trays or bags, and sock aids are often appropriate assistive devices. OTAs play an important role in educating older adults in the proper use of these assistive devices so that the devices themselves do not become fall hazards. OTAs can also help the older adult problem-solve unique situations. For example, they can determine the best way to attach the long-handled reacher to the walker or rearrange items around the living space so they are within reach. Higher electrical outlets also could be recommended to limit the need to reach and bend. Redesigning or rearranging an older adult's environment is often an inexpensive and effective fall prevention technique. However, it is important to consider that rearranging furniture may disorient an older adult, which could increase the possibility of a fall. Environment redesign should occur only with the consent of the older adult, and follow-up visits are recommended to assess the transition.

Difficulty with transfers and mobility during ADL functions may require safety training with the cane, walker, or wheelchair. This is particularly important because many falls occur in transit during transfers. Older adults with nocturia, a normal age change involving increased frequency of urination at night, have a particular need for night-lights and a clear passage to the toilet. A consultation with a physical therapist may help clarify the most appropriate and safe assistive device for ambulation.

Institutional Interventions

Institutional interventions are fall prevention strategies implemented in institutions such as hospitals, nursing homes, and assisted living facilities. Incorporating fall prevention strategies into institutions is necessary as the rate of falls is higher among older adults in institutions than within the community.[84] Hospitals often have screening procedures for all patients, which include assessing patients for their fall risk. Often, these screens include an evaluation of cognition and balance by a physician, nursing staff, and/or occupational therapy. For those patients found to be at high risk for falls, bed or chair alarms, increased supervision (e.g., a sitter in the room or room placement close to the nursing station), low hospital beds, and floor mats are all viable options for keeping the patient safe from falls. Only consider low bed positions for a patient who is resting or if there are concerns about falling out of bed.[125]

Otherwise, for transfers, raise the bed to the correct height.[125] Additionally, early mobilization and participation in familiar ADLs are recommended to address fall risk.

Nursing homes and assisted living facilities can implement programs in addition to those mentioned previously to reduce fall risks. Examples of additional programs or policies to reduce fall risk include dedicated fall-reduction staff who can provide more supervision, multifaceted fall reduction interventions, including walking and other exercise-based programs to improve client factors, and staff education and policies related to fall reduction and reporting.[126-128] Previously discussed in the chapter were methods of restraint reduction and proper seating and positioning; addressing these issues can reduce falls among older adults in institutional settings.

Multifactorial Interventions

Multifactorial interventions are those that identify individual multiple risk factors and incorporate addressment of these risk factors into a coordinated fall prevention program. This is a useful approach for OTAs who want to ensure they are using a holistic, client-centered approach. Included in the occupational therapy plan of care should be referrals to other health professionals who are educated on managing the often complex medical issues of older adults. Older adults who report dizziness with a change in position may be experiencing a decrease in blood pressure that could result in a fall with or without syncope. A referral to the older adult's physician would facilitate medical management of this problem. Meanwhile, the OTA should monitor the older adult's blood pressure, and older adults should be allowed to make slow transitions from supine to sitting or sitting to standing positions. A few minutes may be necessary to allow the blood pressure to accommodate to the change in head position. By teaching older adults different techniques for dressing and bathing and instructing them in the use of long-handle devices, OTAs can help older adults limit and modify their bending. A typical recommendation is that the older adult get dressed while seated to help accommodate for orthostatic hypotension. The rest of the health care team should be informed of reports of dizziness and unstable changes in blood pressure.

OTAs, older adults, family members, and caregivers should work together to identify activities important to older adults that can be modified to prevent falls. Family members should be included because older adults may depend on them to help with preparation and assistance. Older adults may prefer to perform toileting activities independently but may not mind assistance with feeding. OTAs should identify personal and shared spaces in the older adult's living environment. If family members do not want to modify the only bathroom in the home with a raised toilet seat and grab bars, a commode chair by the older adult's bed may be appropriate. OTAs should help older adults and their family members address safety concerns and practice giving assistance in a safe environment.

Additional areas to consider are the frequency and occurrence of falls. If older adults experience repeated falls, their confidence levels may decrease, which could result in a decrease in participation in ADLs and IADLs.[79,129] The time of day that a fall occurs is also important information to obtain. About 64% of older adults in a study reported falls in the afternoon to late afternoon period.[129] The afternoon is generally a time of increased activity for older adults, and the assessment of ADLs and IADLs should address the time factor.

OTAs should make sure that strategies exist for emergency situations. Typical questions include the following:

- If a curtain is not drawn, will the neighbor know that this may be an indication of trouble?
- If an older adult falls, will they know the proper way to get up from the floor if no injuries are apparent?
- Is a telephone within reach?
- Is a list of emergency phone numbers placed by the phone?
- If the older adult is at home alone, are there emergency alert systems available to signal for help?
- Is a telephone reassurance program available in which a volunteer calls daily?
- Is it safer to soil clothes than risk an unassisted transfer to the toilet?

All of these questions should be addressed to ensure the older adult's safety before discharge from occupational therapy. See Box 14.4 for additional safety tips.

OUTCOMES

Identifying outcomes important to the client and that can be measured to demonstrate the effectiveness of occupational therapy intervention is an important step in the occupational therapy process. Ideally, the client and occupational therapy practitioner(s) select client-centered outcomes collaboratively early in the therapy process. OTAs, with guidance from OTs, can contribute to outcomes' identification and use. The *Occupational Therapy Practice Framework*[55] describes broad outcomes for any occupational therapy intervention, any of which may be appropriate, depending on which fall prevention strategy is utilized in the rehabilitation process.

Prevention is an obvious outcome to select in fall prevention programs. The number of falls experienced by the client can be counted during a specified time frame and compared to the number of falls experienced by the client before intervention. These data can provide evidence of the effectiveness of the fall prevention intervention. However, not all clients have experienced falls before occupational therapy intervention but may have risk factors for falls. Therefore, this outcome alone may not be an adequate measure of success.

Adaptation, health, and wellness can be measurable outcomes in fall prevention programs. Secondary effects of such interventions may be a positive change, or adaptation, in body functions and performance skills such as strength, balance, visual acuity, or endurance. If deficits in these functions and skills were intrinsic risk factors for falls, an improvement may help decrease fall risk. For example, if a client had poor muscle strength and balance, and strengthening and balance activities were included in the intervention plan, appropriate outcome measures would be manual muscle testing or a balance or fall-risk assessment. Many valid and reliable balance assessments are available and can be easily administered.

Occupational performance and role competence are commonly used outcomes in occupational therapy practice and may be the client's desired outcomes for fall prevention interventions. For example, if safety with bathing or showering is addressed through environmental modifications, a client's occupational performance may improve from needing assistance with tub transfers to being independent with tub transfers as long as a tub transfer bench is used.

Self-advocacy may be a selected outcome. If a client discovers, through guidance from an occupational therapy practitioner, that he or she is no longer safe to ambulate in the community because of high fall risk, the ability to self-advocate for community transportation services may be an appropriate outcome.

Participation and quality of life should always be overarching outcomes for any intervention, including fall prevention. Simply helping a client improve endurance and balance does not ensure that he or she can safely and comfortably participate in desired life events and believe that he or she has an improved quality of life. OTAs must be sure to carry out interventions in their natural contexts and ensure that clients are able to participate in these contexts. Many standardized measures of participation and quality of life exist as well.

BOX 14.4

Safety Tips

- Consider referrals to others on the health care team. Periodic medication reviews by a pharmacist and medical checkups by a physician are important safeguards against falls.
- Some research has shown that exercise can reduce falls in the elderly but research about exercise is inconclusive. Be sure to proceed with exercise programs that take into account individual elder's comorbidities and functional status.
- Consider issuing and educating on adaptive equipment (e.g., grab bars, tub benches or shower chairs, and bedside commodes) when full remediation is not possible.
- Home safety assessments are beneficial to address occupations in context and to reduce environmental hazards such as poor lighting, excessive clutter, and unsafe walking surfaces.
- Address safety measures and recommend that a cellular or cordless phone always be within reach of an elder at risk for falls (e.g., in a walker bag, fanny pack).

Occupational justice is defined as "access to and participation in the full range of meaningful and enriching occupations afforded to others" (p. S35).[55] Care must be taken to design fall prevention interventions such that clients have a reasonable balance between freedom from falls and participation in meaningful occupations. Fall prevention may be extremely challenging if a client has irreversible risk factors such as dementia or blindness. However, if the only answer to fall prevention appears to be a drastic reduction in physical activities so that falls are minimized, the client may potentially sacrifice or be denied access to meaningful living.

CASE STUDY

Let us revisit the case of Jona. Her daughter finally convinced her to visit with her physician about her recent falls. The physician ordered home health occupational and physical therapy services for Jona. Based on what you know about effective fall prevention, answer the following questions.

■ CASE STUDY QUESTIONS

1 What risk factors does Jona have that contribute to her falling?
2 What further information would you want to have before designing a fall prevention intervention plan? Specifically, what further questions would you want to ask Jona, and what assessments and/or functional observations would you want to observe?
3 Which fall prevention approach(es) would be most appropriate for Jona? Describe two intervention activities for each approach.
4 Finally, consider what outcomes would be most appropriate for Jona. What specific measures would you, along with the OT and client, choose?
5 Which evidence-based programs could you refer Jona to also utilize and include after discharge from therapy services?

SHARON COSPER
(PREVIOUS CONTRIBUTIONS FROM MICHELE LUTHER-KRUG,
MARY ELLEN KEITH, AND CANDICE MULLENDORE)

PART 4 Community Mobility

According to the Occupational Therapy Practice Framework fourth edition (OTPF-4), driving and community mobility are defined as "planning and moving around in the community using public or private transportation, such as driving, walking, bicycling, or accessing and riding in buses, taxi cabs, ride shares, or other transportation systems."[55] Access to transportation for community mobility is vital to participation in many occupations. Without adequate mobility, accessibility diminishes and can impact meaningful engagement in many areas including: ADLs, instrumental activities of daily living (IADLs), health management, education, work, leisure, and social participation. Forms of community mobility include both independent and interdependent options, and often a shift from independent driving to utilization of interdependent transportation occurs for the client as they age. However, a desire for individuals to continue living in their homes and communities increases with age, so ensuring safe options for community mobility are critical to sustain home and community dwelling for older adults.[130] Occupational therapy practitioners can be instrumental in this process, by engaging clients in interventions that promote and restore function or provide compensatory and adaptive strategies that foster safe driving and community mobility through modification and prevention, as well as through client education and advocacy to ensure community-based transportation resources are available that promote access and participation.

DRIVING

By the year 2030, one in five American drivers will be age 65 years or older.[131] Older adults represent 19% of all licensed drivers in the United States.[132] In comparison to younger drivers, 1-year and 10-year trends indicate that more older drivers are involved in fatal crashes than younger drivers.[133] Older adults account for 18% of all traffic fatalities.[132] Older adults may experience age-related changes that can negatively affect their ability to drive. Aging is a highly complex process that varies tremendously among individuals. Factors that can influence driving and mobility include unrecognized disease processes, physical changes, psychosocial issues, medications, cognitive changes, reduction in hearing ability, and environmental issues such as small print on signs.[134] Although driving may seem simple, it is an extremely complex occupation that requires significant use of motor and process skills, as well as integration of sensory, cognitive, and neuromuscular functions. Examples contributing to driving abilities of alder adults more specifically include changes in sensation, range of motion, decrease in reaction time, and decrease in decision-making abilities.[134] Also substantial changes in vision related to decreased visual acuity, color discrimination, depth perception, figure ground and peripheral vision, and increased sensitivity to glare, all have been shown to impact driving performance.[135]

Drivers make about 20 decisions for each mile traveled, demonstrating that the occupation of driving is complex and fast-paced.[136,137] The abilities of sensing, deciding, and acting are critical in operating a vehicle. Drivers must perform a series of coordinated activities with their hands and feet while using input from their eyes and ears. Drivers must make many decisions on the basis of what they see and hear in relation to other vehicles on the road, other drivers, traffic signs, signals, and road conditions. These decisions result in the actions of braking, steering, and accelerating, or a combination of all three to maintain or adjust the position of the vehicle in traffic. Because fluctuations in traffic occur quickly, the coordination between decisions and actions must be smooth. In addition, drivers need to be aware of their surroundings and other drivers who may be engaging in distracted driving activities such as using a cell phone, texting, and eating. Each day in the United States, more than 8 people are killed and 1161 injured in crashes reported to involve a distracted driver.[138]

Age-related or disability-related decreases in motor and process skills, as well as decline in sensory, cognitive, neuromuscular functions may compromise driving safety by reducing the speed with which an older adult can sense, decide, and act in traffic. Some significant sensory perceptual functions used in driving includes visual processing related to visual acuity, visual accommodation, field of vision, dark adaptation, color vision, visual searching, glare, illumination, as well as auditory processing. Impairments with both visual and auditory processing have been shown to associate with a more rapid decline in cognitive function in older adults, demonstrating the interconnectedness of these essential functions on judgment and decision-making.[139] These, along with certain diseases of the eye, may affect the way the driver senses environmental changes. Approximately 60% of all individuals age 65 years and older have a visual impairment.[140] As the size of the older adult population increases, the number of people with visual and auditory impairments will increase significantly. Visual impairments are a primary consideration in safe driving and should be assessed accordingly.

Vision is usually defined as visual acuity or the ability to see fine details. Static acuity (such as looking at an eye chart) is tested in driver licensing examinations. Dynamic acuity (subject or target moving) is more closely related to traffic accidents but is seldom tested. Up to age 40 or 50 years, little change occurs in visual acuity, but visual acuity declines markedly as individuals age.[139] The implications of this decline for driving are that drivers find distinguishing between objects increasingly difficult and need to be closer to objects to clearly perceive them.[141] To compensate for this, older adults may drive slowly to distinguish hazards on the road in time to avoid them. Poor acuity can also result in misinterpretation of objects, therefore resulting in poor judgment or decision-making while driving.

Accommodation is defined as the ability to focus the eyes on nearby objects. With aging, changes in the lenses of the eyes and in the muscles that adjust them decrease their capacity for accommodation. For this reason, many older adults need bifocal or trifocal eyewear, which affects driving because more time is required to change focus from near to distant objects, such as when looking from the instrument panel to the road and vice versa. A younger person can change focus in about 2 seconds, whereas adults older than age 40 years take 3 seconds or more. This delay is potentially hazardous. The retina of the normal eye receives about one-half as much light at age 50 as at age 20 years and about one-third as much at age 60 as at age 20 years.[142] This change is primarily because of a decrease in the size of the pupil. Choosing well-lit highways and instrument panels and keeping headlights, windows, and eyeglasses clean are helpful measures. A driver rehabilitation professional may recommend changes in the enhancement of the instrument panel to improve use such as marking various speeds on the odometer or modifying the speedometer with a magnifier.

Field of vision decreases can contribute to the possibility of collisions. For example, people who can see only directly ahead confront a greater risk for accidents at intersections because they cannot see vehicles approaching from the periphery. Compensation for a decreased field of vision can include the use of special panoramic mirrors and the habit of turning the head more often to check for traffic. Reminders to look over the shoulder before all lane changes may be a helpful strategy to compensate for blind spots on sides of the vehicle.

Dark adaptation is the process whereby eyes adjust for better vision in low light. Older adults not only see less clearly in darkness but also require more time to accommodate to it.[143] This can be a particular problem when driving in and out of tunnels. Many older adults decide on their own not to drive at night for this reason. In addition to adaptation diminishing, older adults may not identify the color of traffic signs or signals as well as younger people, especially when the light is dim or glare is present. This can be a problem because older adults require additional time to read road signs, which diverts their attention from the road and traffic.[144]

Glare occurs when too much light or light from the wrong direction or source is present. If excessive light shines on a highway sign, the older adult may not see it. Quick recovery from oncoming headlights is necessary for safe driving. In the older adult driver, eye recovery may be slower and sensitivity to glare increased. The windshield of a vehicle produces glare, and one way to reduce this glare is to place a black cloth over the dashboard. Uncontrolled glare may mask oncoming traffic and limit the ability to see traffic lights, signs, and brake lights. Not controlling glare can make the driver less safe on the road. Some conditions can require more stringent control of light and glare. A low vision specialist and a driver rehabilitation specialist can help determine the degree of glare problems and appropriate aids, including sun filters, hats, adaptive visors, and other adaptive steps. A driver rehabilitation specialist may advise some individuals to avoid driving just after sunrise and just before sunset when low-lying sun might cause significant glare problems.

According to the AARP, older adults may be able to compensate for some visual limitations.[145] They should have their vision checked at least yearly and avoid eyeglass frames that obstruct peripheral vision. Learning the general meaning of traffic signs by their shapes and colors and avoiding driving at night whenever possible are useful precautions. Various lens tints may be used to improve color recognition or the detection of objects, signs, and road users in low contrast areas.[145]

Another significant sensory function related to driving is auditory processing. Comorbid visual and auditory processing decline has been shown to also correlate with cognitive impairments in older adults, further suggesting the interconnectedness of sensory and cognitive functions.[146] Approximately one-third of older adults between 65 and 74 years of age and one-half over the age of 75 years of age experience some hearing loss.[147] This loss can cause problems during driving because horns, sirens, and train whistles may be difficult to hear, or even if heard, to distinguish the difference and subsequent appropriate response. It may also prevent older adults from realizing that the turn signal indicator is on when no turns are being made. Older adults should have their hearing tested by a qualified professional. When adjusting to any hearing assistive device, it may be helpful for them to keep the volume of the car radio as low as possible, leave the air conditioning or heating units on the lowest possible setting, and visually check turn signals. Alerting systems and mirrors may also be used to improve awareness.

The aging process may also have an effect on muscles and joints in ways that may affect driving, specifically reaction time, as well as general decline in muscle strength and joint integrity as examples. Age has been shown to have a significant effect on hand movement performance, specifically with speed and accuracy showing decline with age.[148] Reaction time is extremely important in safe driving. Reaction time is the time required by the eyes to see and the brain to process, decide what to do, and transmit the information to the proper body parts. For example, after seeing that the traffic ahead has stopped, a driver extends the right leg and pushes on the brake pedal. The ability to respond quickly may decrease with age, but specific safety measures can be used to compensate for the loss. One strategy is to maintain a safe distance from the car ahead. When stopping, the driver should be able to see the tires of the car in front. Other strategies are to avoid rush hour traffic and to take someone else along, especially when traveling to a new destination. Education on compensatory techniques can help older adults change unsafe habits.

Older adults may experience decrease in strength of muscles and joint integrity that contribute to reduced reaction time, as well as other complications to safe driving.

Loss of muscle mass and strength with aging, and a compromised ability to regenerate both is well documented.[149] Emphasis on exercise and physical activity for older adults may be a contributor to maintaining skeletal muscle function and continuing safe engagement in driving.[149] Decline in joint integrity can make it difficult to sit for long periods, due to the pain that can result from prolonged positioning. Arthritis may cause stiffness, for example in the neck region, which can decrease active range of motion (AROM) and make it painful when turning to check for traffic. A wide variety of mirrors are available to compensate for reduced AROM in the neck to improve visibility. Muscle and joint fatigue and discomfort are problems that may distract older adults and lessen their awareness of traffic conditions. Special cushions may be helpful. Using tilt steering and armrests may also help. A driver rehabilitation specialist can help determine whether modifications to their vehicle will help the older adults experiencing a decrease in muscle strength and joint integrity be safer with driving.

OTAs can assist the older adult driver in applying for a disabled parking placard, usually issued by the Department of Motor Vehicles (DMV) of each state. This entitles the driver of the car to park close to buildings and may also include assistance at a gas station. Some older adult drivers do not apply for this placard because they do not understand the application procedure, or because of a perceived social stigma. It is important for the occupational therapy practitioner to help the older adult determine the requirements for a disabled parking placard. In many states, the form must be filled out and signed by a licensed physician.

A behind-the-wheel evaluation is the best method for determining driver safety. A driving evaluation program that specializes in working with persons with disabilities can determine safety and equipment needs. A wide variety of equipment is available to help older adults continue driving. This equipment is available from a variety of sources, including equipment catalogs, vendors, and automobile manufacturers (Table 14.6). The AOTA Older Driver Initiative and the Association of Driver Rehabilitation Specialists (ADED) assist occupational therapy practitioners in locating driver evaluation programs. These programs can also instruct occupational therapy practitioners in the proper procedures for reporting questionable or unsafe drivers to the DMV of each state. OTs and OTAs should clearly document all recommendations to older adults. For example, if the OTA recommends that an older adult's driving ability be evaluated after a stroke, this recommendation must be clearly stated in the medical chart.

The AARP, American Automobile Association (AAA), and American Occupational Therapy Association (AOTA) offer various programs and courses for older drivers. The driver safety course offered by AARP, along with AAA and AOTA, covers many issues, including decreased reaction

TABLE 14.6

Adaptive Equipment Ideas

Difficulty	Effect on driving	Resources to assist elder drivers
Decreased neck ROM or pain when turning head	Limited scope of view of traffic around car	Install panoramic mirrors (Brookstone) or convex mirrors (can be installed by vendors); refer to driving program for evaluation; instruct client in use of head support
Decreased shoulder ROM or pain in shoulders	Difficulty steering, reaching for seat belt, and adjusting rearview mirror	Use arm supports already in vehicle; automobile upholsterer can build up existing arm supports to support elbows, which usually decreases client's shoulder pain; client may need effort of steering reduced, which can be determined by driving evaluation (driving program can refer to appropriate vendor for this modification); instruct elder in use of stick to adjust rearview mirror and tilt steering wheel
Decreased ROM or pain in fingers and hands	Difficulty turning key, opening door, adjusting radio, air conditioning, and so on; possible difficulty holding on to steering wheel safely	A wide variety of key holders and door openers is available from medical supply catalogs; knob extensions can be made by car vendors; refer client for driving evaluation to determine need for steering device or built-up steering wheel
Back pain	Decreased concentration caused by pain; difficulty turning to check traffic	A wide variety of cushions and lumbar supports is available from medical supply companies and vendors; these should be tried before purchase; driving programs can also evaluate and provide resources
Impairment or loss of both lower extremities	Inability to operate gas and brake pedals	Refer to driving program for evaluation of ability to use hand controls
Impairment or loss of right lower extremity	Difficulty using gas and brake pedals	Refer to driving program for evaluation of ability to use left foot accelerator
Impairment or loss of left upper extremity	Difficulty using turn signal and turning	Refer to driving program for evaluation of ability to use right crossover directional and spinner knob
Impairment or loss of right upper extremity	Difficulty steering, shifting gears in automatic or manual cars	Refer to driving program for evaluation of ability to use spinner knob
Hearing impairment	Inability to hear emergency sirens; failure to turn off turn signal	Elder drivers can purchase equipment to amplify sound of blinker; hearing aids can help clients better hear sirens
Cognitive impairment	Decreased judgment and decision-making; slow reaction time; unsafe driving	Refer to driving program for detailed evaluation; discuss concerns with occupational therapist; document recommendations clearly
Visual impairment	Compromised ability to read signs; overly slow driving; generally unsafe driving skills	Refer to optometrist for vision checkup; if elder has low vision, refer to ophthalmologist or neuro-optometrist that specializes in low vision. Neuro-Optometric Rehabilitation Association (NORA) is a good resource for locating this area of specialty.

ROM, range of motion.

Adapted from Lillie S. Evaluation for driving. In: Yoshikawa TT, Lipton E, eds. *Ambulatory Geriatric Care*. St. Louis: Mosby; 1993.

time, visual and hearing losses, the effects of certain medications, and hazardous situations.[150] Many insurance companies will offer a rebate on automobile insurance after successful completion of a driver safety course. However, these classes do not include behind-the-wheel testing. OTAs should discuss any concerns about the older adult's ability to drive safely with the supervising OT and physician whenever possible.

PEDESTRIAN SAFETY

Walking safely is an important factor in community mobility. However, pedestrian fatalities have seen an

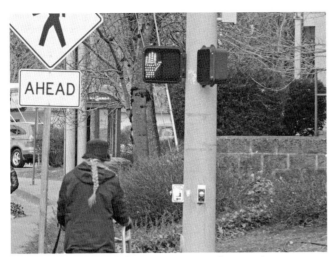

FIG. 14.14 Older pedestrians may need more time to cross streets than other people do.

BOX 14.5

Pedestrian Safety Tips

- Always use a crosswalk.
- Use the pedestrian push button and wait for the WALK sign to appear.
- Before stepping into the roadway, search for turning vehicles, look left-right-left, and keep looking while crossing.
- Wear bright (fluorescent) colors during daylight and wear reflective material and carry a flashlight if walking at night.

Adapted from the American Automobile Association (AAA). Walking through the years. Heathrow, FL: AAA Traffic Safety and Engineering Department; 1993.

annual increase of 3.4% and pedacyclists by 6.3%.[133] Older adults account for 19% of all pedestrian fatalities.[133] Occupational therapy practitioners should observe the ability of older adults to ambulate outdoors in a variety of community contexts and environments before deeming them safely independent in community mobility. Evaluation and intervention occurring in the community setting will allow for authentic determination of ability as well as problem solving to occur for unanticipated issues. The same deficits associated with difficulty driving may also impact negotiation of community environments for the older adult.

Ambulation with visual and auditory deficits, as well as with decline in cognitive and motor skills can greatly impact safety (Fig. 14.14). Sensory deficits may make it challenging to determine the speed of oncoming traffic while attempting to cross the street, for example. Strategies for using crosswalks and environmental sensory cues can be introduced by the occupational therapy practitioner. Strong evidence supports the role of occupational therapy practitioners in providing interventions for older adults with low vision.[151] Difficulty with problem solving or memory deficits can also pose barriers to successful community mobility. Topographical orientation can become challenging and result in an older adult with dementia becoming lost. Occupational therapy practitioners can work with individuals to utilize technology such as GPS and environmental clues to negotiate the community on foot. Motor deficits and the loss of ability to ambulate can result in older adults using assistive devices to continue accessing the community. Box 14.5 lists precautions for safe walking in an older adult's community.

Older adults who use wheelchairs, walkers, and scooters have unique challenges to conquering crosswalks, curbs, and uneven sidewalks. These older adults need training to negotiate cutout curbs because electric scooters or wheelchairs may overturn when descending. A mobility expert should conduct an evaluation to determine the type of equipment needed. This evaluation should take into consideration the older adult's cognitive function, physical ability, seating and positioning needs, home and community environments, and progression of any disease. Whenever possible, OTAs should provide safety training with the exact type of mobility equipment that older adults will be using in the community. OTAs also can help older adults advocate for curb cuts or longer crossing times at various intersections to ensure independence and safety in the community. To this end, the city's Traffic Commission or the Architectural and Transportation Barriers Compliance Board can be of assistance.

Wheeled power mobility devices should be transported only in a van fitted with an electric lift or ramp of the appropriate size and weight. A driver rehabilitation or seating and positioning professional should evaluate each case before a van or lift is purchased to prevent expensive mistakes such as incompatible equipment. These professionals take into account many factors, including the type of wheelchair or scooter that must be transported, whether the person needing the equipment will be a driver or passenger, and the length of time that the equipment will be needed. The occupational therapy practitioner can also determine the ability of the older adult to operate the prescribed equipment. The diagnosis of the older adult is also important. An older adult with a progressive illness has different needs than an older adult without a progressive illness. The driver rehabilitation professional can also provide resources for vendors who install adaptive equipment for vehicles in a particular geographical area. The National Mobility Equipment Dealers Association is a resource for locating these qualified vehicle modifiers/dealers.

ALTERNATIVE TRANSPORTATION

When planning intervention, occupational therapy practitioners must take into consideration the individual's lifestyle and needs.[55] This is especially true for older adults who have never driven, are now unable to drive because of impairments, voluntarily decide not to drive, or want the option of using community transportation in addition to their personal vehicles. Older adults who relied on others for transportation may need to learn to drive, especially if those people are no longer available. Occupational therapy practitioners should help the older adult investigate community transportation resources available where the older adult currently resides or is planning to live. Information on alternative transportation can be obtained by calling or accessing the website for the city, a local senior citizens' center, the local DMV, local transportation agencies, and the local American Association of Retired Persons (AARP) offices. Independent living centers in the community may also be good sources of information. When calling these agencies, occupational therapy practitioners should help the older adult obtain information about application procedures, cost, distance traveled, and eligibility requirements.

Regardless of what form of alternative transportation the older adult is using, their ability to safely exit their homes is of critical importance and must be evaluated to determine whether available services should be used. The older adult may be unable to ascend and descend stairs safely to exit the home, or unlock and lock the door. Occupational therapy practitioners should consider these factors and include them when training in and determining the functional use of alternative transportation services.

Title II of the Americans with Disabilities Act (ADA) addresses many needs of older adults with disabilities.[152] This act states that no qualified individual with a disability shall, by reason of that disability, be excluded from participating in or be denied the benefits of the services, programs, or activities of a public entity. According to the ADA, a qualified individual is defined as a person with a disability who meets the essential eligibility requirements for receiving services or participating in programs or activities provided by a public entity. The individual may meet these qualifications with or without reasonable modifications to rules, policies, or practices. A person may also qualify with or without the removal of architectural barriers or the provision of auxiliary aids and services. Public entity refers to any state or local government or instrumentality of a state or local government.[152] The paratransit and other special transportation services provided by public entities are designed to be usable by individuals with disabilities, whether physical or mental, who need the assistance of another individual to board, ride, or disembark from any vehicle on the system. Individuals for whom no fixed and accessible route transit (usually a public bus) is available are also eligible for paratransit and special transportation services.[152] However, a fixed, accessible route transit should be used if available (Fig. 14.15).[153]

Older adults who have impairments that prevent them from traveling to or from a boarding location for fixed transportation may also be eligible for special services. Under the law, any individual accompanying the person

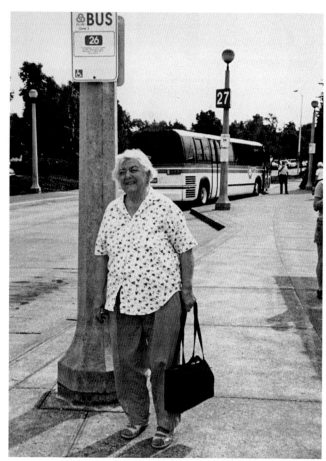

FIG. 14.15 Older adults may need to learn to use community transportation.

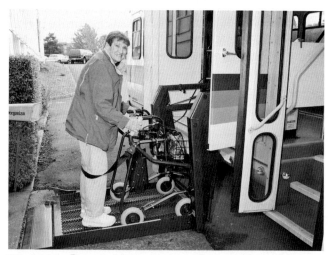

FIG. 14.16 Paratransit services may be a viable option for older adults with limited mobility.

with the disability may be eligible for paratransit services, provided that space is available and other people with disabilities are not displaced (Fig. 14.16).[154] This means that if older adult with a disability cannot use the available bus system, another transportation system that can pick them up directly from their home must be provided. Occupational therapy practitioners working with older adults who have a disability must know the ADA as it relates to transportation and accessibility. They should also become knowledgeable about the paratransit services in the local community.

The process of applying for special transportation services can be complicated and confusing. OTs and OTAs should have applications available and know the eligibility requirements for these services. If possible, an outing should be schedule with the older adult to use particular services and help them resolve any difficulties that arise. Older adults may need encouragement to be assertive when they require assistance. If the outing is successful, older adults are more likely to use the service independently or with a friend or family member.

CASE STUDY

Thomas is 62 years old. One year ago, he had a right cerebrovascular accident and has a nonfunctional left upper extremity. For long distances, he uses a manual wheelchair, which he pushes with his right lower extremity. For short distances, he slowly ambulates using a quad cane. Other medical conditions include a seizure disorder controlled by medication and a left hip joint replacement that causes pain and discomfort with prolonged sitting. A former physical education teacher, Thomas enjoys working with students at the high school level and is anxious to return to work in some capacity. His wife works full time, and he receives occasional assistance in transportation from friends. Thomas believes he is ready to drive, but his wife is very concerned for his safety.

Thomas received a driving evaluation, during which he exhibited difficulties such as weaving out of the lane and forgetting to turn off his turn signal. After driving for 20 minutes, he drifted across two lanes and lost his concentration. The driving instructor had to take over the steering wheel to pull the car over to the side of the road. Thomas stated that his "leg hurt."

After the evaluation, the deficits observed during driving were discussed. Thomas demonstrated insight into his difficulties and expressed the desire to begin training to improve his driving skills. Equipment needs included a spinner knob to allow him to steer with one hand and a right crossover directional device that enabled him to use his right hand for directional use. Training strategies included asking Thomas to tell the driving instructor when he was starting to have pain in his leg and to pull over when it was safe. He was reminded to turn off his directional signal after use and to look ahead while driving. After three training sessions, Thomas was able to demonstrate safe driving skills. He received a driving test from the DMV and passed. He is now able to return to part-time work and independent living.

■ CASE STUDY QUESTIONS

1 Considering the case of Thomas, identify three aspects of this case that indicate Thomas' safety to drive was compromised.
2 Identify alternatives for transportation that may have been necessary while Thomas received driving rehabilitation services.
3 Identify the possible social and emotional impact that not being able to safely drive after his CVA had on Thomas and his family.

■ CHAPTER REVIEW QUESTIONS

1 Explain the reason that Omnibus Budget Reconciliation Act regulations involving the use of restraints were drafted, and discuss related requirements for health providers.
2 Explain the steps to be taken in establishing a restraint reduction program.
3 Explain the role of the OTA in consultations regarding the use of restraints.
4 Describe at least three environmental adaptations that may help reduce the use of restraints.
5 Identify psychosocial approaches to reducing the use of restraints with an older adult who wanders.
6 Explain the ways that activity aids in the reduction of restraints.
7 Discuss the safety and documentation implications if working in a facility that utilizes restraints. How does this impact the therapeutic process?
8 Describe the ideal position in which an older adult should sit in a wheelchair.
9 Describe at least three additional considerations when monitoring the appropriate fitting wheelchair for a person of larger size.
10 List five precautions to consider when monitoring the appropriate fit of a wheelchair for an older adult.
11 Identify three reasons that many falls go unreported.
12 Explain the reason that some older adults and their family members are reluctant to change the environment when personal safety and prevention of falls are a concern.
13 Explain the need for assessment of an older adult's nighttime toileting skills.
14 Describe ways the home can be modified to prevent falls if older adults have vision impairments and poor standing balance.
15 Describe the five broad evidence-based approaches to fall risk intervention.
16 Describe three evidence-based intervention programs and the importance of educating older adults to utilization of such programs.
17 Identify three emergency strategies for an older adult who lives alone and has a history of falls.
18 Discuss the skills and functions that can impact safe driving for older adults.
19 Describe the role of and ways the OT and OTA can assist the older adult in becoming safe with driving and community mobility.
20 Discuss potential barriers that limit the older adult being able to use alternative transportation and ways the OT and OTA can help resolve these access issues.

For additional video content, please visit Elsevier eBooks+ (eBooks.Health.Elsevier.com)

REFERENCES

1. Joanna Briggs Institute (JBI). Physical restraint—part 1: use in acute and residential care facilities. *Best Pract.* 2002;6(3):1-6.
2. Mott S, Poole J, Kenrick M. Physical and chemical restraints in acute care: their potential impact on the rehabilitation of older people. *Int J Nurs Pract.* 2005;11(3):95-101. doi:10.1111/j.1440-172X.2005.00510.x.
3. Berzlanovich AM, Schöpfer J, Keil W. Deaths due to physical restraint. *Dtsch Arztebl Int.* 2012;109(3):27-32. doi:10.3238/arztebl.2012.0027.
4. Omnibus Budget Reconciliation Act, 1987. Pub. L. No. 100-20, 101 Stat. 1330.
5. Centers for Medicare & Medicaid Services. *CMS Publishes Final Patients' Rights Rule on Use of Restraints and Seclusion: Better, More Extensive Training of Staff Required.* 2006. Available at: https://www.cms.gov/newsroom/press-releases/cms-publishes-final-patients-rights-rule-use-restraints-and-seclusion.
6. U.S. Department of Health & Human Services, Centers for Medicare & Medicaid Services. *Release of Report: Freedom from Unnecessary Restraints: Two Decades of National Progress in Nursing Home Care (Ref: S&C-09-11).* 2008. Available at: https://www.cms.gov/Medicare/Provider-Enrollment-and-Certification/Survey CertificationGenInfo/Policy-and-Memos-to-States-and-Regions-Items/CMS1217030.
7. U.S. Department of Health and Human Services. *Nursing Home Data Compendium.* 2015th ed. 2015. Available at: https://www.cms.gov/Medicare/Provider-Enrollment-and-Certification/CertificationandComplianc/downloads/nursinghomedatacompendium_508-2015.pdf.
8. U.S. Department of Health and Human Services, Agency for Healthcare Research and Quality. *National Healthcare Quality Report.* 2009. (AHRQ Publication No. 10-0003). Available at: http://archive.ahrq.gov/research/findings/nhqrdr/nhqr09/.
9. Cosper P, Morelock V, Provine B. Please release me: restraint reduction initiative in a health care system. *J Nurs Care Qual.* 2015;30(1):16-23.
10. Crisis Prevention Institute. *Joint Commission Standards on Restraint and Seclusion/Nonviolent Crisis Intervention® Training Program.* Milwaukee WI: CPI; 2009:1-8.
11. Center for Medicare and Medicaid Services (CMS). *Medicare State Operations Manual Provider Certification: Transmittal 20.* 2000. Available at: https://www.cms.gov/Regulations-and-Guidance/Guidance/Transmittals/downloads/R20SOM.pdf.
12. Center for Medicare and Medicaid Services (CMS). *CMS Manual System: Pub; 2016. 100-07 State Operations Provider Certification: Transmittal 157.* Available at: https://www.cms.gov/Regulations-and-Guidance/Guidance/Transmittals/Downloads/R157SOMA.pdf.
13. Gunawardena R, Smithard DG. The attitudes towards the use of restraint and restrictive intervention amongst healthcare staff on acute medical and frailty wards–A brief literature review. *Geriatrics (Basel).* 2019;4(3):50.
14. Morris K. Issues and answers: restraint use. *Ohio Nurses Rev.* 2007;82(4):14-15.
15. Kleen K. Restraint regulation: the tie that binds: break free of potential litigation by recognizing patient rights related to physical restraints. *Nurs Manage.* 2004;35(11):36-38.
16. Strumpf NE, Evans LK, Wagner J, et al. Reducing physical restraint: developing an educational program. *J Gerontol Nurs.* 1992;18(11):21.
17. Kari N, Michels P. The Lazarus project: the politics of empowerment. *Am J Occup Ther.* 1991;45(8):719.
18. Medicare and Medicaid Programs. *Hospital Conditions of Participation: Patient Rights.* Final Rule. 71 Fed. Reg. 71294 (to be codified at 42 C.F.R. pt. 483.13); 2006.
19. Joanna Briggs Institute (JBI). Physical restraint—part 2: minimization in acute and residential care facilities. *Best Pract.* 2002;6(4):1-6.
20. Brungardt G. Patient restraints: new guidelines for a less restrictive approach. *Geriatrics.* 1994;49(6):43.
21. Janelli LM, Kanski GW, Neary MA. Physical restraints: has OBRA made a difference? *J Gerontol Nurs.* 1994;20(6):17.
22. Strumpf N, Evans L, Bourbonniere M. Restraints. In: Mezey M, ed. *The Encyclopedia of Elder Care.* New York: Springer; 2001:567-569.
23. Reed P, Tilly J. Dementia care practice recommendations for nursing homes and assisted living, phase 2: falls, wandering, and physical restraints. *Alzheimers Care Today.* 2008;9(1):51-59. doi:10.1097/01.ALCAT.0000309016.62587.
24. Saarnio R, Isola A. Use of physical restraint in institutional older adultly care in Finland: perspectives of patients and their family members. *Res Gerontol Nurs.* 2009;2(4):276-286. doi:10.3928/19404921-20090706-02.
25. Voyer P, Richard S, Doucet L, Cyr N, Carmichael PH. Precipitating factors associated with delirium among long-term care residents with dementia. *Appl Nurs Res.* 2011;24(3):171-178. doi:10.1016/j.apnr.2009.07.001.
26. Mamun K, Lim J. Use of physical restraints in nursing homes: current practice in Singapore. *Ann Acad Med Singapore.* 2005;34(2):158-162.
27. Mion LC, Mercurio A. Methods to reduce restraints: process, outcomes, and future directions. *J Gerontol Nurs.* 1992;18(11):5.
28. Rader J. Creating a supportive environment for eliminating restraints. In: Rader J, Tornquist E, eds. *Individualized Dementia Care: Creative, Compassionate Approaches.* New York: Springer; 1995:117-143.
29. Werner P, Koroknay V, Braun J, et al. Individualized care alternatives used in the process of removing restraints in the nursing home. *J Am Geriatr Soc.* 1994;42(3):321.
30. Neufeld RR, Libow LS, Foley WJ, et al. Restraint reduction reduces serious injuries among nursing home residents. *J Am Geriatr Soc.* 1999;47(10):1202-1207.
31. Ericson LL. Restraints in the nursing home environment. *Occup Ther Forum.* 1991;6(4):1.
32. Tideiksaar R. Falls. In: Bonder B, Wagner M, eds. *Functional Performance in Older Adults.* 3rd ed. Philadelphia: FA Davis; 2009.
33. Patterson JE, Strumpf NE, Evans LK. Nursing consultation to reduce restraints in a nursing home. *Clin Nurse Spec.* 1995;9(4):231.
34. Eigsti DG, Vrooman N. Releasing restraints in the nursing home: it can be done. *J Gerontol Nurs.* 1992;18(1):21.
35. O'Rourke K. Maine care center reduces use of bed rails. *Health Prog.* 2004;85(6):32.
36. Evans LK, Forceia MA, Yurkow J, et al. The geriatric day hospital. In: Katz P, Mezey M, Kane R, eds. *Emerging Systems in Long-Term Care.* New York: Springer; 1999.
37. Gallo JJ, Busby-Whitehead J, Rabins PV, et al. *Reichel's Care of the Elderly: Clinical Aspects of Aging.* 5th ed. Philadelphia: Lippincott Williams & Wilkins; 1999.
38. Plautz R, Camp C. Activities as agents for intervention and rehabilitation in long-term care. In: Bonder B, Wagner M, eds. *Functional Performance in Older Adults.* 2nd ed. Philadelphia: FA Davis; 2001.
39. Greenberg D. Geriatric seating and positioning: definitely a therapy task. *Gerontology Special Interest Section Newsletter.* 1996;19(3):1.
40. Jones DA. Seating problems in long-term care. In: Tornquist EM, ed. *Individualized Dementia Care: Creative Compassionate Approaches.* New York: Springer; 1995.
41. *APNA Position on The Use of Seclusion & Restraint.* Apna.org. Available at: https://www.apna.org/i4a/pages/index.cfm?pageid=3730.
42. Guidelines for documentation of occupational therapy. *Am J Occup Ther.* 2018;72(suppl 2):7212410010p1-7212410010p7.
43. *Disability Characteristics: 2019 ACS 1-Year Estimates Subject Tables.* data.census.gov. Published September 10, 2020.
44. Gell NM, Wallace RB, LaCroix AZ, et al. Mobility device use in older adults and incidence of falls and worry about falling: findings from the 2011-2012 National Health and Aging Trends Study. *J Am Geriatr Soc.* 2015;63(5):853-859. doi:10.1111/jgs.13393.

45. LaPlante MP, Kaye HS. Demographics and trends in wheeled mobility equipment use and accessibility in the community. *Assist Technol*. 2010;22:3-17. doi:10.1080/10400430903501413.

46. Koontz AM, Ding D, Jan Y, et al. Wheeled mobility. *Biomed Res Int*. 2015;2015:138176. doi:10.1155/2015/138176.

47. Kaye HS, Kang T, LaPlante MP. *Mobility Device Use in the United States*. Disability Statistics Report 14. Washington, DC: U.S. Department of Education, National Institute on Disability and Rehabilitation Research; 2000.

48. Jones DA, Rader J. Seating and wheeled mobility for older adults living in nursing homes: what has changed clinically in the past 20 years? *Top Geriatr Rehabil*. 2015;31(1):10-18. doi:10.1097/TGR.0000000000000050.

49. Cook AM, Polgar JM. *Assistive Technologies: Principles and Practice*. St. Louis, MO: Elsevier/Mosby; 2015.

50. Chaves ES, Cooper RA, Collins DM, Karmarkar A, Cooper R. Review of the use of physical restraints and lap belts with wheelchair users. *Assist Technol*. 2007;19(2):94-107. doi:10.1080/10400435.2007.10131868.

51. Jones DA, Rader J. Considerations when working with the geriatric population. In: Lange ML, Minkel JL, eds. *Seating and Wheeled Mobility: A Clinical Resource Guide*. Thorofare, NJ: SLACK; 2018:297-315.

52. Ginter E, Simko V. Women live longer than men. *Bratisl Lek Listy*. 2013;114(02):45-49. doi:10.4149/bll_2013_011.

53. Ahmed T, Vafaei A, Auais M, Guralnik J, Zunzunegui MV. Gender roles and physical function in older adults: cross-sectional analysis of the international mobility in aging study (IMIAS). *PLoS One*. 2016;11(6):e0156828. doi:10.1371/journal.pone.0156828.

54. Giesbrecht EM, Mortenson WB, Miller WC. Prevalence and facility level correlates of need for wheelchair seating assessment among long-term care residents. *Gerontology*. 2012;58(4):378-384. doi:10.1159/000334819.

55. American Occupational Therapy Association. Occupational therapy practice framework: domain and process. 4th ed. *Am J Occup Ther*. 2020:74:2.

56. Rosen LE. Manual mobility applications for the person able to self-propel. In: *Seating and Wheeled Mobility: A Clinical Resource Guide*. Thorofare, NJ: SLACK; 2018:149-162.

57. van der Woude LHV, Bouw A, van Wegen J, van As H, Veeger D, de Groot S. Seat height: effects on submaximal hand rim wheelchair performance during spinal cord injury rehabilitation. *J Rehabil Med*. 2009;41(3):143-149. doi:10.2340/16501977-0296.

58. Giesbrecht EM, Ethans KD, Staley D. Measuring the effect of incremental angles of wheelchair tilt on interface pressure among individuals with spinal cord injury. *Spinal Cord*. 2011;49(7):827-831. doi:10.1038/sc.2010.194.

59. Zemp R, Rhiner J, Plüss S, Togni R, Plock JA, Taylor WR. Wheelchair tilt-in-space and recline functions: influence on sitting interface pressure and ischial blood flow in an elderly population. *Biomed Res Int*. 2019;2019:1-10. doi:10.1155/2019/4027976.

60. Babinec M. Power mobility applications: mobility categories and clinical indicators. In: *Seating and Wheeled Mobility: A Clinical Resource Guide*. Thorofare, NJ: SLACK; 2018:165-177.

61. Minkel J. Seating and mobility evaluations for persons with long-term disabilities: focusing on the client assessment. In: *Seating and Wheeled Mobility: A Clinical Resource Guide*. Thorofare, NJ: SLACK; 2018:3-26.

62. Pritchett A. *Best Practice: Houston Methodist Functional Mobility & Wheelchair Assessment Form*. Available at: https://www.numotion.com/blog/october-2017/best-practice-houston-methodist-functional-mobili. Accessed April 20, 2021.

63. Buck SNR. Manual mobility applications for the dependent user. In: *Seating and Wheeled Mobility: A Clinical Resource Guide*. Thorofare, NJ: SLACK; 2018:237-250.

64. Li CT, Chen YN, Chang CH, Tsai KH. The effects of backward adjustable thoracic support in wheelchair on spinal curvature and back

65. Holmes KJ, Michael SM, Thorpe SL, Solomonidis SE. Management of scoliosis with special seating for the non-ambulant spastic cerebral palsy population—a biomechanical study. *Clin Biomech (Bristol, Avon)*. 2003;18(6):480-487. doi:10.1016/s0268-0033(03)00075-5.

66. Papadopoulou S, Exarchakos G, Beris A, Ploumis A. Dysphagia associated with cervical spine and postural disorders. *Dysphagia*. 2013;28(4):469-480. doi:10.1007/s00455-013-9484-7.

67. Smith AE, Molton IR, Jensen MP. Self-reported incidence and age of onset of chronic comorbid medical conditions in adults aging with long-term physical disability. *Disabil Health J*. 2016;9(3):533-538. doi:10.1016/j.dhjo.2016.02.002.

68. Lamb SE, Jorstad-Stein EC, Hauer K, et al. Prevention of falls network Europe and outcomes consensus group. Development of a common outcome data set for fall injury prevention trials: the prevention of falls network of Europe consensus. *J Am Geriatr Soc*. 2005;53:1618-1622. doi:10.1111/j.1532-5415.2005.53455.x.

69. Bergen G, Stevens MR, Burns ER. "Falls and fall injuries among adults aged ≥65 years – United States, 2014". *MMWR Morb Mortal Wkly Rep*. 2016;65(37):993-998.

70. Centers for Disease Control and Prevention. *National Estimates of the 10 Leading Causes of Nonfatal Injuries Treated in Hospital Emergency Departments, United States – 2017*. 2017. Web-based Injury Statistics Query and Reporting System. Available at: https://www.cdc.gov/injury/wisqars/pdf//leading_causes_of_nonfatal_injury_2017-508.pdf.

71. National Council on Aging. *Get the Facts on Fall Prevention*. July 14, 2021. Available at: https://www.ncoa.org/article/get-the-facts-on-falls-prevention.

72. Rubenstein LZ, Solomon DH, Roth CP, et al. Detection and management of falls and instability in vulnerable elders by community physicians. *J Am Geriatr Soc*. 2009;57(9):1527-1531. doi:10.1111/j.1532-5415.2004.52417.x.

73. Alexander BH, Rivara FP, Wolf ME. "The cost and frequency of hospitalization for fall-related injuries in older adults." *Am J Public Health*. 1992;82(7):1020-1023.

74. Sterling DA, O'Connor JA, Bonadies J. "Geriatric falls: injury severity is high and disproportionate to mechanism." *J Trauma*. 2001;50(1):116-119.

75. Parkkari J, Kannus P, Palvanen M, et al. "Majority of hip fractures occur as a result of a fall and impact on the greater trochanter of the femur: a prospective controlled hip fracture study with 206 consecutive patients." *Calcif Tissue Int*. 1999;65(3):183-187.

76. Guzon-Illescas O, Perez Fernandez E, Crespí Villarias N, et al. "Mortality after osteoporotic hip fracture: incidence, trends, and associated factors." *J Orthop Surg Res*. 2019;14(1):203.

77. Haentjens P, Magaziner J, Colón-Emeric CS, et al. "Meta-analysis: excess mortality after hip fracture among older women and men." *Ann Intern Med*. 2010;152(6):380-390.

78. Centers for Disease Control and Prevention. *National Estimates of the 10 Leading Causes of Nonfatal Injuries Treated in Hospital Emergency Departments, United States – 2017*. 2017. Web-based Injury Statistics Query and Reporting System. Available at: https://www.cdc.gov/injury/wisqars/pdf/leading_causes_of_nonfatal_injury_2017-508.pdf.

79. Jung D, Lee J, Lee S. A meta-analysis of fear of falling treatment programs for the elderly. *West J Nurs Res*. 2009;31(1):6-16. doi:10.1177/0193945908320466.

80. The National Institute on Aging. *Prevent Falls and Fractures*. Available at: https://www.nia.nih.gov/health/prevent-falls-and-fractures.

81. Stevens JA, Ballesteros MF, Mack KA, et al. "Gender differences in seeking care for falls in the aged Medicare population." *Am J Prev Med*. 2012;43(1):59-62.

82. Florence CS, Bergen G, Atherly A, Burns E, Stevens J, Drake C. "Medical costs of fatal and nonfatal falls in older adults." *J Am Geriatr Soc*. 2018;66(4):693-698.

83. Frick KD, Kung JY, Parrish JM, et al. Evaluation the cost-effectiveness of fall prevention programs that reduce fall-related

hip fractures in older adults. *J Am Geriatr Soc.* 2010;58:136-141. doi:10.1111/j.1532-5415.2009.02575.x.

84. Rubenstein LZ, Josephson KR. The epidemiology of falls and syncope. *Clin Geriatr Med.* 2002;18:141-158. doi:10.1016/S0749-0690(02)00002-2.

85. Ambrose AF, Paul GP, Hausdorff JM. Risk factors for falls among older adults: a review of the literature. *Maturitas.* 2013;75:51-61. doi:10.1016/j.maturitas.2013.02.009.

86. Carpenter C, Scheatzle M, D'Antonio J, et al. Identification of fall risk factors in older adult emergency department patients. *Acad Emerg Med.* 2009;16(3):211-219. doi:10.1111/j.1553-2712.2009.00351.x.

87. Rubenstein LZ, Josephson KR. Falls and their prevention in elderly people: what does the evidence show? *Med Clin North Am.* 2006;90:807-824. doi:10.1016/j.mcna.2006.05.013.

88. US Department of Helath and Human Services, National Institute on Aging. *Fall-Proofing Your Home.* Available at: https://www.nia.nih.gov/health/fall-proofing-your-home.

89. American Foundation of the Blind. *Special Report on Aging and Vision Loss.* 2013. American Foundation for the Blind. Available at: http://www.afb.org/info/blindness-statistics/adults/special-report-on-aging-and-vision-loss/235.

90. Pollock A, Hazelton C, Henderson CA, et al. Interventions for age-related visual problems in patients with stroke. *Cochrane Database Syst Rev.* 2012;(3):CD008390. doi:10.1002/14651858.CD008390.pub2.

91. Varma R, Vajaranant TS, Burkemper B, et al. Visual impairment and blindness in adults in the United States: demographic and geographic variations from 2015 to 2050. *JAMA Ophthalmol.* 2016;134(7):802-809. doi:10.1001/jamaophthalmol.2016.1284.

92. Light K, Thigpen M. *Geriatric Rehabilitation: Evidence and Clinical Application.* New York: McGraw-Hill; 2010.

93. Naqvi F, Lee S, Fields L. Appraising a guideline for preventing acute care falls. *Geriatrics.* 2009;64(3):10-33. doi:10.1097/NCI.0b013e3181ac2628.

94. Nolte J. *The Human Brain: An Introduction to Its Functional Anatomy.* 6th ed. Philadelphia: Mosby Elsevier; 2009.

95. Ribeiro KMOB de F, Freitas RV de M, Ferreira LM de BM, Deshpande N, Guerra RO. Effects of balance Vestibular Rehabilitation Therapy in older adults with Benign Paroxysmal Positional Vertigo: a randomized controlled trial. *Disabil Rehabil.* 2017;39(12):1198-1206.

96. Costarella M, Monteleone L, Steindler R, et al. Decline of physical and cognitive conditions in the elderly measured through the functional reach test and the Mini-Mental State Examination. *Arch Gerontol Geriatr.* 2010;50(3):332-337. doi:10.1016/j.archger.2009.05.013.

97. Carter ND, Kannus P, Khan KM. Exercise in the prevention of falls in older people: a systematic literature review examining the rationale and the evidence. *Sports Med.* 2001;31:427-438.

98. Mol A, Bui Hoang PTS, Sharmin S, et al. Orthostatic hypotension and falls in older adults: a systematic review and meta-analysis. *J Am Med Dir Assoc.* 2019;20(5):589-597.e5. doi:10.1016/j.jamda.2018.11.003.

99. Montero-Odasso M, Speechley M. Falls in cognitively impaired older adults: implications for risk assessment and prevention. *J Am Geriatr Soc.* 2018;66(2):367-375. doi:10.1111/jgs.15219.

100. Muir SW, Gopaul K, Montero Odasso MM. The role of cognitive impairment in fall risk among older adults: a systematic review and meta-analysis. *Age Ageing.* 2012;41(3):299-308.

101. Payette MC, Bélanger C, Léveillé V, Grenier S. Fall-related psychological concerns and anxiety among community-dwelling older adults: systematic review and meta-analysis. *PLoS One.* 2016;11(4):e0152848.

102. Ang SGM, O'Brien AP, Wilson A. Understanding carers' fall concern and their management of fall risk among older people at home. *BMC Geriatr.* 2019;19(1):144.

103. Woolcott J, Richardson K, Wiens M, et al. Meta-analysis of the impact of 9 medication classes on falls in elderly persons. *Arch Intern Med.* 2009;169(21):1952-1960.

104. Gillespie LD, Robertson MC, Gillespie WJ, et al. Interventions for preventing falls in older people living in the community. *Cochrane Database Syst Rev.* 2012;(9):CD007146. doi:10.1002/14651858.CD007146.pub2.

105. U.S. Department of Health and Human Services, Adminitation for Community Living and Administation on Aging. *2018 Profile of Older Americans.* Available at: https://acl.gov/sites/default/files/Aging%20and%20Disability%20in%20America/2018OlderAmericansProfile.pdf.

106. Phelan EA, Mahoney JE, Voit JC, Stevens JA. Assessment and management of fall risk in primary care settings. *Med Clin North Am.* 2015;99(2):281-293.

107. Tideiksaar R. Geriatric falls: assessing the cause, preventing recurrence. *Geriatrics.* 1989;44(7):57. doi:10.1016/j.amepre.2012.03.008.

108. Peterson EW, Clemson L. Understanding the role of occupational therapy in fall prevention for community-dwelling older adults. *OT Practice.* 2008;13:CE1-CE8.

109. Cameron ID, Gillespie LD, Robertson MC, et al. Interventions for preventing falls in older people in care facilities and hospitals. *Cochrane Database Syst Rev.* 2012;(12):CD005465. doi:10.1002/14651858.CD005465.pub3.

110. Panel on Prevention of Falls in Older Persons, American Geriatrics Society and British Geriatrics Society. Summary of the updated American Geriatrics Society/British Geriatrics Society Clinical practice guideline for prevention of falls in older persons. *J Am Geriatr Soc.* 2011;59(1):148-157.

111. Bergen G, Shakya I. *Center's for Disease Control.* CDC Steadi. Evaluation Guide for Older Adults Clinical Fall Prevention Programs. Available at: https://www.cdc.gov/steadi/pdf/Steadi-Evaluation-Guide_Final_4_30_19.pdf.

112. Elliott S, Leland NE. Occupational therapy fall prevention interventions for community-dwelling older adults: a systematic review. *Am J Occup Ther.* 2018;72(4):7204190040p1-7204190040p11.

113. American Occupational Therapy Association. *Occupational Therapy and Prevention of Falls.* Available at: https://www.aota.org/About-Occupational-Therapy/Professionals/PA/Facts/Fall-Prevention.aspx.

114. Chewning B, Hallisy KM, Mahoney JE, Wilson D, Sangasubana N, Gangnon R. Disseminating Tai chi in the community: promoting home practice and improving balance. *Gerontologist.* 2020;60(4):765-777.

115. *Matter of Balance.* Mainehealth.org. Available at: https://www.mainehealth.org/healthy-communities/healthy-aging/matter-of-balance.

116. Guo JL, Tsai YY, Liao JY, et al. Interventions to reduce the number of falls among older adults with/without cognitive impairment: an exploratory meta-analysis. *Int J Geriatr Psychiatry.* 2014;29:661-669. doi:10.1002/gps.4056.

117. Kim H, Han J, Cho Y. The effectiveness of community-based tai chi training on balance control during stair descent by older adults. *J Phys Ther Sci.* 2009;21:317-323. doi:10.1589/jpts.21.317.

118. Logghe IHJ, Verhage AP, Rademaker ACHJ, et al. The effects of tai chi on fall prevention, fear of falling and balance in older people: a meta-anaylsis. *Prev Med.* 2010;51:222-227. doi:10.1016/j.ypmed.2010.06.003.

119. Swancutt DR, Hope SV, Kent BP, Robinson M, Goodwin VA. Knowledge, skills and attitudes of older people and staff about getting up from the floor following a fall: a qualitative investigation. *BMC Geriatr.* 2020;20(1):385. doi:10.1186/s12877-020-01790-7.

120. University of Michigan Health. *How to Get Up Safely After a Fall.* Available at: https://www.uofmhealth.org/health-library/abl3081.

121. Christenson M, Chase C, eds. *Occupational Therapy and Home Modification: Promoting Safety and Supporting Participation.* American Occupational Therapy; 2011.

122. Centers for Disease Control and Prevention. *Check for Safety: A Home Fall Prevention Checklist for Older Adults*. Available at: https://www.cdc.gov/steadi/pdf/check_for_safety_brochure-a.pdf.

123. Centers for Disease Control and Prevention. Falls and fall injuries among adults with arthritis – United States, 2012. *MMWR Morb Mortal Wkly Rep*. 2014;63:379-383.

124. Centers for Disease Control and Prevention. *Preventing Falls Among Older Adults*. National Center for Injury Prevention and Control; 2009.

125. Quigley P. Tailoring falls-prevention intervention to each patient. *Am Nurse Today*. 2015;8-10. doi:10.1080/17483100903038576.

126. Miake-Lye IM, Hempel S, Ganz DA, et al. Inpatient fall prevention program as a patient safety strategy: a systematic review. *Ann Intern Med*. 2013;158:390-396. doi:10.1002/14651858.

127. Spolestra SL, Given BA, Given CW. Fall prevention in hospitals: an integrative review. *Clin Nurs Res*. 2011;21:92-112. doi:10.1177/1054773811418106.

128. Shimada H, Tiedeman A, Lord S, et al. The effect of enhanced supervision on fall rates in residential aged care. *Am J Phys Med Rehabil*. 2009;88:823-828. doi:10.1097/PHM.0b013e3181b71ec2.

129. Chang J, Ganz D. Quality indicators for falls and mobility problems in vulnerable elders. *J Am Geriatr Soc*. 2007;55(S2):S327-S334. doi:10.1111/j.1532-5415.2007.01339.x.

130. AARP. *Stats and Facts from the 2018 AARP Home and Community Preferences survey*. Available at: https://www.aarp.org/livable-communities/about/info-2018/2018-aarp-home-and-community-preferences-survey.html.

131. Ortman JM, Velkoff VA, Hogan H. *An Aging Nation: The Older Population in the United States*. Washington, DC: US Census Bureau; 2014:25-1140.

132. US Department of Transportation, National Highway Traffic Safety Administration. *Traffic Safety Facts: Older Population 2017 Data*. DOT HS 812 684. March 2019. Available at: https://crashstats.nhtsa.dot.gov/Api/Public/ViewPublication/812684.

133. US Department of Transportation, National Highway Traffic Safety Administration. *Traffic Safety Facts. 2018 Fatal Motor Vehicle Crashes: Overview*. October 2019. Available at: https://crashstats.nhtsa.dot.gov/Api/Public/ViewPublication/ 812826.

134. Borowsky A, Shinar D, Oron-Gilad T. Age, skill, and hazard perception in driving. *Accid Anal Prev*. 2010;42:1240-1249. doi:10.1016/j.aap.2010.02.001.

135. National Institutes on Aging. *Older Drivers*. 2018. Available at: https://www.nia.nih.gov/health/publication/older-drivers.

136. Stav WB. Updated systematic review on older adult community mobility and driver licensing policies. *Am J Occup Ther*. 2014;68(6):681-689. doi:10.5014/ajot.2014.011510.

137. Hoggarth PA, Innes CR, Dalrymple-Alford JC, et al. Comparison of a linear and a non-linear model for using sensory-motor, cognitive, personality, and demographic data to predict driving ability in healthy older adults. *Accid Anal Prev*. 2010;42:1759-1768. doi:10.1016/j.aap.2010.04.017.

138. Federal Communications Commission. *The Dangers of Distracted Driving*. 2020. Available at: https://www.fcc.gov/consumers/guides/dangers-texting-while-driving.

139. Parada H, Laughlin GA, Yang M, Nedjat-Haiem FR, McEvoy LK. Dual impairments in visual and hearing acuity and age-related cognitive decline in older adults from the Rancho Bernardo Study of Healthy Aging. *Age Ageing*. 2021;50(4):1268-1276. doi:10.1093/ageing/afaa285.

140. Centers for Disease Control and Prevention. *The State of Vision, Aging, and Public Health in America*; 2012. Available at: http://www.cdc.gov/visionhealth/pdf/vision_brief.pdf.

141. Esenwah EC, Azuamah YC, Okorie ME, et al. The aging eye and vision: a review. *Int J Health Sci Res*. 2014;4(7):218-226.

142. Schleber F. Aging and the senses. In: Birren J, Cohen G, Sloan R, eds, et al. *Handbook of Mental Health and Aging*. Cambridge, MA: Academic Press; 2013:251.

143. Lockhart TE, Shi W. Effects of age on dynamic accommodation. *Ergonomics*. 2010;53(7):892-903. doi:10.1080/00140139.2010.489968.

144. Ilett G. Functional vision assessment. *Optician*. 2010;240(6260):24-25.

145. AARP. *Vision and Driving*. Available at: http://www.aarp.org/auto/driver-safety/info-2013/vision-and-safe-driving-tips.html.

146. Whitson HE, Cronin-Golomb A, Cruickshanks KJ, et al. American Geriatrics Society and National Institute on Aging Bench-to-Bedside Conference: sensory impairment and cognitive decline in older adults. *J Am Geriatr Soc*. 2018;66(11):2052-2058. doi:10.1111/jgs.15506.

147. National Institute on Deafness and Other Communication Disorders. *Age-Related Hearing Loss*. 2018. Available at: http://www.nidcd.nih.gov/health/hearing/Pages/Age-Related-Hearing-Loss.aspx.

148. Lin CJ, Cheng LY, Yang CW. An investigation of the influence of age on eye fatigue and hand operation performance in a virtual environment. *Vis Comput*. 2020;37:2301-2313. doi:10.1007/s00371-020-01987-2.

149. Distefano G, Goodpaster BH. Effects of exercise and aging on skeletal muscle. *Cold Spring Harb Perspect Med*. 2017;8(3):a029785. doi:10.1101/cshperspect.a029785.

150. Carfit. 2021. Available at: https://www.car-fit.org/.

151. Kaldenberg J, Smallfield S. Occupational therapy practice guidelines for older adults with low vision. *Am J Occup Ther*. 2020;74(2):7402397010p1-7402397010p23. doi:10.7139/2017.978-1-56900-456-2.

152. United States Department of Justice Civil Rights Division. *Information and Technical Assistance on the Americans With Disabilities Act. State and Local Governments* (Title II). Available at: https://www.ada.gov/ada_title_II. htm.

153. Administration for Community Living. *Transportation Options for Older Adults*. 2015. Available at: https://acl.gov/programs/transportation/transportation.

154. Chia D. *Policies and Practices for Effectively and Efficiently Meeting ADA Paratransit Demand: A Synthesis of Transit Practice*. Washington, DC: Transit Cooperative Research Board/Transportation Research Board; 2008.

Working With Older Adults Who Have Vision Impairments

EVELYN Z. KATZ AND MALLORY ROSCHE

(PREVIOUS CONTRIBUTIONS FROM REBECCA BOTHWELL)

KEY TERMS

cataracts, contrast sensitivity, diabetic retinopathy, diplopia, eccentric viewing, glaucoma, hemi-inattention, lens, macular degeneration, oculomotor control, pattern recognition, retina, scanning, scotoma, strabismus, visual acuity, visual attention, visual cognition, visual fields, visual memory

CHAPTER OBJECTIVES

1. Describe typical physiological changes affecting vision that occur with aging.
2. Name and describe the major ocular diseases affecting vision in older adults.
3. Describe common vision deficits resulting from neurological insults in older adults.
4. Describe psychosocial implications of vision impairments in older adults and possible effects on rehabilitation and functional outcomes.
5. Describe the use of the *Occupational Therapy Practice Framework's*, fourth edition, dynamic, interactive process of evaluation, intervention, and outcomes to address

functional deficits in older adult clients resulting from visual impairments.
6. Identify general principles to enhance vision.
7. Identify environmental or contextual considerations and interventions to increase independence and safety in older adults with low vision.
8. Identify general principles in intervention of visual dysfunction after brain insult.
9. Identify team members and community resources that registered occupational therapists (OTs) and occupational therapy assistants (OTAs) may collaborate with to improve functional outcomes in older adults with low vision.

Ellie is an 82-year-old widow who lived alone in the two-story home that she shared with her husband for more than 50 years. At a visit to her ophthalmologist, she was told that her complaints of blurry vision with reading the mail and newspaper were due to dry macular degeneration, and that new glasses would not help her. The ophthalmologist informed her that there was nothing he could do to correct her condition.

Ellie is now at a subacute rehabilitation facility following a recent knee replacement surgery, and the occupational therapist and occupational therapy assistant (OT/OTA) team has been ordered to follow her. She tells them that she is a little afraid to be at home alone. She is having trouble seeing her appliance controls and the phone keypad. Between her new knee replacement and her vision loss, she does not know whether she can navigate the steps in her home. She is nervous about going outdoors because she is having trouble seeing curbs and changes in walking surfaces, especially at dusk or on hazy

days. She feels isolated and lonely. Her children are wondering whether she will be able to return home.

- Do you think someone with partial sight, like Ellie, can function independently?
- What would you do if you, like Ellie, could not read regular print, street signs, or the controls on your appliances?

Visual impairments are common in the older adult population. Over four million American adults age 40 years and older experience irreversible vision loss, and this number is expected to double to close to 9 million by the year 2050.[1] The odds of developing visual impairment worsen with age, as one in four adults age 75 years or older experiences either a moderate or severe visual impairment.[2] In addition to vision loss from ocular disease, many adults are affected by visual impairments resulting from head trauma, stroke, or neurological insult. Between 40% and 75% of individuals with head trauma or stroke are estimated to experience visual impairments requiring rehabilitation.[3]

According to the fourth edition of the *Occupational Therapy Practice Framework: Domain and Process (OTPF-4)*, visual functions are addressed in the Client Factors table as a body function under the sensory functions category, as well as a component of the perception portion of the specific mental functions category.[4] These statistics along with the inclusion of vision in the *OTPF-4* demonstrate the need for OTAs to possess a thorough understanding of the causes of vision loss and appropriate intervention techniques.[4] Regardless of the particular setting, any OTA working with older adults is likely to encounter many clients with visual impairments.

This chapter provides information on the psychosocial effects of vision loss, effects of normal aging on vision, common conditions causing vision loss in older adults, and visual dysfunction after neurological insult. The chapter also addresses the process for assessing older adult clients' occupational performance and outcomes as well as general principles used in planning interventions to help older adult clients achieve their functional goals. OTs and OTAs function as part of a team that includes physicians, other health care providers, family/caregivers, and the older adult client. The chapter addresses the roles of these team members and community resources.

PSYCHOSOCIAL EFFECTS OF VISION IMPAIRMENT

Approximately one-third of older adults with visual impairments experience clinically significant symptoms of depression and anxiety.[5] These percentages are significantly higher when compared to the prevalence of depression in the general older adult population.[5] The thought of losing one's vision is one of the most devastating disabilities imaginable. Without vision, the ability to perform many of the daily activities normally taken for granted is lost. Additionally, social participation is impaired in older adults with low vision, with fewer social interactions and difficulties with interpersonal skills reported.[6] The thought of vision loss conjures up a terrifying world of blackness. However, although most people think of vision loss as total blindness, most individuals with visual impairments are not totally blind. In fact, 85% of all individuals with visual impairments still have some remaining vision, and only about 15% are completely blind.[7] It is often difficult for family members, friends, and the general public to understand the limitations and capabilities of those with partial sight.[8] It is not uncommon for partially sighted individuals to be labeled as "fakes" when others observe that they are capable of one task that requires some degree of vision but are incapable of another task.[8] This confusion about the abilities of those with partial sight may produce more psychological distress than does total blindness.[8]

In addition to the ambiguity associated with being partially sighted, individuals often find it difficult to adjust to their vision loss because of the uncertainty of their condition.

For many, it is difficult to know whether their vision will improve, stay the same, or get worse. There is often an internal struggle with a desire to be independent and the desire to be taken care of. In some situations, older adults may want assistance but feel unable to ask for it. Ball and Nicolle[9] note that, for a person with visual impairment, if a daily activity is not carried out in the normal manner, then it might be avoided as the person does not want to be viewed as different. Furthermore, this attitude may exhibit itself in many ways, most commonly with refusal to use mobility aids or other beneficial equipment.

Older adults struggling with vision loss may experience mood swings and may go through some of the stages of grieving as discussed by Kubler-Ross (denial, anger, bargaining, depression, and acceptance).[10] Many individuals who experience visual loss often are at risk for depression due to their loss of independence.[10] According to Casten and Rovner,[11] if depression is not identified and dealt with, it can interfere with the daily routines of that person and affect the rehabilitation process. Stages of adaptation to the visual impairment identified by Tuttle and Tuttle[12] include trauma (physical or social), shock and denial, mourning and withdrawal, succumbing and depression, reassessment and reaffirmation, coping and mobilization, self-acceptance, and self-esteem.[12]

EFFECTS OF THE NORMAL AGING PROCESS ON VISION

Although older adults are more likely to experience visual impairments because of specific ocular and neurological pathologies, they also experience many age-related changes that affect visual functioning. These normal changes must be taken into consideration when working with this population.

The retina is a multilayered lining of neural tissue on the innermost part of the eye (Fig. 15.1). It receives visual

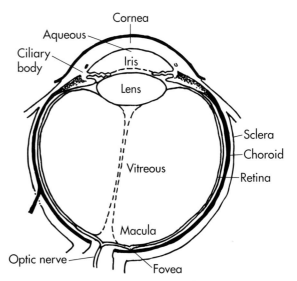

FIG. 15.1 Anatomy of the eye.

messages and transmits them through the optic nerve to the brain.[13] The central area of the retina, or macula, has a concentration of cone cells that enable color vision and fine-detail discrimination. Rod cells are extremely sensitive to light and provide peripheral vision and night vision.[13] As the retina ages, it gradually loses neurons. Central or peripheral vision may be affected, depending on which retinal neurons die. The rate of retinal deterioration and the resultant visual field loss vary among individuals, but, generally, older adults experience shrinkage of the peripheral field and face difficulty with light and dark adaptation. Older adults require increased time to switch from viewing near objects to far objects (accommodation) and to recover from glare. Because pupil size and function decrease with age, older adults require more illumination for fine-detail tasks. Many older adults require three times more light than a person requires in his or her 20s or 30s.[14]

Changes may also occur in the lens of the eye with age (see Fig. 15.1). The lens is responsible for properly focusing the image on the retina.[13] It does this by changing shape according to the distance of the object being viewed.[15] As the lens ages, it loses some of its elasticity, making shape change or accommodation more difficult. This condition, called presbyopia, affects focal ability at near distances, making it difficult to read print or perform close-vision tasks.[16] The greatest change usually occurs between ages 40 and 45 years.[16] Reading glasses or bifocals are often prescribed at this time. In addition to this loss of elasticity, the lens also becomes yellower with age.[17] This deeper yellow can affect the ability to differentiate between colors and discriminate objects with low contrast.[16]

SPECIFIC OCULAR PATHOLOGIES

In addition to the natural aging process, specific pathological eye conditions have a more profound effect on functional visual abilities. Four major conditions that affect an older adult's vision are cataracts, age-related macular degeneration (ARMD; wet or dry), glaucoma, and diabetic retinopathy. Each of these conditions can cause visual impairment when they occur in isolation, but they commonly cooccur in older adults, increasing the challenge to remain functionally independent (Table 15.1). More about general intervention ideas for any ocular condition will be presented later in the chapter.

Cataracts

A cataract is a clouding of the lens, the clear part of the eye that helps focus light, or an image on the retina.[18] This clouding is related to aging and changes in the protein that, along with water, make up the lens. Protein clumps up in the lens, forming cataracts, which make vision blurry and dull by preventing adequate amounts of light from reaching the retina.[19] Cataracts can be treated successfully with surgery and are no longer considered to be a major cause of permanent visual impairment in developed countries. The most common procedure is the removal of the opacified lens followed by the insertion of an intraocular lens implant.[20]

If an older adult is struggling with cataracts before surgery or if the older adult is not a surgical candidate, interventions that control glare, increase lighting, and low levels of magnification can be helpful.

Macular Degeneration or Age-Related Macular Degeneration

Macular degeneration is the leading cause of vision loss in older Americans.[21] The macula is the central portion of the retina where the clearest vision is found. There are two types of macular degeneration: the "dry" (nonexudative or atrophic) type and the "wet" (exudative or hemorrhagic type). Dry ARMD is the result of yellowish deposits, or drusen, forming under the macula. This causes the macula

TABLE 15.1

Changes in Visual System Associated With Age

Structural component	Age-related change	Functional implications
Cornea	Decreased fluid bathing cornea	Dryness, irritation
	Accumulation of lipids	Increased astigmatism with increased blurring of vision
Iris	Decreased permeability	May contribute to glaucoma
Ciliary muscles	Atrophy of muscles	Decreased mobility of lens causing decreased muscle effectiveness
Pupil	Decreased pupil size	Decreased light reaching retina; difficulty seeing dark objects or objects in dim light
	Decreased pupillary reflex	Decreased dark adaptation and recovery from glare
Lens	Lens growth	Decreased accommodative ability
	Decreased refractive index of lenses	Uneven refracture properties can result in double vision in one eye
	Yellowing	Reduced amount of light reaching retina, changes in light composition alters color vision
Vitreous	Contracts	Increased chance of separation from retina or retinal detachment

Adapted from Zoltan B. *Vision, Perception, and Cognition: A Manual for the Evaluation and Treatment of the Adult with Acquired Brain Injury.* 4th ed. Thorofare, NJ: Slack; 2006.

to thin and dry out. As cells on the macula become nonfunctioning, older adults experience a blurry, dark, or blank spot in the center of their visual field. The wet form of ARMD is caused by the rapid growth of small blood vessels beneath the macula. These blood vessels leak and cause scarring on the macula, resulting in vision loss.[21] The wet form of ARMD can sometimes be treated with photocoagulation, laser surgery, or, more recently and effectively, by intraocular injection with Macugen, Lucentis, or Avastin (drugs that dry up the leaking blood vessels and slow their regrowth). Results of the Age-Related Eye Disease Studies suggest that progression of dry ARMD can be slowed by the intake of antioxidant supplements.[19] Current interventions can slow the rate of vision loss; however, there is no known intervention that prevents macular degeneration or that can reverse the loss of vision.[19] Because peripheral visual fields are usually spared, ARMD does not result in total blindness.[21]

Common problems experienced by older adults with ARMD include difficulty distinguishing faces, reading signs, or seeing traffic signals (distance tasks). Other problems are reading regular print, writing, and doing needlework (near tasks). Older adults with wet ARMD often experience distortion of the central visual field that may make straight lines appear wavy (metamorphopsia). This distortion can lead to balance and mobility problems. Visual hallucinations as a result of Charles Bonnet syndrome are sometimes experienced by older adults with ARMD. The hallmark of these hallucinations is that they occur and disappear spontaneously with no known external cause, and they are recognized as unreal by the older adult and are nonthreatening.[22] Visual hallucinations have been described as simple, similar to a grid-like and branching pattern, to more complex hallucinations, which include images of faces, animals, or plants.[22] Older adults experiencing Charles Bonnet syndrome may be reluctant to discuss their visual symptoms, fearing a label of mental instability or decreased cognitive function. They need to be reassured that this is not the case. Charles Bonnet syndrome has been found to affect older adults with ARMD with severe loss of contrast sensitivity in both eyes.[23] OTAs working with older adults who have macular degeneration should be aware of specific interventions for this diagnosis (Box 15.1).

Glaucoma

Glaucoma is a group of serious ocular conditions that involve excessively high pressure inside the eyeball. This increased pressure results from a buildup of excess fluid in the eye.[13] Increased intraocular pressure can eventually cause damage to the optic nerve or the blood vessels that supply the optic nerve.[13] One of the first effects of this optic nerve damage is usually a loss of vision in the peripheral field (Fig. 15.2). This loss of peripheral vision is often not noticed by the individual initially, and the disease frequently progresses substantially before it is noticed.[24] If

BOX 15.1

> ## Interventions for Individuals With Macular Degeneration
>
> Older adults with macular degeneration usually experience problems with loss of detail and central vision early in their vision loss. Peripheral vision is usually spared, even in more advanced stages.
>
> - Lighting—provide training with different types of task lighting: full spectrum incandescent, fluorescent, halogen, and LED as well as positioning of the lighting source so that the older adult can identify which one is preferred for an activity. If using a lamp, light should be positioned over the better-seeing eye.
> - Reduce glare in the older adult's environment by eliminating bare or exposed light bulbs and highly polished or reflective surfaces; use light diffusing shades, blinds, or curtains; and careful placement of furniture.
> - Use color and contrast in the older adult's environment to define objects and surfaces—a contrasting colored towel, draped on a chair can make it easier to see. Eating dark colored foods from a white plate and light colored foods from a dark plate can make it easier to identify foods.
> - Increase object size—large numbered phones, kitchen timers, medicine organizers, large print checks make ADLs and IADLs easier to complete with decreased central or detail vision.
> - Decrease clutter, including visual clutter—clear paths from room to room and in front of furniture, counters, and appliances. Limit the number of items on countertops and tables. Limit use of bold patterns, which create visual clutter.
> - Magnification—when possible, older adults will need referral to a low-vision ophthalmologist or optometrist to prescribe the appropriate magnification devices for near, intermediate, and distance activities. However, magnifying lamps, nail clippers with attached low powered magnifiers, and inexpensive low powered magnifiers for craft and sewing may allow the older adult to complete activities with decreased vision.
> - Transportation options—train older adults in use of alternative transportation. Many communities have paratransit systems for individuals who cannot drive or use conventional public transportation safely. Some communities offer reduced fare taxi programs for the visually impaired.

left undetected and untreated, this loss can lead to total blindness. Older adults should be encouraged to have routine ophthalmological visits so that glaucoma may be diagnosed at an early stage. When the diagnosis is early, individuals respond well to medication and, if necessary, surgery to improve the balance of fluid in the eye.[13]

There are many types of glaucoma, but open-angle is the most common.[13] Other types include closed-angle or

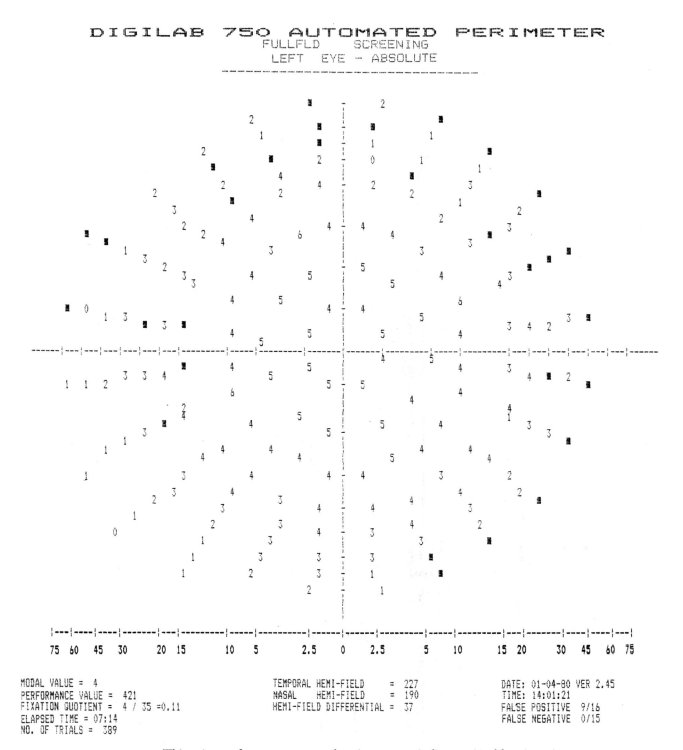

FIG. 15.2 This printout from an automated perimeter test indicates visual loss in points marked with black squares. Note the peripheral distribution.

narrow-angle, traumatic, and low-tension glaucoma.[13] Open-angle glaucoma involves an eye with normal anatomy that, for unknown reasons, is not able to drain the fluid as efficiently as it produces it. This leads to a slow, gradual buildup of intraocular pressure over time.[13]

Closed- or narrow-angle glaucoma is less common. This type of glaucoma progresses rapidly, and symptoms are immediately apparent. Sudden, severe ocular and head pain, blurred vision or sudden loss of vision, nausea, and eye redness may be symptoms of an acute attack of narrow-angle glaucoma.[25] Emergency surgery is often required to reduce the intraocular pressure.

The functional implications of glaucoma vary greatly, depending on the severity of the disease. When diagnosis

BOX 15.2

Interventions for Individuals With Glaucoma

Most individuals with glaucoma do not experience problems with their vision until their disease is relatively advanced.

- Medication management is vital—train older adult in nonvisual techniques, labeling, organization, talking labels, and talking reminders or alarms for self-administering oral medicines and eye drops.
- Mobility problems (due to reduced peripheral vision)—address by use of contrast, reduce clutter/tripping hazards, train for awareness of boundaries and edges when ambulating in the environment; refer to orientation and mobility specialist for long cane (white cane) and nonsighted techniques for community mobility.
- Contrast and glare—use of yellow, amber, or light plum glasses to increase contrast and decrease glare. Reduce reflective surfaces (glass tabletops, mirrors, highly polished floors, or counters), cover exposed light bulbs, windows, and angle task light sources to decrease glare.
- Low-power magnifiers—may help for small print or poor contrast materials.
- Increase object size for ease of identification—use large print medication organizers, telephones, calculators, and calendars to increase success with IADLs.
- Bright colored, high-contrast objects will stand out if the older adult has decreased contrast sensitivity. Using a contrasting color towel underneath grooming tools in the bathroom can increase ability to see the tools.
- Organized scanning patterns—train the older adult to scan in horizontal left to right, zig-zag, and circular patterns to locate obstacles, edges, and objects because of reduced visual field.

is early, glaucoma can be treated, and many people may have little need to adjust their lifestyles. If the disease is allowed to progress, individuals may experience decreased peripheral vision, difficulty adjusting to changing light, fluctuating and blurred vision, shadow-like halos around lights, and an increased sensitivity to glare.[26] If glaucoma goes undiagnosed, a person may lose all of his or her vision beginning with the peripheral field and eventually extending into the central visual field. Mobility and safety can be severely compromised in older adults with advanced glaucoma. Referral to an orientation and mobility teacher may be appropriate for an older adult experiencing decreased mobility because of vision loss at this stage. OTAs working with older adults who have glaucoma should be aware of specific interventions for this diagnosis (Box 15.2).

Diabetic Retinopathy

Diabetic retinopathy, one of the complications of diabetes mellitus, is another leading cause of visual impairment in older adults. Diabetic retinopathy has four stages: (1) mild nonproliferative retinopathy, the earliest stage in which microaneurysms occur as a small ballooning in the tiny vessels of the retina[19]; (2) moderate nonproliferative retinopathy, during which some blood vessels that nourish the retina are blocked; (3) severe nonproliferative retinopathy, during which many blood vessels are blocked, depriving areas of the retina of their blood supply (this causes the growth of new blood vessels to nourish the retina, leading to the next stage); and (4) proliferative retinopathy. In this most advanced stage, new blood vessels grow along the retina and along the surface of the vitreous gel that fills the inside of the eye. The new blood vessels are abnormal, with fragile walls that may leak and cause more severe changes in visual acuity. The new network of vessels and its accompanying fibrous tissue contract, and the vitreous may pull away from the retina causing further hemorrhage into the vitreous. This can also cause a retinal detachment, a serious condition requiring immediate attention and surgery to prevent vision loss.[19] If fluid leaks into the center of the macula, swelling and blurred vision can occur. This condition, known as macular edema, can happen at any stage of diabetic retinopathy, causing a significant distortion and loss of vision.[19]

Diabetic retinopathy may be treated either by photocoagulation, injection (similar to procedures used to treat wet macular degeneration), or a procedure known as vitrectomy, during which blood is removed from the vitreous of the eye with a needle and replaced with saline solution. Many people experience improved vision after these procedures, but they do not cure diabetic retinopathy. The risk of new bleeding and vision loss remains.[19]

Functional implications of diabetic retinopathy, like glaucoma, vary depending on early diagnosis and severity of the disease. Some individuals with mild retinopathy may not need to make adaptations in their performance patterns, whereas others may need to learn adaptive techniques to compensate for vision loss to continue to perform activities of daily living (ADLs) safely and independently. Many older adults who have advanced diabetic retinopathy experience decreased contrast sensitivity, poor night vision, and fluctuating, blurry, or spotty vision. Some older adults may eventually need to learn nonsighted techniques for all ADLs. OTAs working with older adults who have diabetic retinopathy should be aware of specific interventions for this diagnosis (Box 15.3).

VISUAL DYSFUNCTION AFTER NEUROLOGICAL INSULT

The discussion of visual impairments in older adults thus far has focused on impairments as a result of ocular conditions. However, the visual system is not composed of the eyeballs alone. To perceive visual information, the data must travel through a complex nervous system and must be processed by appropriate cerebral centers. In addition, effective control of eye movements depends on proper

BOX 15.3

Interventions for Individuals With Diabetic Retinopathy

Diabetic retinopathy often causes blurriness, fluctuations in vision, and may sometimes result in either central or peripheral field loss.

- Medication management may require referral to a diabetes educator. Consider talking glucometers, prefilled syringes, syringe magnifiers, insulin "pens," large print logs for recording blood glucose readings, insulin dosage counters, and other adaptive equipment.
- Increase contrast in environment, printed materials, writing materials, and on the computer screen.
- Control glare with yellow, amber, or light plum tinted glasses, lighting placement, and limiting reflective surfaces in the environment (see Box 15.8).
- Neuropathy can cause loss of sensation in extremities. Special attention to safety during kitchen and bathroom activities is an essential component of training. Adaptive equipment for kitchen tasks include knife guards that slip over the fingers of the hand that holds the item to be cut, long oven mitts, oven rack guards, oven rack pulls, long handled tongs, can openers that produce a smooth edge, and nonslip cutting boards.
- Magnification or large print materials may make reading, writing, and other near tasks easier.
- Vision substitution—talking books, scales, microwaves, glucometers, and other devices offer options for completing ADLs and IADLs with decreased vision.

BOX 15.4

Interventions for Individuals With Neurological Visual Impairments

It is essential for the OTA to have as complete a picture as possible of the visual, cognitive, and physical deficits of the older adult with neurological visual impairment because they will affect interventions and functional outcomes.

- Train older adults and family/caregiver about the functional implications of visual field loss for safety and ADL performance—make sure they understand how much of the environment the older adult may not see or be aware of.
- For left-sided visual field loss, train the older adult to turn head and eyes toward the "missing" side or area when beginning any activity and more frequently throughout the activity.
- Train the older adult to increase visual search organization and scanning patterns beginning with horizontal left to right, right to left, vertical top to bottom, and circular patterns.
- Use activities that widen boundaries of visual search, and encourage use of appropriate search strategies in a variety of environments: searching for objects/signage on a wall or vacuuming to use left-to-right vertical search.
- Intervention techniques for left-to-right horizontal pattern: dominoes, card search, sweeping, wiping off a counter, and looking for items on a shelf.
- Intervention techniques for left-to-right vertical pattern: reading columns in sports scores or financial pages, reading ingredients in a recipe, and writing a grocery list.
- Intervention techniques for circular patterns: puzzles, walking search, checkers, sorting coins, buttons, sorting laundry, looking for item in refrigerator, grocery store advertising circular.
- Outline doorways, edges of furniture, and closets on side of visual deficit with bright-colored tape for visual cue to scan for.

impulses from the brain. This includes feedback from areas that monitor body and head position and movement.[27] Thus, successful adaptation to the environment through the visual sense requires the proper functioning of both ocular and neurological components (Box 15.4).

Causes of brain insult can include trauma, cancer, multiple sclerosis, and cerebrovascular accidents (CVA) or strokes. The vision system is vulnerable to strokes and other types of brain insult.[28] A host of visual disorders can result from brain insult, including visual field disorders, reduced visual acuity, reduced contrast sensitivity, problems with stereopsis (depth perception), difficulty adapting to changes in light conditions, visual spatial disorders, and oculomotor dysfunction.[29]

WARREN'S HIERARCHY FOR ADDRESSING VISUAL DYSFUNCTION

Because of the complexity of the visual system, a framework for evaluation and intervention of visual impairments, whether ocular or neurological in nature, may be helpful. Warren[28] suggests a developmental model that conceptualizes vision abilities in a hierarchy (Fig. 15.3). The abilities at the bottom form the foundation for each successive level. Higher level abilities depend on the

complete integration of lower level abilities for their development.

The highest visual ability in this model is visual cognition. Visual cognition is the ability to mentally manipulate visual information and integrate it with other sensory information to solve problems, formulate writing, and solve mathematical problems.[28]

Visual memory is the ability directly below visual cognition in Warren's model. Visual cognition depends on visual memory because mental manipulation of a visual stimulus requires the ability to retain a mental picture.[30]

To store a visual image, individuals must be able to recognize a pattern. Pattern recognition, the next ability level, involves identification of the salient features of an

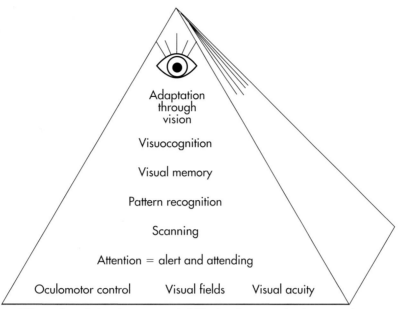

FIG. 15.3   Hierarchy of visual perceptual skills development in the central nervous system. *(Adapted from Warren ML. A hierarchical model for evaluation and treatment of visual perceptual dysfunction in adult-acquired brain injury, Part 1. Am Journal Occup Ther. 1993;47:42-54.)*

object.[31] An individual must not only be able to identify the holistic aspects of an object, such as its shape and contour, but also specific features of an object such as its color detail, shading, and texture.

The ability to scan the environment is necessary for effective pattern recognition. Scanning, therefore, is the fundamental ability required for pattern recognition. The eye must record systematically all of the details of a scene and follow an organized scan path.[28]

The ability directly below scanning is visual attention. Engagement of visual attention is necessary for proper scanning to occur. If individuals are not attending to visual stimuli in a specific space, they will not initiate scanning into that area. A classic example is the older adult with a CVA with left hemi-neglect who requires constant cueing to scan to the left to avoid colliding with objects.[28]

Visual attention and all of the higher level abilities depend on three primary visual abilities that form the foundation for all vision functions: oculomotor control, visual fields, and visual acuity. Oculomotor control enables efficient and conjugate eye movements, which ensure the completion of accurate scan paths and "teaming" of the eyes for binocular vision. The visual field is the extent of view that a person has in front of each eye. Visual acuity describes the sharpness or clearness of vision.[32] Table 15.2 addresses performance skill deficits of all of the discussed visual pathologies, and Box 15.5 addresses performance skills with areas of occupation.

PRINCIPLES OF INTERVENTION

When an occupational therapy visual screen reveals deficits affecting ADLs, the older adult should be referred to an ophthalmologist or optometrist to obtain a comprehensive visual examination. If the available records and clinical observation indicate that the older adult's visual impairment is caused by an ocular disease, it would be best to refer the older adult to a low vision specialist (see later discussion of professionals for collaboration). If, conversely, diagnostic and clinical information indicate that the older adult's visual impairment is caused by a neurological insult such as head injury or stroke, a consultation with a neuro-ophthalmologist or neuro-optometrist is recommended. If either of these scenarios is not possible, a consultation with a trusted ophthalmologist would be the next choice. Ideally, a good working relationship should be established with low vision specialists and neuro-ophthalmologists in the area to facilitate the speed of referral and communication between professionals.

The information provided by an ophthalmologist or optometrist may vary, depending on the condition and the professional's area of specialty. A report from these professionals typically includes many of the following visual functions: visual acuity, visual field, contrast sensitivity function (the ability to distinguish subtle gradations in contrast between an object and its background), and oculomotor control. Reports may also include intraocular pressure (the pressure inside the eyeball), best correction for eyeglass prescription, dates and description of any ocular surgeries or procedures, current prescribed ophthalmic medications, and the general health of ocular structures. Low vision specialists often also make recommendations for special optical devices to access printed materials, computer screens, or detailed eye-guided handiwork if visual acuity cannot be corrected to a functional

TABLE 15.2

Ocular Pathology-Related Functional Performance Skills Deficits With Areas of Occupation

Pathology	Near distance	Intermediate	Far distance	Eye/hand	Mobility
ARMD	Reading continuous print, spot reading	Sewing, knitting, needlework, crafts, computer, handyman tasks	Driving, TV, sporting events	Writing, crafts, sports, musical instruments	Driving, curbs, and steps in low light
Glaucoma	Decreased vision in low light, difficulty with very fine print or poor contrast materials, sensitive to glare	Difficulty finding objects on shelf, difficulty with crafts, computer screens with poor contrast materials	Driving, TV, sporting events, decreased field, depth perception	Sports, crafts, musical instruments	Driving, ambulating on unfamiliar or changing surfaces, steps, difficulty seeing obstacles in peripheral fields
Diabetic retinopathy	Fluctuating/blurry vision may make continuous print reading, regular print difficult	Needlework, crafts, computer, handyman tasks	Driving, TV sporting events, decreased depth perception	Writing, sports, craft, musical instruments	Driving, curbs and steps in low light
Cataract	Decreased or blurry vision for fine detail, in low light/poor contrast, change in color perception	Needlework, crafts, computer, handyman tasks	Driving, sporting events	Crafts, fine needlework, sports, musical instruments	Driving, curbs and steps in low light
CVA/TBI	Hemianopsia or hemi-inattention, may groom or dress only one side, difficulty reading continuous print	Difficulty locating objects on shelf or in part of the room	Driving, sporting events, visual field deficits, depth perception	Writing, self-feeding, crafts, sports, musical instruments	Driving, ambulating, obstacles in area of field deficit, steps and curbs

BOX 15.5

Vision Guided Occupational Survey/Profile

The following are difficult because of vision loss:
- Appliance dial
- Cleaning
- Cooking
- Computer
- Cutting/slicing
- Crafts
- Dressing
- Driving
- Eating
- Grooming
- Identifying money
- Keys/outlets

- Managing finances
- Medications
- Recognizing faces
- Sewing/needlework
- Shopping
- Social activities
- Spiritual participation
- Sports/fitness
- Telling time
- Telephone use
- Television
- Walking/outdoors/indoors
- Other_____

range. This information and that gathered during the occupational therapy evaluation are invaluable in guiding intervention. Box 15.6 is a screening form for the sensory perceptual skill of vision. The following discussion addresses general interventions for many of the deficits that accompany visual loss such as decreased visual acuity,

visual field loss, oculomotor dysfunction, reduced contrast sensitivity, and impaired visual attention and scanning.

DECREASED ACUITY

The input of an eye care specialist is crucial in addressing reduced acuity. Some older adults are simply in need of an

BOX 15.6

Sample Screening Form for the Sensory Perceptual Skill of Vision

1. Do you have trouble seeing?
2. Is part of your visual field missing, blurry, or dark?
3. Does your vision fluctuate?
4. How long have you experienced this difficulty?
5. Has your eye doctor diagnosed or treated you?
6. When was your last eye examination?
7. Which eye is most affected?
8. Can you see newsprint, headlines, computer screen, details on a TV screen, faces, food on your plate?
9. Do you drive?
10. Can you see traffic signals and street signs?
11. Does glare bother you?
12. Can you see curbs, steps, and changes in floor surfaces?
13. Have you ever fallen because of your vision?

Adapted from Kern T, Miller ND. Tools for occupational therapists who work with people with low vision: Vision screening checklist. In: Gentile M, ed. *Functional Visual Behavior in Adults: An Occupational Therapy Guide To Evaluation and Treatment Options.* Bethesda, MD: AOTA Press; 2005:139-140.

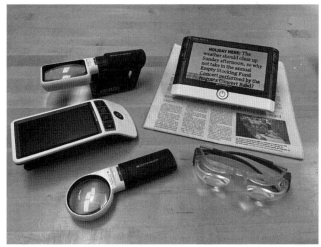

FIG. 15.4 Some common optical aids used by individuals with low vision. *(Courtesy Mallory Rosche.)*

updated eyeglass prescription. In the case of a head injury or stroke, acuity may be reduced initially but often resolves spontaneously in a few months. (See Chapter 19 on the effects of traumatic brain injury [TBI]/stroke [CVA] for a full discussion of more subtle deficits on acuity and intervention.) Reduced acuity secondary to ocular diseases, such as macular degeneration, cannot be improved through a change in eyeglass prescription. Recommendations for special optical devices may be made in this case. Diabetic retinopathy often not only causes reduced acuity but also causes fluctuating acuity. It is important to follow the advice of the eye care specialist when planning intervention related to acuity.

As mentioned earlier, one method to compensate for reduced acuity is to use special optical devices to magnify or enlarge print (Fig. 15.4). It is recommended that OTs and OTAs receive specialized training in optical devices before attempting to train individuals in their use. There are many unique concepts and techniques involved in the proper use of these devices, and older adults typically require very clear instructions and encouragement to become proficient in their use. Other examples of using enlargement to compensate for decreased acuity are the use of large print materials and writing larger letters with a felt tip pen.

When an older adult has decreased acuity, there are other techniques to help maximize function such as the use of proper illumination, reduction of pattern and clutter in the environment, and the use of organizational systems. Proper lighting is usually critical for optimal performance. However, some individuals may be photophobic or sensitive to light, which presents a challenge in finding appropriate lighting. Good, general room lighting (ambient lighting) is necessary for ease and safety in ambulating. Task lighting sources such as a gooseneck lamp or movable track lighting is recommended for fine-detail or low-contrast tasks such as reading, sewing, handyman work, or crafts. Proper positioning of a lamp must be considered to avoid glare. Directing the light from behind the shoulder of the better-seeing eye so that the light source does not create glare often works best. Task lighting with a gooseneck lamp can be positioned closer to the reading material, even in front of it as long as the bulb is not exposed and the shade directs the light downward, concentrating it on the material to be illuminated. Position the light source opposite the dominant hand to avoid shadows when writing.

Patterned backgrounds and clutter in the environment tend to "camouflage" objects that an older adult is seeking (Fig. 15.5). This can be remedied by using solid colors for background surfaces such as bedspreads, place mats, tablecloths, rugs, and furniture coverings. Care should be taken to reduce clutter where possible by limiting the number of objects in the environment and arranging the remaining objects in an orderly fashion. Once the environment is rearranged and simplified, every effort should be made to keep it organized.

There are many national and local services available for those with impaired visual acuity (and other visual impairment). Most of these services are free of charge. They can be found by contacting local state services for the blind and visually impaired (search your state government website). The American Foundation for the Blind and The Lighthouse are examples of services that provide books and magazines to individuals free of charge. There are also catalogs that offer low-tech adaptive devices for the

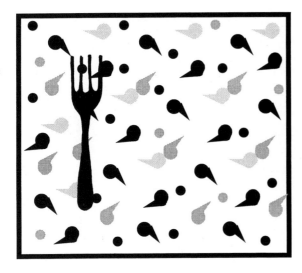

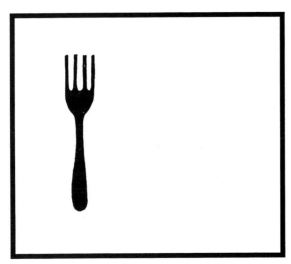

FIG. 15.5 A patterned background can make it difficult to locate objects.

visually impaired such as talking clocks, large print playing cards and Bingo cards, and a variety of other devices for ADLs.

VISUAL FIELD LOSS

Older adults who have a visual field loss may be taught to compensate for this loss in daily activities. The first step, however, is to increase the older adult's awareness of the visual field loss. Having accurate information on the extent and location of the field loss is critical for teaching older adults proper methods of compensation. The exact type and scope of visual field loss will vary depending on the cause of the disorder or disease and on individual presentation. In general, those with ocular conditions experience relatively "spotty types" of field loss, whereas those with a neurological disorder exhibit more uniform or extensive field loss. Of course, there are definitely exceptions to this rule because some ocular conditions can lead to an extensive and even total loss of visual field. Small,

concentrated areas of visual field loss also have been found in those with head injuries.[33]

Older adults who have central field loss, such as that seen with macular degeneration, must learn to compensate by directing their gaze off-center of the target (either slightly above, below, or to the side of) rather than directly at the target. This technique, called eccentric viewing, enables the individual to place the target outside of the blind spot so that it can be seen. This usually requires professional assistance to identify the best area for eccentric viewing, sometimes referred to as the preferred retinal locus (PRL).[34] Additional training and a conscious effort are required on the older adult's part to override the natural tendency to direct the fovea, the most central area of the retina, to the target and instead place the PRL in line with the target. Central field loss usually affects fine-detail tasks but does not significantly interfere with mobility. Those with more peripheral field loss typically require intervention aimed at increasing safety and independence with mobility skills. Older adults with a homonymous hemianopsia occurring after a stroke may be taught to compensate for this loss of half the visual field by systematically training them to turn the head and scan into the impaired field during functional activities such as reading, shopping, and mobility.[35]

OCULOMOTOR DYSFUNCTION

Intervention for oculomotor dysfunction is likely one of the most complex areas for beginning practitioners to comprehend and implement effectively. It is highly recommended that the entry level OTA attend continuing education seminars, develop a mentoring relationship, and establish service competency in this area before attempting any of the intervention strategies suggested. It is also strongly recommended that therapists and assistants work under close supervision of an optometrist or ophthalmologist when treating oculomotor impairments. Oculomotor impairments are seen in individuals who have experienced some type of neurological insult. Ocular conditions do not affect the muscular or neural mechanisms that control eye movements.

A strabismus, or misalignment of an eye,[16] is often seen as a result of extraocular muscle weakness after a stroke or other neurological insult. This misalignment of the eyes results in diplopia, or double vision. The primary intervention methods used to address diplopia include occlusion, eye exercises, application of prisms, and surgery.[3]

Occlusion is essentially the "patching" of an eye to eliminate the double image.[16] Care must be taken to follow an occlusion protocol that optimizes the older adult's comfort and reduces the likelihood of developing contractures in the muscles opposite the weak ones. Occlusion should not be carried out by simply patching the affected eye during all waking hours because this does nothing to encourage the use of the weak muscles. The protocol is typically directed by an ophthalmologist or optometrist.

244

Eye exercises can be used in conjunction with occlusion to help strengthen the affected muscles. One basic method would be to patch the unaffected eye and have the older adult track an object through all ranges of motion.[3] Optometrists may suggest additional exercises to be carried out under their direction.

Another strategy to treat diplopia is the application of prisms.[16] Prisms are sometimes prescribed and used to create a single image in the primary direction of gaze. The prism displaces the image to one side, causing the disparate images created by the strabismus to overlap and fuse into a single image. The prism can be permanently ground into the older adult's eyeglass lens or can be temporarily applied to the eyeglass lens using press-on prisms. If the strabismus is resolving, the older adult should be gradually weaned off of the prism by reducing its strength over time.[16] An ophthalmologist or optometrist determines the strength of the prism and directs the intervention.

In some specific cases, surgery to correct the strabismus may be warranted.[3] This is further testimony to the necessity of consulting with appropriate eye care professionals to obtain optimal intervention for the individual. In most cases, the general approach to the surgery is to make the action of one or more eye muscles weaker or stronger by changing its attachment position. This is done by an ophthalmologist who is specially trained in strabismus surgery.[3]

REDUCED CONTRAST SENSITIVITY

Contrast sensitivity may be affected by both ocular and neurological conditions. This function is different from visual acuity, which reveals only the size of high contrast black and white letters that the individual is capable of seeing. Contrast sensitivity is the capacity to discriminate between similar shades.[13] In daily life, good contrast sensitivity is necessary to see a gray car on a cloudy day, to detect unmarked curbs and steps, and to distinguish subtle contours on people's faces to recognize them. Deficits in contrast sensitivity are typically addressed through environmental adaptation. For persons with low contrast sensitivity, the world often loses its definition. The primary technique to compensate for this deficit is to simply add contrast to the environment whenever possible. Many items used in daily activities can be changed to add more contrast and definition (Box 15.7). Proper illumination (as described earlier under "Decreased Acuity") is also helpful in enhancing contrast. Some individuals find that full-spectrum lighting, either incandescent or fluorescent, provides the best contrast-enhancing illumination. Color filters that may be worn over prescription lenses or alone can also enhance contrast. Light yellow, medium yellow, and light or medium plum are the colors most frequently used to enhance contrast.

IMPAIRED VISUAL ATTENTION AND SCANNING

Deficits in attention and scanning are seen in those with neurological involvement, not commonly in those with ocular conditions. One type of impairment in this area is hemi-inattention, or hemi-neglect. This refers to a lack of awareness of one-half of a person's visual space. Neglect of the left half of visual space is more common, but right hemi-neglect is occasionally seen.[35] Individuals with hemi-inattention are not able to take in visual information in the orderly, sequential, and comprehensive pattern needed to safely complete many daily activities. Grooming, meal preparation, and functional mobility (especially driving) are common examples of affected ADLs and IADLs. Initial intervention of deficits in visual attention and scanning often involves increasing the older adult's awareness of the deficit followed up with appropriate compensation, remediation techniques, or both. Research has shown that individuals with left visual neglect may be trained to reorganize their scanning strategies by beginning the scan path in the impaired space.[36] This is accomplished through intervention strategies similar to those described earlier in treating homonymous hemianopsia. Activities are used that require and encourage a systematic left-to-right scan pattern with a visual anchor (such as a red line or ruler) placed to the left (or right as appropriate) as a visual cue, if necessary. The presence of hemi-neglect also has been associated with poor rehabilitation outcome.[37-39]

HIGHER LEVEL VISUAL-PERCEPTUAL DEFICITS

Warren's[28] proposed intervention for higher level visual deficits includes addressing the foundation visual skills that may affect these areas, education of the client to increase awareness of the deficit, and instruction in the use of compensatory strategies for the deficit. (See Box 15.4; and see Warren[28] for a more detailed description of these techniques.)

BOX 15.7

Examples of Modifications Using Contrast in the Environment

- Use a black felt tip marker for writing.
- Add strips of contrasting tape (usually orange or yellow is best) to the edge of steps.
- Use a white coffee cup so the level of coffee can be seen against the white background when pouring.
- Use a black and white reversible cutting board and slice light-colored items, such as onions, on the black side and vice versa.
- Mark light switches with contrasting fluorescent tape to increase visibility.
- Eat light-colored foods off of a dark plate, and vice versa.
- Use towels that are a contrasting color to the bathroom floor, to make it easier to see a towel that has been dropped to reduce a trip hazard.
- Mark appliances in the kitchen and laundry room with high contrast bump dots or other labels.

SETTINGS IN WHICH VISUAL IMPAIRMENTS ARE ADDRESSED

Low-vision rehabilitation is becoming a specialty field for occupational therapy practicioners. OT/OTAs may provide rehabilitation for diagnoses related to visual impairment when prescribed by an ophthalmologist, optometrist, or other physician. Low vision rehabilitation services provided by occupational therapy practicioners are covered by Medicare.[40] OT/OTAs work in conjunction with other trained professionals to provide comprehensive services to individuals with vision impairments. The majority of individuals treated in low-vision clinics have impairments caused by ocular pathologies. The leading diagnoses resulting in low-vision are macular degeneration, cataracts, glaucoma, and diabetic retinopathy.[41] For this reason, the term "low vision" is typically associated with visual impairments caused by ocular diseases. However, individuals with visual impairments secondary to neurological insult also may seek intervention in some low-vision clinics.

Because visual impairments are a common result of neurological insult, and because ocular diseases are relatively common in the older adult population, OTAs working in any geriatric or neuro-rehabilitation setting should be well educated in visual dysfunction and intervention techniques. Settings may include inpatient and outpatient rehabilitation, subacute rehabilitation facilities, long-term care facilities, and home health agencies.

OTAs working with older adults with visual impairments must have specialized training in areas such as optics and use of optical devices, eccentric viewing techniques, blind techniques for ADLs, and vision enhancement techniques for ADLs. OTAs need a good working knowledge of the extensive adaptive equipment available for clients with low vision. They also must possess a good understanding of available resources to direct clients to appropriate support groups and other services.

There are many other low-vision rehabilitation professionals with whom the OTA can collaborate to provide the best functional outcomes for their clients. Orientation and mobility specialists address travel needs directly related to vision loss. They typically hold master's degrees and have a wealth of knowledge in this area. The goal of their services is to develop independent travel skill within the client's home, neighborhood, or community. These specialists may work in many settings, including public school systems, private agencies, and state-supported programs.

Rehabilitation teachers are professionals who are trained at the university level to address ADLs that have been affected by visual impairment. They provide instruction in using adaptive techniques or equipment to increase independence in areas such as communication, household management, self-care, and other ADLs. Rehabilitation teachers may work in private agencies, itinerant state services, residential schools, and independent living centers. The areas addressed and the knowledge base of these professionals may overlap at times with occupational therapy professionals. As long as there is open communication and collaboration, each profession will likely learn valuable techniques from the other, and the client will receive an optimal rehabilitation program.

Ophthalmologists and optometrists specializing in low vision ensure that comprehensive low-vision services are provided. They evaluate the client's visual function and prescribe optical devices and training to compensate for vision loss. They may see low-vision clients in their own broader-based private practice, or they may work in low-vision clinics. (For more information regarding a program using ophthalmology and occupational therapy to provide low-vision rehabilitation in an outpatient rehabilitation setting, see Warren.[42])

TECHNOLOGY FOR OLDER ADULTS WHO HAVE VISION IMPAIRMENT

Increasing numbers of older adults who have vision impairments are interested in using computers, tablets, smartphones, and electronic magnifiers. These devices can add to the older adult's ability to engage with family and friends and maintain their interests while maximizing independence.

Accessibility features in computer operating systems, such as "Zoom" in Apple computers' IOS and mobile devices, and "Magnifier" for Windows (most currently Windows 7, 8, and 10) in PCs, allow a person with vision impairment to access email, social media, and photographs. Many books, newspapers, and magazines can be downloaded for reading on computer or tablet. This allows the older adult to adjust font size, contrast, and line spacing. Magnification can be used to enlarge the entire screen or a portion of it. An older adult can turn the magnification feature on or off and control the amount of magnification and the view using keyboard shortcuts or "hot keys," or by the computer mouse.

"Voice Over" for Apple devices and "Narrator" for Windows (text-to-speech features) give people with little or no usable vision the ability to access print and Internet-based text by reading selected documents aloud. The older adult can control the rate of speech and volume and choose a masculine or feminine voice. Some individuals with hearing impairment prefer the male voice, as it is usually lower-pitched and easier to distinguish. These text-to-speech features can also "echo" or speak a user's keystrokes as they type.

Special software programs are available to provide more magnification, color choices, and viewing options as well as text-to-speech options, including ZoomText and JAWS. Depending on the older adult's previous level of experience and comfort with computers, additional training may be needed.

Smartphones have applications (apps) that can improve safety for older adults with vision impairment in and away from home. Some of these apps are free. For example, one app identifies the denomination of currency when the phone's camera is held over it. Another app can take a blood pressure reading. Navigation apps can speak walking directions from one destination to another. Many of these apps operate with one touch or gesture and voice command.

Some allow the older adult to access information by interacting with a personal assistant (like Apple's Siri). Some of the functions this personal assistant can complete include dialing a number from a list of contacts, reading emails, and reading and sending text messages.[43] Electronic magnifiers (also referred to as CCTVs or video magnifiers) are good solutions for reading and writing aids when large amounts of magnification or contrast are required. Desktop models provide magnification from $3\times$ to more than $15\times$, as well as contrast enhancement, color viewing options, and other features. Some CCTVs have optical character recognition for text-to-speech and can read text out loud.

The cost of these devices is not covered by insurance. There are, however, assistive technology grants available. As a rehabilitation professional, the OTA may want to become familiar with sources for the devices and funding assistance.

CONCLUSION

Visual impairments in older adults may result from either ocular or neurological pathology. Normal physiological changes that may occur with aging include shrinkage of the peripheral field, increased time required to recover from glare, difficulty with light and dark adaptation, increased need for illumination, loss of elasticity in the lens, and yellowing of the lens. The most common ocular diseases that may occur in older adults are macular degeneration, cataracts, glaucoma, and diabetic retinopathy. Older adults are also at risk for CVAs, which may disrupt any of several neurological components necessary for effective visual functioning.

OTAs can play vital roles in helping older adults with visual impairments learn to function as independently as possible. OTAs can provide sources for information about vision loss to help older adults understand the specifics of their eye conditions. Encouraging older adults to gain knowledge about their eye conditions can be an empowering first step in the process of rehabilitation. OTAs may collaborate with OTs to provide training to compensate for vision loss in daily activities. OTAs can deliver training in community resources and collaborate with other members of the intervention team to provide referrals to appropriate agencies and service providers to facilitate community reintegration. Finally,

BOX 15.8

Environmental Adaptation Basics
■ Increase relative object size—large print, bold labels, or large-sized objects.
■ Lighting—increase ambient and task lighting; add gooseneck lamps for task lighting where activities are completed.
■ Color—light colors for walls and ceilings to reflect and increase light; bright colors for tools and everyday objects to make them stand out.
■ Contrast—floor, walls, counters, furniture, hardware, switch-plates, and doorknobs should contrast with each other.
■ Reduce clutter—limit the number of objects on counters and tabletops, limit bold patterns to decrease "visual clutter," and clear pathways between rooms and around furniture or exits.
■ Reduce glare by eliminating bare bulbs, reflective surfaces, using matte finishes and using light filtering window coverings and lampshades.
■ Texture—use bumpy or rough textured paint, tape or self-adhesive dots to label settings, or define edges and surface changes. Train older adults to notice changes in the feel of carpet versus hard surfaced floors.
■ Audio substitution—use talking clocks, kitchen scales, timers, and other items to substitute for vision when performing ADL and IADL tasks.

OTAs may collaborate with older adults, family members, and/or caregivers to make environmental adaptations, to enhance independence, and to do these safely (Box 15.8).

The loss of vision in older adults is a common occurrence, whether it results from the natural aging process, ocular disease, or disruption of neurological components. Vision loss has significant functional implications and can complicate the older adult's rehabilitation process with other physical impairments. This emphasizes the need for OTAs to familiarize themselves with the causes and types of vision loss and effective intervention techniques, whether they are working in general rehabilitation centers or acute care hospitals.

▌TECH TALK: FOCUS ON LOW VISION

NAME	PURPOSE	APPROX. COST	WHERE TO BUY
Be My Eyes	App designed to connect sighted volunteers to people in need of performing a sighted task via video call	$0	Google Play IOS App Store Bemyeyes.com
Seeing AI	App designed to provide verbal narration of written material including signs, nutrition labels, currency, menus, and settings	$0	Google Play IOS App Store Microsoft.com
Envision AI	App designed to provide audible feedback of visual information including display screens, handwritten notes, environments, objects, colors, QR codes, and friends/family	Free trial then $2/ mo or $20/yr	Google Play IOS App Store

CASE STUDY

John is a 67-year-old widower who lives alone and, following an amputation below the right knee, was just admitted to the rehabilitation unit where you work. He has diabetes mellitus and has had many complications of the disease, including the peripheral vascular disease that led to his amputation and diabetic retinopathy. John states that he did not manage his condition well in the past but wants to do everything he can now to keep these complications from getting any worse. He states that he finds it difficult to see the numbers and lines on his syringes when drawing his insulin. He also has some trouble seeing the blood sugar reading on his glucometer. He needs to check his blood sugar three times a day with this machine and adjust his insulin dosage accordingly. The occupational therapy visual screen reveals that John has moderately decreased visual acuity and decreased contrast sensitivity.

John has good upper body strength and uses his walker well on the unit. He will need to use the walker at discharge while waiting for his leg to heal before being fitted for a prosthesis. Fortunately, you will be able to conduct a home evaluation to make recommendations before discharge.

■ CASE STUDY QUESTIONS

1 What are some specific areas of concern or potential hazards that you would look for on John's home evaluation visit?
2 What are some recommendations you could make to address these concerns and improve safety and ease of functioning in John's home?
3 You would like to increase John's independence in his diabetic management, but you do not know what techniques or adaptive equipment is available to accomplish this. Where could you turn for help? What assistive technology might you inquire about to help John complete his diabetic care?

■ CHAPTER REVIEW QUESTIONS

1 What are some natural age-related changes in the eye, and what implications do they have for function?
2 What are the three primary ocular conditions that account for the majority of referrals to low-vision rehabilitation clinics?
3 Which ocular conditions could potentially lead to total blindness?
4 What are some possible vision problems after a stroke or other neurological insult?
5 What are the primary vision abilities described in Warren's hierarchy that form the foundation for all other vision abilities?
6 Name three environmental adaptation strategies that could be used for older adults with the primary ocular conditions most commonly encountered.
7 Name three other professionals and two community or state agencies with whom the OTA could collaborate regarding a low-vision older adult.

For additional video content, please visit Elsevier eBooks+ (eBooks.Health.Elsevier.com)

EVIDENCE NUGGETS: EFFECTIVENESS OF VISION REHABILITATION FOR OLDER ADULTS

1. Liu CJ, Chang MC. Interventions within the scope of occupational therapy practice to improve performance of daily activities for older adults with low vision: A systematic review. *AJOT.* 2020; 74(1): 1-18.
   - Moderate evidence was found for low vision rehabilitation to increase ADL performance in older adults with low vision. Occupational therapy practitioners should offer comprehensive low vision evaluations and multicomponent services for this population.
   - Low evidence was found for using self-management approach and for the use of tango style dance intervention with older adults with low vision.
   - OT practitioners should be part of multidisciplinary teams that provide comprehensive low vision evaluations and multipronged services to older adults with low vision.

2. Nastasi JA. Occupational therapy interventions supporting leisure and social participation for older adults with low vision: A systematic review. *AJOT.* 2020; 74(1): 1-9.
   - Low strength of evidence was found to support occupational therapy interventions that address leisure and social participation for older adults with low vision.
   - More hours of direct service over a shorter duration resulted in improvements in social participation for older adults with low vision.

   - Group therapy and fittings with low vision devices resulted in improvements in social participation for older adults with low vision.

3. Smallfield S, Kaldenberg J. Occupational therapy interventions to improve reading performance of older adults with low vision: A systematic review. *AJOT.* 2020; 74(1): 1-18.
   - Moderate evidence was found that supports stand-based electronic magnification and eccentric viewing training to improve reading outcomes in older adults with low vision.
   - Strong evidence was found to support the use of multicomponent interventions for older adults with low vision.
   - OT practitioners are encouraged to integrate stand-based electronic magnification, eccentric viewing training, and comprehensive low vision services into routine care with older adults with low vision.

4. van Nipsen RMA, Virgili G, Hoeben M, Langelaan M, Klevering J, Keunen JEE, van Rens G. Low vision rehabilitation for better quality of life in visually impaired adults. *Cochrane Database Syst. Rev.* 2020; 1: 1-36.
   - No evidence of benefit for low vision rehabilitation on improving health-related quality of life.
   - Low certainty of evidence that methods of enhancing vision may improve vision-related quality of life compared to usual care given for older adults with low vision.

REFERENCES

1. Centers for Disease Control and Prevention. *Fast Facts of Common Eye Disorders*. 2020. Available at: https://www.cdc.gov/visionhealth/basics/ced/fastfacts.htm.
2. Alma MA, Van der Mei SF, Groothoff JW, et al. Determinants of social participation of visually impaired older adults. *Qual Life Res*. 2012;21(1):87-97. doi:10.1007/s11136-011-9931-6.
3. Warren ML. *The Brain Injury Visual Assessment Battery for Adults Test Manual*. Lenexa, KS: visABILITIES Rehab Services; 1998.
4. American Occupational Therapy Association. Occupational therapy practice framework: Domain and process fourth edition. *Am J Occup Ther*. 2020;74:1-87. Available at: https://doi.org/10.5014/ajot.2020.74S2001.
5. van der Aa HP, van Rens GH, Comijs HC, et al. Stepped care for depression and anxiety in visually impaired older adults: multicentre randomised controlled trial [published correction appears in BMJ. 2016;353:i1995]. *BMJ*. 2015;351:h6127. doi:10.1136/bmj.h6127.
6. Berger S, McAteer J, Schreier K, Kaldenberg J. Occupational therapy interventions to improve leisure and social participation for older adults with low vision: a systematic review. *Am J Occup Ther*. 2013;67(3):303-311. doi:10.5014/ajot.2013.005447.
7. American Foundation for the Blind. *Fact Sheet: Low Vision and Legal Blindness Terms and Descriptions*. 2020. Available at: https://www.afb.org/blindness-and-low-vision/eye-conditions/low-vision-and-legal-blindness-terms-and-descriptions.
8. Nyman SR, Dibb B, Victor CR, et al. Emotional well-being and adjustment to vision loss in later life: a meta-synthesis of qualitative studies. *Disabil Rehabil*. 2012;34(12):971-981. doi:10.3109/09638288.2011.626487.
9. Ball E, Nicolle CA. Changing what it means to be "normal": a grounded theory study of the mobility choices of people who are blind or visually impaired. *J Vis Impair Blind*. 2015;109(4):291.
10. Kubler-Ross E. *Death and Dying*. New York: Macmillan; 1969.
11. Casten RJ, Rovner BW. Psychiatric and psychosocial factors in low vision rehabilitation. In: Albert D, Miller J, Azar D, eds. Albert & Jakobiec's Principles and Practice of Ophthalmology. St. Louis: Saunders/Elsevier; 2008:5333-5336.
12. Tuttle DW, Tuttle NR. *Self-Esteem and Adjusting with Blindness. The Process of Responding to Life's Demands*. Springfield, IL: Charles C. Thomas; 2004.
13. Mogk LG. Eye conditions that cause low vision in adults. In: Warren M, ed. Low Vision: Occupational Therapy Interventions with the Older Adult: A Self-Paced Clinical Course from AOTA. Bethesda, MD: American Occupational Therapy Association; 2000.
14. Esenwah EC, Azuamah YC, Okorie ME, et al. The aging eye and vision: A review. *Int J Health Sci Res*. 2014;4(7):218-226.
15. Scheiman M. Review of basic anatomy, physiology, and development of the visual system. In: Scheiman M, ed. Understanding and Managing Vision Deficits: A Guide for Occupational Therapists. 3rd ed. Thorofare, NJ: Slack Inc; 2011:9-16.
16. Scheiman M. Management of refractive, visual efficiency, and visual information processing disorders. In: Scheiman M, ed. Understanding and Managing Vision Deficits: A Guide for Occupational Therapists. 3rd ed. Thorofare, NJ: Slack Inc; 2011:119-176.
17. Yang H, Afshari NA. The yellow intraocular lens and the natural ageing lens. *Curr Opin Ophthalmol*. 2014;25(1):40-43. doi:10.1097/ICU.0000000000000020.
18. National Eye Institute (NEI). *Cataracts*. 2019. Available at: https://nei.nih.gov/health/cataract/.
19. Whittaker S, Scheiman M, Sokol-McKay D. *Low Vision Rehabilitation: A Practical Guide for Occupational Therapists*. 2nd ed. Slack: Thorofare, NJ; 2016.
20. American Printing House for the Blind. *An Introduction to Cataracts and Cataract Surgery*. 2020. Available at: http://www.visionaware.org/info/your-eye-condition/cataracts/an-introduction-to-cataracts-and-cataract-surgery/125.
21. American Society of Retina Specialists. *Age-Related Macular Degeneration*. 2020. Available at: https://www.asrs.org/content/documents/fact-sheet-16-amd-2020_2.pdf.
22. Pang L. Visual hallucinations: identifying Charles Bonnet syndrome. *Int J Ophthalmol Eye Sci*. 2015;1:14-22. doi:10.19070/2332-290X-SI01004.
23. Jackson ML, Bassett K, Nirmalan PV, et al. Contrast sensitivity and visual hallucinations in patients referred to a low vision rehabilitation clinic. *Br J Ophthalmol*. 2007;91(3):296-298. doi:10.1136/bjo.2006.104604.
24. American Printing House for the Blind. *Glaucoma: An Overview*. 2020. Available at: http://www.visionaware.org/info/your-eye-condition/glaucoma/an-overview-5932/125.
25. Sprabary A. *Narrow-Angle Glaucoma (angle-closure glaucoma)*. 2020. Available at: https://www.allaboutvision.com/conditions/narrow-angle-glaucoma/.
26. Lopez EF, Karaca EE, Ekici F, et al. Symptoms reported by patients with varying stages of glaucoma: review of 401 cases. *Can J Ophthalmol*. 2014;49(5):420-425. doi:10.1016/j.jcjo.2014.07.014.
27. Zoltan B. *Vision, Perception, and Cognition: A Manual for the Evaluation and Treatment of the Adult with Acquired Brain Injury*. 4th ed. Thorofare, NJ: Slack; 2007.
28. Warren ML. A hierarchical model for evaluation and treatment of visual perceptual dysfunction in adult acquired brain injury, part 1. *Am J Occup Ther*. 1993;47:42-54. doi:10.5014/ajot.47.1.42.
29. Department of Veterans Affairs. *Visual Problems in Traumatic Brain Injury: A systematic Review of Sequelae and Interventions for the Veteran Population*. 2009;1-59. Available at: https://www.va.gov/OPTOMETRY/docs/VISTBI-Vision-tbi-final-report-9-09.pdf.
30. Schurgin MW. Visual memory, the long and short of it: a review of visual working memory and long-term memory. *Atten Percept Psychophys*. 2018;80:1035-1056.
31. Strasburger H, Rentschler I, Juttner M. Peripheral vision and pattern recognition: a review. *J Vis*. 2011;11(5):1-82. Available at: https://doi.10.1167/11.5.13.
32. Cate Y, Richards L. Relationship between performance on tests of basic visual functions and visual-perceptual processing in persons after brain injury. *Am J Occup Ther*. 2000;54(3):326-334. doi:10.5014/ajot.54.3.326.
33. Goodrich GL. *Visual Consequences of Mild to Severe Traumatic Brain Injury: How Screening can Help Rehabilitation*. Paper presented at the XVI L'incapacité Visuelle Et La Réadaptation, Montreal, Canada; 2014. Available at: https://www.researchgate.net/publication/279193096_Visual_consequences_of_mild_to_severe_traumatic_brain_injury_How_screening_helps_rehabilitation.
34. Schoessow KA, Fletcher DC, Schuchard RA. Preferred retinal loci relationship to macular scotomas: a 10-year comparison. *J Vis Impair Blind*. 2012;106(11):745.
35. Grunda T, Marsalek P, Sykorova P. Homonymous hemianopia and related visual defects: restoration of vision after a stroke. *Acta Neurobiol Exp (Wars)*. 2012;73(2):237-249.
36. Dundon NM, Bertini C, Làdavas E, et al. Visual rehabilitation: visual scanning, multisensory stimulation and vision restoration training. *Front Behav Neurosci*. 2015;9:192. doi:10.3389/fnbeh.2015.00192.
37. Kerkhoff G, Reinhart S, Ziegler W, et al. Smooth pursuit eye movement training promotes recovery from auditory and visual neglect: a randomized controlled study. *Neurorehabil Neural Repair*. 2013;27(9):789-798. doi:10.1177/1545968313491012.
38. Kerkhoff G, Schenk T. Rehabilitation of neglect: an update. *Neuropsychologia*. 2012;50(6):1072-1079. doi:10.1016/j.neuropsychologia.2012.01.024.
39. Mödden C, Behrens M, Damke I, et al. A randomized controlled trial comparing 2 interventions for visual field loss with standard occupational therapy during inpatient stroke rehabilitation. *Neurorehabil Neural Repair*. 2012;26(5):463-469. doi:10.1177/1545968311425927.

40. American Occupational Therapy Association. *Occupational Therapy Services for Persons with Visual Impairment*. 2016. Available at: https://www.aota.org/About-Occupational-Therapy/Professionals/PA/Facts/low-vision.aspx.

41. Congdon N, O'Colmain B, Klaver CC, et al. Causes and prevalence of visual impairment among adults in the United States. *Arch Ophthalmol*. 2004;122:477-485.

42. Warren ML. Providing low vision rehabilitation services with occupational therapy and ophthalmology: a program description. *Am J Occup Ther*. 1995;49:877-884. doi:10.5014/ajot.49.9.877.

43. Cantisani Peter. *Twenty-Two Useful Apps for Blind iPhone Users*. 2nd ed. Boston: National Braille Press; 2013.

chapter 16

Working With Older Adults Who Have Hearing Impairments

SUE BYERS-CONNON

(PREVIOUS CONTRIBUTIONS FROM JESSICA HATCH AND SHARON STOFFEL)

KEY TERMS

audiologist, assistive listening device (ALD), cochlear implant,
conductive hearing loss, hearing aid, presbycusis, sensorineural hearing loss
(sensory, neural, mechanical), tinnitus

CHAPTER OBJECTIVES

1. Describe sensorineural and conductive hearing losses.
2. Describe ways that slow, progressive changes in the auditory system interfere with occupations that require communication.
3. List environmental modifications that reduce background noise in homes and institutions.
4. Describe possible safety recommendations for home and institutional environments where hearing-impaired older adults reside.
5. Describe the effect of age-related hearing loss on socialization, communication, and travel, and its possible contribution to feelings of isolation for hearing-impaired older adults.
6. List suggestions for improving communication with hearing-impaired older adults.
7. Describe possible behaviors that may indicate hearing impairment.

The voice of a loved one, the chimes of a grandfather clock, a violin concerto—these are sounds many people not only enjoy but also take for granted. For older adults who have hearing impairments, these sounds may be either misinterpreted or missed altogether.

Hearing impairments may also be associated with the reduced ability to hear warning signals, ambulation difficulties, and difficulties with instrumental activities of daily living (IADLs), balance problems, and increased incidence of falls.[1-3] Hearing impairments can contribute to social isolation. Safety related to hearing impairments may become a concern when older adults are unable to hear alarms and other warning signals.[4]

Among the older adult population, hearing loss is the third most prevalent chronic condition following arthritis and hypertension.[5] In the United States, by the year 2060, 73.50 million people are expected to have hearing loss.[6] Although persons of all ages experience hearing impairments, in terms of a health disparity, older adults are a primary concern.[7] Approximately one-third of older adults between ages 65 and 74 experience hearing loss. This percentage increases to nearly half for those older than 75 years.[8] Furthermore, some studies indicate that 85% to 90% of nursing home residents have hearing impairments that limit function.[4]

Even though hearing impairments are more prevalent than vision loss, they are often more difficult to distinguish. Changes in hearing are often subtle and occur gradually. Many older adults with significant hearing losses often wait as long as 5 years before seeking assistance with their hearing.[9] Older adults, family members, and health care personnel may not recognize hearing losses. Some may accept the loss as an inevitable and unalterable aspect of aging.

According to the *Occupational Therapy Practice Framework: Domain and Process* (fourth edition),[10] hearing function is addressed in Table 9, Client Factors, as a body function under the sensory functions and refers to "sound detection and discrimination; awareness of location and distance of sounds" (p. 52). Hearing loss can have a profound effect on engagement in occupations and activities of daily living (ADLs). Occupational therapy assistants (OTAs) have the opportunity to diminish the effect of hearing loss on functional performance by becoming educated about hearing loss. Learning accommodations that may benefit the patient can make working with hearing-impaired individuals easier and improve performance in functional tasks.[11]

Because older adults seldom seek assistance or plan interventions to enhance their hearing, OTAs must be able to distinguish the various types of hearing impairments. In addition, OTAs should be aware of interventions, services, devices, and activities that can enhance occupational performance for older adults who are hearing impaired.

This chapter provides an overview of the most common types of hearing losses that affect older adults. The possible psychosocial effects that a hearing impairment may have on older adults, their families, and their friends also are addressed. Rehabilitation considerations are discussed, including communicating with an older adult who has a hearing impairment, methods for modifying home, public spaces, and institutional environments, and recommendations for assisting older adults in the use of hearing aids and assistive listening devices (ALDs).

HEARING CONDITIONS ASSOCIATED WITH AGING

If any hearing loss is suspected, individuals should visit their primary care physician to be screened and/or treated for any other underlying pathological processes.[5] The term *presbycusis* is often used when diagnosing older adults with hearing loss. According to the National Institute on Deafness and Other Communication Disorders (NI-DCD),[12] presbycusis is the gradual loss of hearing as an individual grows older. Generally, hearing losses are divided into three areas: sensorineural, conductive, and mixed. These conditions may affect one or both ears.

The most common type of presbycusis or hearing loss in older adults is the result of sensorineural damage to the hearing organ itself or to the body's nervous system.[12] Although older adults rarely have just one type of sensorineural loss, the most common type of loss is caused by hair cell damage or loss of the sensory hair cells of the cochlea. As individuals age, these hair cells are slowly lost, and the ability to hear high-frequency sounds is diminished. One of the most frustrating aspects of this loss is the ways sounds are changed or distorted. Although the older adult may hear someone speaking, the signals that allow him or her to understand what is being said are not clear. Such losses can have serious consequences in both social and therapeutic settings. For example, at a party, someone may say, "How are you?" and the older adult may respond, "Eighty-one." An older adult in a clinic setting who is asked to hand the OTA a "dime" may respond with the correct "time." Such responses often raise questions about mental status and often lead to a loss of confidence in interacting with others.[12,13] In such situations, the OTA should seek assistance to rule out the presence of sensorineural loss before questioning the older adult's orientation or ability to follow directions. If proper audiological services are not available, the older adult can experience decreased mobility, social isolation, and increased cognitive decline.[14] In addition, since women's voices are usually higher pitched than men's, female OTAs must understand that their voices could contribute to decreased comprehension by older adults.

Older adults living in areas with low exposure to loud or high-pitched noise levels may experience less sensorineural hearing loss than those living in noisy, industrial areas. Although those with better overall health seem less likely to experience this type of loss, some sensorineural loss eventually affects older adults regardless of environmental conditions. However, continued exposure to loud noises for long periods may cause permanent damage.[15] For instance, current research indicates that one in six teenagers demonstrates signs of hearing loss, which could be secondary to music players, concerts, sporting events, lawn and farming machinery, or power tools.[16]

Three types of sensorineural hearing loss have been identified: sensory, neural, and mechanical.[13,15] Sensory loss is caused by atrophy and degeneration of the hair cells at the base of the basilar membrane. It produces a loss of high-frequency sounds but does not interfere with the discrimination of speech. Neural loss is caused by the loss of auditory nerve fibers. It affects the ability to distinguish speech sounds, especially in the higher frequencies, but does not affect the ability to hear pure tones. Mechanical loss is characterized by the degeneration of the vibrating membrane within the cochlea. This type of loss leads to the gradual impairment of hearing in all frequencies. In situations where several sounds in various frequencies are present at the same time, the ability to distinguish between the sounds becomes increasingly difficult. Table 16.1 lists common hearing conditions of older adults.

A sensorineural hearing loss may be unnoticed in the early stages because the high-frequency tones that are initially lost are above the functional range used in most environments. As the condition progresses, older adults may notice that they cannot hear the ringing of the telephone, the buzz of the doorbell, the ticking of a clock, or the water dripping from a faucet. With further progression, the sounds of certain consonants such as s, z, t, f, and g become increasingly difficult to distinguish. Eventually, older adults may strain to hear and understand conversations and one-syllable words.[13,15]

A second hearing condition, conductive hearing loss, results in an inability of the external ear to conduct sound waves to the inner ear. Conductive hearing losses may be related to the buildup of cerumen (earwax), fluid accumulation in the middle ear from eustachian tube dysfunction, or an upper respiratory infection. These conductive problems often can be corrected by cleaning the ear, administering medications, or performing surgery. Hearing aids may be effective for persons who have an untreatable or residual conductive hearing loss. A hearing aid amplifies incoming sound and requires functioning hair cells and an intact nerve to transmit the sound to the central auditory pathways. For

TABLE 16.1

Common Hearing Conditions of Older Adults

Condition	Cause	Symptoms
Sensorineural hearing loss	Neural, mechanical, and/or sensory damage to the inner ear or auditory nerves	Impaired hearing, most common is loss of high-frequency sounds
Neural hearing loss	Loss of auditory nerve fibers	Condition affects ability to distinguish speech sounds in higher frequencies; does not affect ability to hear pure tones
Mechanical hearing loss	Degeneration of the vibrating membrane within the cochlea	Condition leads to gradual loss of hearing in all frequencies; ability to distinguish sounds becomes increasingly difficult
Sensory hearing loss	Atrophy and degeneration of the hair cells at the base of the basilar membrane	Condition affects loss of high-frequency sounds but does not interfere with the discrimination of speech
Conductive hearing loss	Inability of the external ear to conduct sound waves to the inner ear; may be related to buildup of earwax, fluid accumulation in the middle ear, or upper respiratory infection	Condition can often be corrected by cleaning the ear, medications, or surgery; hearing aids or cochlear implants may be considered
Tinnitus	May be related to conductive or sensorineural loss, Ménière's, otosclerosis, presbycusis, earwax buildup, lesions, or fluid in middle ear	Buzzing, ringing, whistle, roar in ears, most noticeable at night; may be necessary to rule out underlying conditions before implementing interventions designed to symptoms

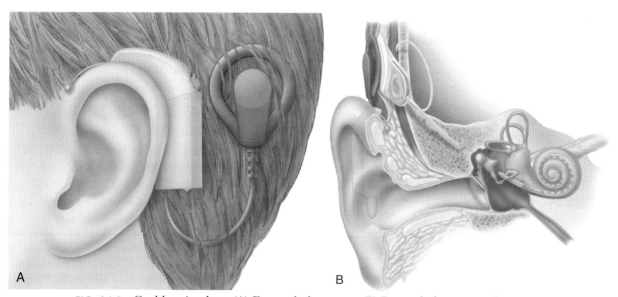

FIG. 16.1 Cochlear implant. (A) External placement. (B) Internal placement. *(Courtesy Cochlear Ltd., Englewood., CO.)*

older adults whose residual hearing is greatly limited because of an absence of hair cells, cochlear implants may be considered.[4] Cochlear implants are appropriate when only minimal or no benefit is possible when a conventional hearing aid is used. Cochlear implants are prosthetic replacements for the functions of the lost hair cells by converting mechanical energy (sound waves) into electrical energy capable of exciting the auditory nerve. Cochlear implants are placed within the inner ear. They bypass the hair cells of the cochlea and directly stimulate the endings of the auditory nerve. The system consists of an external microphone, processor, transmitter, and an internal receiver–stimulator and electrode. Fig. 16.1 shows the external and internal placements for a cochlear implant.

Tinnitus is a subjective auditory problem consisting of a ringing, whistling, buzzing, or roaring noise in the ears. Tinnitus may occur as part of a conductive or sensorineural hearing loss. It may also be associated with Ménière's disease, otosclerosis, sensorineural loss, an accumulation of cerumen pressing on the eardrum, tympanic membrane lesions, and fluid in the middle ear. Medications such as the doses of aspirin prescribed for arthritis or other medical conditions can be additional contributing factors.[15] Before planning interventions to mask the symptoms of tinnitus, possible underlying conditions such as cardiovascular disease, anemia, and hypothyroidism should be ruled out by a physician.

Tinnitus is often most noticeable at night when other noises are reduced. Masking of environment noises may be an effective strategy. A radio, tape recording, or appropriate hearing aid may mask the tinnitus so the individual can fall asleep. Other therapeutic interventions may include relaxation techniques and biofeedback.[2,15]

PSYCHOSOCIAL ASPECTS OF HEARING IMPAIRMENTS

Even though much information about the environment is learned through the sense of hearing, the importance of hearing during travel, while working, and in personal and social situations often goes unnoticed. Some researchers suggest that when hearing loss is the only loss older adults experience, they can adjust well.[13] Others suggest that a hearing loss may lead to isolation and even paranoia.[2,17] Unfortunately, many older adults experience other losses or lifestyle changes at the same time hearing loss occurs. Retirement may lead to a loss of role identity, income, and social contacts. Adjusting to the death of a spouse or undergoing changes in vision or mobility may take priority over a loss of hearing. Older adults who are predisposed to loneliness or have difficulty in initiating or maintaining relationships may become more isolated or avoid interpersonal relationships if they experience a hearing loss. This can result in an increased sense of loneliness or isolation, especially if the hearing impairment is associated with other losses.[13] Early assessment of a perceived hearing loss and recommendations for adaptations may help reduce an older adult's sense of loneliness.

The older adult with a hearing loss often guesses at or misses the content of conversations, is reluctant to ask for clarification, or is embarrassed when mistakes are made because of a misunderstanding. This can occur when an older adult with a hearing impairment is traveling. Studies involving older adult airline travelers have found that misunderstanding or not hearing overhead paging information has resulted in missed flights.[18] Hearing changes also make it difficult to detect and understand speech in crowded and stressful situations. A loss in hearing may decrease an older adult's sense of security and increase feelings of vulnerability, making travel more difficult. As a result, some older adults may either limit their travel or stop engaging in that occupation.[2]

Communication can be exhausting for older adults with a hearing impairment. For example, an 85-year-old man registering for occupational therapy interventions at a rehabilitation clinic will likely be embarrassed if he misinterprets the receptionist's request for his address as a request to undress. He may also experience isolation if his accompanying family member interrupts and answers questions. Repeated frustrating and embarrassing experiences can contribute to feelings of vulnerability, insecurity, and doubts related to self-esteem that can lead to withdrawal from travel, social, cultural, and family contacts.

Some older adults with hearing impairments may hear well at home and only struggle to hear in other social settings. Others may be isolated not only from family and friends but also from the broader world because they cannot get information from television, radio, movies, and even telephone conversations. Older adults may become increasingly frustrated as family, friends, and even health care workers begin to make decisions for them.

An age-related hearing loss may only further complicate the effects of illnesses and mental health conditions such as Alzheimer's disease. Hearing loss in older adults can lead to or exacerbate paranoid ideas, suspicions, and loss of contact with reality and related tendencies.[13] Corso[19] stated that a hearing loss can magnify previously existing paranoid personality attributes. Continued expression of suspicions, hostilities, and accusations of lying may result in friends and family members avoiding the hearing-impaired older adult.

REHABILITATION AND THE HEARING-IMPAIRED OLDER ADULT

Hearing loss usually accompanies other conditions and should be considered in intervention to facilitate a successful experience. Managing hearing loss is about much more than the simple provision of a hearing aid. Rehabilitation for the individual with hearing impairment examines the individual's participation in a variety of activities and functions.[20] The effectiveness of rehabilitation for maximizing occupational independence is based on many factors. Those related to hearing loss may include age-related changes at the time of onset of the hearing impairment, such as vision and mobility losses, retirement, death of a spouse, and loss of clearly defined life roles. Other factors include the severity and rapidity of the loss, the degree of residual hearing, the presence of other medical conditions, and the involvement of the individual and family members in the rehabilitative process.

OTA and occupational therapist (OT) teams may work together along with others on the treatment team to identify older adults who have hearing impairments through an observation of behaviors (Box 16.1). The Self-Rating Hearing Inventory also can be an effective tool for assessing the effects of a hearing impairment on perceived occupational performance.[21] The American Academy of Otolaryngology–Head and Neck Surgery has developed a

BOX 16.1

Observable Behaviors That May Indicate Hearing Loss

- Inappropriate volume increase when speaking—for example, appearing to shout while talking to a person nearby.
- Turning the television or radio volume inordinately high when there is no one else in the room and no noises in the background.
- Turning in a chair or turning the head to get a better hearing position when being addressed.
- Consistently asking for statements to be repeated.
- Not responding to verbal questions or conversation.
- Responding to verbal questions only when there is accompanying visual cueing.
- Looking disoriented or confused or giving inappropriate responses to questions—for example, answering "yes" to a multiple-choice question.
- Answering questions addressed to another person when there are several persons conversing simultaneously in the same room.
- Withdrawing from social situations.
- Exhibiting a short attention span, which is especially apparent when two people are talking simultaneously.

Adapted from Kane RL, Ouslander JG, Abrass IB. *Essentials of Clinical Geriatrics*. 7th ed. New York: McGraw-Hill; 2013.

5-minute hearing test to determine the need for a referral to a hearing specialist (Fig. 16.2). Beyond the scope of therapy practice for more profound hearing losses, a consultation and referral to a hearing specialist regarding the use of a hearing aid, individual or computerized training in speech reading (lip reading), and instruction regarding the use of an ALD may be needed. In addition, referrals for accessing both formal and informal support services through public and community agencies may be beneficial. Individuals for whom none of these interventions are effective may be candidates for cochlear implants.

OTAs are involved in direct interventions for other primary reasons aside from hearing impairment. Regardless, they should address hearing issues as they affect engagement in occupations. OTAs may also assist in adapting environments for individuals, groups, or institutional facilities. The skills and experience of OTAs may be directed toward designing and implementing individual or institutional activities. These recommendations, intended to promote successful adaptation for hearing-impaired older adults, also can assist families, friends, and institutional personnel. As always, safety is a consideration with intervention. Please refer to Box 16.2 for safety tips.

RECOMMENDATIONS FOR IMPROVING OLDER ADULT COMMUNICATION

Psychosocial issues associated with hearing impairments often affect family members and friends, as well as the hearing-impaired older adult. Information and education about the various types of age-related hearing losses and conditions may help OTAs in assisting older adults in developing coping strategies.[15] The OTA should encourage family members and friends to be involved in the education and consultation process so that conversational and environmental adaptations that encourage inclusion of the older adult can be promoted.

Hearing-impaired older adults may need to gain confidence in requesting adaptations that help them adjust to their hearing losses. Having older adults role-play situations in which they request specific needs or adaptations may increase self-confidence for reentering social situations that they may have been avoiding.

Environmental adaptations should first focus on identifying and minimizing the influence of background noises, because competing background noises are considered to be a difficult listening condition.[17] With a hearing difficulty, background noises greatly limit enjoyment of conversations and often contribute to an older adult's avoidance of social gatherings.[22] Common sources of background noise in institutions include music, conversations on television or of persons in the room, dishes being clanked, fans in use, outside traffic, overhead intercoms, and ice machines. Personnel shifts and changes in the institutional environment may also create background noise.

OTAs can recommend environments that reduce background noise. Examples include going to restaurants during times that they are less crowded, requesting to sit in less crowded areas, or sitting away from distracting background noises such as kitchen traffic or music (Table 16.2). When traveling, to help compensate for difficulty in hearing overhead paging systems, older adults can be encouraged to frequently check overhead flight monitors, check in with airport staff, or both. Using theaters and church communities that offer ALDs that amplify specific sounds is another way to reduce interference from background noises in public spaces.

Personal environmental modifications for reducing background noise include adding carpet to floors and acoustical tiles to ceilings, hanging drapes on windows, hanging banners from high ceilings, and replacing wood or metal furniture with upholstered furniture. Although these recommendations are intended to help absorb sound, they also can add esthetic appeal to a home or institution.[22]

Additional interior modifications to reduce background noise within institutions include adding insulated sheetrock around noisy areas such as kitchen, maintenance, and mechanical areas, and tightening window weather seals. OTAs can assist individuals, families, and facility administrators in weighing the benefits of certain recommendations against the expenses of purchasing them. OTAs also can point out that, in some situations, background noises may provide helpful cues to locations of activity rooms, lounges, and beauty shops.

Five-Minute Hearing Test

	Almost always	Half of the time	Occasionally	Never
1. I have a problem hearing over the telephone.				
2. I have trouble following the conversation when two or more people are talking at the same time.				
3. People complain when I turn the TV volume too high.				
4. I have to strain to understand conversations.				
5. I miss hearing some common sounds like the phone or doorbell ringing.				
6. I have trouble hearing conversations in a noisy background such as a party.				
7. I get confused about where sounds come from.				
8. I misunderstand some words in a sentence and need to ask people to repeat themselves.				
9. I especially have trouble understanding the speech of women and children.				
10. I have worked in noisy environments (jackhammers, assembly lines, jet engines).				
11. Many people I talk to seem to mumble (or don't talk clearly).				
12. People get annoyed because I misunderstand what they say.				
13. I misunderstand what others are saying and make inappropriate responses.				
14. I avoid social activities because I cannot hear well and fear I'll reply improperly.				
To be answered by a family member or friend: 15. Do you think this person has a hearing loss?				

Scoring

To calculate your score, give yourself 3 points for every time you checked the "Almost always" column, 2 for every "Half of the time," 1 for every "Occasionally" and 0 for every "Never." If you have a blood relative who has a hearing loss, add another 3 points. Then total your points. The American Academy of Otolaryngology–Head and Neck Surgery recommends the following:
- 0 to 5: Your hearing is fine. No action is required.
- 6 to 9: Suggest you see an ear-nose-and-throat (ENT) specialist.
- 10 and above: Strongly recommend you see an ear physician.

FIG. 16.2   Five-minute hearing test. (*Courtesy American Academy of Otolaryngology–Head and Neck Surgery, Alexandria, VA.*)

Environmental safety issues and concerns could center on the difficulties that hearing-impaired older adults may have in locating the source of sounds in their home. The inability to locate sounds may contribute to a sense of insecurity in an individual's own environment and to the possibility of auditory illusions. This can lead to a decrease in the person's safety. For instance, older adults may not be able to hear alarms or people moving about around them.[15] Fire and smoke alarms tend to have high-pitched sounds that are difficult for persons with

sensorineural losses to hear.[4] Adding visual cues such as flashing lights is recommended for alarms.[17] Flashing lights, lower pitched rings, or low-toned musical chimes are also available options for telephones and doorbells (Fig. 16.3). OTAs should recommend adapting telephones with volume and tone controls for persons who need these modifications. Cell phones, although convenient for many individuals, may add to the confusion and frustration for persons with hearing impairments. The ring of the phone may not be heard or the phone may be difficult to locate

BOX 16.2

Safety Gems for the Hearing Impaired

- Make sure that the older adult's hearing has been properly evaluated.
- Check that hearing aids are working. This would be especially important during activities requiring hearing ability for safety, such as with driving.
- Evaluate the person with a hearing deficit for fall risk. Consider balance and gait, and adapt the environment to prevent falls (e.g., remove clutter, increase lighting).
- Instruct others to be aware that approaching hearing-impaired older adults from the back may startle them and may cause loss of balance.
- Encourage older adults to discuss with their physicians and/or pharmacists' medications that may have side effects related to hearing issues, such as tinnitus.
- Encourage older adults to use vision (if vision is not a problem) as a compensatory safety aid in the environment. Teach scanning of the environment.
- Problem-solve with older adults a safety plan for fires or other issues.
- Use visual alert alarm systems (flashing lights) for awareness that someone is at the door, or that the phone is ringing.
- For fire safety in a home or facility, consider installing visual alarms with strobe lights, lower pitched alarm sounds, and vibration apparatuses. Vibrating beds or pillows can help awaken the person.

Data from National Institute on Aging. *Hearing Loss.* 2018. Available at: https://www.nia.nih.gov/health/publication/hearing-loss; Koorsen Fire & Security. *Fire Protection for the Deaf and Hard-of-Hearing Community.* 2020. Available at: https://blog.koorsen.com/fire-protection-for-the-deaf-and-hard-of-hearing-community; Robinson L, Saisan J, White M. *Age and Driving, Safety Tips and Warning Signs for Older Drivers.* 2016. Available at: http://www.helpguide.org/articles/aging-well/age-and-driving-safety-tips.htm.

if needed for an emergency.[23] Putting a cell phone on a vibration setting or trying text messaging with older adults who can read the screen and have adequate finger dexterity might be a good communication option. Older adults can download their own ring tone and select the ringer volume for recognition. Some cell phones can be adapted for hearing aids and for amplification of sound. Cell phones can also be adapted to be used with a teletypewriter (TTY) or Voice Carry Over device.

Research indicates hearing loss can increase an individual's risk of falling compared with individuals who are not hearing impaired.[3,24] Studies indicate that instruction in ways to substitute visual cues for hearing cues reduces the incidence of falls. OTAs also should make family members and health care providers aware that approaching hearing-impaired older adults from the back and talking to and touching them may startle them and possibly cause them to lose their balance. OTAs should recommend that hearing-impaired individuals be approached from the front, where visual contact can be made before beginning a conversation or expecting a response to a question.

To enhance conversations in areas where groups gather, OTAs should recommend that hearing-impaired individuals stay away from windows and plaster walls. Standing or sitting near soft materials that absorb sound, such as draperies, bookshelves, and upholstered furniture, is also recommended. Sitting in high-backed, upholstered chairs can help shield background noise. Focusing on the speaker's lips during conversation can help increase comprehension. If an individual has more impairment in one ear than the other, the individual can find the position that maximizes hearing with the unaffected ear.[13]

For family members and friends who want to improve communication with hearing-impaired older adults, OTAs should recommend that they position themselves

TABLE 16.2

Environmental Adaptations for the Hearing-Impaired Older Adult

Problem	Intervention
Background noises	Add carpeting to floors, acoustical tiles to ceilings, and drapes on windows, and replace (institutional and home) wood and metal furniture with upholstered furniture. Hang banners from ceilings; add insulating sheetrock around kitchens, maintenance, and (institutional) mechanical areas; tighten window weather seals. In dining rooms, seat no more than four persons at a table and add padded room dividers between tables to absorb sound. On special care units, eliminate ringing telephones, televisions, and intercoms; serve meals in small groups; pass medications at times other than meal times. Go to restaurants at less crowded times; request to sit in areas (public places) away from music and kitchen. Seek out theaters and churches that offer listening devices to amplify specific sounds. Pair emergency alarms, such as smoke alarms, with flashing lights. Rearrange furniture to create a space where all sit at eye level.
Communication	Position to reduce glare, add closed captioning, use ALDs. Use remote controls (television, radio, and music) to select programming, and alternate between music, television, and radio. Sit in a well-lit space with increased contrast. Learn to use technology, such as a computer or tablet, to increase communication.

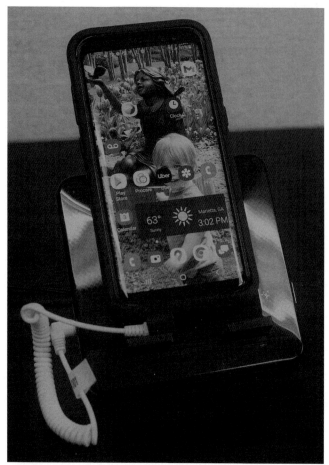

FIG. 16.3 Cell phone flashers incorporate visual cues that a cell phone is receiving a call/notification. *(Courtesy Johnny Barfield)*

BOX 16.3

Communication Tips for Working With the Hearing Impaired

- Face the older adult so that the individual can clearly see your facial features with communication.
- Speak to the older adult in a well-lit area. This helps the older adult with a hearing impairment observe body language and facial expressions, all of which provide clues for understanding communication.
- During conversations, limit background noise by turning off the radio or television.
- In public places, sit far away from the crowded or noisy areas.
- Avoid communication when chewing food.
- Speak in a somewhat louder tone than normal, but avoid shouting because that may distort speech.
- Speak at a regular rate, not faster or slower, and do not overstress sounds.
- Give the older adult with hearing loss clues about the topic of conversation whenever possible.
- Try to keep statements short and simple if the older adult with hearing loss is struggling to understand the conversation. Repeat sentences as necessary.

Adapted from National Institute on Deafness and Other Communication Disorders (NIDCD). *Age Related Hearing Loss.* 2018. National Institute on Deafness and Other Communication Disorders. Available at: https://www.nidcd.nih.gov/health/age-related-hearing-loss#5.

in the older adult's field of vision and get the older adult's attention before speaking. While conversing, they should look directly at the older adult, reduce the rate of speech, and speak distinctly with a low tone. Additional recommendations include asking the older adult to repeat what was said and providing written instructions to reinforce verbal directions. OTAs should stress that a hearing impairment does not reduce an individual's intelligence. Accommodations for the hearing impairment should not be overexaggerated or simplified to the point that older adults with hearing loss feel that their intelligence or judgment is in question.

Since sensorineural hearing loss and its corresponding reduction in the ability to hear high-pitched sounds is the most common hearing disorder in older adults, lowering the voice is especially important for women who address hearing-impaired older adults. Increasing volume only increases tone and contributes to personal and social embarrassment (Box 16.3).

In restaurants and institutional dining rooms, seating no more than four persons at a table, so eye contact can be easily made, can enhance the social aspects derived from conversations during meals. In larger dining rooms, padded room dividers between tables can absorb sounds from surrounding tables. General recommendations regarding reduction of background noises also should be considered.

The effects of glare on the visual and nonverbal cues that enhance auditory communication should be considered when speaking with hearing-impaired older adults. Sources of glare may include windows, lights, and glass surfaces either from behind the person speaking or reflected from eyeglasses. Before beginning a conversation, the OTA, family member, or friend should adjust blinds or shades, adjust lighting, and reposition seating arrangements as needed (see Chapter 15 for more information on visual adaptations with aging).

Entertainment through television, music, websites with sounds on the Internet, and radio offers opportunities for stimulation that are not dependent on other people. When older adults control the times and selections for television, radio programs, and music, the cognitive stimulation can be rewarding. When televisions and radios are on constantly or programs selected are not those the older adult would choose, they become an additional source of background noise rather than a source of stimulation.[4,23] Closed-captioned television is an additional option to suggest. OTAs should identify and reduce sources of glare on the screen when positioning older adults for television viewing. ALDs offer a means of controlling the volume for the hearing-impaired older adult without disturbing others. Adjusting the volume and sound for music for those individuals with sensorineural hearing loss requires increasing the bass and decreasing the treble. Developments in technology have made the cost of these devices quite reasonable when weighed against the potential benefits.[23] Refer to Table 16.2 for ideas for environmental adaptations.

PROVIDING ASSISTIVE HEARING DEVICES

One of the most common assistive devices for persons with a hearing impairment is a hearing aid. An audiologist assists in determining whether a hearing aid would be appropriate. If a hearing aid would be beneficial, the audiologist works with the individual to choose the type of hearing aid that will maximize the individual's hearing and understanding of speech based on the individual's type of hearing loss.[12] Additionally, the audiologist also determines whether other factors associated with aging, lifestyle, and personality are compatible with a hearing aid. OTAs may refer older adults to a physician or audiologist for assessment and evaluation. Advise patients to find out whether insurance will cover the cost of a hearing aid, and tell patients to ask whether a trial period is allowed so that the product can be tried out before it is purchased. Several visits to an audiologist may be required to get everything correct so the device is comfortable and the individual is comfortable using the hearing aid.[25]

Recent improvements in hearing aid technology have made hearing aids more acceptable. The improved devices are smaller and fit in the ear and therefore are more cosmetically appealing. In addition, hearing aids dampen certain frequencies. Some evidence indicates that younger individuals report more satisfaction than older adults with hearing aids.[26,27] This increased satisfaction may result from several factors. The onset of age-related hearing loss is often gradual, and older adults may have accommodated to their hearing loss over an extended period, eventually finding the sudden amplification of all sound to be invasive and disturbing. In addition, the fine finger-and-hand dexterity required to manipulate volume and frequency controls and change batteries may make the hearing aid difficult to operate. The presence of cognitive changes and short-term memory loss may affect the older adult's ability to remember to turn the device on and off. The cost of replacement batteries and the older adult's acceptance of new technologies are the other factors to consider when determining the appropriateness of a hearing aid.[23,28] Goals for an older adult who uses a hearing aid may include identifying alternative ways of operating it, building handles for tools used with the controls, changing or testing batteries with less difficulty, and learning the proper way to insert the device.

Even with improved technology, hearing aids may not be effective for some individuals. For others, sound distortions may be louder with a hearing aid. When hearing aids are not effective, ALDs may be used. ALDs consist of a microphone to capture spoken sounds, an amplifier to increase sound volume, and a headset worn by the hearing-impaired person. Because the amplified sound from an ALD reaches the ear directly, background noises are reduced.[29] ALDs can augment hearing in a noisy clinic or hospital room. When an ALD is plugged into a television, the sound is amplified for the hearing-impaired person only. Use of an ALD also should be considered when visual impairment does not allow the older adult to read lips or to supplement hearing loss by responding to other nonverbal cues. In addition to ALDs, there are some newer options for the hearing impaired such as computer-assisted real-time transcription (CART), visual and tactile alarms, and volume-controlled or caption phones.[30] OTAs can inform the older adult with a hearing impairment about Telecommunications Relay Services. These services, available throughout the United States, allow the person to place telephone calls with the use of computers or other technology. Operators (communication assistants) facilitate these calls by converting text to voice or vice versa. There are a variety of methods available to do this type of telephone communication to meet the needs of the hearing-impaired population.[31]

The ADA established communication rules to create provisions for people with communication difficulty. The provisions ensure on can receive and communicate information within the covered entity by providing aids and services to foster effective communication. Examples include sign language interpreters, Braille, and written material provided by the covered entity. Other auxiliary aids and service technology options covered through the ADA provision includes real-time captioning, closed captioning, telephone handset amplifiers, telecommunication relay services by dialing 711, video relay services, and video remote interpreting. Video relay services and video remote interpreting services are free, but the user must subscribe and obtain the technology with video communication capabilities to use the services.[32] Subtitles, captioning, or alternate audio is available through different technological devices and platforms. Examples include Netflix streaming services or the accessibility features on iPhones and Android devices. To access the captioning service on Netflix, the user should open Netflix, select show or movie, click the dialog icon on screen, and change audio and subtitle sections. Captioning services on the iPhone can be accessed by navigating to and clicking on Settings, Accessibility, Hearing section, Subtitles and Captioning, Closed Captions + SDH turn on, and Style button customize closed captions. To turn on closed captioning on Android devices, the user must navigate to and tap on Settings, Accessibility, Caption preferences, and Show Captions. Other services are available to optimize communication when traveling. One should sign up to receive text messaging updates regarding updates about flights or boarding times and make the attendants on trains or airplanes are aware of any hearing impairments.

Some hearing devices can now connect to Bluetooth-enabled GPS directions for navigation directions.[33]

CONCLUSION

As the number of older adults with hearing impairments increases, the challenges and opportunities for OTAs continue to grow. The occupational performance and psychosocial and environmental issues that surround a hearing impairment demand that OTAs are informed and able to recommend appropriate interventions. OTAs can assist older adults in attaining both performance and quality of life expectations by identifying limitations in hearing, referring older adults for additional evaluation and intervention, and providing appropriate interventions.

CASE STUDY

Joe is an 89-year-old man who has resided at the Garden View Nursing Home for the past 7 years. His diagnoses include dementia (early stages), diabetes, congestive heart failure, and most recently an increase in hearing loss. Until recently, Joe's social history had been active and included participation in recreational activities and daily socializing with staff and other patients. At a recent care conference, the recreation director reported that Joe's participation in activity groups had decreased from five to two groups a week. The nurse working with Joe stated that he was less social during meals and had started to sleep in the afternoons. The social worker shared her current assessments of Joe and stated that he seemed to be isolating himself from others, including his roommate. When the social worker and other staff asked him how he was doing, he seemed to have difficulty understanding the question and changed the subject to talk about the weather. The staff thought his dementia could be contributing to the confusion or perhaps to changes in the level of his hearing loss. The team recommended referrals for a professional hearing evaluation and an occupational therapy assessment. The referral for occupational therapy included an evaluation of Joe's current level of occupational functioning and suggestions for adapting his environment. In addition, staff was seeking suggestions from occupational therapy on how they and others might interact more effectively with Joe. The OT is a new graduate and has been at the Garden View Nursing Home for 2 months only. She has asked the OTA who has worked at the nursing home for 5 of the 7 years that Joe has been a resident at the home to assist her with the assessment.

■ CASE STUDY QUESTIONS

1 Using information from the case study and the chapter, identify why staff would think that Joe's hearing loss might have an effect on his social interaction with others.

2 Describe how Joe's recent decrease in social interaction may be influencing his mood.

3 As the long-standing OTA member of the occupational therapy department, what assistance can you provide for the OT? For Joe?

4 Using information from the chapter, identify assessments that may be useful for Joe.

5 What recommendations would you consider to adapt Joe's environment to make it more purposeful and accommodating for him?

6 What types of assistive devices would be considered for Joe?

7 You have been asked to prepare an in-service on hearing impairments in older adults and provide recommendations that will assist all staff to be more effective when interacting with those who have a hearing impairment.
- How will you organize this in-service?
- What information do you think would be most helpful for staff?
- How will you engage the staff in the learning process?

■ CHAPTER REVIEW QUESTIONS

1 Referring to the chapter, what are some age-related hearing changes in older adults?

2 How do age-related hearing impairments in older adults affect their communication and socialization skills, as well as their safety?

3 How can OTAs contribute to improving communication and socialization skills in hearing-impaired older adults?

4 What safety concerns should OTAs be aware of when working with an older adult who has a hearing impairment?

5 What environmental modifications can OTAs suggest to reduce background noises in an older adult's home?

6 What environmental modifications in an institution might be used to reduce confusion caused by hearing impairments?

7 Why might an older adult prefer not to use a hearing aid?

8 Explain how a cochlear implant would improve the hearing of some older adults.

9 How might an OTA use an ALD to help an older adult in a clinic setting?

REFERENCES

1. Grue EV, Ranhoff AH, Noro A, et al. Vision and hearing impairments and their associations with falling and loss of instrumental activities in daily living in acute hospitalized older persons in five Nordic hospitals. *Scand J Caring Sci.* 2009;23(4):635–643. doi:10.1111/j.1471-6712.2008.00654.x.

2. Garstecki DC, Erler SF. Hearing and aging. *Top Geriatr Rehabil.* 1998;14(2):1-17.

3. Davis A, McMahon CM, Pichora-Fuller KM, et al. Aging and hearing health: the life-course approach. *Gerontologist.* 2016;56(suppl 2):S256-S267. doi:10.1093/geront/gnw033.

4. Hooper CR Sensory and sensory integrative development. In: Bonder BR, Wagner MB, eds. Functional Performance in Older Adults. 3rd ed. Philadelphia: FA Davis; 2001.

5. McKee M, Stransky M, Reichard A. Hearing loss and associated medical conditions among individuals 65 years and older. *Disabil Health J.* 2018;11(1):122-125. doi:10.1016/j.dhjo.2017.05.007.

6. Gomen A, Reed N, Lin F. Addressing estimated hearing loss in adults in 2060. *JAMA Otolaryngol Head Neck Surg.* 2017;143(7):733-734.

7. Crews JE, Campbell VA. Vision impairment and hearing loss among community-dwelling older Americans: implications for health and functioning. *Am J Public Health.* 2004;94(5):823-829. doi:10.2105/AJPH.94.5.823.

8. National Institute on Deafness and Other Communication Disorders. *Hearing Loss and Older Adults.* 2018. National Institute

of Health. Available at: https://www.nidcd.nih.gov/health/hearing-loss-older-adults.

9. Lichtenstein MJ, Bess FH, Logan SA. Screening the elderly for hearing impairment. In: Ripich D, ed. Handbook of Geriatric Communication Disorders. Austin, TX: Pro-Ed; 1991.

10. American Occupational Therapy Association. Occupational therapy practice framework: domain and practice. 4th ed. *Am J Occup Ther*. 2020;74(suppl 2):1-87. doi:10.5014/ajot.2020.74S2001.

11. Meriano C, Latella D. *Occupational Therapy Interventions: Function and Occupations*. Thorofare, NJ: Slack; 2007.

12. National Institute on Deafness and Other Communication Disorders (NIDCD). *Age Related Hearing Loss*. 2018. National Institute on Deafness and Other Communication Disorders. Available at: https://www.nidcd.nih.gov/health/age-related-hearing-loss#5.

13. Cherney LR. The effects of aging on communication. In: Lewis CB, ed. Aging: The Health Care Challenge. 4th ed. Philadelphia: FA Davis; 2002.

14. Pichora-Fuller M, Mick P, Reed M. Hearing, cognition, and healthy aging: social and public health implications of the links between age-related declines in hearing and cognition. *Semin Hear*. 2015;36(3):122-139. doi:10.1055/s-0035-1555116.

15. Hooper CR, Bello-Haas VD. Sensory and sensory integrative development. In: Bonder B.R., Bello-Haas V.D., eds. Functional Performance in Older Adults. 3rd ed. Philadelphia: FA Davis; 2008.

16. Children's Hospital of Philedelphia. *Protecting Your Child Against Hearing Loss*. 2018. Available at: https://www.chop.edu/news/health-tip/protecting-your-child-against-hearing-loss.

17. Bance M. Hearing and aging. *Can Med Assoc J*. 2007;176(7):925-927. doi:10.1503/cmaj.070007.

18. Canadian Transportation Agency, 1997 Location Ottawa-Ontario. *A Look at Barriers to Communication Facing Persons with Disabilities Who Travel by Air*. 2015. Available at: https://www.otc-cta.gc.ca/eng/publication/communication-barriers-look-barriers-communication-facing-persons-disabilities-who-trave.

19. Corso JF. Sensory-perceptual processes and aging. In: Schaie KW, Eisdorfer C, eds. Annual Review of Gerontology. 2nd ed. New York: Springer; 1990.

20. Brodie A, Smith B. The impact of rehabilitation on quality of life after hearing loss: a systematic review. *Eur Arch Otorhinolaryngol*. 2018;275(10):2435-2440. doi:10.1007/s00405-018-5100-7.

21. Janken JK, Cullinan CL, Auditory, sensory, and perceptual alteration: suggested revision of defining characteristics. *Nurs Diagn*. 1990;1(4):147.

22. Christenson MA, Taira E. *Aging in the Designed Environment*. New York: Haworth Press; 1990.

23. Stach BA, Stoner WR. Sensory aids for the hearing impaired elderly. In: Ripich D., ed. Handbook of Geriatric Communication Disorders. Austin, TX: Pro-Ed; 1991.

24. Kamil RJ, Betz J, Powers BB, et al. Association of hearing impairment with incident frailty and falls in older adults. *Aging Health*. 2016;28(4):644-660. doi:10.1177/0898264315608730.

25. National Institute on Aging. *Hearing Loss*. 2018. Available at: https://www.nia.nih.gov/health/publication/hearing-loss.

26. Kane RL, Ouslander JG, Abrass IB. *Essentials of Clinical Geriatrics*. 7th ed. New York: McGraw-Hill; 2013.

27. Rieske RJ, Hostege H. *Growing Older in America*. New York: McGraw-Hill; 1996.

28. Cunningham L, Tucci D. Hearing loss in adults. *N Engl J Med*. 2017;377(25):2465-2473. doi:10.1056/NEJMra1616601.

29. U.S. Food and Drug Administration. *Other Products and Devices to Improve Hearing*. 2018. Available at: https://www.fda.gov/medical-devices/hearing-aids/other-products-and-devices-improve-hearing.

30. Hearing Loss Association of America. *Captioning and CART*. n.d. Available at: https://www.hearingloss.org/hearing-help/technology/cartcaptioning/.

31. Federal Communications Commission. *Telecommunications Relay Services – TRS*. 2021. Available at: https://www.fcc.gov/consumers/guides/telecommunications-relay-service-trs.

32. U.S. Department of Justice. *Effective Communication*. 2014. Available at: https://www.ada.gov/effective-comm.htm.

33. Colino S. *Traveling with Hearing Loss*. AARP; 2018. Available at: https://www.aarp.org/health/conditions-treatments/info-2018/hearing-loss-travel-tips.html.

17

Strategies to Maintain Continence in Older Adults

SARA MUNZESHEIMER

(PREVIOUS CONTRIBUTIONS FROM KRIS R. BROWN, SUE BYERS-CONNON, AND JESSICA HATCH)

KEY TERMS

fecal incontinence, urinary incontinence, urinary frequency,
urinary retention, voiding diary

CHAPTER OBJECTIVES

1. Determine the prevalence and cost associated with incontinence.
2. Indicate common causes of incontinence.
3. Describe the normal anatomy and physiology of urination and defecation.
4. Identify the different types of urinary and fecal incontinence.
5. Explain the Omnibus Budget Reconciliation Act as related to incontinence in nursing homes.
6. Specify the role of each team member, emphasizing the importance of an interdisciplinary approach.
7. Identify the occupational therapy assistant's (OTA's) role in the management of incontinence.
8. List suggestions for the management of incontinence.

Sara is an occupational therapy assistant (OTA) who has been treating Mrs. Smith since her arrival at the nursing home 2 months earlier following a stroke. She works with Mrs. Smith in the morning and after lunch. To start each afternoon session, per Mrs. Smith's usual routine, Sara assists Mrs. Smith with going to the restroom. However, the past few sessions that Sara has worked with her, Sara has noticed that Mrs. Smith has been incontinent each time. When Sara questions Mrs. Smith about it, she states, "I just can't seem to get to the bathroom in time, and lately no one has been helping me go before lunch like they used to do." Additionally, Sara observes that Mrs. Smith's bathroom door is always closed and blocked shut by the bedside table, making access to the restroom difficult. Oftentimes, her call light is not within reach.

Sara is concerned about the noticeable increase in Mrs. Smith's incontinence. She feels that, as an OTA, it is her responsibility to educate both Mrs. Smith and the nursing staff on some tips that may help her decrease her incontinence episodes. Sara screens Mrs. Smith for any medical causes for incontinence. Mrs. Smith reports no burning or foul odor during urination, regular bowel movements, and feels as if she is emptying her bladder completely when she does urinate. "I just have this really strong urge and by the time the nurse helps me to the bathroom it is too late," reports Mrs. Smith. Sara notifies the nurse and physician of her findings. The physician orders a urinalysis, a test to rule out medical cause such as urinary tract infection, which comes back negative. Sara then educates Mrs. Smith about her pelvic floor muscle anatomy and how to use strategic urge suppression techniques to better hold her bladder while waiting for the nurse. "I never knew about this muscle!" exclaims Mrs. Smith. Sara also begins working with the nursing staff to create a timed voiding schedule and a checklist that reminds nursing staff of simple ways to reduce some of the environmental barriers contributing to Mrs. Smith's incontinence. After implementing a few simple techniques and educating both Mrs. Smith and the nursing staff on simple tips regarding incontinence, her episodes of incontinence have decreased.

Urinary and fecal incontinence—the involuntary loss of bladder and bowel control, respectively—is a common problem many older adults face.[1] Bowel and bladder control, toilet hygiene, and clothing management are discussed as occupations in the *Occupational Therapy Practice Framework* (fourth edition). Furthermore, the *framework* highlights management of nighttime toileting needs for improved sleep participation.[2] Incontinence is often considered part of the normal aging process and is therefore accepted but not treated. Society's acceptance of this condition is manifested by the availability of absorbent products found in local stores. Some older adults afflicted with this problem may feel ashamed and embarrassed, which may lead to psychological conditions such as depression and avoidance of social relations or activities. Other older adults may think the problem will correct itself, or they may fear that it will lead to a surgical procedure. Prolonged hospitalizations are common when incontinence is left untreated. Incontinence may even be a primary reason that caregivers decide to place older adults in long-term care facilities. For all these reasons, it is imperative that health care practitioners do their part to address bowel and bladder management in older adults.

URINARY AND FECAL INCONTINENCE

Prevalence

During the normal aging process, bladder capacity and the ability to delay urination and defecation decrease. These changes can increase the risk for incontinence, especially for those with medical comorbidities.

The prevalence of urinary incontinence (UI) in the nursing home setting has been reported to vary from 27.6% up to 43% to 77%.[3] In general, individuals who are female, of older age, and with limited cognition are at higher risk of UI. Overall, UI is thought to be widely underdiagnosed and underreported.[3]

Cost

In the United States, the estimated total annual cost of urinary urgency incontinence was $66 billion per year with projected costs varying between $76.2 and $82.6 billion.[4] For the older adults in nursing homes, managing UI is estimated at $5.34 billion per year.[5,6] This cost can be itemized to include routine care such as labor, supplies, laundry, and diagnostic and medical evaluation; treatment such as surgery and drug costs; incontinent consequences such as skin erosion, urinary tract infection, and falls; and added admissions resulting from incontinence.[7]

The cost of life is just as high as indicated from the results of one study that found a 24% increase in mortality among institutionalized older adults with incontinence after one year as compared to continent cohorts. Risk was graded in the study with a 7% increased risk of mortality for those that had mild incontinence and 44% increased risk of mortality for those with severe incontinence.[6]

ANATOMY AND PHYSIOLOGY

The anatomical structures of the male lower urinary tract primarily responsible for normal urination include the bladder neck, prostate gland, pelvic floor musculature, and urethra. In women, the structures include the bladder neck, proximal urethra (internal sphincter), and the pelvic floor muscles that provide the strength needed to maintain the pelvic floor tone and urethra resistance. These pelvic floor muscles make up the external urethral sphincter in both males and females and are under voluntary control. The pelvic floor musculature is a key anatomical

feature that OTAs can keep in mind when helping their patients.[8]

The bladder fills and empties. The normal bladder capacity averages about 500 mL. The urinary bladder can normally hold between 250 and 350 mL of urine before the individual feels the urge to void. As the urinary bladder reaches its holding capacity, the stretch receptors are activated, which, in turn, causes the muscular wall of the bladder to contract and the internal sphincter to relax. At this point, the individual will be aware of urinary urge. When an individual initiates urination, they voluntarily relax the pelvic floor muscles (which make up the external sphincter). This triggers the muscular walls of the bladder to squeeze, thus emptying the bladder.[8]

The anatomical structures involved with normal defecation include the pelvic floor muscles, anal sphincter mechanisms (internal and external), colon, rectum, and anal canal. A stool of an appropriate consistency is delivered to the rectum and anal sphincter through the gastrointestinal (GI) tract and colon. The normal sensory system acknowledges that the rectum is filling and alerts the structures of the type of rectal content (i.e., solid, liquid, or gas). Once the stool passes the rectum, the internal sphincter relaxes. The individual is able to voluntarily relax the pelvic floor muscles (which make up the external sphincter), allowing the stool to pass.[8] See Figs. 17.1 and 17.2 for images of pelvic anatomy.

ETIOLOGY

Causes of urinary and stool incontinence may be pathological, anatomical, or physiological. The most common potential causes of UI are transient or reversible. These include delirium, infection such as symptomatic urinary tract infection or vaginitis, excessive urine production, and psychological factors such as depression.[9] Hypercalcemia, hyperglycemia, diabetes insipidus, chronic heart failure, lower extremity venous insufficiency, and drug-induced ankle edema are other causes of transient incontinence.[10]

Pharmaceutical causes of transient incontinence are sedative hypnotics (i.e., benzodiazepines); diuretics, leading to polyuria; calcium channel blockers; anticholinergic agents (i.e., antihistamines, antidepressants, antipsychotics, antiparkinsonian agents, and alpha-adrenergic agents); sympathomimetics; and sympatholytics. Potential causes of fecal incontinence include abnormal delivery of feces to the rectum, which may be drug induced, metabolic, or caused by infection; sphincter dysfunction from trauma, diabetes mellitus, or inflammation; reduced rectal compliance such as rectal ischemia or fecal impaction; and anatomical derangement such as from a tumor or from third-degree hemorrhoids or injury. Other causes of fecal incontinence include muscular and neuromuscular disorders such as congenital or hereditary myopathy, behavioral and developmental dysfunction, psychiatric disorders, and neurological impairment such as with the central nervous system, spinal system, or peripheral nervous system.[11]

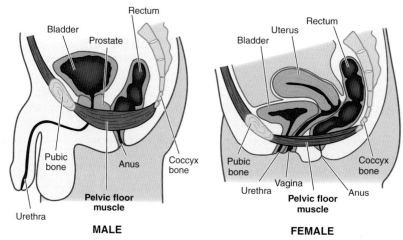

FIG. 17.1   Male and female anatomy, lateral view. *(From Potter PA, Perry AG, et al. Fundamentals of Nursing, 10th ed. St. Louis: Elsevier; 2021.)*

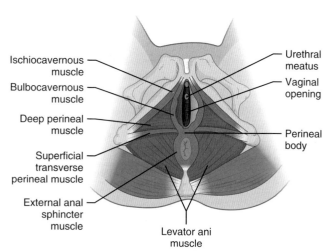

FIG. 17.2   Female anatomy, inferior view. *(From Myers RS. Saunders Manual of Physical Therapy. Philadelphia: Saunders; 1995.)*

TYPES OF URINARY INCONTINENCE

Urge or Urgency Incontinence

Older adults commonly have a combination of types of UI. Urgency urinary incontinence (UUI) is defined as the involuntary leakage of urine accompanied by a sudden urgency to have to go to the bathroom.[3] Urge incontinence is common at night, which would be referred to as nocturnal incontinence. Uncontrolled contraction of the detrusor (bladder muscle), a condition also referred to as neurogenic detrusor overactivity, may be part of the problem.[9]

Stress Urinary Incontinence

Stress urinary incontinence (SUI) is considered more prevalent in women than in men. Older adults with stress incontinence experience uncontrolled loss of urine when intraabdominal pressure is placed on the bladder. This type of incontinence can occur while coughing, laughing, sneezing, exercising, bending, lifting a heavy object, or standing from a chair.[9] Stress incontinence is usually caused by weakened pelvic floor musculature. This can occur as a result of a variety of situations such as childbirth, surgery, trauma, or as a result of immobility and aging.[12]

Overflow Incontinence

An individual with overflow incontinence experiences frequent or constant dribbling of urine, voiding only small amounts at a time. The bladder is always full due to urinary retention, a condition in which a person is unable to empty all the urine from their bladder. The older adult often cannot sense bladder fullness with this condition. The cause is often an underactive detrusor muscle. In men, this type of incontinence is common when there is a blockage in the bladder, such as an enlarged prostate. This type of UI due to urinary retention often requires medical intervention.[3,9] See Fig. 17.3 for a visual of types of UI.

Mixed Incontinence

Mixed urinary incontinence (MUI) is a combination of urge and stress incontinence. In other words, there is involuntary leakage in conjunction with a sense of urgency and increased bladder pressure. Approximately 80% of UI cases are in this category.[9]

Functional Incontinence and Other Types

Functional incontinence is related to impaired cognitive functioning and mobility. With functional incontinence, lower urinary tract function is intact, but decreased cognitive functioning prevents individuals from recognizing the need to use the restroom, or decreased mobility affects the ability to reach the restroom in time.[12] This type of incontinence often warrants occupational therapy (OT) intervention to help with environmental and other adaptations.

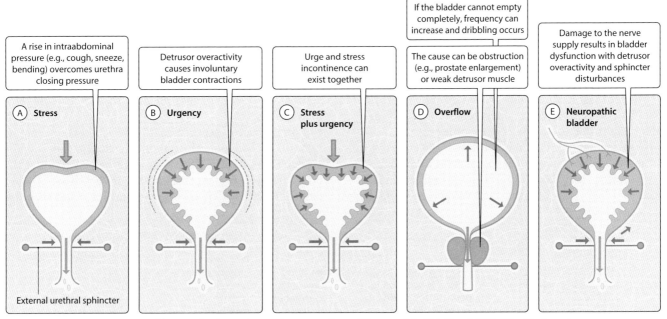

FIG. 17.3 Types of urinary incontinence. *(From Bhangu AA, Keighley MRB. The Flesh and Bones of Surgery. Philadelphia: Elsevier Ltd.; 2007.)*

FECAL INCONTINENCE

Fecal incontinence is often a result of problems with the GI tract and colon. GI problems cause changes in the consistency and volume of stools, leading to problems such as diarrhea and constipation. One study found that one in seven individuals would experience fecal incontinence. Older age is associated with increased risk.[13] Diarrhea is defined as "abnormal looseness of stools and increase in urgency and frequency of defecation."[14] Associated symptoms are abdominal pain and cramping. Diarrhea can be a symptom of problems such as dietary intolerance, malabsorption syndromes, inflammatory bowel disease, fecal impaction, gastroenteritis, and GI tumors.[12]

An individual with constipation will complain of abdominal pain and fullness in the rectum. Defecation usually occurs infrequently, and consistency of the stool is hard and dry. Constipation can result from intestinal obstruction, diverticulitis, tumors, dehydration, lack of exercise, and a poor diet.[13]

OMNIBUS BUDGET RECONCILIATION ACT AND RELATED RESEARCH

In 1987, the Omnibus Budget Reconciliation Act (OBRA) established standards of care in skilled nursing facilities including guidelines for quality of care and older adult rights. These guidelines encompassed many standards, such as identifying and addressing incontinence needs and reducing the incidence of restraint use. Both urinary and fecal incontinence are areas that surveyors look at closely during their annual inspections because of the secondary complications such as skin erosion and falls associated with these problems. Since its passing, a 30-year-survey study found a significant decrease in the use of restraints, but a higher number of reported individuals with UI (62% versus 49%). The authors theorize that this may be due to overall increased needs for nursing home residents and time restrictions for carrying out prompted voiding schedules.[15] OTAs working in skilled nursing facilities using the Minimum Data Set (MDS) Version 3.0 can view results from bladder and bowel assessment by communicating with their nursing coworkers. Section GG of the MDS includes the functional status of toilet hygiene for which therapists may provide input.[16] Refer to Chapter 6 for more information on the MDS.

INTERDISCIPLINARY TEAM STRATEGIES

Only half of older adults residing in the community actually relate incontinence problems to their physicians to receive treatment.[9] When the problem is reported, many health care professionals treat incontinence as a disease rather than determine the underlying cause, often attributing the incontinence to old age or normal body changes. However, incontinence should never be considered normal.[9]

Health care providers involved in the treatment of incontinence in older adults include urologists, gynecologists, psychiatrists, nurses, psychologists, social workers, dietitians, and pharmacists. Other health professionals include OT practitioners and physical and speech therapists. All members of this team work together to determine the most effective plan of care, and each provides a unique role in the interdisciplinary team.

Physicians begin care of older adults with incontinence by taking a thorough medical history, performing a physical examination, and scheduling laboratory tests. They may refer the patient to a specialist such as a gynecologist or urologist if the problem is recurrent. However, a conservative approach is usually initiated. The primary preference is the use of behavioral techniques followed by pharmacological approaches. Surgery may be considered as a third-line treatment for appropriate populations, but is often considered with caution for older adults due to possible complications.[10]

The dietitian can determine hydration or nutrition patterns in the older adult's diet that may be contributing to both urinary and stool incontinence. Recommendations such as a high-fiber diet and fluid recommendations help maintain proper functioning of the bowel and bladder.[7] Caffeine intake should be limited because it acts as a diuretic.

A nurse should complete a bowel (Fig. 17.4A) and bladder (Fig. 17.4B) profile indicating the length of time that incontinence has been present and the frequency and timing of episodes. The nurse usually initiates behavioral approaches and ensures skin integrity in patients with incontinence.[17]

Social service specialists and psychologists are important in determining the family dynamics and support available to older adults. They may help determine the effect that incontinence has on the involvement of older adults in social activities and relationships. They may also

Date and Time	Stimulus to evacuation (digital, suppository, or none)	Response (amount and consistency of stool)	Incontinent episodes (time, amount, and type of leakage)

A

Name_____ Date _____

Time toilet is offered	Leakage (yes or no)	Was client aware of urge? (yes or no)	Did client void? (yes or no)	Comments
0800				
1000				
1200				
1400				
1600				
1800				
2000				

B (2200 and so forth)

FIG. 17.4 Sample recording charts. (A) A diary of bowel function. (B) A diary of bladder function. (*From Doughty DB. Urinary and Fecal Incontinence Nursing Management. St. Louis: Mosby; 2006.*)

provide counseling to assist older adults in expressing feelings about their incontinence problems.

Speech and language pathologists are involved in evaluating older adults' abilities to communicate either verbally or nonverbally to make their needs known in a timely and effective manner. These professionals assist older adults in compensating for impaired communication by providing instruction in the use of gestures and communication aids. Specific training is also provided to the caregiver to ensure proper carryover.

Physical therapists may complete a comprehensive musculoskeletal and functional mobility assessment to ascertain range of motion, muscle strength, bed mobility, sitting balance, and gait. The treatment provided by physical therapists may also include teaching and instruction on the use of an assistive device such as a walker, cane, or brace to improve the older adults' abilities to ambulate to the bathroom. Caregiver training by physical therapists may include the proper use of a mechanical lift or sliding board with transfers or encouraging older adults to carry over a program involving range of motion and strengthening exercises. Electrical stimulation to strengthen the pelvic floor muscles, biofeedback, and Kegel exercises may all be part of the physical therapy intervention, though often the therapist will require specialized advanced education for these interventions. These approaches also may be applied by the OTA with demonstrated service competency and according to any state licensure guidelines.

The OTA's Role

First and foremost, the OTA should know how to screen the patient to determine any need for medical intervention. After the screening questions, the OTA should consult with the OT about providing more thorough evaluation and intervention approaches. See Box 17.1 for example screening questions.

Understanding how incontinence fits in with the *Framework*[2] can be helpful in recognizing the role of OTAs with managing incontinence. According to the *Framework*,[2] bowel and bladder management and toilet hygiene are areas of occupations, or more specifically activities of daily living (ADLs). OTAs have a responsibility to their patients to address ADLs that are important to them.

The following intervention techniques can be provided by members of the treatment team, including OTAs, to help increase independence in ADLs by decreasing the incidence of incontinence.

Education

One of the strongest tools an OTA can use is educating the patient on basic anatomy of bowel and bladder control. Specifically, the OTA can educate the patient about the presence of the voluntarily controlled pelvic floor muscles which are meant to relax when emptying and

---

BOX 17.1

Screening Questions

- For urination:
  - Do you experience any burning or foul odor when you urinate?
  - Are you needing to urinate more frequently than usual?
  - Any cloudiness or blood in the urine?
  - Do you feel you empty your bladder completely when you urinate?

Any of these could indicate need to refer to the doctor to determine presence of urinary tract infection (UTI) or other medical cause.

- For defecation:
  - When was your last bowel movement?
  - Are you having to push and strain to evacuate a bowel movement? What do they look like?

Often if it has been 3 days since the last bowel movement or if the consistency of the bowel movements are overly hard or loose, the patient may need referral to nursing or the doctor.[18]

BOX 17.2

Sample Script for Education on the Pelvic Floor

"Have you ever heard of the pelvic floor? It is a basket of muscles on the bottom of your pelvis that stretches between your tail bone (in the back), your pubic bone (in the front), and your sit bones (on the sides). This is a very important set of muscles as it provides support for our organs and also helps in controlling bowel and bladder function. Have you ever had to squeeze back around the anus because you did not want to pass gas in front of someone? That was you using your pelvic floor muscles. You similarly can squeeze these muscles when trying to hold in your urine before you are able to get to the toilet. When you sit on the toilet, these muscles should be relaxed to let urine and stool out."

---

squeeze when holding. Some studies have demonstrated the efficacy of anatomy education in decreasing cost and incidence of incontinence.[19,20] Refer to Box 17.2 for a sample script. Using simple terms and visual aids may also help the older adult's understanding. Furthermore, the OTA should consider the practicality of such education as this approach may not be effective for an older adult with cognitive deficits.

Timed Voiding and Bladder Training

Timed voiding and bladder training consist of establishing a fixed schedule that requires the patient to attempt to void every so many hours. Every 2 hours may be common for someone who is struggling with urge incontinence or urinary frequency (defined as the need to urinate more often than usual).[3,21] OTAs may help to facilitate communication between the patient, the caregiver, and nursing to create a timed voiding schedule that is personal to each patient/caregiver's daily routine.[20] Toileting is adjusted according to the patient's normal pattern and is determined after approximately 3 days of monitoring. Either the nursing staff or the individual themselves can track these patterns using a voiding diary which can document frequency of output, incidence of incontinence, fluid/food intake, awareness of urge, stimulants used, and many other optional parameters (see Fig. 17.4A and B).[19] To make timed voiding easier, associate the schedule with certain parts of the older adult's daily routine, such as 30–60 minutes after a meal or activity. It is recommended to always include a timed void as soon as the patient wakes up and right before bed.[20]

Bladder training includes the gradual increase of time in between voids while following a timed voiding schedule. Bladder training is recommended as a first step with stress, urge, and mixed incontinence. Some studies have shown a 58%–87% improvement in urinary continence using bladder training for those that have urge incontinence.[20] It should be noted that this approach is not recommended for individuals with significant cognitive impairments as they may not understand the concept of "holding it."[3]

Prompted Voiding

Prompted voiding is recommended for cognitively impaired individuals. Nursing is often responsible for documenting whether the patient is wet or dry on a regular basis, usually every 1 to 2 hours. Nursing, or trained caregivers, are encouraged to ask the patient whether they are wet or dry, check and provide nonjudgmental feedback. The nurse or caregiver then follow up by encouraging a visit to the bathroom or helping them with changing their clothes.[3] Effectiveness may be limited in nursing homes by time restraints among the nursing staff in adequately carrying out the prompted voiding schedule.[15] OTAs can help to address this gap in health care services to better carry out toilet schedules and prompted voiding techniques. They can also provide education to the health care team regarding recommended durable medical equipment, environmental adaptations, and strategies for clothing management and hygiene to decrease burden of care.[20] These interventions can specifically address criteria in Section GG of the MDS.[16]

Pelvic Floor Exercises

Pelvic floor exercises are also known as Kegels. Research indicates that pelvic floor exercises (Kegels) are effective in treatment of SUI in women regardless of age or BMI, often with better outcomes in longer programs.[22,23] Older adults are taught to relax the abdominal muscles while contracting the pelvic floor muscles. Usually a specially trained

occupational or physical therapy practitioner can help to establish a home exercise program for pelvic floor muscle training, which will vary depending on patient tolerance, strength, and coordination.[20] This technique is commonly used to improve fecal incontinence and increase muscle tone in the pelvic floor to prevent stool leakage.

Specialized Technology for Pelvic Floor Training

Some specially trained physical therapy or OT practitioners use technology to help with treatment of bowel/bladder dysfunction, often through training of the voluntarily controlled pelvic floor muscles. Biofeedback offers older adults' visual and auditory information to teach voluntary control of the pelvic floor muscles.[23] If interested in specializing, OTAs can seek out continuing education opportunities for pelvic floor training, specialized technology such as biofeedback, and other interventions.

ENVIRONMENTAL ADAPTATIONS

The ability to be continent resides heavily on being able to reach the restroom or commode. Often, there are environmental barriers that contribute to incontinence. Many residents in long-term care facilities experience incontinence simply because of the inability to obtain help with toileting in a timely fashion. In most cases, changes in the physical environment must be initiated by caregivers.[20] When considering problems with functional mobility, OTAs are encouraged to look at the older adult's environment to determine whether modifications are necessary to facilitate independence and to ensure safety while toileting (Box 17.3). Refer to Table 17.1 for interventions specific to the institutional setting and other more general suggestions that can be applied to the home environment. OTAs

---

BOX 17.3

Considerations for Environmental Adaptations to Help With Incontinence

1. Does the patient need or use side rails to assist with bed mobility?
2. Is the call light easily accessible to the patient?
3. Is the height of the bed appropriate for safe transfers?
4. Is there adequate lighting to and from the bathroom? (A 60-year-old older adult requires three times brighter lighting than a 20-year-old adult.)
5. Are there any obstacles or clutter that would interfere with safe mobility?
6. Is the patient able to manage the door leading into the bathroom?
7. Are the floors highly waxed, which could cause a fall?
8. Is the doorway leading into the bathroom wide enough to allow proper clearance for a wheelchair or walker?
9. Is the height of the toilet appropriate?
10. Are there any grab bars or support to assist with a transfer to the toilet?

TABLE 17.1

Environmental and Safety Adaptations to Help With Incontinence

When implemented appropriately, the following adaptations are ideas that may be used to make it easier for the older adults to manage bowel and bladder needs safely.

Example problem	Environmental modifications
The older adult has an increased risk of falling when accessing the bathroom.	Keep the walkways clear and free of clutter. Provide adequate lighting. Install handrails leading to the bathroom. Place a commode near the bed. Make a urinal or bed pan available. Adjust the height of the bed. Add side rail to the bed for ease with transfers. Eliminate throw rugs or bath mats.
The older adult has difficulty transferring to/from toilet or commode.	Add any combination of a toilet safety frame, elevated toilet seat, and/or grab bars. Add a nonskid material in front of the toilet or commode.
The older adult is not comfortable on the toilet.	If the patient's feet do not reach the floor, the OTA can provide a step or lower the commode. Provide a padded toilet seat for comfort, especially for older adults that have skin integrity issues. Dim the lights, provide privacy as appropriate, or play calming music/toilet meditation as needed. Add grab bars or a toilet safety frame if patient feels unbalanced on toilet or commode.
The older adult has difficulty managing clothing.	Suggest that the older adult wear clothing that is easily removed such as Velcro or elastic waistband pants, skirts, or dresses are another alternative. Trial adaptive approaches to clothing management as appropriate such as use of lateral leans, partial lift offs, transferring to bed for clothing management, use of pant clips, and adding grab bar for ease with standing.

Adapted from Miller C. *Nursing for Wellness in Older Adults*, 5th ed. Philadelphia: Lippincott Williams & Wilkins; 2009.

should make recommendations for improvement where required (see Chapter 14 for more information on fall prevention).

Many environmental modifications can be made in the bathroom. For example, grab bars can be mounted either in a 45-degree horizontal fashion to assist in pushing up or in a vertical position to facilitate pulling up. The length of the bars should be between 24 and 36 inches on the back wall and 42 inches on the side wall.[24] When making adaptations, the OTA should also keep in mind that, per OBRA regulations, restraints are recommended only to encourage more functional independence, to decrease the risk for a life-threatening medical problem, or to promote a better anatomical seating position that is minimally restrictive (see Chapter 14 for more information on restraint reduction).[15,25] The OTA should also consider whether the patient is comfortable sitting on the toilet or commode. Voiding, the process of urination or defecation, is a relaxation reflex, so making the patient comfortable is another way that the OTA can help.[20] See Table 17.1 for recommendations.

CLOTHING ADAPTATIONS AND MANAGEMENT

Clothing management before and after toileting is part of the self-care and mobility items evaluated in treatment.[16]

OTAs can help older adults improve clothing management by providing activities that use fine motor coordination, such as increasing dexterity with manipulation of zippers or buttons. Range of motion and strengthening exercises may facilitate pulling pants over the feet and hips. Another option is to suggest that older adults wear clothing that can be easily manipulated, such as clothing with Velcro or elastic waistbands.[1,20]

ADAPTATIONS FOR PATIENTS WITH FUNCTIONAL INCONTINENCE

An increased incidence of incontinence is often seen in older adults with dementia. In addition to an inability to manage their clothing, these older adults may also have difficulty locating the bathroom and toilet. Some may have problems with their strength, coordination, range of motion, and sense of balance, which affect their abilities to toilet in a timely and safe manner. Older adults with dementia might perform part of the toileting task but become confused at some point and require verbal or physical assistance, or both, to continue. OTAs can encourage maximal functioning by determining what tasks the patient can do and by training caregivers to assist with only those tasks that become difficult. Furthermore, the OTA can use simple verbal cues or visual signage, providing processing time after, for improved patient participation with toileting.[26]

Impaired functional mobility of older adults can be addressed by OTAs in conjunction with physical therapy. The goal is to improve functional mobility skills and train caregivers to provide the proper physical and verbal cues needed for older adults to become successful with safe mobility.

PREVENTION OF SKIN EROSION

One of the secondary effects of incontinence is skin erosion. Caregivers must be educated on a bowel and bladder program, a repositioning schedule, and proper wound care. Skin integrity may be improved by placing a special mattress on the bed or an incontinence cushion on the sitting surface.[9] One study found that interventions such as cleaning skin after each incontinence episode, using gentle disposable wipes, and applying skin barrier cream as needed helped the intervention group to decrease incidence of incontinence acquired dermatitis as compared to the control group (18.2% compared to 54.5%).[17] Adequate nutrition, frequent repositioning of bedridden patients, and early mobilization also aid in improving skin integrity.[17]

FALL PREVENTION AND URGE SUPPRESSION TECHNIQUES

Rushing to the bathroom is one of the leading causes of falls among older adults.[6] Urge suppression techniques are a tool that the OTA can use to educate their patient on controlling their bladder/bowel needs. When the patient feels the urge:

- They should stay calm, breathe, sit, or stand very still. Do NOT rush to the bathroom. If the older adult is in a facility, they may push their call light at this time.
- They should Kegel lightly, raise their heels off the floor if possible. These both send signals to the bladder to "calm down."
- They should use distraction techniques. Think about other things not related to going to the bathroom.
- They should repeat these steps, if necessary.
- Once they feel the urge subside, they can calmly and safely make their way to the bathroom with assistance as needed.[27]

The Knack

Another pelvic floor strategy the OTA can utilize for older adults with stress or mixed incontinence is the "the knack maneuver."[28] This technique is often taught using the term "squeeze before you sneeze," which indicates that the patient should contract their pelvic floor muscle prior to whatever activity tends to precede urinary leakage (standing, sneezing, coughing etc.).[28]

TECH TALK: FOCUS ON CONTINENCE

NAME	PURPOSE	APPROXIMATE COST	WHERE TO BUY
Poop Tracker	Application designed to track bowel movements including time, characteristics symptoms, and custom notes.	$0	Google Play IOS App Store
iUflow	Application designed to track bladder voiding including time, symptoms, characteristics, and custom notes.	$0	Google Play IOS App Store Iuflow.com
Squeezy	Application designed to gamify pelvic floor strengthening exercises such as Kegels. Separate option for males/females.	$3.99 one-time fee	Google Play IOS App Store Squeezyapp.com

CASE STUDY

Ricardo was recently admitted to a skilled nursing facility (SNF) from his home, where his aging husband, Paul, was attempting to care for him. Ricardo's urinary and bowel incontinence was becoming burdensome, and with little support and inconsistent in-home services, the daily routine had become too much for Paul. The situation was also causing a strain on their marriage.

On admission to the SNF, Ricardo was diagnosed with early-stage Alzheimer's-type dementia, rheumatoid arthritis, and long-term low back pain. In addition, Ricardo had the beginning of a pressure sore forming on his coccyx. The nursing home physician reviewed Ricardo's medical history and performed a physical examination. She determined that Ricardo's incontinence was not caused from medications but rather was related to the Alzheimer's disease process and pain associated with movement. Occupational and physical therapies were ordered to evaluate and provide appropriate intervention for Ricardo.

The findings from the OT evaluation were as follows:
1 Working memory deficits.
2 Limited mobility and ambulation secondary to pain.
3 Limited upper extremity range of motion.
4 Weakness in the upper extremities.
5 Ability to follow simple two-step directions.

Josie, the OTA at the SNF, was assigned to provide OT treatment five times a week. She was to assess bed and wheelchair positioning, adaptive equipment needs, fine motor skills, and toileting tasks and transfers. It was determined through the interdisciplinary team process that nursing would assist with pain management, including appropriate medications. Nursing would also implement scheduled toileting and begin intervention to heal the pressure ulcer. The dietitian would provide suggestions for a proper diet, intake, and suggest nutritional supplements to promote healing of the pressure ulcer. Physical therapy would address bed mobility, sitting and standing balance, and safe ambulation.

By the end of the first week of intervention, Josie recommended a higher bed to ease Ricardo's transfer process and to decrease the amount of pain associated with transfers. A bedside commode was placed in Ricardo's room until his ability to ambulate to the bathroom from his room could be evaluated. Because of his dementia, Ricardo was unable to complete pericare; however, with verbal cueing, he was able to assist with clothing management before and after toileting. Josie also recommended a pull-up incontinent undergarment to be used because Ricardo was able to assist with clothing management. She also provided positioning equipment for the bed and wheelchair to assist in the healing of and prevention of further pressure ulcers. This included a bed wedge to help Ricardo maintain side lying during scheduled turning when in bed and a gel cushion with a coccyx cutout for his wheelchair to decrease heat and shear.

Paul began to make regular visits, and the social worker helped them adjust to the changes in their lives.

■ CASE STUDY QUESTIONS

1 Why would a pull-up incontinence product be the most appropriate recommendation for Ricardo?
2 What is the advantage of using a gel cushion?
3 List three possible reasons why a pressure ulcer was developing before Ricardo's admission to the SNF.
4 Identify two reasons why an older adult in Ricardo's situation benefits from scheduled turning.
5 Why would Ricardo's incontinence cause strain on his relationship with his partner Paul?
6 Why is timely pain medication helpful?
7 Identify one reason why improved nutrition is important in Ricardo's situation.
8 Would education on pelvic floor anatomy and urge suppression techniques be appropriate for Ricardo?

■ CHAPTER REVIEW QUESTIONS

1 Identify the members of an incontinence team and their specific roles.
2 Describe how OBRA has affected the management of incontinence in the nursing facility.
3 Discuss whether urinary and fecal incontinence are part of the normal aging process.
4 What type of incontinence is more prevalent in women?
5 Describe the effect of incontinence on nursing home placement.
6 Which behavioral technique is commonly used for incontinence training with an older adult who has dementia?
7 What are some of the secondary complications associated with incontinence?
8 What is the role of the OTA in the management of incontinence?
9 What are some environmental modifications that can improve continence?
10 Discuss the various ways that incontinence with regard to areas of occupation in the OTPF,[2] can be addressed by using Table 17.1. Consider beyond the categories of bowel and bladder management and toilet hygiene to other categories that could be related to incontinence.
11 How would you teach an older adult about urge suppression strategies using pelvic floor anatomy education?

For additional video content, please visit Elsevier eBooks+ (eBooks.Health.Elsevier.com)

REFERENCES

1. Miller C, ed. Urinary function. In: Nursing for Wellness in Older Adults. 8th ed. Philadelphia, PA: Lippincott Williams & Wilkins; 2018:392-417.
2. American Occupational Therapy Association. Occupational therapy practice framework: domain and Process – Fourth Edition. *Am J of Occup Ther.* 2020;74:7412410010. Available at: https://doi.org/10.5014/ajot.2020.74S2001.
3. Huion A, Wtte ND, Everaert K, Halfens RJ, Schols JM. Care dependency and management of urinary incontinence in nursing homes: a descriptive study. *J Adv Nurs.* 2020;77:1731-1740. doi:10.1111/jan.14702.
4. Coyne K, Wein A, Nicholson S, Kvasz M, Chen C, Milsom I. Economic burden of urgency urinary incontinence in the United States: a systematic review. *J Manag Care Pharm.* 2014;20(2): 130-140.
5. Palmer M. Urinary incontinence quality improvement in nursing homes: where have we been? Where are we going? *Urol Nurs.* 2008;28(6):439-444, 453.
6. Damián J, Pastor-Barriuso R, García López F, de Pedro-Cuesta J. Urinary incontinence and mortality among older adults residing in care homes. *J Adv Nurs.* 2016;73(3):688-699.
7. Doughty D. *Urinary and Fecal Incontinence.* 3rd ed. St. Louis: Mosby; 2006.
8. Rocca Rossetti S. Functional anatomy of pelvic floor. *Arch Ital Urol Androl.* 2016;88(1):28-37. doi:10.4081/aiua.2016.1.28.
9. Newman D, Wein A. *Managing and Treating Urinary Incontinence.* Baltimore, MD: Health Profession Press; 2009.
10. Resnick NM. Chapter 23. Urinary incontinence. In: Goldman L, Schafer AI, eds. Goldman-Cecil Medicine. 26th ed. Elsevier, 2020:105-109.
11. Yeong L. What's new in the tool for constipation and fecal incontinence. *Front Med (Lausanne).* 2014;1:5. doi:10.3389/fmed.2014.00005.
12. Kear TM. Chapter 55: Management of patients with urinary disorders. In: Cheever K, Hinkle J, eds. Brunner and Suddarth's Textbook of Medical-Surgical Nursing. 14th ed. Philadelphia: Lippincott Williams & Wilkins, 2018:1650-1621.
13. Mcnees SB, Almario CV, Spiegel B, Chey WD. Prevalence of and factors associated with fecal incontinence: Results from a population-based survey. *Gastroenterology.* 2018;154(6):1672-1681. doi:10.1053/j.gastro.2018.01.062.
14. Stedman TL. (2012). *Stedman's medical dictionary for the health professions and nursing* (7th). Wolters Kluwer Health/Lippincott Williams & Wilkins.
15. Fashaw SA, Thomas KS, McCreedy E, Mor V. Thirty-year trends in nursing home composition and quality since the passage of the Omnibus Reconciliation Act. *J Am Med Dir Assoc.* 2020;21(2): 233-239. doi:10.1016/j.jamda.2019.07.004.
16. Centers for Medicaid and Medicare Services (CMS). *Long-Term Care Facility Resident Assessment Instrument 3.0 User's Manual.* 2019. Available at: https://downloads.cms.gov/files/mds-3.0-rai-manual-v1.17.1_october_2019.pdf.
17. Avşar P, Karadağ A. Efficacy and cost-effectiveness analysis of evidence-based nursing interventions to maintain tissue integrity to prevent pressure ulcers and incontinence-associated dermatitis. *Worldviews Evid Based Nurs.* 2018;15(1):54-61. doi:10.1111/wvn.12264.

18. Jones LF, Meyrick J, Bath J, Dunham O, McNulty CAM. Effectiveness of behavioural interventions to reduce urinary tract infections and Escherichia coli bacteraemia for older adults across all care settings: a systematic review. *J Hosp Infect*. 2019;102(2): 200-218. doi:10.1016/j.jhin.2018.10.013.

19. Diokno AC, Newman DK, Low LK, et al. Effect of group-administered behavioral Treatment on urinary incontinence in older women. *JAMA Intern Med*. 2018;178(10):1333. doi:10.1001/jamainternmed.2018.3766.

20. Cunningham R, Valasek S. Occupational therapy interventions for urinary dysfunction in primary care: a case series. *Am J Occup Ther*. 2019;73(5):7305185040p1-7305185040p8. doi:10.5014/ajot.2019.038356.

21. Booth J, Bliss D. Consensus statement on bladder training and bowel training. *Neurourol Urodyn*. 2020;39(5):1234-1254. doi:10.1002/nau.24345.

22. García-Sánchez E, Ávila-Gandía V, López-Román J, Martínez-Rodríguez A, Rubio-Arias JÁ. What pelvic floor muscle training load is optimal in minimizing urine loss in women with stress urinary incontinence? A systematic review and meta-analysis. *Int J Environ Res Public Health*. 2019;16(22):4358. doi:10.3390/ijerph16224358.

23. Oliveira M, Ferreira M, Azevedo MJ, Firmino-Machado J, Santos PC. Pelvic floor muscle training protocol for stress urinary incontinence in women: a systematic review. *Rev Assoc Med Bras*. 2017;63(7):642-650.

24. US Department of Justice. *2010 Americans with Disabilities (ADA) Standards for Accessible Design*. Washington, DC: 2010. Available at: https://www.ada.gov/regs2010/2010ADAStandards/2010ADAStandards_prt.pdf.

25. Omnibus Budget Reconciliation Act of 1987, HR 3545, 100th Congress (1987-1988). Available at: https://www.congress.gov/bill/100th-congress/house-bill/3545.

26. Allen C, Earhart C, Blue T. *Occupational Therapy Treatment Goals for the Physically and Cognitively Disabled*. Rockville, MD: American Occupational Therapy Association; 1992.

27. Newman D, Borello-France D, Sung V. Structured behavioral treatment research protocol for women with mixed urinary incontinence and overactive bladder symptoms. *Neurourol Urodyn*. 2017;37(1):14-26.

28. Brucker BM, Lee RK, Newman DK. Optimizing nonsurgical treatments of overactive bladder in the United States. *Urology*. 2020;145:52-59. doi:10.1016/j.urology.2020.06.017.

Working With Older Adults Who Have Dysphagia and Oral Motor Deficits

MEGHAN V. HALL

(WITH PREVIOUS CONTRIBUTIONS FROM TERRYN DAVIS, DEBORAH L. MORAWSKI, AND RENÉ PADILLA)

KEY TERMS

alternative means, aspiration pneumonia, bolus, compensations, contraindicated, dehydration, dysphagia, hydration, malnutrition, nutrition, oral intake, positioning, undernourishment, velum

CHAPTER OBJECTIVES

1. Be able to explain the anatomy and sequence of the typical swallow.
2. Be able to identify the signs of aspiration.
3. Be able to gather and interpret assessment data of the most common types of oral-motor deficit and dysphagia in the older adult population.
4. Be able to design and implement intervention for the most common types of oral-motor deficit and dysphagia in the older adult population

5. Discuss the role of the interdisciplinary team in the care of the patient with oral motor deficits and dysphagia.
6. Work with an interdisciplinary team to design a feeding program for older adults.

Eating is essential for survival, a basic activity of daily living (ADL), and often a very meaningful area of occupation.[1] Eating provides an opportunity for regular, meaningful connection to family and culture. In this chapter, we will explore the mechanics of the safe and effective swallow itself, assessment tools available to determine deficits, and the interventions to address associated deficits.

Among older adults residing in care facilities, the prevalence of undernourishment and malnutrition may be as high as 80%. This high prevalence may be explained by the increased numbers of older adults who need assistance with feeding and the lack of sufficient staff to assist them. In assisted living facilities, government statistics show that 23% of residents are reported to need total feeding assistance and 45% require some feeding assistance. In these settings, it has been reported that a nursing assistant may feed from 5 to 20 individuals an hour, with research showing that it may take up to 40 minutes for an assisted living facility resident to complete a meal.[2]

These statistics clearly reflect the growing need for occupational therapy involvement with older adults to help them maintain optimal independence in a home,

hospital, or assisted living setting. Occupational therapy assistance may include training in self-feeding, safe swallowing, positioning, mobility, meal preparation and cleanup, shopping, money management, provision of assistive equipment, and caregiver and nursing education. All of these activities are essential for older adults to adequately maintain nutrition and hydration.

THE ROLE OF THE OCCUPATIONAL THERAPY ASSISTANT IN THE MANAGEMENT OF ORAL MOTOR DEFICITS AND DYSPHAGIA

The level of involvement of the occupational therapy assistant (OTA) in the client's oral motor deficit and dysphagia care depends upon the OTA's level of experience. An entry-level OTA may work on activities that reinforce good nutrition and hydration such as meal preparation, money management, shopping, oral-facial exercises, instruction in assistive devices, and energy conservation during activities. An experienced OTA who has demonstrated competence in this area may participate in videofluoroscopic swallow studies and assist tracheostomized and ventilator-dependent older adults with self-feeding and swallowing. It is recommended that the OTA review the article "Specialized Knowledge and Skills in Feeding, Eating, and Swallowing for Occupational Therapy Practice," developed by the American Occupational Therapy Association.[3]

NORMAL SWALLOW

The swallow response requires a rapid interplay between the brain, 6 cranial nerves, 48 pairs of muscles, the salivary glands, and cartilaginous structures (Fig. 18.1). The OTA working with older adults who have dysphagia must clearly understand the anatomy and physiology of swallowing.[4]

Four phases of swallowing have been defined: oral preparatory, oral, pharyngeal, and esophageal (Fig. 18.2).[5]

1. Oral preparatory phase: The oral preparatory phase includes seeing, smelling, reaching for the item, bringing it to the mouth, and putting it in the mouth. Once the item is placed in the mouth, the lips close to maintain a seal, and the tongue and cheek muscles move the bolus (i.e., the food or liquid) around the mouth in preparation for swallowing. The base of the tongue and the velum (soft palate) also make a seal to prevent the bolus from entering the pharynx prematurely. Saliva mixes with the bolus to aid in swallowing. Taste, temperature, and texture receptors of the tongue also play a part in preparing for the action of swallowing.
2. Oral phase: The oral phase occurs once the bolus is prepared and formed by the tongue. The bolus is then propelled by the tongue to the back of the mouth and over the base of the tongue.

3. Pharyngeal phase: The pharyngeal phase occurs when the bolus passes over the base of the tongue and enters the pharynx. At this time, the soft palate elevates to seal the entrance to the nose, the hyoid bone and larynx elevate upward and anteriorly, the vocal folds close, the epiglottis tilts downward, and the cricopharyngeal sphincter opens to allow the bolus to enter the esophagus.
4. Esophageal phase: The esophageal phase occurs when the bolus passes into the esophagus and is propelled to the stomach.[5]

Changes of Swallowing Structures

When individuals eat and swallow, the oral and pharyngeal structures adapt easily to different liquid and food consistencies and to the texture, temperature, and volume of the bolus. These structures also adapt to the different positions that the head and body may assume while swallowing. Changes in these structures and their adaptability occur in both the typical aging process and in the presence of pathology. In order to maintain functional independence with feeding and swallowing, individuals develop compensations to these changes spontaneously and often unknowingly. In the absence of neurological pathology, some simple compensations may include: smaller bites, longer chewing time, or softer food.[5,6] In the presence of a medical condition or neurological deficit, these simple compensations can be difficult to manage, resulting in an unsafe or ineffective swallow. In addition to understanding the physical changes that occur, OTAs must be attune to the psychosocial effect of swallowing problems on a client's psychosocial wellbeing. OTAs should acknowledge older adults' and caregivers' perspectives regarding changes to the client's diet.

ETIOLOGY OF DYSPHAGIA

Dysphagia is a medical term used to describe any difficulty in swallowing. The definition published by the AOTA is: "dysfunction in any stage or process of eating. It includes any difficulty in the passage of food, liquid, or medicine, during any stage of swallowing that impairs the client's ability to swallow independently or safely."[7] As we have learned, swallowing requires strength, coordination, and endurance, as well as a number of intact anatomical structures. It relies on both voluntary and involuntary muscle control. Therefore, dysphagia may be the result of any pathology that affects those client factors, as well as the typical aging process itself, and may occur at any phase of the swallowing process (Table 18.1). Some examples of these pathologies are cerebrovascular accident, brain tumor, traumatic brain injury, Parkinson's disease, multiple sclerosis, amyotophic lateral sclerosis, or neurocognitive disorder. Additional examples are cancer, diabetes, rheumatoid arthritis, and scleroderma. Dysphagia may also result from prolonged illnesses or from the side effects of medications.[7]

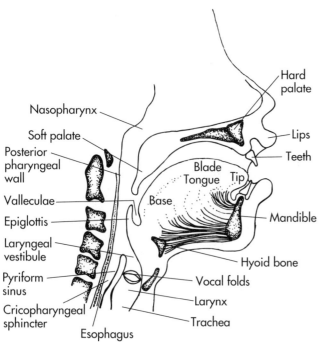

FIG. 18.1 Oral structures and mechanisms at rest.

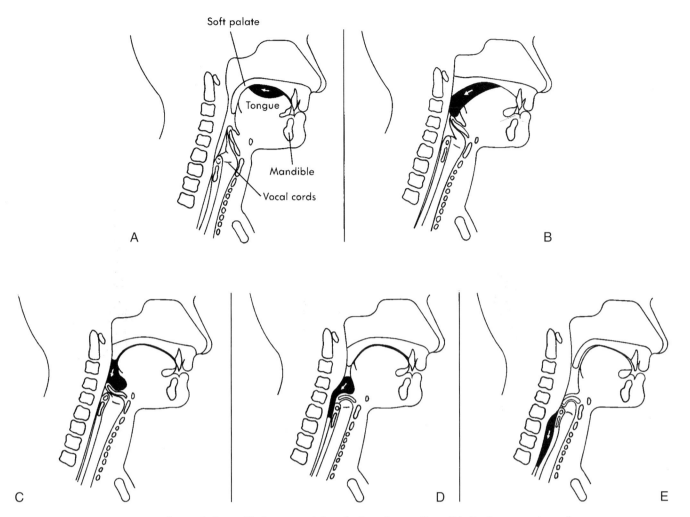

FIG. 18.2 Lateral view of bolus propulsion during the swallow. (A) Oral preparation of the bolus and voluntary initiation of the swallow by the oral tongue. (B) Bolus moves from oral cavity to pharynx, and pharyngeal swallow is triggered. (C) Bolus enters the valleculae and the airway is protected. (D) The tongue base retracts to the anteriorly moving pharyngeal wall. (E) Bolus enters the cervical esophagus and cricopharyngeal area. *(From Logeman G. Evaluation and Treatment of Swallowing Disorders, 2nd ed. Austin, TX: Pro-Ed; 1998.)*

Signs of Possible Aspiration

Indicators of swallowing and nutritional problems may include an increased temperature, lung congestion, and poor intake. Increased temperature and lung congestion may be a sign that the older adult has aspirated food or liquid and that pneumonia is developing. Poor intake may indicate an inability to swallow rather than a poor appetite. All personnel working with older adults with possible swallowing problems must be aware of these indications and be trained in how to assist someone who is choking and in cardiopulmonary resuscitation in the event that an older adult chokes.[8]

Additional signs of aspiration may include coughing during and after eating, a wet or gurgly quality to the clients voice during and after eating, difficulty breathing while eating, and unusual head movements while eating.[8] If swallowing problems are not identified, they can result in aspiration pneumonia, malnutrition, dehydration, and death.[5,9]

CASE STUDY

You are working with a client in an outpatient orthopedic setting as he recovers from a distal radius fracture with ORIF. At the start of your session, he is coughing repeatedly; by about 15 minutes into your session, the coughing subsides. At the end of the session, his wife joins and he reports that he had another one of his "coughing spells." His wife tells you that he "coughs almost every time he eats, even just a little snack in the car." What follow-up questions should you ask? Is it your place to address any feeding concerns in your role as the OTA addressing his wrist?

TABLE 18.1

Possible Deficits at Each Phase of the Swallow

Swallowing phase	Possible deficits
Oral preparatory	Cognitive impairment, such as decreased memory and attention.
	Social isolation, depression, and anxiety that result in decreased food intake and weight loss.
	Missing teeth and/or poor-fitting dentures may result in slow eating and decreased intake.
	Declines in sensory input: vision, smell, taste, hearing, and touch.
Oral	Atrophy of the face, lip, tongue, and jaw musculature.
	Decreased control of oral secretions.
	Altered production of saliva.
Pharyngeal	Duration of the phase lengthens.
	Lag time in the activation of structures.
	Decreases in muscle tone may delay clearing of food residuals.
	The epiglottis may become smaller and move more slowly.
	Cricopharyngeal sphincter remains open for shorter time.
	Upward movement of hyoid and larynx becomes delayed.
Esophageal	Increased time needed for bolus to reach stomach. Food contents may reflux from stomach and reenter esophagus and pharynx.
	Decreased strength of muscles results in increased time for passage of bolus to stomach.

Adapted from Cherney L. *Clinical Management of Dysphagia for Adults and Children*, 3rd ed. 2020. Elsevier.

ASSESSMENT OF ORAL MOTOR DEFICITS AND DYSPHAGIA

To identify oral motor deficits and dysphagia, health care practitioners may use instrumental assessments, noninstrumental assessments, or a combination of both. A client can be considered a candidate for a feeding program assessment if they meet the following basic requirements: alert, able to maintain an upright head and trunk posture with assistance, have developing tongue control, manage oral secretions with minimal drooling, and have a reflexive cough, meaning the client coughs involuntarily and automatically when food or liquid begins to enter the airway.[8] When these basic criteria are met, the OT may move forward with a detailed assessment, as outlined herein.

Instrumental Assessments

Instrumental assessments are those which require advanced training in specialized imaging operation and reading. Two of the most commonly used instrumental assessments in the diagnostic process for oral-motor deficits and dysphagia are videofluroscopic swallowing study (VFSS), aka modified barium swallow study (MBSS), and fiberoptic endoscopic evaluation of swallowing (FEES).[8] To conduct a MBSS, the examiner mixes various consistencies of food/liquid with barium, which allows for real-time visualization of swallow with X-ray. The benefit of MBSS is that the examiner can see not only that aspiration has occurred, but also at which point and to what extent. To conduct a FEES, the examiner passes an endoscope transnasally; the client's swallow is first observed with saliva only, then food or liquid may be introduced to observe the swallow under different conditions.[8] The benefit of the

FEES is its portability: it is a small machine, which means it may be completed at bedside or in the outpatient setting. One drawback of the FEES is the "white-out," which is the result of the reflection of light on pharyngeal and laryngeal tissues, making it impossible to see *during* the swallow. For this reason, the FEES is more commonly used to examine upper gastrointestinal anatomy and tone.[8]

Noninstrumental Assessments

Much information may be gathered through evaluation and skilled observation. These would include:

1. Chart review:
   a. Past medical history
   b. Current medical status and medications
   c. Nutrition/hydration
   d. Respiratory status
   e. Nursing assessment
   f. Cognitive/communicative history
   g. Social history
   h. Other evaluations
2. Clinical exam:
   a. Posture and movement
   b. Alertness, reaction to people in room
   c. Awareness of and control of secretions
   d. Ability to follow directions/answer question (cognitive/communicative status)
   e. Auditory and visual acuity
   f. Caregiver–patient interaction

Based on the findings of the chart review, clinical exam, and any assessment results reported by the OT and other members of the treatment team, the OT will establish a treatment plan to best serve the client.

PREPARATION FOR INTERVENTION

Intervention of swallowing disorders entails attending to both intrapersonal and extrapersonal details (Box 18.1).

Environmental Considerations

There is an ancient saying credited to Apicius, "we eat first with our eyes." Consider the dining environment and experience when preparing for a feeding session. Take care to present food in a palatable manner; for example, if older adults are living in care facilities, food items should be taken off serving trays and put directly on the table to help establish a homelike atmosphere. As deficits in visual acuity, light sensitivity, and color perception are common in older adults, poor lighting can cause undue hardship during feeding. Natural light without glare or soft,

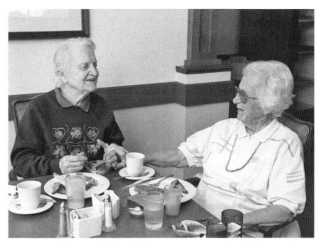

FIG. 18.3 Compatible table mates can make dining a pleasurable experience.

BOX 18.1

Preparation Checklist for Dysphagia and Self-Feeding Interventions

1. Collect information.
   - Evaluate dysphagia.
   - Review medical chart.
   - Consult nursing staff.
   - Assess changes in medical status.
   - Assess changes in diet.
2. Inform older adult.
   - Give evaluation results.
   - Recommend intervention.
   - Discuss intervention goals with client.
   - Provide input.
3. Create environment.
   - Ensure that environment is positive and appropriate.
   - Ensure that environment is conducive to eating.
4. Ensure proper fit.
   - Eyeglasses.
   - Hearing aids.
   - Partial and full dentures.
5. Assess.
   - Arousal and alertness.
   - Safety for eating.
6. Position safely.
   - Trunk.
   - Lower extremities.
   - Upper extremities.
   - Head.
   - Height of table surface.
7. Complete oral preparation as prescribed by the OT.
   - Have client perform oral exercises.
   - Have client perform sensory stimulation.
   - Have client perform tone facilitation or reduction techniques.
8. Check food tray.
   - Correct diet consistency.
   - Provide needed assistive equipment.

diffused overhead lighting is best. A quiet, calm environment excludes television but may allow for age-appropriate dining music. Television may be distracting and detract from social interaction. Compatible tablemates in small groups around a table can add to a positive dining experience (Fig. 18.3). OTAs and other service providers should maintain a therapeutic attitude by allowing older adults plenty of time to eat a meal. Lengthy waiting periods before being served may decrease the older adult's interest in food and may increase fatigue. The table height should be between 28 and 30 inches to accommodate both regular chairs and wheelchairs. The distance between the table surface and an older adult's mouth should be between 10 and 15 inches.[10] Adopting these suggested environmental factors can help provide a pleasurable experience during mealtime and possibly assist older adults to increase their food and fluid intake.

Optimal Seating

Safe positioning is key to reducing the risk of food entering the trachea, avoiding aspiration. Proper positioning of older adults also increases alertness, normalizes muscle tone, provides comfort, and helps with digestion, while allowing dynamic movement for self-feeding.

The preferred seating position for mealtime is sitting in a dining room chair with armrests rather than sitting in a wheelchair. A wheelchair, however, is preferable to a geriatric chair, which is preferable to sitting up in bed. Symmetrical postural alignment is key. The pelvis should be positioned in neutral with a slight anterior tilt. Both upper extremities should be fully supported on a table or lap tray of appropriate height. Finally, the lower extremities should be in a weight-bearing position. Hips and knees should be flexed 80–90 degrees, with ankles in neutral position under the knees and the feet flat on the floor (Fig. 18.4). If the feet do not reach the floor, a stool or wheelchair footrest should be used to provide a secure base of support.[8]

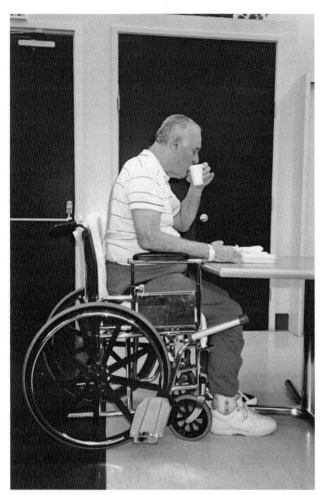

FIG. 18.4 This gentleman is correctly positioned in his wheelchair for self-feeding. This position promotes dynamic trunk movement. *(From Community Hospital of Los Gatos, CA, 1996.)*

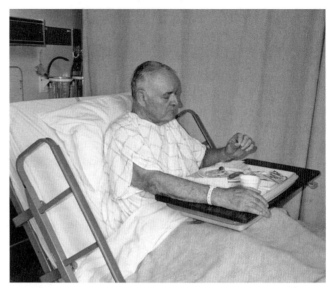

FIG. 18.5 This older adult is correctly positioned in bed for self-feeding. *(From Community Hospital of Los Gatos, CA, 1996.)*

If feeding in bed is essential, older adults should be as close to the headboard as possible before the head of the bed is elevated to 45 degrees or more (Fig. 18.5). A pillow may be placed behind the older adult's back to increase upright trunk posture and hip flexion. To prevent older adults from sliding down in the bed, the knees should be flexed and supported from underneath with pillows if necessary.[10] As with sitting in a chair, older adults should be upright and aligned symmetrically for optimal safety while eating and drinking.

Positioning devices are often required to aid older adults in maintaining a straight midline for a dynamic, upright posture. Padded solid back and solid seat inserts provide better postural support that offsets the slinging seats and backs of wheelchairs. Lumbar and thoracic support can facilitate increased scapulohumeral control for self-feeding. Older adults with low muscular tone may benefit from high-back wheelchairs. Wedges, lateral and forward trunk supports, headrests, pelvic belts, pillows, and towel rolls are often used to obtain proper positioning.

Seating systems must be designed to correct or accommodate postural problems while preventing skin erosion, maintaining comfort, promoting self-feeding, and providing the right position for safe swallowing.

Many variables affect older adults' positioning. If an older adult is sitting in a kyphotic posture, the OTA should have the older adult lean back slightly so the chin is parallel to the floor. Special considerations are also needed for older adults with scoliosis, depending on the curvature of the spine. Older adults with a hemiplegic arm should have the arm placed on the table. The arm/hand should be incorporated as a stabilizer during meals. OTAs also must consider poor sitting tolerance. Older adults with back pain or low endurance need to complete their meal within the time limitations of their upright tolerance.

Assistive Devices

An abundance of options for assistive devices is available to assist older adults in maintaining independence in self-feeding and safe swallowing. Some devices are prefabricated, whereas others are designed by the creative minds of the OTAs. A hole punched in the plastic lid of a cup can hold a straw and will prevent spilling for older adults who have tremors or ataxia. Built-up handles can be used for joint protection or a weak grasp. A universal cuff is available for older adults who have no grasp. A swivel spoon or a long-handled spoon could be used to assist older adults with limited range of motion. Nonslip mats or plates with suction cups can keep items from sliding on the table. Plate guards and plates with lips prevent food from spilling off of the plate. Cutout cups and straws can reduce the need for the older adult to tilt the head back while drinking, thus protecting against aspiration while swallowing.

Straws and cups with spouted lids can also limit the amount of each sip and are helpful for older adults with severe dementia who have a sucking reflex only. Small rubber-coated spoons can help control bite size and prevent older adults from hurting themselves when biting down on utensils. Rocker knives can be used for one-handed cutting. Mobile arm supports can provide stabilization and assist in hand-to-mouth movement.

Assistive devices should be issued if older adults experience a decrease in function. However, older adults should be encouraged toward further independence rather than to continue using assistive devices. Before assistive equipment is issued, the OTA should consult with the OT regarding his or her recommendations.

Diet Modifications

Diet modifications are frequently needed for older adults with dysphagia. These modifications may include different consistencies of liquids (see Table 18.2) and different methods of preparing solid foods (see Table 18.3).[5] If oral intake is limited or impossible, older adults with dysphagia may receive nutrition and hydration through alternative means (such as a nasogastric tube, a gastrostomy, a jejunostomy, or parenteral nutrition). The entire treatment team is responsible for monitoring intake and for ensuring that food and drink are presented in the proper form. OTAs caring for clients residing in care facilities are encouraged to collaborate with kitchen staff when necessary and appropriate. Given the change in palatability of thickened liquids, OTAs should bear in mind that their clients who must drink thickened liquids are at high risk for dehydration due to lower intake.

CASE STUDY

Your client has just been seen for a swallow study, and the client's daughter reports that the SLP recommended thickened liquids. What is one precaution of which you would like to remind the daughter related to thickened liquids and fluid intake during your OTA treatment session?

DIRECT INTERVENTIONS

Oral Preparatory Phase

Various feeding strategies may be used to help older adults with dysphagia to feed themselves and to swallow safely. To ensure that mealtime is a pleasurable experience, the OTA should avoid making infantilizing comments (e.g., use the word *napkin* rather than *bib*). A method of communication must be established with nonverbal older adults so they can indicate when they are ready for another bite or drink. All team members, including family and other caregivers, should use this method consistently. Examples may be a nodding of the head or raising a finger. In addition, the OTA should sit next to the older adults rather than standing over them during meals.

TABLE 18.2

Levels of Thickened Liquids (In Order of Least to Most Intervention)

Thin	No thickener added. Examples include water, juice, coffee, broth, and ice cream.
Nectar thick	Examples include nectars, extra thick milkshake, strained creamed soups, and V-8 juice.
Honey thick	Examples include nectar thickened with banana or pureed fruit, regular applesauce with juice, and creamed soup with mashed potato.
Spoon thick	Achievable only with commercial thickener.

TABLE 18.3

Levels of the Dysphagia Diet (In Order of Least to Most Intervention)

Regular (Level 4)	**No restrictions**
Dysphagia Advanced (Level 3)	Examples include well-moistened cereals, eggs (prepared in any manner), potatoes (prepared in any manner), soups with soft meat or vegetables not exceeding one inch in size, cooked and tender vegetables, thin-sliced and tender or ground meats, soft cakes and desserts (avoid nuts and dried fruit).
Dysphagia Mechanical Soft (Level 2)	Examples include oatmeal, French toast without crust, scrambled eggs, soft canned or cooked fruit (no seeds or peel), soups with easy to chew or easy to swallow soft meats or vegetables not exceeding one half-inch in size, moist macaroni and cheese, moist meatballs, soft fruit pies with bottom crust only, soft and moist cakes with icing.
Dysphagia Pureed (Level 1)	Examples include pureed bread mixes, pureed eggs, pureed well-cooked noodles, mashed potatoes with gravy, soups that have been pureed (note that soups may need thickener), hummus, yogurt.

As noted in the preparation checklist in Box 18.1, oral exercises, sensory stimulation, and tone facilitation or inhibition techniques are often needed before eating. Slow, deep pressure on facial and jaw muscles in the opposite direction to the pull of increased muscle tone may help reduce it.[11] Tongue and facial exercises can increase strength and tone for bolus manipulation. Sensory stimulation may include brushing teeth and icing the cheeks and tongue to increase oral tone and sensation. Brushing teeth also stimulates the salivary glands and helps older adults with dry mouths manipulate the bolus more effectively. These would all be considered preparatory activities for eating.

When there are difficulties in bringing the food from the plate to the mouth, the following strategies may be considered: hand-over-hand guiding, stabilization of the proximal upper extremity, and use of bilateral hands to bring food from plate to mouth. The "clock method" is helpful for older adults with visual deficits to orient them to the position of the plate, cup, eating utensils, and food during mealtimes. Items should be positioned consistently for this method to be most effective. Older adults who are impulsive may require cues for both bite size and pacing of bites. Older adults can be guided or instructed to put the eating utensil down between bites to pace the amount of food entering the mouth. Presenting older adults with one food item at a time may also be helpful. Large food items should be cut into bite-sized portions. Using a spoon for liquids is often helpful. OTAs should coordinate eating with breathing for older adults on ventilators or for those with other breathing difficulties. Energy conservation may also be indicated, including limiting conversation during mealtime. For older adults with low endurance, alternating food textures during the meal, ordering foods that are easy to chew, and/or having six small meals available during the day may be helpful.

For clients with advanced neurocognitive disorder, sitting during mealtime and attending to a meal may be a challenge. For these clients, the OTA may consider frequent small meals as opposed to several large meals and finger foods in lieu of foods requiring utensils. Decreasing environmental stimulation, maintaining consistency in feeding helpers, and reducing verbal communication during the meal may help decrease distractions and permit older adults with neurocognitive disorder to focus longer on eating. When clients with neurocognitive disorders refuse a particular food item, consider presenting the food on a plate of a different color. In the population with altered mental status, the OTA should give extra attention to mealtime safety: nonedible items (e.g., napkins, sugar packets) may need to be removed from the table, as well as knives or other sharp utensils.

Oral Phase

In the oral phase, intervention may be indicated to reduce oral pocketing and clear residue.[8] Tongue sweeps,

performed by sweeping the tongue through the oral cavity, reduce oral pocketing of food. Alternating solids and liquids helps clean the mouth and remove food residue in the oral cavity but may be contraindicated in the presence of dysphagia.

Also in the oral phase, intervention may be indicated to increase sensory awareness of food in the oral cavity. To improve awareness and help with orientation, food should be placed in the center of the tongue. Varying food temperatures with each bite may promote a safer swallow by stimulating the mouth and increasing awareness of the bolus. Cuing may be needed to close the lips fully to form the tight labial seal needed to prevent spillage and create the negative pressure needed for efficient swallow.[8]

Intervention may be indicated for pacing, in which case simply cuing the client to increase the number of times they chew a bite of food may be effective. Older adults should be given sufficient time to swallow between bites. OTAs should learn to observe and palpate swallowing and be able to recognize delays in the swallow response, as these skills help in the ongoing assessment of older adults.

Older adults should be checked for voice clarity after a swallow to make sure that there is no food or liquid residual on the vocal folds.[12,13]

If dentures are used during mealtime, the OTA should ensure proper fit prior to feeding. The OTA should also ensure that the dentures are thoroughly cleaned after each meal to prevent ulcers from developing in the mouth, to prevent chipping of the dentures from hardened food, and to prevent risk for aspiration from food residue under the dentures.[5,6,14]

Pharyngeal Phase

Issues arising during the pharyngeal phase of swallow need special attention and focused intervention, as this is the phase when the food and liquid must pass by the airway. To avoid aspiration, the OTA, in collaboration with the OT, should consider results of the MBSS, as well as any other instrumental assessment date for the patient. Refer to Table 18.4 for indicated positioning and maneuvers. Additional strategies that may be coupled with the strategies above include: coughing or clearing the throat followed by a dry swallow or multiple swallows after each bite.[8]

The OTA should work closely with the OT when feeding older adults with tracheostomies. If approved by the physician, a client with a tracheostomy can be assessed on the same criteria and move forward with a feeding treatment plan. It should be noted that a client who has been on ventilation for any length of time may have significant changes to the swallow anatomy and process, such as muscle atrophy, decreased sensation, and laryngeal damage.[8] During feeding, the tracheostomy may or may not be plugged, and the cuff can be deflated during feeding to increase air pressure for a stronger swallow.

TABLE 18.4

Indicated Positioning and Maneuvers

Intervention	Deficit	How intervention affects deficit	Instructions
Swallowing Posture: Chin tuck	Delay in triggering of swallow, or residue in valleculae after swallow. *Potentially associated diagnoses: CVA, degenerative disease.*	Widens valleculae to prevent bolus from entering airway, pushes tongue base backward.	"Tuck your chin as you swallow."
Swallowing Posture: Head rotated/turned	Unilateral oral and pharyngeal paresis or dysfunction. *Potentially associated diagnoses: CVA, cancer.*	Turning to weaker (damaged) side eliminates the damaged side from the bolus path, allows the bolus to pass through the intact side. Also, increases vocal fold closure by applying extrinsic pressure and narrows laryngeal entrance.	"Turn your head to the weaker side as you swallow."
Rehabilitation Technique: Mendehlson maneuver	Reduced laryngeal movement, uncoordinated swallow. *Potentially associated diagnoses: progressive neurologic diseases (PD, ALS, neurocognitive disorder). Patient must be cognitively intact.*	Improves swallow coordination by teaching some voluntary control of the pharyngo-esophageal segment. Increases tongue base retraction and larynx elevation.	"Place your figures on your voice box and feel it rise up and down when you swallow. Then, try to hold it up and count to three."
Rehabilitation Technique and Swallowing Strategy: Effortful swallow	Reduced posterior movement of the tongue base. Presence of residue in valleculae. *Potentially associated diagnoses: brain stem lesion. Patient must be cognitively intact.*	This increases the tongue driving force by causing exaggerated retraction of the tongue. This helps to get food past the valleculae.	"Swallow with maximal effort," or "Squeeze hard with your throat and neck muscles as you swallow." When used as a rehabilitation technique, the effortful swallow may be completed with or without food.

DIETARY CONSIDERATIONS

A decline in the acuity of taste and smell occurs naturally in the aging process. As this acuity declines, adults often compensate with the addition of sugar and salt to their foods. Other client factors may cause older adults to be more inclined to choose prepared food over fresh ingredients (often resulting in higher sodium intake) and drink less water. All of these factors combine to place older adults at a heightened risk for malnutrition, which can lead to other health problems and decrease the body's efficiency in healing.

Other sensory changes may include a decline in visual acuity, visual field, and hearing,[6,15] which can affect nutritional intake and health status. For example, loss of visual acuity may lead to less activity or a fear of cooking, especially using a stove. Difficulty reading and processing food prices, nutrition labels, or recipes may affect grocery shopping, food preparation, and ultimately eating. Loss of hearing may lead to less eating out or not asking questions to the waiter or store clerk. Slowing of the normal action of the digestive tract plus general physiological changes have a direct effect on nutrition. Digestive secretions diminish

markedly, although enzymes remain adequate. Adequate dietary fiber will maintain regular bowel function and not interfere with the digestion and absorption of nutrients, as may occur with laxative use or abuse.[15] The challenge for older adults is to meet the same nutrient needs as when they were younger, yet consume fewer calories. Choosing nutrient-dense foods (high in nutrients in relation to their calories), reducing overall fat content of the diet, emphasizing complex carbohydrates, enhancing dietary fiber intake, ensuring adequate liquid intake, and consuming a variety of food remain priorities for older adults.[15,16] It may be important for the older adult to be referred to a dietitian to obtain information about optimal nutrition and hydration that does not interfere with medications.

In addition to ensuring safety in eating, the OTA should also consider the client's food preference and the cultural significance of preferred foods. Medical conditions and food allergies may further shape the client's diet. The physician is responsible for finalizing a decision regarding feeding plan recommendations with clients and their families, in collaboration with the treatment team. In the event that an older adult refuses a feeding plan, the team should communicate with one another to offer alternatives that are safe for the client, meet the client's dietary needs, and are palatable to the client.

MEDICATIONS AND DYSPHAGIA

Many older adults receive medications for multiple conditions. Medications must be taken with the correct liquid or semisolid consistency. At least one ounce (30 mL) of liquid should be taken after each pill to ensure adequate transport to the stomach. Older adults should be sitting up and prevented from reclining for 20 minutes after a meal or after taking medication to ensure the safe passage of the food or pill to the stomach.[8] Pills should be taken as specified by the physician. OTAs should consult with the physician or pharmacist to check whether the pills can be halved or crushed because some pills work through time release and crushing them may result in too much medication being absorbed at once. Nursing staff should be present while the medications are taken to ensure that swallowing has actually occurred.

EDUCATION AND COLLABORATION: THE CARE TEAM

OTAs have a vital role in training caregivers to assist older adults with self-feeding and dysphagia management.[7] Caregivers may include spouses, partners, family members, friends, hired attendants, and other health care workers such as nurses and nurses' aides. OTAs must consider the caregiver's culture and lifestyle when making decisions about the most beneficial type of teaching technique to use. Some individuals learn best through observing the OTA. Others may learn best by doing it themselves under the direction of the OTA, and still others may perform best with verbal instruction. Written information and instructions should be provided to older adults and caregivers whenever possible. In general, all of these techniques should be used with each caregiver to ensure the best follow-through.

The education of caregivers must include training in many aspects of self-feeding and swallowing.[7] First, caregivers should understand the feeding strengths and weaknesses of older adults. The need for quality time during the meal and for presentation of a positive attitude to promote older adult motivation and independence should be stressed. Thorough instruction should be given on proper body mechanics required by caregivers when assisting older adults with feeding. Additional instruction should be provided regarding safe positioning, environmental concerns, use and care of assistive equipment, specific intervention techniques, appropriate verbal and nonverbal cueing, dietary modifications, and signs of possible food or liquid aspiration. Caregivers must understand the importance of communicating any problems or changes in an older adult's status to the appropriate team member. Caregivers should also be familiar with choking prevention maneuvers and emergency suctioning procedures.

Problem-solving together with caregivers is useful when dealing with older adults who have difficult feeding behaviors.

Instructing caregivers on the swallowing and self-feeding protocols set up for older adults helps OTAs promote continuity and quality of care. Caregivers should be integrated as soon as possible in the intervention and care of older adults. Training several family members and nursing staff helps to redistribute the responsibility of assisting older adults during mealtime. As with any intervention given to older adults, all training of caregivers should be thoroughly documented. By fulfilling these principles, the OTA abides by the Code of Ethics developed by the AOTA.[17]

A CASE FOR THE IMPLEMENTATION OF FEEDING PROGRAMS

Residents of care facilities who eat their meals in their rooms tend to eat in suboptimal positions and without ample supervision and time to finish the meal. Consequently, their intake, nutrition, and body weight decrease.[5,12,18] A well-organized facility-wide feeding program helps to increase activity in older adults, provide changes in their environment, as well as social stimulation. These measures can promote good nutrition and hydration and increase safety. Although many feeding program formats designed for a variety of settings are available, the following is a generic program that requires adjustments to fit the needs of particular older adults and particular facilities.

An interdisciplinary approach is the most beneficial in a feeding program. Usually the older adult, the OT, OTA, speech and language pathologist, dietitian, kitchen staff, physician, nursing staff, and family are involved. The physical therapist may also be included to assist with positioning, and the respiratory therapist may be included to assist with issues of pulmonary hygiene or coordination of tracheostomy or ventilator equipment. Older adults with self-feeding and dysphagia difficulties are evaluated and referred to a dining group by the OT, the speech and language pathologist, or both. These older adults then are placed in one of several groups organized by the amount of assistance they require. The ratio of older adults to OTAs varies depending on the needs of the group. OTAs should always have a group size that can be safely managed. A written protocol should exist that includes information on the purpose of the program and the format, staffing, size, and site of the group. There also should be criteria for referral to, continuation in, and discharge from the program. Timelines, goals, and responsibilities of the OTA or other leader should be made explicit, and documentation and equipment protocols should be explained. There should also be an established system to maintain communication with the entire team to ensure a successful program.[8]

The feeding program should address all meals. In some settings, OTAs are unable to be present at each meal. In other settings, an OTA may not be needed to assist higher-level groups that require minimal assistance or supervision. In these situations, nursing aides, restorative aides, family members, and volunteers may be best used. However, before volunteers are used in this capacity, the guidelines from regulatory agencies should be consulted. For all individuals to perform effectively and safely, they must receive formal training on leading groups, on therapeutic interventions, and on safety.

CASE STUDY

■ DIAGNOSIS AND PRIMARY SYMPTOMS

Tyrone is a 68-year-old, right-hand dominant man who experienced a left cerebrovascular accident and resulting in right hemiplegia and altered sensation on his right side. In addition, he has apraxia, aphasia, right hemianopsia, and right neglect. One week after his stroke, Tyrone was transferred to a rehabilitation unit in a skilled nursing facility.

■ ASSESSMENT AND RESULTS

A dysphagia evaluation and videofluoroscopy were completed and the following observations were noted: decreased muscle tone with impaired movement and sensation of the face, tongue, and soft palate on the right side resulting in facial droop, poor lip seal, minimal drooling and food spillage, slurred speech, and a nasal quality to his speech. The videofluoroscopy revealed impaired oral control of the bolus and spillage of food and liquid into the pharynx before the swallow was initiated. Initiation of the swallow was delayed up to 5 seconds. Residual pooling was observed in the valleculae and pyriform sinuses after the swallow. Spontaneous clearing of the throat with additional swallows was impaired. Tyrone required verbal cueing to initiate clearing swallows. Aspiration into the trachea was observed while Tyrone swallowed thin and nectar-thick liquids. Tyrone did demonstrate a reflexive cough when aspiration occurred. He had difficulty chewing dry, hard solids (e.g., crackers, cookies) and did better with moist, soft solids (e.g., pasta, soft fruit), although oral pocketing and spillage from the mouth were observed with these consistencies. When Tyrone used the compensation method of turning his head to the right, decreased pooling in the right valleculae and pyriform sinus resulted.

Therapeutic recommendations included one-on-one assistance at meals for self-feeding and a modified diet of honey-liquids by spoon. Soft solids with no mixed consistencies also were recommended. Further suggestions were to provide verbal and tactile cues for Tyrone to turn his head to the right side during the initial swallow and to follow-up the initial swallow with two dry swallows. In addition, Tyrone's caloric and fluid intake were to be closely monitored by the nursing staff.

■ OTA INTERVENTION

The OTA has planned to complete a lunchtime session with Tyrone today. Before the meal, the OTA reviews the chart for any recent orders, as well as for nursing and therapy progress notes. The OTA arranged to meet Tyrone's family in the dining room so that they may observe mealtime strategies. When Tyrone arrives in the dining room, the OTA observes that he is leaning to the right side in his chair. The OTA repositions Tyrone, brings him to

the table, locks the wheelchair, removes Tyrone's feet from the footrests and places them flat on the floor, and helps Tyrone to place his right arm on the table.

Before the meal, the OTA directed Tyrone through several oral-facial exercises. Icing was also used to increase tone and sensation in his right cheek and throat. The OTA iced the outside of Tyrone's mouth with ice wrapped in a washcloth and then iced the inside of his cheeks and tongue with a cold metal spoon that was dipped in a cup of ice. Icing also would be done on the cheek, the anterior part of the neck, and inside his mouth on the right side during the meal.

When the tray with Tyrone's meal arrived, the OTA checked to ensure that the consistencies of both solids and liquids were correct. The liquid on the tray was nectar-thick; therefore, the OTA thickened it with a thickening agent to the prescribed thickness; in this case, honey-thick. No other modifications were needed. A plate guard was put on the plate to prevent food from spilling.

Because Tyrone requires assistance with tray setup and self-feeding, the OTA guided Tyrone's left hand (nonhemiplegic) using the hand-over-hand method to remove the container lids, butter the bread, cut the food with the rocker knife, and bring the food to his mouth. The OTA reduced from hand-over-hand assistance to placing to tactile cues as Tyrone became more motorically adept in the task over the course of the meal. However, when Tyrone moved too quickly and took too large a bite, the OTA resumed the guiding. When Tyrone released excessive oral secretions, the OTA guided him to wipe his face with a napkin. With each bite, the OTA directed Tyrone to double swallow and felt Tyrone's throat for the swallow. The OTA asked Tyrone to speak occasionally to check his vocal quality, and when it was wet-sounding, the OTA asked Tyrone to clear his throat. Whenever Tyrone was unable to clear his throat, the OTA asked him to dry swallow. Throughout the feeding intervention session, the OTA also periodically checked Tyrone's mouth for food pocketing and directed him to clear residuals in his right cheek by using his tongue or left index finger.

After the meal, the OTA guided Tyrone to use a toothette to clean his oral cavity of the food residue. The OTA instructed Tyrone to remain upright for at least 20 more minutes. A nurse then arrived with medications, which were crushed and mixed with the honey-thick liquid and given to Tyrone with a spoon. After he swallowed the medication, Tyrone was given additional honey-thick liquid by spoon to ensure that the medication passed to the stomach.

The OTA then asked the family if they had any questions and provided them with additional instructions. Finally, the OTA documented Tyrone's food consumption (detailing specific foods and liquids, consistencies, and amounts); the level of assistance that was required; duration of time to complete the meal; and the presence of any coughing, vocal changes, or safety concerns. In addition, the OTA documented all instructions given to the family.

In mealtime sessions that followed, Tyrone progressed in his motor control, needing less and less hand-over-hand guiding and verbal instruction from the OTA. The OTA transitioned the role of mealtime aide to the family members as they assisted Tyrone with meals. Tyrone progressed to a group dining scenario. A follow-up videofluoroscopy was done to rule out aspiration of thin liquids and mixed consistencies, and it showed that Tyrone had improved but still had impaired oral control of the bolus and pooling in the pharynx. However, Tyrone now clears this pooling spontaneously, no aspiration is noted, and these items were added to his diet.

Because Tyrone can now set up his tray with minimal assistance, cut the food with a rocker knife, bring the food to his mouth, eat slowly, and check for pocketing independently, he no longer requires occupational therapy supervision at meals, and his family has been trained to provide support as needed during meals upon his return home.

▌▌ CASE STUDY QUESTIONS

1 Why was it important for the OTA to properly position Tyrone before feeding?
2 What might have been the outcome of Tyrone's feeding session if the OTA had not used icing as an intervention?
3 What types of adaptive equipment did the OTA use with Tyrone? What was the purpose of each piece of equipment?

▌▌ CHAPTER REVIEW QUESTIONS

1 What is the definition of dysphagia?
2 What are the four phases of swallowing?
3 What are the four liquid consistencies?
4 Name four signs that may indicate the presence of swallowing problems.
5 Name three common changes that occur during the phases of swallowing as an individual ages.
6 Identify at least two psychological issues that may have an effect on oral intake.
7 Explain why the OTA should be concerned about nutritional balance and amount of oral intake.
8 Why is the dining environment important for nutritional intake?
9 What should the OTA do if an older adult coughs continuously during a meal?
10 Describe how an individual's body should ideally be positioned during a meal.

For additional video content, please visit Elsevier eBooks+ (eBooks.Health.Elsevier.com)

EVIDENCE NUGGETS: EFFECTIVENESS OF BEHAVIORAL TECHNIQUES TO IMPROVE ORAL INTAKE AND SAFE SWALLOWING OF OLDER ADULTS WITH DYSPHAGIA

1. Duncan, S, McAuley DF, Walshe, M, McGaughey, J, Anand R, Fallis, R, Blackwood, B. Interventions for oropharyngeal dysphagia in acute and critical care: a systematic review. *Intensive Care Med.* 2020;46:1326-1338.
   - There is limited evidence on the effectiveness of swallowing treatments on participants with dysphagia.
   - Swallowing treatments showed no evidence for decreasing the time it took participants to return to oral intake, decreasing aspiration, or increasing quality of life scores; however, it did show a reduced risk of pneumonia.
2. Nishinari, K, Turcanu, M, Nakauma, M, Fang, Y. Role of fluid cohesiveness in safe swallowing. *Npj Science of Food.* 2019;3(5):1-13.
   - Cohesiveness of fluids can be increased by adding a thickening agent.
   - This study shows that fluids that are highly cohesive are less fragmented into small particles. This means that highly cohesive fluids are safer for patients with dysphagia than fluids with lower cohesiveness.
   - Cohesiveness is an important component in preventing aspiration in patients with dysphagia.
3. Patel, S, McAuley, WJ, Cook, MT, Sun, Y, Hamdy, S, Liu, F. The swallowing characteristics of thickeners, jellies and yoghurt observed using an in vitro model. *Dysphagia.* 2020;35:685-695.
   - Low oral velocity reduces aspiration and penetration in patients with dysphagia.
   - Fluids with a higher thickener concentration have a higher oral transit time and bolus length. Fluids at high concentrations that are thickened with starch-based thickener have a significantly longer oral transit time that fluids thickened with xanthan gum-based thickener. Nectar-like fluids have a shorter bolus length when thickened with xanthan gum-based thickener versus those thickened with starch-based thickener.
   - Jellies and yoghurt are comparable to fluids with high thickener concentrations.
4. Reyes-Torres, CA, Castillo-Martinez, L, Reyes-Guerrero, R, Ramos-Vazquez, AG, Zavala-Solares, M, Cassis-Nosthas, L, Serralde-Zuniga, AE. Design and implementation of modified-texture diet in older adults with oropharyngeal dysphagia: A randomized controlled trial. *Eur J Clin Nutr.* 2019;73:989-996.
   - Modified consistency and volume diet such as texture modified foods and thickened drinks, improve the total energy intake by 31%, and protein intake by 29% in the intervention group.
   - Participants in the intervention group increased body weight and had a statistically significant increase in BMI.
   - Increase in nutrients improved oral intake, weight, and handgrip strength for participants with dysphagia.
5. Shimizu, A, Fujishima, I, Maeda, K, Wakabayashi, H, Nishioka, S, Ohno, T, Nomoto, A, Kayashita, J, Mori, N. Nutritional management enhances the recovery of swallowing ability in older patients with sarcopenic dysphagia. *Nutrients.* 2021;13:1-10.
   - The higher amount of energy provided to patients with dysphagia may significantly improve swallowing ability and completion of ADLs.
   - Treatments such as swallowing rehabilitation and nutritional management with high provided energy led to improvements in swallowing status.
   - Nutrient intake also leads to an increase in ADL completion in older individuals with dysphagia.

REFERENCES

1. American Occupational Therapy Association. Occupational therapy practice framework: domain and process. 4th ed. *Am J Occup Ther.* 2020;74(suppl 2):S1-S87. Available at: https://doi.org/10.5014/ajot.2020.74S2001.

2. Schnelle J, Bertrand R, Hurd D, et al. The importance of standardized observations to evaluate nutritional care quality in the survey process. *J Am Med Dir Assoc.* 2009;10(8):568-574. Available at: https://doi.org/10.1016/j.jamda.2009.05.004.

3. American Occupational Therapy Association. Specialized knowledge and skills in feeding, eating, and swallowing for occupational therapy practice. *Am J Occup Ther.* 2007;61:686-700. Available at: https://doi.org/10.5014/ajot.61.6.686.

4. McFarland D. *Netter's Atlas of Anatomy for Speech, Swallowing, and Hearing.* 2nd ed. Mosby: St. Louis; 2014.

5. Murray T, Carrau R. *Clinical Management of Swallowing Disorders.* 3rd ed. San Diego, CA: Plural; 2012.

6. Chernoff R. *Geriatric Nutrition: The Health Professional's Handbook.* 4th ed. Burlington, MA: Jones & Bartlett Learning; 2013.

7. American Occupational Therapy Association. Specialized knowledge and skills in feeding, eating, and swallowing for occupational therapy practice. *Am J Occup Ther.* 2007;61:686-700.

8. Smith J. Eating and swallowing. In HM Pendleton, W Schultz-Krohn's, eds. Pedretti's Occupational Therapy: Practice Skills for Physical Dysfunction. 8th ed. Elsevier; 2018:669-700.

9. Nogueira D, Reis E. Swallowing disorders in nursing home residents: how can the problem be explained? *Clin Interv Aging.* 2013;2013(8):221–227. Available at: https://doi.org/10.2147/CIA.S39452.

10. Dewing J. Prioritizing mealtime care, patient choice, and nutritional assessment were important for older in-patients' mealtime experiences. *Evid Based Nurs.* 2009;12(1):30. Available at: https://doi.org/10.1136/ebn.12.1.30.

11. Hägg M, Anniko M. Lip muscle training in stroke patients with dysphagia. *Acta Otolaryngol.* 2008;128(9):1027–1033. https://doi.org//10.1080/00016480701813814.

12. Huang CS, Dutkowski K, Fuller A, et al. Evaluation of a pilot volunteer feeding assistance program: Influences on the dietary intakes of elderly hospitalized patients and lessons learnt. *J Nutr Health Aging.* 2015;19(2):206-210. doi:10.1007/s12603-014-0529-x.

13. Sinclair AJ, Morley JE, Vellas B. *Pathy's Principles and Practice of Geriatric Medicine.* 5th ed. West Sussex, UK: Wiley-Blackwell; 2012.

14. Robnett RH, Chop WC. *Gerontology for the Health Care Professional.* 3rd ed. Burlington, MA: Jones & Bartlett Publishers; 2013.

15. Bales C, Ritchie C. *Handbook of Clinical Nutrition and Aging.* 3rd ed. New York: Humana Press; 2015.

16. Reiser MF, Hricak H, Knauth M. *Dysphagia: Diagnosis and Treatment.* Heidelberg, NY: Springer; 2012.

17. American Occupational Therapy Association. Occupational therapy code of ethics. *Am J Occup Ther.* 2020;74(7413410005). Available at: https://doi.org/10.5014/ajot.2020.74S3006.

18. Manning F, Harris K, Duncan R, et al. Additional feeding assistance improves the energy and protein intakes of hospitalized elderly patients. A health services evaluation. *Appetite.* 2012;59(2):471-477. Available at: https://doi.org/10.1016/j.appet.2012.06.011.

Working With Older Adults Who Have Had Cerebrovascular Accidents

RENÉ PADILLA

(WITH PREVIOUS CONTRIBUTIONS FROM VANESSA JEWELL AND DEBORAH L. MORAWSKI)

KEY TERMS

aphasia, cerebrovascular accident, complex regional pain syndrome (previously known as shoulder-hand syndrome), constraint-induced movement therapy, edema, functional activities, hemiplegia, hypertonicity, hypotonicity, midline alignment, muscle tone, stroke, subluxation, transfers, weight bearing

CHAPTER OBJECTIVES

1. Discuss cerebrovascular accidents by describing the major features of strokes affecting the main arteries of the brain.
2. Discuss at least three considerations in the occupational therapy evaluation of older adults who have had a stroke.
3. Describe the sequence of facilitating midline alignment while older adults are supine, sitting, and standing, and explain the steps to follow when transferring older adults from a supine position to the edge of the bed or from a sitting to a standing position.
4. Explain precautions for handling an older adult's hemiplegic upper extremity.

Virtually every human endeavor is the result of the brain's unceasing activity. The brain is the organ of behavior, cognition, language, learning, and movement. The sophistication of the brain's circuitry is remarkable, if not baffling. Billions of neurons interact with each other to do the brain's work. To appreciate the aging process, occupational therapy assistants (OTAs) must understand the way the brain works.[1,2] Implications of neuropathological disorders for occupational therapy intervention with older adults are described in this chapter. The many biological and behavioral changes that accompany normal aging are explained in other chapters in this book.

Effects of normal age-related changes in the nervous system vary greatly among individuals and are not generally associated with specific diseases. These changes clearly have little detrimental effect on many older adults. Severe cognitive impairment is not an inevitable aspect of aging. However, a number of conditions can be devastating to older adults because they present serious obstacles to the process of normal, healthy aging. Some of these conditions are related to cerebrovascular accidents (CVAs). (Chapter 20 presents the issues related to dementia and Alzheimer's disease, which are additional disorders affecting the brain.)

CEREBROVASCULAR ACCIDENTS

CVAs, or strokes, are lesions in the brain that result from a thrombus, embolus, or hemorrhage that compromises the blood supply to the brain. This inadequate supply of blood results in brain swelling and ultimately in the death of neurons in the area in the brain in which the stroke was located.

There are many different types of strokes an older adult might experience. According to the CDC, the three most common types of strokes are ischemic, hemorrhagic, and transient ischemic stroke[3]. The majority of strokes that occur are ischemic strokes[3]. An ischemic stroke occurs when the flow of blood is blocked in an artery that supplies blood to the brain. A hemorrhagic stroke occurs when an artery in the brain ruptures[3]. There are two types of hemorrhagic strokes. The most common kind is an intracerebral hemorrhage. This is when a ruptured artery directly inside of the brain results in blood flooding to the surrounding tissues. The other type of hemorrhagic stroke is a subarachnoid hemorrhage—bleeding that occurs from a ruptured artery between the brain and the thin layer of tissue that surrounds the brain which puts pressure on brain tissue[3]. A transient ischemic stroke also known as transient ischemic attack (TIA), or "mini stroke," is another, less major type of stroke. A TIA occurs when blood flow to the brain is blocked for less than 5 minutes. While this is considered only a minor stroke, it needs to be taken seriously, and the older adult should receive medical services immediately. A TIA is a warning sign for future, more serious strokes.[3]

Although the incidence of CVA has decreased over the past 50 years, approximately 795,000 individuals experience strokes each year, and nearly 129,000 die as a result, making it the fifth leading cause of death in the United States.[3,4] About 4 million individuals live with varying degrees of neurological impairment after strokes.[5] The incidence of strokes increases with age, with the rate doubling every decade of life after age 55 years, and most strokes occur after age 65 years. Recurrent strokes account for 25% of yearly reported strokes and usually occur within 5 years.[6] Black individuals have a greater risk for disability and death from stroke than other racial and ethnic groups.[3] Men experience strokes more frequently than women until age 55 years, when the risk for women equals that for men; however, more women die of strokes at all ages.[3]

Ischemic strokes, caused by both thrombus and embolus, account for about 87% of strokes. Intracerebral and subarachnoid hemorrhagic strokes account for about 13% of strokes.[3] Mortality rate associated with strokes has declined steadily since the 1950s.[7] While about 40% of people pass away within the year following the stroke, it has been proven that receiving rehabilitation services may extend an individual's life and does improve their quality of life.

Risk factors for stroke can be separated into modifiable and unmodifiable categories. Modifiable factors are those that can be altered by changes in lifestyle or medications, or both. These factors include hypertension, dyslipidemia, carotid artery stenosis, coronary artery disease, atrial fibrillation, congestive heart failure, cigarette smoking, obesity, diabetes mellitus, physical inactivity, and high serum cholesterol, among others.[8] The most preventable of these risk factors is hypertension. Unmodifiable or fixed risk factors include prior stroke, age, race, sex, and family history of stroke. Among these unmodifiable factors, increasing age is by far the most significant because approximately three-fourths of strokes occur in people age 65 years and older.[7]

In older adults, stroke can result in various neurological deficits (Table 19.1). Neurological and functional recovery occurs most rapidly in the first 3 months after a stroke; most older adults continue to progress after that time but at a slower rate.[9] For this reason, predicting functional recovery after stroke and which older adults will benefit from rehabilitation services are difficult. There are typically three types of recovery and rehabilitation indicated poststroke: (1) clients who spontaneously make good recovery without rehabilitation, (2) clients who can make satisfactory recovery through intensive rehabilitation only, and (3) clients with poor recovery of function regardless of the type of rehabilitation.[10] Other factors that complicate prediction of recovery include comorbidity and depression. While there are different types of recovery poststroke, it is important that everyone receive services to

TABLE 19.1

Neurological Deficits After Stroke

Neurological impairment	Definition and impact on functional performance for older adult
Sensory deficits	Impaired sensation leading to potential injury or harm of insensitive area
Dysarthria	Difficulty with speech and other oral and facial motor functions leading to decreased independence in ADLs
Hemiplegia; hemiparesis	Weakness or decreased AROM leading to decreased use of impaired muscles and independence in ADLs and IADLs
Cognitive deficits	Impaired ability to perform mental processes leading to decreased ability to learn new tasks, social interactions, and independence in ADLs and IADLs
Visual-perceptual deficits	Impaired ability to comprehend and make sense of visual input resulting in the difficulty adapting to environments and decreased independence in ADLs and IADLs
Aphasia	Difficulty with speech and ability to understand language (spoken and/or written) leading to decreased communication, social participation, isolation, and self-esteem
Incontinence	Inability to control bowel and/or bladder leading to decreased independence in ADLs, social isolation, and potential skin breakdown
Hemianopsia	Loss of vision in half of visual field leading to difficulty performing ADLs and IADLs, scanning and adapting to the environment, and safety concerns
Ataxia	Decreased ability to coordinate movements resulting in impaired balance and decreased independence in ADLs and IADLs
Dysphagia	Difficulty swallowing leading to possibility of aspiration
Apraxia	Decreased ability to motor plan resulting in difficulty initiating and learning any movements

Adapted from American Stroke Association. *Effects of stroke.* Retrieved from https://www.stroke.org/en/about-stroke/effects-of-stroke.

help them achieve their PLOF—physically, emotionally, socially, etc.

The outcome of a stroke depends greatly on which artery supplying the brain is involved (Table 19.2). Medical treatment of a stroke depends on the type, location, and severity of the vascular lesion. In the acute stages, medical intervention is focused on maintaining an airway, rehydration, and management of hypertension. Measures are often taken to prevent the development of deep venous thrombosis (DVT)—that is, blood clots that form in the veins of the lower extremities after prolonged periods of bed rest or immobility. If such clots are released, they can become lodged in the lungs and can cause death. The OTA must be alert to any sign of DVT and should

request and carefully follow mobilization and activity guidelines set by the physician. Localized signs in the lower extremity that suggest the presence of DVT include abnormal temperature, change in color and circumference, and tenderness. In addition to the use of medications, older adults can prevent DVTs by wearing elastic stockings or intermittent compression garments and through early mobilization. Because of DVT and other potential complications of stroke, the OTA should check the older adult's medical record and communicate with other team members before initiating each intervention session. By doing this, all team members are fully informed and can modify the interventions with the older adult to best serve the older adult's needs.

TABLE 19.2

Impairments Resulting From Cerebrovascular Accidents of Specific Arteries

Artery	Impairment
Middle cerebral artery	Contralateral hemiplegia
	Contralateral sensory deficits
	Contralateral hemianopsia
	Aphasia
	Deviation of head and neck toward side of lesion (if lesion is located in dominant hemisphere)
	Perceptual deficits including anosognosia unilateral neglect, visual spatial deficits, and perseveration (if lesion is located in nondominant hemisphere)
Internal carotid artery	Contralateral hemiplegia
	Contralateral hemianesthesia
	Homonymous hemianopsia
	Aphasia, agraphia, acalculia, right/left confusion, and finger agnosia (if lesion is located in dominant hemisphere)
	Visual-perceptual dysfunction, unilateral neglect, constructional dressing apraxia, attention deficits, topographical disorientation, and anosognosia (if lesion is located in nondominant hemisphere)
Anterior cerebral artery	Contralateral hemiplegia
	Apraxia
	Bowel and bladder incontinence
	Cortical sensory loss of the lower extremity
	Contralateral weakness of face and tongue
	Perseveration and amnesia
	Sucking reflex
Posterior cerebral artery	Homonymous hemianopsia
	Paresis of eye musculature
	Contralateral hemiplegia
	Topographical disorientation
	Involuntary movement disorders
	Sensory deficits
Cerebellar artery	Ipsilateral ataxia
	Nystagmus, nausea, and vomiting
	Decreased touch, vibration, and position sense
	Decreased contralateral pain and thermal sensation
	Ipsilateral facial paralysis
Vertebral artery	Decreased contralateral pain, temperature, touch, and proprioceptive sense
	Hemiparesis
	Facial weakness and numbness
	Ataxia
	Paralysis of tongue and weakness of vocal folds

Bowel and bladder dysfunction are common during the initial phases of recovery from a stroke. Usually, a specific bowel and bladder program that includes fluid intake, stool softeners, and other remedies is ordered by the physician. The OTA may be involved in structuring a scheduled toileting program for the older adult, which is essential for success (Chapter 17 presents a more detailed discussion about bowel and bladder training programs). Other complications during the early phases of recovery from a stroke may include respiratory difficulties and pneumonia caused by the decreased efficiency of the muscles involved in respiration and swallowing. Good pulmonary hygiene, use of antibiotics, and early mobilization are effective prevention measures. Dysphagia, or problems with swallowing, also must be addressed to prevent aspiration pneumonia (see Chapter 18).

OCCUPATIONAL THERAPY EVALUATION

Research evidence and expert opinion suggest that stroke rehabilitation should begin in the acute stage and continue long term, extending several years after onset.[11-13] Occupational therapy is an essential component in this rehabilitation process.[14] The OTA is an active participant in the evaluation process under the supervision of the occupational therapist (OT).[15] As with any client, the occupational therapy evaluation is an ongoing process that occurs during each intervention session. This is particularly true for older adults who have had a stroke because they may experience many changes during the first few months of recovery. These changes may be noted, especially during intervention. Although motor, visual, perceptual, sensory, and cognitive deficits may all contribute to functional impairments, the psychosocial skills and performance skills of older adults and the environment in which they live and perform are critical components of any occupational therapy assessment. In addition, the assessment should always consider older adults' performance skills, past performance patterns, occupational contexts, values, beliefs, and spirituality, not just their deficits.[16] Assessment of performance skills (motor and praxis skills, sensory-perceptual skills, emotional regulation skills, cognitive skills, and communication and social skills) is done simultaneously during the performance of an activity. Although the evaluation of each discrete area may be conducted separately, the interaction of these skills and their effects on occupational participation are of primary importance to occupational therapy.[16] Typical impairments are discussed in the section on intervention, but areas of necessary assessment for OTAs are discussed in the following paragraphs.

In the context of motor assessment, the OTA must understand the older adult's ability to maintain the body in an upright position and in midline against gravity (postural reactions). To do this, the OTA must observe the older adult's degree of hypertonicity or hypotonicity, the presence of abnormal movement patterns, primitive reflexes,

righting and protective reactions, equilibrium, coordination, and range of motion. The OTA should remember that all of these performance skills may be, and often are, affected by posture and endurance, and that the optimal assessment will occur when older adults are upright and not too fatigued. Alignment of the trunk, pelvis, and shoulder girdle should be noted, as well as any voluntary motor control. Assessment of strength has limited benefit in the presence of hypotonicity or hypertonicity and can possibly increase the degree of hypertonicity.[17]

The sensory assessment should include the evaluation of light touch, pressure, pain, temperature, stereognosis, and proprioception. The visual and perceptual areas to be assessed include tracking (smooth pursuits), visual fields, and inattention to the right or left sides. Other areas to be assessed include spatial relations, figure ground, motor planning, and body scheme. In addition, older adults may have other visual impairments that may affect their performance (see Chapter 15 for a review of this topic). Cognitive skills often assessed include attention, initiation, memory, planning, organization, problem-solving, insight, and judgment. The ability to do calculations and make abstractions may also be tested. OTAs should remember that posture can have a significant effect on sensory, visual, perceptual, and cognitive functioning, and the assessment of these areas should occur when older adults are upright.

Assessment of swallowing ability and safety is crucial for all older adults who have experienced a stroke. Swallowing is a complex behavior that results from the simultaneous performance of motor, sensory, perceptual, and cognitive skills. Deficits in any of these areas may result in older adults being at a greater risk for aspirating food into the lungs and subsequent development of pneumonia (see Chapter 18 for a review of this topic).

Depending on the older adult's ability to communicate, an evaluation of psychosocial skills of older adults may need to be completed by interviewing family or other significant people. Knowledge of the occupations or pursuits that the older adult was involved in before the stroke and of the older adult's values and interests is crucial in the selection of intervention strategies. Occupational task considerations should be made at every stage of the occupational therapy intervention.

OCCUPATIONAL THERAPY INTERVENTION

The long-range goal of occupational therapy intervention for dysfunction caused by stroke is to facilitate maximum participation in all contexts of the older adult's life. To reach this goal, intervention is focused on compensatory strategies and/or the restoration of neuromuscular, visual-perceptual-cognitive, and psychosocial skills that support the older adult's ability to perform self-care and engage in all areas of occupation. The degree to which each of these areas is emphasized is determined by the previous physical and social environments of older adult and their plans after hospitalization. Because each older adult's context is unique, the occupational therapy intervention plan is tailored specifically to that individual. By recognizing all of these areas of an older adult's being, the OTA is adhering to the Occupational Therapy Code of Ethics.[18]

The need for tailored intervention programs is illustrated by the cases of Rose and Maria. Both women are in their late 70s and had strokes that left them with a hemiplegic right side and difficulty verbally expressing themselves (aphasia). Their visual, perceptual, and cognitive skills appear to be intact. Rose is a widow who lives in a senior community that provides one meal a day and assists her with laundry and cleaning. Her two sons live in other states. Maria lives at home with her husband and two of her eight adult daughters. Ten grandchildren, whose ages range from ages 3 to 18 years, also live in her home. Both Rose and Maria want to return to their previous living environments. The occupational therapy program for both women will address all their needs, but the emphasis in Rose's program will be on self-care, meal preparation, and light home management tasks because she must be independent in these areas to maintain her apartment at the senior community. Maria, however, is counting on family assistance for her self-care and is more interested in cooking again for her extended family; therefore, her program will focus more on meal preparation, light home management, and social skills. The occupational therapy programs for both women will address their neuromuscular, visual-perceptual-cognitive, and psychosocial skills, but the activities chosen as therapeutic media should reflect their life contexts.

The cases of Rose and Maria illustrate another important principle in stroke rehabilitation: the more familiar an individual is with the activities selected for intervention, the more spontaneous and unconscious are the motor, visual, perceptual, cognitive, and psychosocial reorganization; consequently, changes will last longer.[19] Conscious, attention-focused learning is often necessary in rehabilitation, especially when the likelihood of recovery is small and compensation strategies are more viable. However, these strategies may also slow the rehabilitation process because of the mental effort they require. To illustrate this, OTAs should do the following exercise with partners. Have your partner time you as you write your full name on a piece of paper using your dominant hand, then have your partner time you writing your name again, but this time with your nondominant hand. Focus carefully on your body as you write your name and on the amount of mental control this task requires. The experience of rehabilitation after a stroke is similar to your experience of writing with your nondominant hand. Although clients recovering from stroke may not be learning to use their nondominant hand, they are relearning task accomplishment with different bodily capabilities. The more these clients must concentrate on the task they are attempting, the longer it may take them to complete it. Engagement in automatic activities may take less time and may reinforce the automatic

postural adjustments that support all actions. Consequently, whenever possible, the OTA should approach the intervention for stroke impairments with strategies designed to restore lost function in ways that use the learning and work experiences of older adults before they experienced the stroke. Compensation strategies, particularly those related to the use of assistive equipment or alternative motor patterns, should be evaluated carefully because they require conscious attention and may create habits that may be difficult to break later.

Motor Deficits

Several sensorimotor approaches exist for the treatment of motor dysfunction resulting from stroke. Some of these include Brunnstrom's approach to movement disorders,[20,21,22] Bobath's neurodevelopmental approach to the treatment of neurological disorders,[23-26] constraint-induced movement therapy,[27-29] mirror therapy,[30-32] task-specific training,[33,34] and mental imagery therapy. Regardless of the approach, the goal of intervention is to facilitate normal voluntary movement and use of the affected side of the body. Thus, normal postural mechanisms must also be developed, and abnormal reflexes and movements must be inhibited.

Although hypertonicity is often the most visible sign that a person has a motor dysfunction, this problem is best addressed in the context of postural control rather than in isolation. Abnormal tone in any extremity may drastically change depending on whether the individual is lying, sitting, or standing. Therefore, motor dysfunction should be treated when the individual is in alignment. Alignment means that the individual's pelvis is in a neutral position with no anterior or posterior tilt, that the spine is in midline alignment, and that the upper and lower extremities are in a neutral position.

The correct positioning while the older adult is reclining can have a dramatic effect on muscle tone and pain, especially in the presence of complex regional pain syndrome/shoulder-hand syndrome. (Specific issues with the hemiplegic upper extremity are discussed later in the chapter.) Having older adults lie on the more affected side is most helpful in inhibiting abnormal tone and pain because of the heavy pressure exerted on that side (Fig. 19.1A). However, caution must be taken to determine that the shoulder girdle is correctly aligned, the scapula is slightly abducted, and the humerus is in external rotation. The position of the bed should be rearranged (unless the older adult finds the change too disorganizing) so that the older adult can lie on the affected side and face the side of the bed from which transfers will occur. An added advantage of lying on the affected side is that it frees the less involved upper extremity for functional use while the older adult is in this position (Fig. 19.1B).

Body alignment should be maintained during transitional movements, such as changing from a side-lying position to sitting at the edge of the bed and back to side-lying. This alignment is also maintained when transferring to and

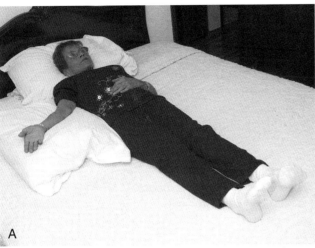 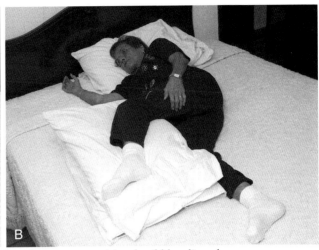

FIG. 19.1 (A) In the supine position, the trunk and upper extremities should be aligned. The hemiplegic upper extremity should be supported on pillows with the palm facing up. (B) Lying on the hemiplegic upper extremity frees the less involved arm for functional use.

BOX 19.1

Sequential Procedures for Changing From a Supine Position to Sitting at Edge of Bed

1. Plan to have the older adult exit bed toward hemiplegic side.
2. Gently provide passive abduction to hemiplegic scapula, and extend hemiplegic arm at side of body so that humerus is in external rotation and palm is facing up; an alternative is to have the older adult clasp hands and hold arms in 90-degree flexion with straight elbows and roll toward side of bed.
3. Have the older adult hook less affected leg under hemiplegic ankle, and slide both legs toward edge of bed.
4. Have the older adult roll on to hemiplegic side, facing side of bed.
5. Have the older adult cross less affected upper extremity in front of body and place on bed at a level slightly below chest.
6. As the older adult lowers legs at the side of the bed, have older adult push up with less affected hand and hemiplegic elbow (if able).
7. Once sitting at edge of bed, have the older adult scoot forward by alternating weight bearing on each thigh and scooting the free thigh forward until both feet are flat on floor.

BOX 19.2

Sequential Procedures for Transfers

1. If transferring from the wheelchair to another chair, toilet, or bed, place wheelchair at no more than 45 degrees (perpendicular) from destination surface; older adult should transfer toward unaffected side whenever possible.
2. Make sure wheelchair is locked and footrests and armrests are out of the way.
3. Place both feet flat on floor.
4. Have older adult sit upright so back is not against back rest.
5. Have older adult scoot forward to front edge of chair by alternately shifting weight on to one thigh and scooting other thigh forward; do not permit older adult to push off back of chair using back extension because this will increase abnormal muscle tone throughout the body.
6. Position older adult's feet so tips of toes are directly below knees; make sure feet remain flat on floor; if ankle dorsiflexion is limited, toes may be placed somewhat anterior to knees.
7. Have older adult lean forward until shoulders are directly above knees.
8. Have older adult push off from knees with both hands, if older adult is able.
9. As older adult leans forward, have older adult stand up; if unable to stand up fully, guide older adult's body toward target chair, toilet, or bed while older adult is partially weight bearing on both feet.

from a chair, wheelchair, toilet, or car; changing from a sitting to a standing position and back to sitting; and while walking. OTAs should follow established sequential procedures when assisting older adults to change from a supine position to sitting at the edge of the bed or when doing transfers (Boxes 19.1 and 19.2). In all of these circumstances, OTAs must remember not to pull on the affected upper extremity to assist older adult. OTAs should assist by holding the older adult from the shoulder with the

OTA's hand on the older adult's scapula. Pulling the arm or supporting the older adult from the axilla can easily cause or worsen any shoulder pain or glenohumeral subluxation. Shoulder subluxation can occur inferiorly, anteriorly, and superiorly. Alignment of the humerus in the glenohumeral fossa is evaluated by the OT. The OTA needs to determine whether the alignment is correct before evaluating range of motion of the shoulder. Shoulder pain is a frequent problem and can occur from malalignment of the trunk, shoulder girdle, and humerus; subluxation; adhesive capsulitis; and trauma.[35] Shoulder subluxation and pain can lead to other complications such as increased hypertonicity, contractures, edema, nerve injury, and complex regional pain syndrome. Before the OTA attempts any intervention for these conditions, service competency should be established with the OT.

OTAs must pay constant attention to the older adult's body alignment during sitting because this is often the older adult's position during most activities, especially during the initial stages of rehabilitation. If the older adult must sit fairly still for long periods, the therapist must ensure that the older adult's pelvis is in a neutral position and is as far back in the chair as possible. Hips should be flexed at no more than 90 degrees. Greater hip flexion will cause posterior pelvic tilt and lumbar and thoracic spine flexion, inhibit breathing and active upper extremity control, and require greater cervical spine extension for the person to look straight ahead. Placing a folded towel or thin pillow in the small of the back to maintain alignment may be helpful. However, too thick a pillow or support can push the lumbar spine into hyperextension, causing anterior pelvic tilt and encouraging the older adult to use back extension as the primary means of posture control. When back hyperextension is the base from which the older adult begins movement in the extremities, hypertonicity throughout the body is likely to increase.

Another concern when the older adult is in the sitting position is lateral pelvic tilt, or lateral flexion of the spine. Because of sensory and tone changes, half of the trunk muscles may not be working well; consequently, the other side of the trunk may be overworking. The resulting misalignment causes the spine to flex toward one side. Because of this lateral flexion, the spine is no longer in midline, and weight bearing on the older adult's thighs is unequal. A pelvic tilt upward toward one side results in the shortening of the trunk on the same side and elongation of the trunk on the opposite side. Weight bearing occurs primarily on the side of the elongated trunk. The OTA must help to actively or passively align the spine toward the midline rather than to simply build up one side of the sitting surface.

When pelvic and spine alignment are achieved, the OTA can focus on placing the feet flat on the floor or on footrests so that knee flexion and ankle dorsiflexion of no more than 90 degrees are present. The OTA should take care that the femurs are in neutral rotation (i.e., there is no external or internal rotation) and that there is little or no hip abduction or adduction. Thus, the heels will be resting directly below the knees, and the knees will be aligned with the hips. Unless the older adult is being pushed in a wheelchair, both feet should be placed on the floor so that they bear weight more evenly. Consequently, hemi-wheelchairs, the seats of which are slightly lower than standard wheelchairs, are recommended so that the older adult's feet can comfortably reach the floor. The use of a padded seat and backboards placed in the wheelchair also improves the older adult's sitting position and midline orientation, thus preventing the problems that may occur from poor positioning in a wheelchair.

After attending to the pelvis, spine, and lower extremities, the OTA can align the older adult's hemiplegic upper extremity. The strategies for positioning are similar for both hypotonic and hypertonic arms. The older adult should be placed in front of a table or outfitted with a full or half lapboard so that the hand can be placed face down on a flat surface to benefit from the normalizing effects of weight bearing. To accomplish this, the OTA should ensure that the older adult's scapula is slightly abducted, the shoulder is flexed so the elbow is anterior to the shoulder, the humerus is in neutral or slight external rotation, the elbow is resting lightly on the lapboard to provide support for the shoulder, the forearm is pronated and positioned away from the trunk, and the hand is resting on the support surface. This permits the hand to bear weight normally. The normal weight-bearing surface of the hand includes the lateral external surface of the thumb, fingertips, lateral border of the hand, and thenar and hypothenar eminences. The OTA should maintain the arch formed by the metacarpophalangeal joints so that the hand is not flattened. The hand should not be fastened in any way to the lapboard except in extreme cases in which clear evidence indicates that the older adult may otherwise be hurt. Restricting normal, spontaneous weight bearing inhibits normalization of muscle tone. In cases of extreme hypertonicity in the hand, the OTA can place a soup bowl or a ball cut in half face down on a square of nonslip material on the lapboard, thus permitting some weight bearing against a hard surface (Fig. 19.2). However, the older adult's hand should never be placed on nonslip material. Such material can contribute to shoulder pain or subluxation because the hand cannot move when repositioning of the shoulder or body occurs. Caution must be made when a lapboard is used with an older adult because it may be considered a form of restraint unless the older adult is independently able to remove it. (See Chapter 14 for a discussion on this topic.)

During intervention sessions that do not require sitting for long periods, the older adult should sit in a chair, on a stool, or at the edge of a mat. The concerns with alignment in this position are similar to those described earlier for sitting, but the focus of intervention will be on the older adult moving into and out of alignment while participating in activities. Sitting on a stool or at the edge of the mat forces active trunk control because there are no back or armrests for support, and the base of support under the thighs is reduced. Concerns regarding lower extremity placement are the same as described previously.

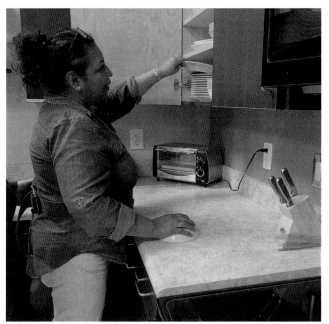

FIG. 19.2 In cases of hypertonicity, the hand with hemiplegia can be placed on an inverted bowl or ball that has been cut in half to bear weight more comfortably during activities. *(Courtesy Amy Shaffer)*

However, as the older adult's ability to control the trunk increases, the height of the mat can be increased, thus gradually increasing and challenging the amount of active weight bearing on the lower extremities. This gradation prepares the older adult for the trunk and postural control required during standing activities. If the older adult has little or no active movement of the hemiplegic upper extremity, the older adult should position the limb on a table following similar guidelines as those described previously. As the height of the mat increases, so should the height of the table or surface that supports the hand.

Although ambulation training does not traditionally fall into the realm of occupational therapy, it should be considered. Functional mobility refers to transitional movements that permits older adults to perform and maneuver from one task or occupation to another. For example, older adults may need to ambulate from the bed to the bathroom and stand to complete toileting tasks, or ambulate from the sink to the stove to the refrigerator and stand to complete a meal preparation task. Consequently, OTAs should assist in maintaining alignment in the same way as described previously. During standing and ambulation, the person's midline shift toward the less affected side is most obvious. This is often accentuated when older adults are taught to walk using a broad-based cane, and they establish the habit of maintaining the midline in the middle of the less affected side rather than in the middle of the body. Because there is less motor control or less sensory feedback, older adults may hesitate to bear weight equally on each leg as they stand or take a step. The OTA should coordinate intervention with the registered physical therapist to understand what standing and ambulation pattern to reinforce with older adults during occupational therapy intervention.

Special attention should be given to the hemiplegic upper extremity. This extremity should be purposefully included in any activity early during the course of intervention, even if little or no active motor control is present, because this will keep the older adult's attention on the extremity and will reduce its neglect and the development of learned nonuse.[27,29] Before any active or passive motion is expected of the older adult, the OTA must first passively mobilize the older adult's scapula to ensure that it glides when the arm is moved. The scapula may not glide sufficiently or may stop altogether because of muscle paralysis or hypertonus. Consequently, the OTA should never flex or abduct the shoulder of the older adult more than 90 degrees unless the OTA can be sure that the scapula is gliding properly. If older adults do not have active scapular control, the OTA can passively move the scapula while ranging the shoulder. When the shoulder is flexed more than 90 degrees, the scapula glides downward on the posterior wall of the rib cage. In addition, the inferior border, or angle, of the scapula rotates slightly upward. When the shoulder is abducted more than 90 degrees, the scapula glides toward the vertebral column and the inferior border rotates slightly downward.

If older adults have minimal or no active movement in the hemiplegic upper extremity, they should be instructed to move it by holding their hands together in one of two ways. If the older adult has any active movement in the hand, clasping the hands with the thumb of the hemiplegic hand on top is recommended. If there is no movement in the hand, the uninvolved hand should be placed on the ulnar side of the hemiplegic wrist and hand and the uninvolved thumb in the palm of the hemiplegic hand. This method will protect the small joints of the hemiplegic hand and will maintain the arches in the palm. While holding on to the hands using either method, older adults should be instructed to extend the elbows and hold the shoulders flexed at approximately 90 degrees. With the arms in this position, older adults can go from a supine to a side-lying position, from a sitting to a standing position, or they can hold on to the knee of the hemiplegic lower extremity to cross it during dressing and bathing and during other functional activities. The OTA's imagination and creativity are essential in assisting older adults to use this two-hand technique to perform numerous functional activities such as picking up a mug to drink and mixing a cake. In addition, older adults can flex or abduct the hemiplegic shoulder themselves by guiding the arm when the hands are held together. This bilateral integration assists with normalizing tone and encourages older adults to actively care for the hemiplegic upper extremity.[23]

Older adults may develop complex regional pain syndrome, previously known as reflex sympathetic dystrophy or shoulder-hand syndrome, if the hemiplegic upper extremity is not managed appropriately. This syndrome is characterized by swelling or edema that is usually observed in the hand but may also be present in the forearm and upper arm, along with tenderness, loss of range of motion, and vasomotor degradation.[22] Pain and subluxation of the glenohumeral joint may not necessarily be present. The OTA should address all of these problems immediately to avoid irreversible atrophy of bones, skin, and muscles.[22] The swelling is best decreased by providing the hemiplegic arm with an ice-bath. Older adults should sit, while maintaining good alignment, placing the hemiplegic hand and wrist in the water for 3–5 seconds. This process should be repeated three times. The OTA should dry the hand gently with a towel. The OTA should ask the older adult to flex the fingers, if possible, or the OTA should provide gentle passive ranging of the fingers and hand. The whole procedure should be done repeatedly during the day until swelling subsides.[22] Other options for reducing swelling are elevation of the extremity positioned on a pillow or usage of an ice pack.[22] While the OTA is providing the range of motion exercise, retrograde massage while the limb is elevated can also be done, and a simple cock-up orthosis can be used to hold the wrist in extension (no more than 30 degrees) to help reduce the build-up of fluid in the hand when older adults are not receiving therapy (Fig. 19.3). Swelling also occurs from decreased muscle activity to move the fluid from the limb, dependent positioning, and trauma.

OTAs can use graded activities to facilitate voluntary control of an older adult's hemiplegic upper extremity. Such activities should be geared toward developing control in a progression from shoulder to elbow to hand. Older adults may develop control in the hand before the more proximal parts of the arm. Despite the apparent control in the hand, the OTA should first facilitate active movement in the shoulder by engaging older adults in activities that emphasize the body moving on the arm while the hand is maintained in weight bearing. The weight-bearing surface of the hand is limited to the lateral surface of the thumb, the thenar eminences, and the fingertips. In this position, the palm of the hand is free and not in contact with the weight-bearing surface. Weight bearing on the hand does not need to be forceful, and older adults should never have the hand completely flattened. Placing weight on a flat hand can lead to loss of the normal and functional arches of the hand and, consequently, can interfere with older adults' abilities to develop grasp later. Placing weight on the hand can be done in both sitting and standing positions. In a sitting position, for example, an older adult's affected hand can be placed in a weight-bearing position on the table or on a stool placed next to the older adult. In a standing position, the older adult should be taught to place the affected hand on a weight-bearing surface such as a table or countertop while performing functional tasks, such as putting away dishes, meal preparation, or folding laundry (Fig. 19.4). As control of the shoulder increases, activities should be introduced that emphasize free movement of the hemiplegic extremity on the more stable part of the body. During all of these activities, the OTA should continue to ensure that good body alignment is maintained and that older adults are not using abnormal movements in one part of the body to obtain control in another.

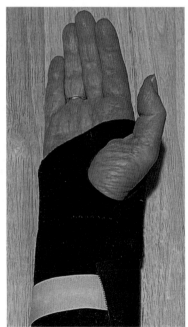

FIG. 19.3   A wrist cock-up orthosis can hold the wrist in slight extension and help reduce fluid build-up in the hand. (*Courtesy Lee Lohman*)

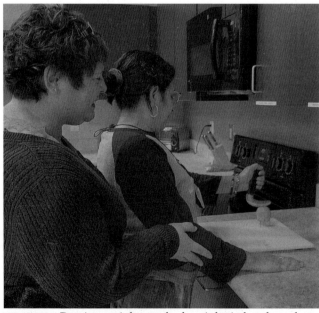

FIG. 19.4   Bearing weight on the hemiplegic hand can be done while standing at the counter performing a functional task. (*Courtesy Amy Shaffer*)

Constraint-Induced Movement Therapy

Constraint-induced movement therapy (CIMT) is one of the most effective rehabilitation interventions for individuals who sustained motor impairments after a stroke. In traditional CIMT protocols, the older adult completes repetitive tasks coupled with shaping from the OTA for 6 hours a day over a 2-week period of time along with functional tasks for 90% of daytime hours.[36] The OTA should work closely with the OT to determine the older adult's eligibility to participate and develop a CIMT protocol. The older adult should have a minimum of 20 degrees of extension in the wrist, 10 degrees of extension at the metacarpophalangeal and interphalangeal joints. In addition, the older adult should have adequate cognition due to potential safety concerns and be able to stand with or without assistance for at least 2 minutes.[36,37]

Examples of assessments to measure outcomes include: Wolf Motor Functional Test or Graded Wolf Motor Function Test, Motor Activity Log, Fugl-Meyer Evaluation of Physical Performance, Stroke Impact Scale, Assessment of Motor and Process Skills, and the Canadian Occupational Performance Measure. Intervention includes massed practice of functional tasks that are meaningful and relevant to the older adult. Examples of interventions include tasks that promote grasp and release, basic self-care activities such as drinking liquids or hair brushing, reaching for functional items, and so on. Shaping is an integral component to the treatment protocol and involves selection of tasks specific to the older adult's needs, physical and verbal assistance to the older adult to promote specific arm-hand movements, and provision of encouragement when the older adult demonstrates improvement in functional tasks.[38] The OTA should provide verbal and tactile feedback to the older adult to promote proper movements and alignment and encouragement and support to the older adult.

Modified versions of CIMT (mCIMT) developed after the emergence of concerns about safety, time, and resources.[37] The mCIMT protocols vary in time from 30 minutes to 6 hours a day, in length from 2 to 12 weeks, in intensity from 2 to 7 times a week, and location of home or clinic.[36,39,40] Both standard CIMT and mCIMT protocols are found to be effective interventions for older adults with extremity motor impairments[36,40]; however, individuals who receive CIMT intervention earlier show a greater recovery curve in hand and arm movement.[41] Results from multiple research studies for both CIMT and mCIMT indicate improvements in the older adults' ability to complete daily activities with their affected extremity (both observed and through self-report) and with improvements in quality of life.[36,42]

Other Techniques

OTAs should instruct older adults in proper one-handed dressing techniques to protect the hemiplegic upper extremity and to avoid falling. Dressing should be done while sitting in a chair and, in general, the hemiplegic extremity should be dressed first and undressed last to avoid pulling on it or twisting it unnecessarily. Front-buttoned shirts or blouses are easiest to don by first dressing the hemiplegic arm and then draping the shirt over the shoulders by holding on to the shirt collar with the other arm. When the shirt is draped over the opposite shoulder, the older adult can reach into the sleeve with the unaffected arm. This procedure is reversed when taking the shirt off. The process is similar when putting on pants, with the exception that the older adult should cross the hemiplegic leg over the opposite leg to dress the hemiplegic leg first. If the older adult is able to stand to pull up the pants, the older adult may do so when both legs are clothed. If standing is not possible, the older adult can shift weight to each side while sitting in the chair and gradually can pull the pants up over the buttocks.

All of the principles mentioned previously should be considered when training older adults in functional activities or selecting assistive equipment. While modifications and compensatory techniques are useful in the beginning, it is important to focus on task-specific training as the older adult regains function of their hemiplegic upper extremity. Task-specific, or task-oriented, training is defined as using the functional activity that is meaningful to the older adult, like washing dishes, as the actual intervention session. When tasks are too difficult, older adults are more likely to use abnormal movement patterns, become fatigued quickly, and become discouraged. The OTA must use good observation and clinical reasoning skills in selecting activities that challenge older adults and grade the activities to the appropriate levels. Although progress may seem slower at the beginning, following these principles can make a marked difference in the quality of movement that older adults develop.

Visual-Perceptual-Cognitive Deficits

Although the motor deficits resulting from a stroke are the most easily observed, many less visible problems can severely hinder the rehabilitation process if not appropriately addressed. Depending on the type of brain lesion, the individual may have sensory disturbances that range from a total absence of sensation to a heightened perception of pain and other distorted sensations. These problems are accentuated when the individual has a body scheme disorder or difficulties planning motor actions, which is known as apraxia. Consequently, the individual has difficulty integrating and using any perceptual input from the hemiplegic side. Visual–perceptual deficits common in strokes include hemianopsia, poor figure–ground perceptions, and difficulty with spatial relationships. Unilateral neglect results from a unique constellation of these symptoms when older adults have no sense that the hemiplegic side of the body even exists, and they fail to visually scan toward that side.[43,44] All of these disorders should be addressed simultaneously during intervention using bilateral functional activities that encourage the use

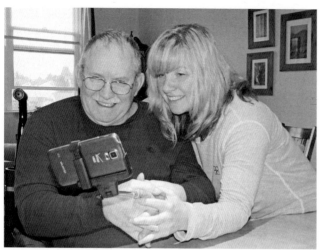

FIG. 19.5   This older adult is using a selfie stick while integrating his hemiplegic arm.

of the hemiplegic side of the body (Fig. 19.5). The use of normal movement will provide repeated sensory stimulation to the hemiplegic side and relay information that will be processed in the brain and used as feedback in determining where each body part is and what it is doing. Consequently, the OTA should grade a variety of motor and sensory activities so that they maximize the older adults' abilities to control movement independently and provide increased sensory input. However, the activities should not be so overwhelming that they cause withdrawal reactions or increases in abnormal tone. Various textures, smells, colors, distances, and depths can be graded during most functional activities. In addition to these remedial approaches, the OTA should teach older adults to compensate for deficits by providing repeated practice in establishing habits of visually scanning the hemiplegic side and methodically protecting and integrating the hemiplegic extremities in whatever activity they may be involved.

Other areas of concern for the OTA include older adults' abilities to comprehend and produce language, and to plan and safely perform activities. As a result of stroke, older adults may not be able to understand what others are saying, a condition known as receptive aphasia; or may not be able to produce the words they intend to utter, a condition known as expressive aphasia; or both disorders may be present, which is known as global aphasia. These disorders may also extend to nonverbal language because older adults may be unable to interpret or appropriately use gestures. Language deficits are usually treated by the speech language pathologist, but strategies must be reinforced during occupational therapy intervention. When talking to older adults, OTAs should keep instructions and explanations simple and concrete, stating them in an empathetic, patient way. Demonstration is usually helpful. The best way to ensure that older adults have understood the instructions is to observe their performance.[43,45]

Cognitive dysfunction is often believed to be a major cause for failure of older adults to reach rehabilitation goals and must be considered, particularly when planning for discharge.[46] Safety may be compromised if older adults cannot plan activities, make judgments, solve problems, or express verbally their needs for emergency care. For example, limited memory may cause older adults to overmedicate themselves or not turn off the stove after cooking. Being unable to remember all of the steps involved in a task may mean that older adults can often be surprised by the outcome. Older adults may get stuck on a step and may be unable to determine what to do next or may neglect to realize that something dangerous could happen if an inappropriate action is taken. Occupational therapy intervention, as mentioned earlier, should involve graded repetition of procedures until older adults can routinely perform them safely. Emphasis should be placed on varying the context or situation in which the procedure is practiced to enhance learning.[47]

Emotional Adjustment

OTAs should consider the emotional adjustment of older adults to the disability caused by the stroke. Depression, a common reaction to any catastrophic event, is one of the most undiagnosed and untreated responses to stroke.[48,49] Depression may be caused from natural grief trying to cope with the loss of function but also may be caused by the location of the lesion in the brain, previous or family history of depression, and social functioning before the stroke. Mild or major depression can develop from 2 months to 2 years after the stroke in up to 33% of clients.[48,49] Stroke survivors in the younger age groups between 25–54 years of age and 55–64 years of age may have higher incidence of depression.[50] Anxiety, poor frustration tolerance, denial, anger, and emotional lability are all signs that older adults are struggling to deal with the reality of their condition. OTAs must listen empathetically and supportively, while sensitively maintaining the focus on areas of realistic recovery. Permitting older adults to control choices in intervention as much as possible can reinforce the sense that they can affect their environments. Although a complete recovery cannot be guaranteed, neither can a lack of recovery. OTAs must honestly explain to older adults that residual limitations will probably be present, but the best chance for recovery will occur by the practice of skills. OTAs should use their creativity and ingenuity skills to help older adults adapt tasks or environments that older adults consider lost, thus instilling new hope and motivation in the rehabilitation process. As with any area of intervention, family and social involvement is crucial for older adults to accept residual limitations and maximize their residual abilities. Ultimately, older adults must see that they can continue to be effective in some measure and can still actively pursue activities and ideals they valued highly before the stroke.

TABLE 19.3

F.A.S.T. Method for Identifying Stroke Symptoms

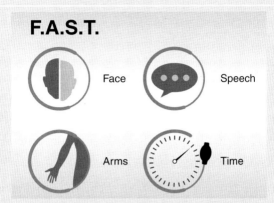

Time is of the essence: These signs and symptoms of a stroke come on suddenly. Treating a stroke quickly (within 3 hours) can reduce the damage that is done to the brain and allow the older adult to have better rehabilitation outcomes. If you recognize any of the symptoms or signs, call 9-1-1 immediately. Acting quickly could save a life.

F—Face: Ask the person to smile. Does one side of the face droop?

A—Arms: Ask the person to raise both arms. Does one arm drift downward?

S—Speech: Ask the person to repeat a simple phrase. Is the speech slurred or strange?

T—Time: If you see any of these signs, call 9-1-1 right away.

Adapted from Center for Disease Control and Prevention. *Stroke signs and symptoms*. Retrieved from https://www.cdc.gov/stroke/signs_symptoms.htm

FAST CAMPAIGN

The Center for Disease Control created the Act F.A.S.T campaign to encourage members of the public to recognize the signs and symptoms of a stroke and take quick action in seeking medical treatment. The F.A.S.T acronym stands for Face, Arms, Speech, Time and is a quick test in which one checks for facial droop by asking the person to smile, looks for arm weakness by asking them to raise both arms, and check their speech for slurring or difficulty. It then encourages one to call 9-1-1 if any of the three-face, arms, or speech are abnormal (Table 19.3)

▌TECH TALK: FOCUS ON TECHNOLOGY

NAME	PURPOSE	APPROX. COST	WHERE TO BUY
Interactive Metronome	Device that can be used in the clinic or at home to facilitate the development of concentration, motor skills, bilateral integration, balance, and processing skills.	$250 for device	Interactivemetronome.com
Music Glove	Device worn like a glove that, when connected to a computer, gamifies finger exercise to encourage ROM, finger isolation, and opposition.	$359 for device	www.flintrehab.com
Saebo Stim One	Wearable device designed to wirelessly stimulate muscles to prevent or reduce muscle weakness by targeting the affected muscles.	$119 for device	www.saebo.com

CASE STUDY

Marcus is a 75-year-old man who recently returned home after having a left middle cerebral artery stroke. He had spent 3 weeks in an acute care hospital followed by 3 weeks in a rehabilitation center. The rehabilitation team concluded that, with the right supports, Marcus would be safe at home. At the time of discharge home, he had some residual weakness of the right side of his body, particularly the leg. He was able to flex the hip and knee against gravity but continued to have the tendency to drag the foot when he walked. He still had some difficulties coordinating his right arm, and he tended to overreach with it, on occasion knocking objects off tables, counters, and shelves. The discharge report from the occupational therapists at the rehabilitation hospital indicated that Marcus was able to feed, toilet, and dress himself independently, although on occasion he became confused about the sequencing of dressing tasks.

York, an OT, and Nikki, an OTA, evaluated Marcus as part of the home-health team and noted that Marcus still had a slight decrease in tactile abilities with his right, dominant hand. They noted a slight droop in the right side of his face was still present, and that his lingual control toward the right side was also reduced. They confirmed that Marcus was able to dress and toilet himself but discovered that, although he had been able to shower himself in the hospital, at home this would require transferring into an old-fashioned bathtub. This tub was higher than the standard tub in which he had been evaluated at the hospital. York and Nikki determined that, without grab bars for safety, Marcus would need minimal to moderate assistance with his shower for safety.

York and Nikki included an analysis of Marcus's home and supports in their intake evaluation. Marcus lived in a first floor apartment that had wooden floors. There were several floor rugs that Marcus had collected in his travels. The furniture was already arranged in a way that York and Nikki believed would not interfere with Marcus's safety. They noted that Marcus lived alone, although his younger brother visited every day and lived only a few blocks away. Up to the time of the stroke, Marcus had been driving his car to get to the grocery store and moved around independently in the community.

■ CASE STUDY QUESTIONS

1 Should York and Nikki conduct any additional evaluations to determine Marcus's needs? What additional information should they consider before finalizing the intervention plan?
2 What interventions should York and Nikki implement to help Marcus continue to make gains in his neuromuscular functions?

3 What strategies should be considered to ensure Marcus's safety in the kitchen considering his remaining neuromuscular deficits?
4 What precautions should be considered given Marcus's facial droop and limited lingual control?
5 What safety measures should be considered in Marcus's home to ensure it is a safe environment for him?
6 What alternatives for community access should be considered with Marcus?

■ CHAPTER REVIEW QUESTIONS

1 Explain the general causes of stroke.
2 Name three modifiable and three unmodifiable stroke risk factors.
3 Why is it important to assess psychosocial skills and performance in addition to motor and cognitive performance of older adults who have had a stroke?
4 What is the sequence in which body parts should be aligned in order to facilitate maximum function for people who have had a stroke?
5 Describe three strategies an OTA may use to reduce shoulder subluxation of a person who has had a stroke.
6 Explain two precautions an OTA should observe when using constraint-induced movement therapy (CIMT).

EVIDENCE NUGGETS: EFFECTIVENESS OF CONSTRAINT-INDUCED MOVEMENT THERAPY AS AN INTERVENTION FOR OLDER ADULTS WHO HAVE SUSTAINED A CVA

1. Doussoulin A, Rivas C, Rivas R, Saiz J. Effects of modified constraint-induced movement therapy in the recovery of upper extremity function affected by a stroke: A single-blind randomized parallel trial-comparing group versus individual intervention. *Int J Rehabil Res.* 2018;41(1):35-40. doi:10.1097/MRR.0000000000000257
    *   Group and individual modified constraint-induced movement therapy (mCIMT) both increase the use and function of the paretic upper extremity.
    *   Group mCIMT showed higher gains than individual mCIMT, with the effects of group mCIMT remaining 6 months postintervention.
    *   Patients in group therapy competitively motivated each other, shared their results with each other, and encouraged each other.
2. Stock R, Thrane G, Anke A, Gjone R, Askim T. Early versus late-applied constraint-induced movement therapy: A multisite, randomized controlled trial with a 12-month follow-up. *Physiother Res Int.* 2018;23(1). doi:10.1002/pri.1689
    *   Constraint-induced movement therapy (CIMT) intervention consisted of 2 hours of shaping tasks, 30 minutes of ADL practice, and 30 minutes of going

over an activity log, a home diary, and an independent assignment, with constraint to be worn 90% of waking hours.
    *   Two weeks postintervention, those who received CIMT within 28 days post-CVA showed greater improvement compared to those who received CIMT 6 months post-CVA, with no statistically significant differences between groups at 1 year follow-up.
    *   Applying CIMT within 28 days post-CVA can lead to faster motor and functional recovery.
3. Baldwin CR, Harry AJ, Power LJ, Pope KL, Harding KE. Modified Constraint-Induced Movement Therapy is a feasible and potentially useful addition to the Community Rehabilitation tool kit after stroke: A pilot randomised control trial. *Aust Occup Ther J.* 2018;65(6):503-511. doi:10.1111/1440-1630.12488
    *   The modified constraint-induced movement therapy (mCIMT) intervention included six 1 hour OT sessions, wearing the constraint 90% of waking hours, and a home exercise program.
    *   At least 40% of participants wore the constraint for an average of 8–12 hours a day, at least 30% wore the constraint for an average of 3–5 hours per day, with at

EVIDENCE NUGGETS: EFFECTIVENESS OF CONSTRAINT-INDUCED MOVEMENT THERAPY AS AN INTERVENTION FOR OLDER ADULTS WHO HAS SUSTAINED A CVA—cont'd

least 50% spending an average of 42 minutes per day on prescribed home exercises.

- The intervention (modified constraint-induced movement [mCIMT]) group and the control (usual occupational therapy) group both experienced a significant increase in the Wolf Motor Function Test (WMFT) time to complete, with the intervention group experiencing a significant increase in the WMFT Functional Scale, Motor Activity Log (MAL), and MAL "How Well" scale.
- This mCIMT intervention can be implemented in a community rehabilitation setting easier than traditional CIMT and can lead to increased function and use of the upper extremity.

4. Kale AA, Kekatpure V, Mahendrakar N. Effect of constraint induced movement therapy versus bimanual task training for improvement of motor hand function in stroke patients. *Indian J Physiother Occup Therap.* 2019;13(1):23-27. doi:10.5958/0973-5674.2019.00005.4
- Patients in the constraint-induced movement therapy (CIMT) group scored higher in the Nine Hole Peg Test and the Action Research Arm Test than the bimanual task training group.

- Interventions that focus on using both the affected and the nonaffected extremity simultaneously are not as effective as interventions that focus solely on the use of the hemiparetic arm.
- CIMT can lead to increased function and dexterity.

5. Mushtaq W, Hamdani N, Noohu MM, Raghavan S. Effect of modified constrain induced movement therapy on fatigue and motor performance in sub acute stroke. *J Stroke Cerebrovasc Dis.* 2020;29(12):105378. doi:10.1016/j.jstrokecerebrovasdis.2020.105378
- Modified constraint-induced movement therapy (mCIMT) resulted in higher statistically significant Wolf Motor Function Test scores than the control group.
- There was not a significant difference between the pretest and the posttest results for levels of fatigue (measured by using the Barrow Neurological Institute scale) for the experimental group and the control group, and there was not a significant difference between groups.
- Modified constraint-induced therapy is not likely to cause fatigue, and it can lead to greater improvements in motor performance than interventions that do not use restraints.

For additional video content, please visit Elsevier eBooks+ (eBooks.Health.Elsevier.com)

REFERENCES

1. Vanderah T, Gould D. *Nolte's the Human Brain: An Introduction to Its Functional Anatomy.* 7th ed. Philadelphia: Elsevier; 2015.
2. Moini J, Piran P. *Functional and Clinical Neuroanatomy: A Guide for Health Care Professionals.* London: Academic Press; 2020.
3. Centers for Disease Control and Prevention. *Stroke Facts.* 2020. Available at: http://www.cdc.gov/stroke/facts.htm.
4. Xu J, Murphy SL, Kochanek KD, Arias E. Mortality in the United States, 2018. *NCHS Data Brief.* 2020;(355):1-8.
5. National Institute of Neurological Disorders and Stroke. *Stroke Rehabilitation Information.* 2016. Available at: https://medlineplus.gov/strokerehabilitation.html.
6. Mozaffarian D, Benjamin EJ, Go AS, et al. Heart disease and stroke statistics—2015 update: a report from the American Heart Association. *Circulation.* 2015;131:e29-e322.
7. Boehme A, Esenwa C, Elkind M. Stroke risk factors, genetics, and prevention. *Circ Res.* 2017;20(3):472-495.
8. Yousufuddin M, Young N. Aging and ischemic stroke. *Aging (Albany NY).* 2019;11(9):2542-2544. doi:10.18632/aging.101931.
9. Lui SK, Nguyen MH. Elderly stroke rehabilitation: overcoming the complications and its associated challenges. *Curr Gerontol Geriatr Res.* 2018;2018:9853837.
10. Cassidy JM, Cramer SC. Spontaneous and therapeutic-induced mechanisms of functional recovery after stroke. *Transl Stroke Res.* 2017;8(1):33-46. doi:10.1007/s12975-016-0467-5.
11. Adeoye O, Nyström KV, Yavagal DR, et al. Recommendations for the establishment of stroke systems of care: a 2019 update. *Stroke.* 2019;50(7):e187-e210. doi:10.1161/str.0000000000000173.
12. Borschmann KN, Hayward KS. Recovery of upper limb function is greatest early after stroke but does continue to improve during the chronic phase: a two-year, observational study. *Physiotherapy.* 2020;107:216-223.
13. Ballester BR, Maier M, Duff A, et al. A critical time window for recovery extends beyond one-year post-stroke. *J Neurophysiol.* 2019;122(1):350-357.
14. Wolf T, Chuh A, Floyd T, et al. Effectiveness of occupation-based interventions to improve areas of occupation and social participation after stroke: an evidence-based review. *Am J Occup Ther.* 2015;69(1):1-11. doi:10.5014/ajot.2015.012195.
15. Moyers PA. *The Guide to Occupational Therapy Practice.* 3rd ed. Bethesda, MD: American Occupational Therapy Association Press; 2020.
16. American Occupational Therapy Association. Occupational therapy practice framework: domain and process fourth edition. *Am J Occup Ther.* 2020;74:1-84. Available at: https://doi.org/10.5014/ajot.2020.74S2001.
17. Wang H, Huang P, Li X, Samuel OW, Xiang Y, Li G. Spasticity assessment based on the maximum isometrics voluntary contraction of upper limb muscles in post-stroke hemiplegia. *Front Neurol.* 2019;10:465.
18. American Occupational Therapy Association. Occupational therapy code of ethics. *Am J Occup Ther.* 2020:74(suppl 3):7413410005.
19. Li S. Spasticity, motor recovery, and neural plasticity after stroke. *Front Neurol.* 2017;8:120. doi:10.3389/fneur.2017.00120.
20. Sawner K, Lavigne G. *Brunnstrom's Movement Therapy in Hemiplegia: A Neurophysiological Approach.* Hagerstown, MD: Lippincott Williams & Wilkins; 1992.
21. Pan B, Sun Y, Xie B, et al. Alterations of muscle synergies during voluntary arm reaching movement in subacute stroke survivors at different levels of impairment. *Front Comput Neurosci.* 2018;12:69.
22. Mayo Clinic. *Complex Regional Pain Syndrome.* 2020. Available at: https://www.mayoclinic.org/diseases-conditions/crps-complex-regional-pain-syndrome/symptoms-causes/syc-20371151.
23. Renner CIE, Brendel C, Hummelsheim H Bilateral arm training vs unilateral arm training for severely affected patients with stroke: exploratory single-blinded randomized controlled trial. *Arch Phys Med Rehabil.* 2020;101(7):1120-1130.

24. Michielsen M, Vaughan-Graham J, Holland A, Magri A, Suzuki M. The Bobath concept - a model to illustrate clinical practice. *Disabil Rehabil*. 2019;41(17):2080-2092.

25. Haripriya S, Eapen SS, Raghu SR. Improving upper limb function in a person with stroke using proprioceptive neuromuscular facilitation approach: a case study. *Indian J Physiother Occup Ther*. 2020;14(1):217-220. doi:10.5958/0973-5674.2020.00039.8.

26. Vaughan-Graham J, Cott C, Wright V. The Bobath (NDT) concept in adult neurological rehabilitation: what is the state of the knowledge? A scoping review. Part I: conceptual perspectives. *Disabil Rehabil*. 2015;37(20):1793-1807. doi:10.3109/09638288.2014.985802.

27. Corbetta D, Sirtori V, Castellini G, et al. Constraint-induced movement therapy for upper extremities in people with stroke. *Cochrane Database Syst Rev*. 2015;(10):CD004433. doi:10.1002/14651858.CD004433.pub3.

28. Abdullahi A, Truijen S, Saeys W Neurobiology of recovery of motor function after stroke: the central nervous system biomarker effects of Constraint-Induced Movement Therapy. *Neural Plast*. 2020;2020:9484298.

29. Maier M, Ballester BR, Verschure PF MJ. Principles of neurorehabilitation after stroke based on motor learning and brain plasticity mechanisms. *Front Syst Neurosci*. 2019;13:74.

30. Arya K. Underlying neural mechanisms of mirror therapy: implications for motor rehabilitation in stroke. *Neurol India*. 2016;64(1):38-44. doi:10.4103/0028-3886.173622.

31. Gandhi DB, Sterba A, Khatter H, Pandian JD. Mirror therapy in stroke rehabilitation: current perspectives. *Ther Clin Risk Manag*. 2020;16:75-85.

32. Kim J, Lee B. Mirror therapy combined with biofeedback functional electrical stimulation for motor recovery of upper extremities after stroke: a pilot randomized controlled trial. *Occup Ther Int*. 2015;22(2):51-60. doi:10.1002/oti.1384.

33. Thant AA, Wanpen S, Nualnetr N, et al. Effects of task-oriented training on upper extremity functional performance in patients with sub-acute stroke: a randomized controlled trial. *J Phys Ther Sci*. 2019;31(1):82-87.

34. Rowe VT, Neville M. Task oriented training and evaluation at home. *OTJR (Thorofare N J)*. 2018;38(1):46-55.

35. Kumar P. Hemiplegic shoulder pain in people with stroke: present and the future. *Pain Manag*. 2019;9(2):107-110.

36. Kwakkel G, Veerbeek J, van Wegen E, et al. Constraint-induced movement therapy after stroke. *Lancet Neurol*. 2015;14:224-234. doi:10.1016/S1474-4422(14)70160-7.

37. Baldwin CR, Harry AJ, Power LJ, Pope KL, Harding KE. Modified Constraint-Induced Movement Therapy is a feasible and potentially useful addition to the Community Rehabilitation tool kit after stroke: a pilot randomised control trial. *Aust Occup Ther J*. 2018;65(6):503-511.

38. Etoom M, Hawamdeh M, Hawamdeh Z, et al. Constraint-induced movement therapy as a rehabilitation intervention for upper extremity in stroke patients: systematic review and meta-analysis: systematic review and meta-analysis. *Int J Rehabil Res*. 2016;39(3):197-210.

39. Barzel A, Ketels G, Stark A, et al. Home-based constraint-induced movement therapy for patients with upper limb dysfunction after stroke (HOMECIMT): a cluster-randomized, controlled trial. *Lancet Neurol*. 2015;14:893-902. doi:10.1016/S1474-4422(15)00147-7.

40. Yadav RK, Sharma R, Borah D, Kothari SY. Efficacy of modified Constraint Induced Movement Therapy in the treatment of hemiparetic upper limb in stroke patients: a randomized controlled trial. *J Clin Diagn Res*. 2016;10(11):YC01-YC05.

41. Stock R, Thrane G, Anke A, Gjone R, Askim T. Early versus late-applied constraint-induced movement therapy: a multisite, randomized controlled trial with a 12-month follow-up. *Physiother Res Int*. 2018;23(1):e1689.

42. Kelly KM, Borstad AL, Kline D, Gauthier LV. Improved quality of life following constraint-induced movement therapy is associated with gains in arm use, but not motor improvement. *Top Stroke Rehabil*. 2018;25(7):467-474.

43. Grotta JC, Albers GW, Broderick JP, Stroke, et al. Pathophysiology, Diagnosis, and Management. Amsterdam: Elsevier - Health Sciences Division; 2015:373–390. 6th ed.

44. Smith TM, Pappadis MR, Krishnan S, Reistetter TA. Stroke survivor and caregiver perspectives on post-stroke visual concerns and long-term consequences. *Behav Neurol*. 2018;2018:1463429.

45. American Stroke Association. *Effects of Aphasia*. 2018. Available at: https://www.stroke.org/en/about-stroke/effects-of-stroke/cognitive-and-communication-effects-of-stroke/effects-of-aphasia.

46. Vluggen TPMM, van Haastregt JCM, Tan FES, Kempen GIJM, Schols JMGA, Verbunt JA. Factors associated with successful home discharge after inpatient rehabilitation in frail older stroke patients. *BMC Geriatr*. 2020;20(1):25.

47. Ahn SN, Yoo EY, Jung MY, Park HY, Lee JY, Choi YI Comparison of Cognitive Orientation to daily Occupational Performance and conventional occupational therapy on occupational performance in individuals with stroke: a randomized controlled trial. *NeuroRehabilitation*. 2017;40(3):285-292.

48. Robinson R, Jorge R. Post-stroke depression: a review. *Am J Psychiatry*. 2016;173(3):221-231. doi:10.1176/appi.ajp.

49. Hildebrand MW. Effectiveness of interventions for adults with psychological or emotional impairment after stroke: an evidence-based review. *Am J Occup Ther*. 2015;69(1):1-17. doi:10.5014/ajot.2015.012054.

50. McCarthy M, Sucharew H, Alwell K, et al. Age, subjective stress, and depression after ischemic stroke. *J Behav Med*. 2016;39:55-64. doi:10.1007/s10865-015-9663-0.

20

Working With Older Adults Who Have Dementia and Alzheimer's Disease

RENÉ PADILLA

(PREVIOUS CONTRIBUTIONS FROM CARLY R. HELLEN)

KEY TERMS

activity-focused care, Alzheimer's disease, bridging, chaining, cognitive impairment, creative reality, mild cognitive impairment, person-centered care, personhood, rescuing, Therapeutic Fibs

CHAPTER OBJECTIVES

1. Understand that older adults with cognitive impairments (CI), Alzheimer's disease (AD) are persons first; they are not their disease. Therefore, person-centered care (personalized) focuses on overall well-being, reflecting the older adults' remaining strengths and abilities.
2. Describe person-centered care and personhood.
3. Gain awareness and sensitivity to the cognitive, physical, and psychosocial needs of older adults with AD.
4. Describe occupation-focused care.
5. Relate suggestions to promote wellness through task simplification and modification.
6. Identify caregiving techniques, approaches, and interventions that can be used to help empower older adults who have AD to participate in daily living tasks.
7. Suggest appropriate communication responses to older adults with AD.
8. Problem-solve antecedents and approaches to refocus unwanted behavioral responses.

Micah is an occupational therapy assistant (OTA) who works in a skilled nursing facility (SNF). One of their responsibilities is consulting with staff at a special care unit for persons with Alzheimer's disease (AD). John, the charge nurse on the unit, contacts Micah. "We are having problems with Grace. She is wandering in and out of others' rooms and taking their possessions, which is irritating the other residents. She is also having difficulty communicating her needs. Her performance with activities of daily living (ADL) functions seems variable. We are also having problems with increased agitation with Grace and all of our residents, especially at shift change. Do you have any ideas?"

Hilde is an OTA working on a subacute unit. Ruth, one of the older adults, was admitted after a total hip replacement. After reviewing her chart, Hilde finds out that Ruth has a history of AD. Both Micah and Hilde can provide practical suggestions to better help these older adults with AD function. This chapter provides background information about AD and occupational therapy interventions.

An estimated 5.8 million Americans have AD. AD is the sixth leading cause of all deaths in the United States, and the fifth leading cause of death among Americans age 65 and older.[1] Between 2000 and 2018, heart disease deaths

decreased nearly 8%, stroke deaths decreased 12%, and prostate cancer-related deaths only increased 1.3%, whereas deaths attributable to AD increased 146.2%.[1] Every 65 seconds, someone in the United States develops AD, and, by 2050, this time is expected to decrease to every 33 seconds.[2] It has been projected that the Baby Boomer population would add 25 million people to these numbers.[3] In 2050, the incidence of AD in the United States is expected to approach 14 million people.[1]

From a worldwide standpoint, in 2010, it was projected that the incidence of AD would be expected to nearly double every 20 years. With 35.6 million people having the disease in 2010, the incidence was expected to rise to 65.7 million and 115.40 million by 2030 and 2050, respectively, if a cure was not found.[4] The projection for 2050 has already increased. With 50 million people having the disease in 2020, the 2050 projection has climbed to 152 million people if a cure is not found.[1]

Dementia does not follow a uniform or single predictable course. Dementia syndrome includes unpredictable fluctuations in basic memory, judgment, and performance.[5] Although delirium, depression, medications, and metabolic dysfunction may cause a reversible dementia, nonreversible dementia may be caused by small strokes (vascular dementia), dementia with Parkinson's disease, dementia with Lewy bodies, frontal lobe dementias, and AD.[1] AD is the most common form of dementia and accounts for 60%–70% of cases.[6] AD is a progressive, degenerative, and fatal disease of brain tissue that leads to memory loss and problems with thinking and carrying out daily life activities. Participation in routine occupations, using good judgment, being aware of surroundings, communicating effectively, and coping with life become more difficult as the disease progresses. Problems start gradually and become more severe over time, leading to a total disruption in performance patterns and the inability to participate in most areas of occupation.[7] Although the rate of change varies, the usual stages of Alzheimer's dementia are mild, moderate, and severe (Table 20.1).[7,8]

Individuals 65 and over on average survive with AD for 4–8 years but some have lived as long as 20 years. Most people die after 8 years, often from pneumonia or other systemic problems. Causes of AD are not known, but current research suggests the involvement of two abnormal structures called plaques and tangles as prime suspects in damaging and killing nerve cells.[6] Plaques are deposits of a protein fragment called beta-amyloid that build up between nerve cells. Tangles are twisted fibers of another protein called tau that form inside dying brain cells. Although most people develop some plaques and tangles as they age, those with AD tend to develop far more. These plaques and tangles tend to form in a predictable pattern, beginning in areas important in learning and memory, and then spreading to other regions.[1] With the help of standardized diagnostic criteria, physicians can now diagnose AD with an accuracy of 85%–90% once symptoms occur.[9] Intervention is based on the combination of medical and psychosocial support.[1] Two types of medications are often used (cholinesterase and memantine) to support communication among nerve cells and delay problems with learning and memory.[10] Concerns have been raised about the growing number of herbal remedies, vitamins, and other dietary supplements being promoted as memory enhancers or interventions for AD. Claims of their effectiveness and safety are based mostly on anecdotal evidence.[11] Because of unknown side effects or potentially dangerous interactions with prescribed

TABLE 20.1

Three Stages of Alzheimer's Disease	
Early/mild impairment stage	Average 2–4 years, possibly longer
	Memory loss, especially with recent or new events
	Difficulty with complex cognitive tasks
	Difficulty performing tasks in social settings
	Misplacing or losing valuable items
	Lack of spontaneity and lessening of initiative
	Impaired word-finding skills
	Difficulty with planning and organization tasks
Mid/moderate impairment stage	Average 2–10 years, possibly longer
	Chronic recent memory loss
	Difficulty remembering personal history and information
	Tendency to withdraw from mentally challenging situations
	Difficulty with written and spoken language
	Possible delusions, hallucinations, and agitation
	Increasing difficulty with familiar objects and tasks
	Assistance with ADL functions necessary
	Tendency to wander, pace, and rummage
	Changes in sleep patterns
Late/severe impairment stage	Average 1–3 years
	Dependent on others for daily personal care
	Unaware of their surroundings
	Difficulty with walking and sitting
	Difficulty with chewing and swallowing
	Incontinence
	Difficulty communicating
	Vulnerable to infections
	Impaired ambulation/gait, increased falls
	Repetitious movement or sounds

medications, the OTA should encourage the older adult and/or caregivers to consult a physician before beginning use of any alternative or complementary medicine approaches. The National Center for Heath Statistics of the CDC[12] reported that 47.8% residents of nursing homes in the United States have AD or some other form of dementia. OTAs work with older adults who have AD and related dementia in hospitals, nursing homes, assisted living facilities, adult day programs, special care units, and homes. Occupational therapy interventions for these older adults usually focus on participation in the various areas of occupation by concentrating on performance skills and patterns or modifying activity demands in considerations of various client factors and, within the older adult's context and environments, to the highest degree possible.[13]

PERSON-CENTERED AND OCCUPATION-FOCUSED CARE FOR OLDER ADULTS WITH COGNITIVE IMPAIRMENTS

Like all human beings, older adults who have AD or related dementia continue to seek meaningful participation in life. Although sometimes the behavior brought on by AD may make it appear as though they no longer are the same person they once were, it is important to remember that they are not defined by the dementia.[14,15] Personhood, as described by Kitwood,[16] refers to one's sense of self, the "I am" within each person. Kitwood described indicators of personhood and well-being for individuals with dementia, including the assertion of desire or will, the ability to experience and express a range of emotions, initiation of social contact, self-respect, humor, creativity, and self-expression. Person-specific or person-centered daily care supports older adults with dementia and enhances and promotes their sense of personhood and meaning in life.[17]

The OTA developing a therapeutic program for older adults with dementia individualizes care that supports wellness, strengths, and abilities. This personalized, or person-centered, care also supports the components of activity-focused care that recognizes that all of life is an activity of being and doing or, as occupational therapy philosophy articulates it, of seeking meaning through occupation.[18] The tasks of life, therefore, are interconnected. The objectives of occupation-focused care include concentrating on abilities, not limitations; promoting the purposeful and meaningful use of time; supporting the sense of belonging; and enabling verbal and nonverbal communication skills. Occupation-focused care encourages positive behaviors and the development of interventions to refocus unwanted behaviors.[18,19]

Occupation-focused care redefines interventions, especially in long-term care settings and special care units. Success is achieved through augmenting the client's strengths by reframing expectations and relating to all daily life tasks as parts of meaningful occupation. It involves the willingness to enter the client's world with sensitivity, flexibility, and the provision of holistic support. In this process, the OTA must remain mindful that the goal is for the client to find meaning, not for the caregivers, staff, or occupational therapy personnel to understand such meaning.[20]

Communication: Understanding and Being Understood

Communicating with people who have AD is often challenging. As the disease progresses, verbal abilities decrease and communication continues through nonverbal gestures and sounds. Verbal and nonverbal communication reflects the same objectives: expressing thoughts and needs, and supporting the older adults' self-image and sense of worth. Other objectives for communication include improving socialization, maximizing quality of life, increasing involvement in a supportive community, understanding others, and promoting safety and comfort. OTAs must care enough to listen carefully. During the early stages of AD, changes that occur in language and communication include the onset of difficulty with using nouns. Substituted words are sometimes used for the noun.[21,22] For example, Mary was asked to identify an object (a comb). Her response was, "Oh, honey, you know," as she ran her hand through her hair. She was unable to use the noun *comb* but the gesture denoted she knew what the object was.

Reality orientation is usually embarrassing for older adults with AD because of their inability to remember and retrieve words to answer questions. One type of response that maintains the dignity of older adults with disorientation is to refrain from confronting them with corrections, especially if the confrontation would increase agitation. Caregivers should use creative reality with older adults by focusing on the emotions being expressed and responding appropriately by validating feelings. Improvements in orientation and subjective sense of quality of life may result from verbal cues that encourage the person to use information processing rather than factual knowledge.[23]

A strategy called "therapeutic fibs" can be used as illustrated by the following story. Jim states, "My wife is taking me home in 5 minutes." In reality, the intervention session has an additional 30 minutes remaining. Sue, the OTA, agrees with him, stating that he and his wife will soon be together and he has a wonderful, caring wife. Sue realizes that a discussion of the amount of remaining time would increase Jim's agitation. Sue, having validated Jim's desire for his wife, can then redirect him to do a meaningful task. Older adults asking for their mothers or wanting to go home may be seeking acceptance and the need to feel connected. They may also be expressing the need for safety, purposeful use of time, or the company of others. Telling them that their mother is dead or the facility is now their home can upset them. Instead, the OTA may say, "You are safe with me, and I will be here today with you. If you are like your mother, she must have been wonderful. I miss my mother too; we used to have fun folding the laundry; perhaps you and I can work together." The purpose of such communication is to acknowledge the meaning or emotion behind an older adult's statement.[22]

As the disease progresses, the ability to speak and understand decreases. Some older adults become more intuitive, often with increased awareness of people's attitudes and the environment.[24] Therefore, caregivers should be aware of their nonverbal messages such as acting rushed, looking at the clock, sighing, or raising one's voice. In time, older adults with AD lose almost all language skills, but they may still occasionally utter a perfectly appropriate statement.[25] For example, Juan talked a lot, but his words were just sounds that made no sense. When a caregiver impatiently spoke to him in an abrupt and firm tone, saying "Juan, time out; go to your room," Juan responded, "In the military, I was in solitary confinement, and I can do that standing on my head." The family later confirmed that Juan had indeed been in the military and the story was true. The caregiver's "drill sergeant" tone and body posture triggered Juan's response.

People with AD need to experience acceptance and success, especially as their language skills diminish. OTAs can keep the dialogue going even when the words are few (Box 20.1).[22]

Behavior and Psychosocial Aspects

People with dementia are not "stupid"; they are forgetful and often maintain an inner wisdom. Like anyone else, they have needs and should be approached and cared for with respect. They also should have opportunities for proud and meaningful involvement. Knowledge of the older adults' life story often becomes the basis for OTAs to plan and carry out therapy. A "Life Story" book can be used for this purpose. This book can include pictures with captions, lists, favorite recipes, family traditions, schools attended, and military history. Using the book is an excellent tool for connecting with older adults and as an intervention to refocus difficult behaviors and to reduce agitation.[26,27]

The behaviors of people with dementia are often attempts to communicate. For example, increased agitation may be the client's way of communicating illness. Rapid pacing might be a sign of an inability to cope with others, escape from excessive noise, or environmental factors.[22]

Some of the typical behaviors displayed by people with AD include wandering, pacing, and rummaging or redistribution of personal belongings. Combativeness and aggression also can occur. Catastrophic reactions are explosive responses to distress.[22] These reactions result from the inability to understand, interpret, and cope with real or imagined situations, people, the environment, or

---

BOX 20.1

Suggestions for Improving Communication and Connectedness

- Attract the client's attention by using touch and talking to them at eye level.
- Use short, simple sentences to express one thought at a time. Be willing to repeat as needed, allowing time for the older adult to respond. Do not appear rushed; offer the older adult your full attention. Assess and limit distractions from the environment, such as the television, vacuum cleaners, and loud nearby conversations.[22]
- Be aware that asking questions can be frustrating for people with AD, who often have difficulty finding the right words for the answer. Instead, help them respond by giving as many multisensory verbal or nonverbal cues as possible. If asking a question, offer two choices. For example, ask Ella if they would like to shower before breakfast or after breakfast, showing them the towel and clean clothing that you are holding. Allow the individual plenty of time to respond to the question.
- Do not try to apply logic or to give long explanations. Ignore the need to be right, to argue, or to confront. At times having information written down for older adults helps them focus and understand, especially when they ask the same question repeatedly. For example, providing Richard with a business type letter with their name on it that states that their apartment has been paid in full and that they have a place to spend the night helps them retain the information. Be willing to supply this letter as often as he needs for reassurance of having a place to stay.
- State requests with positive words ("Please sit here" rather than "Don't sit there").
- Listen carefully to all of the words, gestures, and facial expressions that the person uses. Validate feelings behind the words. For example, if Henry's words seem to make no sense but sound angry and upset, say, "You sound upset, Henry. I know when I feel that way I like a hug. Can I give you a hug?" However, be aware that some people are tactile defensive and become agitated when touched.
- Realize that older adults with AD often respond literally to words (because the fire alarm says "pull," Hazel pulls it).
- Consider supplementing your words with your nonverbal communication strategies such as gesturing, touch, smiles, and nods.[22]

---

oneself. "Sundowning" results from a combination of increased behavioral responses occurring in the mid-to-late afternoon. These responses often reflect physical problems such as dehydration and physical/emotional exhaustion. Screaming, yelling, and calling often reflect fear, a need for acceptance, and a lack of active participation and connectedness during the day. Other behavioral manifestations may include inappropriate sexual conduct, hitting or pushing staff or other older adults, accusing or demanding speech, withdrawal from activities, and apathy. Older adults with AD might also show perseveration in their actions by repetitious movement or sounds, such as wiping or patting the table surface, pulling on clothing, and shouting.[28]

Difficult behaviors are usually not done on purpose as a method of making care more difficult; rather, they are often part of the disease. At times, behaviors can be a problem to others but not to the older adult.[22] For example, Betty, who lives in a special care unit, goes into other people's rooms. She looks through their closets and takes clothing and items from their drawers. This behavior suggests that Betty likes to feel in control and is "cleaning up the house." Whose problem is it? Carmen, the owner of these possessions, is angry and feels that her privacy has been invaded. The facility staff meets the challenge of working with both people in a supportive way by identifying acceptable places for Betty to rummage, such as a bureau or desk in the social center and "busy boxes" or baskets filled with safe items. Examples of items to include in a "busy box" are balls of yarn, greeting cards, small scrapbooks, car brochures, maps, catalogs, fabric pieces, and carpet samples. Having Betty participate in the purposeful activity of carrying safe items can help address her need to feel connected.

A respectful response exists for every behavior. In some cases, attempting to reason with people with AD may not work, especially if they mistake others for people whom they do not like. Logic also may not work, especially with people who are having visual or auditory hallucinations.[22,29] Usually, OTAs can identify the event that precipitated the unwanted behavior and make adjustments that might prevent it, stop it, or decrease the likelihood of

BOX 20.2

Behavior Profile
■ WHAT exactly is happening?   ■ WHY has the behavior happened?   ■ WHAT was the antecedent?   ■ WHO is involved?   ■ WHERE is the behavior exhibited?   ■ WHEN does the behavior usually occur?   ■ WHAT now?

recurrence. Three problem-solving tools can help refocus unwanted behavior: the behavioral profile, the behavioral analysis, and the behavioral observation form.

The behavioral profile is a tool used to examine the situation. OTAs can ask themselves the following thought-provoking questions: What exactly is happening? Why has the behavior happened, and what was the antecedent? Who is involved, and where is the behavior exhibited? When does the behavior usually occur? What now? (Box 20.2)

The behavioral analysis outlines the specific behavior by focusing on the client's actions and defining the antecedent or possible causes. In addition, it outlines acceptable approaches and interventions with attention to the effect on the family, environment, and activity (Table 20.2).

The behavior observation form is used to determine a behavioral pattern involving the time of day and possible antecedents. This form can help OTAs and other health care workers make appropriate changes for reducing or refocusing difficult behaviors (Fig. 20.1).

The challenge of identifying the source of the difficult or unwanted behavior and a solution to the problem also requires critical reasoning. The following

TABLE 20.2

Problem: Pacing, Wandering, or Both (Behavior Analysis Approach)	
Behaviors exhibited	Pacing with increases in speed, intensity, and length of time; unable to respond to normal fatigue. Trying to exit area without supervision. Displaying increased agitation, anxiety, frustration, pushing, or kicking. Seemingly lost; packing and leaving. Searching behavior for something unattainable (e.g., mother). Inappropriately going into areas/rooms not their own.
Possible cause or antecedent	May have feelings of fearfulness, insecurity. May be reflecting on a past life role such as being in the workforce or being a parent. May want to escape. May be feeling out of control or sensing overmanipulation by others. May be searching for something familiar or something lost. May be acting consistent with former habits (always "on the go") or doing a stress-reducing activity. May reflect need for self-stimulation as a method to reestablish sense of well-being. May be expressing a physical need such as hunger, constipation, or illness. May result from anxiety, boredom, hyperenvironmental or hypoenvironmental stimulation.

Continued

TABLE 20.2

Problem: Pacing, Wandering, or Both (Behavior Analysis Approach)—cont'd

Interventions with the resident	Ask what the wandering is "telling" you: whether the client is hungry, needs to void, feels uncomfortable, is really lost.
	Identify positive aspects of the pacing/wandering.
	When attempting redirection, use a calm approach with eye contact.
	Use distraction techniques to break up the pacing pattern (offer to sit with the older adult, have a glass of juice).
	Monitor older adults for unwanted weight loss and excessive fatigue.
	Monitor older adults for increased risks for falls and compromised safety.
	Have older adults wear Medic-Alert ID bracelet of Alzheimer's Association's "Safe Return" program.
	Take photographs for the police, if elopement is a factor.
	Avoid stressful situations such as excessive environmental stimulation, too many people present, or overwhelming demands.
	Provide regular and consistent routines with familiar staff and caregivers.
	Develop a "head count" system for at high risk for elopement.
Family/caregiver focus	Discuss treatment approaches.
	Provide information on policies and procedures.
	Provide information such as the phone number of the local Alzheimer's Association chapter and their "Safe Return" program.
	Instruct not to contradict the older adult's stories; instead, they should assure the older adult that everything will be all right. This helps facilitate a sense of security and reduces feelings of fearfulness.
	Recommend to not overdramatize entrances, exits, and promises to return.
	Encourage walks with the older adult and usage of walking areas, "discover" paths, or fitness trails.
	Inform of possible risks for elopement even when the treatment area has a security system.
	Encourage use of local support groups for discussions with others.
Facility adaptations	Provide environmental changes and sensory stimulation to decrease stress and restlessness, and to increase physical well-being, gross motor skills, appetite, and healthy fatigue.
	Allow for environmental changes that promote purposeful ways to spend time.
	Remove environmental cues that suggest leaving the facility, such as coats and suitcases.
	Use familiar objects in rooms that facilitate a sense of comfort and security.
	Install Dutch doors, if permitted by regulations.
	Design walking areas, "discover" paths, or fitness trails within the care setting that offer safe, monitored spaces for pacing.
	Develop procedures to follow such as periodic unit safety checks and checks for missing persons.
	Provide routine orientation and escorts for new admissions.
	Alert visitors to facility procedures. For example, when leaving an area, visitors should turn around and check that wandering older adults have not followed them out of the door.
	Employ experienced, trained staff who know the older adults.
	Introduce the older adult to all staff, especially those near the doors (e.g., switchboard operators and receptionists).
	Write problems/interventions on a Kardex after identifying any positive aspects from the physical activity of pacing and wandering.
Activity	Support physical exercise to promote overall wellness.
	Offer to walk with the older adult as a meaningful activity. Suggest that the older adult help out by taking letters to be mailed, visiting a friend, or picking up laundry.
	Establish a walking club, keep track of miles walked, and provide club t-shirts.
	Provide supervised outings with a focus on safety and the reduction of elopement risks.
	Offer expressive arts that include large muscle groups and movement or dancing activities.
	Present routine, familiar, normalized activities that promote sense of connectedness, respect, and meaningfulness.
	Set up a fitness trail that includes repetitive upper and lower extremity movements such as doing pulley activities, finger climbing ladders, and deep knee bends. Train volunteers and family members to involve the older adults with the trail's activities.

Name:							
Date	Time	Observed activity and behavior	Behavior				Observer
			Trigger (What started it)	Intervention (What stopped it)	Time elapsed •Before stopping •Stayed stopped		

FIG. 20.1 Behavioral observation form.

are some questions that OTAs can ask themselves to help with the critical reasoning process: What is this behavior "saying"? Whose problem is it? What are some environmental factors that might be contributing to the behavior?

The story of Alfonso, an older adult in an AD special care unit, illustrates the importance of critical reasoning in addressing difficult or unwanted behaviors. Alfonso tries constantly to go out the door because he thinks it is time to go to work. Possible reasons for his attempts to leave include the time of day, that he sees visitors leaving with their hats and coats, and lack of involvement in meaningful activities. The staff may not be trained to redirect him when his anxiety and agitation increase, the day room may be too noisy, or he may believe that the intercom voice is calling him to the phone. The OTA might consider the following options: asking him to help with a project (he might forget his need to leave), painting the exit door the same color as the walls on either side so it appears less obvious, involving Alfonso in a meaningful activity (drawing ideas from his life story), and spending some quality time with Alfonso.

Audrey is another person in the same unit. She often becomes combative when performing ADL functions, especially showering. In fact, she strikes the OTA during an assessment of showering. The OTA considers possible causes for this behavior: Did Audrey formerly take baths, and is she unhappy with the change in her routine? Is Audrey a very private person, and is she embarrassed that

someone is helping her? Did she react to the OTA's tone of voice? Is Audrey getting sick and unable to report it? Is she too tired when the shower is scheduled? Is she experiencing chronic pain such as arthritis, which may be upsetting her? Does she feel rushed? Has the showering task been simplified enough so that she can participate and feel in control? The OTA then considers the following behavioral interventions: asking Audrey to help wash down the shower, singing Audrey's favorite hymn with her while she showers, postponing the shower for another time, and allowing Audrey to bathe with some of her clothes on or wrapping her in a bath blanket during the bathing process.

As illustrated by the preceding examples, handling the behavioral difficulties of older adults who have AD can be a trial-and-error process until OTAs identify solutions that work. Each older adult will respond differently. Different techniques, based on the person's abilities, can succeed one time and fail the next. Even when OTAs cannot ascertain the exact reason for the behaviors, they can try the following intervention techniques. Distraction is a helpful technique, especially if the person is agitated. OTAs can be creative with ideas for distraction that involve the person in a meaningful activity, such as listening to music or offering a snack. Rescuing is another distraction technique: When one caregiver is in conflict with the client, a second caregiver responds by "rescuing" that person. This technique is illustrated by the following example. Sally, a nursing assistant, says to Theresa, the resident, "Don't go out the door." If Amy, the OTA, approaches Theresa in the same fashion, Theresa might feel outnumbered. Conversely, if Amy says, "Sally, Theresa and I want to be alone; please leave us," Theresa might feel "rescued" and go with Amy.

Inappropriate timing, attempts to manipulate the older adult to fit a schedule, and unrealistic performance expectations can cause negative behavior such as hitting. Consequently, caregivers must be aware of the older adult's mood before approaching with an ADL or social event.

INTERVENTION

Observations, Screening, and Assessment

As with any occupational therapy client, the first step in the occupational therapy process is assessment and development of the client's occupational profile. The profile helps to provide the OT/OTA team with an understanding of why the client is seeking services, what the client's current concerns are to engaging in occupations, as well as provides the team with the client's occupational history and experiences, patterns of daily living, interests, values, and needs. From the occupational profile, the client's priorities are determined.[13] Later, the OT/OTA team should analyze the older adult's occupational performance to identify the individual's problems, or potential problems more specifically. During this phase of the evaluation, the individual's actual performance is observed, often in context, to identify what supports performance and what hinders performance. The team may also be "selecting and using specific assessments to measure client factors that influence performance skills and performance patterns."[13] Performance skills, performance patterns, context or contexts, activity demands, and client factors are all considered, although in some situations not all of them are specifically assessed.[13] This helps the team identify targeted outcomes.

The OT/OTA team may collaborate in the administration of the following evaluations among others. The Folstein Mini-Mental State is a short and simple quantitative measure of cognitive performance. This measure is a questionnaire in five areas of cognition, including orientation, registration (memory), attention, and calculation, as well as recall and language (following oral and written instructions).[30] The Global Deterioration Scale measures clinical characteristics at seven levels based on the progressive stages of AD.[31]

The Allen Cognitive Performance Tests and the Routine Task Inventory examine cognitive function through the completion of tasks.[32] The levels of function help predict behavior and effects on ADL functions. These levels range from the ability to use complex information and perform ADL functions accurately and safely to severe deficits in recognition and use of familiar objects. This assessment includes information on communication, response to tasks, and need for task simplification. It also addresses the role of the therapist during intervention. (See Chapter 7 for a more detailed explanation of these tests.)

The Cognitive Performance Test is a standardized functional assessment instrument designed for the evaluation of Allen cognitive levels.[33] Six functional tasks—dressing, shopping, making toast, making phone calls, doing laundry, and traveling—comprise the test. This test also looks at the person's abilities to process information in relation to functional performance.

The importance of the OTA being an integral part of the overall treatment team with other disciplines cannot be stressed enough.[34,35] The continuous development of dementia-specific assessments provides the treatment team with sensitive, appropriate tools that not only bring together information about the older adult's challenges, but also encourage the recognition of the client's personhood and how to build on current strengths and abilities.[36,37] For example, the Person, Environment, Occupation measurement model helps determine how AD affects the function of both the person with this disease and his or her family.[38]

Intervention Planning

Occupational therapy for people with AD most often involves attention to participation in self-care and leisure occupations, consideration of communication and functional mobility, and careful regard for safety. Areas to address in intervention planning include decreased attention span, the inability to initiate tasks, difficulty with sequencing tasks, impaired judgment, and overall wellness. Intervention planning begins with establishing a cognitive and functional baseline and includes ability-based goals. These goals should identify functional capacity and the need to restore, maintain, or improve skills. The goals should focus on abilities and opportunities for participation in activities that support cognitive, physical, and psychosocial wellness. These goals should include interventions that enable person-centered caregiving and refocus difficult behaviors in a supportive and safe environment.

Intervention planning should include the use of assessment and observation to measure changes in functional status. The process of intervention planning includes providing and suggesting continuous modifications and adaptations of approaches, such as task simplification and cueing. The older adult's life story may be used as the basis for intervention that focuses on past (and present) wisdom and experiences. Intervention planning also involves assessing all aspects of intervention support and factors that lead to negative responses, including environmental components.[17,39] For example, Andrew's limited attention span prohibited him from eating more than a few mouthfuls of each meal. He was seated in a large dining room with five other people at his table. Music was played on the tape deck, and the staff often talked loudly with each other. When the OTA suggested relocating Andrew to a small dining area where the tables seated two and reducing the environmental stimulation, he was able to focus on his food and complete his meal.

Intervention Implementation

Occupational therapy interventions consider the effects of dementia on the older adult's cognitive abilities and well-being. Success with interventions entails many crucial components, including the OTA's flexibility and creativity. Success may need to be redefined, as exemplified by Beverly, a resident of a special care unit. Beverly liked to wear a yellow floral blouse and her favorite orange and black plaid skirt. She was proud of her ability to select and dress independently, although some disapproved of her choices.

Equally important for successful intervention is the OTA's nonverbal approach. It should reflect acceptance and respect for the older adult with AD. To ensure success, intervention should not place older adults in situations in which their inabilities may lead to failure. For example, Clara had always been a talented knitter of lovely sweaters. Her ability to do intricate stitches became impaired as her dementia progressed. The OTA set up the stitches on large needles and helped her get started knitting squares using a basic stitch. Clara was able to knit the simple squares for a baby blanket and was delighted in the recognition of her success. This activity could be further adapted by involving Clara in winding yarn as her knitting abilities diminish.

Applying life history and experiences to functional abilities also is meaningful. For example, Sara, a 78-year-old mother of five, responds to normalization activities such as washing dishes, hanging laundry, and sweeping floors. These activities provide tactile stimulation, lower and upper body range of motion, strengthening, trunk stabilization, and fine hand motor skills.

OTAs can use their skills in analyzing activities to identify steps toward task simplification. Harry was able to dress himself independently when each item of clothing was placed on his bed in the appropriate sequence for dressing. Successful intervention also should focus on working with older adults to promote active participation and collaboration. Charles had lost interest in feeding himself but accepted the OTA's suggestion to have the caregiver place a hand over his hand. That way he could continue to feed himself with assistance rather than being fed by others.

When possible, intervention should be provided in appropriate and familiar settings.[40] For example, Millie was unable to experience success with simple dressing tasks when she attempted them in the clinic. However, when the OTA arrived at Millie's bedside early each morning, Millie was able to use visual cues found in her bedroom, including the bureau and closet, to trigger self-dressing skills.

Activities of Daily Living

OTAs can make a significant contribution to the well-being of older adults with AD and enhance their quality of life by supporting ADL occupations. Understanding the activity's demands, breaking down and simplifying tasks, and so on enable these older adults to become involved in performing familiar skills. Understanding can be facilitated by using one-step commands and visual cueing, including objects or gestures. The use of the Allen's stage levels can be a helpful measure of the older adult's level of functioning.[41]

Difficulties with ADL occupations associated with dementia include a decreased attention span, limited ability to follow directions, and increased length of time to complete tasks. Other difficulties include problems with sequencing, perception, and body awareness. Emotional responses of fear, paranoia, and reactions to excessive environmental stimulation that are real or imagined also can influence ADL functioning. Aggressive behavior of older adults with cognitive impairments can significantly affect ADL outcomes.[22]

Modifications in the ways in which people with AD carry out daily activities can help maintain their independence longer and even regain some lost function. Further maintaining engagement in meaningful activities for longer periods of time reduces dementia-related behaviors such as screaming, wandering, and physical aggression. The consistent use of directed verbal prompts and positive reinforcement maximizes ADL functional status, particularly with feeding.[22,42] OTAs working on ADL functions will be most successful when they use creative problem-solving. Therapy requires working with older adults, not doing to or for them.[22,43] OTAs should do everything possible to make ADL functions meaningful. The use of distraction techniques (e.g., singing and holding items such as costume jewelry, scarves, and neckties) should be part of daily care. The OTA's attitude, approach, and direct involvement are key components in supporting the older adult's quality of life.

OTAs should consider the timing when working on ADL functions. Often, these decisions are based on knowing the older adult and responding to nonverbal language that suggests the best and worst times for these activities. Sometimes, OTAs must come back several times because many older adults with AD are sensitive to being rushed. For example, Charles appeared agitated when the OTA wanted to work on dressing skills. After several attempts, the OTA decided to return later. At that time, Charles was calmer and accepting of the activity.

Assisting with ADL functions can also provide opportunities for OTAs to monitor the older adult's physical well-being and safety. Older adults with AD often do not report bruises, rashes, and blisters. Decreased cognitive ability and judgment, combined with an unawareness of perceptual difficulties, may lead to unsafe situations. Older adults may eat dirt or plants, walk on wet floors, put their shoes on the wrong feet, forget necessary items such as glasses, misjudge a chair seat and fall, or scald themselves in the shower because they do not know how to turn on the cold water—all of these are examples of potential dangers.

When working with older adults on ADL functions, OTAs should always focus on abilities by encouraging active involvement. The techniques of hand-over-hand guidance, chaining, and bridging can be used. Hand-over-hand guidance may help the older adult complete the ADL task. With chaining, the caregiver begins a task by putting one hand over the older adult's hand and continuing until the older adult can take over and complete the task. For example, Astrid had no idea what a toothbrush was or how to use it. However, when the OTA placed it in her hand and guided it to her mouth to start the brushing action, Astrid was able to complete the task independently. With these techniques, the palmar surfaces of the hand or the surface receiving touch during a handshake can be a more "accepting" surface than the back of the hand. OTAs should establish contact with the older adult's palm before moving their hand around to the dorsal surface if needed for assisting the older adult during activities.

With bridging, older adults who are unable to perform any part of the daily living task can focus their attention by holding the same object the caregiver is using. This technique also can help to decrease anxiety. For example, Allan could not shave. The OTA demonstrated to the caregivers a bridging technique to try with Allan. The OTA placed a turned-on electric razor in his hand so he could feel the vibration while the OTA shaved him with another electric razor. By holding a razor, Allan was better able to focus attention on the task.[22]

The creativity and flexibility of OTAs can promote the remaining abilities of older adults and their willingness to be actively involved in daily life tasks (Table 20.3). Knowledge of the client's past routines is helpful during ADL functions.

Using Adapted Equipment

Older adults with AD often refuse or misuse adapted equipment. Improper use may affect the older adult's safety, especially if the item does not look familiar. For example, a plate guard may appear so strange that the older adult with AD might spend the mealtime trying to remove it from the plate. Sometimes, large, built-up handles on eating utensils may feel so different that clients do not use them. Reachers and other metal devices used for ADL functions can be used as weapons. Flatware with large handles and scoop dishes can be helpful because they closely resemble their ordinary counterparts. Adapting the environment by using color contrast between objects, pictures, words, labels, and

TABLE 20.3

	Suggestions for Provision of Activities of Daily Living Support for Older Adults With Alzheimer's Disease
Bathing	Know whether client prefers a bath or shower; use handheld shower head.
	If privacy is an issue, older adult can bathe with some clothing on or with a bath blanket.
	If needed, older adult may wash one part of the body per day until able to accept total bathing.
	Consider safety by using adaptations such as bath seats, grab bars, and floor mats.
	Create a warm and homelike bathing environment. Placing colorful beach towels on the walls can help reduce the room's echo and loud water sounds. The towels also can be used to wrap older adults if they become agitated during clothing removal.
	Consider alternatives such as having a family member present to assist with bathing to help reduce the older adult's anxiety.
Shaving	Use a mirror unless older adults do not recognize themselves or feel that they are being "watched."
	Use a bridging technique with older adults incapable of actually shaving. Have them hold an electric razor that they can see, feel, and hear while shaving them with another electric shaver.
Oral care	Use a child-sized tooth brush.
	Pretend to be brushing your own teeth and encourage older adults to mirror the activity.
	Use bridging technique of asking the older adult to hold an extra set of dentures while removing the older adult's dentures.
	Set up a simulated dental chair and announce that the dentist has sent you to assist with dental care.
	Set up a monitor system so that presence of dentures are checked after each meal in case older adults have wrapped them up in a napkin for disposal.
Dressing	Suggest clothing one size larger for dressing ease. Keep the clothes appropriate to the older adult's past lifestyle.
	Use verbal and visual cues to simplify each step, and always thank the older adults for helping.
	If older adults become anxious, ask them to show you how the clothing items are put on.
	If possible, use washable shoes with Velcro closures.
	Use 100% cotton clothing because it does not retain the odor of urine.
	Ask the older adult to sit when dressing, especially if balance is a concern.

TABLE 20.3

Suggestions for Provision of Activities of Daily Living Support for Older Adults With Alzheimer's Disease—cont'd

Toileting	Be aware of older adult's past toileting routines and habits.
	Use pictures of toilets with the word "toilet" on the bathroom doors.
	Determine whether the bathroom mirror prohibits older adults from using the toilet because they do not recognize their image and think someone else is there.
	Be sure the toilet seat color contrasts with the floor. Change the seat or use a washable rug around the toilet base.
	Use key words to remind the older adult about the task. Often, the words they used when toilet training their children work well.
	Offer the older adult something (e.g., a magazine) to hold or do while seated on the toilet.
	Never refer to pads for incontinence as "diapers" (use terms such as panties or shorts).
	Have different types of incontinence products available. Do not assume that a full-sized item is needed immediately. For example, a pad placed within a panty can be used if urine is leaked.
	Use suspenders to keep full-sized incontinence products in place.
Eating[a]	Observe eating for safety problems such as overstuffing the mouth, not chewing before swallowing, and eating nonedibles (napkins, foam cups). If the older adult is storing food in the mouth, check for a clear swallow. Obtain a swallowing evaluation if a problem is apparent.
	Offer the meal in a quiet area to decrease distractions and to improve attention span. If the food needs to be set up, always do that out of the older adult's sight. This prevents reinforcement of the older adult's inability to perform certain simple tasks.
	Provide color contrast between the food and the plate and the plate and the table.
	Avoid plastic utensils, which are easily bitten and broken.
	Obtain, if appropriate, a dietary order for variation in food textures.
	Simplify the meal by serving one item and one utensil at a time.
	If older adults will not sit to eat, use finger foods or have a small bowl that can be easily carried.
	Incorporate food into a sandwich. Pureed food can be put into an ice cream cone to assist older adults who want to continue self-feeding.
	If older adults are not eating and no medical reasons prohibit it, use sugar or honey on the food to increase palatability.
	After a swallowing evaluation, if deemed appropriate, provide nonsalty chicken or beef broth that can be poured over the food for a more "slurpy" consistency to facilitate an appropriate swallow.
	If the older adult needs to be fed, bridge the task by having the older adult hold a spoon or plastic cup.
	If the older adult is disinterested in eating, alternate bites of hot and cold foods and sweet and nonsweet food.
	When the older adult appears to stop eating or has lost all interest in food, ask the family to identify the older adult's "comfort foods" to facilitate reinterest in eating.
	Foods such as mashed potatoes and gravy, pizza, and macaroni give a sense of well-being.
	If weight loss is a problem, double the older adult's breakfast.
	Try to avoid commercial food supplements, if possible, by allowing time for the meal to be eaten and providing protein-enriched foods such as milkshakes.
	Sit with the older adult. Have something to eat or drink to reduce the older adults' anxiety that they need to share some of their food with you.
	If older adults refuse to eat because of not having money, provide a letter stating that their dues to your association (the name of your facility or place of practice) have been paid in full and meals are included in their membership.

[a]See discussion of dysphagia in Chapter 18 for more specific information about safe eating.

arrows is often the best way to cue for successful involvement in ADL functions.

Using Activities to Promote Well-Being

Activities can be adapted for individuals and groups. The objectives of therapeutic activities are enhancing meaning, encouraging active participation, and ensuring success. All of life's activities can be used as intervention modalities. Suggestions for cognitive activities are adapted trivia games, word puzzles, rhyming games, singing of familiar songs, and reminiscence. Others include spelling games, simple crafts, clothes-sorting, cards, and Life Story "book clubs." Suggestions for physical activities include parachute exercises; dancing; and tossing, hitting, and kicking balls and balloons. An exercise program may include the use of handheld wands, light weights, scarves,

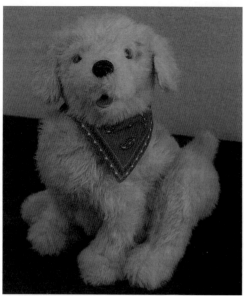

FIG. 20.2 This battery-operated puppy "companion" assists older adults with memory impairments enjoy the psychosocial benefits of owning a pet without the required care. *(Courtesy Johnny Barfield)*

and fabrics. Psychosocial activities include parties, service projects, grooming tasks, celebrations of special days, field trips, and real or stimulated pet care (Fig. 20.2). Worship and related spiritual activities may offer older adults with dementia a sense of the familiar, well-being, and security. Recommendations for normalizing activities are folding and hanging up laundry, dusting and sweeping, sorting silverware, and shining shoes.[22,43]

Environment-based interventions appear to have some positive effect on reducing agitation of people with dementia. Simulations of a natural environment (e.g., use of recorded sounds of babbling brooks, birds, and other small animals; large pictures of the outdoors) during bathing reduce agitation and can improve the relationship between caregivers and the individual.[44] There is some evidence that ambient, nonvocal music has some calming effect on people with AD.[44,45] The OT/OTA team should consider this intervention as part of a multisensory stimulation program or as part of the background feature of a dining room, for example. However, music selection may need to be matched to the person's taste. Because of the low cost, these types of interventions could be implemented in institutional, community, or home settings.

Communication With and Teaching Caregivers

Occupational therapy intervention with older adults who have AD focuses on maintaining functional abilities and preventing secondary complications. These objectives can be achieved by tailoring communication and education to caregivers. About 16 million family members, friends, and neighbors provide 18.6 billion hours of unpaid care for persons with AD each year.[1] This care is estimated to

make an annual contribution to the nation valued at $244 billion.[1] About two-thirds of unpaid caregivers are wives, daughters, daughters-in-law, granddaughters, and other female relatives, friends, and neighbors. At any one time, 86% of family and other unpaid caregivers of people with AD have been providing help for at least the past year, 57% have been providing care for 4 or more years, and 49% expect to continue having caregiving responsibility for the next 5 years.[1]

Caregivers benefit from a variety of techniques, including written instruction and demonstration. The instructional method of requiring a "return demonstration" allows OTAs to observe first-hand that caregivers follow through with activities. Afterward, the OTA can make necessary suggestions or corrections. As the dementia progresses, caregivers provide more and more care, until they can no longer manage their caregiving responsibilities on their own. Caring for a person with AD is often very difficult, and caregivers have high rates of anxiety, stress, and burnout.[1] Their life expectancy is reduced, and 30%–40% are depressed.[1,46] Encouraging caregivers to strengthen their social support system for the long term should be a basic component of OT intervention.[47] A basic occupational therapy plan for people with AD should include providing caregivers with information about progression of disease, referral to community resources, practical ideas for caregiving, and understanding of how the caregiving role is different from other family roles.[47,48]

The OTA/OT team can formulate a maintenance program.[49,50] Contributing to a maintenance program may require OTAs to sensitize caregivers to the nature and progression of AD. An understanding of task breakdown and simplification, activity modification, behavioral interventions, supportive communications, and the need for flexibility is essential in maintenance programs.

MILD COGNITIVE IMPAIRMENT

Mild cognitive impairment (MCI) is estimated to affect 15%–20% of older adults over age 65.[51] MCI is a classification of cognitive impairment at its early stages. Cognitive impairment, like many other disorders, can be associated with a spectrum. In this way, MCI lies on one end of the spectrum, end stage dementia or Alzheimer's disease lies on the other end, with various levels between the end points. At its heart, MCI is a disorder in the thinking or memory processes of a person that are outside the normal level for their age.[52] MCI does not have a specific cause; however, advancing age, along with other medical conditions (i.e., diabetes, CVA, sleep apnea) have been attributed to increasing risk of MCI.[51]

MCI, AD, and dementia have similar symptoms; however, MCI symptoms are less severe and are not attributed to the personality changes seen in dementia/AD.[52] Older adults with MCI exhibit symptoms of memory lapse such as misplacing items, forgetting events or appointments, word finding problems, and increased frustration with their "forgetfulness."[53] The symptoms are still mild enough that the older adult is able to complete the majority of their ADLs and other daily occupations independently. The completion of occupations does take both more cognitive and physical energy for completion.

Research has indicated that older adults with MCI are more likely to develop dementia or AD.[51,52] Though MCI is a stand-alone diagnosis in the DSM-V, the OTA treating the older adult with MCI relies on their training for all cognitive impairments. Occupational therapy interventions for MCI are based on the individual symptoms exhibited by the older adult and are rooted in their occupational profile, goals, and interests. Occupational therapy practitioners can also take a health and wellness approach for the client with MCI. OTAs can facilitate appropriate wellness strategies for the client regarding exercise, healthy eating, and monitoring of other comorbidities as well as strategies for scheduling with members of their care team for follow-up care every 6–12 months.[51]

LATE STAGE ISSUES

Severe dementia, or late-stage, is exhibited when the older adult is oriented only to person and depends entirely on others for self-care. Defining the exact time of terminal, or end-stage, AD is difficult because of changes and variations in the disease process.[8,54] For example, Vernon appeared to have entered the terminal stage because he had been refusing food for 2 weeks. When offered familiar "comfort" foods from his past and sweet foods, he suddenly started to eat again.

Many older adults at the late stage of AD are kept in bed or positioned in wheelchairs or recliners. Unfortunately, those kept in bed often lie in the fetal position. These older adults are dependent on others for basic life functions and display an almost total loss of communication skills or the ability to express pain.[8,55] To help make them more comfortable, OTAs may provide positioning suggestions and passive range-of-motion exercises. A caring touch, hand-over-hand movement, and various sensory activities may produce a response. Some people become ill with symptoms leading to pneumonia or other systemic problems shortly before death. This is an important time for supporting family members and staff caregivers.[7,56]

REIMBURSEMENT FOR SERVICES

A functional outcome must be meaningful, utilitarian, and sustainable over time. Currently, the maintenance of remaining abilities of older adults with dementia, or any chronic illness, is not usually covered by third-party payers such as Medicare unless there is a need for "skilled" therapeutic coverage. (See Chapter 6 for more details on reimbursement for services under the Medicare Part A system in Skilled Nursing Facilities.) For older adults on Medicare Part B, the OTA/OT team may address cognitive and physical impairment related to functional performance. Medicare will reimburse for cognitive disabilities that require "complex and sophisticated knowledge to identify current and potential capabilities."[57] All levels of assistance from total to standby address both physical and cognitive components. Table 20.4 outlines the cognitive components

TABLE 20.4

Medicare Cognitive Levels of Assistance	
Assistance level	**Cognitive assistance**
Total assistance	Total assistance is the need for 100% assistance by one or more persons to perform all cognitive assistance to elicit a functional response to an external stimulation. A cognitively impaired patient requires total assistance when documentation shows external stimuli are required to elicit automatic actions such as swallowing or responding to auditory stimuli. Skills of an OT are needed to identify and apply strategies for eliciting appropriate, consistent automatic responses to external stimuli.
Maximal assistance	Maximum assistance is the need for 75% cognitive assistance to perform gross motor actions in response to direction. A cognitively impaired patient, at this level, may need proprioceptive stimulation and/or one-to-one demonstration by the OT because of the patient's lack of cognitive awareness of other people or objects.
Minimum assistance	Moderate assistance is the need for 50% assistance by one person or constant cognitive assistance to sustain/complete simple, repetitive activities safely. The records submitted should state how a cognitively impaired patient requires intermittent one-to-one demonstration or intermittent cueing (physical or verbal) throughout the activity. Moderate assistance is needed when the OT/caregiver needs to be in the immediate environment to progress the patient through a sequence to complete an activity. This level of assistance is required to halt continued repetition of a task and to prevent unsafe, erratic, or unpredictable actions that interfere with appropriate sequencing.

Continued

TABLE 20.4

Medicare Cognitive Levels of Assistance—cont'd	
Assistance level	**Cognitive assistance**
Standby assistance	Standby assistance is the need for supervision by one person for the patient to perform new procedures adapted by the therapist for safe and effective performance. A patient requires such assistance when errors are demonstrated or the need for safety precautions is not always anticipated by the patient.
Independent status	Independent status means that no physical or cognitive assistance is required to perform functional activities. Patients at this level are able to implement the selected courses of action, demonstrate lack of errors, and anticipate safety hazards in familiar and new situations.

Note: The Physical Levels of Assistance are not included in this chart.
From Centers for Medicare and Medicaid Services (CMS). *Medicare program integrity manual.* Retrieved from http://www.cms.hhs.gov/manuals/downloads/pim83c06.pdf.

only. Behavioral issues with cognitive impairment can be focused on if they require skilled occupational therapy services.[57]

The OTA/OT team may suggest a short-range program on the basis of continuous functional support, especially if a change in functional status has occurred. Often, older adults with AD who receive Medicare reimbursement for care have an initial evaluation from occupational therapy. A maintenance program is then developed by the therapists and carried out by facility staff. Medicare will reimburse if skilled occupational therapy is needed to evaluate a "complex" patient to increase function or safety, and then to train staff to carry out the program.[57] The OT evaluates the older adult and establishes the plan of care. The OTA may train caregivers to carry out the plan. Occupational therapy practitioners may manage the older adult for re-evaluation when significant changes occur in functional status. As discussed in Chapter 6, memorandums from Medicare prevent automatic denials just because a person has the diagnosis of AD and mentions benefits for therapeutic intervention with this diagnosis.[57]

CONCLUSION

OTAs can make a unique contribution to older adults with AD. OTAs can treat these older adults from the initial stages of forgetfulness and poor judgment by offering strategies for continuing independence. OTAs may also provide advice about late-stage care by focusing on positioning, feeding, and responses to sensory activities. Understanding the changes that occur as dementia progresses challenges older adults, caregivers, and families to pursue creative and supportive solutions for daily care. The holistic programs and care provided by OTAs support the abilities and well-being of older adults. When offered occupation-focused care, older adults with dementia can have meaningful lives.

TECH TALK: FOCUS ON PRESERVING MEMORY

NAME	PURPOSE	APPROX. COST	WHERE TO BUY
Digital Story Book	Various products designed to lead the user through the process of developing a personalized digital story book of memories for a person with dementia.	Varies by device and service	Various
Day and Date Clock	Clock with display of digital time and date as well as details including "morning," "afternoon," or "evening" and the day of the week to facilitate orientations.	~$59.99	Amazon
Jitterbug	Cell phone designed with simplified menus and larger format for ease of use by persons with visual or cognitive impairments. Flip phone and smart phone options available.	~$49.99 to ~$79.99	Livelydirect.com

CASE STUDY

Mildred is 78 years of age and has mid-stage AD. Mildred was formerly a teacher and experienced a happy family life with her husband of 58 years and their two sons. She has been widowed for the past 5 years. Mildred was originally brought to the special care unit where she currently resides when she was found wandering outside during the cold winter months.

At the special care unit, the OTA helps to assess Mildred's functional status. The OTA identifies the following abilities: Mildred follows one-step directions, responds to multisensory cueing, maintains strong socialization skills, and refers to her former profession by often mentioning her past role as a teacher. She also mentions her past interest in the activities of cooking and sewing.

Mildred functions at Allen's Cognitive Level 3. The OTA observes that she is forgetful, with limited instructional carryover. Mildred experiences problems with sequencing ADL functions. She often becomes anxious, which leads to combativeness during ADL functions, especially bathing. Other assessment findings include the inability to toilet independently and use multiple utensils with meals. Communication challenges included receptive and expressive understanding of words, especially nouns.

The OTA instructs all staff members who work with Mildred to consider her strengths, as well as their attention span deficits and feelings of depression, as she attempts to cope with her disease.

■ CASE STUDY QUESTIONS

1 Considering Mildred's case, how can visual triggers and written phrases be used to help Mildred be as independent as possible?
2 What anxiety-reducing approaches can be explored? What specific interventions can be used during bathing?
3 How can the OTA develop a system for sequencing Mildred's clothing?
4 What environmental issues might need to be addressed, especially in the bath/shower room?
5 What suggestions can be incorporated as mealtime interventions for promoting successful dining?
6 If Mildred can find the toilet, what strategies can enable her to remain continent?
7 How can the OTA use ADL functions as therapeutic modalities for reducing feelings of depression and helplessness?
8 How can the OTA make Mildred's care "person-centered" and "activity-focused"?

■ CHAPTER REVIEW QUESTIONS

1 In reference to the entire chapter, what are the basic symptoms of AD, and how do they affect older adults with the disease and their caregivers?
2 Identify six ways to facilitate communication with older adults who have dementia.
3 How can a functional assessment be used to develop intervention goals?
4 List three guidelines for the provision of ADL support to older adults functioning at the moderate level of AD.
5 Outline six specific mealtime adaptations for older adults with a short attention span.
6 List steps for getting dressed using task simplification.
7 What are possible antecedents and appropriate interventions for agitation?
8 Why do people with dementia wander, and how can the risk for elopement be decreased?
9 Give specific examples of ways that activity-focused care supports OTAs' interventions.
10 Describe strategies to adapt the activity of folding laundry to address the older adult's cognitive, physical, psychosocial, and normalization needs.

EVIDENCE NUGGETS: EFFECTIVENESS OF INTERVENTIONS TO REDUCE AGITATION AND WANDER OF OLDER ADULTS WITH ALZHEIMER 'S DISEASE OR DEMENTIA

1. Bennett S, Laver K, Voigt-Radloff S, et al. Occupational therapy for people with dementia and their family carers provided at home: a systematic review and meta-analysis. *BMJ Open.* 2019;9(11):e026308. Published 2019 Nov 11. doi:10.1136/bmjopen-2018-026308
   - OT services provided at home significantly decreased the number of behavior problems and psychological problems for older adults with dementia.
   - OT services provided at home significantly improved function during ADLs and IADLs and improved the quality of life for older adults with dementia.
   - Caregiver distress due to behavioral issues can be improved by occupational therapy services provided in the home with older adults who have dementia.
2. Jensen L, Padilla R. Effectiveness of Environment-Based Interventions That Address Behavior, Perception, and Falls in People With Alzheimer's Disease and Related Major Neurocognitive Disorders: A Systematic Review. *American Journal of Occupational Therapy.* 2017;71(5):1-10. doi:10.5014/ajot.2017.027409
   - Ambient music was found to decrease agitation, wandering, and overall behavior for those with Alzheimer's disease and other neurocognitive disorders except at mealtime.

- In 1 study, proprioceptive input provided by an air mat led to a short-term reduction in wandering behaviors.
   - Moderate evidence was found to support individualized environmental modifications and multisensory environments led to a decrease in agitation for older adults with Alzheimer's disease and other neurocognitive disorders.
3. Gage H, Hamilton L, Goodman C, et al. Managing behavioural and psychological symptoms in community dwelling older people with dementia: 1. A systematic review of the effectiveness of interventions. *Dementia (14713012).* 2019;18(7/8):2925-2949. doi:10.1177/1471301218762851
   - In 2 studies, training of caregivers did not have an effect on agitation or quality of life for older adults with dementia.
   - An intervention focused on both behavior and training on communication, coping, and lifestyle improved behavioral and psychological symptoms of dementia in one dyadic study examining older adults.
   - Tailored activity programs (TAP) provided by occupational therapists, which included six 90-minute home visits and two sessions by phone, led to decreased agitation in patients with dementia in one pilot study.

Continued

EVIDENCE NUGGETS: EFFECTIVENESS OF INTERVENTIONS TO REDUCE AGITATION AND WANDER OF OLDER ADULTS WITH ALZHEIMER 'S DISEASE OR DEMENTIA—cont'd

4. Gitlin LN, Arthur P, Piersol C, et al. Targeting Behavioral Symptoms and Functional Decline in Dementia: A Randomized Clinical Trial. *Journal of the American Geriatrics Society*. 2018;66(2):339-345. doi:10.1111/jgs.15194
   - Tailored activity programs for veterans (TAP-VA) consisted of 8 sessions with occupational therapists who performed assessments then educated caregivers about dementia and about implementing activities tailored for each specific client.
   - 4 months after the implementation of the TAP-VA program, veterans showed a statistically significant improvement in behavioral problems.
   - 4 months after the implementation of the TAP-VA program, caregivers experienced a statistically significant decrease in stress related to veterans' behavioral symptoms.
5. Oliveira AM, Radanovic M, Homem de Mello PC, et al. An intervention to reduce neuropsychiatric symptoms and caregiver burden in dementia: Preliminary results from a randomized trial of the tailored activity program-outpatient version. *International Journal of Geriatric Psychiatry*. 2019; 34(9):1301-1307. doi:10.1002/gps.4958
   - The Tailored Activity Program – Outpatient (TAP-O) intervention consisted of an assessment of the older adult with dementia, education on dementia and on stress-reduction techniques, 3 activities tailored to the patient, and generalization of communication strategies to daily activities.
   - After the TAP-O intervention, there was a statistically significant decrease in the Neuropsychiatric Inventory-Clinician rating scale (NPI-C) agitation scores (14.73 to 9.73; p =0.03) for older adults with dementia.
   - After the TAP-O intervention, there was a statistically significant decrease in the NPI-C aberrant motor behavior scores (7.45 to 4.30; p=0.02) for older adults with dementia.

REFERENCES

1. Alzheimer's Association. *2020 Alzheimer's Disease Facts and Figures*. 2020. Available at: https://www.alz.org/media/Documents/alzheimers-facts-and-figures.pdf.
2. Bright Focus Foundation. *Alzheimer's Disease: Facts & Figures*. 2019. Available at: https://www.brightfocus.org/alzheimers/article/alzheimers-disease-facts-figures.
3. Thompson D. *As Baby Boomers Age, Alzheimer's Rates Will Soar*. WebMD; 2015. Available at: https://www.webmd.com/health-insurance/news/20150720/as-baby-boomers-age-alzheimers-rates-will-soar#1.
4. Alzheimer's Disease International. *World Alzheimer's Report 2009: Executive Summary*. London: Author; 2009.
5. National Institute on Aging. *Alzheimer's Disease Fact Sheet*. 2019. Available at: https://www.nia.nih.gov/health/alzheimers-disease-fact-sheet.
6. The University of Queensland. Types of Dementia. Queensland Brain Institute. https://qbi.uq.edu.au/brain/dementia/types-dementia n.d.
7. Ellis ME. *The Progression of Alzheimer's Disease: What Are the Stages?* Healthline; 2017. Available at: https://www.healthline.com/health/stages-progression-alzheimers#stage1.
8. Alzheimer's Association. *Stages of Alzheimer's Disease*. 2018. Available at: https://www.alz.org/media/documents/alzheimers-stages-early-middle-late-ts.pdf.
9. Texas Health and Human Services. *Diagnosing Alzheimer's Disease*. 2020. Available at: https://www.dshs.texas.gov/alzheimers/diagnose.shtm.
10. Alzheimer's Association. *Medications for Memory*. 2021. Available at: https://www.alz.org/alzheimers-dementia/treatments/medications-for-memory.
11. Alzheimer's Association. *Alternative Treatments*. 2021. Available at: https://www.alz.org/alzheimers-dementia/treatments/alternative-treatments.
12. Harris-Kojetin L, Sengupta M, Lendon JP, Rome V, Valverde R, Caffrey C. Long-term care providers and services users in the United States, 2015-2016. National Center for Health Statistics. *Vital Health Stat*. 2019;3(43). https://www.cdc.gov/nchs/data/series/sr_03/sr03_43-508.pdf.
13. American Occupational Therapy Association. Occupational therapy framework: domain and process fourth edition. *Am J Occup Ther*. 2020;74(suppl 2):1-87.
14. Wilkins JM. Dementia, decision-making, and quality of life. *AMA J Ethics*. 2017;19(7):637-639.
15. Mayo Clinic. *Dementia*. 2019. Available at: https://www.mayoclinic.org/diseases-conditions/dementia/diagnosis-treatment/drc-20352019.
16. Kitwood T. Toward a theory of dementia care: ethics and interaction. *J Clin Ethics*. 1998;9(1):23-34.
17. Fazio S, Pace D, Flinner J, Kallmyer B. The fundamentals of person-centered care for individuals with dementia. *Gerontologist*. 2018;58(1):S10-S19.
18. Wood W. *Activity-Focused Dementia Care: Meaningful Activities*. Alzheimer's Research & Resource Foundation; 2020. Available at: https://ararf.org/lesson/activity-focused-dementia-care-meaningful-activities/.
19. Fazio L. *Developing Occupation Centered Programs for the Community*. 3rd ed. Thorofare, NJ: Slack Incorporated; 2017.
20. Alzheimer's Association. *A Guide to Quality Care from the Perspective of People Living with Dementia*. 2020. Available at: https://www.alz.org/getmedia/a6b80947-18cb-4daf-91e4-7f4c52d598fd/quality-care-person-living-with-dementia.
21. Salehi M, Reisi M, Ghasisin L. Lexical retrieval or semantic knowledge which one causes naming errors patients with mild and moderate Alzheimer's disease. *Dement Geriatr Cogn Disord Extra*. 2017;7:419-429.
22. Alzheimer's Association. *Family Care Guide: A Guide for Families Caring for Someone with Alzheimer's Disease or a Related Dementia*. 2021. Available at: https://www.alz.org/media/manh/documents/alzheimer_s-family-care-guide-(fcg).pdf.
23. Heerema E. *Using Reality Orientation in Alzheimer's and Dementia*. Verywell Health; 2020. Available at: https://www.verywellhealth.com/treating-alzheimers-disease-with-reality-orientation-98682.
24. Novy C. Life stories and their performance in dementia care. *Arts Psychother*. 2018;57:95-101.

25. Banovic S, Zunic LJ, Sinanovic O. Communication difficulties as a result of dementia. *Mater Sociomed.* 2018;30(3):221-224.

26. Elfrink TR, Zuidema SU, Kunz M, Westerhof GJ. The effectiveness of creating an online life story book on persons with early dementia and their informal caregivers: a protocol of a randomized control trial. *BMC Geriatr.* 2017;17:95.

27. Elfrink TR, Zuiderna SU, Kunz M, Westerhof GJ. Life story books for dementia: a systematic review. *Int Psychogeriatr.* 2018; 30(12):1797-1811.

28. Druan J, Julian MK. A look at sundown syndrome. *Nursing Made Incredibly Easy!* 2020;18(6):42-50.

29. Chiaravalloti ND, Goverover Y. *Changes in the Brain.* New York: Springer; 2017.

30. Rotstein A. Network analysis of the structure and change in the mini-mental state examination: a nationally representative sample. *Soc Psychiatry Psychiatr Epidemiol.* 2020;55:1363-1371.

31. Mougias A, Christidi F, Kontogianni E, Skaltsounaki E, Politis A, Politis A. Patient-and caregiver-related factors associated with caregiver assessed global deterioration scale scoring in demented patients. *Curr Gerontol Geriatr Res.* 2018;2018:9396160.

32. Earhart CA, Elgas K. *Brief History of the Cognitive Disabilities Model and Assessments.* Allen Cognitive Network; 2017. Available at: http://www.allen-cognitive-network.org/index.php/allen-cognitive-model.

33. Burns T, Lawler K, Lawler D, Mccarten JR, Kuskowski M. Predictive value of the cognitive performance test (CPT) for staging function and fitness to drive in people with neurocognitive disorders. *Am J Occup Ther.* 2018;72(4):7204205040.

34. Foster S, Balmer D, Gott M, Frey R, Robinson J, Boyd M. Patient-centered care training needs to health care assistants who provide care for people with dementia. *Health Soc Care Community.* 2019;27(4):917-925.

35. Cleveland University. *What Do OTAs Do...for Those with Alzheimer's and Dementia.* 2020. Available at: https://www.cleveland.edu/blog-post/~post/what-do-otas-dofor-those-with-alzheimers-and-dementia-20200612/.

36. Jarry C, Osiurak F, Baumard J, et al. Daily life activities in patients with Alzheimer's disease or semantic dementia: multitasking assessment. *Neuropsychologia.* 2021;150:107714. https://doi.org/10.1016/j.neuropsychologia.2020.107714.

37. Toyoshima K, Araki A, Tamura Y, et al. Use of dementia assessment sheet for community-based integrated care system 8-items (DASC-8) for the screening of frailty and components of comprehensive geriatric assessment. *Geriatr Gerontol Int.* 2020;20(12):1157-1163.

38. Wong C, Leland NE. *Applying the Person-Environment-Occupation Model to Improve Dementia Care.* AOTA CEU. Available at: https://www.aota.org/~/media/Corporate/Files/Publications/CE-Articles/CE-Article-May-18.pdf.

39. Kudlicka A, Martyr A, Bahar-Fuchs A, Woods B, Clare L. Cognitive rehabilitation for people with mild to moderate dementia. *Cochrane Database Syst Rev.* 2019;2019(8):CD013388.

40. Gramegna SM, Biamonti A. Environments as non pharmacological intervention in the care of Alzheimer's disease. *Des J.* 2017;20(1):S2284-S2292.

41. Allen CK. *Occupational Therapy for Psychiatric Diseases: Measurement and Management of Cognitive Disabilities.* Boston: Little Brown; 1985.

42. Prizer LP, Zimmerman S. Progressive support for activities of daily living for persons living with dementia. *Gerontologist.* 2018;58(1):S74-S87.

43. National Institute on Aging. *Adapting Activities for People with Alzheimer's Disease.* 2017. Available at: https://www.nia.nih.gov/health/adapting-activities-people-alzheimers-disease.

44. Eggert J, Dye CJ, Vincent E, et al. Effects of viewing a preferred nature image and hearing preferred music on engagement, agitation, and mental status in persons with dementia. *SAGE Open Med.* 2015;3:2050312115602579.

45. Abraha I, Rimland JM, Trotta FM, et al. Systematic review of systematic reviews of non-pharmacological interventions to treat behavioural disturbances in older patients with dementia. The SENATOR- OnTop series. *BMJ Open.* 2017;7(3):e012759.

46. Avargues-Navarro ML, Borda-Mas M, Campos-Puente AM, Perez-San-Gregorio MA, Martin-Rodriguez A, Sanchez-Martin M. Caring for family members with Alzheimer's and burnout syndrome: impairment of the health of housewives. *Front Psychol.* 2020;11:576.

47. Whitlatch CJ, Orsulic-Jeras S. Meeting the informational, educational, and psychosocial support needs of persons living with dementia and their family caregivers. *Gerontologist.* 2018;58 (suppl 1):S58-S73.

48. Eden SR. *Family Caregiving Roles and Impacts. Families Caring for an Aging America.* National Academies of Sciences, Engineering, and Medicine. 2016.

49. American Occupational Therapy Association. Guidelines for supervision, roles, and responsibilities during the delivery of occupational therapy services. *Am J Occup Ther.* 2020;74(suppl 3): 7413410020. Available at: https://doi.org/10.5014/ajot.2020.74S3004.

50. American Occupational Therapy Association. *Enhanced CMS Training and Education Required to Support Maintenance Therapy.* Federal Regulatory Affairs News; 2017. Available at: https://www.aota.org/Advocacy-Policy/Federal-Reg-Affairs/News/2017/Enhanced-CMS-Training-Education-Required-Support-Maintenance-Therapy.aspx.

51. American Psychological Association. Spotting the signs of Mild cognitive impairment. *Monit Psychol.* 2019;50(8). Available at: https://www.apa.org/monitor/2019/10/ce-corner-impairment.

52. United States Department of Health & Human Services National Institute on Aging. *What Is Mild Cognitive Impairment? Basics of Alzheimer's Disease and Dementia.* 2021. Available at: https://www.nia.nih.gov/health/what-mild-cognitive-impairment.

53. Alzheimer's Association. *Mild Cognitive Impairment (MCI).* 2021. Available at: https://www.alz.org/alzheimers-dementia/what-is-dementia/related_conditions/mild-cognitive-impairment.

54. Alzheimer's San Diego. *Recap: Preparing for the Late Stage of Alzheimer's Disease.* 2018. Available at: https://www.alzsd.org/recap-preparing-late-stage-alzheimers-disease/.

55. Alzheimer's Association. *Late-Stage Care. Providing Care and Comfort During the Late Stage of Alzheimer's Disease.* 2019. Available at: https://www.alz.org/media/Documents/alzheimers-dementia-late-stage-care-b.pdf.

56. Alzheimer's Association. *Late-Stage Caregiving.* 2021. Available at: https://www.alz.org/help-support/caregiving/stages-behaviors/late-stage.

57. Centers for Medicare & Medicaid Services. *Patient Driven Payment Model.* 2021. Available at: http://www.cms.hhs.gov/Manuals/.

chapter 21

Working With Older Adults Who Have Orthopedic Conditions

BRENDA M. COPPARD, RENÉ PADILLA, AND PATRICIA J. WATFORD

(PREVIOUS CONTRIBUTIONS FROM KAROLINE D. HARVEY AND TYROME HIGGINS)

KEY TERMS

arthroplasty, boutonnière deformity, closed reduction, comminuted fracture, compound fracture, delayed union, orthopedic, energy conservation, external fixation, fracture, joint protection, malunion, nonunion, open reduction internal fixation, orthoses, osteoarthritis, rheumatoid arthritis, spiral fracture, swan-neck deformity, thromboembolic deterrent hose, total hip replacement, transverse fracture, ulnar drift, wrist subluxation, work simplification

CHAPTER OBJECTIVES

1. Explain the causes of fractures in the older adult population.
2. Identify terminology related to fractures and their management.
3. Describe the precautions required after an ORIF and implications of such a procedure relative to occupational performance.
4. Describe the precautions required after a total hip replacement and the implications of such a procedure relative to occupational performance.
5. Identify adaptive equipment and modified methods of performance that benefit older adults with hip fractures.
6. Identify the signs and symptoms of osteoarthritis, rheumatoid arthritis, and gout.
7. Describe the effects of osteoarthritis, rheumatoid arthritis, and gout on occupational performance.
8. Explain the principles of joint protection, work simplification, and energy conservation.

The 2 weeks I spent in rehab were tough, but I had to learn how to walk all over again, just like a baby! Not only did the physical therapist teach me how to walk, the occupational therapist taught me how to dress, and how to do things around the house. They presented me with all sorts of new gadgets that would help me in my daily living.

—Linda, age 69, after her left hip arthroplasty.

Fractures of older adults 65 years of age and older are escalating in occurrence and are becoming a major health concern. The most common types of fractures found among older adults in the United States are lower trunk (pelvis, hip, and lower spine) accounting for 34% of fractures followed by upper trunk (upper spine, clavicle, and ribs) accounting for 13% of fractures (data from 2014).[1] With adults over 65, women are about two times more likely to suffer a fracture than men. In 2012, women accounted for approximately 71% of fracture cases.[2] Orthopedic problems may result in older adults

being hospitalized for a surgical procedure, rehabilitation, and possibly being placed temporarily or permanently in a long-term care facility. Older adults who sustain a hip fracture as a result of a fall have a 22% mortality rate within 1 year of the fracture.[3] The most common complications of older adults who undergo orthopedic surgery include possible stroke, cardiac failure, and severe infection.

The role of the occupational therapy assistant (OTA) and occupational therapist (OT) team is to help maximize the occupational performance of older adults who have orthopedic problems. Older adults who would otherwise need to enter an extended care facility are often able to go home as a result of occupational therapy intervention. OTAs must be familiar with orthopedic conditions and their effects on occupational performance to ensure that appropriate evaluation and intervention are carried out. This chapter addresses orthopedic problems and conditions that contribute to these problems.

FRACTURES

Causes of Fractures

Causes of fractures include falls, trauma from automobile accidents, osteoarthritis (OA), and metastatic carcinoma.[4] Other factors such as a current or previous smoking habit, alcohol abuse,[5] diabetes,[6] psychological dysfunction,[7] income,[8] and decreased level of physical activity also correlate with the incidence of fractures.[9]

The majority of fractures in older adults result from falls.[10] Factors associated with falling include vision impairment, postural hypotension, poor balance, side effects of medication, and muscle weakness.[11] Other factors include neurological and other chronic diseases, reduced alertness, incontinence, home hazards, fear of falling, and dementia.[11] (An in-depth examination of the causes of falls in older adults is provided in Chapter 14.)

The number of older adult drivers is increasing. In 2018, there were 45 million licensed drivers age 65 and older in the United States.[12] Despite their growing numbers, older adult drivers are involved in fewer fatal collisions than in previous years.[13] However, older adults have greater rates of fatal crashes per mile traveled than younger drivers due to age-related declines in cognitive, visual, and physical function.[14] Trauma resulting from auto accidents accounts for a portion of the fractures seen in the older adult population.

Older adults are more likely to sustain fractures after a fall because of osteoporosis and deficits in bone geometry and material properties, leading to bone fragility.[15] Stress fractures and other injuries also can occur in older adults who, for example, suddenly increase their levels of activity by walking farther and faster than usual or walking on a different terrain. However, many studies found this to be a general risk, not necessarily an increased overall risk for injury.[16] A very common fracture often related to osteoporosis that occurs with older adults is called a Colles' fracture. These wrist fractures of the distal radius result in "dorsal displacement of the distal fragment and radius shortening"[17] and usually occur because of a **fall on** an **o**utstretched **h**and (FOOSH).

Fractures may also be caused by cancer that has metastasized to bone. Although any cancer may metastasize to bone, metastases from carcinomas, particularly those that arise in the breast, lung, prostate, kidney, and thyroid, are most common. Metastatic lesions weaken the strength of bones and may lead to fractures.[18]

Types of Fractures

A fracture is a break in a bone. Although radiographs are used to diagnose the fracture, it does not reveal damage to soft tissues or cartilage. Fracture sites can disrupt the intraarticular, epiphyseal, metaphyseal, or diaphyseal portions of the bone. If a fracture occurs and dislocates a joint, it is a fracture-dislocation.[19]

Various terms are used to categorize fractures. A fracture is considered to be compound or open if the bone

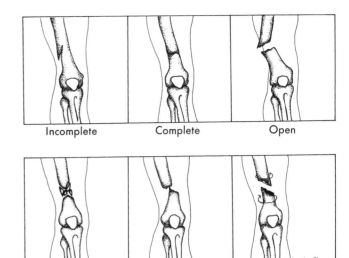

FIG. 21.1 TYPES OF FRACTURES. *(Modified from Garland JJ. Fundamentals of Orthopedics. Philadelphia: WB Saunders; 1979.)*

protrudes through the soft tissue and skin. If the soft tissue and skin are undamaged, the fracture is considered to be closed or simple. Different physical forces can result in certain types of fractures. A transverse fracture occurs as a result of a direct force, whereas a spiral fracture results from a circular or twisting force. A fracture that results in more than two bone fragments is a comminuted fracture. Fig. 21.1 shows these various types of fractures.

Medical Intervention for Fractures

The goals of medical management of a fracture are to reduce pain and align the fracture for proper healing.[19] The fracture can be aligned with or without surgery. The process of manually realigning (sometimes using traction devices) and then casting a fracture is termed closed reduction. The open reduction is a surgical procedure used to internally fixate the fracture site. Internal fixation is performed with the use of orthopedic nails, screws, pins, rods, or plates. When external fixation is used to align or reduce a fracture, the fixator device is attached with pins or wire inserted through the soft tissues and into the bone (Fig. 21.2). This device usually involves the use of screws and rods removed after the fracture has healed. The skin around placement sites of the rods or screws must be kept clean to prevent infection.

OTAs also should be familiar with terminology relating to the healing of fractures. Three terms used to describe fractures that do not heal well are delayed union, nonunion, and malunion.[19] Delayed union describes a fracture that heals at an abnormally slow rate. Nonunion describes a fracture that has not healed within 4–6 months. Malunion describes a fracture in which the bone heals in a normal length of time but with an unsatisfactory alignment.

Complications After Fractures

Several complications can occur after fractures.[19] Edema can lead to joint stiffness, and joint contractures often are

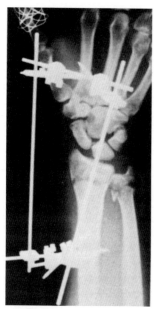

FIG. 21.2 External fixator in place to maintain reduction. *(From Hunter J, Mackin E, & Callahan A, eds. Rehabilitation of the Hand: Surgery and Therapy. 4th ed. St. Louis, MO: Mosby; 1995.)*

caused by adhesions or prolonged immobilization. After fractures, posttraumatic arthritis can occur in joints associated with or near the fracture site. Complex regional pain syndrome is a syndrome that often occurs after minor injuries. The condition is believed to affect the peripheral and central nervous system and presents with severe pain, increased sensitivity, edema, stiffness, muscle atrophy, muscle spasms, contractions, and loss of bone mineralization. Other symptoms include changes with skin temperature and color.[20] Myositis ossificans is the formation of heterotopic ossification near a traumatized area. The most common joints where heterotopic ossification forms are the arms, thighs, and hips.

Factors Influencing Rehabilitation

Several factors affect the outcome of rehabilitation efforts in older adults who sustain fractures. Age is a predominant factor in rehabilitation.[21] Older adults may need more time than younger persons to achieve their greatest levels of independence. For example, in older adults, a comminuted fracture of the proximal humerus should be immobilized for the shortest period possible to reduce the chances of development of adhesive capsulitis or frozen shoulder. With a younger person, the threat of such a complication may not always be a concern.

The general condition of older adults also affects the course of rehabilitation. For example, older adults who are in shock or are unconscious require different intervention than those who are alert and oriented. In addition, past and current medical conditions may affect the rehabilitation of older adults who have fractures. Older adults

with congestive heart failure or chronic obstructive lung disease may be limited in their abilities to participate in endurance and strengthening activities. Furthermore, a large percentage of older adults with fractures also have associated medical problems such as heart disease, cancer, diabetes, and hypertension.[22,23]

The presence of dementia often affects rehabilitation outcomes for older adults with fractures. For example, teaching the integration of hip precautions or joint protection methods while engaging in self-care tasks to an older adult with short-term memory deficits is difficult, and engaging the caregiver is important for effective intervention. (A detailed discussion of intervention considerations for older adults who have dementia is presented in Chapter 20.)

Although hip fractures are the most common type of fracture sustained by older adults, fractures of other bones also occur, such as Colles' fractures. OTAs should know the common fractures and general recommended intervention techniques (Table 21.1).

Colles' Fractures

Colles' wrist fractures are considered the most typical fracture in postmenopausal women reaching a peak incidence at 65 years of age and older.[24] Because these fractures are so common, OTAs may follow older adults with this condition in general practice. As previously discussed, various surgical approaches may be utilized to stabilize this fracture and other fractures although commonly plates and screws are inserted for unstable Colles' fractures.[17] If external fixators or pins are utilized, OTAs must be very careful with infection control procedures and provide clear education with their older adult clients. OTAs need to be in communication with the older adult's physician about wound control protocols. OTAs should be aware that there may be general decreases in upper extremity movement of noninvolved joints if older adults are being protective of their extremity. Therefore, while still stabilized, postsurgery older adults may be referred for range of motion of noninvolved joints. Many other complications can occur with Colles' fractures, such as complex regional pain syndrome, soft tissue damage, damage to the distal radioulnar joint (DRUJ), median nerve involvement, tendon rupture, or extensor and intrinsic tightness.[17] Postsurgery, after the immobilization period is over, getting back functional wrist extension is a key therapeutic goal, and fabricating a serial orthosis (an orthosis that is regularly adjusted to gradually increase range of motion) may be beneficial.[25] Other therapeutic approaches are edema control, scar management, and addressing pain and range of motion (especially wrist and forearm motions) to prevent stiffness. Because Colles' fractures are very common yet so complicated, it is important for OTAs to be in good communication with their OT partner and the physician.

TABLE 21.1

General Recommended Intervention Techniques for Upper Extremity Fractures

Fracture location	Precautions and/or contraindications	Acute injury treatment techniques	Treatment postimmobilization
Humeral	Keep elbow, wrist, and finger joints mobile or per physician's order; monitor for signs of edema; position upper extremity above heart if edema occurs and is not contraindicated for cardiac conditions; begin PROM with physician approval usually after radiographic confirmation of adequate healing; discontinue immobilizer or brace with physician's order.	Use shoulder immobilizer or plaster cast to immobilize; after removal, a humeral cuff brace can be used; immobilization period varies based on type of humeral fracture.	For stable fractures with no major displacement, work on controlling distal edema and tightness and begin early AROM at the shoulder; for nondisplaced (unstable) fractures, do AROM of wrist and hand immediately after immobilization and follow physician guidance for beginning AROM and PROM of the shoulder and elbow; generally with humeral fractures, consider doing isometric exercises during and after immobilization; Codman's exercises should be encouraged only in the absence of edema; some humeral fractures may require ORIF, so earlier active and passive ROM may be allowed with physician approval.
Elbow	Keep shoulder, wrist, and finger joints mobile or per physician's order; monitor for signs of edema; position upper extremity above level of heart if edema occurs and is not contraindicated for cardiac condition; PROM is contraindicated; discontinue immobilizer(s) with physician's order.	A plaster cast or elbow orthosis can be used to immobilize the elbow. The angle is based on which structures need to be protected.	Begin gentle, nonresistive AROM after removal of cast; perform AROM in a gravity-eliminated plane; PROM in the early stage is not advised; person may have difficulty regaining full elbow extension, but a functional arc should be regained for ADL.
Wrist (scaphoid)	Keep shoulder, elbow, and finger joints mobile or per physician's order; if an external fixator is in place, monitor sites for infection; clean pin sites per physician guidance; discontinue any orthoses with physician's order.	A plaster cast may be worn for 2 weeks to 2 months depending on the physician; a thumb spica orthoses can be used after cast removal to position thumb in CMC palmar abduction and MCP in 0–10 degrees flexion with the wrist in neutral.	When stabilized and cast is removed, AROM should begin doing wrist motions with physician guidance.
Colles' (distal radius)	Keep shoulder, elbow, and finger joints mobile or per physician's order; if an external fixator is in place, monitor sites for infection; clean pin sites per physician guidance; monitor for complex regional pain syndrome, soft tissue damage, damage to the distal radioulnar joint (DRUJ), median nerve involvement, tendon rupture, and extensor and intrinsic tightness; get hand and wrist moving once the wrist is no longer immobilized; discontinue any orthoses with physician's order.	A wrist orthosis is used after the wrist is no longer immobilized. Orthosis is positioned in the maximal wrist extension that the person can tolerate (up to 30 degrees) and is discontinued when appropriate to encourage functional wrist movement.	Begin ROM of wrist and forearm once bony union has occurred and wrist is no longer immobilized with physician guidance.

ADL, activities of daily living; *AROM*, active range of motion; *CMC*, carpometacarpal; *MCP*, metacarpophalangeal; *PROM*, passive range of motion; *ROM*, range of motion.
Note: Physicians may vary these protocols.
Adapted from Coppard BM, Lohman H. *Introduction to Orthotics: A Clinical Reasoning & Problem-solving Approach.* 5th ed. St. Louis: Mosby/Elsevier; 2019; Dutton M. *Dutton's Orthopedic Examination, Evaluation, and Intervention.* 3rd ed. New York: McGraw Hill Medical; 2012; Daniel MS, Strickland LR. *Occupational Therapy Protocol Management in Adult Physical Dysfunction.* Gaithersburg, MD: Aspen; 1992; Moscony AMB, Shank T. Wrist fractures. In: Wietlisbch, CM, ed. *Cooper's Fundamentals of Hand Therapy: Clinical Reasoning and Intervention Guidelines for Common Diagnoses of the Upper Extremity.* 3rd ed. St. Louis: Mosby; 2020.

Hip Fractures

At least 300,000 hip fractures occur annually in people older than age 65 years, and women experience three-quarters of all hip fractures.[26] Fractures of the hip are classified by the type and direction of the fracture line.

Hip fractures usually require an open reduction internal fixation (ORIF) or pinning procedure. The ORIF of the involved hip usually must be protected from excessive force through weight-bearing restrictions (Table 21.2).

The amount of time required for a hip fracture to heal depends on the older adult, the fracture site, the fracture type, and the severity of the injury. In the past, most incisions for hip surgeries were 12–18 inches in length; however, now, more common surgical approaches involve less cutting of muscle, tendons, and ligaments.[27]

Many health care providers in hospitals follow a protocol or clinical pathway that outlines the timeframe for each professional's rehabilitation tasks.[28] Out-of-bed therapy activities for persons with an ORIF may be initiated 2–4 days after surgery.[21] Most function returns within 6 weeks to 6 months after the fracture occurs; most persons experience little improvement in function from 6 months to 1 year after sustaining a fracture.[29]

Weight-Bearing Restrictions

Depending on the type and severity of the fracture, the physician may restrict the amount of weight bearing allowed on the involved hip while the person is walking. Most weight-bearing restrictions are observed for 6–8 weeks, during which time the person may use crutches or a walker to ambulate.[21] OTAs must be aware of any weight-bearing precautions before initiating therapy and should know the terminology related to weight-bearing restrictions (see Table 21.2).

JOINT REPLACEMENTS

Total Hip Arthroplasties

Total hip arthroplasties (THAs), or total hip replacements (THRs), are often elective surgeries indicated for reducing pain and restoring motion for older adults who have severe OA, rheumatoid arthritis (RA), or ankylosing spondylosis. Emergency THAs frequently follow traumatic injuries to the hip, such as after a motor vehicle accident or fall. A hip replacement, or arthroplasty, may be full or partial. During a full hip arthroplasty, the hip's ball and socket are replaced with metal or metal and plastic prosthetic implants.[30] During a partial joint replacement, which is commonly used for fractures of the femoral neck and head, the femoral neck and head are replaced with a prosthesis. Hip prostheses last approximately 15–20 years or longer in three-quarters of older adults.[31] When radiographs show evidence of loosening of the cement and the client is experiencing pain, a hip revision arthroplasty may be performed.

The two basic surgical approaches for THAs are the anterolateral approach and the posterolateral approach.[32] When an anterolateral approach of surgery is used, older adults must avoid adduction, external rotation, and extension of the operated hip. If a posterolateral surgical approach is used, older adults should avoid flexion beyond 90 degrees, adduction, and internal rotation of the operated hip.[32] OTAs must be aware of which type of surgical approach was used to properly carry out OT intervention. OTAs also should note the position precautions for each surgical approach.

The movement precautions are usually observed for 6–12 weeks as indicated in a physician's order (Table 21.3).[32]

TABLE 21.3

Motion Precautions for Clients Who Have Had a Total Hip Replacement	
Approach	**Position precautions**
Anterolateral[a]	1. Hip external rotation 2. Hip adduction 3. Hip extension
Posterolateral	1. Hip flexion beyond 90 degrees 2. Hip internal rotation 3. Hip adduction

[a]Some surgeons perform anterior hip replacements with no precautions. Consult with the surgeon for specific precautions.

TABLE 21.2

Weight-Bearing Terminology	
Term	**Definition**
Nonweight bearing (NWB)	No body weight is borne on the involved side.
Toe-touch weight bearing (TTWB)	No weight is borne on the heel; weight is borne on the toes only.
Partial weight bearing (PWB)	A partial amount of the body weight can be borne on the involved side; usually a percentage of body weight (e.g., 50% PWB) or pounds (PWB with 50 lb) is stated.
Weight bearing as tolerated (WBAT)	Weight bearing is allowed to the extent that it does not cause the older adult too much pain; the older adult tolerates the weight bearing.
Full weight bearing (FWB)	Full body weight is borne on the involved side.

Cemented THAs usually have no weight-bearing restrictions. When cement is not used, bony ingrowth is used to secure the prosthesis to the older adult's bone. Often, 6–8 weeks of weight-bearing restrictions are required when this type of prosthesis is used.[32]

After THA surgery, physicians often instruct clients to wear thigh-high thrombo-embolic deterrent (TED) hose when out of bed. Clients are instructed to wear this type of hosiery because it assists with blood circulation, prevents edema, and reduces the risk for deep vein thromboses. If an older adult has not been instructed to wear TED hose and complains of pain or swelling in the affected leg, the physician should be consulted immediately because it could be a sign of the presence of a thrombus. OTAs should be skilled in donning and doffing antiembolus hosiery because they may need to assist older adults before bathing. If the hose are to be worn for a length of time, caregiver training should occur because it is often difficult for older adults to perform this task independently.

Researchers show that there are several milestones during rehabilitation, including adherence to hip precautions; ambulating 100 feet with a mobility aid; independence with home exercise program; and requiring supervision only with toileting, transfers, and activities of daily living (ADL).[33]

Three areas reported in research studies that are important concerns for clients with THA are sexual activity, driving, and work return.[34] In a study of 86 clients with THA, 50% of preoperative clients reported experiencing difficulties with sexual activities because of hip problems, and 90% of these clients reported a desire for more information about sexual functioning after THA. The majority of clients (55%) resumed sexual activity within 2 months of the THA with physician approval and following positioning precautions. Most people report that the supine or missionary position during intercourse is the most comfortable,[34] and evidence supports this position as the safest one.[35] (A detailed discussion of addressing sexuality including THA with older adults is presented in Chapter 12.)

After surgery, driving reactions normalize between 3 and 8 weeks if older adults resume good leg control. Return to work activities is dependent on the amount of stress and torque on joints. Typically, older adults must take off from work for 3–6 weeks after surgery.

A number of studies exist on appropriate leisure activities after a THA.[34] A survey of 28 orthopedic surgeons from the Mayo Clinic recommended that activities such as cycling, golfing, and bowling are acceptable after a THA.[34] Generally, many physicians counsel well older adults to avoid participation in sports that impart high torque or stress on the hip joint, such as jogging. Often, active older adults resume activities and athletics regardless of physician or therapist warnings.

Psychosocial Issues After Total Hip Replacement

A number of psychosocial issues may surface during an older adult's rehabilitation after a hip replacement. Dealing with a chronic condition such as arthritis can be stressful and frustrating; many older adults are required to cope with pain, swelling, and mobility limitations on a daily basis. Providing information on support groups may be beneficial to the older adult.

After a THA, some older adults find it difficult to abide by the position precautions. They may view these precautions as impediments to resuming the lifestyles they had before the procedure, especially when they had no predisposing medical conditions that limited activities. OTAs should be empathetic to the older adult's concerns, but they must also help older adults understand the rationale for adhering to hip precautions. The OTA also should address the consequences of not following these precautions. OTAs may need to reassure older adults that healing takes time and that involvement in activities may continue but usually with some modifications.

Many older adults feel guilty or become anxious when they require assistance from family or friends.[36] Older adults who are temporarily placed in an extended care facility while they heal may also find it difficult to accept assistance from nursing staff in the facility. Feelings of guilt are sometimes accompanied by financial worries about the cost of care. In addition, relocation to a new environment such as a hospital, extended care facility, or long-term care facility can be stressful.[37] OTAs should encourage older adults to talk about their feelings. When possible, discussing the situation with older adults before they are moved to a new facility is beneficial. In addition, the older adult should be thoroughly oriented to the new facility.

Occupational Therapy Interventions

The specific intervention strategies and techniques used with an older adult who has had a THA vary depending on whether the anterolateral or posterolateral surgical approach was used (Table 21.4). Adaptive equipment is typically supplied to patients regardless of approach. The most suggested piece of adaptive equipment tends to be the raised toilet seat, which often is used for at least 6 months after THA. Other pieces of equipment that can be helpful include the long-handled reacher, long-handled shoehorn, and sock aid; however, they did experience some difficulties in using them. OTAs are involved in educating older adults and their caregivers about proper and safe usage of adaptive equipment, observing hip precautions during functional activities, and making environmental adaptations.

Stephanie is an OTA who works in an acute care hospital and is involved in patient education. Before having a hip replacement, older adults and their primary caregivers attend a class to prepare them to return home. Stephanie reviews the precautions for both the posterolateral and

TABLE 21.4

Occupational Therapy Interventions for Posterolateral and Anterolateral Approaches to Total Hip Replacement

Bed mobility Walking	▪ Abduct legs with wedge or pillows to prevent hip rotation and adduction. ▪ Avoid pivoting on the leg that has been operated on. ▪ When approaching corners, take small steps in a circular fashion. ▪ If possible, take 10- to 15-minute walks four times per day 6–8 weeks after the operation. ▪ Walk at a slow, comfortable pace.
Chair transfers	▪ Sit on chairs with firm seats, preferably with arm rests. ▪ Avoid low, soft chairs and rocking chairs. ▪ Extend leg that has been operated on, reach for arm rests, and bear some weight through arms when trying to sit down.
Commode chair transfers	▪ Use a chair with a height that accommodates for hip flexion precaution. ▪ Wipe between legs while seated or wipe from behind while standing with caution to avoid internal rotation.
For posterolateral approach	▪ Stand and face the toilet to flush.
For anterolateral approach	▪ An over-the-toilet commode is usually used initially in the hospital and on discharge; older adults usually have enough hip mobility to use a standard toilet seat. ▪ Avoid external rotation while wiping. ▪ Stand and face the toilet to flush.
Shower stall transfer	▪ Use a nonskid mat to avoid slips and falls. ▪ Use a shower chair and grab bars.
Car transfer	▪ Avoid bucket seats in small cars. ▪ Back up to passenger seat, hold on to a stable part of the car, extend the leg that has been operated on, and slowly sit in the car. ▪ Increase the seat height with pillows, if necessary. ▪ Avoid prolonged sitting in the car.
Lower extremity dressing	▪ Sit on a chair or the bed's edge when dressing. ▪ Use assistive devices, if necessary, to observe precautions. ▪ Use a reacher or dressing stick in donning and doffing pants and shoes. ▪ Dress the leg that has been operated on first using a reacher or dressing stick to bring pants over the foot and up to the knee. ▪ Avoid crossing the operated lower extremity over the nonoperated lower extremity. ▪ Use a sock aid to don socks or knee-high nylons and a reacher or dressing stick to doff these items. ▪ Use a reacher, elastic shoe laces, and a long-handled shoehorn, if necessary.
Hair shampooing	▪ Use a long-handled sponge or back brush to reach the lower legs and feet safely, and use soap on a rope to prevent the soap from dropping (drill a hole into a bar of soap and thread a cord through the hole). ▪ Wrap a towel around a reacher to dry the legs. ▪ If a bath bench is used, place a damp towel on the seat to avoid sliding off of the bench. ▪ Consider a handheld shower extender. ▪ Shampoo hair while seated until able to shower.
Leisure interests	▪ Adapt and use long-handled tools when appropriate. ▪ Use stools when appropriate to avoid bending, squatting, and stooping.
Home management	▪ Avoid heavy housework (e.g., vacuuming, lifting, and bed making). ▪ Practice kitchen activities; keep commonly used items at countertop level. ▪ Carry items in large pockets, a walker basket, a fanny pack, or a utility cart. ▪ Use reachers to grasp items in low cupboards, or pick up items off of the floor. ▪ Move frequently used items located low in cabinets and shelves to counter level. ▪ Keep a cell phone close by at all times. ▪ Carry a water bottle with a belt holster. ▪ When initially recovering, place the television remote control, radio, telephone, medication, tissues, wastebasket, and water glass in the most convenient location. ▪ Consider usage of smart technology to voice activate items in the house, such as turning on and off lights. ▪ Before surgery, stock up on food that can be easily prepared or reheated. Or consider meal delivery services.

anterolateral approaches. The older adults bring clothing to practice using a dressing stick, reacher, sock aid, and long-handled shoehorn. Stephanie has the older adults practice transferring to and from a chair, couch, commode, and raised toilet seat. They also practice using reachers to retrieve items from the floor. During one question-and-answer session, several older adults expressed that they enjoy feeding their pets. Stephanie asked a volunteer from her church to make pet feeders that could be easily lifted from the floor to the counter so that the older adults could fill them with water and food without bending over. Stephanie also reviews information in a notebook with older adults and their caregivers that will be used as their home programs. After surgery, Stephanie works with older adults to review the dressing techniques and reinforces the information that they learned earlier in class. Stephanie makes recommendations for bathroom equipment that the older adults may need to return home. Some older adults have stated that it was helpful to be exposed to the information before surgery because it was harder for them to concentrate after surgery.

Knee Replacements

The knee joint has a large amount of synovium fluid, and thus is often affected by rheumatoid and OA.[22] Chronic knee pain may cause difficulty in ascending and descending stairs, squatting, walking, and jogging, thus affecting one's quality of life.

Nonsurgical intervention may include a variety of approaches, including medication, activity modification and exercise, braces, and weight reduction.[22] Nonsteroidal antiinflammatory drugs (NSAIDs) are often prescribed to reduce swelling and pain. Intraarticular injections are sometimes used when oral NSAIDs are ineffective.

Activity modification is targeted to minimize symptoms by avoiding high-impact activities. Maintaining a healthy body weight is difficult for people with knee pain because it often decreases their activities without changing their intake of calories. If possible, older adults with knee pain should try to maintain a regular exercise program to maximize aerobic conditioning.

Physical therapists may provide braces to help active older adults regain a sense of knee stability during activities. Such knee braces are helpful in the short term, but people tend not to use them on a day-to-day basis.[22] Surgical intervention includes a total knee joint arthroplasty (TKA) or total knee replacement (TKR). Total knee arthroplasties seem to last longer in adults older than 50. Adults ages 65–74 years have been found to have the greatest number of TKA revisions overall, while those older than 75 years typically have less revisions.[38]

Rehabilitation After Knee Replacement

After a TKA, the knee is bandaged and changed 2–4 days after surgery. To promote blood flow and decrease the chance of blood clot formation, the older adult will likely wear knee-high TED hose. Early movement is encouraged by all involved with care.

Occupational and physical therapy services will work with older adults to meet the following goals: transfer independently to and from bed, walk with crutches or a walker on a level surface, independently ascend and descend three stairs, independently carry out one's home exercise program, flex affected knee to 90 degrees, and extend knee to neutral. Other rehabilitation concerns of clients with TKAs include sexual activity, driving, and return to work. Many physicians do not discuss sexual activity related to the TKA. However, clients should be counseled to avoid sexual intercourse for 4–6 weeks after TKA. (See Chapter 12 for more specific information about resuming sexual activity after a TKA.) Resuming driving can occur as early as 3 weeks for some older adults, whereas others are not ready to drive until 8 months after surgery. The ability to return to driving is dependent on exhibiting good leg control, limiting the use of narcotic pain relievers, and whether the overall recovery is unremarkable.[39] Returning to work is more difficult to predict and is dependent on the type of work. Typically, patients return to work 3–6 weeks after their surgery.[39] Keep in mind these are generic timeframes; physicians may instruct their clients with different timeframes on the basis of the clients' conditions. Finally, OTAs should pay attention to payment initiatives in the health care environment related to total hips and knees, such as bundled payments.

ARTHRITIS

Arthritis affects about 54.4 million adults in the United States and is prevalent in nearly half of the older adult population, projecting to affect 78.4 million by 2040.[40] The self-reported prevalence of arthritis is greater among women than men, and there is a 44% prevalence of arthritis-attributable activity limitation for those over 65.[41] Arthritis is also a leading predisposing condition for injury after a fall including fractures.[42] Arthritis causes bone demineralization. The pain from arthritis limits people's activity, thus causing weight gain. These factors combined with environmental factors often result in falls or fractures. More than 100 types of arthritis have been identified; the three most common types in the older adult population are OA, RA, and gout.[43] Descriptions, causes, and symptoms of these three forms of arthritis are presented in Table 21.5.

Treatment for arthritis in older adults can consist of any combination of therapy, medication, and surgery. Therapy may consist of the provision of physical therapy and occupational therapy. Medications commonly prescribed to older adults who have arthritis are NSAIDs and cyclooxygenase-2 inhibitors (similar to NSAIDs but with fewer side effects). Performing surgery to replace joints is often a last resort. OTAs must be aware of the physical restrictions and limitations that arthritis imposes

TABLE 21.5

Description of Osteoarthritis and Rheumatoid Arthritis

Condition	Definition	Cause	Symptoms
Osteoarthritis (degenerative joint disease)	A degenerative disease of cartilage with a secondary degeneration involving underlying bone	Possible biomechanical, inflammatory, and immunological factors; secondary factors include congenital defects, trauma, inflammation, endocrine and metabolic disease, and occupational stress	Progressively developing pain, stiffness, and enlargement with limitation of motion; crepitus with PROM; commonly affects weight-bearing joints (hips, knees, cervical and lumbar spine, PIPs [enlargements or osteophytes in PIPs are often referred to as Bouchard's nodes], DIPs [enlargements or osteophytes in DIPs are often called Heberden's nodes], CMCs, and MTPs); joints appear red, tender, swollen; asymmetrical presentation; deformities of joints; pain often follows periods of overuse or extended inactivity
Rheumatoid arthritis	Chronic, systemic disease characterized by inflammation of the synovial tissue of joints; may involve the heart, lungs, blood vessels, or eyes	Unknown; seems to be of an unknown immune reaction in synovial tissue	Characterized by exacerbations and remissions; commonly affects weight-bearing joints (hips, knees, cervical and lumbar spine, PIPs, DIPs, CMCs, and MTPs); joints appear red, tender, swollen, and hot; usually a symmetrical presentation; deformities of joints (i.e., swan-neck, boutonnière); fusiform swelling in PIPs
Gout	Painful rheumatic disease affecting connective tissue, joint spaces, or both, caused by uric acid	Caused by deposits of needle-like crystals of uric acid in the connective tissue, joint spaces, or both	Characterized by swelling, redness, heat, pain, and joint stiffness; commonly affects the toes, ankles, elbows, wrists, and hands

CMC, carpometacarpal; *DIP*, distal interphalangeal; *MTP*, metatarsophalangeal; *PIP*, proximal interphalangeal; *PROM*, proximal range of motion.

on older adults' activities. Interventions by the OTA/OT team should focus on helping older adults manage their symptoms more effectively in addition to modifying occupational tasks.

Common Problems Associated With Arthritis

Incidence for OA of the knee increases after age 50, with about twice as many knee OA cases than hand and hip combined.[44] Limitations caused by knee OA include difficulty using stairs, walking, rising from chairs/bed, getting in and out of cars, and limiting participation in community and leisure activities.[45] These activities can be quite painful and can reduce the quality of life for an active older adult.

Upper extremity deformities caused by OA can be problematic. Osteophytes form in the fingers and base of the thumb. Although osteophytes are not painful, they are seen at the distal interphalangeal (DIP; Heberden's nodes) and proximal interphalangeal (PIP) joints (Bouchard's nodes). Such nodes result in difficulty and pain during pinching. In advanced stages, the thumb's carpometacarpal (CMC) subluxations can occur with joints and result in instability.

The hands are the most severely affected joints in RA. Often, the PIP joints present with fusiform swelling or spindle-like shape. Boutonnière and swan-neck deformities are also finger deformities that may result from RA. Ulnar drift is often present in the metacarpophalangeal (MCP) joints of the hand and volar subluxation of the wrist.

Gout commonly affects the toes, ankles, elbows, wrists, and hands. Swelling can cause the skin to become taut around the joint and make the area appear red or purple and be tender. These presentations, in turn, reduce joint mobility.[43]

Occupational Therapy Intervention

The primary goal of OT intervention is to improve the quality of life of older adults with arthritis. Specific goals may include maintaining joint mobility or joint stability, preventing joint deformity, maintaining strength, and maintaining or improving functional ability. Other goals include maintaining a healthy balance of rest and activity, modifying performance of activities, and improving psychosocial acceptance and coping mechanisms.

Maintenance of Joint Mobility and Stability

OTAs may develop an exercise program for the older adult to keep arthritic joints moving. Such an exercise program should seek to minimize stress to all involved joints. Older adults with arthritis often find that taking a warm bath or shower after waking up in the morning relieves joint stiffness, thereby making it easier to exercise and engage in other activities. Older adults with arthritis may also find it helpful to use a paraffin bath before engaging in wrist and hand exercises. OTAs should demonstrate service competency when using physical agent modalities and follow any state regulatory requirements.

Joints requiring stability may warrant orthotic intervention. A carefully designed orthosis (splint) may provide stability to a joint and improve function. For example, discomfort in the CMC joint may be reduced by fabricating a hand-based thumb spica orthosis to support the CMC joint in a functional position.[46]

Prevention of Joint Deformity

OTAs must be aware of the common types of joint deformities that may develop as a result of arthritis. Deformities include wrist subluxation, ulnar drift of the MCP joints, swan-neck deformity, and boutonnière deformity. Volar subluxation of the wrist frequently occurs in older adults who have arthritis. A wrist cock-up orthosis may aid the older adult in maintaining better wrist alignment, which will promote function and reduce pain.[25] Ulnar drift, or ulnar deviation, of the MCP joints is another common deformity caused by RA. Ulnar drift is caused when the carpal bones deviate ulnarly and the metacarpals deviate radially, usually due to loosening of ligaments. Some experts suggest that the use of an ulnar drift orthosis may prevent further deformity. However, such orthosis cannot correct the deformity.[25]

A swan-neck deformity of the finger results in PIP hyperextension with DIP flexion. A boutonnière deformity results in PIP flexion with DIP hyperextension. Both deformities can be provided an orthosis or surgically repaired with varying results.[47,48] An orthosis for swan-neck deformity places the PIP in slight flexion, while an orthosis for boutonnière deformity places the PIP in extension.[47,48]

To prevent further deformity, older adults should be evaluated to determine whether they need orthoses (splints) that are appropriate for the deformity and activity level. In addition, older adults should be taught joint protection techniques (Box 21.1).

Maintenance of Strength

OTAs may be asked to develop graded strengthening programs for older adults who have arthritis. These programs should include the principles of joint protection discussed previously. During periods of acute exacerbation of arthritis, older adults should not engage in strengthening programs.

BOX 21.1

Joint Protection Principles

- Respect pain. Monitor activities and stop to rest when discomfort or fatigue develops. For example, if kneeling or stooping to garden causes pain and stiffness, stop and rest. Next time try sitting on a stool.
- Reduce stresses on joints. Use the largest joint possible for activities. For example, when using hands to push up from a seated position, push up with the palms, not the back of the fingers.
- Wear orthoses as prescribed to protect joints. For example, wear resting hand orthoses during exacerbation periods to reduce pain.
- Hand movements should be done in the opposite direction of deformity. For example, when wringing out a wash cloth, twist toward the radial side rather than the ulnar side.
- Avoid sustaining a strong, tight grasp. For example, use foam or a cloth wrapped around handles to relax the grip needed to manipulate an object.
- Avoid carrying and lifting heavy objects. For example, use a cart to move heavy objects.
- When handling a heavy object distribute the weight evenly over the joints. For example, use both hands to handle a carton of milk.
- Limit the amount of time spent climbing, walking, and standing. For example, take an elevator or escalators; drive or use a walking aid; sit whenever possible.
- Avoid sustained flexion of the finger joints. For example, use a large sponge for cleaning; work with the fingers extended over the sponge rather than squeezing it.
- Avoid using heavy objects. For example, cook with lightweight pots and pans rather than heavy cast-iron pots and pans.

Improvement of Functional Ability

Functional ability can be improved through careful collaboration between the OTA, OT, and the older adult. This collaboration can help determine whether assistive equipment works well and is accomplishing the goal for which it was intended. For example, a rocker knife may allow the older adult to continue to cut meat during meals. OTAs must observe how the older adult handles the knife to ensure that the involved joints are protected as the knife is used and to ascertain that the knife actually cuts the meat.

Maintenance of Life Balance

Graded strengthening programs for older adults who have arthritis are developed by OTs and may be administered by OTAs. Assisting older adults in achieving a balance between rest and activity is paramount. For example, older adults are often tempted to schedule all activities during the morning hours with the hope of resting in the afternoon. However, a better balance is achieved when activities are scheduled throughout the day and an appropriate period of rest is incorporated after each activity. This type of schedule will help decrease the fatigue of older adults and is less likely to lead to an exacerbation of their conditions. In addition, older adults will likely accomplish more during the day.

Modification of Activity

Work simplification and energy conservation techniques often benefit older adults who have arthritis (see Chapter 23). These older adults must attempt to distribute their energy output evenly over the number of tasks to be accomplished. Incorporating energy conservation and work simplification techniques into the older adults' daily routines can assist them in maintaining a functional lifestyle.

Improvement of Psychosocial Well-Being and Coping Mechanisms

The combination of acute and chronic pain, coupled with joint stiffness and immobility, can result in limitations of ADL such as dressing, and recreational and social outlets such as dancing. The population of older adults who experience pain is challenged daily to use strategies that will enhance productive living. Older adults who do not have coping and support systems will need assistance in developing such systems. OTAs may assist by linking older adults who have arthritis with community resources that can provide support and help older adults develop coping mechanisms. Self-help courses sponsored by the Arthritis Foundation can provide social interaction. Alternative methods of pain control may include relaxation training, cognitive restructuring and modification, medication fading, and social assertiveness training. The process of helping older adults cope with arthritis must involve a multidisciplinary approach for chronic pain management to be successful.

CASE STUDY

Michael and Deanna are meeting with a builder to design their retirement condominium. In planning the space, they decide to consult with an agency that aids with home design and modification for older adults. They are awaiting a contact from the agency to schedule a meeting to begin plans for the new condominium.

One month previously, Michael fell during the nighttime in an attempt to go to the bathroom and sustained a hip fracture.

Subsequently, he underwent an ORIF his right hip. Also, last year, Deanna had a total knee arthroplasty. Deanna has considerable pain from RA. They hope to plan their ranch-style condominium to meet their current and future needs in relation to their health.

■ CASE STUDY QUESTIONS

1 List the precautions that Michael might need to follow after his ORIF procedure.
2 List the ADL functions that will be directly affected by Michael's hip ORIF procedure.
3 Describe the problems that Deanna may be dealing with as a result of RA.
4 Name the wrist and hand deformities associated with RA that may be afflicting Deanna.
5 Describe some possible causes for Michael's fall that should be investigated.
6 Describe the ways in which Michael's performance of ADL functions and his environment will need to be modified.
7 List appropriate recommendations for the living room, kitchen, bathroom, and bedroom for their new condominium.

■ CHAPTER REVIEW QUESTIONS

1 Identify the most common causes of fractures in older adults.
2 Why do older adult women have a greater occurrence of orthopedic problems than older adult men?
3 Why is it important for the OTA to understand the anterolateral and posterolateral approaches related to total hip replacements?
4 Identify two psychosocial issues that may have an effect on an older adult after a total hip replacement.
5 Using joint protection techniques, explain how you would teach older adults with arthritis in their hands to do the following:
   a Wash delicate clothing in the sink
   b Lift a child from a playpen
   c Use a computer
   d Start a car with a push button system
6 Explain how you would teach an older adult energy conservation techniques during the following activities:
   a Removing groceries from the trunk of a car and taking them in the house
   b Vacuuming the floor
   c Cleaning the kitchen after a meal

EVIDENCE NUGGETS: EFFECTIVENESS OF INTERVENTIONS FOLLOWING TOTAL HIP REPLACEMENTS

1. Aftab A, Awan WA, Habibullah S, Lim JY. Effects of fragility fracture integrated rehabilitation management on mobility, activity of daily living and cognitive functioning in elderly with hip fracture. *Pak J Med Sci.* 2020;36(5):965-970. doi:10.12669/pjms.36.5.2412
   • The Fragility Fracture Integrated Rehabilitation Management (FIRM) intervention was administered

15 days after hip replacement surgery and involved 10 PT sessions and 4 OT. OTs provided training on ADL and adaptive equipment during their sessions.
   • Older adults who received the FIRM intervention following hip replacement surgery experienced higher statistically significant functional improvements than the control group in the stair climbing portion of the

EVIDENCE NUGGETS: EFFECTIVENESS OF INTERVENTIONS FOLLOWING TOTAL HIP REPLACEMENTS—cont'd

Modified Barthel Index and in ambulation or walker use.
- Participants in the FIRM intervention showed significant improvement in cognitive function as measured by the mini mental status examination (MMSE).

2. Dorsey J, Bradshaw M. Effectiveness of occupational therapy interventions for lower-extremity musculoskeletal disorders: a systematic review. *Am J Occup Ther*. 2017;71(1):7101180030p1-7101180030p11. doi:10.5014/ajot.2017.023028
   - Participants with hip replacements experienced greater independence, increased mental health scores, less pain, and less disability after receiving occupational therapy focused on education, adaptive equipment, compensatory strategies, and joint protection strategies.
   - Participants who went through hip surgery experienced a lower length of stay and higher quality of life scores when occupational therapists were involved in the early mobilization process.
   - Posthip replacement surgery, participants experienced higher confidence levels and better performance with community-related tasks after completing a community reintegration program provided by occupational therapists.

3. Jogi P, Zecevic A, Overend TJ, Spaulding SJ, Kramer JF. Force-plate analyses of balance following a balance exercise program during acute post-operative phase in individuals with total hip and knee arthroplasty: A randomized clinical trial. *SAGE Open Med*. 2016;4:2050312116675097. Published 2016 Nov 7. doi:10.1177/2050312116675097
   - Participants completed 10 reps of strengthening, joint range of motion, and balance exercises three times per day for 5 weeks following a total hip arthroplasty (THA).
   - Following a THA or TKA, older adults who added balance exercises to regular joint ROM and muscle-strengthening exercises had improved balance when compared to those who only performed joint ROM and muscle-strengthening exercises.

4. Jame Bozorgi AA, Ghamkhar L, Kahlaee AH, Sabouri H. The effectiveness of occupational therapy supervised usage of adaptive devices on functional outcomes and independence after total hip replacement in Iranian elderly: A randomized controlled trial. *Occup Ther Int*. 2016;23(2):143-153. doi:10.1002/oti.1419
   - OTs provided skilled instruction in the use of adaptive devices and education in the advantages they provide to participants who had total hip replacement (THR) surgery.
   - Participants who received training from the occupational therapist experienced statistically significant improvements with large effect sizes in the Western Ontario and McMaster Universities Osteoarthritis Index, the Barthel Index, the Visual Analogue Scale, hip flexor strength, hip extensor strength and hip abductor strength.
   - The group who received supervision in the use of adaptive devices experienced less pain and higher functional independence than the control group.

5. Jogi P, Overend TJ, Spaulding SJ, Zecevic A, Kramer JF. Effectiveness of balance exercises in the acute post-operative phase following total hip and knee arthroplasty: A randomized clinical trial. *SAGE Open Med*. 2015;3:2050312115570769. Published 2015 Feb 11. doi:10.1177/2050312115570769
   - Participants in the intervention group completed 10 repetitions of balance, joint range of motion, and strengthening exercises three times a day for 5 weeks during home visits following a THA or TKA.
   - Following the intervention, participants who underwent a THA or TKA experienced statistically significant improvements in the Berg Balance Scale (BBS), Timed UP and Go Test (TUG), Western Ontario and McMaster Universities Osteoarthritis Index physical function subscale (WOMAC-function), and Activities-specific Balance Confidence Scale after completing the 5-week program.
   - Participants who underwent a THA or TKA and followed the exercise program experienced significantly better improvements on the BBS and the TUG than the group who did not complete the exercises.

For additional video content, please visit Elsevier eBooks+ (eBooks.Health.Elsevier.com)

REFERENCES

1. Baidwan NK, Naranje SM. Epidemiology and recent trends of geriatric fractures presenting to the emergency department for the United States population from year 2004-2014. *Public Health*. 2017;142:64-69.
2. Cauley JA. Public health impact of osteoporosis. *J Gerontol A Biol Sci Med Sci*. 2013;68(10):1243-1251. Available at: https://doi.org/10.1093/gerona/glt093.
3. Downey C, Kelly M, Quinlan JF. Changing trends in the mortality rate at 1-year post hip fracture—a systematic review. *World J Orthop*. 2019;10(3):166-175. Available at: https://doi.org/10.5312/wjo.v10.i3.166.
4. Woolf A, Akesson K. Preventing fractures in elderly people. *Br Med J*. 2009;338(7685):89-96. Available at: https://doi.org/10.1136/bmj.327.7406.89.
5. Sahni S, Kiel DP. Smoking, alcohol, and bone health. In: Holick MF, Nieves JW, eds. Nutrition and Bone Health. 2nd ed. New York, NY: Humana Press; 2014.
6. Schneider A, Williams EK, Brancati FL, et al. Diabetes and risk of fracture-related hospitalization: the atherosclerosis risk in communities study. *Diabetes Care*. 2013;36(5):1153-1158. Available at: https://doi.org/10.2337/dc12-1168.
7. Court-Brown CM, McQueen MM. Global Forum: fractures in the elderly. *J Bone Joint Surg Am*. 2016;98(9):e36. Available at: https://doi.org/10.2106/JBJS.15.00793.

8. Taylor AJ, Gary LC, Arora T, et al. Clinical and demographic factors associated with fractures among older Americans [published correction appears in Osteoporos Int. 2011;22(4):1275-1276]. *Osteoporos Int.* 2011;22(4):1263-1274. Available at: https://doi.org/10.1007/s00198-010-1300-8.

9. Thibaud M, Bloch F, Tournoux-Facon C, et al. Impact of physical activity and sedentary behavior on fall risks in older people: a systematic review and meta-analysis of observational studies. *Eur Rev Aging Phys Act.* 2012;9(1):5-15. Available at: https://doi.org/10.1007/s11556-011-0081-1.

10. Uusi-Rasi K, Karinkanta S, Tokola K, Kannus P, Sievänen H. Bone mass and strength and fall-related fractures in older age. *J Osteoporos.* 2019;2019:5134690. Available at: https://doi.org/10.1155/2019/5134690.

11. Centers for Disease Control and Prevention. *Risk Factors for Falls [Brochure].* 2017. Available at: https://www.cdc.gov/steadi/pdf/Risk_Factors_for_Falls-print.pdf.

12. Insurance Information Institute. *Background on: Older Drivers.* 2021. Available at: https://www.iii.org/article/background-on-older-drivers.

13. Insurance Institute for Highway Safety. *Older Drivers.* 2021. Available at: https://www.iihs.org/topics/older-drivers.

14. Cox AE, Cicchino JB. Continued trends in older driver crash rates in the United States: data through 2017-2018. *J Safety Res.* 2021;77:288-295. Available at: https://doi.org/10.1016/j.jsr.2021.03.013.

15. Binkley N, Blank RD, Leslie WD, Lewiecki EM, Eisman JA, Bilezikian JP. Osteoporosis in crisis: it's time to focus on fracture. *J Bone Miner Res.* 2017;32(7):1391-1394. Available at: https://doi.org/10.1002/jbmr.3182.

16. Stathokostas L, Theou O, Little RMD, et al. Physical-activity related injuries in older adults: a scoping review. *Sports Med.* 2013;43(10):955-963. Available at: https://doi.org/10.1007/s40279-013-0076-3.

17. Seeley E, Baier S, Szekeres M. Wrist fractures. In: Wietlisbach CM, ed. Fundamentals of Hand Therapy: Clinical Reasoning and Intervention Guidelines for Common Diagnoses of the Upper Extremity. 3rd ed. St. Louis: Mosby; 2020:254-269.

18. Macedo F, Ladeira K, Pinho F, et al. Bone metastases: an overview. *Oncol Rev.* 2017;11(1):321. Available at: https://doi.org/10.4081/oncol.2017.321.

19. Egol K, Koval K, Zuckerman J. *Handbook of Fractures.* 6th ed. Hagerstown, MD: Lippincott Williams & Wilkins; 2019.

20. NIH National Institute of Neurological Disorders and Stroke. *What Is Complex Regional Pain Syndrome?* 2020. Available at: https://www.ninds.nih.gov/Disorders/Patient-Caregiver-Education/Fact-Sheets/Complex-Regional-Pain-Syndrome-Fact-Sheet.

21. Sueki D, Brechter J. *Orthopedic Rehabilitation Clinical Advisor.* St Louis: Mosby; 2010.

22. Brotzman B, Wilk K. *Handbook of Orthopedic Rehabilitation.* 2nd ed. St. Louis, MO: Mosby; 2006.

23. Administration on Aging. *2019 Profile of Older Americans.* Washington, DC: U.S. Department of Health and Human Services; 2020. Available at: https://acl.gov/sites/default/files/Aging%20and%20Disability%20in%20America/2019ProfileOlderAmericans508.pdf.

24. Azad A, Kang HP, Alluri RK, Vakhshori V, Kay HF, Ghiassi A. Epidemiological and treatment trends of distal radius fractures across multiple age groups. *J Wrist Surg.* 2019;8(4):305-311. Available at: https://doi.org/10.1055/s-0039-1685205.

25. Lohman H. Orthoses for the wrist. In: Coppard BM, Lohman H, eds. Introduction to Orthotics. 5th ed. St. Louis, MO: Mosby; 2020:116-155.

26. Centers for Disease Control and Prevention. *Hip Fractures Among Older Adults.* 2016. Available at: http://www.cdc.gov/homeandrecreationalsafety/falls/adulthipfx.html.

27. Brun OCL, Månsson L, Nordsletten L. The direct anterior minimal invasive approach in total hip replacement: a prospective departmental study on the learning curve. *HIP Int.* 2018;28(2):156-160. Available at: https://doi.org/10.5301/hipint.5000542.

28. Parker M, Handoll H. Replacement arthroplasty versus internal fixation for extracapsular hip fractures in adults. *Cochrane Database Syst Rev.* 2006;(2):CD000086. Available at: https://doi.org/10.1002/14651858.CD000086.pub2.

29. Tang VL, Sudore R, Cenzer IS, et al. Rates of recovery to pre-fracture function in older persons with hip fracture: an observational study. *J Gen Intern Med.* 2017;32(2):153-158. Available at: https://doi.org/10.1007/s11606-016-3848-2.

30. Hozak W, Parvisi J, Bender B. *Surgical Treatment of Hip Arthritis: Reconstruction, Replacement, and Revision.* Philadelphia: WB Saunders; 2009.

31. Evans J, Evans J, Walker R, Blom A, Whitehouse M, Sayers A. How long does a hip replacement last? A systematic review and meta-analysis of case series and national registry reports with more than 15 years of follow-up. *Lancet.* 2019;393(10172):647-654. Available at: https://doi.org/10.1016/S0140-6736(18)31665-9.

32. Lawson S, Murphy LF. Hip fractures and replacement. In: Pendleton HM, Schultz-Krohn W, eds. Pedretti's Occupational Therapy. 8th ed. St. Louis, MO: Mosby; 2017.

33. Khan F, Ng L, Gonzalez S, et al. Multidisciplinary rehabilitation programmes following joint replacement at the hip and knee in chronic arthropathy. *Cochrane Database Syst Rev.* 2008;(2):CD004957. Available at: https://doi.org/10.1002/14651858.CD004957.pub3.

34. Brander VA, Mullarkey CF, Stulberg SD. Rehabilitation after total joint replacement for osteoarthritis: an evidence-based approach. *Am J Phys Med Rehabil.* 2001;15(1):175-197.

35. Neonakis EM, Perna F, Traina F, et al. Total hip arthroplasty and sexual activity: a systematic review. *Musculoskelet Surg.* 2020;104(1):17-24. Available at: https://doi.org/10.1007/s12306-020-00645-z.

36. Robnett R, Chop W. *Gerontology for the Health Care Professional.* 4th ed. Sudbury, MA: Jones & Bartlett; 2020.

37. Alkema G, Wilber K, Enguidanos S. Community- and facility-based care. In: Blackburn J, Dulum C, eds. Handbook of Gerontology: Evidence-Based Approaches to Theory, Practice, and Policy. Hoboken, NJ: John Wiley & Sons; 2007.

38. Delanois RE, Mistry JB, Gwam CU, Mohamed NS, Choksi US, Mont MA. Current epidemiology of revision total knee arthroplasty in the United States. *J Arthroplasty.* 2017;32(9):2663-2668. Available at: https://doi.org/10.1016/j.arth.2017.03.066.

39. Mullarkey CF, Brander V. Rehabilitation after total knee replacement for osteoarthritis. *Phys Med Rehabil.* 2002;16:431-443.

40. Hootman JM, Helmick CG, Barbour KE, Theis KA, Boring MA. Updated projected prevalence of self-reported doctor-diagnosed arthritis and arthritis-attributable activity limitation among US adults, 2015-2040. *Arthritis Rheumatol.* 2016;68(7):1582-1587. Available at: https://doi.org/10.1002/art.39692.

41. Barbour KE, Helmick CG, Boring M, Brady TJ. Vital signs: prevalence of doctor-diagnosed arthritis and arthritis-attributable activity limitation—United States, 2013-2015. *MMWR Morb Mortal Wkly Rep.* 2017;66(9):246-253. Available at: https://doi.org/10.15585/mmwr.mm6609e1.

42. Bergen G, Stevens MR, Burns ER. Falls and fall injuries among adults aged ≥65 years—United States, 2014. *MMWR Morb Mortal Wkly Rep.* 2016;65(37):993-998. Available at: https://doi.org/10.15585/mmwr.mm6537a2.

43. MedlinePlus. *Gout.* April 13, 2021. Available at: https://medlineplus.gov/gout.html.

44. Lespasio MJ, Piuzzi NS, Husni ME, Muschler GF, Guarino A, Mont MA. Knee osteoarthritis: a primer. *Perm J.* 2017;21:16-183. Available at: https://doi.org/10.7812/TPP/16-183.

45. White DK, Master H. Patient-reported measures of physical function in knee osteoarthritis. *Rheum Dis Clin North Am.* 2016;42(2):239-252. Available at: https://doi.org/10.1016/j.rdc.2016.01.005.

46. Lohman H. Thumb immobilization orthoses. In: Coppard BM, Lohman H, eds. Introduction to Orthotics. 5th ed. St. Louis: Mosby; 2019:156-186.

47. Cooper C, Deshaies L. Orthotics for the fingers. In: Coppard BM, Lohman H, eds. Introduction to Orthotics. 4th ed. St. Louis: Mosby; 2015.

48. Valdes, K. Orthotics for the fingers. In: Coppard BM, Lohman H, eds. Introduction to Orthotics. 5th ed. St. Louis: Mosby; 2019:251-273.

chapter 22

Working With Older Adults Who Have Cardiovascular Conditions

TONYA BARTHOLOMEW AND LAURIE VERA

(PREVIOUS CONTRIBUTIONS FROM JANA K. CRAGG, JEAN T. HAYES, AMY MATTHEWS, RENÉ PADILLA, AND CLAIRE PEEL)

KEY TERMS

angina, blood pressure, cardiac rehabilitation, cardiovascular disease, dyspnea, energy conservation, heart rate, maximum heart rate, metabolic equivalents, tachypnea, work simplification

CHAPTER OBJECTIVES

1. Identify the signs and symptoms of cardiac dysfunction.
2. Describe the phases of cardiac rehabilitation.
3. Recognize the role of occupational therapy in cardiac rehabilitation.
4. Describe assessments, intervention techniques, and precautions used with older adults who have cardiac conditions.
5. Describe intervention approaches for older adults with cardiac conditions in various treatment settings.

Sarah is an occupational therapy assistant (OTA) who specializes in cardiac rehabilitation. She works closely with the cardiac team as she provides occupational therapy interventions. Logan is an OTA employed by a skilled nursing facility (SNF). He works with older adults who have a variety of conditions. Many of his clients are admitted for specific reasons, such as rehabilitation after a total hip replacement or stroke. Most have accompanying chronic illnesses, including cardiac conditions. Logan often informally consults with Sarah when he has an intervention question about cardiac conditions because he does not have the same specialty experience that she has, and he values her expertise. This chapter focuses primarily on the role of OTAs in cardiac rehabilitation settings. However, intervention with older adults who have cardiac conditions in other settings is also addressed.

Cardiovascular disease is an overarching term that refers to several types of heart conditions, which include (1) diseases that primarily affect the heart such as coronary artery disease and congestive heart failure, (2) circulatory problems involving peripheral vessels such as peripheral vascular disease, and (3) circulatory problems involving the cerebral circulation. This chapter focuses primarily on diseases in the first category: the heart. Heart disease is the leading cause of death in the United States[1] and one of the most prevalent chronic conditions among older Americans.[2]

BACKGROUND INFORMATION

During the aging process, the body experiences gradual changes. Although many of these changes are inevitable, studies show that some of the changes are less pronounced in older adults who do not have cardiovascular diseases and associated risk factors.[2] This is especially true for older adults who have lifestyles that include regular physical activity. However, most older adults experience age-related changes in their cardiovascular systems, including changes in the heart muscle and vessels, peripheral vascular disease, and an increase in systolic pressure, which makes the heart work harder and less efficiently.[3] Most coronary diseases are related to lifestyle and family history, as well as age. Chronic cardiac conditions include hypertension, angina pectoris, congestive heart failure, atrial fibrillation (AFib), and peripheral vascular disease. Heart disease often accompanies other illnesses or conditions such as diabetes or chronic obstructive pulmonary disease (COPD); therefore the OTA should be aware of any additional precautions or contraindications associated with these diagnoses and cardiovascular disease.

Medical treatment varies according to the condition and other individual health factors. Thrombolytic drugs are used to prevent muscle damage from heart attacks. Other common drugs are those used to treat hypertension, angina, heart failure, and dysrhythmias. The OTA should be aware of the medications that the patient is taking and the associated side effects. If conservative treatments involving medications are not effective, then surgical interventions may be necessary. Surgical treatments may include angioplasty or a bypass for damaged arteries. In rare cases, treatment may involve a heart transplant to replace heart muscle that is irreversibly damaged. Cardiac management may include a cardiac ablation, or the implantation of electromechanical devices such as pacemakers or defibrillators to achieve a normal heart rate (HR) and rhythm.

Heart disease may begin with a loss of elasticity in the small vessels, causing the heart to work harder to maintain blood flow to organs. A change in the temperature in the extremities, cyanosis, or an increase in systolic blood pressure (BP) may indicate circulatory insufficiency.[4] Atherosclerosis is a condition in which lipid deposits accumulate on the walls of large and medium vessels.[5] This narrows the lumen of these vessels, which restricts blood flow. Atherosclerosis of coronary vessels can produce ischemia, which causes angina (chest pain), a myocardial infarction (MI), or both, which damages the heart muscle. Atherosclerosis of cerebral vessels can lead to a cerebrovascular accident or stroke. A change in the structure of the heart valves, either from viral illness or aging, may result in heart failure, a condition in which the heart cannot deliver enough oxygen to peripheral tissues.

Valvular disease may be identified by detecting a murmur during a routine examination. When the left side of the heart fails, fluid accumulates in the lungs, causing exertional dyspnea, paroxysmal nocturnal dyspnea, dyspnea at rest, pulmonary edema, tachycardia, weakness, bronchospasm, and fatigue.[4,6] When the right side of the heart fails, blood backs up in the periphery, causing an impairment in systemic venous drainage, dependent edema, abdominal pain, anorexia, nausea, bloating, and fatigue.[6] Many older adults with cardiovascular disease lose the ability to perform physical activities and have decreased independence in their daily skills.[2]

PSYCHOSOCIAL ASPECTS OF CARDIAC DYSFUNCTIONS

Cardiac dysfunction can have profound psychosocial implications on older adults and their significant others. Everyone reacts differently to a cardiac event, experiencing a wide range of emotions including anxiety, depression, denial, and helplessness,[7] but most progress through the stages of adjustment. Initially, the anxiety produced by fear of death, discomfort, dependence, and disability can have a profound effect and produce overwhelming feelings. Some clients may demonstrate this anxiety in behavioral changes and may act out or become agitated. This level of anxiety places a physiological demand on the cardiac system at a time when rest is important. Older adults experiencing a rapid change in their care status may also have difficulty with anxiety; as a result, antianxiety medications are often used to assist them. However,

antianxiety medications can have unwanted side effects and lead to additional stress. Clients with these concerns should be encouraged to voice their feelings and work with the health care team to alleviate their fears about the course of events. Good communication and supportive staff members are the key elements in reducing anxiety levels.[8] Fear of another cardiac event can impair functional levels, especially in the early rehabilitation phase. Education and therapeutic intervention can help alleviate these fears. Once stable, they should be encouraged to begin incorporating activities of daily living (ADL), self-care, and functional mobility following the guidelines established by the occupational therapist (OT). This helps to eliminate the helplessness these clients may feel after a cardiac event. The longer that these two elements are delayed, the more helpless the client may feel, which can reinforce the disability.[7,8] (Chapter 12 includes a discussion of ways to address the sexual concerns of older adults with heart disease.)

As older adults begin to regain some strength and control over their activity after adjusting to a new or different cardiac condition, the denial of risk related to the disease may become evident. Denial gives some the mechanism necessary to cope with the cardiac event. This particular phase may be more prevalent in older adults with coronary disease because the symptoms and characteristics associated with this disease are vague. OTAs must not try to break through the denial phase too soon. Facing the realities of the situation may be overwhelming and may create stress-related physical and emotional complications. OTAs can help these clients by instructing them to monitor their performance carefully, thus reducing the risk for another cardiac event.

Some older adults become depressed after a cardiac event. Inactivity and anxiety may trigger depression. Depression and anxiety combined can have a long-term effect on the client's physical and emotional well-being. Patients with depression are less likely to resume normal activity and are at an increased risk for death.[7]

OTAs can play a strong role in addressing the psychosocial aspects of cardiac disease by educating older adults about the expected outcomes after a cardiac event. Relaxation training and lifestyle education are key elements in achieving emotional well-being. Informing the family of risks and precautions can assist older adults in the transition to the home environment and ensure that they have the best chance to regain their status in the home and community.[9]

EVALUATION OF OLDER ADULTS WITH CARDIAC CONDITIONS

OTAs working with older adults who have had cardiac events or who have chronic cardiac conditions should be able to monitor vital signs. It is important that OTAs accurately determine HR and take BP during activities. Physician-directed guidelines for HR and BP responses are typically written as treatment precautions, but OTAs should be aware of standard guidelines as well. To determine the HR, OTAs should palpate the client's pulse at the wrist, count the number of beats felt for 15 seconds, and then multiply this number by 4. This will provide a baseline HR in beats per minute (bpm) before the client engages in activity. Although HRs vary, a normal baseline HR ranges between 60 and 100 bpm.[9] Maximum HR corresponds with performing maximal levels of exertion that involve large muscle groups in rhythmic activities, such as walking and cycling. One method of predicting maximum HR is by subtracting the client's age from 220. This figure is multiplied by 0.6, which represents the percentage of desired exercise intensity, to predict the appropriate HR response for normal activity.[10] For example, a 78-year-old woman's predicted maximum HR would be 142 bpm (220 − 78 = 142). Her HR appropriate for activity would be 85 (0.6 × 142 = 85 bpm). Signs and symptoms, such as dyspnea, must be considered when using formulas to predict activity HR values. Older adults should perform activities in a symptom-free range. Some medications (beta-blockers, verapamil, and diltiazem) blunt the usual HR in response to exercise, especially in older adults; therefore, watching for symptoms is especially important.[4] In the first phase of cardiac rehabilitation, patients are often on continuous pulse oximetry. The OTA should be careful to ensure that the patient is maintaining pulse and oxygen saturation levels within the range set by the physician.

Likewise, the BP should be taken if a physician has so ordered or if the client has symptoms of distress such as shortness of breath, dizziness, weakness, or cyanosis. Older adults with hypertension should be monitored for excessive increases in the BP, or orthostatic hypotension, which may occur as a side effect of medications. BP values greater than 140/90 mmHg indicate moderate stage 1 hypertension, and those greater than 160/100 mmHg indicate severe stage 2 hypertension.[11] BP is considered hypotensive if the systolic BP is less than 90 mmHg. Hypotension can be associated with dizziness and lightheadedness or, in severe cases, circulatory inadequacy of the extremities.[9] In the presence of a shunt for renal dialysis, an arterial line, lymphedema, or postmastectomy, the BP should be read on the opposite limb. Some implanted medical devices and tissue following surgical intervention are fragile, and cannot withstand the pressure produced by the BP cuff (sphygmomanometer) during monitoring. For training, OTAs should practice monitoring HR and BP with an instructor before performing care.

The OTA/OT team should be able to perform basic bedside ADL evaluation as part of the initial evaluation. This might include having the older adult perform oral care, grooming tasks, washing of the upper body, and dressing. OTAs working with older adults who have decreased endurance and low activity tolerance caused by cardiac disease may use metabolic equivalents (METs) as a basis for estimating the energy expended when performing an activity. The MET table provided along with HR and BP responses can help OTAs determine the cardiovascular stress and amount of work performed for specific tasks (Table 22.1).[12,13] Further areas to be assessed are grip strength, muscle strength, and bed mobility. The OT should also assess the patient's cognitive abilities to ensure that the patient will be able to comprehend the education and interventions that the OTA is teaching.

An important consideration for occupational practitioners when working with older adults with cardiovascular conditions is understanding and teaching the client precautions following surgery that requires a medial sternotomy. A sternotomy is required in some cardiovascular surgeries to allow access to thoracic cavity.[16] Procedures that involve a medial sternotomy include coronary artery bypass surgery (CABG), heart or lung transplant, and heart valve replacement or repair.[16] See Table 22.2 for a

TABLE 22.1

Santa Clara Valley Medical Center's Metabolic Equivalents After Myocardial Infarction and After Open Heart Surgery and the 2011 Compendium of Physical Activity

Cardiac rehab stage	Occupational therapy intervention
In ICU	General mobility (bed mobility, transfers to the commode, and position changes) with energy conservation techniques (environmental setups, equipment, and pacing)[12]
1.0–1.9 METs	Sedentary leisure tasks with arms supported (reading, writing, playing cards)[12]
	Standing tasks (seconds to 2 minutes)[12]
	Simple hygiene, semirecline sitting position[12]
	Standing tasks (3–5 minutes)[12]
	Bedside bathing (assist with feet and back)[12]
	Bathroom privileges[12]
	Light leisure tasks such as keyboarding at a computer[12]
	Writing[13,14]
	Ironing[13]
	Needlework[14]

TABLE 22.1

Santa Clara Valley Medical Center's Metabolic Equivalents After Myocardial Infarction and After Open Heart Surgery and the 2011 Compendium of Physical Activity—cont'd

Cardiac rehab stage	Occupational therapy intervention
2.0–2.9 METs	Standing tasks (5–30 minutes)[12,13] Sustained upper extremity (UE) activity (2–30 minutes)[12,13] Total body bathing at sink[12,13] Total hygiene, bathing, dressing at sink[12,13] Total body mobility: bending for small objects, retrieval training[12,13] Moderate leisure tasks[12,13] Billiards[13] Walking at a slow or moderate pace, 2.0 mph[13,14] Driving[13,14] Playing the piano or other musical instrument[14,15] Using a sewing machine[14,15]
3.0–3.9 METs	Shower transfers[12] Total showering task (hair washing, total body washing, drying, and dressing)[12] Simple homemaking tasks such as meal preparation[12] Energy conservation techniques with activity such as cleaning windows[12] Walking at a pace of 3.0 miles per hour[13] Fishing[13] Doing laundry[14] Vacuuming[14]
5.0–7.0 or 5 or more/5 + (many of these are listed as greater than 6) METs	Digging in a garden[12] Sex[12] Hiking[13] Jogging[13] Leisurely swimming[13] Shoveling snow[13] Most sports involving running (e.g., basketball, softball)[14]

TABLE 22.2

Precautions Following Surgical InterventionRequiring a Median Sternotomy

Timeline: 8–12 weeks following surgical intervention; modifications per physician clearance only

Precaution	Notes
No pushing or pulling	This includes opening or closing a heavy door, using the upper extremities to push up from the sitting position, using the upper extremities to get in and out of the car, using the upper extremities to assist in bed mobility, etc. For sitting and standing, encourage patients to cross arms over chest, or to loosely hold a small pillow at the chest level.
Avoid lifting >5–10 pounds	A good reference for clients is to avoid lifting anything heavier than a half a gallon of milk.
Do not perform activities that require shoulder flexion >90 degrees	Some precautions may allow for movement within a "pain free range," or for a short period of time such as to wash or style hair.
Do not reach behind the back	This includes reaching for toilet hygiene and perineal care, to adjust the waistband of pants, to get something in/out of a back pocket, etc.
Driving, and other activities that could require quick, sudden upper extremity use	Encourage patients to complete activities requiring upper extremity use in a careful and controlled environment.

Note: Precautions may vary due to client need and physician preference. Always confirm any precautions with the surgeon prior to evaluation or intervention.
Adapted from Cahalin LP, LaPier TK, Shaw DK. Sternal precautions: Is it time for change? Precautions versus restrictions - A review of literature and recommendations for revision. *Cardiopulm Phys Ther J.* 2011;22(1):5–15.

TABLE 22.3

	The Four Functional Categories of Cardiac Disease
Class I	Clients with cardiac disease but without resulting limitations of physical activity. Ordinary physical activity does not cause undue fatigue, palpitation, dyspnea, or anginal pain.
Class II	Clients with cardiac disease resulting in slight limitation of physical activity; comfortable at rest. Ordinary physical activity results in fatigue, dyspnea, palpitation, or anginal pain.
Class III	Clients with cardiac disease resulting in marked limitation of physical activity; comfortable at rest. Less than ordinary physical activity causes fatigue, dyspnea, palpitation, or anginal pain.
Class IV	Clients with cardiac disease resulting in inability to perform any physical activity without discomfort. Symptoms of cardiac insufficiency or of anginal syndrome may be present even at rest. If any physical activity is undertaken, discomfort increases.

From New York Heart Association. *Nomenclature and Criteria for Diagnoses of Diseases of the Heart and Great Vessels.* 8th ed. Boston: Little, Brown; 1979.

TABLE 22.4

	The Three Phases of Cardiac Rehabilitation
Phase I	This phase occurs in the acute phase of hospitalization for the cardiac event. Clients qualifying for cardiac rehabilitation must be stable after event as determined by physician(s).
Phase II	Client enters a program designed to regain former functional and performance level. Focus is on increasing duration and intensity of physical activity to achieve health benefits and to increase cardiorespiratory fitness.
Phase III	Client enters a maintenance phase of cardiac rehabilitation. This phase is indefinite in length and involves periodic evaluations.

list of common sternal precautions prescribed following a medial sternotomy. Visual cues, such as a handout and demonstration, are often helpful in ensuring patient understanding and carryover of these restrictions. The precautions found in Table 22.2 are common, but note that each surgeon has their own precautions that may vary by procedure and/or patient. Always contact the surgeon for specific restrictions for your client.

INTERVENTIONS, GOALS, AND STRATEGIES

For interventions to be effective, OTAs must understand the functional levels used to classify older adults with cardiac disease. There are four functional categories for cardiac disease (Table 22.3). Knowing the categories allows OTAs to make adjustments in rehabilitation programs. In addition, there are four phases of cardiac rehabilitation which describe where the patient is in the recovery process (Table 22.4).

OTAs need to be aware of activities that can be stressful to the heart. Such activities include isometric and upper extremity activities, especially if performed at a level above the heart. The stress on the heart is reflected by the patient's HR and BP responses, as well as other signs and symptoms. Consequently, any activity that produces excessive increases in HR and BP may overstress the heart (Box 22.1).

The primary goal of any cardiac rehabilitation program is to return older adults to their maximum functional capacities. The OTA/OT team must design an individualized rehabilitation program for each patient.

BOX 22.1

When to Stop Activity and Seek Medical Help

If any of the following symptoms lasts more than a few minutes before, during, or after the activity program, the client should stop activity and seek medical help:

- Nausea
- Tachypnea (rapid breathing)
- Uncomfortable pressure, squeezing, fullness, or pain in the center of the chest that lasts more than a few minutes
- Severe fatigue
- Extreme sweating
- Discomfort in the upper body (arms, neck, jaw, or stomach) during activity
- Lightheadedness
- Unexplained low heart rate or dramatically higher rate than the target heart rate
- Drop in systolic blood pressure or failure of systolic blood pressure to rise
- Excessively high blood pressure (over 240/100 mmHg)

Adapted from Streuber S, Amsterdam E, Stebbins C. Heart rate recovery in heart failure patients after a 12-week cardiac rehabilitation program. *Am J Card.* 2006;97(5):694–698.

Although the phases of rehabilitation follow certain key steps, each patient's progress will be different. Psychosocial aspects, family support, age, medical status, and the desire to participate in the rehabilitation program all affect progression. A rehabilitation intervention plan for occupational therapy with MET allowances for specific activities is useful (see Table 22.1).

Phase I

Phase I consists of the period of inpatient hospitalization. Most referred older adults are in the acute phase after undergoing surgery or experiencing MI. Others are referred for atypical chest pain. In phase I, patients are evaluated by an OT. During the evaluation, the OTA/OT team reviews the medical chart to obtain information on medical history and current cardiac status, and they interview the patient to determine lifestyle and personal goals for rehabilitation. During phase I, occupational therapy practitioners and patients work toward developing a discharge plan on the basis of the older adult's individual needs and lifestyles. Goals for meeting each of the stages in phase I are discussed (see Table 22.4). Activities and educational information are introduced as the rehabilitation process begins. Activities and exercises are initially low level. Early in phase I, OTAs educate patients regarding the need for balancing their lifestyles, which includes stress reduction techniques. Patients are also educated to accommodate for changes in their health status. Using the occupational behavioral model of work, rest, and play, OTAs can introduce the concepts of energy conservation and work simplification while providing bedside intervention.[15] This gives older adults the ability to regain some independence with self-care and dignity while learning to work within limitations after a cardiac event. OTAs can build rapport and support continued rehabilitation by carefully monitoring physiological responses, signs and symptoms, and structuring activities to prevent older adults from feeling fatigue.

METs help establish parameters for functional activities. One MET, the oxygen consumed by the body at rest, is equal to approximately 3.5 mL O_2/kg body mass per minute. To translate this concept into an activity level, it takes 1.5 METs to write a letter in bed with the arms supported.[17] Most self-care activities range from 1.5 to 3.5 METs, and, although this may seem to be light work, it can be physically demanding for some older adults. In some rehabilitation settings, occupational therapy does not intervene in cardiac rehabilitation until the older adult is able to perform light work (1.5–2 METs) without symptoms of dyspnea, palpitation, or angina during or after activity. Once patients are at this level, they can attempt activities required to return home and can independently perform most self-care activities. See Table 22.1 for a list of common activities and associated MET levels. During phase I, older adults are reevaluated to determine whether additional equipment or education is necessary so that they are able to return home and conduct functional activities with safe and appropriate HR, electrocardiogram (ECG), and BP responses.

Phase II

Phase II, often referred to as the recovery or healing phase, is the period immediately after hospitalization.[18] In this phase, older adults typically receive rehabilitation through home health or outpatient clinic services. For medically complicated patients or those having difficulties with ADLs, short-term admission to a subacute rehab facility or a SNF could be indicated. A patient's functional performance during self-care activities is evaluated by monitoring the resting pulse and peak pulse during a task, and then measuring the recovery time to a resting pulse once the activity is terminated. The patient's status is monitored during the activities by measuring HR, BP, ECG, and respiratory responses before, during, and after task completion. The course of treatment and the patient's progress are determined by the physiological responses during activities and the estimated MET level for activities. During this phase of rehabilitation, education and training continue for modifications of risk factors and monitoring of the older adult's general health.[19]

Phase III

Once older adults are able to tolerate increased MET activities at greater than 3.5 METs with safe and appropriate HR, BP, and ECG responses, they are ready to move into phase III of rehabilitation. At this level of function, older adults ideally have been under the care of a cardiac rehabilitation team for 2–3 months. Goals of phase III programs include increasing activity duration and intensity to a level sufficient to elicit cardiorespiratory training adaptations while assisting patients in making necessary lifestyle changes.[19] Phase III of cardiac rehabilitation requires older adults to be more responsible for self-monitoring and to react appropriately if signs or symptoms of a recurring cardiac event become evident. Patients in phase III programs typically attend outpatient programs 2–3 times per week. These sessions provide opportunities for therapists to evaluate function and performance and to facilitate progression of activity programs. Providing patients with the education and techniques necessary to maintain their new lifestyles allows them to be more successful at self-monitoring. Patients are often counseled to make dietary changes, to stop smoking, and to increase physical activity levels. OTAs are in a position to reinforce lifestyle changes. Continued training in energy conservation and the use of assistive devices is provided to older adults at functional levels III and IV. In outpatient clinics, older adults can also receive training in a simulated work environment to provide guidelines for returning to a job or for avocational interests.

ENERGY CONSERVATION, WORK SIMPLIFICATION, AND OTHER EDUCATION

During occupational therapy intervention, patients receive education on energy conservation, work simplification, and cardiac status monitoring.[15] Energy conservation is not only important for overall well-being, but it is also a safety monitor for routine tasks. In the acute portion of cardiac rehabilitation, this component allows patients to set the pace of their self-care routines. Energy conservation begins with basic task analysis, which includes identifying the main steps in the task, analyzing the way the task is performed, and determining the tools or skills needed to perform the task. Once analyzed, the next component of work simplification is added. Having patients perform basic grooming in sitting at the bedside is an example of ADL energy conservation. Using the bedside table with arms propped, the patient can perform grooming with all of the supplies and a basin of water on the table (Fig. 22.1). Patients may need to be directed to take rest breaks during the task if they experience dyspnea or an increase in HR beyond the established parameters. The task can be simplified with a complete setup of supplies, including the removal of all caps from grooming supplies, for example. With the patient in the semireclined position in bed, this task can be accomplished with no more than 1.5 METs. Other ADL functions are analyzed in the same manner, with the therapist identifying ways to reduce the energy expenditure (energy conservation) and minimize steps to perform the task (work simplification). The addition of assistive devices may be an

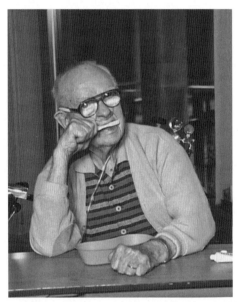

FIG. 22.1 Older adults can perform oral care seated with arms propped on a table to conserve energy.

added benefit (Table 22.5). (See Chapter 12 to learn about addressing sexuality aspects of ADL with heart disease.)

Patients should be educated to pace themselves during activities to reduce fatigue. The work–rest–work principle is important to maintain in the acute phase, especially when denial is an issue. Patients in denial about their cardiac disease may want to prove they are well by overworking or pushing themselves, placing unnecessary stress on their cardiopulmonary systems.

INTERVENTION FOR OLDER ADULTS WITH CARDIAC CONDITIONS IN OTHER SETTINGS

The chapter has focused primarily on cardiac rehabilitation when cardiac disease is the primary diagnosis. However, OTAs may encounter older adults who have cardiac problems in addition to any number of other chronic conditions in settings such as skilled nursing and assisted living facilities, outpatient clinics, or at home. Older adults with acute cardiac conditions eventually may be transferred from the cardiac rehabilitation setting to another setting for further rehabilitation. In these settings, OTAs who are not formally trained in cardiac rehabilitation need to be aware of treatment approaches and precautions. Patients with cardiac conditions in any setting need to be educated on work simplification and energy conservation. The optimal approach is to demonstrate work simplification and energy conservation during the performance of meaningful tasks.

The primary recommendation for all patients with cardiac conditions is to monitor responses to activity by measuring HR, BP, and respiratory rate at rest, during activity, and during recovery. Activities that elicit excessive changes in HR, BP, or any other abnormal signs and symptoms should not be performed or should be modified to ensure appropriate responses. Patients who have had coronary artery bypass graft (CAGB) surgery are often given lifting restrictions. Recommendations vary by physician and often include not lifting more than 10 pounds for at least 1 month after surgery. Lifting precautions may also be recommended for patients who have had a procedure involving catheterization of the femoral artery, such as angioplasty and stent placement. Lifting guidelines for these

TABLE 22.5

Assistive Devices and Rationale for Use	
Item(s)	**Rationale**
Long-handle reacher Long-handle shoehorn Sock aid Elastic shoelaces Long-handle bath sponge	These items prevent the need to bend more than 90 degrees forward flexion in trunk. This may be a precaution for bypass surgery to reduce strain over incision. Limiting trunk flexion to 90 degrees facilitates breathing by allowing full excursion of the diaphragm.
Bath bench	Allows patient to sit during bathing.
High stool	Allows patient to sit during household tasks, such as food preparation and ironing.

TABLE 22.6

Examples of Common Medications and Potential Side Effects

Condition	Medication category (examples)	Side effects
Angina pectoris	Nitrates (nitroglycerin, isosorbide dinitrate)	Headache, orthostatic hypotension, dizziness
	Beta-blockers (atenolol, propranolol)	Bradycardia, depression, fatigue
	Calcium channel blockers (verapamil, diltiazem)	Peripheral edema
Heart failure	Cardiac glycosides (digitalis, digoxin)	Cardiac dysrhythmias, GI distress, CNS disturbances
	Diuretics (furosemide)	Electrolyte disturbances, volume depletion
	ACE inhibitors (enalapril, captopril)	Skin rash
Hypertension	Beta-blockers (atenolol, metoprolol)	Bradycardia, depression, fatigue
	Diuretics (hydrochlorothiazide)	Volume depletion, electrolyte imbalance
	Calcium channel blockers (verapamil, diltiazem)	Peripheral edema
	ACE inhibitors (enalapril)	Skin rash
	Alpha-blocker (prazosin)	Reflux, tachycardia, orthostatic hypotension
	Centrally acting SNS antagonists (clonidine)	Dry mouth, dizziness, drowsiness
	Vasodilators (hydralazine)	Reflux, tachycardia, dizziness, orthostatic hypotension, weakness, headache
Dysrhythmias	Sodium channel blockers (quinidine, lidocaine)	Cardiac rhythm disturbances
	Beta-blockers	Bradycardia
	Drugs that prolong repolarization (amiodarone)	Pulmonary toxicity, liver damage
	Calcium channel blockers (verapamil)	Bradycardia, dizziness, headache
Acute MI	Narcotic analgesic (morphine)	Sedation, respiratory depression, GI distress
	Platelet-aggregation inhibitors (aspirin)	GI distress
	Thrombolytics (streptokinase, tissue plasminogen activator)	Excessive bleeding

ACE, angiotensin-converting enzyme; *CNS*, central nervous system; *GI*, gastrointestinal; *MI*, myocardial infarction; *SNS*, sympathetic nervous system.

procedures are determined by the physician and based on the patient's lifestyle, physical status, and the specific procedures performed.[9]

Recognition of distress signals is vital in any setting when working with clients with cardiac dysfunction. Primary signs and symptoms are chest pain, shortness of breath, cyanosis, sweating, fatigue, weakness, and confusion. Clients with cardiac dysfunction often complain of burning or pressure in the chest, or of upper extremity, jaw, or neck pain. These symptoms may occur with clients who have congestive heart failure, dysrhythmias, or a history of MI or angina.[20] If clients demonstrate or report any of these symptoms, the OTA should monitor their BP, HR, and ECG readings for changes in medical status. Any abnormal sign or symptom should be documented and discussed in a timely manner with the OT and other health care professionals such as nursing and/or the physician.

Another key area of consideration is the type of medication that clients with cardiac or BP problems are taking. Anticoagulants are commonly used for clients who have hypertension, who have had a cerebrovascular accident, or who have had joint replacement surgery. Nitroglycerin is a common medication for clients with angina pectoris. Table 22.6 lists commonly prescribed medications. Knowledge of common medications and side effects is important to any therapy practitioner, but especially to those who perform therapy services through a home health agency or in a community setting due to isolation from easily and quickly discussing concerns with other health care providers.

CASE STUDY

Adelle, who is 79 years old, is receiving occupational therapy in an acute care hospital setting after a coronary bypass graft (CABG). Her medical history includes type 2 diabetes mellitus, hypertension, peripheral vascular disease, and iron-deficiency anemia. Her occupational history includes interests in growing tomatoes and volunteering at her church, where she answers the telephone and sends welcome letters to new members. She lives alone in a home with three stairs. Some adaptations have been made in the home environment such as a tub/shower combination on the main level next to her bedroom. Adelle would like to remain independent with self-care and light homemaking tasks, managing her health, and gardening. Her son and daughter live nearby and drive her to appointments, shopping, and social activities. Her friends from her church visit weekly, and they tend to her garden together. Adelle's niece helps her with vacuuming and cleaning the bathroom.

Trina, the OTA, has been educating Adelle on energy conservation and work simplification techniques. They have practiced pacing with bed-level self-care activities and have discussed techniques for gardening and cooking simple meals when she returns home. Trina has also provided Adelle with handouts and a home program. Adelle will be receiving home health occupational therapy, and Trina will be communicating with the home health OT to update her on Adelle's progress and goals in the acute care hospital program.

CASE STUDY QUESTIONS

1 Describe how the goal HR range for rest versus activity should be determined in Adelle's case.
2 How would Adelle's endurance for dressing be calculated? Discuss when it can be increased.
3 What tools or equipment could be provided to simplify her self-care and home-making tasks?
4 What are three activities that Adelle should avoid? Why are these activities contraindicated?
5 What would be important for Trina to report to the home health OT?
6 What recommendations should the OTA make for home health?
7 How does Adelle's support affect her overall health?
8 What health management techniques would be important for Adelle to engage in?

CHAPTER REVIEW QUESTIONS

1 Describe the effect that anxiety may have on an older adult's ability to perform occupations.
2 Explain the role that OTAs play in addressing the psychosocial aspects of cardiac disease.
3 Describe how maximum HRs and activity HRs are determined.
4 Describe what is involved in the evaluation of older adults with cardiac conditions.
5 Describe why evaluating cognition is important.
6 Describe the four functional categories of cardiac disease.
7 Describe the four phases of cardiac rehabilitation.
8 What is an MET, and how can the MET system be used in cardiac rehabilitation?
9 Describe how energy conservation and work simplification are used in older adults with cardiac conditions.
10 What should OTAs do for older adults who report symptoms of angina pectoris while completing an ADL or treatment activity?
11 Identify a method of energy conservation that older adults can use during lower body dressing.

For additional video content, please visit Elsevier eBooks+ (eBooks.Health.Elsevier.com)

EVIDENCE NUGGETS: EFFECTIVENESS OF STRESS MANAGEMENT IN IMPROVING FUNCTION OF OLDER ADULTS WITH HEART CONDITIONS

1. Blumenthal JA, Sherwood A, Smith PJ, et al. Enhancing cardiac rehabilitation with stress management training: A randomized, clinical efficacy trial. *Circulation.* 2016;133(14): 1341-1350. doi:10.1161/CIRCULATIONAHA.115.018926
   - Both cardiac rehabilitation (CR) groups showed reductions on each stress component following treatment.
   - CR + SMT (Stress Management Training) group showed greater reductions on stress compared to CR alone.
   - CR + SMT showed greater improvements in anxiety and distress and greater reductions in perceived stress.
2. Sherwood A, Blumenthal JA, Koch GG, et al. Effects of coping skills training on quality of life, disease biomarkers, and clinical outcomes in patients with heart failure: A randomized clinical trial. *Circ Heart Fail.* 2017;10(1):e003410. doi:10.1161/CIRCHEARTFAILURE.116.003410
   - Coping Skills Training (CST) participants displayed a lower rate of heart failure hospitalizations and death during the 3-year follow-up.
   - CST participants experienced significantly greater improvements in QoL global score when compared to education alone.
   - Individuals exhibiting clinically elevated depressive symptoms at baseline showed reductions in depressive symptoms that were greater among individuals in CST relative to education alone.
3. Norlund F, Olsson EM, Pingel R, et al. Psychological mediators related to clinical outcome in cognitive behavioural therapy for coronary heart disease: A sub-analysis from the SUPRIM trial. *Eur J Prev Cardiol.* 2017;24(9):917-925. doi:10.1177/2047487317693131
   - Stress management had a small protective effect on somatic anxiety.
   - There was no effect in psychological outcomes for stress, vital exhaustion, and depression.
   - An association was found between somatic anxiety, depression, and vital exhaustion and the risk of fatal or nonfatal cardiovascular events.
4. Schneider RH, Grim CE, Rainforth MV, et al. Stress reduction in the secondary prevention of cardiovascular disease: randomized, controlled trial of transcendental meditation and health education in Blacks. *Circ Cardiovasc Qual Outcomes.* 2012;5(6):750-758. https://doi.org/ 10.1161/CIRCOUTCOMES.112.967406
   - There was a significant net difference in systolic BP for the transcendental meditation (TM) group compared to the education group.
   - There was a significant net difference in heart rate for the TM group compared to the education group.
   - There was a decrease in primary clinical events the more frequently individuals practiced TM at home.
5. Dehbarez NT, Lynggaard V, May O, Søgaard R. Learning and coping strategies versus standard education in cardiac rehabilitation: a cost-utility analysis alongside a randomised controlled trial. *BMC Health Serv Res.* 2015;15:422. https://doi.org/10.1186/s12913-015-1072-0
   - There was an improved quality-adjusted life years (QALY) from baseline during 5 months of follow-up for the learning and coping (LC) group.
   - Participants in the LC group utilized more resources such as primary health care, prescriptions, and outpatient visits than the control group, but only outpatient visits were statistically significant.
   - There was a lower rate of admissions to the hospital for the (LC) group.

REFERENCES

1. Centers for Disease Control and Prevention. *Deaths and Mortality.* 2019. Available at: http://www.cdc.gov/nchs/fastats/deaths.htm.

2. Federal Interagency Forum on Aging-Related Statistics. *Older Americans 2016 Key Indicators of Well-Being.* Washington, DC: US Government Printing Office; 2016.

3. Forman DE, Fleg JL, Wenger N. Cardiovascular disease in the elderly. In: Zipes DP, Libby P, Bonow RO, et al., eds. Braunwald's Heart Disease: A Textbook of Cardiovascular Medicine. 11th ed. Philadelphia: Elsevier/Saunders; 2018.

4. Jugdutt B, ed. *Aging and Heart Failure: Mechanisms and Management.* New York: Springer; 2014.

5. Libby P. The vascular biology of atherosclerosis. In: Zipes D, Libby P, Bonow RO, et al., eds. Braunwald's Heart Disease: A Textbook of Cardiovascular Medicine. 11th ed. Philadelphia: Elsevier/Saunders; 2018.

6. Kemp C, Conte J. The pathophysiology of heart failure. *Cardiovasc Pathol.* 2012;21(5):365-371.

7. Bennett P. Psychological care of cardiac patients. In: Niebauer, ed. Cardiac Rehabilitation Manual. London: Springer; 2017.

8. Anderson L, Sharp G, Norton R, et al. Home-based versus centre-based cardiac rehabilitation. *Cochrane Database Syst Rev.* 2017;(1): CD007130.

9. Hobbs M. Cardiac and pulmonary diseases. In: Radomski M, Latham C, eds. Occupational Therapy for Physical Dysfunction. 8th ed. Baltimore, MD: Lippincott Williams & Wilkins; 2020.

10. Riebe D, Ehrman J, Liguori G, et al. General principles of exercise prescription. In: ACSM's Guidelines for Exercise Testing and Prescription. 10th ed. Baltimore: Lippincott Williams & Wilkins; 2017.

11. Kotchen TA. Hypertensive vascular disease. In: Jameson J, Fauci A, Kasper D, et al., eds. Harrison's Principles of Internal Medicine. 20th ed. New York: McGraw-Hill; 2018.

12. Reed K. *Quick Reference to Occupational Therapy.* 3rd ed. Austin, TX: Pro-Ed; 2014.

13. Ainsworth B, Haskell W, Herrmann S, et al. *The Compendium of Physical Activities Tracking Guide.* Healthy Lifestyles Research Center, College of Nursing & Health Innovation, Arizona State University; 2011. Available at: https://sites.google.com/site/compendiumofphysicalactivities.

14. Adams A, Hubbard M, McCullough-Shock T, et al. Myocardial work during endurance training and resistance training: a daily comparison, from workout session 1 through completion of cardiac rehabilitation. *Bayl Univ Med Cent.* 2010;23(2):126-129.

15. LaPier T, Wintz G, Holmes W, et al. Analysis of activities of daily living performance in patients recovering from coronary artery bypass surgery. *Phys Occup Ther Geriatr.* 2008;27(1):16-35.

16. Huntley N. Cardiac and pulmonary diseases. In: Radomski M, Trombly C, eds. Occupational Therapy for Physical Dysfunction. 7th ed. Baltimore, MD: Lippincott Williams & Wilkins; 2014.

17. Cahalin LP, LaPier TK, Shaw DK. Sternal precautions: Is it time for change? Precautions versus restrictions - a review of literature and recommendations for revision. *Cardiopulm Phys Ther J.* 2011; 22(1):5-15

18. Pinto B, Goldstein M, Papandonatos G, et al. Maintenance of exercise after phase II cardiac rehabilitation: a randomized controlled trial. *Am J Prev Med.* 2011;41(3):274-283.

19. Wu S, Lin Y, Chen C, et al. Cardiac rehabilitation vs. home exercise after coronary artery bypass graft surgery: a comparison of heart rate recovery. *Am J Phys Med Rehabil.* 2006;85(9):711-717.

20. Silverstein A, Silverstein V, Nunn L. *Heart Disease.* Minneapolis, MN: Twenty-First Century; 2006.

Working With Older Adults Who Have Pulmonary Conditions

ANGELA M. PERALTA, SHERRELL POWELL, AND PATRICIA J. WATFORD

(PREVIOUS CONTRIBUTIONS FROM SUE BYERS-CONNON AND DAVID PLUTSCHACK)

KEY TERMS

bronchiectasis, chronic bronchitis, chronic obstructive
pulmonary disease, chronic pulmonary emphysema, dyspnea,
energy conservation, work simplification

CHAPTER OBJECTIVES

1. Define chronic obstructive pulmonary disease.
2. Identify common symptoms of chronic obstructive pulmonary disease.
3. Explain the impact of pulmonary conditions on older adults' daily function.
4. Identify the psychosocial effect of pulmonary conditions on older adults.
5. Describe assessments and interventions for older adults with pulmonary conditions.

Caroline is an occupational therapy assistant (OTA) who works in a large rehabilitation hospital in the South Bronx section of New York City. Her clients are from lower socioeconomic backgrounds. Many of them are factory workers and manual laborers. Caroline has noticed a marked increase in the number of referrals to occupational therapy of older adults who have chronic obstructive pulmonary disease (COPD) as a secondary diagnosis. These older adults are finding it difficult to carry out their activities of daily living (ADL) because of the debilitating effects of COPD. On reviewing their social histories, Caroline found that many of these older adults worked with a variety of chemicals and were heavy smokers. Some of the major problems these older adults deal with include difficulty engaging in self-care activities, a decreased level of endurance, chronic fatigue, and an inability to engage in leisure activities. Like many older adults with COPD, some of them report a fear of not being able to breathe because of frequent episodes of shortness of breath.

COPD, along with other respiratory conditions, can be seen in older adults, usually as a secondary diagnosis. OTAs working with older adults who have COPD and other respiratory diagnoses must be aware of the causes, symptoms, and occupational therapy interventions. When addressing older adults with pulmonary conditions or issues related to respiratory system function, OTAs should consider the *Occupational Therapy Practice Framework* (4th ed.)[1] for all aspects of the person's life.

CHRONIC OBSTRUCTIVE PULMONARY DISEASE

COPD is a common disorder that can include chronic pulmonary emphysema and chronic bronchitis. COPD affects the upper and lower respiratory tracts and is characterized by cough, wheezing, sputum production, and dyspnea. These symptoms occur first with exercise and later when the older adult is at rest.[1,2] COPD is associated with airflow obstruction, which may be accompanied by airway hyperreactivity, and may be partially reversible.[2,3] Clinical symptoms of COPD vary, depending on the severity and duration of the disease. Those with COPD may experience exacerbations, worsening of the symptoms during an acute event, in response to respiratory infections or pollutants. COPD can be caused by exposure to lung irritants, with most cases associated with smoking, although one-fourth of all individuals with COPD have never smoked.[2-4]

CHRONIC BRONCHITIS

Chronic bronchitis is defined as the presence of a chronic productive cough and sputum production for at least 3 months out of a year for a 2-year period.[2] One symptom of chronic bronchitis is hypersecretion of mucus in the respiratory tract in individuals for whom other causes, such as infection, have been ruled out.[2,5,6] The sputum of a person with chronic bronchitis is usually thick yellow to gray. A deep, productive cough is the main symptom of this disease. Other symptoms include shortness of breath, wheezing, a slightly elevated temperature, and pain in the upper chest that is aggravated by cough.[2]

A person may have a mild form of chronic bronchitis for many years. Individuals with mild chronic bronchitis may have only a slight cough in the morning after being inactive at night. This cough can become aggravated after the person has an acute upper respiratory tract infection. As the condition progresses, obstructive and asthmatic symptoms appear, together with dyspnea. Chest expansion becomes diminished, and rhonchi (gurgling sounds) and wheezing are frequently heard.[7]

Bronchiectasis, a permanent dilation of the bronchi, is the most common complication of bronchitis. Bronchiectasis is often associated with bronchiolectasis, a dilation of the bronchiole.[8] Such dilation occurs as a result of persistent inflammation inside the airways. The dilated bronchi and bronchiole are filled with mucopurulent material that stagnates and cannot be cleared by coughing. Infection then spreads into the adjacent alveoli, and recurrent episodes of pneumonia are common. Clubbing of the fingers often develops in older adults with this condition.[8]

CHRONIC PULMONARY EMPHYSEMA

Emphysema is a chronic condition characterized by the permanent enlargement of the air spaces distal to the terminal bronchioles. Emphysema is accompanied by the destruction of the alveolar walls and causes the lungs to lose elasticity, resulting in decreased airflow.[1] This decreased airflow results in dyspnea. Older adults with emphysema have no bronchial obstruction or irritation that would cause them to expectorate.[7,9] The inability to exhale the carbon monoxide trapped in the lungs causes the chest to overexpand, a condition referred to as barrel chest.[10] The older adult must hunch forward while holding on to a stable object to engage the auxiliary respiratory muscles during breathing. These older adults manage to oxygenate their blood by hyperventilating, which prevents cyanosis and anoxia.[7]

ASTHMA

Asthma is defined as a reversible airway disease characterized by an increased responsiveness of the trachea and the bronchi to various stimuli. Asthma is displayed by a widespread narrowing of the airways that changes in severity either spontaneously or as a result of therapy.[11] During an acute attack, pronounced wheezing occurs because of difficulty in inhaling and exhaling air. Dyspnea, tachypnea, and chest tightness may also occur. In severe cases, the older adult experiencing an asthmatic attack may also perspire profusely.[11]

PSYCHOSOCIAL EFFECT OF CHRONIC PULMONARY CONDITIONS

Rehabilitation of older adults with pulmonary conditions should include both medical management and assistance in coping with the debilitating effects of these conditions.[12] As with any chronic condition, older adults adapt in different ways. Some older adults accept and adapt to the changes in energy level and other accompanying symptoms. For other older adults, coping with symptoms may be a frustrating and depressing experience. Furthermore, older adults with pulmonary conditions often have additional stressors in their lives, such as the loss of a spouse and close friends, changes in their living situation, a decrease in financial status, the loss of productivity, a lack of family support, the inability to perform ADL functions, and the loss of general body function.[12]

A common psychosocial effect of pulmonary conditions is anxiety. Anxiety is often associated with dyspnea and concern about the future with a chronic lung diagnosis. Anxiety associated with lung conditions can create a negative circle of events. The person may experience dyspnea, which leads to anxiety about being short of breath, which leads to increased dyspnea and a feeling of being out of control. In addition, anxiety can lead to inactivity, which can lead to increase weakness which can worsen pulmonary symptoms.[13,14]

Weakness and fatigue associated with pulmonary conditions may require changes in living situations, including a move to a higher level of assistive living. As with any move, emotional adaptations are required. Often older adults with these conditions seek to live in a different environment where they believe the air is cleaner or they can breathe better; however, they may find that such a move is not the solution to their problem because it cuts them off from a social support network. A sense of isolation may cause an increase in anxiety and may lead to depression.

Additional problems related to decreases in finances may arise for older adults. The primary source of income for some older adults is Social Security payments. Funds obtained from this source may not be sufficient to pay for medications or home health services, if needed. However, the prescription medication benefit available from Medicare (Part D) with improvements made with health reform may provide some assistance with medication purchases. The situation can be particularly frustrating for older adults with pulmonary conditions who are insured by Medicare because they will not be reimbursed for rehabilitation care unless they have a change in functional status.

In addition, older adults with pulmonary conditions may have a sense of loss of productivity if they are unable to engage in activities that provided enjoyment in previous years. Social isolation because of concerns about a decreased energy level, shortness of breath, oxygen usage, coughing, and sputum production may contribute to depression. Older adults may become afraid that engaging in any type of physical activity may cause an increase in shortness of breath. This can lead to a cycle of fear and ultimately a need for more oxygen. Some older adults with pulmonary conditions also experience frustration because of a decline in their abilities to perform ADL functions as a result of a decreased level of endurance. Finally, some older adults with these conditions may have other chronic problems such as decreased vision, or perhaps a general decline in other body systems. All of these stressors could contribute to anxiety and depression.

Over time, some older adults with pulmonary conditions begin to realize that a change in emotional status, whether positive or negative, has a direct effect on the respiratory system. Fear of expressing any type of emotion becomes a reality. This situation can further perpetuate a state of isolation. These older adults may rationalize, "If I cannot express my emotions, then I will stay by myself." This position may be misinterpreted by others as hostility or aloofness, thereby creating more isolation.

OCCUPATIONAL THERAPY ASSESSMENT AND INTERVENTION PLANNING

OTAs contribute to the evaluation process of older adults with pulmonary conditions and collaborate with registered occupational therapists (OTs) in intervention planning. ADL functions and productive and leisure activities are often the primary areas of concern because of the disabling effects of these conditions.[1] A qualitative study of 72 individuals with COPD found that the most commonly reported symptom from COPD was shortness of breath. In addition, the participants reported that COPD impacted their life by affecting their ability to sleep and socialize and by contributing to emotions such as embarrassment and anxiety/depression.[15] Older adults may experience the most disabling symptoms of pulmonary conditions, such as dyspnea and fatigue, when engaging in ADL and leisure activities. These symptoms, together with anxiety and depression related to the chronic illness, perpetuate the vicious cycle of inactivity. The deconditioning and muscle weakness that occur from inactivity make it increasingly difficult for older adults to perform necessary ADL functions to be independent in the home and community.[12]

The OT and OTA consider client factors when assessing the effects of pulmonary conditions on function.[1] Client factors such as sensory function and pain are assessed to determine tactile impairment. Perceptual skills are assessed to determine an older adult's response during episodes of dyspnea, particularly if they become dizzy. Neuromuscular and movement-related functions are assessed to determine physical tolerance and endurance, shortness of breath on exertion, muscle strength, range of motion, and posture. Higher-level cognition is assessed to determine the older adult's knowledge of the disease and accompanying problems. The older adult's judgment, problem-solving skills, ability to generalize learning, and

BOX 23.1

Safety Considerations

- Individuals with COPD are often unconditioned and present with muscle weakness, which puts them at risk for injuries and falls. Be very observant during intervention and think of safety.
- Strenuous activity and overexertion can be life threatening to older adults with COPD or asthma. Stop activities that cause nausea, dizziness, fatigue, dyspnea, or chest pain.
- Engaging in exercise and activity may activate debilitating effects of COPD and asthma, such as dyspnea, fatigue, and wheezing. OTAs must be aware of these symptoms and monitor the patient accordingly. Asthmatic attacks are life-threatening occurrences, and precautions must be taken when dealing with these patients.
- Recognize the effect that the environment may have on the older adult. Smoke, pollution, dust, and other environmental irritants can trigger COPD symptoms and asthmatic attacks.

---

awareness of safety hazards are evaluated. Global mental functions such as energy and drive, temperament, and personality are considered. Psychosocial ability is assessed to determine the older adult's psychological, social, and self-management skills. Older adults with pulmonary conditions may experience feelings of hopelessness, anxiety, depression, withdrawal from social activities, and dependency on a spouse or caregiver.[16] Impairment in any of these areas directly affects the older adult's ability to engage in self-care, work, and leisure activities.

OTAs must be aware of certain precautions during intervention (Box 23.1). Knowing the various symptoms associated with pulmonary conditions is important, such as shortness of breath and asthma, as well as the environmental irritants that can affect the older adult's ability to breathe. These irritants can include cigarette smoking, dust from woodworking activities, and fumes that arise from activities such as copper tooling. Other irritants include talcum powder, certain perfumes, and poor air quality in the clinic.

Occupational therapy intervention is geared toward increasing independence in functional activities by improving strength and endurance through resistive activities (Box 23.2). Reconditioning programs such as the metabolic equivalents (METs) used with individuals who have cardiac conditions are often also used with patients with pulmonary conditions.[12,17] (A more in-depth discussion of the use of METs to guide activity prescriptions is provided in Chapter 22.) Low-impact exercise places minimum stress on joints and is easier to perform than high-impact activities. Exercise programs should include functional activities that target the upper body, and they should be

BOX 23.2

Interventions for Clients with COPD

- Collaborate with the older adult and the OT to formulate an intervention plan that will be beneficial for the individual. Intervention should focus on increasing the older adult's independence in everyday activities. Consider client functions as you make your intervention plan.
- Reinforce the use of energy conservation and work simplification techniques during ADL. Have the older adult demonstrate these techniques. The older adult will need to take breaks during and between ADL tasks. Environmental modifications and adaptive equipment can also be used by the older adult to successfully complete ADL tasks.
- Reconditioning through strengthening and exercise is a necessity with older adults who have COPD. The METs program is a valuable reconditioning program. Low-impact exercise can be used with patients with COPD as a precursor to meaningful occupations.
- Demonstrate and educate the older adult on the effectiveness of the two breathing techniques described in the chapter, pursed-lip breathing and diaphragmatic breathing. Recognize and address psychosocial issues that the older adult may have in relation to the COPD.

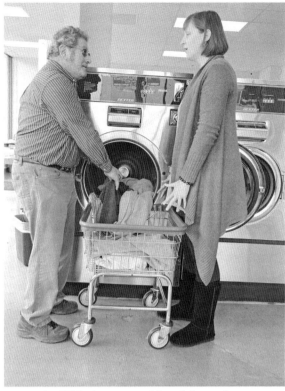

FIG. 23.1 An OTA observes an older adult practice energy conservation and work simplification techniques as he does laundry.

designed to increase the strength of respiratory muscles. Activities should be stopped if nausea, dizziness, fatigue, increased shortness of breath, or chest pain develops.

Energy conservation and work simplification techniques are used with older adults predisposed to fatigue (Fig. 23.1). See Box 23.3 for basic principles of energy conservation and work simplification and Table 23.1 for energy conservation tips. OTAs should actually try these techniques with older adults rather than simply provide them with education sheets. Energy conservation and work simplification techniques should include scheduling rest periods between activities, sitting whenever possible, reducing or eliminating steps, pushing rather than pulling, and analyzing an activity before starting it. Having all of the supplies for ADL functions within easy reach to avoid unnecessary trips is also beneficial. Time management is a technique that teaches older adults to plan daily activities so that rest periods are "built in" to avoid some of the complications of COPD. Good time management skills may make the difference between a full, active life and a sedentary one.

Older adults must develop the problem-solving skills needed to identify that they are no longer able to perform a task in the customary way and when to change the process. Adaptive equipment such as a reacher, a cart to carry heavy items, and a motor scooter for outdoor activities

BOX 23.3

Basic Principles of Energy Conservation and Work Simplification

1. Plan your schedule.
   - Schedule rest breaks between tasks.
   - Alternate days of heavy and light tasks.
   - Minimize steps in any task.
   - Eliminate unnecessary tasks
   - Delegate tasks to others when possible.
2. Pace yourself
   - Work at a slow to moderate pace.
   - Relax. Don't rush. Breathe.
   - Take frequent short rest breaks.
3. Environment
   - Gather all items before starting a task.
   - Reduce clutter.
4. Position
   - Sit during tasks.
   - Use good body posture and body mechanics.
   - Keep items within easy reach.
   - Avoid reaching up or bending over.
5. Techniques and Equipment
   - Push items rather than carry them.
   - Use adaptive equipment when possible.
   - Use carts when transporting items.

Adapted from Advocate Aurora Health. Energy Conservation techniques. For Your Wellbeing. https://ahc.aurorahealthcare.org

TABLE 23.1

		Energy Conservation Tips During ADLs, IADLs, and Leisure
ADLs	Bathing, showering	▪ Sit down to bathe and dry off.
		▪ Put on a terry cloth robe instead of drying off.
		▪ Use a shower/bath organizer to decrease leaning and reaching.
		▪ Use long-handled sponges and brushes.
		▪ Install and use grab bars.
	Dressing	▪ Lay out clothes before dressing.
		▪ Sit down to dress.
		▪ Use sock aides, long-handled shoe horns and reachers to decrease bending.
	Functional mobility	▪ Place chairs or benches along long pathways
		▪ Wear comfortable, low-heeled, slip proof, slip on shoes.
		▪ Wear button front shirts rather than pullovers.
	Grooming	▪ Sit in front of the sink to perform grooming.
		▪ Rest your arms on the sink if needed.
IADLs	Home management	▪ Alternate days of heavy and light tasks.
		▪ Do housework sitting down.
		▪ Use long-handled dusters, mops, etc.
		▪ Use a wheeled cart to carry supplies.
		▪ Delegate heavy housework when possible.
		▪ Stop working before becoming overly tired.
	Meal preparation	▪ Use healthy convenient and easy-to-prepare foods.
		▪ Use small appliances that take less effort to use.
		▪ Arrange the preparation environment for easy access to frequently used items.
		▪ Prepare meals sitting down.
		▪ Soak dishes instead of scrubbing.
		▪ Let dishes air dry.
		▪ Prepare double portions and freeze half.
	Shopping	▪ Organize shopping list by aisle.
		▪ Use a grocery cart to carry items and for support.
		▪ Shop during less busy times.
		▪ Ask for help in getting to the car.
	Work	▪ Plan workload to take advantage of your peak energy times.
		▪ Alternate physically demanding tasks with less demanding tasks.
		▪ Arrange work environment for easy access to commonly used equipment and supplies.
Leisure		▪ Do activities with a companion.
		▪ Select activities that match your energy level.
		▪ Balance activity and rest. Don't get overtired.

Adapted from University of California San Francisco Health. Tips for Conserving Your Energy. https://www.ucsfhealth.org

can assist with function. In addition, OTAs can encourage older adults to become involved in social activities. Teaching stress reduction techniques can help encourage older adults to have a sense of independence.

The OTA/OT team may also reinforce breathing techniques taught in the respiratory therapy program, such as pursed-lip breathing and diaphragmatic breathing (Fig. 23.2). According to Roberts et al. "Pursed lips breathing is carried out by exhaling through partially closed lips, i.e. through pursed lips as if making the flame of a small candle flicker. It has also been described as "moderately active expiration through half opened lips."[18] OTAs working with older adults who have COPD must become efficient at administering oxygen and must be prepared to assist with controlled coughing, breathing, and other procedures.

CONCLUSION

Pulmonary conditions are very common in the United States, especially among older adults. OTA/OT teams are becoming increasingly proactive in the intervention of this debilitating disease. They provide intervention to older adults with pulmonary conditions in a variety of settings. Occupational therapy intervention is geared toward the restoration of self-care skills, instruction in the pacing of daily activities, and the restoration of physical capabilities. OTAs are instrumental in teaching compensatory techniques to be used in the performance of ADL

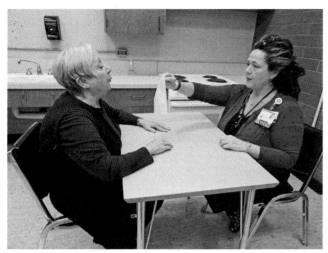

FIG. 23.2 OTAs often must reinforce techniques such as pursed-lip breathing during activity.

functions and in the selection and use of assistive devices and adaptive equipment. OTAs may also become involved in teaching energy conservation and work simplification techniques. Addressing stress management may be a part of therapy; this may also help reinforce respiratory therapy breathing techniques. Ultimately, the goal of OT with older adults who have pulmonary conditions is to maximize their level of independence as they adjust to living with a chronic condition.

CASE STUDY

Linda is a 70-year-old woman who was recently discharged from the hospital after being treated for pneumonia. She has a 20-year history of COPD. Linda's most current hospitalization greatly compromised her health. Linda has been a widow for 25 years. She has one son who lives in the area but is not very involved in her life. "He is afraid that I may need him to fix something. I wish that I would see him more often as I do enjoy his company," Linda stated.

Linda enjoys needlework, and her concern for the environment is evident in the extensive recycling she does in her home. She previously went out into the community three or four times a month for doctor appointments, shopping, and socializing with friends. She does not drive and relies on others for transportation.

Linda was independent in ADL and in instrumental activities of daily living (IADL) before her hospitalization. Her primary care physician ordered home health at discharge, and the OT completed the initial evaluation. Isabella is an OTA who has been working in home health for 5 years and will work with Linda twice a week for 3 weeks. Initially, Linda is concerned about how she will be able to complete her daily routine now that she is on oxygen 24 hours a day and her endurance is severely limited.

Isabella and Linda discuss the occupational tasks that Rose wants to complete independently. They identify that it would be best to start with basic self-care activities incorporating

energy conservation. Isabella reviews handouts on energy conservation for Rose to refer to later. She then has her practice the techniques while engaged in activities. For example, she places a chair in the bathroom for her to sit in while undressing, dressing, and for resting. Isabella instructs Linda in using pursed-lip breathing techniques during self-care tasks. Isabella saw photos of Linda posted in her home and observed that she took pride in her appearance. Low endurance and a fixed income have prevented Linda from visiting the beauty salon, so Isabella suggests that she purchase a wig. Linda embraces the idea.

Isabella provides a commode that Linda can use over the toilet and next to her bed at night. Other bathroom equipment includes a handheld shower and a tub transfer bench. The shower doors are removed and replaced with a shower curtain to help Linda transfer safely to the tub.

Linda becomes independent in ADL using energy conservation techniques. She figures out ways to get around safely in her home while managing the oxygen hose. She reports difficulty with food preparation and the desire to address that area in intervention. Subsequently, Isabella completes a kitchen evaluation and finds that cooking is difficult and unsafe. Linda tires easily, forgets about food in the oven, and leaves food out to spoil. She has lost interest in eating nutritious meals. Isabella suggests that Linda receive Meals on Wheels.

Linda expresses an interest in continuing her recycling activities. The recycling bins are located on the porch floor, and she has difficulty reaching them. Isabella moves a small picnic table close to the door, places the recycling bins on top of it, and labels the bins for easy identification. The picnic table allows Linda to work at a proper work height. A neighbor boy who visits frequently volunteers to take the bins to the curb on a weekly basis. At discharge, Linda is able to function safely in her environment and plans to pursue public transportation so she can move about the community because she is interested in taking a needlepoint class at a local craft store.

■ CASE STUDY QUESTIONS

1 Why did Isabella instruct Linda in pursed-lip breathing techniques while transferring?
2 What are the physical and psychological benefits of Linda wearing a wig?
3 Why is it important to practice energy conservation techniques during activities?
4 Describe how Linda could use energy conservation during two other activities.

■ CHAPTER REVIEW QUESTIONS

1 Describe several physiological factors that may affect older adults with pulmonary conditions.
2 Describe several psychosocial facts that may affect older adults with pulmonary conditions.
3 What ADLs and IADLs may be difficult for older adults with pulmonary conditions to complete?
4 Describe precautions to be aware of when working with older adults with pulmonary conditions.
5 Describe community resources that would be useful for older adults with pulmonary conditions.

EVIDENCE NUGGETS: EFFECTIVENESS OF INTERVENTIONS WITHIN THE SCOPE OF OCCUPATIONAL THERAPY TO TREAT OLDER ADULTS WITH COPD

1. Papp ME, Wändell PE, Lindfors P, Nygren-Bonnier M. Effects of yogic exercises on functional capacity, lung function and quality of life in participants with obstructive pulmonary disease: a randomized controlled study. *Eur J Phys Rehabil Med*. 2017;53(3):447-461. doi:10.23736/S1973-9087.16.04374-4
   - The study found significant improvements on the Chronic Respiratory Disease Questionnaire fatigue and emotional domains for the conventional training program (CTP) group after the 12-week program.
   - There were significant improvements for the 6-minute walk distance after the 12 weeks intervention for both the hatha yogic group and the CTP.
   - After 12 weeks, the CTP group showed significantly lower diastolic BP.

2. Hansen H, Bieler T, Beyer N, et al. Supervised pulmonary tele-rehabilitation versus pulmonary rehabilitation in severe COPD: A randomised multicentre trial. *Thorax*. 2020;75(5):413-421. doi:10.1136/thoraxjnl-2019-214246
   - More participants completed the pulmonary tele-rehabilitation (PTR) compared to the pulmonary rehabilitation (PR).
   - There was no difference between PTR and PR for 6MWD after the intervention or at the 22-week follow-up.
   - After the intervention, the PTR group had a significant decrease in depression and anxiety scores compared to the PR group.

3. Kaminsky DA, Guntupalli KK, Lippmann J, et al. Effect of yoga breathing (pranayama) on exercise tolerance in patients with chronic obstructive pulmonary disease: A randomized, controlled trial. *J Altern Complement Med*. 2017;23(9):696-704. doi:10.1089/acm.2017.0102
   - The pranayama group showed significant improvements with the 6MWD at 12 weeks, while the control group did not.

- There were small, nonsignificant improvements in inspiratory capacity and air trapping for the pranayama group.
- The pranayama group had lower COPD symptom scores, including less shortness of breath and increased time spent on breathing exercises.

4. Schaadt L, Christensen R, Kristensen LE, Henriksen M. Increased mortality in patients with severe COPD associated with high-intensity exercise: a preliminary cohort study. *Int J Chron Obstruct Pulmon Dis*. 2016;11:2329-2334. Published 2016 Sep 26. doi:10.2147/COPD.S114911
   - There were high mortality rates (30%) among the participants who participated in a high-intensity rehabilitation course, with 4/5 deaths attributed to COPD exacerbation, but not during the 8-week course.
   - There were no differences in the hospitalizations rates for the high-intensity exercise group or the regular intensity group.
   - This study raises concerns about possible serious risks associated with high-intensity exercise rehabilitation of severe COPD patients.

5. Jiang Y, Liu F, Guo J, et al. Evaluating an intervention program using WeChat for patients with chronic obstructive pulmonary disease: Randomized controlled trial. *J Med Internet Res*. 2020;22(4):e17089. Published 2020 Apr 21. doi:10.2196/17089
   - The effect of Pulmonary Internet Explorer Rehabilitation (PeR) combined with behavioral strategy intervention was the same as the face-to-face intervention in helping patients with COPD relieve dyspnea symptoms, improve quality of life, and improve self-efficacy.
   - The COPD assessment test score showed significant improvements in both the face-to face group and the PeR group over the 6-month period.

For additional video content, please visit Elsevier eBooks+ (eBooks.Health.Elsevier.com)

REFERENCES

1. American Occupational Therapy Association. Occupational therapy practice framework: domain and process fourth edition. *Am J Occup Ther*. 2020;74:1-87. doi:10.5014/ajot.2014.682006.
2. Global Initiative for Chronic Obstructive Lung Disease (GOLD). *Global Strategy for the Diagnosis, Management, and Prevention of Chronic Obstructive Pulmonary Disease*. 2021. Available at: https://goldcopd.org/wp-content/uploads/2020/11/GOLD-REPORT-2021-v1.1-25Nov20_WMV.pdf.
3. Senior RM, Pierce RA, Atkinson JJ. Chronic obstructive pulmonary disease: epidemiology, pathophysiology, pathogenesis, and α 1-antitrypsin deficiency. In: Grippi MA, Elias JA, Fishman JA, et al., eds. Fishman's Pulmonary Diseases and Disorders. 5th ed. New York: McGraw-Hill; 2015:613-635.
4. National Institutes for Health & Centers for Disease Control and Prevention. *COPD National Action Plan*. 2017. Available at: https://www.nhlbi.nih.gov/health-topics/all-publications-and-resources/copd-national-action-plan.
5. Shibata Y. Epidemiology of COPD: Why is the disease so poorly recognized? In: Nakamura H, Aoshiba K, eds. Chronic Obstructive Pulmonary Disease. 1st ed. Singapore: Singer; 2017:17-28.
6. Mosby. *Mosby's Dictionary of Medicine, Nursing & Health Professions*. 10th ed. St. Louis, MO: Elsevier; 2016.
7. Weinberger SE, Cockrill BA, Mandel J. *Principles of Pulmonary Medicine*. 6th ed. Philadelphia: Elsevier; 2014.
8. Damjanov I. *Pathology for the Health Professions*. 5th ed. Philadelphia, PA: Elsevier Saunders; 2017.
9. Silverman EK, Crapo JD, Make BJ. Chronic obstructive pulmonary disease. In: Jameson JL, Fauci AS, Kasper DL, Hauser SL, Longo DL, Loscalzo J, eds. Harrison's Principles of Internal Medicine. 20th ed. New York, NY: McGraw-Hill; 2018.
10. Piper T, Lukens R, Dirckx J, et al., eds. *Stedman's Medical Dictionary for the Health Professions and Nursing*. 7th ed. Philadelphia: Lippincott Williams & Wilkins; 2012.
11. Patadia MO, Murrill LL, Corey J. Asthma: symptoms and presentation. *Otolaryngol Clin North Am*. 2014;47(1):23-32. doi:10.1016/j.otc.2013.10.001.

12. Dean E. Cardiopulmonary and cardiovascular function: health conditions. In: Bonder BR, Bello-Haas VD, eds. Functional Performance in Older Adults. Philadelphia, PA: FA Davis; 2018.

13. European Lung Foundation & European Respiratory Society. Mental wellbeing and lung health. *Breathe*. 2020;16(2):1-8. doi:10.1183/20734735.ELF162.

14. Farris SG, Abrantes AM, Bond DS, Stabile LM, Wu WC. Anxiety and fear of exercise in cardiopulmonary rehabilitation: patient and practitioner perspectives. *J Cardiopulm Rehabil Prev*. 2019;39(2):E9.

15. Svedsater H, Roberts J, Patel C, Macey J, Hilton E, Bradshaw L. Life impact and treatment preferences of individuals with asthma and chronic obstructive pulmonary disease: results from qualitative interviews and focus groups. *Adv Ther*. 2017;34:1466-1481. doi:10.1007/s12325-017-0557-0.

16. American Psychiatric Association. *Diagnostic and Statistical Manual of Mental Disorders*. 5th ed. Washington, DC: American Psychiatric Association; 2013.

17. Matthews MM. Cardiac and pulmonary disease. In: McHugh Pendleton H, Schultz-Krohn W, eds. Pedretti's Occupational Therapy: Practice Skills for Physical Dusfunction. 8th ed. St. Louis, MO: Elsevier; 2018:1117-1133.

18. Roberts SE, Stern M, Schreuder FM, et al. The use of pursed lips breathing in stable chronic obstructive pulmonary disease: a systematic review of the evidence. *Phys Ther Rev*. 2009;14(4): 240-246. doi:10.1179/174328809X452908.

24

Working With Older Adults Who Have Oncological Conditions

SUE BYERS-CONNON

(WITH PREVIOUS CONTRIBUTIONS FROM CHRISTY WALLOCH AND LESLIE BRUNSTETER-WILLIAMS)

KEY TERMS

alopecia, anemia, cachexia, cancer, dignity therapy, end-of-life care, energy conservation, fatigue, hospice, lymphedema, metastasis, myelosuppression, oncology, pathological fracture, palliative care

CHAPTER OBJECTIVES

1. Identify four common oncological diagnoses associated with aging.
2. Discuss treatment provided to older adults with cancer and the associated side effects.
3. Describe the role of occupational therapy with the older adult with cancer and list three different approaches that might be used with them.
4. Identify three common complications that older adults receiving cancer treatment often face and discuss the effect of these on the OT intervention process.
5. Describe modified approaches to daily occupations that might be used by the occupational therapy assistant (OTA) when working with an older adult who has cancer.
6. Discuss the role of the OTA in hospice and end-of-life care.

INTRODUCTION

Jenna is an occupational therapy assistant (OTA) who works at a university medical center in a large city. The occupational therapy (OT) department cross trains all the therapists. Jenna is beginning a rotation on the oncology and palliative care/hospice units. After being oriented to the units, she is introduced to the team members serving each of the units. She reviews the charts of the older adults with whom she will be working. Her caseload includes five older adults who are on the oncology unit and one older adult who is on the palliative care/hospice unit. Of those on the oncology unit, three are currently undergoing chemotherapy for cancer. She learns those receiving chemotherapy have limited tolerance to activity and greater susceptibility to infections; thus, she plans to allow time before her intervention to review the special precautions with this group of older adults and to collaborate with the other team members to provide the best intervention possible, all while ensuring the older adults' safety.

After reviewing the medical record, Jenna learns of the older adult on the palliative care/hospice unit whose cancer has reoccurred for the third time and now has metastasized to other organs. In concert with the supervising OT, Jenna will meet with a representative of the palliative care/hospice team to ensure her intervention approach is consistent with the team's philosophy of palliative and end-of-life care.

OVERVIEW OF CANCER WITH THE OLDER ADULT POPULATION

Nearly 16% of the total US population is age 65 years or older.[1] At the current rate of population growth, by 2030, this age group is predicted to increase to over one-fifth of the US population, in other words, to a total of 73.1 million people.[2] With the expanding population of older adults, it is important to look at diseases directly associated with the process of aging. The incidence of cancer in older adults is larger than in any other age group and ranks second only to heart disease as the leading cause of death in the United States.[3] Although heart disease still ranks first in terms of national mortality, the gap between heart disease and cancer deaths is closing; between 2000 and 2014, 22 states reported cancer as the leading cause of death in 2014 compared to heart disease in 2010.[4] Health care providers must become adept at recognizing and dealing with health problems and treatment issues faced by older adults with cancer. OTAs have a valuable role in contributing to improved quality of life of the older adult with cancer. Specific strategies and interventions will follow in this chapter.

Age is the single highest risk factor for the development of cancer. From ages 60 to 69, one in eight men and one in ten women have the probability of developing cancer; however, the risk increases after age 70 to one in three for men and one in four for women.[5] According to a report by the American Cancer Society,[5] an estimated 1,806,590 new cases of cancer will be diagnosed in 2020. Although this reflects a large number of people who are dealing with cancer, it is important to note that the current national trend in cancer incidence and death rates appears to be declining.[5–7] The decrease in incidence of all cancers appears to be the result of changes in screening, diagnostic techniques, the reduction in exposure to environmental risk factors, and changes in behaviors, such as smoking cessation and more healthful lifestyle.[5–7] In addition, the decrease in death rates is reflective of greater availability to, increased public awareness about, and development of more effective disease treatment options.[5,6]

COMMON CONDITIONS

In this chapter, four types of cancers (i.e., lung, colorectal, breast, and prostate cancers) associated with aging will be considered. In Table 24.1, the four types of cancer are listed in relation to their 5-year survival rates and the median age at diagnosis.[3]

Lung Cancer

Since the early 1950s, lung cancer has been the most common cause of cancer deaths among men and women and causes more deaths than colorectal, breast, and pancreatic cancer combined.[7,8] According to the Surveillance Epidemiology and End Results (SEER) survey, between 2014 and 2018, the median age at diagnosis for cancer of the lung and bronchus was 72 years.[9] As one ages, the risk of developing lung cancer increases, rising to a high of 32.4% between ages 65 and 74.[9]

The two major categories of lung cancer are small cell lung cancer (SCLC) and nonsmall cell lung cancer (NSCLC). The categories are defined by the type of cells identified. The two types of SCLC are small cell carcinoma

(oat cell cancer) and combined small cell lung carcinoma (c-SCLC). Although c-SCLC has cell characteristics of both small cell and large cell lung cancer, it is classified as a SCLC because its expression and treatment are similar to that of SCLC. SCLC is the more aggressive of the two categories of cancer and is often found in multiple organs at the time of diagnosis. SCLC is almost always caused by smoking.[8] NSCLC accounts for 80%–85% of total lung cancers and tends to metastasize to other parts of the body more slowly.[8] The types of NSCLS are adenocarcinoma, squamous cell (epidermoid) carcinoma, and large cell (undifferentiated) carcinoma.[8]

Smoking continues to be the major cause of all lung cancers in both men and women.[10] Although women have a higher rate of both categories of lung cancer, a greater number of risk factors other than smoking have been associated with the lung cancer, such as behavioral and environmental exposures (e.g., obesity, radon in the home, and second-hand smoke). Occupational exposures including radon, asbestos, diesel exhaust, and uranium have been shown to cause lung cancer as well.[8]

Upon the initial diagnosis of lung cancer, the oncologist determines the prognosis and the best course of treatment available according to a process called staging, which determines whether the cancer has metastasized to other parts of the body. Generally, three levels are described: localized (within lungs), regional (spread to lymph nodes), and distant (spread to other organs).[8] Unfortunately, lung cancer cases are not diagnosed at an early or localized stage, which would increase the probability of an improved 5-year survival (see Table 24.1).[7] The difficulty in an early diagnosis is that the symptoms associated with lung cancer, such as coughing with mucous production, do not occur until the advanced stages of the disease. Frequently, the symptoms are mistakenly assumed to be allergies, lung infections, or long-term effects of smoking.[8] Currently, the only screening tool that has shown to be effective in detecting cancer at a stage that will increase the survival rate is low-dose computed tomography.[8]

The type of treatment is dependent on the type of cancer, stage of cancer, and treatment goals. The treatment options vary greatly and include surgery, radiation therapy (RT), chemotherapy, target therapies, immunotherapy, supportive/palliative care, and complementary and alternative lung cancer therapies. Often, various treatment options will be combined (e.g., chemotherapy with or without RT, surgery, and targeted therapies, etc.).[8,11]

It is becoming more common to complete a geriatric assessment that addresses the specific strengths and weakness of older adults. Understanding the older adult's fitness, including level of independence in activities of daily living (ADL) and instrumental activities of daily living (IADL), cognitive status, and social support system are imperative in assisting the older adult in setting treatment goals.[11]

TABLE 24.1

5-Year Relative Survival Rates of Common Cancer Diagnoses, 2020

Diagnosis/site	5-Year relative survival rates (2010–2016)	Median age at diagnosis
All sites	67.4%	66
Lung/bronchus	20.5%	71
Colorectal	64.6%	67
Breast	90.0%	62
Prostate	97.8%	66

Adapted from *SEER cancer statistics review 1975 to 2017*. National Cancer Institute; 2020. Retrieved from https://seer.cancer.gov/crs/1975_2017/.

Breast Cancer

With the exception of skin cancer, breast cancer is currently the most common type of cancer in women and is second to lung cancer as the cause of cancer-related deaths in American women.[12] The SEER survey database shows the incidence of breast cancer in all women to be approximately 15.3%, a rise from 12% in 2015.[13,14] Although the incidence of new breast cancer cases has increased over the past few years, 89% of patients diagnosed with breast cancer were still alive 5 years postdiagnosis. The median age of a breast cancer diagnosis is 62 years old, and women between the ages of 54 and 74 make up approximately 48% of individuals with new breast cancer diagnoses.[13] However, as women age, the risk for developing invasive breast cancer increases.[13,15]

Disparities exist regarding survival rate of older adult women from breast cancer, which may be due to a variety of factors (e.g., less aggressive treatment, less use of the latest state-of-art treatment technology/protocols, exclusion from clinical trials, finances, etc.). Or the fragility of the older adult can influence survival rate. It is imperative that treatment goals are developed on an individual basis and the assumption of fragility is not just assumed, so the best options available are offered.[16,17]

At the time of diagnosis of breast cancer, the specific type of breast cancer involved will be determined with a biopsy done either through a fine-needle aspiration of the mass or lumpectomy (removal of the mass). At that point, the pathology and the stage of disease can be determined and decisions can be made regarding recommended treatment. Surgery, radiotherapy (RT), cytotoxic chemotherapy, and hormonal therapy are all treatment choices with potential side effects that may compound already present comorbidities. Hormonal therapy is a treatment option often used with older adults with breast cancer. This has been shown to be of particular benefit with tumors that are estrogen-receptor positive (ER-positive), meaning that the tumor is likely to be stimulated to grow by the presence of estrogen. A common endocrine or antiestrogen drug used with breast cancer patients is tamoxifen, which has been studied extensively in older women with breast cancer. Some studies have reported a complete or a partial response in 73% of those women treated with this drug alone.[16,17]

Prostate Cancer

Other than skin cancer, prostate cancer is currently the most common cancer diagnosed in men age 70 years and older; however, because tumors confined to the prostate are often diagnosed early, the 5-year survival rate is high in this group (see Table 24.1).[18,19] Between 2009 and 2013, the median age at the time of diagnosis of prostate cancer was 66 years old.[19] It is estimated that there just over 3 million men living in the United States with prostate cancer.[18] The high 5-year survival rate in this group appears to be a result of the use of the prostate specific antigen blood test as well

as other improved treatments of the disease itself.[19] Nonmodifiable risk factors for prostate cancer include age, African American race, and a positive family history of prostate cancer.[19] There are also risk factors that men can control or modify, thus reducing the risk, such as diet, smoking habits, exercise, and large body size.[19]

The treatment of prostate cancer may include radiation, surgery, hormonal (or androgen deprivation therapy), and cytotoxic chemotherapy.[19] All types of treatment carry with them a potential for adverse side effects, and when determining the best option for each older adult, the oncologist considers each individual's quality of life and anticipated longevity in the decision-making process.[19]

Colorectal Cancer

Colorectal cancer is currently the third most common cancer in both men and women in the United States when excluding skin cancer.[20] Between 2009 and 2013, the median age at the time of diagnosis was 67 years old.[21] The overall rate for colorectal cancer survival is improving because of enhanced screening, which yields earlier diagnoses with localized disease staging.[20] The screening procedure for this disease can include detection and removal of colorectal polyps before they become cancerous, thus helping reduce the mortality and advanced-stage diagnosis.[20] The greatest predictor of survival and treatability of this cancer is finding the cancer at an early stage.[20] Surgery, which can be curative but sometimes results in a colostomy, is commonly part of the treatment regimen.[20] However, the presence of comorbidities in the older adult population may preclude this option.[22] There is increasing evidence that, although older adults maintain higher function than in prior decades, they often are not treated with the same surgery as younger groups, and they receive less aggressive treatment based on their age alone.[22]

Adjuvant chemotherapy, either alone or in combination with radiation, may be used before or after surgery in cases where the cancer has spread locally to the bowel wall or metastasized to the lymph nodes.[20] As in other types of cancer associated with aging, there is a need to expand clinical studies for colorectal cancer to include people over age 65 to make the best treatment available to them and to those people for whom it will most likely prove successful.[22]

The risk factors for colorectal cancer include increased age, family history, the presence of inflammatory bowel disease, or a personal history of colorectal neoplasms.[20] Screening for this disease in persons with an average risk may include flexible sigmoidoscopy, in which the left side of the colon is visualized. The fecal occult blood test, in which a specimen is taken from three consecutive stools to detect the presence of blood, can indicate early presence of the disease. Finally, a colonoscopy, which allows a view of the entire colon, is the most effective screening tool. The American Cancer Society currently recommends that a colonoscopy be done once every 10 years beginning at age 50 for people with an average risk of the disease.[20]

CANCER METASTASIS

Metastasis occurs when malignant or cancerous cells spread from the primary site (or site of origin) to other organs or systems in the body. This spread may be local, occurring in tissues or organs adjacent to the primary tumor site, or distant, traveling to another site in the body. This movement takes place through blood vessels and the lymphatic system at a microscopical level. Common sites of metastasis include breast cancer to bone, lungs, or brain; lung cancer to brain, liver, or bone; prostate cancer to bone; and colorectal cancer to the liver or lungs.[23]

Lung metastasis may be seen secondary to breast cancer and is sometimes found in progressed colorectal cancer.[23] When the lungs are involved in either primary cancer or metastasis, pulmonary functions may change, altering the older adult's functional capacity and respiratory potential during daily activities and functional mobility.[24] Rehabilitation efforts can be of benefit in these situations, working to maximize the older adult's functional abilities with adaptive approaches, pacing, and the utilization of correct body mechanics.

Skeletal or bone metastasis may occur secondary to breast, prostate, or colorectal cancers.[24] If weight-bearing bones are affected, the structures become weakened, thus resulting in the potential for breaking.[25] This is referred to as pathological fracture. A pathological fracture may occur with very little actual weight or pressure applied to the bone, but, because of its weakened support system, a break occurs.[26] For example, if the older adult's humerus has a metastatic lesion, performing a daily task such as emptying the trash or picking up a grocery bag could precipitate a fracture at that site. Immobilization, surgical reduction, or RT may be used to improve bone healing and function if the upper extremity is affected by a fracture.[26] During this time, the older adult may have only one upper extremity available for use and will require training in one-handed ADL.

If the hip or femur is involved, surgical repair or total hip replacement may be necessary to restore joint integrity and enable the person to resume weight bearing on the hip joint (Chapter 21 further describes orthopedic interventions).[26] Depending on which surgical approach is used in the hip surgery, there may be postsurgical precautions in movement, such as hip flexion, adduction, or abduction, and limited weight bearing, which must be followed for proper healing to occur. Therefore, the OTA's intervention should include instruction in ADLs with needed adaptive equipment to achieve modified independence in lower extremity activities such as dressing and bathing, while adhering to the necessary hip precautions. If metastasis involves the spinal column, pain can limit reaching and bending during ADLs.[26] Medical treatments may include epidural nerve blocks, radiation treatments, or surgical stabilization of the spine.[26] In these cases, OT efforts should include teaching correct body mechanics in ADLs and IADLs to protect the spine and to prevent further damage.

Brain metastasis is a common complication of late-stage breast cancer and is also sometimes seen in lung cancer.[23] The symptoms may include headache, nausea, vomiting, mental status changes, seizures, or motor paresis similar to that seen in persons who have had a stroke. Medical approaches used to manage this problem include RT, surgery, and chemotherapy. Impaired balance or ataxia, upper or lower extremity weakness, and impaired cognition may become apparent in these older adults, and OT should include one-handed, self-care tasks and safety in ADLs through fall prevention strategies and strengthening exercises.[27]

CANCER TREATMENT AND SIDE EFFECTS

Advances in treatment protocols are constantly being made based upon clinical trials. However, data from these trials do not always represent the older adult population.[28] If chronological age is used as the criteria for subjects in these trials, older adults with cancer are often excluded by virtue of their age alone.[17] This seems ironic in that the most common diagnoses of cancer are age-related. However, there are assessments that oncologists and other health providers use in cancer settings that more clearly identify older adults with cancer who are appropriate for certain types of cancer treatment and determine the best course of action available for them. Some assessments consider a holistic perspective such as the Comprehensive Geriatric Assessment, which looks at function, physical performance, comorbidity, nutrition, social support, cognition, and depression.[22] Another assessment example that considers function is the Barthel Index, which is an observational tool frequently used with stroke patients but may also be applied with cancer patients.[29] The Karnofsky Performance Status Scale measures functional ability of patients with cancer, requiring the oncologist's assessment of the patient's abilities.[29] A disadvantage of using assessments such as these is that they are time-consuming to complete. Further, not all assessments have been validated for use with older adults with cancer.[29] Hopefully, inclusion of the aging population into more clinical trials will increase as these screenings are further used and results extrapolated.

Currently, standardized treatment protocols established from clinical trials are devised for the younger population who inherently have less comorbidities and are less susceptible to the complications from cancer treatment than older adults. Comorbidities that may be present with older adults, such as hypertension, arthritis, gait imbalance, or chronic lung disease. Other comorbidities include visual, cognitive, or hearing impairments and all make aggressive treatment a challenge.[22] There are also changes that take place in the body during the normal aging process, such as declines in peripheral nerve functioning, muscle strength, and muscle mass.[30] Because of these issues, the older adult's tolerance to established protocols can be impaired,[30] further supporting the need for inclusion of these considerations when protocols are created.

Surgery, RT, and cytotoxic chemotherapy are frequently applied cancer treatments. The side effects of each vary, depending on which part of the body is involved and the dosage administered. Body image changes or loss of bodily functions may result from surgery, requiring that attention be focused on the older adult's ability to adapt or modify activities that are affected. RT is a common cancer treatment that can be used to target localized cancer cells at multiple stages of the disease.[31] RT can be used alone or in conjunction with surgery or chemotherapy. If used preoperatively, RT can lessen the extent of surgery required, a helpful option for older adults with cancer. It may also be used as a curative treatment in the early stages of a disease or as a palliative treatment, improving comfort and control of adverse symptoms in more advanced stages of cancer.[32]

Recent studies show that RT is beneficial and generally well tolerated by most older adults, and age should not be a reason to avoid its use.[16] Systemic chemotherapy may be used for any of the previously mentioned cancer diagnoses.

When making decisions about which chemotherapeutic agents to use with this population, the oncologist considers factors such as quality of life, costs to the older adult, management of potential toxicities, and associated physiological changes that take place with aging in older adults. The side effects of chemotherapy will depend on the drug used and dosage given. They may include nausea/vomiting, peripheral neuropathy, alopecia (loss of hair), body image changes, fatigue, and myelosuppression (impairment of the body to produce normal white blood cells, red blood cells, or platelets). Other side effects may include mouth, tongue, and throat problems resulting in possible pain with swallowing, urine/bladder changes, mood changes, and changes in sexual functioning.[33] Table 24.2 describes some of the cancer treatment side effects and the implications for OT intervention.

TABLE 24.2

Complications Related to Cancer and Its Treatment

Complication	Clinical symptoms	OT intervention implications
Granulocytopenia (decreased white blood cells)	Increased susceptibility to infection	Adhere to universal precautions; good hand washing technique, frequent cleaning of equipment, wearing of mask if in reverse isolation; treatment in older adult's room
Thrombocytopenia (decreased platelets)	Easily bruised, potential for bleeding, CNS bleeding	Avoidance of sharp objects, resistive exercises, participation in less strenuous activities
Anemia (decreased red blood cells)	Easy fatigue, shortness of breath	Frequent rest periods, older adult monitored for fatigue, treatment modified according to persons tolerance
Fatigue	Mild to moderate shortness of breath; decreased tolerance with task completion; poor interest in initiating activities	Pacing techniques in all activities; gradation of physical activities or strengthening exercises as tolerated
Hypercalcemia (excessive calcium in blood; normal level: 8–10.5 mg/dL Ca)	Confusion, giddiness, mental status changes, drowsiness, polyuria, polydipsia	Consultation with physician before beginning activity
Hyperkalemia (abnormally high level of potassium)	Weakness, paralysis, ECG changes, renal disease if severe	Decrease in physical demands of treatment
Airway obstruction (emergent situation caused by tumor impingement on trachea)	Coughing, SOB, acute difficulty breathing	Immediate notification of medical staff
Increased intracranial pressure (caused by primary tumor or metastatic lesion in the brain)	Headaches, blurred vision, nausea or vomiting, seizure	Avoidance of physically active tasks requiring fine vision, quiet environment for treatment
Spinal cord compression (caused by tumor impingement on spinal cord)	Back pain, leg pain or weakness, sensory loss, bowel or bladder retention	Consultation with physician before treatment, avoidance of resistive exercise, extreme care in older adult transfers, immediate notification of any changes in sensation or strength
Skin desquamation (breakdown of outer layer of skin)	Open ulcers on skin, fragile epidermis	Protection of skin surfaces during treatment, avoidance of abrasive contact

TABLE 24.2

Complications Related to Cancer and Its Treatment—cont'd

Complication	Clinical symptoms	OT intervention implications
Cardiac toxicity (decreased cardiac output or function)	Limited cardiovascular tolerance, SOB, dizziness	Selection of activities that do not exceed older adult's tolerance, monitoring of older adult's pulse and blood pressure during treatment
Peripheral neuropathy (impaired sensory pathways in upper or lower extremities)	Impaired sensation; loss of coordination; unsteady gait, foot-drop	Adaptive equipment, orthoses, compensation techniques
Mood changes	Anxiety, depression, irritability, mood swings, increased alcohol usage	Awareness of possible mood changes, encourage the older adult to contact their physician, provide a supportive treatment environment allowing the older adult to communicate feelings, foster involvement in meaningful occupations

CNS, central nervous system; *ECG*, electrocardiogram; *OT*, occupational therapy; *SOB*, shortness of breath.

PSYCHOSOCIAL ASPECTS OF ONCOLOGICAL CONDITIONS/IMPLICATIONS FOR OCCUPATIONAL THERAPY

Psychosocial issues arise as the older adults with cancer begin the process of dealing with the diagnosis of cancer and enter the initial phase of treatment. These issues should be acknowledged by all health professionals involved in the older adult's care.[34] Fear of the unknown, depression, and worry about the effect of the disease on the ability to maintain one's previous level of activity and function often come with the diagnosis of cancer. Anger over having to experience cancer at all may also arise. It is not uncommon for older adults with cancer to be fearful of the pain associated with cancer, which in some cases of advanced disease may have precipitated the diagnosis. Uncontrolled pain can limit activity tolerance and accelerate feelings of loss of control.[35] A sense of control is a basic human need, which, if lost, can negatively affect an older adult's quality of life. OTAs are in a unique position to use active listening, develop a trusting relationship with the older adult, and give supportive responses while encouraging the older adult to express concerns, anxieties, and fears.

As a trusting relationship develops, it is important that the OTA, along with members of the treatment team, provides information to the older adult and family, as appropriate, about the treatment and potential side effects because it can alleviate anxieties and fears. If older adults sense they have greater knowledge about the illness and treatment, they may also feel empowered during this potentially very difficult life experience.

Although financial implications may not be the first concern that comes to mind when one receives the diagnosis of cancer, it soon becomes an important one for many older adults. Some older adults who have modest incomes are eligible to receive Medicaid and may have the majority of their costs covered; however, many people and populations remain who must face cancer without adequate health insurance coverage, especially if the person is not quite old enough to qualify for Medicare. Inadequate insurance can result in delays or limited access to treatment and a significant financial burden. Sadly, if older adults had consistent coverage for adequate screenings, or better access to health care throughout their lives in the first place, the need for cancer treatment could be prevented altogether or diagnosed at an earlier stage, reducing financial burden and struggle. Communication between the physician and older adult may allow costs of cancer treatment to be transparent and increase the likelihood that an older adult openly discusses any financial concerns.[36]

Adverse side effects may bring about changes in the older adult's body image and self-confidence. If alopecia occurs because of chemotherapy or total brain irradiation, the older adult may tend to avoid social situations because of a decreased comfort level around other people. Avoidance of previous social opportunities that gave the person a sense of fulfillment may create a void in life and remove opportunities for receiving emotional support during this difficult time. However, some older adults with adequate finances may desire to purchase a wig. Women may have difficulty adjusting to the loss of a breast after a mastectomy and experience changes in their feelings about femininity and sexuality.[15] The OTA may want to refer these older adults to community- or hospital-based support groups for breast cancer survivors.

If myelosuppression occurs because of cytotoxic chemotherapy, the bone marrow is limited in production of necessary white and red blood cells and platelets. This, in turn, results in increased susceptibility to opportunistic infection, anemia (which can cause increased fatigue), or easy bruising and bleeding.[37] In the case of decreased white blood cells (granulocytopenia), older adults may

355

need to limit their contact with other people to prevent infection. In doing this, feelings of isolation may increase. OTAs should adhere to universal precautions during intervention, including frequent hand washing and using antibacterial wipes on equipment during intervention and wearing a face mask. OTAs can work with older adults to explore interests and encourage solitary activities such as putting photos in albums, which promotes reminiscence, communicating with friends and family through email or letter-writing, or developing a new meaningful hobby that can be done at home. With the growth of Internet-based communities, online support groups may be a practical option for socialization. Impaired platelet production (thrombocytopenia) makes a person prone to bleeding, and activities with sharp tools or resistive strengthening exercises should be limited to protect skin and maintain muscle integrity. If there is a decrease in red blood cells (anemia), activities will need to be paced well throughout the day because the older adult's physical tolerance to activity will be limited. Because of these blood count-related issues, it is important that the OTA check the older adult's daily blood counts in the medical record for changes that may preclude intervention or require modifications to the plan.

Fatigue is the most common side effect of cancer treatment.[38] The American Cancer Society defines cancer-related fatigue as a "distressing side effect of cancer and its treatment,"[38] as it is worse than normal fatigue, is unpredictable, and affects all aspects of one's life. When fatigue occurs, it can result in significant limitations in an older adult's ability to engage in the occupations of value in their life, limiting mobility, working ability, and social interactions, thus eroding their physical, social, and spiritual well-being.[31] These areas directly affect one's quality of life. Providing social support and referring to community resources that help in daily activities may be of benefit.

As the cancer treatment continues, the chronic nature of the disease and the effect it has on the entire family system become evident. Daily routines and schedules may require changing to include required medical appointments for treatment and blood work. Periodic radiographic scans and tests are necessary to assess one's response to treatment. Older adults often face problems with transportation to and from clinics for regular treatment, which compounds the already present stress and anxiety about the potential recurrence of the disease.

If the cancer recurs, feelings of denial, anger, and loss of control resurface. Uncertainty about the future may become a concern and fear of dying can reappear. If the disease recurrence results in the loss of functional ability, family roles may require change. Cancer affects the entire family, and its consequences on the family and caregiver are clearly evident throughout all stages of the illness.[39] It is important to recognize the caregiver's needs and provide support and assistance as changes are made in family roles. An example of how this change can occur is the case

of an older adult female with breast cancer and metastasis to the lumbar spine with subsequent pain while lifting or bending. Up to this time, maintaining laundry duties and shopping were her responsibilities at home, while her husband performed the meal preparations and clean up. She may now need her husband to assume parts of the laundry and shopping duties that require lifting and carrying loads. In exchange, she may have to perform some meal preparation and clean up (see Chapter 11 for a discussion of caregiver and family issues).

In most communities, there are cancer support and self-help groups that can benefit older adults with cancer, their caregivers, and their families. One of the most effective means of support given to older adults dealing with the chronic nature of cancer comes from others who are dealing with the same issues. The health care team should provide information and referrals to community groups and support options. Examples include the American Cancer Society, American Cancer Society programs, such as Road to Recovery (provides transportation to and from cancer treatment) and Reach to Recovery (for persons facing breast cancer), the local YMCA or YWCA (for supervised indoor exercise, swim programs, and support groups), and hospital-based exercise programs and support groups. There are many online support websites that offer connections with other survivors. Support websites for cancer survivors include The American Cancer Society, The Cancer Survivors Network, Cancer Hope Network, CanCare, and the Pink Ribbon Survivors Network.

Quality of life is a concept that has increasingly been studied by professionals from diverse perspectives, often in search of definitive parameters to better assess an older adult's appropriateness for treatment, tolerance to treatment, and outcome success when considering a cancer diagnosis. Studies show that quality of life is compromised over the course of potentially life-saving cancer treatment.[39] Older adults' perceptions of their functional status can influence their feelings of self-worth and emotional adjustment and, therefore, affect their ability or desire to seek out needed social support. It is because of this dynamic that achieving the highest functional level possible becomes a primary goal in OT intervention.

Family support and education are critical when older adults reach the end stage of the cancer process. The team must identify needed home care services, including therapies, a home attendant if indicated, and possible respite care for the primary caregiver. It is important the OTA include the caregiver(s) as contributing team-member(s) in the assessment of the older adult's needs and in the planning of care. At the end stage of the disease, referral to hospice/palliative care should be made to help alleviate suffering while maintaining the older adult's dignity. All services provided should be coordinated to be ever-mindful of maintaining the emotional adjustment and support of the entire family. Table 24.3 provides ideas for questions that help establish rapport, and from

TABLE 24.3

Dignity Therapy Question Protocol

Tell me a little about your life history; particularly the parts that you either remember most or think are the most important. When did you feel most alive?

Are there specific things that you would want your family to know about you, and are there particular things you would want them to remember?

What are the most important roles you have played in life (family roles, vocational roles, community-service roles, etc.)? Why were they so important to you and what do you think you accomplished in those roles?

What are your most important accomplishments, and what do you feel most proud of?

Are there particular things that you feel still need to be said to your loved ones or things that you would want to take the time to say once again?

What are your hopes and dreams for your loved ones?

What have you learned about life that you would want to pass along to others? What advice or words of guidance would you wish to pass along to your (son, daughter, husband, wife, parents, other[s])?

Are there words or perhaps even instructions that you would like to offer your family to help prepare them for the future?

In creating this permanent record, are there other things that you would like included?

From Chochinov HM, Kristjanson LJ, Breitbart W, et al. The effect of dignity therapy on distress and end-of-life experience in terminally ill patients: A randomized controlled trial. *Lancet Oncol.* 2011;12(8): 753-762. doi:10.1016/S1470-2045 (11)70153-X.

these questions, OTAs can develop intervention ideas for the person leaving a legacy.

OCCUPATIONAL THERAPY INTERVENTION

Evaluation and Intervention Planning

Jenna, an OTA, prepares for her day by first reviewing the OT evaluation and history information for each older adult, which was gathered at the time of the initial visit. This helps her familiarize herself with any obstacles or safety concerns that may inhibit the older adult's functional independence and will need to be addressed by her intervention. Jenna will need to keep in mind as she instructs the older adult in self-care tasks with the use of adaptive equipment, if necessary, to work toward achieving their prior level of function.

When beginning the evaluation process with older adults with cancer, a holistic approach is ideal. As stated earlier, health and well-being are directly affected by the physical, functional, emotional, and social domains. OT intervention should be personally tailored to the stage of the disease—early diagnosis, treatment phase, or recurrence—and in the end stage for the palliation of symptoms.

The first step is a thorough review of the older adult's medical/surgical records. This should include past medical history to identify comorbidities, current medical progress notes, treatments being provided, laboratory results (checking blood values to monitor possible myelosuppression), and radiographic reports (checking for potential skeletal or other organ metastasis).

After reviewing the medical record, the OT, the OTA, and the older adult collaborate to perform the evaluation. The focus of the assessment is the older adult's functional status; incorporated into this must be their emotional level of adjustment, perceptions of that functional status, and areas of concern/distress that may affect functional status. Family or caregiver concerns should also be assessed as early as possible. This process provides an understanding of the older adult's occupational history and experiences, patterns of daily living, values, beliefs, habits, roles, and routines.[40] With this information, the older adult, OT, OTA, and caregivers, as appropriate, collaborate to identify priorities of intervention. Participation in daily occupations suitable for the older adult is included, and through observation, the activity demands can be noted, problems that hinder success are recognized, and targeted outcomes are identified. For example, the older adult may be observed ambulating to the bathroom with a walker, performing a toilet transfer, demonstrating toileting skills, attending to hygiene, managing clothing, and returning to a chair. Areas that may be assessed are an incorporation of safety, fine-motor performance in daily activities, balance, cognitive sequencing, and functional tolerance. As deficits are noted in the older adult's performance of the activity, they are included in the intervention plan. Throughout the evaluation process, it is important to communicate with the older adult's family and/or caregivers. This communication provides assurance that the details of the home environment and prior occupational history are accurate and enable the OT and OTA to have a clear understanding of all durable medical equipment (DME) or adaptive equipment that may be present in the home, including information about usage before the referral to OT. Standardized, objective assessments such as sensorimotor assessments may be helpful in the evaluation process and should be used whenever possible. Shortened length of stay and increasing time constraints in the acute-care settings require a general functional assessment of the strength, range of motion, or cognitive abilities needed for the performance of daily occupations.

As noted earlier, the OT, OTA, older adult, and caregivers collaborate to develop the intervention plan. The plan includes objective and measurable goals, a timeframe for planned achievement, and specific OT interventions that will be implemented to achieve these goals. The therapy team considers appropriate Medicare standards for skilled care in their documentation (see Chapter 6). Communication with other team members is important to provide the most comprehensive plan possible. As the intervention progresses, the OTA and the OT have ongoing communication to discuss complications and the older adult's tolerance to intervention, thus making modifications or changes as needed. It is important with this population that, each day before OT intervention, the OTA reviews the medical record, checking laboratory and radiology tests, physicians' orders, and progress notes, to ensure that the older adult's blood counts continue to allow for active involvement in intervention. This medical record review, ensures that there are no new developments in disease spread that may compromise the older adult's abilities and safety during OT intervention. During the course of therapy, involvement and education of the family members and caregivers is important to provide them with an increased understanding of the older adult's capabilities and level of assistance that will be needed after discharge. Whenever possible, instruction and inclusion of family members within the intervention session are helpful. This provides the family with education about proper body mechanics, giving them increased comfort in their assistance of the older adult and safe use of needed adaptive equipment or DME to be used at home. If it becomes apparent during this process that changes in family roles may be necessary, the OTA can provide support to all as this unfolds, or suggestions can be provided of places for support. The OTA may consult with the social worker or case manager for such suggestions.

From the beginning of the evaluation process throughout intervention provision, the OTA must be mindful of the discharge plan and anticipate home care needs, equipment needs, and assistance required in the older adult's care. To ensure interdisciplinary communication, it is important to identify what the best "next step" is from the OT perspective in the older adult's discharge destination. Discharge written recommendations should be made in the daily progress notes for which the OT will document and the OTA can contribute information. These recommendations can delineate, for example, "Home with home health" or "Skilled nursing stay is needed for..." or "Inpatient rehabilitation stay is recommended." It is understood that this recommendation is from the perspective of OT, incorporating safety issues and the current functional performance capacity of the older adult as observed in the OT intervention sessions. The format for this type of recommendation will vary depending on the setting and documentation guidelines used there and, of course, the ideal is a team decision for the best setting.

Goals and Interventions

Jenna is treating a 75-year-old man with prostate cancer that has metastasized to his spine and pelvis, resulting in pain with forward flexion and prolonged standing. By instructing him in the use of a shower bench and long-handled sponge, he is now able to bathe seated, reaching his lower body without bending, thus limiting stress on his skeletal system. Because this intervention occurred in the hospital, Jenna knows it is important to coordinate home health efforts with the interdisciplinary team, recommending grab bars in his shower at home and referring to home health OT follow-up with training after the needed equipment is in place. Jenna and the OT confer about local equipment source options to help decrease out-of-pocket expenses incurred by the older adult, and this information is relayed to the older adult and caregiver.

The purpose of OT intervention is to help the client, "achieve health, well-being, and participation in life through engagement in occupations."[40] Considering these concepts with older adults who have cancer, therapy practitioners should be cognizant about the importance of achieving maximal functional independence in meaningful daily occupations, as allowed within the limits of the disease. It is through this process that goals are established for improving the older adult's quality of life. To meet these goals, OTAs focus on improving the older adult's abilities in areas of meaningful occupations through training in ADLs such as bathing, showering, toileting and toilet hygiene, dressing, eating, swallowing, feeding, functional mobility, personal hygiene, and grooming. Other areas of ADL training may include personal device care (such as hearing aids, orthotics, and adaptive equipment) or sexual activity. IADLs addressed may involve care or supervision of others at home, care of pets, communication management (such as the use of a computer), meal preparation and clean up, shopping for groceries, or driving and community mobility. If adaptive equipment or an orthotic device is needed as part of the intervention, education of the family and the older adult is important to ensure appropriate fit and compliance with the use of the device. If muscle weakness prevents progress in intervention, OTAs may include strengthening exercises to increase functional capacity.

As noted, fatigue is a common problem among older adults with cancer, being found almost universally in older adults receiving chemotherapy.[38] With the identification of fatigue as a major impairment, the use of energy conservation techniques becomes an important component of OT intervention. OTAs may issue a written handout for energy conservation and work simplification in daily activities to the older adult, provide instruction, and observe the older adult demonstrate these principles. It is through performance in daily activities, while using the modified pacing techniques, that the older adult can learn how to better tolerate those activities required during their day. Adaptation of body mechanics in performing daily activities is important in the case of an older adult with bone disease, which increases his susceptibility to pathological fractures (see Box 24.1). Educating the older adult and family in modified positions for daily activities can increase tolerance for the activities, decrease pain during

BOX 24.1

Body Mechanics to Decrease Stress on Bones and the Skeletal System

- Pain may arise from sitting in one position for prolonged periods, therefore change positions frequently.
- While working at a desk or table, make sure the work surface is the correct height so your shoulders are not raised or lowered, and your neck is not bent forward.
- While sitting for activities, place a small pillow or rolled towel at your lower back for added support. Also, keep your knees higher than your hips by using a low stool to slightly raise your feet.
- Stooping and bending are not advised, but if you must perform a task in a bent position, interrupt the position at regular intervals before the pain starts. This may be done by standing upright or sitting down briefly.
- Avoid bending your neck backward; you may need to rearrange your kitchen to prevent reaching and looking up for items on high shelves.
- While driving, move the seat forward enough to keep your knees bent and back straight. Using a small pillow or supportive roll behind your lower back may be helpful while sitting in the car.
- When moving from lying to a sitting position, use a log-rolling technique: roll on your side, bring your legs up toward your chest, then as you swing your legs off the bed, push up with your arms.
- Usually a good firm bed with support is desirable. If your bed is sagging, slats or plywood supports between the mattress and base will help add firmness.
- Slide objects rather than lifting or carrying, and push instead of pull objects when able.
- When performing daily tasks with equipment or tools, use lightweight tools. Stand near the work, rather than reaching for the activity.
- Avoid sitting or lying on low surfaces. Use foam or pillows to raise the seat with chairs or beds.
- Sit rather than stand while working whenever possible. Any activity longer than 10 minutes should be done sitting.
- Whenever lifting, follow these rules:
  - Stand close to the object.
  - Concentrate on using the small curve, or lordosis, in your lower back.
  - Bend at your knees and keep your back straight.
  - Get a secure grip and hold the load as close to you as possible.
  - Lean back slightly to stay in balance, and lift the load by straightening your knees.
  - Take a steady lift, and do not jerk.
  - When upright, shift your feet to turn and avoid twisting the lower back.

the activities, and lower the risk of sustaining a fracture during the task.

It is well known that, as one ages, the risk of falls increases.[41] Because of their age, older adults with cancer are at increased risk for falls. Falls are associated with intrinsic factors, such as arthritis, depression, muscle weakness, or cognitive impairments. Falls can result from extrinsic factors including uneven walking surfaces, inadequate lighting, throw rugs, improper footwear, or clothing.[41] OTAs have an opportunity to intervene in both intrinsic and extrinsic areas to help prevent falls. Maximizing the older adult's tolerance to daily activities through energy conservation techniques and modified body mechanics with adaptive equipment use can help modify intrinsic fall risk. Working to adapt the home environment by improving lighting, removing throw rugs, and repositioning furniture to make a clear path can aid in modifying extrinsic fall risk (see Chapter 14). Providing the older adult with strengthening exercises, thus improving proprioception, can also aid in decreasing fall risk. Chapter 14 contains a discussion of fall prevention with older adults.

Sometimes OT intervention may necessitate the use of orthotic devices designed to protect and support joints, maintain functional position, alleviate pain, support fractures, promote healing, and improve functioning. Examples of devices frequently seen are lumbosacral supports, arm elevators, slings, arm immobilizers, orthoses (splints), and braces. OTAs may need to fabricate an upper or lower extremity orthosis, which positions the extremity in a functional position while providing needed joint support. After making the orthosis and fitting it, the OTA should instruct the older adult regarding the purpose of the device, proper fit, techniques for donning and doffing, wearing schedule, skin inspection techniques, and care of the device or support. If caregivers are needed to assist the older adult in donning the orthosis or device, it is important to include them in the teaching, allowing their participation for proper fit and wearing after discharge. There are many prefabricated orthoses available on the market, and it is important that the OTA have knowledge of cost-saving options or sources when recommending these devices to provide the best care at the lowest possible cost to the older adult.

If and when the disease progresses, changes can occur that limit the older adult's physical capacity to perform previously accomplished daily activities, and, at this time, alterations in family roles may be needed. For example, if an older adult female with breast cancer has a new onset of metastasis found in her femur, she may need to learn the proper techniques for ambulating with a cane or walker and incorporate the use of this assistive device in her daily activities. It may be important to get assistance in grocery shopping and housework from family members while she is able to maintain her role as menu planner, grocery list compiler, and checkbook manager for the family. Throughout this process of role adaptation, it is very important that the older adult and family all are involved in discussing potential changes and everyone is aware of the older adult's abilities and limitations. With the use of empathetic listening, respect for the family's dilemma, and a trusting relationship during this period, potentially difficult situations can be resolved.

An integral part of the OTA's perspective includes recognition of the older adult's emotional needs while meeting his or her physical challenges. OTAs draw from their psychological and supportive perspectives as well as problem-solving skills when helping their older adults manage change. It is in recognizing the emotional needs of older adults and caregivers that we can truly serve older adults with cancer and their families. Psychological issues, including feelings of fear, lack of self-confidence, loss of control, and stress, have been reported as having a major effect upon older adults with cancer.[34] With the use of relaxation exercises, such as visual imagery or deep breathing, older adults can achieve increased feelings of control and manage their fear and anxiety in a positive manner (see Chapter 4). The therapeutic use of touch reaffirms acceptance and counters potential feelings of rejection that may be triggered by alopecia or loss of hair following chemotherapy or total brain irradiation. Before instituting this intervention, the OT/OTA team must verify the cultural appropriateness of touch for the older adult. The OTA may provide or suggest a scarf, cap, turban, or wig and help supply the older adult with local source options for these products. The use of such items can minimize decreased self-esteem, enabling the older adult to continue much needed social connections, thus receiving support from friends and family.

Jenna is seeing an older adult with breast cancer who had a recent right humeral pathological fracture diagnosed on X-ray. The orthopedist's recommendation was to immobilize the older adult's upper extremity with an orthotic immobilizer for 8 weeks during which time the older adult will also receive RT to the area. The older adult is right-handed, very frightened, and anxious about the potential for further damage if she moved her arm "in the wrong way." Jenna instructs the older adult in adaptive dressing and bathing techniques, teaching one-handed techniques, using her nondominant hand to perform these tasks. Jenna realizes that reassurance and psychological support are important throughout this process to alleviate the older adult's anxiety, increase her attention on the task, and enable her to retain the information she is learning. Jenna allows the older adult time to express her fears, listening and responding with gentle support and encouragement. Jenna includes the older adult's husband in her intervention, instructing both of them in the method of donning and doffing the immobilizer for bathing, the care of the immobilizer, proper fit, and skin inspection techniques.

Special Considerations in Intervention Planning and Implementation

One of the older adults on Jenna's caseload is a 64-year-old man with a recent diagnosis of lung cancer who is recovering from a surgical thoracotomy for the removal of the tumor. As Jenna enters his room, she finds him sitting on the edge of the bed, on 8 L of oxygen per nasal cannula. He is very short of breath and appears quite anxious. He states he is "tired of not being able to do anything," and that he has been unable to walk 20 feet to the bathroom for toileting and bathing tasks because of his poor endurance and breathing difficulties. He states he has lost control of his life and is so nervous he "wishes he would just die now." Jenna maintains good eye contact with him, listening to his fears, and acknowledging how frightening his situation must be. She discusses with him the option of using pursed-lip breathing techniques and muscle relaxation techniques to decrease feelings of anxiety and gain control over his breathing (refer to Chapter 23). They then perform the relaxation exercise, with the older adult seated in a chair at bedside. She provides him with energy conservation techniques in writing to use in his daily routine, incorporating frequent rests, using modified body mechanics, and the use of adaptive devices, such as a bath bench, to maximize his tolerance during bathing. Through the demonstration of the relaxation exercise and performance of the proper transfer technique with the bath stool, the older adult learns that he is able to accomplish these tasks and feels an increased sense of control in his life. After completing this intervention, Jenna communicates to the nurse and the social worker what the older adult has stated about his death so that all of the team members can maintain an awareness of this older adult's emotional needs.

There are unique considerations that one should be mindful of while working with older adults with cancer. Cachexiais sometimes seen with this population during the course of the disease and intervention. This condition presents itself with malnutrition, muscle atrophy, weakness, and loss in body mass, and occurs because of biochemical abnormalities and loss of appetite. With decreased nutritional intake, there is less energy, inactivity, and a downward spiral begins. In this situation, it is difficult to increase the older adult's activity level, and the OTA should be aware of the current nutritional status of the older adult during the intervention course. Strategies used to help cope with fatigue, such as lifestyle management, planning, and energy conservation techniques, are useful approaches in these situations.

The presence of depression with fatigue is common in older adults with cancer, and sometimes depression can prevent participation in the intervention process or contribution to establishing goals of intervention. It is important that the OTA recognize when additional psychological support/counseling is needed and help facilitate formal psychological interventions, if indicated.

Inactivity may occur because of the cancer process itself or to the treatment of the disease. In the normal aging process, there is a decrease in muscle mass and strength as well as reduced peripheral nerve functioning.[30] Certain chemotherapeutic agents are known to bring with them the potential for neurotoxicity and myotoxicity, which results in impairments of muscles and the sensory nerves. Issues such as peripheral neuropathy and muscle weakness can have devastating consequences for older adults who may no longer be able to perform their daily living activities without assistance.[30] Recent evidence suggests that increasing physical activity of older adults with cancer can decrease cancer fatigue, improve physical functioning, and enhance the quality of life.[42] The OTA can institute a supervised exercise program to carefully progress the older adult's activity as tolerated, incorporating seated ADLs and pacing techniques with the activities.

Lymphedema sometimes develops following lymph node resections in older adults with breast cancer but can also occur with lymph node removal in the inguinal area in other types of cancer. Swelling takes place because of an abnormal collection of protein-rich fluid and may be present in the upper or lower extremities (Fig. 24.1). The retrieval of

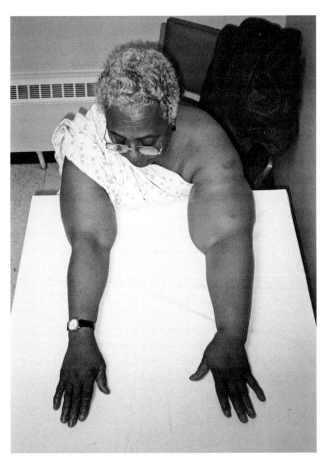

FIG. 24.1 Lymphedema is the swelling resulting from the abnormal accumulation of protein-rich fluid. This condition is sometimes seen after lymph node removal or radiation treatment for breast cancer.

lymph nodes following the diagnosis of breast cancer is important to accurately identify the stage of the cancer, thus affording the older adult the best options for treatment. However, the interruption of the normal lymph system and fluid drainage increases the risk of lymphedema. When present, this condition may also bring pain, chronic inflammation, or fibrosis. At any degree of severity, lymphedema can impair the older adult's ability to wear certain types of clothing, and it often reduces self-esteem and body image, and thus quality of life. Some practitioners specialize in lymphedema intervention and become certified. OT interventions may include applying pressure to the extremity with compression garments or bandages, exercise, massage therapy (known as manual lymph drainage), and sequential pumps. Treatment can improve skin texture and sensation, overall appearance, decrease limb girth, and increase functionality. In conjunction with the physical interventions, OT intervention should include education of the older adult about lymphedema prevention strategies, skin protection techniques, and early identification of potential infection. It is hoped that, with the recent use of sentinel node dissection (a surgical technique that results in fewer lymph nodes being removed) and new surgical and radiation techniques, there will be a reduction in the presence of lymphedema.

It is important for the OTA to collaborate with the OT during the intervention process and modify or advance goals as the older adult progresses. However, if disease progression causes loss of function, the intervention goals may need to be modified to accommodate changing needs with additional adaptations. It can be empowering to the older adult to have the opportunity to make decisions about daily routines or activity adaptations, thus restoring a sense of control during a difficult time. Encouragement, reassurance, and effective communication with both the older adult and family members are essential in this process to ensure a therapeutic transition.

Following an intervention session with a 70-year-old older adult with prostate cancer, Jenna realizes that his tolerance was limited and prevented the completion of the planned upper extremity strengthening program. The older adult's medical record shows that he has completed his second course of chemotherapy and although the prognosis is hopeful, his level of physical tolerance has diminished in the past several days. Jenna discusses this with the OT and together they modify the plan of care to include progressively more strenuous activities, working toward increasing his tolerance. They put together a written program beginning with sitting activities and eventually toward standing and then activities that include walking and carrying household items. They instruct the older adult to follow the program at home and discuss how and when he can progress the activities on his own after discharge. Jenna also communicates the recommendation to the social worker for OT follow-up at home, which provides ongoing monitoring of the older adult's progress and strengthening after discharge. Table 24.4

TABLE 24.4

OT Intervention Gems

Problem	OT intervention option
Inability to reach lower extremities for dressing due to spinal metastasis or joint replacement surgery	■ Instruct in use of a reacher, long-handled shoehorn, sock aid for dressing ■ Have the older adult demonstrate modified techniques in dressing
Limited use of one upper extremity for bathing, dressing, cooking tasks	■ Instruct in adapted long-handled sponge for bathing ■ Teach one-handed techniques for dressing ■ Use adapted cutting board, rocker knife, or Dycem matting for cooking tasks
Anxiety or fear inhibiting the older adult's attention/participation in therapy	■ Deep breathing techniques ■ Visual imagery or relaxation exercises ■ Therapeutic use of touch ■ Active listening techniques
Increased susceptibility to infection; decreased immune response	■ Universal precautions and frequent hand washing ■ Develop interest in solitary activities (photo album development, needlework, computer games)
Upper extremity weakness	■ Occupation-based strengthening program using household items ■ Thera-Band exercise program ■ Progressive resistive exercise as tolerated
Decreased endurance in ADL and IADL	■ Participation in functional tasks while standing, such as meal preparation, grooming tasks at the vanity ■ Progress time as tolerated
Fall history; risk of falls/fractures	■ Issue/instruct in Fall Risk Reduction handout ■ Performance in bathing, dressing, or kitchen task while using techniques ■ Modify extrinsic fall risk factors at home by including family/caregiver in education ■ Strengthening exercises
Shortness of breath, weakness in ADL	■ Pursed-lip breathing techniques ■ Energy conservation techniques
Upper extremity lymphedema	■ Compression bandaging ■ Manual lymphatic drainage ■ Lymphedema prevention strategies in ADL ■ Skin protection techniques ■ Sequential pumps

provides intervention ideas for the OTA to apply with different problems that may arise when working with an older adult who has cancer.

Discharge Planning

Because of the current short length of stays in hospitals and the push for early discharge, the process of discharge planning begins at the time of evaluation and continues with each subsequent OT intervention session. There should be an ongoing discussion with the older adults, their families, and the interdisciplinary team members about the older adult's abilities, need for assistance, and recommendations for postacute rehabilitation, discharge, or home health care follow-up. It is helpful to have an interdisciplinary team meeting to discuss the older adult's progress and for the care team to effectively communicate to one another concerns or issues that may need to be addressed before discharge. The OTA should anticipate home equipment needs of the older adult and with the older adult, family, and DME provider to ensure that important equipment is in place for the older adult's safety

at home. Provision of any needed equipment should include thorough written and verbal instructions by the OTA to both the older adult and caregiver on the set up, use, and care of the equipment. If a caregiver will be needed to assist the older adult with any daily activities, practice of the caregiver in the task, such as bathing or transfers, is helpful during a therapy session before discharge. Referral to home health OT services may be made to ensure a seamless transition to home, providing the family and older adult with supervised instruction within the home. Strengthening programs may be used, and adaptations of the home environment should be recommended as needed to improve safety of the older adult.

CASE STUDY

At the end of the day, Jenna has one more older adult to work with. Carol is a 68-year-old woman who was diagnosed with small cell carcinoma of the lung 1 month ago. At that time, she underwent left lower lung lobectomy for removal of the primary tumor and has been recovering well from that surgery, although she continues to have shortness of breath with exertion in activities. She has now been readmitted to the hospital with left-sided weakness and behavior changes as reported by her husband, including poor attention span and occasional impaired judgment. An MRI scan of the brain reveals a right hemispheric lesion, and a stereotactic brain biopsy shows it to be a metastatic lesion secondary to the primary lung cancer. Carol has begun RT treatments to the brain, and her oncologist has ordered "OT to evaluate and treat as indicated."

During the OT assessment, the OT and Jenna learned that Carol and her husband live in a two-story home. The master bedroom and bath are on the second floor, although there is a guest bedroom and bath on the main level. Before her illness, Carol had been the primary cook and housekeeper. She had also maintained the family finances while her husband managed the yard, was the primary driver, and worked part time as a consultant for a nonprofit agency. During the brief time she was home after her initial lung surgery, Carol fell once while getting out of the shower. Fortunately, she was not injured. She continued to perform her own self-care tasks but with increasing difficulty due to a recent one-sided weakness on her dominant left side. Her husband had begun to assist her with her daily activities intermittently, and she was walking without an assistive device.

A functional sensorimotor assessment of Carol's upper extremities shows that her right upper extremity function is within functional limits with both strength and active range of motion (AROM). Her left upper extremity appears to have 3+/5 muscle strength throughout with AROM within functional limits. Sensation appears intact, but mild left neglect is present throughout functional activities. During toileting and shower transfers, Carol moves impulsively and has two episodes of loss of balance in which she catches herself, preventing a fall. When discussing her behavior during transfers, Carol denies any imbalance, stating she really "does just fine." She also denies any previous falls at home. With the evaluation of her ADL performance, Carol exhibits increased shortness of breath, requiring frequent rest periods. However, she is able to maintain her blood oxygen saturation level above 90% without additional oxygen throughout the tasks. She requires minimal assistance for dressing and bathing because of decreased left upper extremity strength and increased fatigue. Carol is very anxious to return home with her husband and is cooperative but minimizes the need for therapy.

■ CASE STUDY QUESTIONS

1 In this case study, identify daily occupations that Jenna should include in the OT intervention to help with improving Carol's independence and endurance.

2 What adaptations could be incorporated in the bathroom to improve Carol's safety at home while bathing, toileting, and performing grooming tasks?

3 What techniques could be used to maximize Carol's independence and tolerance to her daily occupations and leisure activities at home?

4 What instructions and/or suggestions need to be provided to Carol and her husband to help prevent falls in the future? Are there any suggestions related to the home architecture to consider?

5 How can Jenna assist Carol and her husband in modification of their roles at home to allow Carol to maintain a contributory family role now and in the future?6What needs of Carol's should Jenna communicate to the other team members during discharge planning to ease the transition from hospital to home?

7 What other special considerations in intervention apply to Carol?

■ CHAPTER REVIEW QUESTIONS

1 What precautions should an OTA use when working with an older adult who has prostate cancer with bone metastasis to his spine?

2 What should an OTA suggest to help an older adult female who has recently lost her hair from chemotherapy?

3 If cancer-related fatigue is preventing an older adult from performing their own bathing without assistance, what approaches could be used to improve independence?

4 What information should an OTA gather before treating an older adult with cancer?

5 Why is the older adult's participation in daily activities important in achieving the OT intervention goals?

6 What is the ultimate goal of OT intervention with an older adult who has cancer?

7 What approaches can the OTA use to help the older adult who is experiencing anxiety, depression, or fear of the unknown?

8 At what point in the intervention process should the OTA be contributing to the discharge process with the other team members?

EVIDENCE NUGGETS: EFFECTIVENESS OF NONPHARMACOLOGICAL INTERVENTIONS IN THE MANAGEMENT OF LYMPHEDEMA

1. Melam GR, Buragadda S, Alhusaini AA, Arora N. Effect of complete decongestive therapy and home program on health-related quality of life in post mastectomy lymphedema patients. *BMC Womens Health*. 2016;16:23. Published 2016 May 4. doi:10.1186/s12905-016-0303-9
   - After 6 weeks of treatment, both the Conventional Therapy (CT) group and Complete Decongestive Therapy (CDT) group showed decreased pain and improved quality of life.

- The CDT group had significantly higher improvement in the QLQ BR-23 (Functional Scale) and the QLQ BR-23 (Symptom Scale) compared to the CT group.
- The greatest reduction of pain and therefore improved quality of life were found in the CDT group in the first 4 weeks of the treatment.

Continued

EVIDENCE NUGGETS: EFFECTIVENESS OF NONPHARMACOLOGICAL INTERVENTIONS IN THE MANAGEMENT OF LYMPHEDEMA—cont'd

2. Vafa S, Zarrati M, Malakootinejad M, et al. Calorie restriction and synbiotics effect on quality of life and edema reduction in breast cancer-related lymphedema, a clinical trial. *Breast*. 2020;54:37-45. doi:10.1016/j.breast.2020.08.008
   - Edema volume significantly decreased in both the calorie-restricted diet plus a symbiotic supplement (CRS) and a calorie-restricted diet plus a placebo (CRP) groups compared to the beginning of the study.
   - A greater reduction of BMI was noted for both the CRS and CRP groups in comparison to the control group.
   - The CRS and CRP groups showed a significant difference on the Lymphedema Life Impact Scale compared to the control group for the mean total, psychosocial, and functional scores.

3. Mayrovitz HN, Ryan S, Hartman JM. Usability of advanced pneumatic compression to treat cancer-related head and neck lymphedema: A feasibility study. *Head Neck*. 2018;40(1):137-143. doi:10.1002/hed.24995
   - A single treatment session was associated with a small but statistically and clinically significant reduction in the head and neck lymphedema.
   - For the subjective questions regarding treatment comfort, how the subject feels posttreatment, and the likeliness of the patient to use the treatment device at home; positive responses were statistically greater compared to the nonpositive responses.

   - 42 out of the 44 subjects were able to independently doff the pneumatic compression garments appropriately, demonstrating its ease of use.

4. Ochalek K, Gradalski T, Partsch H. Preventing early postoperative arm swelling and lymphedema manifestation by compression sleeves after axillary lymph node interventions in breast cancer patients: A randomized controlled trial. *J Pain Symptom Manage*. 2017;54(3):346-354. doi:10.1016/j.jpainsymman.2017.04.014
   - After 1 month of treatment, only the compression group displayed a reduction in the postoperative swelling.
   - In the compression group, significantly less edema was seen after 3, 6, and 9 months of treatment.
   - There was no difference in health-related quality of life between the compression group and group without compression.

5. Tugral A, Viren T, Bakar Y. Tissue dielectric constant and circumference measurement in the follow-up of treatment-related changes in lower-limb lymphedema. *Int Angiol*. 2018;37(1):26-31. doi:10.23736/S0392-9590.17.03843-3
   - There was a significant reduction in the circumference along all nine measurement sites of the lower limb after complex decongestive physiotherapy (CDP).
   - Percentage skin water content measurements displayed a significant decrease of skin tissue water for the ankle, calf, and thigh measurement sites after CDP.
   - CDP demonstrated a significant increase in overall quality of life.

For additional video content, please visit Elsevier eBooks+ (eBooks.Health.Elsevier.com)

REFERENCES

1. US Department of Health and Human Services. *Administration on Aging: A Profile of Older Americans*. 2020. Available at: https://acl.gov/about-acl/administration-aging.
2. Vespa J, Medina L, Armstrong DM. *Demographic Turning Points for the United States: Population projections for 2020 to 2060, P25-P114*. Washington, DC: US Census Bureau; 2018. Available at: https://www.census.gov/content/dam/Census/library/publications/2020/demo/p25-1144.pdf.
3. Howlander N, Noone AM, Krapcho M, et al., eds. *SEER Statistics Review, 1975-2017*. Bethesda, MD: National Cancer Institute; 2020. Available at: https://seer.cancer.gov/csr/1975_2017/.
4. Xu J, Murphy, SL, Kochanek, et al., eds. *National Center for Health Statistics: Mortality in the United States, 2018*. NCHS Data Brief; 2020. Available at: https://www.cdc.gov/nchs/products/databriefs/db355.htm
5. American Cancer Society. *Cancer Facts & Figures*. 2020. Available at: https://www.cancer.org/content/dam/cancer-org/research/cancer-facts-and-statistics/annual-cancer-facts-and-figures/2020/cancer-facts-and-figures-2020.pdf.
6. Arias E, Xu J. *United States Life Tables, 2018. National Vital Statistics Reports, 69(12)*. National Center for Health Statistics, Centers for Disease Control and Prevention. Available at: https://www.cdc.gov/nchs/data/nvsr/nvsr69/nvsr69-12-508.pdf.
7. American Lung Association. *Trends in Lung Disease*. 2020. Available at: https://www.lung.org/research/trends-in-lung-disease.
8. American Cancer Society. *Learn about Lung Cancer*. 2020. Available at: cancer.org/cancer/lung-cancer/about.html.
9. National Cancer Institute. *Cancer Stat Fact: Lung and Bronchus Cancer*. 2020. Available at: https://seer.cancer.gov/statfacts/html/lungb.html.
10. American Lung Association. *Trends in Lung Cancer Morbidity and Mortality*. 2014. Available at: http://www.lung.org/our-initiatives/research/monitoring-trends-in-lung-disease/.
11. Weiss J, Langer C. Treatment of lung cancer in the elderly patient. *Semin Respir Crit Care Med*. 2013;34:802-809. doi:10.1055/s-0033-1358560.
12. American Cancer Society. *Cancer Statistic Center*. 2018. Available at: https://seer.cancer.gov/archive/csr/1975_2017/#contents.
13. National Cancer Institute. *Cancer Stat Facts: Female Breast Cancer*. 2020. Available at: http://seer.cancer.gov/statfacts/html/breast.html.
14. Centers for Disease Control and Prevention. *U.S. Cancer Statistics: Breast Cancer Stat Bites*. 2020. Available at: https://www.cdc.gov/cancer/uscs/about/stat-bites/stat-bite-breast.htm.
15. American Cancer Society. *About Breast Cancer*. 2021. Available at: https://www.cancer.org/cancer/breast-cancer/about.html.
16. Karuturi M, VanderWalde N, Muss H. Approach and management of breast cancer in the elderly. *Clin Geriatr Med*. 2016;32(1):133-153.
17. Tang J, Tang S, Cheung K. Optimizing care of elderly women with primary breast cancer. *Eur J Clin Med Oncol*. 2012;4(3):45-53.
18. National Cancer Institute. *Cancer Stat Facts: Prostate Cancer*. 2020. Available at: https://seer.cancer.gov/statfacts/html/prost.html.

19. American Cancer Society. *About Prostate Cancer*. 2021. Available at: https://www.cancer.org/cancer/prostate-cancer/about.html

20. American Cancer Society. *About Colorectal Cancer*. 2021. Available at: https://www.cancer.org/cancer/colon-rectal-cancer.html.

21. National Cancer Institute. *Cancer Stat Facts: Colorectal Cancer*. 2020. Available at: https://www.seer.cancer.gov/statfacts/html/colorect.html.

22. Ugolini G, Pasini F, Montroni I, et al. How to select elderly colorectal cancer patients for surgery: a pilot study in an Italian academic medical center. *Cancer Biol Med*. 2015;12(4):302-307.

23. National Cancer Institute. *Metastatic Cancer: When Cancer Spreads*. 2020. Available at: https://www.cancer.gov/types/metastatic-cancer.

24. University of Rochester Medical Center. *Lung Metastasis*. Available at: https://www.urmc.rochester.edu/encyclopedia/content.aspx?contenttypeid=22&contentid=lungmetastasis.

25. American Cancer Society. *Advanced and Metastatic Cancer*. 2021. Available at: https://www.cancer.org/treatment/understanding-your-diagnosis/advanced-cancer.html.

26. Agarwal MG, Nayak P. Management of skeletal metastases: an orthopaedic surgeon's guide. *Indian J Orthop*. 2015;49(1):83-100. doi:10.4103/0019-5413.143915.

27. American Brain Tumor Association. *Metastatic Brain Tumors*. 2020. Available at: https://www.abta.org/tumor_types/metastatic-brain-tumors/.

28. Schiphorst A, Ten Bokkel Huinink D, Breumelhof R, et al. Geriatric consultation can aid in complex treatment decisions for elderly cancer patients. *Eur J Cancer Care (Engl)*. 2016;25(3):365-370. doi:10.1111/ecc.12349.

29. Gosney MA. Clinical assessment of elderly people with cancer. *Lancet Oncol*. 2005;6(10):790-797.

30. Kneis S, Wehrle A, Freyler K, et al. Balance impairments and neuromuscular changes in breast cancer patients with chemotherapy-induced peripheral neuropathy. *Clin Neurophysiol*. 2016;127(2):1481-1490. doi:10.1016/j.clinph.2015.07.022.

31. American Cancer Society. *Radiation Therapy*. 2021. Available at: https://www.cancer.org/treatment/treatments-and-side-effects/treatment-types/radiation.html.

32. Gore E, Movsas B, Santana-Davila R, et al. Evaluation and management of elderly patients with lung cancer. *Semin Radiat Oncol*. 2012;22:304-310.

33. American Cancer Society. *Chemotherapy Side Effects*. 2021. Available at: https://www.cancer.org/treatment/treatments-and-side-effects/treatment-types/chemotherapy/chemotherapy-side-effects.html.

34. Rennie H, MacKenzie G. The psychosocial oncology learning assessment: a province-wide survey of cancer care providers' learning needs. *J Cancer Educ*. 2010;25:206-210. doi:10.1007/s13187-010-0112-z.

35. Batioglu-Karaaltin A, Binbay Z, Yigiy O, et al. Evaluation of life quality, self-confidence and sexual functions in patients with total and partial laryngectomy. *Auris Nasus Larynx*. 2017;44(2):188-194. doi:10.1016/j.anl.2016.03.007.

36. Shih YT, Chien C. A review of cost communication in oncology: patient attitude, provider acceptance, and outcome assessment. *Cancer*. 2016;123(6):928-939. doi:10.1002/cncr.30423.

37. Goodman CC, Fuller KS. *Pathology: Implications for the Physical Therapist*. St. Louis: Elsevier; 2015.

38. American Cancer Society. *Fatigue and Weakness*. 2021. Available at: https://www.cancer.org/treatment/treatments-and-side-effects/physical-side-effects/fatigue.html.

39. Hwang EJ, Lokietz NC, Lozano RL, et al. Functional deficits and quality of life among cancer survivors: implications for occupational therapy in cancer survivorship care. *Am J Occup Ther*. 2015;69:6906290010. doi:10.5014/ajot.2015.015974.

40. American Occupational Therapy Association. Occupational therapy practice framework: domain and process fourth edition. *Am J Occup Ther*. 2020;74(suppl 2):1-96. Available at: https://research.aota.org/ajot/article/74/Supplement_2/7412410010p1/8382/Occupational-Therapy-Practice-Framework-Domain-and.

41. Centers for Disease Control and Prevention. *Important Facts about Falls*. 2017. Available at: https://www.cdc.gov/homeandrecreationalsafety/falls/adultfalls.html.

42. Banzer W, Bernhorster M, Schmidt K, et al. Changes in exercise capacity, quality of life and fatigue in cancer patients during an intervention. *Eur J Cancer Care (Engl)*. 2014;23:624-629. doi:10.1111/ecc.12201.

OTHER RESOURCES

Callanan M, Kelly P. *Final Gifts: Understanding the Special Awareness, Needs, and Communications of the Dying. (Reprint Edition)*. New York: Simon & Schuster; 2012.

Gawande A. *Being Mortal: Medicine and What Matters in the End*. New York: Metropolitan Books; 2014.

Gutkind L, ed. *At the End of Life: True Stories About How We Die*. Pittsburg: In Fact Books; 2012.

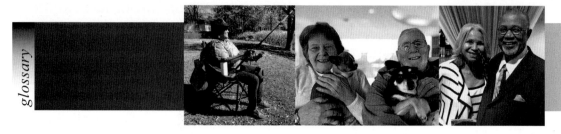

Glossary

A

abstractive: Having an abstracting nature or tendency; tending to be withdrawn or separate.

abuse: To use something for the wrong purpose in a way that is harmful or morally wrong.

activity-focused care: Part of person-centered care, which focuses on individual needs and wants. In person-centered care, caregivers interact with care recipients based on knowledge of and deep respect for them as unique human beings.

adaptations: The state of being adapted; adjustments.

adult day care: Services consist of planned programs and activities that provide supervised care and companionship to older adults during the day in a professional care setting. These programs are designed to promote well-being through health and social-related services.

adult foster home: Single-family residences that offer 24-hour care in a home-like setting. Adult foster homes provide the opportunity for residents to reside in a safe and caring family-like environment.

advance directives: A legal document that states a person's wishes about receiving medical care if that person is no longer able to make medical decisions because of a serious illness or injury. An advance directive may also give a person (such as a spouse, relative, or friend) the authority to make medical decisions for another person when that person can no longer make decisions.

adverse drug reactions: An appreciably harmful or unpleasant reaction, resulting from an intervention related to the use of a medicinal product, which predicts hazard from future administration and warrants prevention or specific treatment, or alteration of the dosage regimen, or withdrawal of the product.

advocacy: The act or process of supporting a cause or proposal: the act or process of advocating.

ageism: Prejudice or discrimination against a particular age group, particularly the elderly.

aging in place: Living where the elders have lived for years, typically not in a health care environment, using products, services, and conveniences that allow them to remain home as circumstances change. Elders continue to live in the home of their choice safely and independently as they get older. Livability can be extended through the incorporation of universal design principles, telecare, and other assistive technologies.

aging stereotypes: Beliefs concerning features of the aged population; they could be refined and amplified across the life span and could be manifested in both positive (e.g., wise and generative) and negative forms (e.g., unproductive and forgetful).

alopecia: A condition that causes hair to fall out in small patches.

alternative means: Different from the usual or conventional.

alternative transport: Community transportation other than individual motor vehicle use.

Alzheimer's disease: A brain disorder that slowly destroys memory and thinking skills and, eventually, the ability to carry out the simplest tasks.

American Occupational Therapy Association (AOTA) Ethics Commission (EC): The Ethics Commission (EC) is responsible for developing the Occupational Therapy Code of Ethics and Ethics Standards for the profession, which apply to occupational therapy personnel at all levels and in all professional and societal roles.

anemia: A lack of healthy red blood cells, resulting in an inability to carry adequate oxygen to the body's tissues.

angina: Chest pain caused by reduced blood flow to the heart.

aphasia: A disorder that results from damage to portions of the brain that are responsible for language.

aspiration pneumonia: The infectious pulmonary process that occurs after abnormal entry of fluids into the lower respiratory tract.

assessment: The process of considering all the information about a situation or a person and making a judgment.

assisted living: A system of housing and limited care that is designed for senior citizens who need some assistance with daily activities but do not require care in a nursing home.

assistive listening device (ALD): Any device, except hearing aids, which help a deaf or hard of hearing person communicate more effectively through direct sound amplification or visual or vibrotactile alerts.

associative: Dependent on or acquired by association or learning.

audiologist: An expert who can help to prevent, diagnose, and treat hearing and balance disorders for people of all ages.

autonomy: The ability to make your own decisions without being controlled by anyone else.

B

benefits: A helpful or good effect, or something intended to help.

blood pressure: The force of circulating blood on the walls of the arteries. Blood pressure is taken using two measurements: systolic (measured when the heart beats, when blood pressure is at its highest) and diastolic (measured between heart beats, when blood pressure is at its lowest). Blood pressure is written with the systolic blood pressure first, followed by the diastolic blood pressure (e.g., 120/80).

bolus: Food or liquid placed in the mouth for swallowing.

boutonnière deformity: A medical condition in which the finger is flexed at the proximal interphalangeal joint (PIP), and there is hyperextension at the distal interphalangeal joint (DIP).

bridging: The existence or formation of a physical connection, normal or abnormal, between two structures.

bronchiectasis: Lung tissue around the end of the breathing tube becomes infected.

burdens: Something difficult or unpleasant that you have to deal with or worry about.

C

cachexia: A wasting disorder that causes extreme weight loss and muscle wasting.

cancer: Group of diseases involving abnormal cell growth with the potential to invade or spread to other body parts.

cardiac rehabilitation: An important program for anyone recovering from a heart attack, heart failure, or other heart problem that required surgery or medical care.

cardiovascular disease: A type of disease that affects the heart or blood vessels.

caregivers: A person who gives care to people who need help taking care of themselves. Caregivers may be health professionals, family members, friends, social workers, or members of the clergy. They may give care at home or in a hospital or other health care setting.

case mix groups: Patient classification as a tool to improve financial and clinical management in a clinical facility.

cataracts: A condition in which the lens of the eye becomes cloudy. Symptoms include blurred, cloudy, or double vision; sensitivity to light; and difficulty seeing at night.

cerebrovascular accident: A loss of blood flow to part of the brain, which damages brain tissue. Cerebrovascular accidents are caused by blood clots and broken blood vessels in the brain.

chaining: Learning related behaviors in a series in which each response serves as a stimulus for the next response.

chronic bronchitis: A type of chronic obstructive pulmonary disease (COPD) that is defined as a productive cough of more than 3 months occurring within a span of 2 years.

chronic illness: Conditions that last 1 year or more and require ongoing medical attention or limit activities of daily living or both.

chronic obstructive pulmonary disease (COPD): Refers to a group of diseases that cause airflow blockage and breathing-related problems.

chronic pulmonary emphysema: A chronic lung condition. It's often part of COPD, a group of lung diseases that cause airflow blockage and breathing problems. It develops very slowly over time. It's most often caused by smoking. It causes shortness of breath that often gets worse with activity and many other symptoms, such as wheezing, cough, anxiety, and heart problems.

client-centered practice: Individual autonomy and choice, partnership, therapist and client responsibility, enablement, contextual congruence, accessibility, and respect for diversity.

clinical models of practice: Provides practitioners with terms to describe practice, an overall view of the profession, tools for evaluation, and a guide for intervention.

closed reduction: A procedure to set (reduce) a broken bone without cutting the skin open.

cochlear implant: A device that can help someone with hearing loss perceive sound.

cognition: A range of mental processes relating to the acquisition, storage, manipulation, and retrieval of information.

cognitive style: A person's characteristic mode of perceiving, thinking, remembering, and problem solving.

cohort: A collection or sampling of individuals who share common characteristics, such as individuals of the same age or sex.

collectivism: A social or cultural tradition, ideology, or personal outlook that emphasizes the unity of the group or community rather than each person's individuality.

community: The people living in one particular area or people who are considered as a unit because of their common interests, social group, or nationality.

community mobility: Planning and moving around in the community using public or private transportation, such as driving, walking, bicycling, or accessing and riding in buses, taxi cabs, ride shares, or other transportation systems (OTPF-4).

compensations: The counterbalancing of any defect of structure or function.

complex regional pain syndrome: A chronic pain condition. It causes intense pain, usually in the arms, hands, legs, or feet. It may happen after an injury, either to a nerve or to tissue in the affected area.

comminuted fracture: A fracture of a bone in which the separated parts are splintered or fragmented.

compound fracture: A bone fracture resulting in an open wound through which bone fragments usually protrude.

conductive hearing loss: When sounds cannot get through the outer and middle ear. It may be hard to hear soft sounds. Louder sounds may be muffled.

confidentiality: The ethical principle or legal right that a physician or other health professional will hold secret all information relating to a patient, unless the patient gives consent permitting disclosure.

constraint-induced movement therapy: An innovative, scientifically supported method of upper extremity rehabilitation for clients with neuromotor impairments.

context: The interrelated conditions in which something exists or occurs.

continued competency: The demonstration of specified levels of knowledge, skills, or ability not only at the time of initial certification but throughout an individual's professional career.

contraindicated: Anything (including a symptom or medical condition) that is a reason for a person to not receive a particular treatment or procedure because it may be harmful.

contrast sensitivity: The ability to distinguish between an object and the background behind it.

coping skills: The methods a person uses to deal with stressful situations. These may help a person face a situation, take action, and be flexible and persistent in solving problems.

creative reality (augmented reality): A technology that integrates digital information into the user's real-world environment.

cultural competence: The ability to understand, appreciate, and interact with people from cultures or belief systems different from one's own.

cultural context: The environment or situation that is relevant to the beliefs, values, and practices of the culture under study.

cultural norms: A societal rule, value, or standard that delineates an accepted and appropriate behavior within a culture.

cultural pluralism: A condition in which minority groups participate fully in the dominant society, yet maintain their cultural differences.

culture: The customary beliefs, social forms, and material traits of a racial, religious, or social group.

D

dehydration: A condition that occurs when the body loses too much water and other fluids that it needs to work normally. Dehydration is usually caused by severe diarrhea and vomiting, but it may also be caused by not drinking enough water or other fluids, sweating too much, fever, urinating too much, or taking certain medicines.

delayed union: A delay in the healing of the ends of a fracture and healing of a fracture that takes longer than expected.

demography: The statistical study of human populations especially with reference to size and density.

diabetic retinopathy: An eye condition that can cause vision loss and blindness in people who have diabetes. It affects blood vessels in the retina (the light-sensitive layer of tissue in the back of your eye).

dignity therapy: Therapy preserving end of life through asking questions regarding life history, work, and ultimately defining the patient's legacy.

diplopia: Double vision.

distributive justice: The justice that is concerned with the apportionment of privileges, duties, and goods in consonance with the merits of the individual and in the best interest of society.

driving: The ability to operate a motor vehicle safely and independently for travel within the community.

drug interactions: A change in the way a drug acts in the body when taken with certain other drugs, herbals, or foods, or when taken with certain medical conditions. Drug interactions may cause the drug to be more or less effective, or cause effects on the body that are not expected.

dysfunction: Impaired or abnormal functioning.

dysphagia: Difficulty with swallowing.

dyspnea: Shortness of breath; difficult or labored breathing.

E

eccentric viewing: A technique in which a person views objects by directing his or her gaze to an area just adjacent to the target object to compensate for a scotoma involving the fovea or macula. This position allows the desired target to be focused on a healthy area of retina.

edema: The abnormal accumulation of fluid in interstitial spaces of tissues, such as in the pericardial sac, intrapleural space, peritoneal cavity, and joint capsules.

education: The process of teaching or learning, especially in a school or college, or the knowledge that you get from this.

elder abuse: Any knowing, intentional, or negligent act by a caregiver or any other person that causes harm or a serious risk of harm to a vulnerable adult.

emerging practice: Responding to changes in the health care system by expanding the contexts and models for service provision.

end-of-life care: Support or treatment given during the time surrounding death.

energy conservation: Using less energy by adjusting behaviors and habits.

environment: The circumstances, objects, or conditions by which one is surrounded.

ethical dilemma: A situation in which two moral principles conflict with one another.

ethical distress: When one knows the ethically correct action to take but feels powerless to take that action.

ethics committee: Offer assistance in addressing ethical issues that arise in patient care and facilitate sound decision making that respects participants' values, concerns, and interests.

ethnicity: A particular ethnic affiliation or group.

ethnocentricity: Believing that the people, customs, and traditions of your own race or nationality are better than those of other races.

explicit bias: Conscious beliefs one has regarding a person, group, or population.

external fixation: May be used to keep fractured bones stabilized and in alignment. The device can be adjusted externally to ensure the bones remain in an optimal position during the healing process.

F

fall prevention: Instituting special precautions with the patient at risk for injury from falling.

fall protocol: A sequential process to assess immediate care needed following a fall; including but not limited to; current health status, safety of the scene for fall recovery, environmental needs to promote fall recovery, implementation of a fall recovery strategy to regain an upright position.

fall recovery: Techniques utilized by a person following a fall that enable them to regain an upright position.

fall reduction: Active strategies that can be implemented into a person's daily routine to help avoid or reduce falls from occurring, including, but not limited to managing internal factors to a person (such as medication management), as well as external factors (such as environmental modifications.)

falls: An event resulting in an unexpected, inadvertent descent to the ground or lower surface area.

family: A group of two or more persons related by birth, marriage, or adoption who live together; all such related persons are considered as members of one family.

fatigue: Feeling tired with low energy or a strong desire to sleep.

fecal incontinence: Involuntary loss of bowel control.

fracture: A break, usually in a bone.

function: Any of a group of related actions contributing to a larger action especially the normal and specific contribution of a bodily part to the economy of a living organism.

functional activities: Actions associated with basic daily home and work requirements: an umbrella term encompassing both activities of daily living and instrumental activities of daily living.

G

generational cohort: The group of individuals born within a similar time period who experience the same events within the same time or historical interval.

geriatrics: The care of elderly people based on the integration of knowledge of gerontology and chronic disease.

gerontology: The comprehensive study of aging and how it affects individuals—physically, socially, psychologically, and economically.

geropsychiatric unit: Units are departments of hospitals or nursing facilities that focus on treating mental health and psychiatric disorders in older adults, usually 60 years and older.

glaucoma: An abnormal condition of increased pressure inside the eyeball, often leading to damage to tissues of the eye and vision loss if untreated.

H

habits: A behavior pattern acquired by frequent repetition or physiologic exposure that shows itself in regularity or increased facility of performance.

health: The condition of being sound in body, mind, or spirit; also a general condition of well-being or flourishing.

health behaviors: Behaviors that affect health; can have a positive or a negative impact.

health belief model: A model for health education with a core tenet that individual beliefs about health conditions predict individual health-related behaviors.

health education: The process and strategies to educate people, groups, and populations about health.

health literacy: The degree to which a person has the capacity to understand, process, use, and obtain health information and services in order to make health decisions.

health management: One of the occupations identified in the OTPF-4. "Developing, managing and maintaining routines for health and wellness by engaging in self-care with the goal of improving or maintaining health, including self-management, to allow for participation in other occupations."

health promotion: Process of enabling people to increase control over, and to improve, their health. To reach a state of complete physical, mental, and social well-being, an individual or group must be able to identify and to realize aspirations, to satisfy needs, and to change or cope with the environment.

hearing aid: An electronic device for amplifying sound that is usually worn in or behind the ear of a person with hearing loss.

heart rate: The number of times the heart beats within a certain time period, usually a minute.

hemi-inattention (also referred to as hemi-neglect, neglect syndrome, unilateral neglect syndrome): A disregard or lack of attention for one side of a person's visual space. Inattention to the left visual space is much more common than inattention to the right.

hemiparesis (hemiplegia): Paralysis of one side of the body.

HIPAA The Health Insurance Portability and Accountability Act of 1996 (HIPAA) is a federal law that required the creation of national standards to protect sensitive patient health information from being disclosed without the patient's consent or knowledge.

home health: Includes skilled nursing care, as well as other skilled care services, like physical and occupational therapy, speech language therapy, and medical social services. These services are given by a variety of skilled health care professionals at home.

hospice: End-of-life medical care given to someone with a terminal illness.

hydration: The process of combining with water. In medicine, the process of giving fluids needed by the body.

hypertonicity: Excessive tone, tension, or activity.

hypotonicity: Lower or lessened tone or tension in any body structure, as in paralysis.

I

illness: An unhealthy condition of body or mind.

implicit bias: Unconscious beliefs one has regarding a person, group, or population.

individualism: A theory maintaining the political and economic independence of the individual and stressing individual initiative, action, and interests.

informed consent: Patients have the right to receive information and ask questions about recommended treatments so that they can make well-considered decisions about care.

inpatient rehabilitation: Free standing rehabilitation hospitals and rehabilitation units in acute care hospitals. They provide an intensive rehabilitation program and patients who are admitted must be able to tolerate 3 hours of intense rehabilitation services per day.

inpatient rehabilitation facility patient assessment instrument (IRF-PAI): The assessment instrument IRF providers use to collect patient assessment data for quality measure calculation and payment determination in accordance with the IRF Quality Reporting Program (QRP).

intergenerational: Being or occurring between generations.

intervention: The action of becoming intentionally involved in a difficult situation, in order to improve it or prevent it from getting worse.

J

joint protection: A technique for minimizing stress on joints, including proper body mechanics and the avoidance of continuous weight-bearing or deforming postures.

justice: A core value of occupational therapy that promotes occupational therapists to provide services to all persons who require services and remain objective.

L

learned helplessness: Occurs when an individual continuously faces a negative, uncontrollable situation and stops trying to change their circumstances, even when they have the ability to do so.

least restrictive environment: To the maximum extent appropriate, children with disabilities, including children in public or private institutions or other care facilities, are educated with children who are not disabled, and that special classes, separate schooling or other removal of children with disabilities from the regular educational environment occurs only when the nature or severity of the disability is such that education in regular classes with the use of supplementary aids and services cannot be achieved satisfactorily.

leisure: Activities include socializing, pleasure, meditating, painting, sports, etcetera.

lens: A clear part of the eye behind the colored iris. It helps to focus light on the retina so you can see.

LGBTQ+ An acronym for "lesbian, gay, bisexual, transgender, and queer" with a "+" sign to recognize the limitless sexual orientations and gender identities used by members of our community.

loss: The fact that you no longer have something or have less of something.

lymphedema: Swelling that generally occurs in one upper or lower extremity.

M

macular degeneration: A progressive deterioration of the macula of the retina and choroid of the eye.

malnutrition: A condition caused by not getting enough calories or the right amount of key nutrients, such as vitamins and minerals, that are needed for health. Malnutrition may occur when there is a lack of nutrients in the diet or when the body cannot absorb nutrients from food.

malunion: A bone heals, but not in the right position.

managed care: A health care delivery system organized to manage cost, utilization, and quality.

maturation: The process of becoming mature.

maximum heart rate: The age-related number of beats per minute of the heart when working at its maximum, that is usually estimated as 220 minus one's age.

Medicaid: Provides health coverage to millions of Americans, including eligible low-income adults, children, pregnant women, elderly adults, and people with disabilities.

Medicare: The federal government program that provides health care coverage (health insurance) if you are 65+, under 65 and receiving Social Security Disability Insurance (SSDI) for a certain amount of time, or under 65 and with end-stage renal disease (ESRD).

Medicare administrative contractures (MACs): Multi-state, regional contractors responsible for administering both Medicare Part A and Medicare Part B claims.

medication therapy management: A distinct service or group of services provided by health care providers, including pharmacists, to ensure the best therapeutic outcomes for patients. MTM includes five core elements: medication therapy review, a personal medication record, a medication-related action plan, intervention or referral, and documentation and follow-up.

metabolic equivalents: The amount of oxygen consumed while sitting at rest and is equal to 3.5 mL O_2 per kg body weight $\times$ min. The MET concept represents a simple, practical, and easily understood procedure for expressing the energy cost of physical activities as a multiple of the resting metabolic rate.

metastasis: Development of additional growths and tumors from a primary cancer site.

midline alignment: All midline anatomy is arranged on the straight line of the median plane and the body is balanced.

mid old: Elderly adults between the ages of 75 and 84 years.

minimum data set (MDS): Part of the federally mandated process for clinical assessment of all residents in Medicare and Medicaid certified nursing homes. This process provides a comprehensive assessment of each resident's functional capabilities and helps nursing home staff identify health problems.

minority: Any small group in society that is different from the rest because of their race, religion, or political beliefs, or a person who belongs to such a group.

mobility and seating assessment: The physical, functional, and environmental assessment of the wheelchair user to determine the most optimal seating and mobility solution.

motor action: Based on the neural structures within the spinal cord that produced a basic pattern of muscle activation.

muscle tone: The continuous and passive-partial contraction of the muscle or the muscle's resistance to passive stretch during the resting state.

myelosuppression: Impairment of the body to produce normal white blood cells, red blood cells, or platelets.

myths: A commonly believed but false idea.

N

National Board for Certification in Occupational Therapy (NBCOT): A national not-for-profit organization that provides certification for occupational therapy professionals. NBCOT develops, administers, and continually reviews its certification process based on current and valid standards that provide reliable indicators of competence of occupational therapy practice.

neglect: To not give enough care or attention to people or things that are your responsibility.

nonunion: The failure of a broken bone to heal.

nursing facilities: Provided by Medicaid certified nursing homes, which primarily provide three types of services: skilled nursing, rehabilitation, or long-term care.

nutrition: The taking in and use of food and other nourishing material by the body.

O

OBRA Omnibus Budget Reconciliation Act or the Nursing Home Reform Act of 1987; assisted in creating a national standard of care and rights for those living in nursing facilities.

occupation: An activity in which one engages.

occupational engagement: The degree to which a person is able to participate in occupations or occupational activities that are meaningful and the person connects to at a deeper level.

occupational justice: A virtue that is categorized within the value of Justice. Occupational justice promotes fair access of occupations for all people.

occupational therapy practice framework: An official document of the American Occupational Therapy Association (AOTA). Intended for occupational therapy practitioners and students, other health care professionals, educators, researchers, payers, policymakers, and consumers, the OTPF-4 presents a summary of interrelated constructs that describe occupational therapy practice.

oculomotor control: The ability to move the eyes together in a coordinated fashion.

old: Of or relating to the latter part of the life or term of existence of a person or thing.

older Americans act: Supports a range of home and community-based services, such as meals-on-wheels and other nutrition programs, in-home services, transportation, legal services, elder abuse prevention, and caregivers support. These programs help seniors stay as independent as possible in their homes and communities.

omnibus budget reconciliation act of 1987 (OBRA): Set forth new provisions for Medicare and Medicaid sections related to new standards for care in the nursing home setting.

oncology: The study of cancer.

open reduction internal fixation (ORIF): Puts pieces of a broken bone into place using surgery. Screws, plates, sutures, or rods are used to hold the broken bone together.

oral intake: Administration of food, liquid, or medication taken through the mouth.

organization health literacy: The degree organizations equitably enable people to find, understand, and use health information and services in order to make health decisions.

orthopedic: The treatment or study of bones that have not grown correctly or that have been damaged.

orthoses: An orthopedic appliance or apparatus used to support, align, prevent, or correct deformities or to improve function of movable parts of the body.

osteoarthritis: A form of arthritis in which one or many joints undergo degenerative changes, including subchondral bony sclerosis, loss of articular cartilage, and proliferation of bone and cartilage in the joint, forming osteophytes.

OTA/OT partnership: An OT works independently and is responsible for developing and carrying out treatment plans to help a person increase their independence in daily activities. Their work is higher level and more strategic in nature. It can be done in a variety of settings. An OTA does similar work to an OT, but they work under the supervision of an occupational therapist in carrying out the treatment plan. An OTA can decide when treatment needs to be modified according to patient/client progress. There is ongoing collaboration with the OT and OTA from the time the person is assessed through discharge.

outcome and assessment information set (OASIS): A group of standard data elements designed to enable systematic comparative measurement of home health care patient outcomes at two points in time in adult skilled Medicare and Medicaid, non-maternity home health care patients.

over-the-counter: Drugs that are bought over the counter are bought in a store without first visiting a doctor.

P

palliative care: Specialized medical care for a person living with a serious illness.

pathological fracture: A bone fracture which occurs without adequate trauma and is caused by a preexistent pathological bone lesion.

patient-driven groupings model (PDGM): A patient-centered payment system that places home health periods of care into more meaningful payment categories while eliminating the use of therapy service thresholds for adjusting payment for home health episodes. The system also moves payment from a single 60-day episode to 30-day periods of care, still retaining the 60-day certification and plan of care requirements.

patient-driven payment model (PDPM): To improve payment accuracy by addressing each patient's circumstances independently and classifying patients into payment groups based on specific, data-driven patient characteristics. PDPM redefines the relationship between payment and quality measures, realigning payment incentives and quality incentives.

pattern recognition: Identifying salient features of an object and using these features to distinguish the object from its surroundings.

pedestrian: An individual navigating the community near streets and roads, on foot or with alternative forms of mobility.

performance: The execution of an action: the ability to perform.

person-centered care: Individuals' values and preferences are elicited and, once expressed, guide all aspects of their health care, supporting their realistic health and life goals. Person-centered care is achieved through a dynamic relationship among individuals, others who are important to them, and all relevant providers. This collaboration informs decision-making to the extent that the individual desires.

personal health literacy: The ability to a person to find, understand, and use health information and services in order to make health decisions.

personhood: The state or fact of being an individual or having human characteristics and feelings.

physiological changes: A change in the normal function of a living organism. Occur with aging in all organ systems.

play: An imaginative, intrinsically motivated, interactive and rigorous activity. Play is fun-oriented, socially motivated, and guided by rules and regulations.

PLISSIT model: Offers a succinct method for introducing sex into a clinical conversation, narrowing the scope of a patient's concern and offering effective counseling and treatment.

polypharmacy: The concurrent use of multiple medications by a patient to treat usually coexisting conditions and which may result in adverse drug interactions.

positioning: A deliberate placement of the patient or a body part to promote physiological and/or psychological well-being.

prejudice: An unfair and unreasonable opinion or feeling, especially when formed without enough thought or knowledge.

presbycusis: A loss of hearing sensitivity and speech intelligibility associated with aging.

prevention: Education or health promotion efforts designed to identify, reduce, or prevent the onset and decrease the incidence of unhealthy conditions, risk factors, diseases, or injuries.

primary aging: The process of individuals aging that is not caused from a particular condition, instead it is caused by time impacting the physical, genetic, and molecular factors of an individual.

R

recovery model: An approach to care that is client centered, and holistic with a focus on building resilience and living a meaningful life despite any ongoing symptoms.

rescuing: To help someone or something out of a dangerous, harmful, or unpleasant situation.

resources: A useful or valuable possession or quality of a country, organization, or person.

rest: A state where the mind and body are calm and muscles are relaxed in order for the body to rejuvenate or recover.

restraint reduction: A goal for schools, hospitals, and human services organizations that are: committed to safely managing agitated behavior, dedicated to providing person-centered care, and bound by policies, licensing requirements, or state or federal rules, laws, or standards.

restraints: Any method, drug or medication, physical or mechanical devise, material or equipment, that immobilizes or reduces the ability of an individual to move any part of the body freely, particularly when used to restrict or manage a client's behavior or movement.

retina: Internal lining of the eyeball, functions much like film in a camera.

rheumatoid arthritis: An autoimmune and inflammatory disease, which means that your immune system attacks healthy cells in your body by mistake, causing inflammation (painful swelling) in the affected parts of the body.

role changes: A change in the shared conception and execution of typical role performance and role boundaries.

roles: The position or purpose that someone or something has in a situation, organization, society, or relationship.

S

scanning: Use of saccadic eye movements that move the eye to the object of interest.

scotoma: An area of the retina where vision is depressed or absent.

seating component: The parts and accessories that provide for the custom fit of a wheelchair and its seating system.

secondary aging: The process of individuals aging due to conditions that impact health and unhealthy lifestyle choices.

section GG: Includes admission and discharge self-care and mobility performance (GG0130 and GG0170) data elements.

self-care: Taking care of yourself so that you can be healthy, you can be well, you can do your job, you can help and care for others, and you can do all the things you need to and want to accomplish in a day.

self-management: Taking charge of one's own health to manage chronic conditions and complications that arise including treatment, symptom management, and necessary lifestyle changes.

self-medication: The act or process of medicating oneself, especially without the advice of a physician.

sensorineural hearing loss: Happens when there is damage in your inner ear.

service competency: The determination made by various methods that two people performing the same or equivalent procedures will obtain the same or equivalent results.

sexual activity: Means the oral, anal, or vaginal penetration by, or union with, the sexual organ of another or the anal or vaginal penetration of another by any other object; however, sexual activity does not include an act done for a bona fide medical purpose.

sexually transmitted diseases: Infections that are passed from one person to another through sexual contact.

side effects: Any effect of a drug, chemical, or other medicine that is in addition to its intended effect, especially an effect that is harmful or unpleasant.

skilled nursing facility (SNF): A facility (which meets specific regulatory certification requirements) which primarily provides inpatient skilled nursing care and related services to patients who require medical, nursing, or rehabilitative services but does not provide the level of care or treatment available in a hospital.

skilled services: Those services provided directly by a licensed professional for the purpose of promoting, maintaining, or restoring the health of an individual or to minimize the effects of injury, illness, or disability.

skills: The ability to use one's knowledge effectively and readily in execution or performance.

sleep: A state of mind and body that typically occurs for several hours at a time when the nervous system has minimal activity, eyes are closed, and the body and muscles are relaxed. There is minimal consciousness during this state.

sleep hygiene: Habits, practices, and routines that promote sleeping well on a regular basis.

social cognitive theory: Describes the influence of individual experiences, the actions of others, and environmental factors on individual health behaviors.

social support system: The provision of assistance or comfort to others, typically to help them cope with biological, psychological, and social stressors. Support may arise from any interpersonal relationship in an individual's social network, involving family members, friends, neighbors, religious institutions, colleagues, caregivers, or support groups.

spiral fracture: Occurs due to torsion or twisting force that produces a fracture that circles or spirals around the shaft.

stakeholders: A person such as an employee, customer, or citizen who is involved with an organization, society, etc. and therefore has responsibilities toward it and an interest in its success.

state regulatory board (SRB): The key bodies in state government responsible for setting licensing requirements, reviewing licensee applications, investigating complaints against licensees, and carrying out disciplinary measures.

stereotypes: Rigid concepts, exaggerated images, and inaccurate judgments used to make generalizations about groups of people.

strabismus: A condition in which an eye is deviated from its normal position and is not aligned with the other eye.

stress: The body's response to physical, mental, or emotional pressure. Stress causes chemical changes in the body that can raise blood pressure, heart rate, and blood sugar levels. It may also lead to feelings of frustration, anxiety, anger, or depression. Stress can be caused by normal life activities or by an event, such as trauma or illness. Long-term stress or high levels of stress may lead to mental and physical health problems.

stressors: Any event, force, or condition that results in physical or emotional stress. Stressors may be internal or external forces that require adjustment or coping strategies on the part of the affected individual.

stroke: Happens when there is a loss of blood flow to part of the brain. Your brain cells cannot get the oxygen and nutrients they need from blood, and they start to die within a few minutes. This can cause lasting brain damage, long-term disability, or even death.

subluxation: A partial abnormal separation of the articular surfaces of a joint.

subsystem: A system that is part of a larger system.

successful aging: An individual that ages and maintains a healthy mind, body, and is able to interact with others and their environment. The individual also does not develop a serious disease.

swan-neck deformity: Characterized by proximal interphalangeal (PIP) joint hyperextension and the distal interphalangeal (DIP) joint flexion. There is also reciprocal flexion noted of the metacarpophalangeal (MCP) joint. This is a result of an imbalance of the extensor mechanism of the digit.

T

tachypnea: Rapid breathing.

task: A usually assigned piece of work, often to be finished within a certain time.

teach-back method: A technique used by health care providers to ensure that patients are understanding the health information provided. This method is based on having the patient repeat or teach the health information or technique to the health care provider as a way to verify understanding.

therapeutic fibs: Lying, or bending the truth, in order to avoid increased agitation from a person with dementia.

thrombo-embolic deterrent (TED) hose: Also known as Compression Stockings or Anti-Embolism Stockings and are specially designed stockings that help reduce the risk of developing a deep vein thrombosis (also referred to as a DVT) or blood clot in your lower leg after your surgery, while you are unwell or while you are less active than normal.

tinnitus: A sensation of noise (such as a ringing or roaring) that is typically caused by a bodily condition (such as a disturbance of the auditory nerve or wax in the ear) and usually is of the subjective form which can only be heard by the one affected.

total hip replacement: Also called total hip arthroplasty, the damaged bone and cartilage is removed and replaced with prosthetic components.

transfers: To move someone or something from one place, vehicle, person, or group to another.

transtheoretical model of health behavior change: Health behavior change involves progress through five stages of change: precontemplation, contemplation, preparation, action, and maintenance.

transverse fracture: A type of broken bone. Transverse fractures run horizontally perpendicular to your bone (opposite the direction of your bone). You might see them referred to as complete fractures. This means the line of the break goes all the way through your bone. Transverse fractures usually affect long bones in your body.

trends: The general movement over time of a statistically detectable change.

U

ulnar drift: A hand deformity, seen in chronic rheumatoid arthritis and lupus erythematosus, in which swelling of the metacarpophalangeal joints causes the fingers to become displaced to the ulnar side.

undernourishment: The condition of not eating enough food to continue to be in good health.

unskilled services: Do not require the special knowledge and skills. Skilled services that are not adequately documented may appear to be unskilled.

urinary frequency: The need to urinate more often than usual as identified by the individual.

urinary incontinence: Involuntary loss of bladder control.

urinary retention: A condition in which a person is unable to empty all the urine from their bladder.

V

values: The principles that help you to decide what is right and wrong, and how to act in various situations.

velum: The soft area at the top in the mouth.

visual acuity: The clearness or sharpness of vision, typically measured in Snellen equivalents, such as 20/20.

visual attention: Ability to shift from object to object. Critical prerequisite for cognitive processing.

visual cognition: Product of the brain's ability to interpret patterns of visual input from the retina, commit the pattern to memory, recall pattern, and combine with other sensory information.

visual fields: The visual surround that can be seen when one looks straight ahead.

visual memory: Ability to use working memory to interpret a new pattern or recognize a familiar one and formulate a response.

voiding diary: A daily record of the patient's bladder and bowel activity. Records can also include the type of fluid intake and the frequency and volume of voids.

W

weight bearing: Any activity that one performs on one or both feet. It requires that one carry bodyweight on at least one lower extremity. Weight-bearing is an activity that the skeletal system does against gravity.

wheeled mobility devices: Medical devices that provide mobility and function for persons who have limited or no ability to ambulate without assistance from technology.

work: Exertion or effort directed to produce or accomplish something.

work simplification: The making of daily tasks easier in order to reduce strain or to decrease the amount energy required to complete an activity.

wrist subluxation: A condition that causes the joint to "snap," "pop," or "click" with rotation.

Y

young old: Elderly adults between the ages of 65 and 74 years.

BIBLIOGRAPHY

American Academy of Ophthalmology. For Public and Patients. American Academy of Ophthalmology. San Francisco, California. 2022.

American Occupational Therapy Association. Occupational Therapy Practice Framework: Domain and Process 4th Ed. *Am J Occup. Ther.* 2020; 74(suppl 2), 7412410010p1–7412410010p87. https://doi.org/10.5014/ajot.2020.74S2001.

American Psychiatric Association. *Diagnostic and Statistical Manual of Mental Disorders.* 5th ed. Washington, DC: The Association; 2013.

American Psychological Association. *APA dictionary of psychology.* Washington DC: The Association; 2022. Available at: https://dictionary.apa.org/.

Anderson DM(ed) Mosby's Medical, Nursing, and Health Dictionary. 11th ed. St. Louis: Elsevier; 2022.

Cambridge University Press. *Cambridge dictionary.* Cambridge: Cambridge University Press; 2022. Available at: https://dictionary.cambridge.org/.

Centers for Medicare & Medicaid Services. *Glossary.* Baltimore, Maryland: Centers for Medicare & Medicaid Services; 2022. Available at: https://www.cms.gov/glossary.

Centers for Medicare & Medicaid Services. *Medicaid.* Baltimore, Maryland: Centers for Medicare and Medicaid Services; 2022. Available at: Medicaid.gov.

Chan SCY, Au AML, Lai SMK. The detrimental impacts of negative age stereotypes on the episodic memory of older adults: does social participation moderate the effects? *BMC Geriatr.* 2020;20:452. Available at: https://doi.org/10.1186/s12877-020-01833-z.

Epstein EG, Haizlip J, Liaschenko J, Zhao D, Bennett R, Marshall MF. *Moreal Distress Mattering and Secondary Traumatic Stress in Provider Burnout: A Call for Moral Community.* AACN Advanced Critical Care. 21 (2). 146-157. 2020. Doi: https://doi.org/10.4037/aacnacc2020285

Goodman C, AGS Expert Panel of Person Centered Care. Person Centered Care: A definition and essential elements. *J Am Geriatr Soc.* 2016;64:15. doi:10.1111/jgs.13866.

Health Resources and Services Administration. *Data warehouse.* Rockville, Maryland: HRSA; 2021. Available at: https://www.hrsa.gov/.

Human Rights Campaign. *Resources.* Washington DC: Human Rights Campaign; 2022. Available at: https://www.hrc.org/resources.

Lee SB, Oh JH, Park JH, Choi SP, Wee JH. Differences in youngest-old, middle-old, and oldest-old patients who visit the emergency department. *Clin Exp Emerg Med.* 2018;5(4):249-255. Available at: https://doi.org/10.15441/ceem.17.261.

Merriam-Webster Incorporated. *Merriam Webster Collegiate Dictionary.* Springfield, Massachusetts: Merriam-Webster Incorporated; 2021.

Miller BF, Keane CB. *Miller-Keane Encyclopedia & Dictionary of Medicine, Nursing, and Allied Health.* 7th ed. Philadelphia: WB Saunders. 2005

National Board for Certification in Occupational Therapy. *Certification exam handbook.* Bethesda, Maryland: NBCOT; 2021.

National Institute of Health National Cancer Institute. *Dictionary of cancer terms.* Bethesda, Maryland: National Institute of Health; 2022. Available at: https://www.cancer.gov.

National Institute of Health National Institute on Deafness and Other Communication Disorders. Bethesda, Maryland: National Institute of Health; 2022. Available at: https://www.nidcd.nih.gov/.

National Institute of Health National Eye Institute. Bethesda, Maryland: National Institute of Health; 2022. Available at: https://www.nei.nih.gov/.

Stedman TL. *Stedman's Concise Medical Dictionary.* 28th ed. Baltimore: Lippincott Williams & Wilkins; 2006.

American Journal of Occupational Therapy. Occupational Therapy Practice Framework: Domain and Process—Fourth Edition. *Am J Occup Ther.* 2020;74(suppl 2):7412410010p1-7412410010p87. Available at: https://doi.org/10.5014/ajot.2020.74S2001.

United Stated Department of Health and Human Services Centers for Disease Control and Prevention. *Diseases & Conditions.* Washington DC: CDC; 2022. Available at: https://www.cdc.gov/Diseases Conditions/.

Venes D. *Taber's Cyclopedic Medical Dictionary.* 24th ed. Philadelphia: FA Davis; 2021.

Index

Note: Pages number followed by "*b*" indicate boxes; "*f*" figures; "*t*" tables.

THE DRAGON AND THE SNAKE

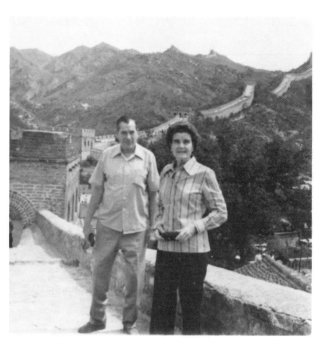

Thomas S. and Anne Gates at the Great Wall

THE DRAGON
& THE SNAKE

*An American Account of the
Turmoil in China 1976–1977*

*by Millicent Anne Gates
and E. Bruce Geelhoed*

With a Foreword by Gerald R. Ford

uɒɒ UNIVERSITY OF PENNSYLVANIA PRESS
Philadelphia · 1986

Permission is hereby acknowledged to reprint material from the following sources.

Michel Oksenburg and Sai-cheung Yeung, "Hua Kuo-feng's Pre-Cultural Revolution Years, 1949–1960: The Making of a Political Generalist." China Quarterly 69 (March 1977). Reprinted by permission of the United States Information Agency.

Henry Kissinger, Years of Upheaval. *Reprinted by permission of Little, Brown and Company.*

Harrison Salisbury, China: A Century of Revolution. *Reprinted by permission of Henry Holt and Company.*

Ross Terrill, The White-Boned Demon. *Reprinted by permission of William Morrow & Company, Inc.*

Library of Congress Cataloging-in-Publication Data

Gates, Millicent Anne.
  The dragon & the snake.

  Bibliography: p.
  Includes index.
    1. China—Politics and government—1976–
I. Geelhoed, E. Bruce, 1948–   .   II. Title.
III. Title: Dragon and the snake.
DS779.26.G38   1986   951.05'7   86-19218
ISBN 0-8122-8036-9

Printed in the United States of America
Designed by Adrianne Onderdonk Dudden

To Thomas S. Gates III

Contents

Foreword

The Dragon and the Snake: An American Account of the Turmoil in China, 1976–1977 recounts the story of Thomas S. Gates's leadership of the United States Liaison Office to the People's Republic of China during a crucial period in recent Chinese-American relations. It is also an account of one aspect of Tom Gates's distinguished career of service to America, in a post which played an important part in the foreign policy of my administration.

I first met Tom Gates during the early years of World War II when we were shipmates aboard the *U.S.S. Monterey (CVL 26)* in the Pacific. The relatively brief time which we served together in the Pacific was only the prelude, however, to a friendship which grew and lasted between us for the next four decades. We became especially close during the 1950s when I served in the United States House of Representatives as a member of the Subcommittee on Defense Appropriations of the House Committee on Appropriations, and Tom Gates regularly testified before our committee in his capacity as secretary of the navy, and then later as secretary of defense, in the administration of Dwight D. Eisenhower. As a result of our many experiences together, I came to admire and greatly respect Tom as a man who was totally dedicated to his country and who also possessed the high degree of sound judgment so necessary to effective leadership in our nation's Department of Defense.

In 1976, as president I faced the decision of appointing a successor to George Bush as the chief of the United States Liaison Office in Peking and, in surveying the list of possible candidates for this post, I immediately remembered my long friendship with Tom Gates. In my mind, Tom met every qualification which I considered vital for the successful performance of this responsibility. More importantly, Tom was a person of impeccable personal and public integrity who epitomized honesty in everything that he said and did. He proved to be an outstanding presidential envoy and a most worthy representative for our country in China.

Seen now through the perspective of Anne Gates, Tom Gates's widow, and Bruce Geelhoed, his research associate, *The Dragon and the Snake* explains the dynamics of being an American who was living and working in China during a critical period in recent Chinese history. The book also reveals the great importance which those of us in the Ford administration attached to the essential improvement of relations between the United States and the People's Republic of China.

GERALD R. FORD

Preface

In the autumn of 1981, Thomas S. Gates began work on a historical account of his experiences in government which included his service as secretary of the navy and secretary of defense in the Eisenhower administration, and chief of the United States Liaison Office to the People's Republic of China during the Ford administration. Tom was also a life trustee of the University of Pennsylvania, and his decision to undertake a published account of his public career occurred, in good measure, in response to the rather persistent encouragement which he received from the university's senior administrators.

After analyzing the sizable task which lay ahead of him in organizing a large quantity of official records, spending many hours before a tape recorder in recollecting the important events and decisions in which he had participated, and then in composing draft after redraft of a manuscript, Tom Gates asked his friends at the University of Pennsylvania to retain a historian to work with him as his research assistant and partner on the project. In response to that request, Bruce Geelhoed, a historian of the defense policy of the Eisenhower administration, took a leave of absence from his responsibilities at Ball State University in Muncie, Indiana, to assist Tom Gates in his endeavor.

The project's original objective was a historical account of Tom Gates's experiences in the Pentagon during the Eisenhower administration as well as his service as presidential envoy to China in the Ford administration. In fact, after some discussion with several scholars at the University of Pennsylvania, Tom even chose a prospective title for his study, "From the Pentagon to Peking: Memoirs, 1953–1977." After more than a year's research, however, both Tom Gates and Bruce Geelhoed concluded that the experience in China between 1976 and 1977 merited a separate volume, and so they agreed to publish two separate studies. The Chinese account was to appear first with the story of Tom's tenure in the Eisenhower administration to come later.

Tom Gates and Bruce Geelhoed reached this decision in the summer of 1982. Less than a year later, unexpected complications of a chronic illness would claim Tom's life, on March 25, 1983. Following Tom's passing, Millicent Anne Gates, his widow, agreed to work with Bruce Geelhoed in continuing the project to completion. Anne Gates had, of course, been in Peking with Tom during his important period as chief of USLO. She witnessed first-hand the dramatic events which occurred in China at that time as the Chinese began a social, political, and economic transition which continues to this day. More important, she became acquainted with the members of the USLO staff, the Peking diplomatic community, and the various personalities in the Chinese leadership who crossed the paths of the Americans in China. To a considerable extent, therefore, *The Dragon and the Snake* reflects the observations of both Tom and Anne Gates as they encountered a Chinese nation in a period of critical change. The forces in China which they analyzed during the mid-1970s would become more evident in the mid-1980s as both the United States and China continued to build upon the diplomatic framework established a decade earlier.

Acknowledgments

We wish to thank a great number of helpful people who have supported this project in many important ways. President Emeritus Martin Meyerson of the University of Pennsylvania, during his tenure as president of the university, initially encouraged Thomas S. Gates to undertake a published account of his years in government. President Meyerson also obtained valuable research grants from the SmithKline Beckman Foundation and the INA Foundation in support of this project.

In addition to President Meyerson, Dr. Vartan Gregorian, then the provost of the University of Pennsylvania, and Dr. Robert H. Dyson, Jr., the first Thomas S. Gates Dean of the Faculty of Arts and Sciences at the university, were instrumental in coordinating many of the details associated with this project in 1981–82. Without the support of these three outstanding scholar-administrators and that of the University of Pennsylvania, this book would not have been possible.

Several of Thomas S. Gates's distinguished colleagues also agreed to be interviewed for this study. Former President Gerald R. Ford kindly took time to comment on his relationship with Tom Gates. David Dean, currently the executive director of the American Institute in Taiwan, and Richard Mueller of the United States Department of State, served with Tom Gates in China and spent several hours with the authors, recounting their experiences in Peking between 1976 and 1977. James H. Douglas, whose tenure in Washington paralleled that of Tom Gates during the 1950s, also provided an interview for this study.

We also wish to acknowledge the assistance of Frank Machak, Jessie Williams, James Anderson, Jack Friedman, and Ivan Izenberg of the Classification/Declassification section of the State Department. Their assistance in the identification of important diplomatic records and cheerful cooperation were critical to the completion of this study. We also wish to thank the staff of the Special Collections Department at the University of Pennsylvania Library and particularly James Dallett, the university archivist, for their assistance.

Finally, our families were supportive of our efforts throughout the entire project. They patiently interrupted their own plans and schedules in order to assist in the research and writing tasks of the study. We love them all and thank them for their interest and encouragement.

E. Bruce Geelhoed
Muncie, Indiana

Millicent Anne Gates
Devon, Pennsylvania

December 1985

"Everything Seemed to Happen in 1976 and 1977"

On May 6, 1976, Thomas Gates arrived in Peking to begin his tenure as chief of the United States Liaison Office (USLO) to the People's Republic of China (PRC). Nominated to this post the previous March by President Gerald R. Ford and subsequently confirmed by the Senate with the rank of ambassador, Tom thus became America's official representative to the largest nation on earth. His service as the presidential envoy to China lasted until May 1977, when President Jimmy Carter replaced him with Leonard Woodcock. Tom's year of diplomatic experience in the PRC therefore included a good portion of both 1976 and 1977, the Year of the Dragon and the Year of the Snake, respectively, in the Chinese lunar calendar.

Tom Gates had been very active in public life prior to his departure for China in the spring of 1976, although he had not held a full-time position in Washington since leaving the Eisenhower administration in 1961. Throughout the 1950s, he occupied several high-level posts in the Defense Department, first as under secretary of the navy (1953 to 1957), then as secretary of the navy (1957 to 1959), deputy secretary of defense (May to December 1959), and finally as secretary of defense (1959 to 1961). As secretary of defense during the last fourteen months of Dwight D. Eisenhower's presidency, Tom sat on the National Security Council and served as the president's principal adviser on military affairs. When combined with his other duties at the Pentagon, these responsibilities brought him into frequent contact with Secretary of State Christian Herter; Gordon Gray, Eisenhower's national security adviser; Allen Dulles, the director of the Central Intelligence Agency; and other representatives of the diplomatic community and the national security establishment. As a result, Tom became vitally involved in the national security planning process during the 1950s and retained a strong interest in international affairs even after he left the Cabinet in 1961 to return to his banking career with the Morgan Guaranty Trust Company in New York.

By virtue of his experience in the Eisenhower administration, Tom Gates felt no professional reluctance in accepting Gerald Ford's offer to serve as chief of the United States Liaison Office in China. By agreeing to serve as presidential envoy to the PRC, he became responsible for keeping both President Ford and Secretary of State Henry A. Kissinger informed on developments in China which affected American foreign policy and, in addition, working for improved relations between the two countries. In that regard, the chief of USLO "worked for the president" in addition to overseeing the operation of the American mission in China. Indeed, the opportunity to represent President Ford, rather than the administrative responsibilities of supervising the USLO operation, ultimately became the determining factor in Tom's decision to re-enter public service.

Between the time of his Senate confirmation and the date for the actual departure to China, Tom Gates conscientiously studied the history, culture, and political traditions of the People's Republic of China as part of a cram course in Sinology administered to him by the State Department. No amount of study, however, could have sufficiently prepared anyone for the events which unfolded in China during his tenure. Between January 1976 and August 1977, the People's Republic of China witnessed the most tumultuous period in its history. During this short time, the PRC withstood a virtually incomparable series of political, economic, and social dislocations. Three heroes of the Chinese Revolution, Premier Zhou Enlai, veteran Field Marshall Zhu De, and Chairman Mao Zedong, all died in 1976. Their deaths left gaping holes in the Chinese national psyche and, just as important, in the apparatus of the state and the Chinese Communist Party. The deaths of Premier Zhou and Chairman Mao accelerated the intense power struggle then under way between the PRC's rival political factions for control of post-Mao China, a struggle which took what to most Western observers were completely unpredictable turns. This fascinating struggle began with Deng Xiaoping's purge from his posts in the Party and government and the subsequent elevation of the almost-unknown Hua Guofeng as premier in the winter-spring of 1976. Then, amazingly, the struggle continued with the purge of Deng's radical foes, the Gang of Four, in October and ended with Deng's rehabilitation (for the second time in his career) in the spring of 1977. It has since become clear that the deaths of Zhou and Mao, and the purge of

Deng, in 1976 provided an opening for the entrance of other Chinese leaders onto the stage of China's political drama. More specifically, three relatively unknown Chinese leaders, Hua Guofeng, Marshall Ye Jianying, the PRC's veteran defense minister, and Li Xiannian, one of China's respected civilian vice premiers, dominated the politics of the Year of the Dragon and the Year of the Snake. After two and one-half decades of analyzing Chinese policy from the standpoint of the pronouncements of Mao and Zhou, officers of the USLO and Western observers in general began to get a glimpse of how the PRC would conduct its affairs in the absence of its historical giants.

Economically, China continued in 1976 and 1977 to wrestle with the gigantic tasks of feeding its population and modernizing its industry. But severe drought in some regions of China, and cold, wet weather in others, combined to produce poor harvests in both years. Industrial production also suffered as political factionalism and provincial strife resulted in strikes, sabotage, and even violence at several vital factory complexes. To further complicate the Chinese economy, the worst earthquake in history devastated the industrial city of Tangshan in late July 1976, taking a terrible toll in human life and also disrupting transportation, coal, iron, and steel production, and communications throughout north China. In meeting the herculean task of providing relief and reconstruction assistance to the beleaguered Chinese in Tangshan and Tianjin, the central authorities diverted resources from other provinces, a necessary action but nevertheless one which created shortages and economic bottlenecks throughout the country.

Socially, the Year of the Dragon and the Year of the Snake witnessed the emergence of a genuine, visible expression of public opinion in China which rival Chinese political factions sought to manipulate for their own purposes. When Tom Gates arrived in Peking, the radical campaign to "deepen the criticism" of Deng Xiaoping had exploded with great ferocity throughout China. The radical faction's control of the media reflected this attempt by Deng's foes to turn the Chinese masses against the individual widely believed to be the late Premier Zhou's choice for a successor.

In early April, however, one month before Tom's arrival, tens of thousands of Chinese in Peking and across the country indicated their displeasure with the anti-rightist campaign. During the days of the Qing Ming festival, from March 30 to April 5, throngs of Chinese assembled in Tienanmen Square to place memorial wreaths at the Martyr's Monument in honor of the beloved Premier Zhou. More pro-Zhou, and by extension pro-Deng and anti-Mao, demonstrations also occurred simultaneously in other parts of China. Knowledgeable Chinese observers immediately grasped the significance of these demonstrations; they were not only a tribute to the late premier but also a warning to the radicals that China's masses "well understood" their ill treatment of Zhou during his final years and also disapproved of the anti-Deng campaign. When Peking's authorities sought to disperse the demonstrators in the capital on April 5, a riot broke out which resulted in considerable mayhem, several deaths, and scores of injuries. American officials who reported the scene to Washington even recalled seeing the almost unheard-of sight of several demonstrators assaulting an armed officer of the People's Liberation Army (PLA).[1] The PLA responded to these so-called Tienanmen riots by restoring order in a display of force which remained effective for the remainder of the year and well into 1977.

Six months later, in October, China witnessed an outpouring of relief, celebration, and sheer joy when the Party Center, nominally led by Hua Guofeng, arrested and thereby purged the leaders of China's radical faction, the so-called Gang of Four which included Jiang Qing, Mao's widow, and her Shanghainese cohorts Zhang Chunqiao, Wang Hongwen, and Yao Wenyuan. Huge demonstrations, both spontaneous and organized, again erupted in Peking, Shanghai, and at provincial levels throughout the country. The downfall of the "Shanghai clique" meant the end of the Cultural Revolution, experienced Chinese observers again assumed. Yet, even with the Gang of Four imprisoned, the Hua regime maintained a decidedly neo-Maoist profile in November and December. Once again, the Chinese masses expressed their displeasure with the leadership and pressed for the prompt rehabilitation of Deng Xiaoping. A well-organized campaign by Deng's supporters to rehabilitate the twice-deposed vice premier climaxed during the winter and early spring of 1977 and resulted in the Politburo's decision to restore Deng to the posts which he had held prior to his ouster by the radicals almost a year earlier.

In summarizing all these remarkable events, Tom Gates once wrote that "everything seemed to happen in 1976 and 1977" in China. Indeed the Chinese, who possess a legendary ability to take the historically long view, considered this period the most eventful of any in several centuries.[2] The dramatic events of the Year of the Dragon and the Year of the Snake possessed their own singular importance but, more important, collectively represented the transition from a China governed by revolutionary heroes preoccupied with questions of ideology to one managed by Communist administrators who confronted the domestic and international problems of a major world power as it attempted to adjust to the realities of the last quarter of the twentieth century. The breakup of the Long March generation in 1976 and 1977 ushered in a new era in the PRC's history.[3] In a real sense, Hua Guofeng, Ye Jianying, and Li Xiannian faced the immense task of carrying the initial burden of Chinese leadership during a period in which the entire nation was beginning a process of transformation.

Watching the unfolding drama in China proved fascinating for Tom Gates and the other Americans living in Peking in 1976 and 1977. Reporting

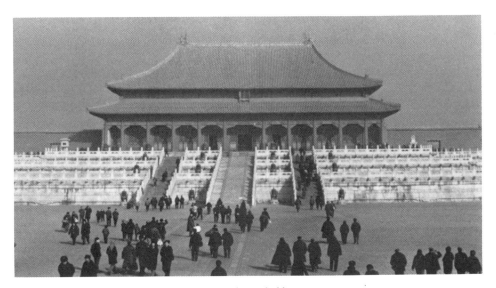

Entrance to the Forbidden City

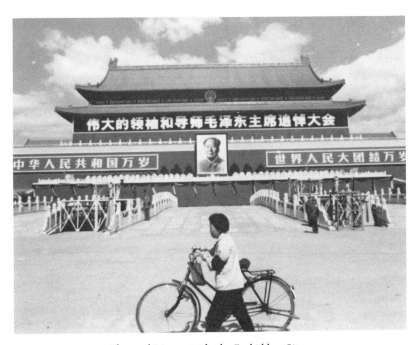

Photo of Mao outside the Forbidden City

these events to Washington and trying to interpret their significance, however, represented only one aspect of the American responsibility in Peking.
A greater concern involved the future of the Chinese-American relationship
and the degree to which the USLO could promote progress in this vital area
of foreign policy. By 1976, this concern loomed large indeed in the minds of
America's China-watchers, especially since the relationship had developed
some worrisome strains over the previous three years.

For a variety of complex reasons, America and China had made little
progress between 1973 and 1976 in resolving the outstanding issues which
blocked each country's diplomatic recognition of the other. The dramatic initiatives which had occurred in Chinese-American relations between 1971
and 1973—Henry Kissinger's secret visit to China in 1971, Richard Nixon's
trip to Peking and his meetings with Mao and Zhou in 1972 which resulted
in the issuance of the Shanghai Communique, and the agreement in 1973
reached by Kissinger and Zhou to establish respective liaison offices in
Washington and Peking—all belonged to the past.[4] The momentum gener-
ated between 1971 and 1973, which many knowledgeable observers believed
would lead to normalization within a relatively brief time, slowed to a virtual snail's pace by 1976 as difficult international differences between America and China and, more significantly, domestic upheavals in each country,
prevented the kind of diplomatic progress contemplated just five years earlier
by both American and Chinese leaders.

Despite these problems, neither nation had retreated from the objective
of full normalization, a goal which Tom affirmed upon his arrival in China.
When he announced his intention to "work for the normalization of relations between the United States and the People's Republic of China," he correctly described the Ford administration's China policy[5] but did not ignore
the unsteady diplomatic situation which then existed between the two countries. Tom was not in Peking long before he discovered the extent of China's
impatience and even disapproval of the direction of American foreign policy
since 1973. The Chinese reserved most of their frustration for America's
continued reluctance to recognize the PRC, and not the Republic of China
(ROC) on Taiwan, as the legally constituted government of China. In that
regard, the Chinese insistently demanded that America withdraw its troops
and recall its ambassador from Taiwan, in addition to abrogating the 1954
defense treaty with the ROC, as the price for any future diplomatic progress. Discreet suggestions to PRC officials that they might help American
policy-makers on this issue by resolving to settle their Taiwan dispute by
"peaceful means" and "without the use of force" inevitably produced the
curt response that such remarks constituted an unacceptable American attempt to meddle in China's internal affairs.

The Chinese behavior on the Taiwan issue continued to fascinate Tom
Gates and the USLO officials throughout their tenure in China. Undeniably,

the matter became a point of contention between the Americans and their hosts. More curiously, though, the Chinese appeared content to make their position clear on this subject without prescribing any particular timetable for a favorable American response. While the Chinese insisted that they had spelled out their position on the Taiwan issue in the Shanghai Communique (and thus no further clarifications were necessary) and regarded America's refusal to break with the ROC as irresponsible, the PRC's officials repeatedly indicated a willingness to "wait" and show "patience" until the United States found a convenient time to meet China's conditions. Tom soon grew accustomed to the strange policy ambiguity whereby the Chinese insisted for the record that America sever its relations with Taiwan immediately as the price of complete normalization at the same time that they were conducting a semi-normal practice of diplomacy with USLO officials. The PRC appeared willing to wait indefinitely for the United States to see what it considered the reasonableness of the Chinese position, but indefinitely did not mean forever. As one Chinese radical reputedly said, "How can Kissinger be sure we will have patience?"[6] On another occasion, Tom encountered a similar expression as one senior Chinese diplomat reminded him that the PRC "had been waiting for twenty-seven years" for the United States to break with Taiwan. To emphasize their concern, Chinese officials frequently informed Tom that "Taiwan is an American problem" and the United States should not expect to enjoy the luxury of a two-China policy permanently.[7]

Continued American involvement in Indochina between 1973 and 1975 also complicated the Chinese-American relationship in 1976. Had not Premier Zhou informed President Nixon in 1972 that future progress in relations between America and China depended upon a resolution of the conflict in Indochina? Chinese officials inquired. Yet after signing the 1973 Paris accord, the United States continued to support the Thieu regime in South Vietnam. When added to the lack of progress on the Taiwan issue, continued American involvement in Southeast Asia created internal political difficulties for both Mao and Zhou, both of whom attached much importance to China's new relationship with the United States. The "American opening" represented a profound break with the course of the PRC's foreign policy, and if the initiative proved to be too great a domestic political liability for Mao and Zhou, who could predict the future course of relations between the two countries?[8]

The Chinese also reacted strongly to the recent course of Soviet-American relations and, on this matter, they showed no ambiguity. Chinese distrust, and even contempt, of the Soviet Union appeared limitless, even reaching the point where the PRC prohibited any of its people from working in the Soviet Embassy. According to PRC officials, the Soviets were "paper tigers" and "social imperialists." Unlike the Chinese who practiced "self reliance" in order to feed, house, and clothe their population, the Soviets humiliatingly crawled to the West and begged for grain, technology, and capital. "We stand for independence and self-reliance," the Chinese repeatedly stated. "This does not mean we decline to study foreign experience, neither does it mean we lock the door against the world and refuse to develop foreign trade or to introduce from abroad certain techniques and equipment really useful to China. But this is entirely different from . . . depending on foreign technologies and equipment for developing China's economy."[9]

Anxious to assert their own influence with the developing nations of the Third World, the Chinese always renounced any ambitions to reach "superpower" status and were therefore critical of the direction of Soviet foreign policy in the mid-1970s. Was America willing to stand by helplessly while Cuban proxies of the Soviet Union undermined the stability of emerging African nations? Chinese officials repeatedly asked. What about the Helsinki Declaration and the so-called Sonnenfeldt Doctrine; did these not signify a "Munich mentality" and "appeasement"? Did the United States not realize that the Soviet Union sought global "hegemony" and was attempting to intimidate Western Europe and Japan with its military buildup? Throughout his year in Peking, Tom repeatedly reassured the Chinese that the United States government fully intended to fulfill its diplomatic commitments and also maintain a strong national defense. Despite such assurances, the Chinese continued to warn virtually every visiting American Congressional delegation about their assessments of Soviet intrigue, with the parallel assertion that the United States would become a "declining power" and the Soviet Union a "rising power" if the current international trend continued.

Differences in outlook between China and the United States over the international situation, serious though they were, did not constitute the major barriers to normalization, however. In retrospect, it became apparent that both nations could have moved more rapidly toward normalization between 1973 and 1976 if domestic factors in both countries had not greatly hampered the effective conduct of foreign policy. In the United States, progress toward improved relations with China became stalled when the Watergate scandal, and then the presidential campaign of 1976, made any continuation of the strong initiatives of 1971–73 too politically risky for Presidents Nixon and Ford. In China, Chairman Mao and Premier Zhou fell into steadily deteriorating health after 1972, the year in which Zhou's physicians informed him that he had cancer of the bladder. In the autumn of 1973, Zhou himself came under vigorous attack from the radical faction within the Politburo, especially for his conduct of foreign policy.[10] Nor did the radicals cease their campaign against Zhou once he fell ill; in fact, they intensified their efforts to gain control of China's political apparatus in anticipation of his demise, and when Zhou died in January 1976, the radical faction used its control of the national media to sharply limit the extent of the masses' mourning for the late premier. According to one account, Yao Wenyuan (the radical Politburo member who controlled the media) personally forbade the nation's propaganda organs to broadcast the list of names on Zhou's funeral committee, to televise any popular expressions of grief over the premier's death, or to broadcast any pictorial history of Zhou's life. In addition, the radicals organized the mourning in such a fashion that Zhou's body, as it lay in state, was placed in a room where any television cameraman would encounter difficulty recording scenes of the leadership paying its respects to Deng Yingchao, Zhou's widow.[11] Thus, both American and Chinese domestic considerations prevented diplomatic progress more than did any major international differences between the two countries.

To a great extent, Tom Gates realized that domestic factors in the United States strongly affected the diplomatic environment in which he operated. At first glance, one would not suspect that the Watergate scandal exerted much influence on America's policy toward the PRC. But when Watergate exploded in full fury during the summer and autumn of 1973, it exposed Richard Nixon's political weakness and invited attack on all the policies of his administration, including his foreign policy.[12] The carefully prepared achievements of Nixon's first term—the opening to China, the SALT I Treaty with the Soviet Union, indeed the entire policy of detente—became objects of attack once Watergate embraced his presidency. By the middle of 1974, Nixon faced the likelihood of impeachment by the House of Representatives and conviction by the Senate, an action which would have meant removal from office. Confronting that dilemma, Nixon sought to preserve the full extent of his conservative support in Congress throughout the Watergate crisis. He well understood that if he raised the China issue, he was certain to alienate his conservative backers, and therefore, wishing to avoid the charge of "selling out Taiwan," he relegated progress on normalization with the PRC to a lesser role.

Gerald Ford's accession to the presidency in August 1974 briefly changed the foreign policy environment as it affected America's future relations with the PRC. Shortly after taking office, Ford addressed a joint session of Congress and reaffirmed his support of the objectives of Nixon's foreign policy. China-watchers, both in the Ford administration and elsewhere, presumably applauded the course laid out by the new president. Not forced to govern under the burden of a major scandal, Ford stood on firmer ground than his Watergate-stricken predecessor on the question of improved Chinese-American relations. Furthermore, Ford's knowledge of foreign policy extended well beyond the range assumed by his critics. With over two decades of experience on the House Subcommittee on Defense Appropriations, Ford had followed the trend of America's postwar foreign and defense commitments. On the matter of America's policy toward China, Ford strongly supported improved relations with the PRC and was one of the few Americans (along with Nixon and Kissinger) to meet personally with both Mao and Zhou in the 1970s. That meeting occurred in July 1972 when he visited China while he was minority leader of the House of Representatives.[13]

Gerald Ford's best intentions to normalize relations with the PRC, however, soon ran afoul of the 1976 presidential primaries and the general election campaign. The conservative challenge to the Ford presidency is a familiar story but parts of it bear repeating because of their impact upon the administration's China policy. As the primaries unfolded in February and March 1976, Ford won close victories over Ronald Reagan, his conservative challenger, in New Hampshire and Florida. He followed that with a more substantial victory in Illinois and seemed well on the way to locking up the GOP nomination. With his campaign in some disarray, Ronald Reagan badly needed a victory over Ford in the North Carolina primary on March 23. After well over two months of active campaigning, Reagan had discovered that a surefire way to energize his audiences was to attack the Ford administration's foreign and defense policies. Reagan reserved most of his ammunition for charges that Ford and Kissinger intended to "give away the Panama Canal." Yet, he was also sharply critical of detente ("placating our adversaries") and skeptical about America's improved relations with the People's Republic of China.[14] Reagan's critique of the Ford/Kissinger foreign policy struck an especially responsive chord with conservative voters in the South and West. When Reagan won an upset victory over Ford in North Carolina, his campaign received the lift which galvanized his candidacy and guaranteed a continuation of the attack on the administration's foreign policy right up to the Republican National Convention in August. In April and May, published reports also began circulating that the State Department was considering the discussion of possible arms sales to the PRC. Reagan immediately saw this development as detrimental to the interests of Taiwan, although he conceded that it may have been an example of "our developing relationship" with the PRC.[15] Reagan's comments on the issue, however, proved that China policy was a potential political liability for the Ford administration and the entire discussion soon collapsed.

Gerald Ford successfully overcame Ronald Reagan's challenge at the Republican Convention in Kansas City in August 1976. Even so, Reagan's conservative followers still prevailed in writing an essentially anti-administration foreign policy plank into the GOP platform. The Party's position on Chinese-American relations supported a continuation of the two-China policy which had been in effect since 1972.

Tom Gates considered these partisan political developments unfortunate and often asked himself whether real progress in Chinese-American relations was possible when the two nations remained far apart on the Taiwan issue and domestic controversies raged on in each country. Yet he soon discovered, early in 1976, primarily in conversations with President Ford, that America and China still had much of a worthwhile nature to say to each other. In December 1975, Ford himself had visited China for the second time. On that occasion, he met again with Mao Zedong but, more important, held extensive discussions with Vice Premier Deng Xiaoping. Because of the uncertain domestic situations in each country, Ford's visit failed to produce either the substantive results or the boost to public relations that the Nixon trip had three years earlier. Even Kissinger described the second Ford visit as a holding action.[16]

For some valid reasons, however, the president did not share the pessimistic assessments of his trip. First, every presidential visit to a foreign nation is a high-level affair. When compared to the effort which the Chinese put forth for Nixon in 1972, their treatment of Ford was well in keeping with the importance which they attached to relations with the United States. Second, Ford's journey to Peking underscored a sense of continuity in America's China policy. In briefing the press on December 4 after Ford's meetings with Mao and Deng, Kissinger noted that the "visit served to put the relationship of 1972 into a more mature" framework. In that sense, each country took another step forward in dealing positively with the other.[17]

Ford's discussions with Deng, moreover, clarified the extent of existing Chinese-American disagreements as well as the areas of common interest. Both countries were concerned about recent examples of Soviet adventurism, both sides were interested in keeping Western Europe and Japan economically strong and militarily secure, and both sides continued to be divided on the Taiwan issue. In his discussions with Deng, however, Ford pressed for an expansion of the various bilateral arrangements which existed between America and China in such areas as trade, science, and cultural exchanges. Deng backed off; he wanted the Taiwan issue settled first before agreeing to progress in the other fields.[18] In retrospect, one suspects that Deng's hesitation to pursue a new negotiating path stemmed from his knowledge of the recent radical attacks on Zhou's foreign policy as well as his own then-precarious position within the Chinese hierarchy. Not wishing to risk his place in the leadership on any new initiatives toward the United States, Deng kept strictly to the record of the Chinese position as outlined in the Shanghai Communique. Even so, Ford left Peking with an admiration for Deng and the belief that America's interests in China were better served with him in power than with a member of the radical faction.[19]

In conclusion, Tom Gates soon realized that America's new relationship with China was of great strategic importance. The Ford administration acknowledged this point publicly; in September 1975, Kissinger had declared that "there is no relationship to which the United States assigns greater significance than its new ties with the People's Republic of China." After his visit to Peking, Ford considered "America's relationship with China a permanent part of the international political landscape."[20] Since 1972, the Americans and the Chinese had shown their interest in each other's policies, recognized that their problems with the Soviet Union outweighed their respective differences, and dramatically reduced the danger of war with each other.[21] Yet by 1976, each nation found itself devoting much of its public energy to the resolution of internal, partisan, and highly emotional political matters. As presidential envoy to China during the Year of the Dragon and the Year of the Snake, Tom Gates bore the responsibility for maintaining the thread of America's relations with the People's Republic during a difficult period for both nations. Tom's tenure in Peking occurred after a startling series of diplomatic spectaculars; his challenge was to preserve the new relationship through the diligent application of workman-like diplomacy. Such a task was completely necessary, although considerably less glamorous than the presidential summitry to which the American public had grown accustomed during the early to mid-1970s. In that context, Tom's job of "holding the fort in Peking," of preserving the Chinese-American relationship and not permitting it to deteriorate, proved to be a truly fascinating, intellectually challenging experience.[22] To his credit, Tom Gates understood that *both* America and China benefited from a time when improved relations were possible only if acrimonious foreign policy issues did not complicate the domestic political environments. In that regard, Gerald Ford summarized Tom's contribution to American diplomacy during the mid-1970s by noting that not only was he the right choice for America's representative *to* China at the time but also he was the right American to be *in* China in 1976 and 1977.[23]

Notes

1. United States Department of State, Official Files, Peking to Washington, 5 April 1976. Hereafter cited as OF, date.

2. Thomas S. Gates, "On China," *Pennsylvania Gazette* 76, no. 8 (September 1978): 29. See also Ross Terrill, *The Future of China: After Mao* (New York: Delacorte Press, 1978), pp. 8–23; Roger Garside, *Coming Alive: China After Mao* (New York: McGraw-Hill, 1981), pp. 13–17, 18.

3. Terrill, *Future of China*, pp. 1–25. We are also indebted to Jack Friedman of the United States Department of State for his description of the political struggles in the PRC in 1976 and 1977 as evidence of "the breakup of the Long March generation."

4. See Henry A. Kissinger, *White House Years* (Boston: Little, Brown, 1979), pp. 736–55, 1049–53; and Richard Nixon, *RN: The Memoirs of Richard Nixon* Vol. II (New York: Warner, 1978), pp. 7–52, for a discussion of the Sino-American diplomatic initiatives of the early 1970s. Kissinger, *Years of Upheaval* (Boston: Little, Brown, 1981), pp. 60–63, covers the Kissinger/Zhou discussions which led to the establishment of diplomatic liaison offices.

5. *New York Times*, 7 May 1976.

6. See Senator Mike Mansfield, "China Enters the Post-Mao Period," *Report Number Three*, Senate Foreign Relations Committee, U.S. Congress, Senate, 94th Congress, 2d Session (Washington: Government Printing Office, 1976), pp. 4–10; also Terrill, *Future of China*, pp. 182–83.

7. Terrill, *Future of China*, p. 190.

8. Richard Nixon, *The Real War* (New York: Warner, 1980), pp. 126–49. The bitter war in Cambodia, and the role of the Americans and Chinese in it, was an especially sore point between the two nations. See William Shawcross, *Sideshow* (New York: Simon and Schuster, 1979), pp. 360–61.

9. OF, "Basic Policy, 1976," n.d., 1976.

10. Kissinger, *Years of Upheaval*, pp. 678–99. Kissinger also discusses how domestic controversies in both America and China during the mid-1970s presented obstacles to normalization between the two countries. See his essay, "Mr. Schultz Goes to China," in *Observations* (Boston: Little, Brown, 1985), pp. 139–49.

11. OF, Peking to Washington, 12 December 1976.

12. Kissinger, *Years of Upheaval*, p. 582; Nixon, *RN*, 2: 583–84.

13. Gerald R. Ford, *A Time to Heal* (New York: Harper and Row/Reader's Digest Press, 1979), pp. 96–98.

14. Lou Cannon, *Reagan* (New York: G. P. Putnam's Sons, 1982), pp. 210–18; Rowland Evans and Robert Novak, *The Reagan Revolution* (New York: E. P. Dutton, 1981), pp. 54–55, 57; Ford, *A Time to Heal*, pp. 373–74; Jules Witcover, *Marathon* (New York: Viking Press, 1977), pp. 401–3.

15. *New York Times*, 27 May 1976; "U.S. Arms for Red China?" *Forbes* 119, no. 11 (1 June 1976): 21–22.

16. Kissinger, *Years of Upheaval*, p. 698; see also Terrill, *Mao: A Political Biography* (New York: Harper and Row, 1980), pp. 397–99, and *Future of China*, pp. 28–29.

17. OF, "Highlights of Secretary Kissinger's Press Conference," 4 December 1975, Peking; Gerald R. Ford, interview with the authors, 6 May 1983, Grand Rapids, Michigan; David Dean, interview with the authors, 7 December 1982, Rosslyn, Virginia.

18. Thomas S. Gates Oral History, 30 October 1982. Hereafter cited as Gates OH, date.

19. Interview, Gerald R. Ford.

20. OF, "US-PRC Relations," Briefing Paper, 21 August 1976.

21. Terrill, *Future of China*, pp. 174–77.

22. Gates OH, 30 October 1982.

23. Interview, Gerald R. Ford.

CHAPTER **I**

"Tell the President We'll Go"

On January 16, 1976, Thomas Gates received a telephone call in his office at the Morgan Guaranty Trust Company in New York from Vice President Nelson Rockefeller. Close personal friends since the 1930s, the two men enjoyed a warm relationship which included an occasional business association before World War II as well as service together in the Eisenhower administration during the 1950s. The vice president wasted little time describing the purpose of his call. "Tom, are you sitting down?" he asked. "President Ford wants you to go to China as chief of the United States Liaison Office in Peking. If you agree, the president will send your name up to the Senate for confirmation as ambassador."

Taken completely by surprise, Tom Gates asked Rockefeller to explain the circumstances which had brought his name to the president's attention. Patiently, Rockefeller related that the China post had stood vacant since late in 1975 when Ford had summoned George Bush, then the chief of the USLO, back to the United States to assume the directorship of the CIA. Early in November, the Ford administration had undergone a major personnel shake-up, referred to by Washington's political pundits as the Halloween Massacre; Bush had replaced William Colby as director of the CIA, Ford had fired James Schlesinger as secretary of defense and appointed Donald Rumsfeld to fill that post, Richard Cheney had replaced Rumsfeld as the White House chief of staff, and Henry Kissinger remained secretary of state while relinquishing his duties as the president's national security adviser to

Brent Scowcroft.[1] When Rockefeller telephoned Tom Gates in mid-January, therefore, the administration had not yet found a suitable replacement for Bush as the chief of the USLO and, considering the importance of America's new relationship with the PRC, Ford wanted to fill the vacancy expeditiously.

After Ford recalled George Bush, he received an extensive list of potential candidates to fill the post of chief of the United States Liaison Office in Peking. Ford was dissatisfied with the qualifications of the individuals recommended to him for this post. But then he thought of Tom Gates, with whom he had had a long personal and professional relationship. The two men had first met during World War II as fellow naval officers aboard the *U.S.S. Monterey* in the Pacific. (Tom outranked Ford during the war, a point Ford loved to bring to Tom's attention in the years thereafter.) During the 1950s, Tom often testified before the House Subcommittee on Defense Appropriations in his capacity as secretary of the navy and then as secretary of defense; Ford was a leading Republican on this subcommittee and therefore played a key role in the formation of the defense budget.

For several reasons, Tom met the important criteria which both Gerald Ford and the Chinese considered necessary for the person who served as chief of the United States Liaison Office in Peking. First, the chief functioned as the personal envoy of the president and the secretary of state in addition to handling the administrative responsibilities of the mission in China. The Chinese expected the chief to possess direct personal access to both the president and the secretary of state and not simply be a functionary of the foreign policy bureaucracy. Both David Bruce and George Bush, Tom's two predecessors as chief of the USLO, enjoyed such access to Nixon, Ford, and Kissinger. Considering Tom's longstanding friendship with Ford, the Chinese could be certain of Tom's freedom to talk directly with the president about the status of Sino-American relations.

A second factor working in Tom Gates's favor for this post was his record in the Department of Defense during the 1950s, especially his tenure as secretary of defense between 1959 and 1961. By virtually every account, Tom's performance as secretary of defense was highly regarded; he had skillfully dealt with several difficult defense policy issues and served faithfully as Eisenhower's principal military adviser during the last year of his presidency.[2] The Chinese preferred that the United States appoint a chief of the USLO who already owned a proven record in government, a person with acknowledged stature, not an individual who received the post on the basis of past political service. Not only did such an appointment underscore the importance which America attached to its relationship with the PRC, but it also, so the Chinese believed, prevented an American diplomat from developing his professional reputation at their expense.

Furthermore, American relations with the Soviet Union had recently taken a turn for the worse during the mid-1970s. In that regard, Ford envisioned a second importance to Tom Gates's past experience in the Pentagon as it related to the USLO post. In appointing Tom as chief of the USLO, Ford effectively served notice to the Soviets that the United States took its new relationship with the PRC seriously and that he was qualified to discuss any matter with the Chinese which the two sides considered appropriate. The Soviets possessed an extreme sensitivity to any hint of possible military co-operation between the United States and China and, while Tom's appointment did not reflect any plan by the administration for a Chinese-American defense effort, it nevertheless effectively kept the Russians off-balance in making an assessment of the depth of the relationship between the United States and the PRC.[3]

Finally, Tom would celebrate his seventieth birthday on April 10, 1976, and his age represented another factor in his favor as the prospective chief of the United States Liaison Office. The Chinese leadership, comprised of men mostly in their seventies and even eighties, regarded advanced age as a sign of wisdom and experience. Tom's stature as an elder statesman made it more likely that he would be able to gain the respect of the Chinese. For those reasons, Rockefeller summarized on the telephone, the president wanted Tom to take the post. Considering the sudden nature of the request and the fact that he was unaware that the administration was even considering him for this position, Tom asked the vice president to allow him a couple weeks to consult with his colleagues and family before giving his final answer. Rockefeller found this suggestion agreeable and promised to inform the president accordingly.

Although highly flattered by Gerald Ford's offer, Tom Gates was initially inclined to refuse it. In January 1976, Tom was actively contemplating retirement from a professional career which began almost fifty years earlier after his graduation from the University of Pennsylvania in 1928. During the 1930s and 1940s, he developed a profitable investment banking practice in both Philadelphia and New York with the well-established firm of Drexel and Company, Incorporated (now Drexel, Burnham, Lambert, Incorporated). When the United States entered World War II in 1941, Tom enlisted in the navy and served as an air combat intelligence officer in both the Mediterranean and the Pacific, ultimately rising to the rank of lieutenant commander.

After the war, Tom returned to Philadelphia to continue his investment banking career until September 1953, when Secretary of the Navy Robert B. Anderson asked him to join the Defense Department as under secretary of the navy. Tom expected to stay at the Navy Department for only two or three years or possibly until the end of Eisenhower's first term. As it happened, however, he became totally involved in the civilian management of the Pentagon and remained in Washington until Eisenhower left office in 1961.

After stepping down as secretary of defense, Tom Gates joined the Morgan Guaranty Trust Company of New York as the chairman of its executive committee in April 1961. In August 1962, he succeeded Dale Sharp as Morgan's president and in June 1965 became chairman of the bank's board of directors and chief executive officer. He concluded his tenure as chairman in 1969, although he continued to chair Morgan's executive committee and also remained a director of the bank until 1976. Even without daily operating responsibilities at the Morgan Guaranty Trust Company after 1969, however, Tom stayed active as a director of several large corporations in Pennsylvania and also served as a trustee of both the University of Pennsylvania and the College of the Atlantic in Bar Harbor, Maine.[4] For obvious reasons, Tom warmly anticipated a return to a less-hectic life at our permanent home in Devon, Pennsylvania, after spending most of the past quarter-century in either Washington or New York. Full retirement also held out the attractive prospect of being close to two of our three daughters and their families, both of whom lived nearby in suburban Philadelphia.

To further complicate the decision, Tom never possessed any desire to be an ambassador and, as he recalled later, "my own frustration with the State Department from the outside [during the 1950s] did not encourage me to be on the inside."[5] Like many of his other Pentagon colleagues, Tom often grew discouraged with the perception of a slow pace of decision-making at the State Department as well as the endless meetings and mountains of paperwork which seemed to ensnarl its senior officers. "At State, they all write novels to each other," he once moaned. Furthermore, Tom also sensed a trend developing in the 1960s and 1970s where government-to-government business moved increasingly between Washington and other foreign capitals. As a result, ambassadors seemed all too often to be shunted to the diplomatic sidelines or left with only routine administrative and protocol matters. For all these reasons, when President Nixon offered Tom an appointment as ambassador to West Germany in 1971, he declined.

In declining Nixon's offer, however, Tom Gates discovered the extraordinarily difficult task of refusing a presidential request. During the 1950s, Tom proved exceptionally unsuccessful in this regard; on two separate occasions, Dwight D. Eisenhower talked him out of returning to private life in order to fill important Pentagon vacancies, first as secretary of the navy in 1957 and then as deputy secretary of defense in 1959.[6] In refusing the ambassadorship to West Germany, Tom spent three days drafting a letter to Secretary of State William Rogers, another close friend from the Eisenhower administration, explaining the reasons for his inability to accept Nixon's offer. Tom quickly realized the personal difficulty of declining an important position offered by Jerry Ford, whom he not only admired as president but also valued as a friend.

In giving the entire matter further thought, moreover, Tom Gates became intrigued with the possibility of going to China, for several important reasons. First, ever since leaving the Eisenhower administration, he had been concerned about the perilous state of relations between the United States and the People's Republic of China. It seemed a particular act of folly on the part of the United States government to ignore diplomatically the nation which comprised one-quarter of the earth's population. In addition, the People's Republic certainly intended to grow stronger, both economically and militarily in the years ahead, and any attempt to keep it isolated was bound to create strategic problems for the United States in the Far East. In May 1965, shortly before becoming chairman of the Morgan Guaranty Trust Company, Tom gave a speech in New York in which he advocated pressing the military campaign against the Viet Cong to a victory, followed by a strong initiative to establish diplomatic relations with the PRC. Coming as it did during a critical time in America's involvement in the Vietnam War, Tom's speech won him few admirers. Public opinion in America simply was opposed to improved relations with the PRC at this particular time.[7] After Nixon and Kissinger completed the American opening to China between 1971 and 1973, however, Tom was correctly credited as one of the first Americans to recognize the potential advantages to the United States of better relations with the PRC.

Second, Tom also considered the unique responsibilities of the chief of the USLO and the operation of the liaison office itself, concluding that the chief was not an ambassador in the normal diplomatic sense nor was the USLO a typical embassy. In 1976, the USLO was only three years old, established as a result of an agreement negotiated by Kissinger and Zhou Enlai. Both the USLO and the Liaison Office of the People's Republic of China in Washington served a specific diplomatic purpose; they were created in recognition that "the Sino-American dispute over Taiwan" should not negate the fact that "common concerns . . . required regular and intimate contact" between the two nations.[8] Otherwise, the liaison offices were "embassies in all but name," administered in the normal diplomatic fashion with each country's personnel enjoying diplomatic immunity.[9] The head of each liaison office held the title of chief, instead of ambassador, although that distinction was more semantic than substantive. Both David Bruce and George Bush held ambassadorial rank and functioned in that capacity by conducting the normal flow of diplomatic exchanges between Peking and Washington. Their appointments also revealed the Nixon administration's (and later the Ford administration's) desire to send outstanding men to China; the chief of the USLO was no mere political appointee. The position held a special place within America's foreign policy network during the mid-1970s, and Tom discovered the possibility of serving as the presidential envoy to China and, in the extraordinary way in which the liaison offices conducted their business, also avoid much of the diplomatic routine which characterized the work of other embassies. Indeed, the prospect of engaging in "regular and intimate contact" with the Chinese, on behalf of the president, within this highly unusual and less prescribed environment ultimately became the determining factor in Tom's decision to accept Ford's offer. In that important respect, the China opportunity had no parallel; as Tom said, China *was* different.

Thus with mixed feelings about Gerald Ford's offer, Tom spent the last two weeks of January consulting with members of his family, his business associates, and former colleagues from the Eisenhower administration about whether to become the next presidential envoy to China. For the Gates family, the prospect of serving the administration in China seemed like a tremendous opportunity and well worth delaying our return to Devon for one to two years. (Once we were in China, we felt it was a privilege to be there. With the Ford administration strongly committed to normalization with the PRC, Tom was prepared to stay in China as long as the president desired. Had Ford been reelected in 1976, Tom most likely would have remained in Peking until full normalization occurred.) Our three daughters, Anne (Mrs. Joseph Ponce), Patsy (Mrs. William Norris), and Kathe (Mrs. Charles McCoy) all strongly encouraged their father to accept the position. Two of Tom's close business associates, Elmore (Pat) Patterson, then the chairman of J. P. Morgan and Company, and Lewis Preston, then an executive vice president and now the chairman of Morgan, also argued strongly for acceptance. "Sitting around on the fringe of things at the golf club isn't good enough, Tom," Preston advised. Dr. Thomas Langfitt, chief of neurosurgery at the University of Pennsylvania Hospital and Tom's longtime physician, informed him that *no* medical reason existed for *not* accepting the post. In fact, Langfitt explained that he understood Tom's formal retirement was only a short time away and, if he was concerned about his health, he should remain as active as possible (that is, go to China) after such a busy working life.

In Tom's mind, the major drawback to accepting the post was his own self-confessed lack of knowledge about Chinese affairs. To be sure, he was well-acquainted with the strategic importance of the Far East to America's national security. But absorbing the tremendous amount of information necessary to function as chief of the USLO seemed an overwhelming task, especially in view of the short amount of time left before the president wanted the next envoy nominated, confirmed, and at work in Peking. At the end of January, therefore, Tom began consulting some of his colleagues from the Eisenhower years to get their advice on the matter. In separate conversations with Amory Houghton, Douglas Dillon, General George Brown, then the chairman of the Joint Chiefs of Staff but also Tom's military aide when he served as secretary of defense, and with Robert Lovett, President Harry S. Truman's secretary of defense, Tom received variations of the same message: as important as China had become to the foreign policy of the United States since 1971, its importance was certain to grow in the future. If Tom thought he could make a strong contribution to better relations between the two countries, he should accept the post.

Finally in late January, Tom Gates spoke with both David Bruce and George Bush to discuss his concern about a knowledge of Chinese affairs as a prerequisite for taking the post. Both men agreed that Chinese-American relations had changed rapidly in the past half-decade and few individuals could responsibly consider themselves expert in this field. The State Department's officers at the China desk in Washington, as well as the Foreign Service contingent in Peking, were experienced and diligent, however. Tom could therefore expect competent support from both sources and should feel confident about taking the assignment. Given his previous experience at the Pentagon and knowledge of foreign policy, he would encounter little difficulty adapting to the new responsibility.[10]

Somewhat reassured but not entirely convinced that he should accept Ford's offer, Tom finally called Nelson Rockefeller in early February and asked him to thank the president for considering him but, given his present circumstances, he felt it necessary to decline the post. The vice president was not surprised by Tom's response, agreeing that he had performed more than his share of public service and was entitled to a full retirement. Neither Tom nor I, however, was pleased with this decision but believed that it was the only responsible course. Knowing that the president needed to fill the post quickly, we did not wish to further delay his selection process.

On February 9, 1976, Tom and I left Philadelphia for what we assumed would be a two-month vacation at the El Dorado Club in Palm Springs, California. Five years earlier, we had begun a custom of spending February and March in Palm Springs, visiting with old friends from the Eisenhower administration who also vacationed there, playing golf, and enjoying the beautiful weather. More than anything else, El Dorado meant visiting with Amory and Laura Houghton, two close friends whose home was usually overflowing with guests. Amory Houghton had served as ambassador to France under President Eisenhower during the late 1950s and he and Tom became well-acquainted at that time. A gracious hostess, Laura Houghton also ran something of a salon for the retired Cold Warriors of Ike's presidency at her "Pink House" in Palm Springs.

At the time of our visit in 1976, the Houghtons' sole house guest was Robert D. Murphy, former under secretary of state to both John Foster Dulles and Christian Herter, and an individual who exerted a great influence on America's postwar foreign policy. Bob Murphy and Tom Gates had also worked closely as members of the National Security Council's 5412 Committee, which oversaw intelligence matters and other aspects of NSC policy. One evening, Am Houghton raised the subject of Ford's offer to appoint Tom as chief of the USLO, and Murphy immediately brightened up. "You're going, aren't you?" he asked. Shaking his head, Tom replied that he had declined the post. With considerable emotion, Murphy responded, "I think you should reconsider. Zhou just died, Mao's ill, China's going to change. You ought to be there. You'll be useful to the administration and, besides, it's a once-in-a-lifetime opportunity."

The next day, Tom, Am Houghton, and Murphy were joined by Robert Lovett and James Douglas, who had served as deputy secretary of defense under Tom at the end of the 1950s. The five men sat around the pool at the Houghtons' residence, talking about China and whether Tom should reconsider his decision, fully mindful that Ford may already have offered the post to another person. Tom especially valued the advice of Bob Lovett and Jim Douglas, although Douglas's views on the subject were a bit surprising. "Forget all this policy business, Tom," he said. "You'll reach an understanding of that part of the job soon enough. If you think going to China will mean a richer life for you and Anne, go ahead and take the position." [11]

Then chance played a trick. While Murphy was in Palm Springs, he received a telephone call from President Ford asking him to come to Washington to discuss accepting the chairmanship of the newly created Intelligence Oversight Board. Murphy left California apparently convinced that Tom had changed his mind about accepting the USLO post. On February 16, President Ford telephoned Tom directly and asked him to take the USLO position, reiterating the reasons why he was the administration's first choice. But Tom still hesitated and requested another two to three days to consider the offer. "Tom, you've always been a lousy bridge player so quit playing games with me and take the job," Ford demanded. At that point, I called out (loudly enough, presumably, for Ford to hear), "Tell the president we'll go." After that comment, Tom agreed to accept the nomination, to the everlasting amusement of Ford, who believed his wife had apparently made the difference in the decision. But Tom and I always suspected that when Bob Murphy returned to Washington, he personally informed Ford about Tom's change of thinking about the China post and encouraged him to contact him again.

II

Once Tom had decided to accept the nomination as chief of the United States Liaison Office to Peking, we spent a relaxing time in California until March 15, when we returned east to begin the process of preparing for our departure to China at the end of April. Tom resigned from all of his directorships and trusteeships in accordance with federal conflict-of-interest regulations. He would have to have confronted these decisions anyway, since the mandatory retirement age for most directors was seventy and he celebrated that particular birthday on April 10.

After two days in Devon, Tom spent most of the next two weeks in Washington, beginning with a 10:15 A.M. meeting with the president on March 19. News of Tom's nomination as chief of the USLO had leaked prematurely, as usually happens in Washington, and his session with Ford officially confirmed the administration's action.[12] Kissinger and Scowcroft also attended the meeting, which included a brief review of America's China policy and the kind of expectations which Tom held for the position. After the meeting concluded, the White House formally released the news of Tom's nomination. President Ford described the position of chief of the Liaison Office as a "very, very important post," one essential to America's improved relations with the PRC.[13]

Tom Gates's nomination as chief of the United States Liaison Office received a positive reception in Washington but, more important, revealed the extent of America's newfound interest in China. Major newspapers, small newspapers, and radio and television reports carried the story of the nomination. During the Eisenhower years, Tom had received considerable publicity, especially as secretary of defense, but the story of his nomination as chief of the USLO claimed considerably more attention from the press than had any of his actions during the 1950s.[14]

Between March 20 and 23, Tom Gates began his briefings at the State Department in preparation for his confirmation hearings before the Senate Foreign Relations Committee, scheduled for the end of the month. "The China desk took charge of me," he later recalled. Tom reviewed the status of Chinese-American relations between 1971 and 1976, examining in particular the significance of the Nixon, Ford, and Kissinger visits and the tenures of Ambassadors Bruce and Bush. He held numerous discussions with his fellow China-watchers about the current political and economic turmoil in China. These briefings provided him with his first serious examination of the political factionalism which occupied the Chinese leadership in the spring of 1976. The interplay of personalities who were contending for Mao's throne was also the special preoccupation of America's China-watchers during the Year of the Dragon, although it proved exceptionally difficult to describe the intense factional strife which existed in China at that time. Indeed, only recently have scholars of Chinese politics been able to untangle with some degree of accuracy the complicated political environment which prevailed in the PRC between Zhou's death in January and Mao's in September 1976.[15]

So fluid and delicate was China's internal political situation throughout

1976 that anyone trying to explain this uniquely confusing picture could have chosen from a variety of possibilities. Since that time, China scholars have advanced several interpretations which have shed further light on, if not completely revealed, the depths of China's leadership struggle in 1976. The most common interpretation holds that three factions, the Maoist radicals, moderate pragmatists, and neo-Maoist "centrists," contended for power in anticipation of Mao's demise. Since none of the factions possessed enough strength to govern by itself, each engaged in an unending series of compromises with the others in an attempt to build a lasting coalition which might prove capable of ruling the country. The radicals were Mao Zedong's ideological disciples, believers in rapid, comprehensive, and even violent change. They had unleashed the ill-fated Great Leap Forward in the 1950s and the fury of the Cultural Revolution in the 1960s.

Primarily oriented toward mobilizing China's urban masses, the radicals controlled the Shanghai and Shenyang municipalities, had numerous allies throughout China at the provincial levels, retained some support within the PLA, and most important, dominated the structure of China's media and propaganda apparatus. Furthermore, the radicals controlled a vocal group of students and intellectuals at the universities in Peking. In addition to Mao, the radical leadership consisted primarily of Jiang Qing, his estranged wife, and three other vice premiers, Zhang Chunqiao, Wang Hongwen, and Yao Wenyuan. The influence and strength of the radicals was immediately visible because they had a majority on the Standing Committee of the Politburo, the highest governing body in China.

By controlling the PRC's media apparatus, the radicals had also invented the country's dominant political vocabulary, a partisan language which Tom soon confronted in China. According to the radicals, their archenemy Deng Xiaoping was an "unrepentant capitalist roader" who was stirring up a "right deviationist wind to reverse the correct verdicts" of the Cultural Revolution by attempting to promote production through the increased usage of economic incentives. Deng was also guilty of trying to overturn the "newborn socialist things," the radicals' Cultural Revolutionary reforms in educational and cultural affairs.[16]

By contrast, the moderate pragmatists had embraced Zhou Enlai and his program for China's economic and political modernization. One year before his death, Zhou spoke of his plans to "make China a modern state by the year 2000." The moderates who espoused Zhou's program believed in the modernization of China's industry and agriculture, as well as political reforms accomplished through the party bureaucracy rather than through ideological struggle. Although Deng Xiaoping was the individual most closely associated with the pragmatist viewpoint, he had other strong colleagues, including Li Xiannian, a vice premier and Politburo member who

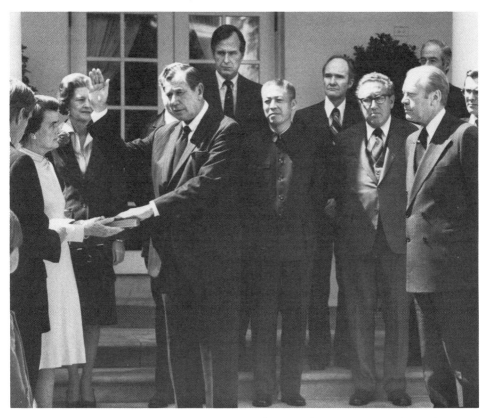

Thomas S. Gates being sworn in as chief of the United States Liaison Office to the People's Republic of China, April 14, 1976. L-R: *Gates grandchildren; Henry Catto; Anne Gates; Betty Ford; Vice President Nelson Rockefeller (partially hidden); Thomas S. Gates; George Bush, director of the Central Intelligence Agency; Han Hsu, chief, Liaison Office, People's Republic of China; National Security Adviser Brent Scowcroft; Secretary of State Henry Kissinger; President Gerald R. Ford; UN Ambassador William W. Scranton; Secretary of Defense Donald Rumsfeld.*

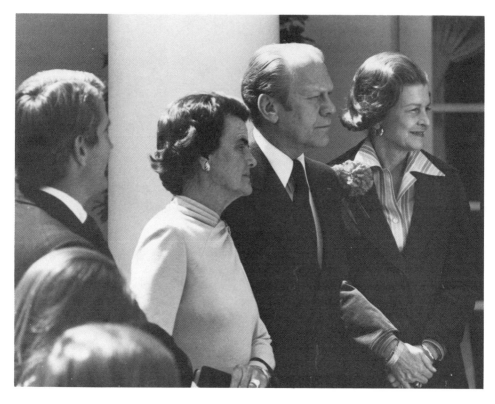

During Tom Gates's speech following the swearing-in ceremony. L-R: Gates grand-children; Henry Catto; Anne Gates; President Gerald R. Ford; Betty Ford. (Courtesy Diana H. Walker.)

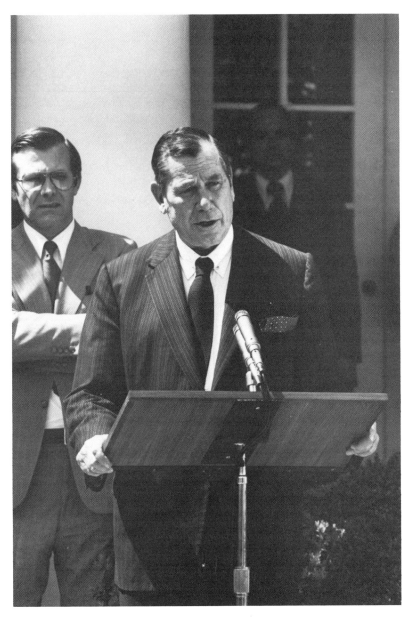

Tom Gates speaking following the swearing-in ceremony. Secretary of Defense Donald Rumsfeld is to the left. (Courtesy Diana H. Walker.)

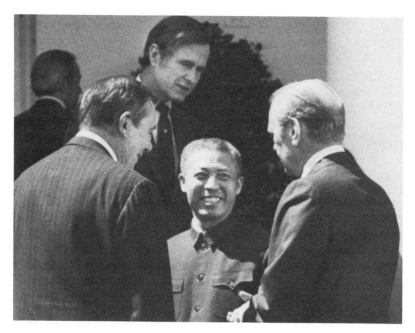

L-R: *Tom Gates, George Bush, Han Hsu, and President Ford visit informally following the swearing-in ceremony.*

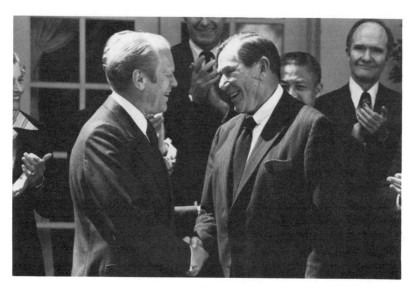

President Ford congratulates Tom Gates after his appointment. (Courtesy Diana H. Walker.)

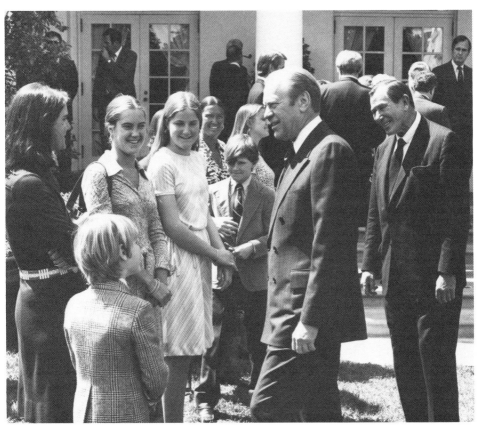

President Ford greets the Gates children. L-R: *Gates Scott, Kathe McCoy, Sandra Norris, Sara Scott, Christopher Scott, Patsy Norris, Polly Norris, Ford, and Tom Gates. (Courtesy Diana H. Walker.)*

was the PRC's chief economic planner (now president of the PRC); Marshall Ye Jianying, China's veteran defense minister; Xu Shiyou, the commander of the Guangdong military region; and Wei Guoqing, the Party's provincial first secretary in Guangdong.

Between the radical and moderate factions stood the so-called centrists, individuals whose careers profited from the Cultural Revolution but who were not linked with Jiang Qing, Zhang Chunqiao, Wang Hongwen, and Yao Wenyuan. Sometimes labeled as neo-Maoists, the centrists belonged to a second generation of Chinese Communist leaders (few of them had participated in the Long March, for example) and were most notably led by Premier Hua Guofeng; Wu De, the mayor of Peking; Chen Xilian, the commander of the Peking military region; and several other vice premiers who were also Politburo members including Ji Dengkuei and Chen Yonggui, an uneducated sixty-five-year-old vice premier personally selected by Mao and Zhou to represent the peasants on the Politburo. Interestingly enough, some knowledgeable China-watchers placed Zhang Chunqiao in this faction, although subsequent events changed that view entirely.[17]

A second assessment of China's political hierarchy tended to discount questions of ideology and concentrate more on the organizational aspects of the PRC's government. According to this view, power in China was distributed throughout four clusters: the personnel system which controlled appointments in the Party and the state bureaucracy; the propaganda network which controlled the media; the coercive apparatus of the military and public security forces which kept order throughout the country; and the economic/production apparatus which governed the allocation of material goods, energy, and capital. The "cement" which held each network together was the Chinese concept of *guan-xi*, the relationship or connection between Chinese which guaranteed loyalty and a sense of mutual obligation. Thus, according to this view, the Chinese leadership was not particularly influenced by ideology or political philosophy but instead by an occupational or social network which preeminently valued personal loyalty. Zhou, Deng, and their allies controlled the personnel system; Li Xiannian was the primary leader in the economic/production realm; Jiang Qing, Wang Hongwen, and Yao Wenyuan controlled the media; and Hua, Ye, and Wang Dongxing controlled the public security apparatus. Wang Dongxing, Mao's bodyguard, also commanded the elite 8341 Unit of the Communist Party's Central Committee, which protected the leadership.[18]

Tom Gates discovered in China that the Japanese essentially subscribed to a variation of this second interpretation. In their view, power in China was split into four clusters but those clusters included the Communist Party, then under radical control; the state bureaucracy, essentially loyal to Deng and his Zhouist supporters; the military, divided at the time between its moderate and radical factions; and the police, controlled by Hua and other centrists.

The most in-depth exploration of the PRC's factionalism revealed as many as seven political factions, each looking for support from other groups in order to form the coalition that could effectively govern China. The first faction included veteran civilian cadres who remained in office during the Cultural Revolution. Represented on the Politburo by Li Xiannian and possibly Wu De, this group rallied around Premier Zhou when he came under vigorous radical attack in 1973. Originally consisting of more than forty-five full members of the Central Committee, this faction had been reduced to thirty-eight or thirty-nine members by the mid-1970s because of the deaths of several members. These veteran cadres usually found support from a second faction, another group of civilians, who had been rehabilitated in the Party after the Cultural Revolution. Deng Xiaoping symbolized and led this faction, which included fourteen or fifteen members of the Central Committee by late 1976.

The third faction in the PRC consisted of the central military organization, and the fourth, of the regional military commanders. Defense Minister Ye led the central military machine, although the ailing Marshal Liu Bocheng and Su Zhenhua, an alternate Politburo member who commanded the PLA Navy, were considered influential members of this faction. In 1976, the central military held approximately thirty full members of the Central Committee and maintained strong support among professional military officers and China's increasingly influential scientific/technical establishment. Like Ye Jianying, most members of the central military organization appeared sympathetic to the moderates' policies. The loyalty of the regional military leaders was another matter, however. Considered the most fluctuating of all the factions, the regional military commanders included such diverse individuals as Xu Shiyou, an acknowledged Deng supporter, and Chen Xilian and Li Desheng, the commanders of the Peking and Shenyang regions, both presumed loyal to the radicals.

With moderate cadres divided along two lines, and the military also split two ways, China's leftists found themselves rent with factionalism in 1976. Three separate groups, the so-called Cultural Revolution Left, the Mass Organization Left, and the Secret Police Left, could all be considered opposed to moderate rule in China but also distrustful of each other. The Cultural Revolution Left rallied around Jiang, Zhang, Wang, and Yao, the so-called Gang of Four (at least until their downfall; see chapter 5). The Mass Organization Left included a group of civilians, such as Politburo member Chen Yonggui, who rose to power during the Cultural Revolution. This faction drew its support from the rank and file of the Party, or from "model peasants" and "labor heroes," and could count on at least thirty to thirty-five of its members within the Central Committee. The Secret Police Left, potentially the most critically important of the seven factions, included Hua Guofeng, Ji Dengkuei, and Wang Dongxing on the Politburo and another fourteen or fifteen members in the Central Committee. Hua, Ji, and Wang had supported Mao on several controversial decisions, including his suppression in 1971 of the alleged coup attempt by Lin Biao. As a result, their leverage and influence within the Party increased markedly during the half-decade between 1971 and 1976.[19]

In the spring of 1976, Tom Gates and the rest of America's China-watching contingent had ample reason to be concerned about the future direction of Chinese politics. From all indications, it appeared that a leftist, or possibly Center-Left, coalition was on the verge of taking political control of the PRC.[20] Zhou's death in January had removed one voice in support of improved relations with the United States. Furthermore, the radicals succeeded in ousting Deng, a move which presumably made it easier for China to reestablish relations with the Soviet Union. Would Mao's impending demise open the way for a radical initiative to draw closer to the Soviets and a marked decline in America's relations with the PRC?

The answers to these questions notwithstanding, Tom Gates found himself concerned above all with the reasons why the Chinese had reached such a divisive internal situation. Was it a dispute over ideology or simply a quest for power which drove the factions? Was it a conflict between separate generations of Chinese leaders or simply personal animosities which had accumulated over several decades of intense political strife? Was it a conflict between the rural-oriented northern Chinese based in Peking who considered themselves more revolutionary than their southern, urban-oriented brethren who had a more conservative vision for China?[21] Whatever the answers to those difficult questions, it was certain that Tom Gates would spend much of his China-watching time in Peking following the path of the PRC's internal turmoil.

After the briefings at the State Department between March 20 and 23, Tom Gates spent the next few days in Washington attending a series of working luncheons in preparation for his appearance before the Senate Foreign Relations Committee on March 30. On March 23, we (I had joined Tom in Washington on March 20) had lunch with David and Evangeline Bruce. This event proved to be a welcome reunion; the four of us had been neighbors in Washington during the 1950s, and Tom again profited from learning about the Bruces' experiences in Peking in 1973 and 1974. The next day, Secretary Kissinger gave a luncheon in Tom's honor at the State Department. Han Hsu, the acting chief of the PRCLO, attended this event, and Tom welcomed the opportunity to meet his Chinese counterpart. On March 26, Tom visited the Pentagon for a luncheon with Secretary Rumsfeld and

General George Brown which also included a briefing on China's military capabilities and the individuals involved in leading the PRC's defense establishment. Finally, on March 27, we had lunch with George and Barbara Bush and received their keen observations about the Chinese officials whom Tom could expect to encounter and the nature of the Peking diplomatic community.

On Monday, March 29, Tom spent the morning at the State Department reviewing his China material in preparation for his confirmation hearing scheduled for the next day with the Foreign Relations Committee. In the afternoon, he called on Senator John Sparkman (D-Alabama) and Senator Hugh Scott (R-Pennsylvania), the committee's chairman and ranking Republican, respectively. Scott especially shared Tom's interest in Sino-American relations and, as a fellow Pennsylvanian, was delighted to recommend him for confirmation. Both Sparkman and Scott indicated that the committee would most likely center their questioning on four topics: the prospects for normalization with the PRC and the future of American ties with Taiwan, the current status of the Sino-Soviet dispute and its effect on America's China policy, the effect of China's internal situation on China's policy toward the United States, and the significance of Tom's record as secretary of defense as a potential signal of a hardening of the administration's attitude toward the Soviet Union. By that time, Tom felt adequately briefed on each point and expected little trouble in winning confirmation.

Tom's advisers at the State Department expected his hearing on March 30 to be brief and routine, with a high probability that several members of the Foreign Relations Committee would be absent. To their surprise (and Tom's), the entire committee was present for the hearing, perhaps as a gesture of support since many of the senators knew Tom personally. Tom was especially touched when his old friend Senator Hubert Humphrey (who was not well at the time) came into the hearing room to offer a few words of encouragement. Tom took some questions from the committee, asked mostly by Senator Charles Percy (R-Illinois), and the hearing progressed satisfactorily. The Foreign Relations Committee subsequently recommended Tom's confirmation unanimously, and the full Senate followed suit shortly thereafter.[22]

After a two-week break spent in Devon, we returned to Washington once again on April 12 for more briefings at the State Department. On April 14, President Ford officially appointed Tom as chief of the USLO at swearing-in ceremonies on the South Portico of the White House. Rockefeller, Rumsfeld, Bush, United Nations Ambassador William Scranton, another close friend and fellow Pennsylvanian, and several Cabinet members also attended the ceremony. In addition, the White House had invited Ambassador Han Hsu to the swearing-in ceremony, and Ford addressed several of his remarks to Han, especially his statement that "our two countries have differences which neither side attempts to hide, but we also share many, many important interests which provide the foundation for a durable and growing relationship."[23]

When President Eisenhower had officially appointed Tom as secretary of defense on December 6, 1959, I attended the swearing-in ceremony at the White House with our three daughters. Now, over a quarter century later, at another swearing-in ceremony at the White House, not only were our daughters present, but also, as Tom noted in his remarks to the president, "a healthy sample of our grandchildren."

Before leaving for China, we fulfilled one last social obligation on April 26 by attending a banquet held in our honor at the Liaison Office of the People's Republic in Washington. An incident that occurred during the evening revealed to us how extremely sensitive the Chinese were about the Taiwan question. After the dinner, Han Hsu took Tom aside and informed him that the Chinese had read the transcript of his confirmation hearing before the Senate Foreign Relations Committee. Several officers of the PRC Liaison Office had also attended the hearing. Did Tom realize that he had spoken of Taiwan as a "country"? inquired Ambassador Han. Then reaching in his pocket and pulling out a copy of the Shanghai Communique, Han reminded Tom: "There is only one China, of which Taiwan is a part." Han's "clarification" did more than reveal the seriousness with which the Chinese approached the Taiwan issue and the Shanghai Communique; it demonstrated the remarkable attention to detail which characterized the work of the Chinese diplomats.

III

With time now running out before our departure to Peking, we finished up some assorted business and personal details in Philadelphia and New York during the last two weeks of April. On April 29, we began the long journey to China aboard a 10 A.M. flight from New York to San Francisco and on April 30, flew on to Hawaii. In Honolulu, we were met by Admiral Noel Gayler, USN, then commander-in-chief, Pacific. In the mid-1950s, Gayler had served as Tom's military aide when he was secretary of the navy and was, according to Tom, "about as fine a naval officer as one could imagine." Gayler had earned two navy crosses for bravery as a naval aviator in World War II and, after the war, went on to several high-level posts in the navy and in Washington. He had commanded the *U.S.S. Ranger* and directed the National Security Agency before being appointed commander-in-chief, Pacific. For us, it was another fond reunion.

The reunion with Noel Gayler also provided Tom with the opportunity for a frank discussion about American strategic interests in the Far East and his potential role in that area. Gayler had strongly encouraged Tom to accept the USLO position, although he realized that it was, in his words, a "tough and lonely post." Even so, he regarded the chief of the USLO as having both an important and sensitive assignment, especially since the evolution of America's policy toward the PRC had clearly not stopped. Gayler considered Chinese-American cooperation crucial to America's interests in the Far East. China represented the "keystone of the arch" for America's policy in Asia, and no one should underestimate the importance to the United States of a period of stability in the Far East.[24] By coincidence, Gayler was scheduled to attend a military commanders' conference in South Korea at the same time that our itinerary called for us to leave for Japan. As a result, the long flight provided Gayler with an additional opportunity to brief Tom about the military situation in the Pacific and the Far East.

America and China had experienced an enormous degree of change in their relations since Tom Gates had served in the Eisenhower administration. When he entered the Navy Department as under secretary, in 1953, the United States and the PRC had just ended their period of hostilities during the Korean War. One year later, in September 1954, Tom and I accompanied Secretary of Defense Charles E. Wilson on a tour of American and Allied military installations in the Far East which was publicly described as a review of America's military capability in the Pacific and Asia. Tom and Wilson also met with Philippine President Ramon Magasaysay, South Korean President Synghman Rhee, and Generalissimmo Chiang Kai-Shek on Taiwan in an effort to reinforce America's defense commitment to its allies in the Far East. Wilson's taking Tom with him on this trip underscored the importance of the United States Navy in protecting American interests in the Far East, especially against any possible military action by the PRC.

Throughout the 1950s, America and China were undeniably enemies. American military planning reflected that assumption. Most Americans referred to the PRC as either mainland China, Communist China, or more often, simply as Red China. In this war of words, the Chinese also reciprocated, denouncing the United States as a "paper tiger," and the world's "chief imperialist." Both countries came perilously close to war twice in the post-Korean period, once in 1955 when the PRC shelled the offshore islands of Quemoy and Matsu, threatening a possible invasion of Taiwan, and then again in 1958 when that situation almost repeated itself.[25] Eisenhower responded to both crises by using the navy to provide the military muscle necessary to support the diplomatic effort which defused each crisis. Both as undersecretary and as secretary of the navy, Tom played an instrumental role in managing both crises (a fact certainly known by the Chinese in 1976) and completely understood the military stakes involved in the Far East.

Twenty years later, instead of casting a wary eye toward potential Chinese military action in the Far East, Tom Gates, as America's official representative to the PRC, was preparing to work to promote improved relations between America and China through diplomacy, rather than the application of military power.

We landed in Tokyo on May 4 and spent the next day at the American Embassy in Japan, guests of Ambassador and Mrs. James Hodgson. Hodgson arranged for us to dine on May 5 with Akio Morita, the chairman of SONY corporation and one of Japan's leading businessmen. Morita's comments on the current scene in the PRC and his extensive knowledge of the people and politics involved in the relationships between Japan, China, and the United States proved extremely helpful.

At 9 A.M. on May 6, we left Tokyo for Peking. All the briefings and preparations were over, all the packing and farewells. Tom was as ready as any American could be to work in a country which few Americans had ever either visited or studied. As soon as we arrived in Peking, we knew that a memorable adventure was in store. The scene that confronted us in the capital of the People's Republic was astonishing—wide streets, hundreds of thousands of bicyclists, multitudes of people, and beautiful architecture. It was the beginning of what Henry Kissinger later called our "brief and dramatic stay in China." [26]

Notes

1. Ford, *A Time To Heal*, pp. 315, 316, 326; Robert T. Hartmann, *Palace Politics: An Inside Account of the Ford Years* (New York: McGraw-Hill, 1980), pp. 370–74; Ron Nessen, *It Sure Looks Different from the Inside* (Chicago: Playboy Press, 1978), pp. 155–59.

2. C. W. Borklund, *Men of the Pentagon* (New York: Praeger, 1966), pp. 184–205; Dwight D. Eisenhower, *Waging Peace: White House Years, 1956–1961* (Garden City, N.Y.: Doubleday, 1965), p. 294.

3. Interview, Gerald R. Ford; Thomas S. Gates Oral History, 31 August 1982. Hereafter cited as Gates OH, date. Coincidentally, the discussion of possible arms sales to the PRC by the United States government occurred at precisely the time when Tom Gates was under consideration as the next chief of the USLO. See "U.S. Arms for Red China?" *Forbes* 119, no. 11 (1 June 1976): 21–22; *New York Times*, 12 April 1976, p. 5; *New York Times*, 14 April 1976, p. 21; *New York Times*, 15 April 1976, p. 6.

4. See John R. Wadleigh, "Thomas Sovereign Gates," in *American Secretaries of the Navy*, edited by Paolo Coletta, vol. 2 (Annapolis: Naval Institute Press, 1980), pp. 877–93. Thomas Gates served as a director of the Bethlehem Steel Corporation, the Campbell Soup Company, the INA Corporation (now CIGNA Corporation), the SmithKline Corporation (now the SmithKline Beckman Corporation), and the Scott Paper Company. He was also a trustee of the College of the Atlantic and a life trustee of his alma mater, the University of Pennsylvania. In addition, he was the honorary chairman of the Eisenhower Exchange Fellowship Program, and a director of the Blue Cross/Blue Shield program of Pennsylvania for many years.

5. Gates OH, 31 August 1982.

6. Eisenhower, *Waging Peace*, p. 294.

7. "New Man at Morgan," *Newsweek*, 17 May 1965, p. 74.

8. Kissinger, *Years of Upheaval*, pp. 60–63.

9. Ibid.; Terrill, *Future of China*, p. 29.

10. Thomas S. Gates Papers, University of Pennsylvania, Philadelphia, Notes of Telephone Conversations, January 1976. Hereafter cited as Gates Papers, source.

11. James H. Douglas, interview with the author, 10 August 1980, Chicago.

12. *New York Times*, 28 February 1976.

13. Gates Papers, "Exchange of Remarks Between the President and Thomas Gates upon His Designation As Chief of the United States Liaison Office in the People's Republic of China," The White House, 19 March 1976.

14. *New York Times*, 20 March 1976; *Washington Post*, 20 March 1976.

15. For excellent discussions of the political factionalism which existed in China in 1976–77, see Jurgen Domes, "The 'Gang of Four' and Hua Kuo-feng: An Analysis of Political Events in 1975–1976," *China Quarterly* 71 (June 1977): 473–97; and Michel Oksenberg and Richard Bush, "China's Political Evolution, 1972–1982," *Problems of Communism* 31 (September–October 1982): 1–19.

16. Fox Butterfield, "Mapping the Capitalist Road," *New York Times*, 24 April 1976, p. 6.

17. U.S. Department of State, Official Files, Peking to Washington, 11 May 1976; ibid., 27 July 1976.

18. Oksenberg and Bush, "China's Political Evolution," pp. 3–8.

19. Domes, "The 'Gang of Four' and Hua Kuo-feng," pp. 494–97; see also Immanuel C. Y. Hsu, *China Without Mao: The Search for a New Order* (New York: Oxford University Press, 1983), p. 41.

20. Gates Papers, Memorandum to Ambassador Gates from Thomas S. Brooks, "Political Section Briefing," 5 May 1976; Garside, *Coming Alive*, pp. 9–24.

21. Garside, *Coming Alive*, pp. 171–79; Terrill, *Future of China*, pp. 41–67.

22. U.S. Congress, Senate, 94th Congress, 2d Session, Committee on Foreign Relations, Hearings on Nomination of Thomas S. Gates, Jr., as Chief, United States Liaison Office to the People's Republic of China (Washington: Government Printing Office, 1976).

23. Gates Papers, "Exchange of Remarks Between the President and Thomas S. Gates at His Swearing-In As Chief of the United States Liaison Office, the People's Republic of China," The White House, 14 April 1976.

24. Gates Papers, Admiral Noel Gayler, USN, to Thomas S. Gates, 19 March 1976.

25. Eisenhower, *Mandate for Change: White House Years, 1953–1956* (Garden City, N.Y.: Doubleday, 1963), pp. 459–83; Eisenhower, *Waging Peace*, pp. 292–304.

26. Gates Papers, Secretary of State Kissinger to Ambassador Gates, 7 January 1977.

CHAPTER **2**

The Work of a China-Watcher

Before Thomas Gates left the United States to become the chief of the United States Liaison Office in Peking, several of his friends advised him, "Take along your Shakespeare" for leisure reading when diplomatic life in China becomes routine. But Tom was in China only a few weeks before discovering that the complexity of his China-watching task left little time for reading Shakespeare or indulging in any other form of recreation. Indeed, as a former student of English literature, he often lamented that his official duties rarely provided him with time to relax with Hamlet or King Lear.

As chief of the United States Liaison Office, Tom had three primary responsibilities: administering the work of the mission as it related to personnel and general operations, maintaining (and cultivating) contacts with Chinese officials and other members of the diplomatic community, and most important, keeping abreast of the changes then occurring in the PRC's political, social, and economic environments. Closely related to that third responsibility was the necessity of sending accurate reports of the situation in China back to Washington. The job was a China-watcher's delight, especially since events in the PRC moved so rapidly and unpredictably during the late spring and summer of 1976.

Once in the PRC, Tom developed an immediate understanding of the USLO's singular importance to American diplomacy during the mid-1970s and also an appreciation for the concession which Zhou Enlai apparently made in 1973 when he permitted the establishment of the United States Liaison Office without also demanding the closure of the American Embassy in Taiwan.[1] Richard Mueller, one of the USLO's Economic officers, aptly described the contribution of the Liaison Office to America's foreign policy during that period: "USLO was the American way of listening to what was going on in China. We were essentially the eyes and ears of the United States government in the PRC."[2]

As Henry Kissinger explained in *Years of Upheaval,* both the United States Liaison Office in Peking and the Liaison Office of the People's Republic of China in Washington were "embassies in all but name."[3] The organization of each liaison office reflected the typical structure of an official embassy except that the officer in charge, who held ambassadorial rank, was labeled chief instead of ambassador. These semantic distinctions were inconsequential in China; all of Tom's diplomatic acquaintances—USLO colleagues, Chinese officials, and foreign diplomats—routinely referred to him as Ambassador Gates. Moreover, his status as a presidential envoy gave added importance and visibility to his position. The USLO's special status as a quasi-embassy therefore presented no obstacle to the advancement of America's relationship with the PRC, or to its reception by other foreign embassies stationed in Peking.[4]

In many respects, the unique status of the United States Liaison Office enhanced its standing within the diplomatic community but also gave the officers some social latitude. The Chinese occasionally invited American officers to attend cultural events before they sent formal invitations to other embassies, but they were not offended if an American representative did not attend every diplomatic event they sponsored, since America and China still lacked formal diplomatic relations. By contrast, many of the other embassies were woefully understaffed in view of the social obligations imposed by the PRC's extensive diplomatic calendar. One hundred twenty-five nations maintained embassies in the PRC. As a result, the diplomatic community engaged in what seemed to be an everlasting round of receptions, courtesy calls, National Day festivities (every nation had one), welcoming parties, farewell parties, and just plain parties. Tom and his American colleagues sympathized, for example, with their Swedish and Finnish counterparts, who often appeared to be in a constant parade between their embassies and the Great Hall of the People in order to be represented at a particular reception or dinner.[5] As officers of an "unofficial" embassy, the Americans enjoyed the luxury of being able to concentrate more on their substantive reporting responsibilities, and less on social or protocol matters.

Once Tom had confronted the major problems of living and working in Peking, he quickly developed a strong respect for the dedication of the USLO's Foreign Service contingent and their families. The acute shortage of living and work space which the Americans encountered in Peking must have contrasted sharply with the conveniences available in other posts. The USLO's thirty-three staff members worked in the mission compound, a pleasant but not particularly spacious Mediterranean-style building in Peking's diplomatic district. The USLO residence itself was a lovely, comfortable house built by the Chinese in 1973 and completely adequate for our needs. (We later learned that the house had been built using a series of joints which could adjust to earthquake shocks.) The USLO officers and their families, however, lived nearby in small apartments or temporary quarters at the Peking Hotel. The apartments, which generally had one or two bedrooms, would be considered small by Western standards but quite acceptable to the Chinese. Like the Chinese, the Americans bought and prepared their food fresh daily; packaged food in the American tradition was not available. The children of USLO officers attended an international school located near the diplomatic sector of Peking.

In an attempt to improve the quality of the living quarters for the American families stationed in Peking, Tom made one of his first official calls on Ding Guoyu, the PRC officer who handled much of the daily administration for the Peking municipality. Tom had initially requested a meeting with Wu De, the mayor of Peking and an influential Politburo member, only to be informed that Wu was "too busy" for such an appointment. (Wu had also been "too busy" for appointments with Ambassadors Bruce and Bush.) Ding listened patiently to Tom's explanation of the USLO's housing and space problems but then launched into a completely irrelevant discussion of his efforts to reduce pollution and bicycle traffic congestion in Peking. He gave no indication whatsoever that USLO's space needs represented any kind of priority.[6]

Despite the inconveniences, the seventy Americans who lived and worked in Peking during Tom's tenure as chief of the United States Liaison Office adapted remarkably well to life in this unique environment. Part of the explanation for their adaptability was that the USLO attracted an exceptionally competent and sought-after corps of officers. An assignment in Peking was highly coveted by China-watchers in the Foreign Service, many of whom had spent a decade or more studying China from the outside.

America's Foreign Service contingent in Peking, Tom Gates found, was superb. He especially admired Harry Thayer and David Dean, the two men who served as deputy chief of the mission during his tenure. Both Thayer and Dean spoke excellent Chinese and had accumulated a wealth of experience at other posts in the Far East before taking their assignments at the USLO. By coincidence, Harry Thayer's parents were our neighbors in Philadelphia, although we did not become acquainted with Thayer himself until he took the responsibility for introducing Tom to the diplomatic community in Peking. David Dean had previously served in both Taiwan and Hong Kong;

he and his wife, Mary, understood Chinese and thoroughly immersed themselves in the USLO's work. Thayer was deputy chief when Tom arrived in Peking, and in July Dean succeeded him and remained in Peking until 1978. Tom enjoyed a close, collegial relationship with both men and considered them more qualified than he, in many ways, to serve as chief of the USLO.

The USLO functioned much like a typical embassy. The work of the Liaison Office was divided into four sections: the Economic and Commercial, the Political, and the Consular units, each of which had three officers, and the Administrative unit, which had four. William Thomas supervised the Economic unit; Stan Brooks, the Political; Jerry Ogden, the Consular; and first Jerry Levesque and later Hal Vickers, the Administrative.[7]

In addition to the Americans in Peking, the USLO also employed a sizable contingent of Chinese who handled such various tasks as interpreting, cooking, gardening, and maintenance. These individuals also were industrious and dependable. One Chinese employee so impressed Tom that he made a point of complimenting his work when he met with Ding Guoyu. "If [this particular individual] had been born in America," Tom told Ding, "I'm sure that he'd already be a millionaire. He's extremely capable and his personality matches his competence." For Tom, making such a compliment to an individual's superior was natural, and after returning home, he explained to the employee how he had praised his work in his conversation with Ding. To Tom's astonishment, the man reacted, not with gratitude, but with horror. "Ambassador, you do not understand China!" he exclaimed. "I am here to work, to learn, to improve. This is the same for all of us. We are all equal. Saying I am better than others is not so—and it will do me no good. [The leaders] will think I have stopped trying, stopped learning." This episode always served as a ready reminder of how little the American experience prepared someone for the absolute egalitarianism which the Maoists had attempted to create in the PRC.[8]

II

Between May and July, Tom Gates settled into his responsibilities as a China-watcher and soon encountered the legendary subtlety and seriousness which the Chinese attach to their political life and the unparalleled depth of secrecy which pervades the PRC's political system. Events in China are "not a mystery, just a secret," an American diplomat once observed.[9] Confronted with that secrecy, Tom and his colleagues spent hours trying to place the information which they received, from a multitude of sources, into a coherent framework for reporting and analysis. China-watching was an exercise in listening, watching, analyzing, and most important, speculating on events in the PRC. J. Raoul Schoumaker, the Belgian ambassador to China, warned Tom shortly after his arrival of the inherent difficulty of becoming a China-watcher and forming judgments which might later prove to be inaccurate or in need of modification. "There are two equally competent experts on China—the man who had spent three hours at the airport and the other who had lived in China for thirty years," Schoumaker explained. Kissinger put the point more bluntly in one of his conversations with Tom: "Anyone who makes predictions about China is either a fool or a liar." [10] Indeed, Tom's experience in the PRC revealed the profundity of both comments, so mystifying were the PRC's forthcoming events.

In addition to the secrecy which covered the political life of the PRC, Westerners were also handicapped by the exceptionally subtle, indirect method of communication employed by the PRC's officials. Ding Guoyu, for example, did not refuse Tom's request for additional housing space for the USLO families; he simply changed the conversation to a discourse on the problems he faced in administering the city, leaving Tom to form his own opinion about the reasons why the Chinese refused to assist him in solving this particular problem. As a result, Tom and the other Americans relied on at least four different sources for acquiring and analyzing information about the PRC. The first source was the personnel in other American diplomatic missions in the Far East, such as the American Consulate General in Hong Kong, and the American Embassies in Japan, Taiwan, Malaysia, and Australia. Charles Cross, the American consul general in Hong Kong, was an experienced China hand who occupied a pivotal point in acquiring knowledge about events in the PRC. He had access to many Chinese officials stationed in Hong Kong and was able to obtain valuable "traveler's tales" from people who were about to enter, or had just left, China. In addition, the independent Hong Kong newspaper *Ming Pao* regularly published stories, based on its own sources of information, about the PRC which proved indispensable for their timeliness and accuracy. The USLO's officers also worked closely with their counterparts at the American Embassy in Japan. Tom Gates and James Hodgson became close friends, a development which undoubtedly strengthened the working relationship between the two missions.

The second source of information for Tom and his USLO colleagues was their discussions with other members of Peking's diplomatic community, primarily the ambassadors to China from other NATO countries and Japan. Tom spent much of the first few weeks in China making the normal diplomatic rounds in Peking, meeting other ambassadors and embassy officers, and also attending the routine of lunches, receptions, and dinners given for a new member of the foreign diplomatic community. "The game around here is usually lunch," Tom wrote home, to describe how the diplomatic community conducted a good deal of its business. [11] These occasions quickly became regular events for the exchange of information as well as, unfortunately, misinformation.

Like the United States, virtually every nation sent outstanding people to China, but the USLO's contacts primarily involved an informal network of embassy personnel from New Zealand, Australia, Canada, England, and Japan. Tom wasted no time in becoming acquainted with the ambassadors from those countries. He found Richard Atkins, the ambassador to China from New Zealand, to be a fine individual, thoroughly knowledgeable about China, and he and his wife, Jill, became two of our closest friends. Stephen Fitzgerald, the Australian ambassador, possessed a wealth of experience in Asia, spoke Chinese fluently, and probably enjoyed the most extensive political contacts with the Chinese of any ambassador. John Small, the Canadian ambassador, was a quiet, sensible, and reserved man with exceptional judgment about Chinese affairs. Several times when Tom needed advice or assistance about a particular matter, he conferred with Small. Sir Edward Youde, the British ambassador, likewise was a man of fine judgment who, like Tom, served in the Pacific during World War II. Finally, Heishiro Ozawa, the ambassador from Japan, was an exemplar of hard work and diplomatic expertise. Ozawa proved valuable as a source of information not only about the PRC but also about the entire political and economic situation in the Far East.[12]

Foreign journalists stationed in Peking occasionally provided a third source of information. Lacking formal relations with the United States, the PRC refused to allow American journalists in Peking, although Fox Butterfield of the *New York Times* and Jay Mathews of the *Washington Post* covered Chinese affairs from their posts in Hong Kong. Tom read their stories regularly, usually finding them useful as a measure of life in China. Otherwise, the reporting which USLO officers found most accurate appeared in Reuters, the Agence France Press, and the *Toronto Globe and Mail.* The USLO enjoyed good relations with the journalists from each of these organizations and found them all to be particularly competent and professional: David Rogers, the bureau chief for Reuters, and his assistant, Peter Griffiths; Rene Flipo, bureau chief for Agence France Presse, and his assistant, Georges Biannic; and Ross Munro of the *Toronto Globe and Mail.* Munro knew both the Chinese and the American political scenes, having served previously as a Washington correspondent for his newspaper.[13] On May 19, the USLO hosted a reception for these and several other foreign correspondents, an event memorable for its lively discussion of the current political scene in the PRC.

The most important source of information about China was the Chinese themselves. The USLO's officers had many opportunities to meet with PRC officials at either high or specialized levels as a means of advancing the relationship between the two countries. Even so, when Tom first arrived in Peking, he found the Chinese conspicuously aloof, reserved, and official in their discussions with Americans. Always polite and courteous, the Chinese nevertheless maintained a certain detachment which made the task of developing contacts and sources of information difficult. This attitude changed somewhat over the course of 1976 and into 1977; yet the fact remained that the Chinese were obviously wary of engaging in direct conversations with USLO officials. As a result, once in Peking, any Westerner grew immediately alert to signals emanating from the PRC leadership which either clarified or indicated a possible change in a given situation. Tom and his associates paid special attention to the PRC media, the wall posters which appeared throughout Peking, and eye-witness observations of such public events as gatherings of China's political leadership.

Any discussion of the PRC media must first assume that the *People's Daily*, the New China News Agency, *Liberation Army Daily* (the publication of the PLA), *Red Flag* (the official voice of the Chinese Communist Party), and the state radio and television were extensions of the Party's propaganda apparatus, then considered to be controlled by the radicals. Members of Peking's diplomatic community read these publications regularly (although the *Liberation Army Daily* was especially difficult to acquire), always remaining mindful of the need to interpret their contents as an expression of the radical faction's current orthodoxy. In reading the *People's Daily*, Tom and his colleagues always speculated on the reasons behind the appearance of a given story; the actual story itself may have had far less significance than the circumstances which caused the leadership to publish it at a particular time. To cite one particular case, the major challenge confronting Tom Gates during the early summer of 1976 involved making an assessment of the direction of China's internal political power struggle. Formulating such an assessment, however, proved difficult; China's radical faction controlled the flow of information to the population and were filling it daily with anti-Deng, anti-rightist propaganda. Every morning at 5 o'clock, the residents of Peking awoke to the sounds of loudspeakers blaring out the latest call to "deepen the criticism of Deng Xiaoping." Nowhere was the criticism of Deng Xiaoping more evident, however, than in the editorials which appeared in the *People's Daily*. Tom and his American colleagues gained something of an understanding of the PRC's internal leadership struggle and where it was leading, not by analyzing these editorials, but by finding out about the process by which the Party composed and released them. The responsibility for preparing these editorials lay with the editorial department of the *People's Daily*, which was composed of a group of young (between 30 and 34 years of age), highly talented theorists and writers. After composing an editorial, the writers sent it to Yao Wenyuan, then assumed to be responsible for the Central Committee's Propaganda Department. Yao reviewed the editorial and made any desirable changes prior to its publication. If Yao determined that the editorial was a major policy statement, he referred it to the members of the Standing Committee of the Chinese Communist Party.[14] At that time, the Standing Committee included Chairman Mao; Premier Hua Guofeng; Marshall Zhu De, the aging military hero of the Chinese Revolution who was also chairman of the Standing Committee; Defense Minister Ye Jianying; Marshall Liu Bocheng, another ailing military officer; Jiang Qing; and three radical vice premiers, Yao, Zhang Chunqiao, and Wang Hongwen. Given the poor physical health of the military men represented on the Standing Committee, one could effectively determine that the radicals controlled the committee and with it the Party's propaganda. The three military leaders were all presumed moderates, but Zhu was dying, Liu ailing, and Ye, thoroughly alienated from the radicals, absent from Peking much of the time. Mao also was gravely ill but nevertheless a source of protection for the radicals while he remained alive.

The posters which appeared on buildings, fences, and at other public places in Peking and throughout the country were another source of information about the political life of China. When the Party's central authorities (Party Center) wished to convey a certain message, they put it on posters which were displayed throughout the capital. Roger Garside, an officer in the British Embassy during the mid-1970s, interpreted the poster campaigns as the vehicles by which rival Chinese factions attempted to consolidate national public opinion to their respective sides.[15] When Tom arrived in Peking, posters urging the Chinese to "deepen the criticism of Deng Xiaoping" were ubiquitous, especially at the leftist-controlled Peking and Qinghua universities, a vivid reminder of the radical campaign to banish Deng to the wilderness of the PRC's political life. Several months later, however, when the radicals' opponents overthrew Deng's foes, posters calling for the Chinese to "rally closely around the Party Center led by Comrade Hua Guofeng" appeared almost instantly and by the thousands throughout China. The diplomatic community discovered this dramatic political change first by reading the posters, and then by reading the newspapers.

America's China-watchers in Peking also gave much attention to observing the Chinese leadership when it appeared in public. The PRC hierarchy generally gathered in rank order, and if one member of the Chinese Politburo or another important official, for example, failed to appear at an official gathering, his absence immediately set off speculation within the diplomatic community about his health (both physical and political). In one such instance, Tom and his USLO colleagues watched closely over a three-week period in early July when Foreign Minister Qiao Guanhua and Defense Minister Ye Jianying were absent from Peking. Both Qiao and Ye suffered from occasional periods of poor health; Qiao was recovering from tuberculosis at the time but continued to chain-smoke and maintain a sizable workload. For his part, Ye Jianying was seventy-seven years old and ap-

peared to be growing increasingly frail, often being shown assisted by attendants as he moved about Peking. Perhaps their illnesses accounted for their
absences. Yet, Qiao and Ye were generally considered moderates (although
Qiao subsequently was purged in the autumn after the Gang of Four); had
the radicals succeeded in turning them out-of-favor? Eventually, both men
reappeared and so their absence from official duties indicated that their positions were not in jeopardy.[16]

Tom Gates's more experienced China-watching colleagues searched for
more subtle signals, besides simple absences, when the PRC hierarchy
gathered in public. Was one member of the leadership standing too close, or
too far, from another member? Did this stance indicate a possible political
realignment or estrangement? Photographs in the PRC media also occasionally revealed a change in an individual's political fortunes. The Chinese per-
fected the technique of deleting a deposed comrade's picture from the media
as a signal to the population (as well as to foreign observers) of a political
change. After Jiang Qing's arrest in October, for instance, it became virtually
impossible to obtain any photographs of her, even the celebrated one of her
riding on horseback beside Mao at Yanan in 1937. Prior to her arrest Jiang's
photographs were available everywhere in China.

Despite this varied collection of sources, the task of accurately reporting
events in China still involved placing the isolated pieces of information into
the right framework. Given the complexity of that period of Chinese history, that process of puzzle-assembly was no simple task, as Tom Gates
learned once he became directly involved in reporting on the PRC's internal
events during the summer of 1976.

III

Three separate but obviously interrelated issues occupied Tom Gates's attention and that of the entire diplomatic community during the early summer
of 1976: the apparent breakdown of China's political and social discipline, the
precarious state of Mao Zedong's health, and finally, the character and political savvy of Hua Guofeng, China's recently installed and virtually unknown
premier. Amid all the bustle of daily life in Peking, with millions of Chinese
going about their daily tasks, one still could not escape the impression that a
great drama was building, a drama soon to unfold before everyone's eyes.

Tom first felt a sense of drama in the tense, uneasy situation he found in
Peking when we arrived on May 6. The PRC leadership was still preoccupied
with the aftermath of the Tienanmen riots which had erupted in early
April. Although the Center managed to suppress these demonstrations, the
hierarchy still found it difficult to reassert its authority over the course of
the next six weeks. PLA troops patrolled the streets and shopping districts of

Peking, and there were reports that several "struggle sessions" in the style of the Cultural Revolution had recently occurred at Peking University where alleged "counter-revolutionaries" had experienced verbal humiliation and even physical abuse from their radical foes.[17]

Before Tom's arrival in Peking, USLO officers had noticed an unusual display of security precautions at the various activities on May Day. Normally a festive, lighthearted holiday of national celebration, May Day in Peking in the Year of the Dragon was anything but a jubilant occasion. In the wake of the Tienanmen riots, an air of foreboding hung over the city. The urban militia and other security personnel kept a large gathering of Chinese far from the sports stadium where the hierarchy viewed an impressive fireworks display. Those Chinese who entered the stadium were searched prior to entrance, and once inside, they found their freedom to move freely about the stadium sharply restricted by the authorities.[18]

In the two weeks following May Day, security continued to remain tight in Peking. The presence of PLA soldiers, standing guard with fixed bayonets along the busy thoroughfares, was a constant reminder of the tensions which existed between the Chinese people and their leadership. Apparently such precautions failed to halt the demonstrations of discontent in the capital, however; the USLO heard background reports of over "48 separate counter-revolutionary incidents" occurring in Peking around May Day.[19] In other parts of China, demonstrations of discontent continued into the summer. Vandals ransacked newspaper offices in Shanghai and attacked a military arsenal in Hebei province. In early July, robbers held up a bank in Zhengzhou, killing a guard and escaping with the American equivalent of $100,000. The bank robbery was an extraordinary event, especially in a nation which claimed to have abolished crime. The robbers, who brazenly called themselves the "July 7 Counter-revolutionary Assassin Group," taunted the provincial authorities whose efforts to apprehend them proved completely futile. Wall posters that jeered "You can dig up all of Zhengzhou and all of Honan to a depth of three feet and you will never find us" signified the robbers' arrogance in confounding their pursuers. More important, perhaps, the robbers became virtual Jesse James or John Dillinger-like folk heroes in the region and (as far as USLO could determine) the provincial authorities received no cooperation from other Chinese in their attempt to locate the criminals.[20]

Amidst these demonstrations of internal division, the Chinese leadership attempted to present an image of harmony and continuity to its people throughout the early summer of 1976. The PRC hierarchy appeared en masse at the various festivities on May Day and sought to assure foreign diplomats that a "collective leadership" comprised of Premier Hua Guofeng, Vice Premier Zhang Chunqiao, and Defense Minister Ye Jianying (sometimes included on this list was Vice Premier Wang Hongwen) handled China's daily political responsibilities. Simply the admission of "collective leadership," however, indicated a departure from the normal state of affairs in the PRC. In truth, the PRC's hierarchy found itself divided and torn by indecision in the early summer of 1976. The anti-Deng campaign had paralyzed the government, and Hua Guofeng lacked the stature to provide the decisive leadership characterized by Zhou Enlai. According to several reports, Hua Guofeng acted with considerably more deliberation and less direction than his predecessor. Unlike Zhou, who acted expeditiously in administering the business of his office, Hua preferred to write out in longhand his solutions to the problems which were brought to his attention. Hua then circulated these expressions throughout the leadership, and if he encountered no opposition, instituted his measures. If several of his colleagues disagreed with his proposed course of action, however, Hua would call a meeting of the Politburo to decide upon a particular solution to the problem under consideration. For their part, Jiang Qing and her radical followers, sensing the end of Mao's life drawing near, insisted on being consulted on any major decision, a further impediment to orderly government.[21]

On July 6, 1976, Marshall Zhu De died at the age of ninety. His death, while not as traumatic for the nation as that of Zhou Enlai, nevertheless removed from the leadership another veteran of the Long March generation, as well as a voice of moderation. Although Zhu had been ailing for several years, he had retained two key positions, chairman of the Standing Committee of the National People's Congress and member of the Politburo. Of the individuals who remained on the Standing Committee after Zhou's death, only Ye and Mao were members of the pre-Cultural Revolution Old Guard. Undeniably, Zhu's death represented another setback for China's moderate faction, which had already lost several key members to either death or purge within the past seven months. Perhaps just as important, Zhu's death reduced the influence of the PLA within the Party. Since the 1930s, Zhu had been either a chief officer or commander of the PLA, a symbol of the importance and power of the military within China.

The commemoration of Zhu De's death presented the PRC hierarchy with another opportunity to present its facade of harmony to the populace, despite the fact that the passing of another leader added more uncertainty to the leadership situation. The official farewell to Zhu De on July 8 was a dignified event; the leadership paid its last respects to the Old Hero at the Capital Hospital and then accompanied his remains to the Peking crematorium. Thousands of Chinese assembled along the route to witness silently the procession. Once more, security personnel were highly conspicuous, perhaps evidence that the radicals hoped to keep the commemoration for Zhu as undemonstrative as possible. (In a similar effort at the time of Zhou Enlai's death, the radicals had failed miserably. Only the prompt, dignified intervention of Zhou's widow, Deng Yingchao, prevented Zhou's funeral procession from turning into an anti-radical demonstration.) On the afternoon of July 9, Tom Gates led a twelve-member USLO delegation to sign the memorial book and pay last respects to Zhu's remains at the Great Hall of the People.[22] The PRC leadership, to its credit, handled the public ceremony honoring Zhu De in a capable and serious manner. The passing of this Old Hero, however, so soon after the death of Zhou Enlai in January, drew more attention to the physical condition of the last major survivor of China's Communist Revolution, Chairman Mao Zedong, now lying gravely ill himself in a Peking hospital.

Tom Gates knew many of the details of Mao Zedong's precarious health even before he left for China. In conversations with President Ford, he learned that Mao had seemed only "on the fringe" of political life in China when he met with the president the previous December.[23] In early 1976, however, the chairman apparently summoned enough effort to purge Deng Xiaoping (for a second time), but the anti-Maoist tone of the Tienanmen riots reportedly drove him into an increasingly despondent state. When Tom began his China-watching assignment, therefore, virtually everyone in the diplomatic community was searching for clues about the status of Mao's health. By late spring of 1976, Mao no longer spoke intelligibly and moved only with the help of aides. Few diplomatic observers doubted that he was failing rapidly. In late April and then in early May, he held formal appointments with Robert Muldoon, prime minister of New Zealand; Lee Kuan Yew, premier of Singapore; and Ali Bhutto, prime minister of Pakistan, but each meeting proved both physically debilitating and personally embarrassing to Mao. Photographs of these sessions showed the chairman slumping noticeably in his chair, apparently having only minimal muscular control. Muldoon left his meeting with the chairman visibly shaken; Mao appeared so frail that the prime minister was convinced that his life could not last much longer.[24] In early June, the PRC's Foreign Ministry issued the important announcement that, while Mao was busy with his work, he would not be receiving any more foreign visitors. The diplomatic community immediately interpreted this notice as a signal that the chairman's condition had grown worse, probably much worse.[25]

Mao Zedong's physical decline inevitably prompted widespread speculation about the extent of his ailments. In mid-May, one reliable diplomatic source reported that he had suffered another stroke (perhaps an explanation for the slack jaw and lack of muscular coordination visible in the last photographs taken of him) which aggravated the ailments caused by his Parkinson's disease. Further information which the USLO officers managed to acquire about Mao's condition led to the conclusion that any additional complication, such as a bout with influenza, could prove fatal.[26]

As early as mid-May and continuing until the end of June, the concern about Mao's steadily deteriorating health led to numerous rumors that the chairman had indeed died. Powerless to prevent these rumors, the PRC leadership nevertheless did its best to prevent such stories from making an extensive circulation. Much more offensive from the leadership's standpoint, however, was the bizarre rumor that "Mao was wired up" to life-support machinery, thereby leaving the PRC's ship of state dangerously adrift.[27]

Discussions of Mao's imminent death also led to conversations about his potential successor as chairman of the Chinese Communist Party. Considering the factional power struggle then under way in China, no shortage existed of prospective heirs-apparent to Mao's throne. Most knowledgeable China-watchers narrowed the list of prospective candidates to three: Premier Hua Guofeng, Vice Premier Zhang Chunqiao, and Jiang Qing. From the USLO's perspective in the early summer of 1976, none of these three was particularly attractive because none seemed likely to place a high priority on improving Sino-American relations. In terms of their careers, each had profited directly from the Cultural Revolution; Zhang and Jiang were acknowledged leftists and Hua was a member of the Left-leaning neo-Maoist group of younger Communist leaders. As a result, Tom and the other USLO officers spent countless hours assessing the relative prospects of each of these three people as Mao's successor, believing that within a relatively short time, they would be dealing with a government presided over by one of them.

Tom directed much of his attention to analyzing the leadership capability of the mysterious Hua Guofeng, who had been picked by Chairman Mao from relative obscurity and named acting premier after Zhou Enlai's death. On April 7, after the suppression of the Tienanmen riots, Mao went a step further: he designated Hua premier and first vice chairman of the Party. (Interestingly enough, first vice chairman was a new position, created by Mao to block the upward mobility of Wang Hongwen, who outranked Hua at the time within the Party.)[28] The question asked most often in the diplomatic community about Hua Guofeng was whether he was a "survivor" or merely a transitional figure in a long political drama which would see the rise and fall of many Chinese leaders. During the early summer of 1976, the diplomatic community tended to view Hua as "an independent actor," an individual with real ability, because of his considerable experience in the Party, his control of the Party apparatus in Hunan (Mao's home province), the fact that at various times in the past Mao, Zhou, and even Deng had praised his work, and most important, because of his control of the Party's internal security machine between 1973 and 1976.[29] If Hua possessed one shortcoming, it appeared to be that his rise to power had occurred so quickly that he had been unable to develop a suitable power base within the Party. But if Mao lived long enough, Hua would gain the necessary time in which to consolidate his power and could emerge as China's leader for well into the future.

Such an analysis of Hua Guofeng's prospects did not overlook, however, the other uncertainties in his future. Unlike Mao, Zhou, or Deng, Hua lacked the dynamism, assertiveness, and even charisma which the Chinese have come to expect in their leaders. Ross Terrill, an eminent scholar of China, analyzed Hua's career and concluded that the new premier "was a modest man with every reason so far to be." He "specialized in not making enemies" and possessed "all the charisma of an insurance clerk."[30] In a curious way, Terrill also reasoned, Mao may have been attracted to Hua because he bore a physical resemblance to his own son, Mao Anying. Furthermore, the simple fact that Mao had chosen Hua for a position of prominence was not necessarily a source of comfort; Mao had frequently turned on his presumed heirs-apparent (Liu Shaoqui, Lin Biao, even Deng Xiaoping) and purged them from the leadership.

Zhang Chunqiao was considered next as a prospective successor to Mao Zedong if Hua Guofeng faltered. A person of considerable ability, Zhang had held several high positions in the Party and commanded a strong power base from his home city of Shanghai. At that time, Zhang also served as the general secretary of the PLA's General Political Department, a post which appeared to give him access to the military. In the summer of 1976, Zhang's star was clearly on the rise and he was widely (though erroneously) rumored to be functioning in the same capacity under Hua that Deng had held under Zhou. Most China-watchers considered that Zhang had cast his lot with Hua (for reasons of pure expediency) and, even if not named Mao's successor, stood to be appointed premier if Hua eventually assumed the chairmanship.

Even so, the diplomatic community found itself divided on the question of Zhang Chunqiao's prospects for higher office. In the first place, Zhang was known to be deeply embittered about being passed over for the premiership after Zhou's death and apparently made little effort to establish more than an official relationship with Hua Guofeng. Much more the ideologue than Hua, Zhang reportedly chafed under the new premier's quasi-pragmatic approach to governance, especially at a time when the future leadership of China was at stake.[31]

In such a confusing and unsettled political environment, there existed the possibility that Mao's wife, Jiang Qing, might attempt to succeed him when he finally died. If the radicals possessed a definite strategy for taking over the PRC's leadership, most observers believed that Jiang would make a bid for the Party chairmanship which, if successful, would also lead to the installation of Zhang Chunqiao as premier and Wang Hongwen as chairman of the Standing Committee. Indeed, little doubt existed about Jiang Qing's ambitions to succeed Mao; "even under communism, there can be an empress," she once remarked. More to the point, she also claimed that Mao (in a highly disputed comment) even planned for her succession. "Help Jiang Qing," Mao allegedly said to his comrades as he entered his final weeks.[32] As the chairman's health steadily deteriorated throughout the summer, Jiang reportedly traveled extensively throughout northern China, attempting to consolidate her supporters for a possible assumption of power in the immediate post-Mao period.

In reality, Jiang Qing's prospects for power were poor. A shrewish, devious, and polemical woman, Jiang thrived on conspiracy and intrigue at a time when all of China had grown weary of ideological, Cultural Revolutionary-style campaigns and struggles. Jiang had powerful enemies within the Party and the state bureaucracy, and she was also widely despised by the Chinese masses. As long as Mao lived, however, she had a protector. After Mao's death, her political fortunes were destined for a free fall, a development which the chairman himself foretold. Jiang also realized that her position in the PRC hierarchy depended upon her estranged husband's survival. "Within a month of the chairman's death, my enemies will come for me," she predicted.[33]

Mao's impending death meant that the radicals were in a race against time to consolidate their power before the loss of their protector deprived them of indispensable sources of support within the Party and the state. Despite Mao's unquestioned achievements as a revolutionary, he had proven far less adept and even ill-suited for the more complicated task of leading China into a period of economic and political modernization.[34] In fact, Mao's fear that a Soviet-style revisionism had crept into the Chinese Communist Party drove him to increasingly irrational measures as he grew older, even though the Chinese people repeatedly made it clear that they had grown weary of ideological campaigns. By 1976, Mao and his radical supporters had achieved the unpleasant result of alienating most of the Party cadres with the Cultural Revolution, the criticism of Zhou, and the anti-Deng campaign; most of the industrial work force with their rigid insistence on an inflexible wage scale; a good portion of the scientific/technical establishment with their cultural and educational reforms; and prominent sectors of the PLA with the anti–Lin Biao campaign. As Mao lay dying in July and August, he probably drew little comfort from the knowledge that most of his support came from the ideologues who controlled the media, the worker-peasant-soldier students who dominated the campuses, and young leftist cadres who had no power base. Without question, Mao had failed to develop an orderly, institutionalized means of succession, and the anti-Deng campaign, if anything, revealed the weakness of his supporters. Tom and his colleagues wondered if it was simply a matter of time before the combined anti-radical forces triumphed over a leftist faction mortally wounded by the loss of Mao Zedong. Most knowledgeable China-watchers considered Zhou Enlai's death more damaging to China's political stability; had Mao died before Zhou, Zhou would still have possessed sufficient stature as a "protector of the people" to unify the country.

The role of the PLA was another factor to be considered in speculations about any future power struggle. Throughout the summer of 1976, the Americans in Peking sensed an increase in the power of the military. Defense Minister Ye was considered, in some minds, a peer of Premier Hua and Vice Premier Zhang during this period of so-called collective leadership in the PRC. Such a position was curious; had Mao not decreed that "the Party controls the gun"? How then could the Party exercise such control when the professional military counted its senior officer as an equal in the group then managing China's political affairs?[35] In any future political showdown, was it possible that the PLA held the balance of power? Was it possible that the PLA could even determine the outcome of the struggle? If the military supported the radicals, Chinese-American relations were clearly in jeopardy.

IV

Tom Gates began his own contacts with Chinese officials in mid-May 1976. Several of his early calls were courtesy visits with Chinese officials such as Lin Ping, director of the Foreign Ministry's Bureau of Americas and Oceania (the PRC's counterpart to the Department of East Asian Affairs at the State Department), who had met us at the airport in Peking, and Li Chiang, minister of foreign trade. Tom also met with Foreign Minister Qiao Guanhua and Vice Foreign Minister Wang Hairong. These visits resulted in substantive discussions of Chinese-American relations.

Tom's meeting with Qiao on May 15 occurred as a result of a request which he made through the PRC's diplomatic channels shortly after his arrival in Peking. Citing past experience, the USLO's officers had warned Tom to expect a considerable delay before the Chinese scheduled his appointment with the foreign minister, but the Foreign Ministry surprised them by scheduling the appointment for May 15, less than two weeks after the request.

Tom Gates's first meeting with Qiao Guanhua had two purposes, to discuss the current status of Chinese-American relations and to request formally a meeting between Tom and Premier Hua Guofeng. If Qiao felt any tension over the PRC's then-uncertain political situation, he certainly did not reveal it during this meeting. An urbane, intellectually oriented individual,

Qiao obviously enjoyed life and relished his role as the PRC's chief diplomat. During the conversation, he twice referred to the Shanghai Communique, first, as the basis upon which he and Tom might expect to center their relationship, and second, as the focus of future relations between the United States and China, regardless of the outcome of the 1976 presidential election in America.

After disposing of those formalities, Qiao then queried Tom extensively on the subject of the presidential primaries then under way in the United States. Qiao appeared especially concerned about Jimmy Carter's discussion of a possible withdrawal of American troops from South Korea and also his plans to reduce the defense budget by $7 billion in the next fiscal year. He left Tom with the clear impression that the Chinese considered the American military presence a stabilizing force in the Far East. When Qiao stated that America's elections are "very confusing to foreigners," Tom responded by discounting the importance of campaign rhetoric on the defense issue, especially every candidate's practice of introducing numerical comparisons of Soviet and American force levels and weapons systems into the political debate. From his own experience, Tom assured Qiao that the formulation of defense policy was an inexact science and the Chinese should not be concerned about any long-term decline in American military power. Furthermore, improved Chinese-American relations would be a priority for any presidential administration, regardless of the outcome of the elections, and specifically for a second Ford administration in light of the president's own public stance on the issue.

Qiao concluded the meeting by explaining that he and Tom could expect to have a productive association, like the ones he had had with Ambassadors Bruce and Bush, by "adhering to the principles laid down" (a poignant phrase as future events proved) in the Shanghai Communique. Throughout the meeting, Qiao remained relaxed and conversed easily. Except for a brief query about whether American military resolve had weakened since the 1950s (possibly a reference to the two Taiwan Straits crises which occurred while Tom served in the Navy Department), Qiao appeared to enjoy his session with Tom.[36]

On May 22, Vice Foreign Minister Wang Hairong held a dinner in Tom Gates's honor at the old United States legation's compound in Peking. Unlike Qiao Guanhua, who took the diplomatic high road and in statesmanlike fashion tried to point out the common interests between the United States and China, the redoubtable Wang Hairong apparently had been assigned the task of reminding Tom of the differences which existed between the two countries. Indeed, Wang Hairong was eminently suited for such a task. A small and rather shy woman, she was nevertheless direct and determined. Many USLO officers found her difficult; she did not have the sense of humor which Qiao possessed, and she always sprinkled her conversations with a healthy dose of Communist ideology. She was widely rumored to be Mao's niece (she was actually the great granddaughter of Mao's older sister) [37] and was also considered at that time to be close to Jiang Qing. That analysis was later proved incorrect when Jiang aggressively set out to weaken Wang's position in the Party.

Before the dinner, Wang Hairong asked to meet with Tom for an "informal talk." At that time, she came quickly to her point of indicating displeasure with the direction of Sino-American relations, particularly with America's refusal to break with Taiwan. "If America cannot remove the Taiwan albatross from its neck, we shall sever it with the bayonets of the PLA," Wang stated. [38] Tom withstood Wang's stern demeanor for several minutes and then inquired if, considering his recent arrival in Peking, the vice foreign minister had not raised such a complex issue too quickly. "We have a record to maintain, and that's a serious matter," Wang shot back. [39] Tom's future attempts to penetrate the tough, strait-laced, ideological exterior of Miss Wang proved equally unsuccessful.

Early in June, Tom received the startling news from the Chinese Foreign Ministry that he was scheduled for a thirty-minute appointment with Premier Hua Guofeng on June 10. The diplomatic community reacted to this news with some amazement; high-level contacts with members of the Chinese hierarchy were exceptionally rare. Most bilateral discussions with PRC officials occurred at the Foreign Ministry level.

In all likelihood, the Chinese arranged for this meeting because of a letter which President Ford wrote to Premier Hua requesting that the premier grant this appointment with Tom. Tom had presented Ford's letter to the foreign minister at their meeting on May 15, but officials at both the USLO and the State Department were pleasantly surprised that the Chinese acted so quickly in responding. The quick response was taken as a positive signal that the Chinese continued to desire improved relations with the United States, despite the changes then occurring in their own midst.

Tom received immediate instructions to report back to both President Ford and Secretary Kissinger about the results of his meeting with Hua. Most important would be his personal assessment of Hua who, even then, had only been the premier (or acting premier) of the PRC since early February. The major questions about Hua were why Mao had selected him as Zhou's successor, and whether he appeared to have the ability to govern China indefinitely.

One rather intriguing view of Hua's rise to power held that Deng Xiaoping had engineered Hua's appointment to the premiership after discovering that he lacked the necessary support to acquire the post himself. That argument rested on the assumption that Deng concluded that Hua would be easier than one of the radicals to move aside in a future showdown.[40] That hypothesis assumed, however, that Deng held considerably more power in the spring of 1976 than he actually did. In reality, it was the radicals who compromised on the selection of Hua, rather than holding out for Zhang Chunqiao, and accepted him as premier in the belief that *they* could oust him in the future. Indeed, the radicals' belief that they could manipulate Hua later proved to be one of their most fateful miscalculations.[41] In retrospect, Hua Guofeng was attractive to Mao Zedong in the spring of 1976 because he had demonstrated his loyalty to the chairman and his policies since the mid-1950s. And as Ross Terrill has noted, loyalty was a quality in short supply among Chinese politicians during that time.[42]

Tom Gates faced the responsibility, in his meeting with Hua Guofeng on June 10, of ascertaining the role which Hua played in the PRC's current political drama. Quite an undertaking, it seemed, especially for a meeting scheduled to last only thirty minutes. The assignment was serious, however. Just where exactly did Hua fit in with the other members of the PRC hierarchy? Was he, for example, a true Maoist, someone who would attempt to rule China according to ideology? Or, since former Premier Zhou Enlai had found Hua to be a capable administrator in dealing with agricultural, industrial, and other economic matters at the provincial level, was Hua an example of the more bureaucratic, procedurally oriented officials associated with the moderates? Since his place in the PRC's factional lineup seemed confusing, was Hua possibly a balance wheel between China's rival factions? Or was Hua simply an opportunist, a career politician primarily concerned about advancing his own interests and doing so by alienating as few people as possible?[43]

Tom was the second American to meet with Premier Hua Guofeng; the first was Richard Nixon, who had met with him in late February. When Tom sat down with the premier on June 10, he found him to be a cordial but somehow quite uncommunicative individual, even though their session stretched on for two hours. Hua covered most of the same subjects which Tom had discussed with Qiao Guanhua, including the Shanghai Communique and Chinese concern over the Soviet threat. The premier's conversation, however, impressed Tom more as a rote recitation of the Party's official line than a businesslike discourse between two diplomats. Furthermore, throughout the meeting, Hua assiduously took notes of the remarks, even though an interpreter and note-taker sat nearby. (The interpreter for most of Tom's official conversations with Chinese leaders was Tang Wensheng, known to Americans as Nancy Tang. She was born in Brooklyn and had moved to the PRC at the age of twelve. At the time of the meeting, she held the title of deputy director, Bureau of Americas and Oceania, in the Chinese Foreign Ministry and without doubt was the best interpreter in China. Like Wang

Hairong, her constant companion and diplomatic colleague, Tang Wensheng was very ideological in her conversations and undoubtedly a dedicated Marxist. Unlike Wang, however, Tang had an extremely pleasant personality and many USLO officers found their dealings with her to be quite useful.) Was this note-taking an example of self-consciousness, attention to detail, or simply a personal characteristic? Tom left the meeting with a vague sense of unease about this man who was the de facto leader of the largest nation on earth.

After returning to the United States Liaison Office, Tom spent several days with his colleagues arguing over the contents of the cable which they intended to send back to President Ford and Secretary Kissinger describing the meeting with Hua Guofeng and assessing his degree of influence within China. Was this admittedly modest man capable of governing a nation in the midst of a power struggle, resolving that struggle, and then fashioning a political program which led to a degree of national stability? Tom doubted that Hua possessed those talents, mostly because he seemed to lack Mao's charisma, Zhou's *gravitas*, or Deng's blunt determination. Tom's assessment of Hua Guofeng was in the minority, however; most American China-watchers (as well as others in the diplomatic community) felt that, since Hua had risen so rapidly, he must have had the stature and even ruthlessness to govern China. Tom Gates conceded that Hua Guofeng did enjoy considerable power in China, but only at that moment; what remained at issue was his capacity to influence events well into the future. The cable that was eventually dispatched to Washington concluded that Hua's prospects for long-term leadership of the PRC were not promising. As a result, America's policy-makers could expect further shake-ups in the Chinese hierarchy.[44]

V

Many of the varied aspects of China-watching came into sharper focus in mid-July when Senator Hugh Scott led a delegation to visit the People's Republic between July 10 and July 24. Tom had known Scott since their boyhoods together in the Chestnut Hill section of Philadelphia. Hugh Scott and his wife, Marian, were longtime friends of ours who also shared our strong interest in Chinese history and civilization. In addition, Scott had visited the PRC once previously in 1973, and the Chinese regarded him as an "old friend."

Senator Scott did not intend to run for re-election in 1976 and thus his visit to China served as something of a farewell from public life. Because of his position as the ranking Republican on the Foreign Relations Committee, the Chinese knew of Scott's views on improving Chinese-American relations and took the necessary steps to welcome him to the PRC. Before leaving the

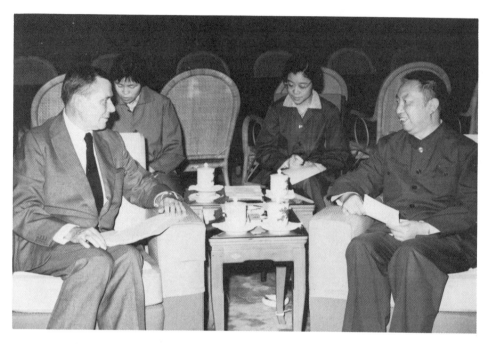

In conference with Premier Hua Guofeng, June 10, 1976. L-R: *Tom Gates, Wang Hairong, Tang Wensheng, Premier Hua.*

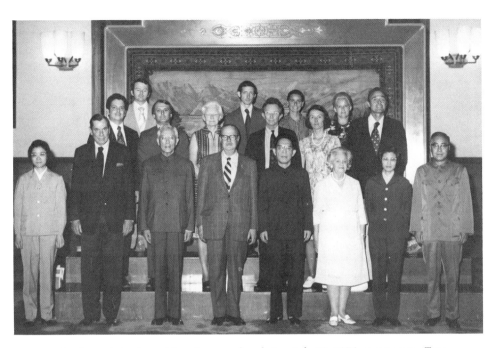

Members of the Scott delegation pose for photos, July 13, 1976. FRONT, L-R: *Tang Wensheng, Tom Gates, unidentified Chinese official, Senator Hugh Scott, Vice Premier Zhang Chungiao, Marian Scott, Wang Hairong, unidentified Chinese official.*

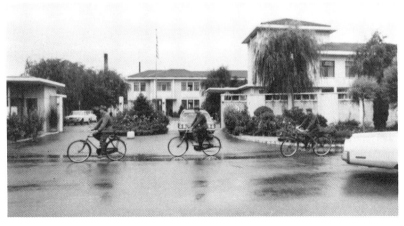

The USLO compound, June 1976; now the American Embassy in China.

United States, Scott talked with the president and was also briefed by Kissinger at the State Department, an indication that the administration also took his visit seriously.

Hugh Scott arrived in Shanghai with his delegation on July 10 and flew on to Peking from there. In addition to Hugh and Marian Scott, the delegation included Robert Barnett, head of the Washington office of the Asia Society, and his wife, plus several members of the senator's official staff and their spouses. While in Peking, Scott was scheduled for a series of discussions with Foreign Minister Qiao Guanhua and other officials, although the Foreign Ministry did not tell the USLO's officers in advance which members of the leadership would be meeting with the senator's delegation.

On July 12, Tom met with Scott and Barnett in the Peking Hotel prior to their meeting with Qiao Guanhua on July 13. Tom spoke at length with both men about the best manner in which to proceed with the Chinese, and Scott asked Tom whether he should raise the subject of Taiwan as the major obstacle to normalization between the two countries. Tom advised against such an approach unless the Chinese introduced the subject. "I hope you don't bring up the Taiwan issue in your discussions with the Chinese because they will shut you off and say the Shanghai Communique is the way the matter stands and that will be your answer. We've all received that answer a hundred times and the Chinese won't appreciate your bringing it up again and I doubt that you'll get them to change their position at all," he explained.[45] Scott agreed to follow Tom's advice, although Barnett was somewhat skeptical about such an approach. Reminding the senator of the importance of his visit and that he would be reporting back to the president, Barnett encouraged Scott not to ignore such important subjects as normalization and the problem of Taiwan when he met with Qiao. Tom repeated his earlier warning and Scott again indicated his approval of the cautious approach. (Sometime later, Kissinger told Tom that he had also advised Scott not to raise the subject of Taiwan.)

Thus on Monday July 13, Senator Hugh Scott and Robert Barnett, accompanied by Tom Gates, met with Foreign Minister Qiao Guanhua between 4 and 6 P.M. at the Foreign Ministry. The meeting began routinely, with the foreign minister welcoming Scott and taking him "on a trip around the world" (the USLO euphemism for the Chinese review of their foreign policy) and explaining the usual orthodoxy of Chairman Mao. Nothing of any particular substance developed except that Qiao commented again on the American elections ("troublesome for foreigners to observe") and the Chinese view of Soviet "hegemony" with the parallel assertion that the Helsinki Conference represented another Munich for the West.

Apparently believing that the meeting was proceeding smoothly, Scott and Barnett cautiously raised the subject of normalization, explaining their desire to make progress on the Taiwan issue but also expressing the opinion that the American public desired a peaceful resolution of the matter. Qiao stiffened immediately. "The responsibility for failure to normalize relations lies with the United States government," he declared. "Your [government's] position on Taiwan is illegal. In 1949, Secretary of State [Dean] Acheson declared to the world that the Taiwan matter was an internal affair of China. No foreign country has a right to interfere in the internal relations of China." In response, Scott explained, "We understand your views entirely. The problem, however, involves American public opinion. The American government needs evidence to assure the American people that one China can be brought about without resorting to force. Without wishing to intrude in your internal affairs, we need to believe that any solution will be peaceful." Qiao retreated not an inch. "Your [government's] position is self-contradictory in principle. On the one hand, you recognize one China of which Taiwan is a part. On the other, you ask China to do this and do that. That is an interference in China's internal affairs. You want us to do this and do that with regard to Taiwan. That position does not conform. If the United States government has difficulties at present, we won't press you. But it is an issue of right and wrong. Can we shift to another subject?" [46]

Whatever the other results of this meeting, Senator Scott and Robert Barnett at least received a better view of the Chinese position on normalization with the United States after their meeting with Qiao Guanhua. The following day, Scott's delegation kept an appointment with Vice Premier Zhang Chunqiao who, much to everyone's surprise, was the person selected by the PRC hierarchy to meet with the senator. The USLO's officers had assumed that Scott and Barnett would meet with Vice Premier Li Xiannian, who usually handled protocol matters and conferences with foreign guests. Zhang Chunqiao arrived for the meeting accompanied by Wang Hairong, Tang Wensheng, and Shi Yanhua, who acted as interpreter (apparently much to Tang's chagrin, since she repeatedly corrected Shi).

Throughout the meeting, Zhang maintained a demeanor totally consistent with the assessment the USLO's officers had made of him. Although Zhang was a physically slight individual, he nevertheless gave the impression of being a decidedly tough member of the hierarchy. Self-confident, uncompromising, and unmistakably shrewd, Zhang seemed unconcerned about establishing any personal rapport with the Americans. He arrived without notes and consulted neither Wang Hairong nor Tang Wensheng during the session. Zhang relied completely on his memory in explaining the Chinese position on various international issues, and it must be said that his memory never failed him.

Zhang's discussions with Scott proceeded acceptably for a considerable length of time with the vice premier responding easily but forcefully to the senator's questions. When Scott inquired when the United States and the People's Republic might expect to settle the issue of normalization, Zhang's conversation, which had already been marked by considerable sarcasm, took a distinctly menacing tone. "As the Foreign Minister explained to you yesterday at 4 P.M., our position on Taiwan is unchanged," he replied.[47] Scott found no reason not to try to get Zhang's views on the subject, however, and asked the vice premier for further comments. His reply was emphatic: "If the Americans insist on settling the issue, we shall settle it with bayonets. We will not permit interference by the U.S. or anyone." With that remark, everyone's pencils stayed poised in the air, and Tom expected Zhang to bolt from the room. Zhang remained firmly seated, however, as the Americans quickly terminated their conversation, posed for pictures, and ended the session.[48]

Tom and his USLO colleagues considered the Zhang/Scott meeting a momentary setback in their attempt to promote improved relations between the United States and China. One particular objective of USLO diplomacy at that time was to work with the Chinese over the matter of disavowing the use of force as a means of settling the Taiwan issue. With this assurance that the PRC intended to resolve its dispute with Taiwan by peaceful means, China and the United States could have normalized relations in reasonably short order. But the entire matter was extremely sensitive to the Chinese, and again the PRC's internal situation was a major factor in its attitude about Taiwan. "What few Americans realized," Richard Mueller once observed, "was that the generation of leaders then governing the PRC had fought against the Nationalists in the Chinese Revolution. For such people as Deng Xiaoping, the Revolution was not over until the Communists completely defeated the Nationalists. It was an exceptionally personal matter with them." Scott and Barnett, however, apparently believed it possible to obtain a constructive answer from the Chinese and clearly did not expect the emotional response which they received from Zhang Chunqiao. Instead of even gesturing toward the possibility of renouncing the use of force in settling the Taiwan dispute, Zhang clearly held out the PRC's option of military action against the Republic of China. Whether Zhang was making an implicit threat or whether he was simply repeating standard partisan rhetoric made little difference to Tom at the time. The fact remained that the American session with Zhang Chunqiao was a discouraging affair.[49] Regardless of Zhang's private attitude toward Americans and Chinese-American relations, his public approach and apparent inflexible views on Taiwan were worrisome, especially as a barrier to constructive discussions with the Chinese in the future. Moreover, the consensus within the diplomatic community in 1976 held that Zhang was a strong prospect for survival in the PRC hierarchy. The fact that he met with Scott (and in 1972 had escorted Richard Nixon on his visit to Shanghai) suggested that Zhang indeed might play a prominent role in future negotiations between the United States and the People's Republic. Facing the inflexible Zhang in future negotiations was not a pleasant prospect, especially since the vice premier appeared very comfortable in his role as an ideologue. [50]

Another major question for American diplomats was whether Zhang's performance was an indication of an increase in radical power in China. Scott believed that Zhang's actions indeed demonstrated that the radicals had "grabbed the Party machinery" from the moderates and were now in a decidedly anti-American mood. [51] Tom disagreed somewhat with that assessment but could hardly quarrel with the prevailing view that radical influence outweighed that of the moderates. The PRC media distributed daily samples of anti-Deng propaganda, the diplomatic grapevine contained rumors of Zhang's expanding influence, and China's cultural and educational life appeared to reflect the radicals' policies.

Not all of Tom Gates's China-watching, however, consisted of observations about the PRC's political situation. On July 4, the staff of the Liaison Office held a Bicentennial celebration which was open to the Chinese and the entire diplomatic community. Two hundred and fifty Chinese attended the festivities in the morning and remained for a showing of *Hello Dolly* in the afternoon. Later in the day, another six hundred people from the diplomatic community came to help the Americans celebrate the nation's two hundredth birthday. Handling the logistics for over eight hundred people proved to be a considerable undertaking, but the USLO family again demonstrated its great resourcefulness. There was a fine art exhibit of material from the American Revolution; many of the illustrations were copies of Birch's Views of Philadelphia. American flags from the revolutionary era flew throughout the compound, including a Betsy Ross on the USLO flagpole and "Don't Tread on Me" draped over the residence staircase. Throughout the day, Tom kept three projectors going with films about famous moments in American history. The USLO staff searched all over the Far East for the turkeys and hams to make a Bicentennial buffet, which they served with Cokes and American beer in cold cans. People loved it! The next day, the USLO staff gathered the remains of the food and went out for an office picnic alongside a lake near the Ming Tombs. [52]

Tom Gates's first two months in Peking were memorable. The Liaison Office's work was undoubtedly a vital aspect of America's diplomatic effort in the Far East. After meeting with several Chinese diplomats and observing the pattern of events in the PRC, he had grown accustomed to expecting the unexpected as it related to his China-watching chores. Events in the months to follow were to prove equally unexpected.

Notes

1. Terrill, *Future of China,* p. 29.
2. Interview, Richard Mueller, 17 February 1983.
3. Kissinger, *Years of Upheaval,* pp. 60–63.
4. Interview, David Dean, 7 December 1982; Richard Mueller, interview with the author, 17 February 1983, Washington, D.C.
5. Ibid.
6. United States Department of State, Official Files, Peking to Washington, 14 May 1976 (hereafter cited as OF, date); Thomas S. Gates Oral History, 31 March 1982 (hereafter cited as Gates OH, date).
7. Gates Papers, "United States Liaison Office-Peking" (Official Roster, May 1976). The USLO staff during Tom Gates's early months consisted of the following personnel: Harry T. Thayer (who was followed by David Dean), deputy chief; William W. Thomas, Jr., Foy J. Neeley, Frank P. Wardlaw, Lucille Sargent, and Caryn M. Solomon, Economic/Commercial Section; Thomas S. Brooks, B. Lynn Pascoe, Christopher H. Ballou, Pamela H. Moore, and Sue Quenan, Political Section; Gerard J. Levesque (followed by Hal Vickers), Mary Walsh, Roger E. Burgess, and Roberta A. Florkey, Administrative Section; Jerome C. Ogden, Consular Section; Joseph F. Acquevella, Marvin A. Konopik, Warren L. Salzer, Peter S. Quenan, and Catherine E. Dick, Communications Section; Evan L. Dewire, John P. Chornyak, Robert D. Booth, and David Bocskor, Security Section; Diana L. Pascoe and Patricia Chornyak, Receptionists; and thirty-seven local Chinese.
8. Gates OH, 1 January 1979.
9. *New York Times,* 13 February 1976, p. 4.
10. Gates, "On China"; Gates Papers, Thomas S. Gates to Anne Ponce et al., 9 July 1976.
11. Gates Papers, Thomas S. Gates to Anne Ponce et al., 9 July 1976.
12. Gates OH, 31 March 1982.
13. Gates Papers, Memorandum to Ambassador Gates from B. Lynn Pascoe, "Foreign Correspondents in Peking," 5 May 1976.
14. OF, Peking to Washington, 7 July 1976.
15. Garside, *Coming Alive,* pp. 110–14; OF, Peking to Washington, 29 November 1976.
16. OF, Peking to Washington, 23 July 1976.
17. OF, Peking to Washington, 10 June 1976.
18. OF, Peking to Washington, May–June, 1976.
19. OF, Peking to Washington, 11 May 1976.
20. Fox Butterfield, "Robbers of Bank Seem to Be Folk Heroes," *New York Times,* 23 August 1976.
21. OF, Peking to Washington, 27 July 1976.
22. OF, Peking to Washington, 7 July 1976; OF, Peking to Washington, 9 July 1976.
23. Interview, Gerald R. Ford.
24. OF, Reuters Dispatch, 5 May 1976.
25. Garside, *Coming Alive,* p. 137; Terrill, *Mao,* pp. 417–19.
26. OF, Peking to Washington, 20 May 1976. See also Theodore H. White, "Burnout of a Revolution," *Time,* 26 September 1983, pp. 31–32.
27. OF, Peking to Washington, June 1976.
28. OF, Peking to Washington, 7 February 1976.
29. Gates Papers, Memorandum to Ambassador Gates from Thomas S. Brooks, "Political Section Briefing," 5 May 1976.
30. Terrill, *Future of China,* p. 13; Terrill, *Mao,* pp. 407–8; Terrill, *The White-Boned Demon: A Biography of Madame Mao Zedong* (New York: William Morrow, 1984), p. 367.
31. OF, Peking to Washington, 19 July 1976.
32. OF, Peking to Washington, 10 February 1977; Terrill, *Mao,* p. 419.
33. Fox Butterfield, "The Intriguing Matter of Mao's Successor," *New York Times Magazine,* 1 August 1976, pp. 12, 37, 46, 48.
34. OF, Washington to Peking, 1976–77; Garside, *Coming Alive,* pp. 9–22.

35. OF, Peking to Washington, 11 May 1976; Fox Butterfield, "Hua May Be Chairman but Peking Rule Is Becoming a Two-Man Show," *New York Times*, 21 June 1976.

36. OF, Peking to Washington, 8 May 1976; OF, Washington to Peking, 10 May 1976; OF, Peking to Washington, 15 May 1976; Gates OH, 31 October 1982.

37. OF, November–December 1976.

38. Gates OH, 31 October 1982.

39. Ibid.

40. OF, General Reports and Statistics, July–August 1976; OF, Peking to Washington, 7 October 1976.

41. Interview, David Dean, 9 February 1983.

42. Terrill, *Mao*, pp. 407–9.

43. Domes, "The 'Gang of Four' and Hua Kuo-feng," pp. 483–88; Michel Oksenberg and Sai-cheung Yeung, "Hua Kuo-feng's Pre-Cultural Revolution Years, 1949–1960: The Making of a Political Generalist," *China Quarterly* 69 (March 1977): 3–53; Gates Papers, Thomas S. Gates to Anne Ponce et al., 9 July 1976.

44. Gates OH, 31 October 1982.

45. Ibid.

46. OF, Peking to Washington, 12 July 1976; Gates OH, 31 October 1976.

47. Gates OH, 31 October 1982. Tom developed a high degree of respect for the junior officers in the PRC's Foreign Ministry. They had obviously briefed Zhang Chunqiao intensively before his meeting with Hugh Scott. "The grapevine in China is very prompt," Tom once declared. "I don't think the junior people at the Foreign Ministry ever sleep."

48. Ibid.

49. Ibid.

50. Ibid.; OF, Peking to Washington, 15 July 1976.

51. *New York Times*, 3 August 1976; *Washington Post*, 3 August 1976.

52. Gates Papers, Thomas S. Gates to Anne Ponce et al., 9 July 1976.

CHAPTER **3**

Coping with Calamity: The Tangshan Earthquake

At 3:40 on the morning of July 28, 1976, Thomas Gates and I were sleeping peacefully in the residence of the United States Liaison Office in Peking when suddenly we were awakened by a tremendous jolt which shook the house and lifted our bed off the floor. The tremor lasted for ten to fifteen seconds (although it seemed to us much longer), and it was followed by a second shock. Then we felt nothing for the next several minutes except an ominous silence. It is perhaps an element of human subconsciousness that when confronted with the horrible and unexpected, one's mind races to an event in the past to help it regain its bearing. Not completely awake, Tom found his mind flashing back to his years in the Pacific during World War II aboard the *U.S.S. Ranger* when the carrier was hit by kamikaze attacks in the Okinawa campaign. I immediately flashed back to an experience in Washington during the 1950s when I did weekly physical exercise on a "Slenderella," a vibrating machine used by weight watchers. "What am I doing in Washington now?" I asked myself.

Within moments, both Tom and I realized that we were not in the Pacific or in Washington but in the midst of an earthquake, an immensely powerful one which we learned later was ripping apart north China. A strange and overwhelming force seemed to hold us in its grasp. Following advice I had heard years before, I jumped out of bed and called to Tom to get under a door jamb. But fortunately the quaking stopped, and within moments, the telephone rang. John Chornyak, a member of the USLO security detail, had called to determine our condition. I assured him that we were fine and then went downstairs to see if any damage had occurred to the residence. There was no major damage in the house; pictures, chairs, and ornaments were upset but structurally the house was in good order. Outside, the Chinese guard stood on duty by the USLO gates acting as if nothing had happened.

David Dean took the responsibility for calling the USLO personnel. Of particular concern were the several USLO families who had taken temporary quarters high up in the Peking Hotel, but Dean soon reported, to everyone's relief, that all the staff members and their children were safe and unharmed. At 4 A.M., the USLO community gathered on the small grass plot outside the compound and awaited further information. Tom raised Old Glory to the top of the USLO flagpole as a signal to the rest of the diplomatic community that we were in no imminent danger. Elsewhere in Peking, however, the earthquake produced confusion and panic. The first tremor brought hundreds of anxious people in the diplomatic quarter out into the streets. In Peking's residential sections, hundreds of thousands of Chinese, some reportedly screaming in fright, came streaming from their homes and out into the early morning darkness.[1]

Those who experienced the earthquake in Peking will never forget it, even though it did considerably less damage in the capital than in the rest of north China. David Dean later remembered awakening early that morning and seeing a strange, eerie light in the east and hearing a menacing, "keening" sound moments before the quake struck. The earthquake was completely unexpected and left everyone with feelings of fear compounded with confusion and anxiety. After the first tremors, the Chinese authorities issued an earthquake alert: all residents of Peking, both Chinese and foreign, were encouraged to remain outdoors. Shortly after 4 A.M., we received a telephone message from the Foreign Ministry which confirmed that an "abrupt eruption" earthquake had struck north China, with the epicenter being 150 kilometers southeast of Peking. "For the sake of safety," the Chinese instructed, USLO was "reminded to stay alert."[2] Despite the warnings, however, many people returned to their homes after the two early morning tremors. At 7:25 A.M., though, another quake hit north China and this tremor increased the sense of fear and panic in the city. Those Chinese and foreigners who had returned inside before the latest sharp tremor again fled to safety outdoors, some completely terrified.

Tom was particularly concerned about the members of a large American Congressional staff delegation which was then visiting Peking. The delegation had been housed in the Peking Hotel, and shortly after daylight, Tom received word that all of the delegation's members were unhurt. The Congressional staffers deserted the Peking Hotel, however, and joined the group at the USLO compound. Those who had been on the higher floors of the hotel were thoroughly frightened. One staff member spent the next twenty-four hours trying to telephone his mother back in the United States and became furious with Tom, the United States government, and the Chinese authorities because he could not complete his call. Another staffer hugged our best sofa as his territory, refusing to leave it for any reason.

When daylight arrived it was clear that Peking's taller buildings had suffered damage. The cracks in the buildings caused by the first tremors had widened considerably after the later shocks. Many homes in the capital, especially the older ones, had crumbled and collapsed under the force of the quake. In other buildings, most of the elevators were out of order. Peking's main stores on Wang Fu Ching Avenue were partly demolished. In the city's countless high-rise buildings, balconies had fallen off and lay crumbled on the streets below. Peking was in a state of emergency. As the early morning hours passed, the USLO staff members and their families (sixty-two adults and twenty children), plus the American Congressional staff delegation, gathered at the mission compound to await further developments.

While the residents of Peking and the foreign diplomatic community experienced their own emergency on the morning of July 28, another group of Americans, not far away in Tianjin, was also coping with this massive earthquake. Located in the northeast coastal region, Tianjin was China's fourth largest city and, in late July, the site of an elaborate trade fair exhibition. Sol and Rose Salz and Samuel and Beatrice Steinberg, two American couples from New York City, were then visiting the city as part of a touring labor delegation scheduled to attend the trade exhibition. These four Americans also awoke to the enormous jolt of the first tremors early on July 28 and discovered that their hotel was swaying back and forth. Beatrice Steinberg jumped into her husband's bed, grabbed him, and exclaimed, "If we're going to go, let's go together." Samuel Steinberg only recalled saying, "Babe, this is it. It's the end."[3] After the first shocks ended, the four Americans were located by their Chinese guides. "American friends, are you all right?" the guides inquired from the hallway of the hotel. "Please put [your] shoes on, leave everything and come with us. Stay calm. Trust us. We are prepared."[4] Following these instructions, the Salzes and Steinbergs left their hotel for the relative safety of the streets of Tianjin and were then taken to a nearby athletic stadium where the Chinese were organizing the visiting foreign groups then in the city. Later that day, the Americans left Tianjin for Peking and shortly afterward returned to the United States.

The Americans in Peking later discovered that Tianjin suffered considerably more damage than Peking. Stephen Fitzgerald, the Australian ambassador to China, also happened to be in Tianjin at the time of the earthquake and reported that the Chinese had confirmed several deaths in the city but refused to provide additional information about the number of fatalities.[5]

Fitzgerald was accompanying Gough Whitlam, the former prime minister of Australia, on a visit to China, and Whitlam later provided an exceptionally revealing account of his experiences on the night of July 28. Whitlam recalled that he and his wife were awakened by the earthquake in their room on the second floor of the Tianjin Guest House. "The hotel was lunging and tearing," Whitlam explained. A chest of drawers toppled over on his wife and cut her leg. The Tianjin Guest House, a new, modern building, was "split down the middle with a one-foot gap separating the two parts. We had to walk over the gap going down the corridor and [were] evacuated from the hotel. Luckily a Chinese official accompanying us found a flashlight." Ambassador Fitzgerald also described the earthquake as literally "throwing [the hotel] around."[6] "It was not just a kind of swaying around but it was moving very heavily in all directions, punctuated by extreme jolts which flung me around in the bed. For some time after, the building swayed in a way that suggested it was undecided about whether to fall over, but it would get to each end of the arc and then just kind of teeter there for awhile and then swing to the other end and teeter there for awhile. I felt a building could not possibly survive being thrown around this way."[7]

Once out of their hotel, the Whitlams and Fitzgerald noticed that most of Tianjin's residents were already out in the streets. "Some old houses had completely collapsed," Whitlam recalled. "Some modern houses stood up very well. The people were gathered in open spaces."[8] Chinese physicians attended to Mrs. Whitlam and then other officials escorted the Australians to the stadium and eventually drove them to Peking over a route which had been examined for its safety. Once in Peking, Whitlam observed that the situation in the capital was nowhere near as serious as that in Tianjin. In fact, the earthquake which struck north China on the morning of July 28 did such enormous damage and caused such immense destruction that the full extent of the catastrophe will probably never be known. This earthquake, which measured an astonishing 8.2 on the Richter scale, inflicted its worst damage in Hebei province where it completely leveled the industrial city of Tangshan, a city of over one million people. In addition to inflicting a great loss of life (estimates of which conflict up to this day), the quake severely disrupted the industrial and technological infrastructure of north China and undoubtedly contributed to the PRC's poor economic performance in 1976.

The earthquake alert in the capital lasted from August 1 to August 16. During that time, Tom Gates decided to evacuate several of the USLO's staff members and a majority of its dependents to safer posts throughout the Far East. In Peking, however, over four million Chinese lived outside in makeshift tents, huts, and other shelters until the authorities became sufficiently convinced that the period of danger had passed.

Coping with the calamity of the earthquake occupied everyone's attention in August 1976. The Chinese authorities concentrated their efforts on the overwhelming task of providing relief and other forms of humanitarian assistance to the beleaguerèd residents of Tangshan and Hebei province. The matter of relief also created controversy within the Chinese hierarchy which ultimately enhanced the power of Premier Hua Guofeng and the influence of the PLA within China's political establishment. The Chinese leadership reaffirmed the unusual fact that even a natural disaster (at least in 1976) could not be handled in a nonpolitical way. The earthquake, and the Party Center's response to it, also became part of the succession struggle during the Year of the Dragon.

The earthquake was one more important event in China's unending drama during 1976. First, the death of Zhou Enlai, then the Tienanmen riots and the ouster of Deng Xiaoping, then the death of Zhu De; when taken with the natural disaster of the earthquake, such a trail of tragedy convinced the Chinese people that the end of the Maoist regime was drawing near. The aged and ill Mao Zedong would soon die, and what then?[9] Tom Gates and the other Americans found their China-watching activities diverted in August from speculating on the course of the PRC's internal power struggle to observing how the leadership dealt with the natural disaster.

In several ways, the earthquake represented a turning point in the events of the Year of the Dragon, for both the Chinese and the foreign diplomats stationed in Peking. First, the absolute requirement of providing relief for the victims of the quake brought Hua Guofeng and the leadership of the PLA closer together while also deflating the power of China's radical faction. Correctly so, the radicals viewed the relief effort as an obstacle in their desire to keep public opinion firmly riveted on the anti-rightist, anti-Deng campaign. Second, the calamity resulted in increased cooperation between various members of the diplomatic community as the USLO officers and their counterparts in other embassies met daily (sometimes hourly) to exchange information and develop contingency plans for meeting the safety requirements of their staffs and dependents. Tom was instrumental in establishing an informal "earthquake committee" comprised of the ambassadors and senior staff of the United States Liaison Office and the Australian, British, Canadian, French, New Zealand, and Japanese embassies, an association which grew as a result of the shared experience of the earthquake emergency. Tom also noticed that Chinese officials became more forthright and less official in their dealings with the USLO and the rest of the diplomatic community. For both the Chinese and the USLO's diplomatic colleagues, a closeness and informality replaced the stiffer, more formal, and more serious relationships which existed before the earthquake. A common concern for each other's welfare became more apparent. Since the earthquake had such a significant

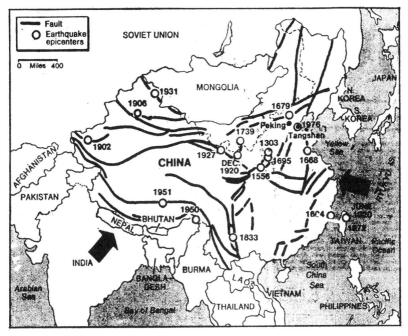

Incidence of earthquake activity in China over the last several centuries. Historic records show that earthquakes equivalent to magnitude 8 or greater on the Richter scale were centered at places designated by circles and in years indicated. Arrows indicate pressures that may have been responsible for the tremors. (The New York Times, July 31, 1976, by Woodrow W. Wilson. Copyright © 1976 by the New York Times Company. Reprinted by permission.)

impact on the USLO's China-watching activities, its effect on the American and Chinese experiences in Peking during the Year of the Dragon demands closer scrutiny.

Although the Chinese have certainly had experience with earthquakes, the available evidence suggests that the Tangshan quake caught the PRC almost totally by surprise. China itself lies across two fault lines, one running north to south, and the other east to west. The Tangshan earthquake occurred along the north-south line and, despite the great damage which it inflicted, Chinese seismologists considered that any quake along the east-west fault line (which passes through Peking) would result in considerably greater destruction and loss of life than the one which occurred in late July 1976. Even so, informed scientists still would contend that the Tangshan earthquake was the strongest and most violent tremor, and probably the worst natural disaster in recorded history.[10]

Earthquakes have plagued China throughout its history. In 1556, according to Chinese seismologists, the quake which hit Shanxi province resulted in over 830,000 deaths. On July 12, 1720, China witnessed another severe earthquake, with damage so great that estimates placed the magnitude of the shock at 6.75 on the Richter scale. With such catastrophes historically possible, the Chinese developed an intricate (though technologically simple) seismological system designed to detect the imminence of an earthquake so that the authorities could warn the people accordingly. In 1976, the Chinese employed over ten thousand scientists, engineers, and technicians (ten times the number of Americans engaged in such work) at seventeen seismological stations and auxiliary stations, all at work attempting to detect any evidence of earthquake activity. In addition, the Chinese augmented their professional watch system by instructing the civilian population about observing natural peculiarities which might indicate future earthquakes. Over centuries, sometimes by fact and sometimes by legend, strange phenomena have become part of earthquake lore. Did the water level in wells rise unexpectedly? Did snakes refuse to go underground or horses refuse to enter barns? Were turtles agitated; did pandas hold their heads and scream? Did birds flock and chatter incessantly?[11] (Sometime after the Tangshan earthquake, Tom recalled that immediately before the earthquake the cicadas around the USLO compound had kept up a constant chirping.) The Chinese tended to view all of these natural phenomena, when noticed consistently over a length of time, as indications of an impending earthquake.

The earthquake of July 28 proved to be an embarrassment to both the amateur and professional seismologists in China. The earthquake happened with sudden intensity and virtually no warning to the Chinese people. The tragedy is that professional seismologists knew the earthquake was imminent but chose not to alert the population in north China. On the evening of July 27, several provincial and municipal officers in the Tangshan-Fengnan region met with their seismologists, then closely occupied with observing the geologic situation. The seismologists expected a quake of the magnitude of 4 or 4.5 on the Richter scale. The scientists remained uncertain, however, about the true size of the quake or when it might occur. This meeting, which began early in the evening, lasted for several hours as the officials debated whether to alert the population and take other precautions. Finally, the provincial leaders decided not to alarm the population by calling an earthquake alert; such a warning might be premature and lead to unnecessary fears. Instead, they agreed to resume their meeting at *10 o'clock the following morning.* The earthquake struck at 3:45 A.M., however, and presumably these officials were among the several hundred thousand people who perished while lying asleep on that terrible morning.[12]

The first reports out of Tangshan bespoke a tale of almost unspeakable human misery. The city itself was "ruined totally, 100%; it looked like Hiroshima after the atomic bomb," according to one observer.[13] Since the earthquake was of the "abrupt eruption" type, people had been hurled against the ceilings of their homes as it struck. It left the huge coal, steel, and industrial complex which the Chinese had erected in Tangshan during the mid-1960s in ruins. It caused the collapse and immediate destruction of an enormous building which housed two recently constructed generators which supplied electrical power to the city. Not only were the Chinese in Tangshan without electrical power, the railroad line leading into the city was broken, as were bridges along the route leading northward. After the quake, fires broke out in Tangshan, further complicating the disaster. Nor was the destruction limited to the first day of the earthquake and the awful moments when the initial shocks tore the city apart; over the next five days, a hundred more aftershocks were reported in Tangshan (some measuring over 5 on the Richter scale), and these smaller quakes caused still more damage. In addition, the earthquake damaged reservoirs, dams, and irrigation projects and caused heavy flooding; the Chinese were especially concerned about the stability of a large dam on the nearby Luan He River. Many large-scale government construction projects, especially those along the Hai He River, were destroyed. The pipeline to China's oil fields in Manchuria was inoperable.

Most important, Tangshan was the site of China's critically important Kailuan Coal Complex, the PRC's largest coal mining operation. Serious concern existed about the fate of the miners who may have been trapped underground (all the mines were underground) when the earthquake struck. The information which the USLO received led Tom to believe that, especially because of the suddenness of the quake, as many as ten or twelve thousand miners may have been trapped. For their part, the Chinese insisted through the PRC media that while some miners had perished, the "great majority" either were rescued or otherwise found their way to safety.[14]

The damage to property, great as it was, did not raise as much concern among America's China-watchers in Peking as the number of human casualties inflicted by the earthquake. First reports indicated that perhaps 100,000 Chinese either perished, or were severely injured, in the quake. Following those reports, the estimates of casualties began to rise; at various intervals, USLO officers heard that as many as 900,000 Chinese (out of a population of approximately 1,500,000 in the greater Tangshan area) had been killed. In 1979, the Chinese released an official account of the loss of life in the quake, listing the number of dead at 240,000, with 160,000 listed as injured or missing. Even from the perspective of several years, however, those estimates appeared to be low. For example, six months after the earthquake, Tom received two items of information which placed the casualty figures higher than the later published version. First, the independent newspaper *Ming Pao* in Hong Kong published a letter written by a Tangshan resident who claimed that 900,000 casualties (both dead and injured) resulted from the quake. The author of that letter, who lost his entire family in the calamity, supported his conclusions by claiming as his source a relative who had been involved in earthquake relief work. The same letter also spoke of an outbreak of cholera in the devastated area.

This report in *Ming Pao* appeared to confirm the accuracy of information received by a foreign journalist in Peking which estimated the number of casualties in the neighborhood of 800,000 fatalities. Another observer cautioned against such estimates, however, explaining that "given the great damage and loss of life which resulted, it may take years to get an approximately complete account."[15] USLO officials later in 1976 received more information that the death and casualty toll may have exceeded the preliminary estimates issued by the PRC leadership. Provincial authorities in Hebei province apparently completed a report which they dispatched to the Party Center, late in 1976, listing the extent of human suffering exacted by the earthquake. According to a key part of this document (which was apparently leaked to the editorial offices of *Ming Pao*), "Material for the Study of the Conference on Resisting Earthquakes and Relieving Disaster Among Third Echelon Cadres," 655,237 Chinese perished in the earthquake, another 79,000 suffered serious injuries which required emergency treatment, and 700,000 received minor injuries.[16] The precision with which that report appeared to be written, combined with Hua Guofeng's later public statement that "such damage has seldom before been seen in history," leads one to believe that the actual number of deaths greatly exceeded the PRC's official reports.

When the earthquake struck north China, the PRC authorities immediately clamped a news blackout on the situation in Tangshan and forbade any foreign travel into the region. (Since most of the transportation arteries into Tangshan were destroyed, this prohibition was largely unnecessary.) The authorities admitted that the situation in Tangshan was "very serious" but put forth no further details. The accounts which the USLO received about the earthquake, therefore, were mostly second-hand, from Chinese who were willing to discuss the disaster or members of the diplomatic community who had knowledge of the event. For example, one of the USLO's Chinese employees had a brother living in Tangshan at the time of the earthquake. Apparently unable to sleep in the early morning hours before the earthquake struck, this man went for a walk outside of his home. Sensing that an earthquake was imminent, he immediately ran back to his home, awakened his wife and children, piled his family into a nearby truck, and sped for Peking. While they were en route, the earthquake struck, and the man was later able to give a precise description of the tremendous horror and destruction which accompanied the tremors in north China.

II

A major question in the minds of Tom Gates and the USLO officers was the extent to which the earthquake would damage China's economic performance in 1976. The area affected by the quake, the Peking-Tianjin-Tangshan triangle, was the third most important industrial region in China, ranking only behind Manchuria and Shanghai. More important, the economic activity in this region ranged from coal mining to power generation to textile production. The region also included the large Dagang oil field and was connected to Manchuria and the rest of north China by a rail network which also linked the area with several important sea ports.[17]

The earthquake tragedy, combined with political turmoil and worker apathy, put an end to the hope that 1976 would be the springboard in the PRC's Fifth Five Year Plan and that the nation would make strong, early strides in Zhou Enlai's ambitious program of political and economic reform. Throughout the early summer, the radical-controlled media had kept up a drumbeat of criticism about Deng Xiaoping's economic views, a demoralizing influence on anyone concerned with orderly production. Furthermore, evidence existed to support the conclusion that the radicals were actively involved in fomenting labor unrest and trying to slow production. For instance, eight factories in Hangzhou, as well as the heavy machinery works at Wuhan, had suffered either "full or semi-stoppage of production" since January. Factional violence at other industrial sites caused hundreds of other factory workers to stay away from work, rather than become drawn into life-threatening situations.[18]

In addressing the impact of the earthquake upon China's economic performance in 1976, Tom Gates first needed to examine the effect of the disaster upon the Tangshan region and then assess how the relief and reconstruction effort might affect the rest of China. Reports the USLO received about the damage in Tangshan indicated a staggering degree of economic destruction. Tangshan was a relatively new city, constructed in the late 1940s and early 1950s in an attempt by the PRC leadership to develop the economy of north China. By 1976, the city numbered over one million residents and was an important center for coal and steel production as well as a critical link in north China's rail network. When the earthquake struck Tangshan, it virtually flattened the city. The large Hitachi generating complex in Tangshan, built with foreign investment, was badly damaged, and the city's power supply was cut off, with no indications about when it might be restored. The Tangshan Iron and Steel Plant, according to one report, suffered "heavy losses." [19]

The area immediately surrounding Tangshan, which included the Kailuan coal complex, China's largest, also suffered serious damage. At the coal mines in and around Tangshan, electrical failures cut off power to both elevators and pumps, trapping miners and allowing water to enter the pits, some of which were over eight hundred meters deep. Production at the mines stopped completely, and within days there was a shortage of coking coal for the PRC's steel industry.

The earthquake also seriously disrupted transportation in the north China region. The Peking-Harbin railroad was broken at dozens of points, completely shutting down service into Tangshan. The Jinan-Peking line continued to function, although damage to the line and rolling stock was extensive. The rail bed had been cracked and tracks sank throughout the length of the line; rails were twisted and broken; dozens of bridges were damaged, including the large ones over the Ji Canal and the Yongding River in Tianjin. The devastation also disrupted shipping; China's already crowded harbor at Hsinkang became even more congested in the weeks ahead. Later, the congestion proved to be such a problem that the Chinese diverted shipping to other ports, principally to Dalien, Qingdao, and Shanghai.

In the economic realm, probably the greatest concern to the Chinese involved the status of the coal mines and the electric generating plant around Tangshan. China was the world's third largest coal producer, and the Chinese operated eight large mines in the Tangshan region with a combined annual output of more than twenty-five million metric tons. Any disruption in coal production reverberated throughout the Chinese economy because coal played an overwhelmingly predominant role in meeting the PRC's fuel requirements, and because coal production was essential for the manufacture of coke and therefore an integral factor in the PRC's production of steel. When the earthquake struck Tangshan, the PRC leadership immediately sent in rescue teams from as far away as Anhui, Zhejiang, and Shandong to assist in the relief effort. Even so, estimates at the time concluded that full production in the mines would not resume for at least one year. One observer reported that he foresaw no prospect for restoring production at Tangshan's coal mines any time in 1976 since the mines "were full of water." [20]

The immediate outlook for the restoration of electric power around Tangshan was equally dismal. The city's electrical power facility, which supplied 15 percent of China's total output, sustained considerable damage, and the two major thermal plants around Tangshan lost 95 percent of their capacity. Repair of such destruction would take months, at the minimum. These electrical plants were also part of the important Peking-Tianjin grid; their loss undoubtedly affected all of north China. Tom Gates and the other Americans had good reason to suspect that the official report that "the damage [around Peking] was severe but localized" may have been wishful thinking. The Americans knew that the quake had caused the near-total destruction of housing around Tangshan, and it was difficult to believe that any productive activity could occur under these circumstances, so extensive was the destruction.

III

During the days immediately after the earthquake, on everyone's mind was concern about the possibility of another earthquake, or of damaging aftershocks. After the PRC authorities announced the earthquake alert, millions of Chinese in Peking continued to remain outdoors as a safety precaution, but there was hardly any sign of disrupted services; transportation and utilities functioned as though no state of emergency existed. Compounding the feeling of uncertainty, however, was a heavy rainstorm in Peking which lasted for the next two days. Yet despite fears that the storm might indicate a possibility of renewed earthquake activity, the residents of Peking massed on the sidewalks, holding their umbrellas and attempting to go about their daily business.

Peking's municipal authorities advised the foreigners in the diplomatic community to "be watchful" and remain out of their buildings. At the same time, the Chinese began a systematic, building-by-building examination of the structures in Peking. With the entire city in this state of alert, the USLO officers observed the remarkable transformation which occurred in Peking on July 28. After the second series of tremors struck the city at 7:25 A.M., Peking became a tent city, almost by magic. Shanties and pieced-together shelters sprang up everywhere in response to the earthquake alert. The Chinese were highly organized and disciplined; some showed remarkable ingenuity in constructing their temporary shelters on the sidewalks and in the parks of Peking. Throughout July 28, Peking remained in a sensitive alert status, although many of the USLO personnel eventually concluded that it was safe to return inside for a brief period. Tom had scheduled a reception for the members of the Congressional staff delegation and some Chinese guests, and everyone agreed to proceed with it. Ke Bonian, vice president of the Chinese People's Institute on Foreign Affairs, and Tang Wensheng led the group of Chinese visitors.

At 6:50 that evening, during the reception, with the USLO residence full of American and Chinese guests, a second strong earthquake jolted Peking, the third powerful tremor in just a little over twelve hours. Later recorded at 7.9 on the Richter scale, this quake again swayed Peking's taller buildings and destroyed more homes. Although shorter than the earlier tremors, this severe quake was followed by more aftershocks, causing the Chinese and the diplomatic community to wonder if the worst of the earthquake activity still lay ahead.

This third earthquake proved to be of critical importance to the leadership of the People's Republic. Throughout the day on July 28, the Chinese authorities were noticeably restrained in their discussions of any future danger. After the third quake, however, they moved with considerably greater dispatch. Not only were all Chinese in Peking ordered out of their dwellings, but the leadership also began closing off access to the taller buildings in the city, forbidding any entry into most of the structures until an assessment had been made of their condition. The authorities immediately prohibited entrance to any building in Peking which was over five stories tall, including the Peking Hotel, which they sealed off on the morning of July 29. When several apartment buildings in the diplomatic community were closed, many USLO families were forced to seek temporary quarters within the American compound. Other embassies followed the Americans and began using their official headquarters for temporary lodgings. The Chinese also began suggesting that foreign diplomats consider evacuating their personnel until the earthquake alert and emergency had passed.

Despite these developments, the main problem confronting the USLO and the other embassies in Peking was the lack of available information about the real extent of the danger which the city faced. Typical of the Chinese in 1976, the PRC authorities said as little as possible about the situation in the capital. An accurate assessment of the situation proved virtually impossible to obtain. On July 29, the *People's Daily* admitted that "violent quakes" had struck north China, resulting in "serious damages and loss," but the article provided no further details. At the time, the USLO heard nothing from the State Department or from the American Embassy in Japan. Both American and Japanese seismologists apparently agreed that the Chinese knew more about earthquakes in China than they; the USLO would simply have to await word from the Chinese. (In the following week, we began to receive considerably more information from Washington about the potential for more earthquake activity in China.)[21] To help keep the diplomatic community informed, Tom became instrumental in forming the "Earthquake Committee," an informal group which met daily to share information about the situation in Peking. Comprised of the ambassadors and key embassy personnel from Australia, England, New Zealand, Canada, France, and Japan, plus Tom and several other USLO officers, the Earthquake Committee began a practice of meeting daily at 11 A.M. Following each meeting, the group prepared an "Earthquake Update," a report on the current situation based on the information acquired in each meeting.

The next two days, July 29 and 30, were critical for our entire experience in China. On July 29, Tom sent a letter to Foreign Minister Qiao Guanhua offering American humanitarian assistance in the PRC's effort to deal with the calamity. Based on instructions from President Ford, Tom informed Qiao that the United States was "prepared to be helpful in whatever way you think would be useful. This assistance can be provided through whatever channels you consider appropriate."[22] The offer of assistance was presented in a decidedly low-key manner. Many nations had offered aid to China; some foreign governments even passed formal resolutions to that end. By July 29, however, Tom had observed (although he never completely understood) the Chinese attitude toward the earthquake as one almost of embarrassment or even shame that the quake had chosen to strike China. Given that attitude, as well as a number of other factors to be mentioned later, it became highly unlikely that the Chinese would accept foreign assistance of any kind, regardless of the source. The Japanese, for example, made a much more public offer of assistance to the People's Republic and, to their discomfiture, received a prompt refusal.

On July 30, the Foreign Ministry issued a polite refusal to the American offer of humanitarian assistance. The Chinese message dwelt on the value given to the concept of self-reliance exhibited in China since the Communists assumed power in 1949. The message read in part: "Thank you for your sympathy for the strong earthquake which occurred in the Tangshan-Fengnan area of our country not long ago. But the Chinese have always overcome various natural disasters through self-reliance, and the same holds true in the case of the current earthquake. We believe that under the leadership of Chairman Mao and the Party Central Committee, the people of the stricken area, with the support of the people of the whole country, will certainly be able to prevail over the losses sustained in the recent earthquake."[23]

Even with this careful explanation, the Americans found a great deal of difficulty understanding why the Chinese chose to reject such generous offers of assistance and sincere gestures of friendship, not only from the United States and other countries, but also from international rescue and relief organizations such as the Red Cross. Gerald Ford, for example, was astonished that the People's Republic would refuse the American offer, particularly in view of the magnitude of the human emergency which it then confronted.[24] The American government historically offers humanitarian assistance to countries struck by natural disasters, regardless of their political philosophy. And yet, given the Maoist tenor of this period in China, combined with the fact that Mao apparently insisted on knowing every detail about the tragedy in Tangshan, it is not surprising that the Chinese rejected all foreign assistance. "Since the revolution, China has stood up," Mao once declared.[25]

Tom Gates did make a last attempt to penetrate the official Chinese exterior of self-reliance, however. On the evening of July 31, Tang Wensheng led a delegation of Chinese officials to the USLO compound, ostensibly an inspection tour of the buildings but in reality a goodwill mission. This gesture was typical of the Chinese, who were exceptionally conscientious about being polite hosts. The delegation inspected the compound, talked with the USLO officers, and generally inquired about our welfare. Tang thanked Tom for the American offer of assistance and explained the Chinese refusal: "As for your message, thank you very much for your sympathy but, as you know, our people have always relied on our own efforts and this is the case now." By this time, Tom had become well acquainted with Tang Wensheng and chose this occasion to ask her a question. In time of great trouble, he explained, people everywhere rely on their friends for aid; why do the Chinese stay so rigidly with the doctrine of self-reliance and refuse all help? Tang did not resent the question or respond merely in an official way. Instead she thought for a moment and then replied: "You understand our policies more than most [people]. We have talked many times. You have talked also with our leaders. You know our position. We can *only* thank you for your offer and your consideration of our difficulties" (emphasis added).[26] To Tom, Tang's response appeared to reveal a vague sense of change, perhaps even a behind-the-scenes questioning of Mao's philosophy. If so, forces did exist which were moving China toward becoming a more open nation, forces which in fact emerged only ten weeks later with the arrest of the Gang of Four.

IV

By July 30, the situation at the USLO compound had clearly grown serious. Once the Chinese authorities declared the earthquake alert and began closing off access to the apartment complexes and other residences in the diplomatic community, large numbers of diplomatic personnel, including a great many wives and children of USLO officers, found it impossible to return to their homes. As a result, the USLO became a refugee camp for the families of the Americans stationed in Peking. Jerry Levesque managed to acquire several dozen mattresses (how he happened to find them remained a mystery) which we laid wall-to-wall in each room of the residence and office. These mattresses, plus the beds already in the residence, and later a tent pitched on the grassy plot outside the residence provided enough temporary quarters. The Chinese staff at the USLO continued to perform yeoman work. They seemed to be working around the clock dishing up army-mess style meals three times a day. These conditions were not easy or comfortable for the USLO officers and their families, especially when they realized that they faced a long wait before being able to return to their residences.

Given these inconvenient circumstances, the Earthquake Committee continued to hold its meetings. With a shortage of hard news, the members of the committee met to share information on the topics of most interest to everyone: food, water, the possibility of epidemics, and the likelihood of more aftershocks. Between July 29 and July 31, the alert, rumbling aftershocks, gloomy forecasts, and wicked mid-summer heat continued.

On July 31, Tom Gates received the first visible expression of hard news from the Chinese since the earthquake had occurred. On that day, the Protocol Department of the Ministry of Foreign Affairs confirmed the extent of the earthquake activity which had occurred on the morning of July 28 as well as the imminence of more aftershocks in the vicinity of Peking. In part, the Protocol Department's message read:

[The] aftershocks [have] been going on continuously since the quake which took place at the Tangshan and Fengnan area. There might be a strong earthquake within this month in Peking. The earthquake centre is likely to move near the Peking area. Considering the safety of foreign diplomats and families, the Ministry of Foreign Affairs would like to inform them of the following: (1) The Ministry would provide any convenience possible for those diplomats and their dependents who wish to leave China temporarily; (2) Those wishing to leave Peking may go through formalities as usually done when having trips within the land of China; (3) The Ministry advises all diplomats and their dependents to stay outside of buildings.

The message concluded with the ominous warning to "take into great account your own safety."

The Protocol Department's message and warning confirmed the information which the USLO's other sources had already reported. Another fault running east and west just outside of the center of Peking at the site of the Ming Tombs apparently had given signs that it might rupture sometime in August. Confronted with this information, Tom believed that he had no alternative but to evacuate the USLO families. In addition to the dangers involved in remaining in Peking, the USLO staff could not continue to live in such a confined space for a prolonged period. The "campout" in the USLO compound was resulting in fatigue and unhappiness among mothers and children as well as frustration for the staff officers who found it difficult to perform their duties while their offices were being used as playpens and bedrooms.[27] Furthermore, the Chinese authorities had clearly concluded that the alert would last indefinitely and preferred that nonessential foreign personnel leave the capital until the danger period had passed.

After almost thirty-six hours of consultation with the State Department, Tom decided to evacuate the American dependents on August 1, one day after the British, Canadian, and New Zealand embassies evacuated their personnel. The decision received a mixed reaction from the USLO personnel. Some families were glad to be alive, glad to get away, and glad to receive a break from the tension in Peking. Some wives, especially those without their children, did not want to leave Peking without their husbands. If another major earthquake were to hit Peking while the families were separated, in all likelihood they would never see each other again. And at that point, no one could be absolutely certain about the degree of danger then confronting the residents of the capital. The only choice open to Tom, however, was to determine the essential staff needed to handle an expected reduced workload for the next thirty days and then evacuate the remainder of the Americans. The only women who remained behind were Tom's executive secretary Henrietta Norris, Sara Thomas, and me; we stubbornly refused to leave Peking, and Tom concluded that this was no time to confront three determined ladies.[28]

On August 2, the American evacuation from Peking began, with fifteen women and twenty-five children departing for Tokyo, Hong Kong, Seoul, and Manila. The USLO received excellent cooperation from these other posts in the Far East, all of whom had their own problems with space limitations.[29] These other embassies proved extremely helpful in arranging for accommodations in American government facilities in their area. Jerry Levesque coordinated the USLO's transportation requirements with the Chinese authorities, a process which took considerable arrangement but one which Jerry nevertheless performed to perfection. By August 4, when Stan Brooks's family left Peking, the evacuation was complete.

For the rest of August, the USLO handled its reduced workload with a skeleton staff consisting primarily of Tom Gates, David Dean, Bill Thomas, Jerry Levesque, Jerry Ogden, and Stan Brooks. The Chinese authorities explained that it would be "very inconvenient" for the Americans to have visitors during that time, so we invited no one. To those who stayed behind, the first two weeks of August were memorable mostly for the remarkable display of discipline which the Chinese exhibited while living outdoors on the streets of Peking.

The Chinese method of coping with their calamity was indeed a spectacle. Early on July 30, the Chinese literally created an exodus to the main streets and parks of Peking, leaving the clear impression that they intended to be there for a considerable length of time. By late afternoon on July 30, the streets were jammed with Chinese families, many of whom settled in the middle of the city's major thoroughfares. The Chinese built lean-tos of wood and brick in the city's parks and along its sidewalks. Within days, many of these shelters had spilled out into the streets, transforming them into a gigantic encampment sheltering some three million inhabitants. An inextricable sprawl of tents and shanties, improvised from planks and sheeting, appeared to cover the city. Makeshift beds constructed from chairs set side by side in the "residences" provided the only furniture for sleeping. After the heavy rains on July 29 and 30, the Chinese slung mosquito nets over the tree branches in the parks as a way of providing some protection against the onslaught of insects which passed through after the storms.

Everywhere one looked were people, including hundreds stretched out on the ground along the Great Avenue of Eternal Peace (Changan Avenue). The large square opposite the central railway station was crowded with old men and young women, children and babies, all living there side by side while other young people performed various "housekeeping" tasks. The Chinese had established health clinics at frequent intervals throughout the city, and teams of nurses moved slowly through the tents and shelters on bicycles, stopping to give aid where needed. By 4 p.m. on July 30, the family shelters had sprung up even on the southern edge of Tienanmen Square and the approaches to the National Historical Museum. Although some work in the city had resumed, a considerable proportion of Peking's labor force still appeared to be idle, presumably because of safety considerations at factories and offices located in multi-story buildings. Yet, based on the reports which the USLO had already received about the situation in Tangshan, the residents of Peking probably considered themselves fortunate in having to experience only relatively little destruction and massive personal inconvenience.

For the next week, Tom Gates and his USLO colleagues attempted to acquire as much information as possible about the extent of the earthquake damage in China and also the length of the earthquake alert. Over the weekend of July 31–August 2, the general situation in Peking changed very little. The Chinese who were living outside on the streets of the capital continued to appear calm and in reasonably good spirits; many even seemed to be enjoying the curbside camping life. The erection of the shelters was largely a matter of family and individual enterprise; the Chinese displayed considerable resourcefulness in both the design and composition of the huts, tents, lean-tos, and other accommodations. Tom noticed that many of the shelters lacked mosquito netting, and the absence of protection from the insects probably created much discomfort. On August 3, the Chinese authorities took the initiative in supplying tents to a number of diplomatic missions that did not already have them. As a result, the Chinese sent the USLO a drab, olive-gray tent which could sleep eight to ten adults; we placed it in front of the compound beside the other two which were already standing there. The PRC authorities also began constructing screened-in outdoor latrines in a number of neighborhoods throughout Peking, an action which considerably eased concern about potential sanitation problems in the city.[30]

On August 4, Tom received word from the Foreign Ministry that the period of maximum danger may have passed. In an announcement distributed throughout the diplomatic community, the Foreign Ministry declared that, while "we have not discovered any full premonitory indication for tremors in the coming days, the possibility still cannot be excluded. It is still necessary to maintain vigilance."[31] Further inquiries to the Foreign Ministry nevertheless caused the USLO officers to believe that it would be at least a full week before the Chinese authorities allowed any relaxation in precautions. The August fourth announcement had an immediate impact, however, upon the Chinese in Peking. The capital seemed much more relaxed and considerably less tense after this announcement than at any time since July 28.

On August 8–9, Peking again experienced some mild tremors of noticeably less intensity than those of the previous week. The PRC authorities immediately alerted the diplomatic community to a "possible intensification of seismic activity," and the USLO again went into an alert status.[32] But the earthquake activity never reappeared in Peking, although Tianjin reportedly received some fairly heavy aftershocks.

On the night of August 15, Tom Gates received a telephoned message from the Ministry of Foreign Affairs that the period of the earthquake alert was almost finished.

According to the report from the State Seismological Bureau on earthquake activity in the Tangshan and Fengnan area, the general tendency is that aftershock activities are diminishing. But there will be ups and downs in the process. There may be fairly strong aftershocks. The abnormal phenomena that existed in the Peking area in the last several days have in the main disappeared, and no strong earthquakes will occur in the near future.[33]

Promptly the next morning, thousands of Chinese started dismantling their shelters and moving back into their regular homes and apartments. This early homecoming by no means applied to all the residents of Peking, however; only those Chinese whose dwellings were found safe for re-entry were allowed to return inside. The Chinese residents of Peking whose homes needed repair and reconstruction found themselves living out on the streets for another six weeks. By 4 o'clock on the afternoon of August 16, however, the major thoroughfares in Peking were almost clear of temporary structures. Some parks still retained their tent-city characteristics, and temporary housing continued to be evident around some parts of Peking's athletic fields.

Once the Chinese evacuated many of Peking's streets, the PRC authorities began the enormous task of repairing the damage in the capital. During the last two weeks of August, this work proceeded with a vengeance. The Chinese removed huge quantities of rubble from the city's afflicted areas, especially in the small lanes between Peking's main arteries, and began loading the debris onto trucks. Everywhere, night and day, the Americans in the USLO watched as numerous front-end loaders worked around-the-clock to accelerate the clean-up process. Damage from the earthquake seemed to have resulted mainly in collapsed or severely cracked walls which required extensive repairs rather than full-scale reconstruction. As the Chinese began picking up the pieces, they demonstrated superb discipline and overall coordination. Large numbers of people, including many PLA soldiers, were organized into work teams which labored late into the night. As the repair work proceeded, the USLO officials began to encounter numerous wall posters with messages expressing gratitude to the PLA for its assistance in the relief effort.[34]

Probably few Americans have witnessed such an exercise in discipline which the Chinese in Peking displayed during the earthquake alert in August 1976. From July 29 to August 16, four million Chinese lived on Peking's busy streets, in the hottest part of the year, under complete discipline and total order, with the necessary supplies of food, medical care, and sanitation facilities. Several weeks later, when the alert period formally ended and the Chinese returned to their homes, they left not a trace behind; not a newspaper or even a cigarette could be found in sight. The entire spectacle was a visual display of China's extraordinary discipline.[35]

V

Perhaps the most astonishing and startling discovery which Tom Gates made about China's attempt to cope with the calamity of the Tangshan earthquake was that the earthquake relief effort became the subject of a bitter, behind-the-scenes dispute within the PRC hierarchy. The dispute was over the question of whether the leadership should mobilize relief on a broad, national scale or simply leave the beleaguered residents of Tangshan and Hebei province to handle their own evacuation and reconstruction tasks. In the final analysis, it became inconceivable that the leadership simply turn its back on Tangshan, and in typical Chinese fashion, an immense effort was forthcoming to assist the suffering victims of the earthquake. More important, however, that effort signified a noticeable shift in the political balance of power in China toward Premier Hua Guofeng and the PLA and away from the radicals.[36] Without question, Hua Guofeng and the leadership of the PLA became much better acquainted during the period of the earthquake relief effort in August 1976, and this association proved to be extremely critical in the political events of the next six months in China.

China's radical faction viewed the earthquake relief effort with what can only be described as an inhumane cynicism and skepticism. Even in the in-

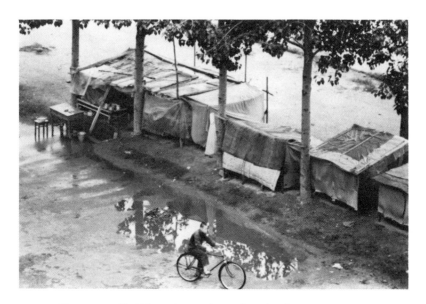

Tents erected in Peking during the earthquake alert, August 1976.

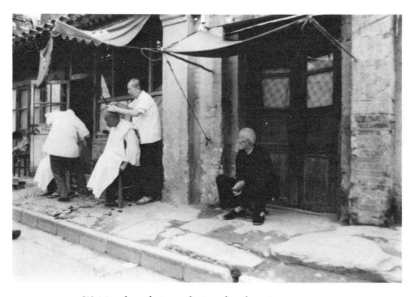

Waiting for a haircut during the alert, August 1976.

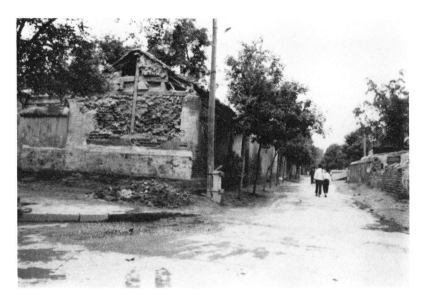

Earthquake damage in Peking, August 1976.

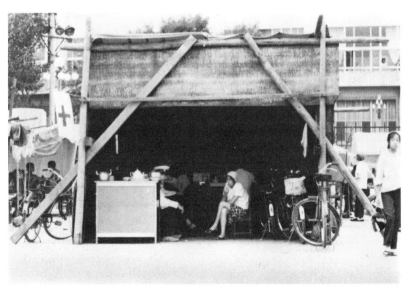

Makeshift medical station during the earthquake alert, Peking, August 1976.

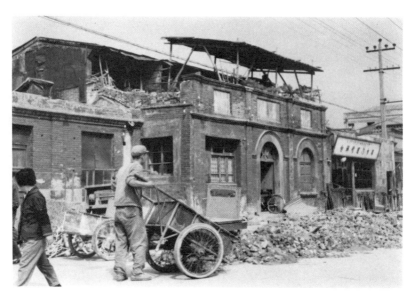

A Chinese laborer involved in clean-up following the earthquake, Peking, August 1976.

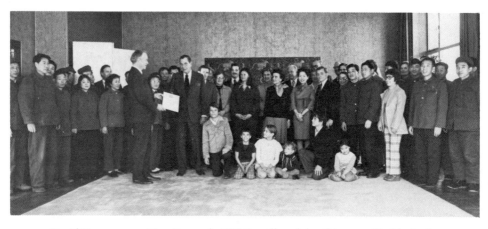

David Dean presents Tom Gates, the USLO staff, and the Chinese staff with citation from the State Department for work during the earthquake alert, September 1976.

terests of national unity, the leftists ruled out any temporary truce with their foes. By late July and early August, the anti-rightist campaign in the PRC had reached a critical point, with the radical-controlled media issuing daily denunciations of Deng Xiaoping. On July 29, for example, an editorial in one of Hebei's provincial newspapers emphatically demanded that the people continue their campaign to criticize Deng. In addition, always concerned about the loyalty of the PLA, the radicals issued a call through the *People's Daily* as early as August 3 for the Army to purge itself of Deng's influence and support the Left.

During the next two weeks, the anti-rightist tone of the media increased, probably much to the displeasure of millions of Chinese. On August 12, the editors of *People's Daily* exhorted the nation "to deepen the criticism of Deng Xiaoping in anti-quake relief work." The editorial praised the "heroic efforts of the people, cadres, and PLA in organizing and carrying out relief for the stricken area" and went on to point out that "opportunists have used natural calamities since 1949 to divert people's attention." [37] In a remark of almost unutterable cynicism, Jiang Qing reportedly described the radical's attitude toward the earthquake relief effort by exclaiming, "The Tangshan earthquake involves only one million people. What's so terrific about several hundred thousand people dying in Tangshan? There are people who are using the anti-quake relief efforts to suppress the anti-Deng campaign. Criticizing Deng involves 800 million people." [38]

Other evidence pointed to the fact that the radicals may even have attempted to use the self-reliance theme to strengthen their own position. Certainly little doubt existed that the Chinese intended to solve the earthquake relief problem by themselves; around the beginning of August, the Nationalist government on Taiwan had sent some relief supplies in balloons across the Taiwan Strait which PRC fighter aircraft intercepted and destroyed. Some diplomatic observers believed that the disaster was tailor-made as an object lesson for driving home the importance of Mao's doctrines, particularly that of self-reliance. For example, Mao had often spoken about the ability to triumph over nature. [39] In that regard, the doctrine of self-reliance was suitable for a radical-style campaign, a "means of getting people off their bottoms," according to one report. [40]

After the earthquake struck Tangshan, the PRC leadership exited from public view for almost nine days. During that time, probably on July 30, Premier Hua Guofeng led a leadership delegation to the stricken area. Prior to that visit, and after a few stormy Politburo meetings on the subject of earthquake relief (some of which the radicals reportedly refused to attend), Hua had authorized the airlift of several thousand PLA troops into Tangshan as a relief task force. On August 1, the *People's Daily* published a story which described the Party Center's response to the crisis.

A grave natural calamity has tempered and tested our people. The PLA rapidly organized [and] rushed to the rescue of the people and their property. Some workers and lower-level cadres have sacrificed their own lives to save their class brothers. Some injured cadres at all levels have plunged into the anti-quake battle right after being rescued. A large number of PLA commanders and fighters have rushed to the heavily afflicted area, braved perils without fear, and rescued the people. Though heavily injured themselves, some medical personnel have persisted in rescuing the injured people. Large quantities of medicine, food, clothing, building materials, and other materials and equipment are flowing in an endless stream to the quake-stricken area from all parts of the motherland.

In total, Hua Guofeng rushed eleven PLA divisions into Tangshan, and, because the damage prevented close-in landings, the troops were forced to run much of the final distance to the devastated city. Within eight hours of their arrival on July 29, the PLA rescued approximately 630,000 people who were trapped in the city, and another 70,000 were rescued by civilians. The wounded people were then carried by PLA aircraft to safety. On August 7, relief shipments of medical supplies, food, and water began arriving in Tangshan in great amounts, and several thousand medical personnel, including 800 from as far away as Shanghai, began working in the stricken city.

The "comfort" delegation which Hua Guofeng led to Tangshan was a unique mixture of neo-Maoist politicians and PLA veterans. Along with Hua, the delegation included Chen Yonggui, a Politburo member; Ulanfu, a vice chairman of the National People's Congress; Ruo Yufeng, director of the Organizational Department of the Party's Central Committee; Fan Ziyu, the PRC's minister of commerce; Zhang Zongxun, who directed the PLA's logistics department; and Huang Yukun, the PLA's deputy chief of staff. When Hua and the delegation arrived in Tangshan, they must have recoiled in horror at the sight of such suffering and destruction. The quake had damaged irrigation ditches and drainage projects, leaving large areas of arable land swamped with sand or "foul liquids," according to Li Xiannian, who later briefed Tom on the extent of the destruction.[41] The major problem, however, was the hundreds of thousands of bodies which the PLA had "stacked like cordwood" on ice, in the words of one observer.[42] On the southern edge of Tangshan stretched mile upon mile of refugee camps. Everywhere, tents and makeshift shelters provided the only means of housing. Amazingly, a sizable number of people continued to live amidst the rubble. Their homes destroyed, these victims apparently had picked up the stones and bricks of their dwellings and built them back up again. More than thirteen provinces throughout China sent medical teams and relief groups to assist the beleaguered city.

Early reports from Tangshan revealed the continuing stranglehold which the radicals exercised over the provincial media. One dispatch from the provincial newspaper commented:

People in the stricken area feel incomparable warmth and happiness and have been greatly encouraged. People who are armed with Marxism-Leninism-Mao Zedong thought can never be intimidated or discouraged by any difficulty. In 1963, our province encountered a particularly great flood. In 1966, a strong earthquake took place in Xingtai prefecture in our province. Today the people, who have been tempered in the Great Proletarian Cultural Revolution, the movement to criticize Lin Biao and Confucius, and the struggle to criticize Deng Xiaoping and rebuff the right deviationist wind to reverse the verdicts, have a heart like fire, their fighting morale is as firm as steel.[43]

The effort to rescue the survivors of the earthquake in Tangshan had its own dynamics. The shipments of relief cargoes to the stricken city took priority over all other goods moved along north China's railroad system, at least that which remained operable. As tons of emergency medical supplies and food made their way to Tangshan, the Chinese economy underwent a severe disruption. The costs involved in diverting national resources to Tangshan must have been enormous. For the Chinese, meeting the emergency in Tangshan was not a matter of resupplying the city with surpluses from other parts of the country; the decision to resupply meant depriving other regions of China of their own limited resources. This decision made it absolutely certain that the Chinese would tighten their belts even further during the Year of the Dragon.

VI

It is almost impossible to summarize the impact which the Tangshan earthquake exerted on China in 1976. First, the city of Tangshan was evacuated and its reconstruction put off considerably into the future. The expense must have been enormous; one observer estimated that the Chinese were confronted with a $10 billion reconstruction project.[44] Moreover, the earthquake occurred during a time when the People's Republic was experiencing economic difficulties; the earthquake compounded the problems faced in virtually every sector of the economy.

Second, the earthquake relief effort may have marked the high point of Hua Guofeng's leadership of the PRC. Before the earthquake, the PRC media referred to Hua as Hua Guofeng Zongli or Premier Hua Guofeng. In the post-quake period, the New China News Agency referred to him as Hua Zongli; ordinarily only Mao was described in such a respectful manner.[45] Indeed, once the earthquake struck Tangshan, Hua Guofeng did move quickly to consolidate his power. His visit to the quake-stricken area was viewed as a positive gesture of leadership; the state-controlled television repeatedly showed film clips of his visit as a way of informing the Chinese that Hua was no longer simply the first among equals but the de facto leader of

China. The films portrayed Hua as a determined leader, fully equal to the challenge of leadership, and, like Zhou Enlai and Mao Zedong, concerned about the welfare of the people.

Hua Guofeng had demonstrated during the period of the earthquake that he was capable of building a coalition with the PLA. Reportedly a key participant in the earthquake relief meetings was Ye Jianying; certainly no doubt existed that the PLA acted decisively in dealing with the national emergency. The results of a closer collaboration between Hua and the PLA were immediately visible in Peking. By September 1, the PRC media had taken a decidedly moderate tone, stressing unity and production and the heroic efforts of the PLA, and pushing the anti-rightist campaign into the background.[46] This speedy assertion of authority came at a time when the Chinese desperately needed such action, beset as they were by popular protest, political turmoil, economic setbacks, natural disasters, and the impending death of Chairman Mao Zedong.

Notes

1. United States Department of State, Official File, Peking to Washington, 29 July 1976. Hereafter cited as OF, date.

2. Ibid.

3. *New York Times*, 31 July 1976, pp. 1, 2.

4. Ibid.

5. OF, Peking to Washington, 28 July 1976.

6. OF, Peking to Washington, 28 July 1976; *Washington Post*, 29 July 1976, p. 4.

7. Ibid.

8. OF, Peking to Washington, 28 July 1976; interview, David Dean, 14 December 1982; Thomas S. Gates Oral History, 31 March 1982 (hereafter cited as Gates OH, date).

9. OF, Peking to Washington, 12 August 1976; Gates OH, 31 March 1982; Garside, *Coming Alive*, p. 138; Terrill, *Future of China*, p. 8; Terrill, *Mao*, p. 420.

10. Interview, Richard Mueller, 23 February 1983. It is important to understand this point: the entire northern sector of China is still susceptible to an immense earthquake, one which conceivably could devastate Peking. See also OF, USLO-Peking, 1976–1977; Garside, *Coming Alive*, p. 138; Hsu, *China Without Mao*, pp. 3, 9.

11. Gates OH, 31 March 1982; interview, Richard Mueller, 23 February 1982; Terrill, *Mao*, p. 420.

12. OF, Peking to Washington, 11 August 1976; OF, Peking to Washington, 12 October 1976; interview, David Dean, 14 December 1982.

13. OF, Peking to Washington, 29 July 1976; OF, Peking to Washington, 5 August 1976; OF, USLO-Peking, 1976–77.

14. OF, Peking to Washington, 11 August 1976; Gates OH, 31 March 1982; interview, David Dean, 14 December 1982; *New York Times*, 31 July 1976.

15. OF, Peking to Washington, 11 August 1976; OF, Peking to Washington, 10 September 1976.

16. *New York Times*, 5 January 1977, p. 4; see also Andrew H. Malcolm, "Chinese Disclose that 1976 Quake Was Deadliest in Four Centuries," *New York Times*, 2 June 1977.

17. OF, USLO-Peking, 1976–77.

18. For accounts of the impact of the Tangshan earthquake upon China's economic performance in 1976, see "The Chinese Economy in 1976," *China Quarterly* 70 (June 1977): 355–58.

19. OF, Peking to Washington, 11 August 1976.

20. OF, Peking to Washington, 21 October 1976; OF, USLO-Peking, 1976–77.

21. OF, Peking to Washington, 29 July 1976; OF, Peking to Washington, 29 July 1976; Gates OH, 31 March 1982; interview, David Dean, 14 December 1982.

22. OF, Secretary of State Kissinger to Ambassador Gates, 29 July 1976; Gates OH, 31 March 1982.

23. OF, Peking to Washington, 31 July 1976.

24. Interview, Gerald R. Ford.

25. Interview, Richard Mueller, 23 February 1983; Terrill, *Mao*, p. 420.

26. Gates OH, 31 March 1982.

27. Ibid.; see also OF, Washington to Peking, "Disaster and Disaster Relief," 1 August 1976.

28. Ibid.

29. OF, Peking to Washington, 30 July 1976; OF, Peking to Washington, "Disaster and Disaster Relief," 1 August 1976; see also *Philadelphia Evening Bulletin*, 2 August 1976, for a discussion of the evacuation of embassy families from Peking. Tom Gates's statement regarding the evacuation of American dependents read as follows: "Given the circumstances, I have decided to evacuate all wives and dependents unless they specifically choose to remain. I also intend to reduce staff to essential members. Names of those who are to leave will be forthcoming." See also Gates OH, 31 March 1982.

30. OF, Peking to Washington, 2 August 1976; OF, Peking to Washington, 3 August 1976.

31. OF, Peking to Washington, 4 August 1976.

32. OF, Peking to Washington, 9 August 1976; OF, Peking to Washington, 10 August 1976.

33. OF, Peking to Washington, 16 August 1976.

34. OF, Peking to Washington, 16 August 1976; OF, Peking to Washington, 9 September 1976.

35. Gates, "On China," pp. 29–30.

36. Interview, Richard Mueller, 23 February 1983.

37. OF, Peking to Washington, 29 July 1976; OF, Peking to Washington, 12 August 1976.

38. OF, Peking to Washington, 13 December 1976; OF, Peking to Washington, 1 December 1976.

39. Fox Butterfield, "Notes on China," *New York Times*, 21 August 1976.

40. *Washington Post*, 4 August 1976; see also Frank Ching, "China Looks for a Silver Lining," *Wall Street Journal*, 2 September 1976.

41. OF, Peking to Washington, 12 December 1976; OF, USLO-Peking, 1976–77; OF, 19 October 1976; Ching, "China Looks for a Silver Lining."

42. OF, 29 July 1976; OF, Peking to Washington, 7 August 1976.

43. OF, 29 July 1976.

44. Ibid.

45. *New York Times*, 22 August 1976, p. 3.

46. OF, USLO-Peking, 1976–77; OF, Peking to Washington, 13 August 1976; OF, Peking to Washington, 1 September 1976; OF, Peking to Washington, 3 September 1976.

CHAPTER **4**

"Mao's Dead!"

Late in August 1976, Thomas Gates and I left China for a three-week visit to the United States. Tom had scheduled three days of consultations in Washington with President Ford and officials at the China desk in the State Department for August 25–27. Considering the experiences of the past three months—the meeting with Premier Hua Guofeng, the impact of the Tangshan earthquake upon China, and the unending power struggle within the hierarchy of the People's Republic—Tom found no shortage of information to bring before his diplomatic colleagues. After these consultations, we left Washington for our summer home in Northeast Harbor, Maine, where we remained through the first week of September. Spending summers in Maine had been a tradition in the Gates family for at least forty years; Tom often declared that going to Maine had become almost a religion with us.

At 7 A.M. on the morning of September 9, the telephone rang and Tom took a call from Bridie Homsher, our housekeeper in Devon. "Mao's dead!" she exclaimed. That was Tom's first notice of the death of Mao Zedong. Shortly thereafter, Tom received another call from the State Department, confirming the news of Mao's death. Tom immediately dispatched a message of sympathy to Foreign Minister Qiao Guanhua and made plans for an immediate return to the People's Republic.[1] On September 11, Tom left New York for the return flight to China, while I remained behind in Northeast Harbor for another two weeks before returning to the People's Republic.

In 1976, the events in China developed in such a fashion that each month appeared to possess its own unique development. In May and June, Tom's attention centered on the nature of the factional political power struggle in the PRC. In early July, the death of Zhu De served as a reminder of the deaths that seemed to be stalking the heroes of the Chinese Revolution. In late July and early August, the Tangshan earthquake occupied the nation's attention. And now in September, it became clear that Mao's death had taken center stage, at least until another dramatic event emerged to take its place.

Mao Zedong's death in early September was an event of enormous significance for the People's Republic of China. First, his death signalled the beginning of the end of the Maoist era. Second, his death intensified the factional struggle then being waged by the radicals and their enemies. More important, Mao's death deprived Jiang Qing and her supporters of the measure of protection from their enemies which they enjoyed while the chairman was alive. The door was at last opened for the resolution (by whatever means) of the internal political turmoil which had afflicted the People's Republic for the past decade. Third, in China itself, Mao's death was met with a strange mixture of grief and apprehension, grief for the passing of a man of such stature that he had become a symbol of Chinese nationhood (even though he was feared and even hated by millions of Chinese) and apprehension over the future course of Chinese political life. Would China's radical faction take control of the PRC, or somehow, would the more pragmatic moderates manage to prevail in the inevitable jockeying for power which lay ahead? Earlier in the year, the Tienanmen riots indicated that the Chinese masses would not tolerate a prolonged period of radical rule, and yet Jiang Qing and her cohorts *had* succeeded in deposing several moderate leaders in the past year and the pragmatists appeared further weakened by the deaths of Zhou Enlai and Zhu De. The future outlook was certainly questionable, as the Chinese undoubtedly understood. Tom and the other USLO officers determined that Mao's death indeed brought the curtain down on the Cultural Revolution, but they reached that conclusion only after seeing how the Chinese people responded to the news of the chairman's death in September 1976 and how the Chinese people commemorated his passing, and only after seeing how Mao's death affected the next stage in the PRC's political life.

Rumors of Mao's impending death were evident throughout the Far East when Tom Gates arrived in China in early May 1976. Mao had last appeared in public in 1971 and, over the course of the next five years, the Chinese saw him only in photographs or on television in his meetings with foreign leaders. Even in those appearances, Mao often looked as "fragile as a piece of porcelain," according to one reporter.[2] Suffering from Parkinson's disease (or perhaps Alzheimer's disease) and afflicted by several strokes, Mao obviously found life physically difficult as he entered his eighty-second year in 1976.

In May and June, Tom heard numerous stories, all of which proved to be inaccurate, claiming that Mao's life was quickly drawing to a close. On May 18–19, for example, a rumor circulated within the diplomatic community that Mao had suffered a stroke in the early evening on May 18 and died about twenty-four hours later. The American diplomats immediately grew watchful and tried to detect any sign of unusual activity in the strategic locations around Peking. The PRC leadership had suppressed the news of Zhou Enlai's death for eighteen hours; was the same thing happening in Mao's case? Although the report of Mao's death proved untrue at that time, it is possible that Mao suffered another stroke around the middle of May. Another rumor which also made the rounds of the diplomatic community at this time maintained that the PRC authorities had alerted lower- and middle-level officials within the Party that Mao would not live much longer and that they should be prepared to notify the people of his death. According to this report, Mao had recently taken a turn for the worse and was existing with the help of life-support machinery. On June 15 the Chinese leadership announced that Mao would not be receiving any more foreign visitors.[3]

The leadership's decision to close off access to Mao Zedong created some difficulties for Tom and the American China-watching contingent in Peking. Mao had scheduled an appointment in late May with Malcolm Fraser, the prime minister of Australia, and Fraser intended to take Stephen Fitzgerald, Australia's ambassador to China, with him to the meeting. Fitzgerald was one of the most highly regarded China experts within the diplomatic community. He spoke excellent Chinese and would have been in a position to assess correctly the status of Mao's health. The PRC hierarchy apparently decided, however, that Mao's physical decline was too embarrassing, both to him and to China, to permit any additional potentially risky encounters with foreign leaders. Predictably, the Chinese canceled the Fraser-Fitzgerald appointment with Mao and the diplomatic community thereby lost a critical opportunity to gauge the full extent of the chairman's ailments.[4]

Between June 6 and June 21, the diplomatic community received word that Walther Birkmeyer, a Viennese physician world-renowned as a specialist on Parkinson's disease, was in China ostensibly on a tourist visa. News of Birkmeyer's visit, despite being conducted in great secrecy, nevertheless leaked out and touched off a flurry of speculation within the foreign press and the diplomatic community that he had come to treat the chairman. Once Birkmeyer's presence became known, both he and the officials at the Austrian Embassy denied that his visit involved any additional prescription of treatments for Mao, even though Birkmeyer had ministered to him previously. In all likelihood, Birkmeyer did not see Mao personally but probably met with a team of Chinese physicians, explaining his special treatments and also recommending a regimen for the chairman. Birkmeyer was also reportedly pessimistic about any prospect for improvements in Mao's health, believing that the chairman had only a few months left, at the most.[5]

By July, Mao's health had begun to deteriorate even more rapidly; one Chinese spokesman even allowed himself to voice the sentiment that the chairman was so enfeebled that the Chinese people might never see him again. Later in the month, according to another story, Mao summoned several influential Politburo members to his bedside. "Few live beyond 70," Mao reminded his visitors, "and as I am more than 80, I should have died already." Mao was dying, and he knew it. "Are there not some among you who hoped I would go to see Marx sooner?" he asked his listeners. The burden of responding to that particular question fell to Premier Hua Guofeng who reportedly answered, "None." "Really, no one? I don't believe it," Mao shot back.[6] In early September, the chairman of the Communist Party of the People's Republic of China lapsed into the coma from which he never emerged.

In the last weeks and months of Mao's life, the power struggle within the ranks of the PRC hierarchy intensified. Jiang Qing and her radical followers understood completely what Mao's death meant to their political fortunes and earnestly set about to bolster their supporters throughout China. Despite their efforts, the supporters of the moderates at the provincial levels proved especially adept at preventing any purges of their followers. In addition, reports from the PRC's provincial media outlets demonstrated some independence from radical control, encouraging the people to show "unity" and "promote production," two appeals of the PLA and their pragmatic allies.[7] The details of these and other intrigues which occurred within the PRC leadership during August and early September are still somewhat unclear but two facts have emerged. First, Mao had assembled a group of radicals who remained close to him during the last months of his life in order to retain a record of his final thoughts and instructions for the future of post-Mao China. Apparently this "Mao office" consisted of Jiang Qing, Mao Yuanxin (Mao's nephew and close confidant who became the chairman's de facto chief of staff), and possibly Wang Hairong and Tang Wensheng, both of whom interpreted for Mao in his meetings with foreign leaders. This group was far from unified internally; Jiang and Mao Yuanxin were rumored to be close, but Jiang distrusted and even despised Wang Hairong. Second, the radicals attempted to increase the tension between themselves and their neo-Maoist critics and moderate foes in the last weeks of Mao's life.[8] Such actions had the effect of further isolating the radicals, a development which became evident once the USLO discovered that attempts by the radicals' provincial supporters to purge rehabilitated moderate cadres was meeting stiff resistance throughout the country. When Mao finally died on September 9, the stage was set for a critical round of reshuffling within the PRC hierarchy, an excruciatingly delicate and sensitive period as each faction sought to increase its support by either entering into or refraining from entering into coalitions with other groups.

II

The death of Mao Zedong presented the bitterly divided PRC hierarchy with a fresh set of challenges as well as the need to make a number of major decisions. One immediate matter was the official announcement of the chairman's death; the wording of that statement would be an indication of the status of the current political balance of power in China. Another problem was how Mao's death would be observed and commemorated, a sensitive subject since it involved the public's first glimpse of the PRC's post-Mao, political hierarchy. A third problem was what to do with Mao's remains: Was the body to be preserved, in the tradition of Lenin, as an everlasting reminder to the Chinese of Mao's role in founding and leading the People's Republic, or was the body to be cremated in the tradition of Zhou Enlai and Zhu De? Since Mao apparently had never left clear instructions about the disposition of his remains, this subject promised to be an especially difficult one. Considering the stakes involved in the resolution of these issues, one tended to sympathize with the unfortunate position of Hua Guofeng. While Hua undoubtedly possessed the opportunity to emerge as the "man in charge," he also faced the possibility that if political strife in China went out of control while the nation was mourning its founder, his fall from power would certainly be swift and sure. As Andres Onate observed, "In China, there is no such thing as death for its own sake. As everything else, death too is political." [9]

The Chinese leadership announced the chairman's passing almost sixteen hours after he died at ten minutes past midnight on September 9. To a Westerner, this delay in announcing Mao's death was inexplicable; by Chinese standards, the announcement came with great haste. Within minutes of the announcement, however, the Chinese in Peking immediately began the preparations for commemorating Mao's death. The spontaneous response suggested to some of the USLO officers that the Chinese knew of Mao's death well before the official announcement. The Chinese instantly turned to wearing black armbands, and the government lowered the state's flags to half-staff. Mao commemorative badges became an item of apparel, a sign of respect for the departed leader. [10] By 7 that evening, a quiet, orderly crowd had gathered in Tienanmen Square, with many people weeping and laying funeral wreaths at the Martyr's Monument. Somber, serious music played from the city's loudspeakers and presumably throughout China. Mao's passing also increased the visibility of the PLA, much more so than had the deaths of Zhou Enlai and Zhu De. The PLA's heightened presence projected a sense of military responsiveness to the interim leadership, a fact which the Chinese in Peking understood completely.

The Americans who witnessed the scene in Peking upon the occasion of Mao's death retain poignant memories of the time. According to both David

Dean and Richard Mueller, the atmosphere in Peking was oppressive. Most Chinese did not know a China without Mao at the helm and naturally wondered about the future of their country, and the direction of their lives, under a new regime. Coupled with this sense of loss was a high degree of anxiety and apprehension. The Chinese realized that the resolution of the nation's political power struggle was certainly at hand, although the outcome of that struggle remained in doubt.[11]

Despite the expressions of grief, however, one could not escape the conclusion that the Chinese had been more grieved by the death of Zhou Enlai the previous January. "Few Chinese," Ross Terrill has commented, "felt strong enough affection for Mao to move them to tears," not after a decade of Cultural Revolutionary strife and political turmoil, as well as an even longer period of economic stagnation.[12]

On September 9, the day of Mao's death, the PRC leadership issued two important statements. First, mourning services for Mao would take place at the Great Hall of the People between September 11 and September 17, to be followed by a solemn memorial rally on September 18. Flags were to remain at half-staff through September 18, and no foreign delegations were to be permitted to attend the memorial rally, although representatives from the diplomatic community were permitted to pay their respects at the Great Hall of the People according to a prescribed schedule.[13] The second announcement contained the statement given to notify the Chinese people of Mao's death, a statement notable for the obvious compromises in its content made by the PRC's rival factions. According to one account, the statement was not released until after the Politburo had met to discuss the nature of the announcement. Jiang Qing and her radical supporters were represented at the meeting but apparently contributed little to the discussions. The statement itself, a joint announcement by the Party Central Committee, the Standing Committee of the National People's Congress, the State Council, and the Military Commission of the Central Committee, stressed several points. It noted Mao's role as the founder of the Chinese Communist Party, the People's Liberation Army, and the People's Republic of China. Mao, the statement read, would always be honored as the Great Helmsman and also as the Great Teacher of the Chinese Masses. Undoubtedly to please the radicals, the statement exalted Mao as "the greatest Marxist of the contemporary era" and praised his efforts in criticizing Liu Shaoqui, Lin Biao, and Deng Xiaoping (certainly a "must" for that particular time in Chinese history although the Americans nevertheless wondered why the supreme ruler of China needed to be praised for his part in undermining his critics). For China's moderates, the announcement spoke of "turning grief into determination," almost the identical statement used by Deng Xiaoping in his eulogy for Zhou Enlai.[14]

The leadership of the various provinces also issued statements on the occasion of Mao's passing. Whereas the announcement from Peking stressed unity and the need for all Chinese to "rally closely around the Party Center," the statement issued by Shanghai's provincial leadership emphasized Mao's personal role in leading the "Party, the Army, and the people in weathering the tempest of class struggle . . . and vanquishing the interference and sabotage by the opportunist and revisionist lines." In the absence of Chairman Mao, the Shanghai Municipal Revolutionary Committee vowed to "continue the criticism of Deng Xiaoping and consolidate the victories of the Great Proletarian Cultural Revolution." By contrast, the statement issued by the municipal leadership in Tianjin largely ignored ideological rhetoric and concentrated on Mao's "benevolent role" in the earthquake relief effort and the city's commitment to "self-reliantly restore industrial production to pre-earthquake levels." [15]

III

Between September 11 and September 17, the Chinese instituted a period of national mourning over the death of Mao Zedong. The events of these seven days proved to be another fascinating period for the American China-watching contingent in Peking. They were especially interested in the composition of the funeral committee (which would reveal who was currently in and who was currently out of favor), any photographs of the Party leadership as they attended the various memorial functions (which would reveal whether the Party hierarchy was affording any particular treatment to Jiang Qing or simply treating her as another member of the Politburo), and, finally, whether the messages of condolence which the Central Committee received from the provincial party committees contained any gestures of sympathy for Jiang Qing. [16]

The fact that Mao's body went on public view almost immediately after his death answered one particular question: the Politburo had decided to preserve Mao's remains rather than to cremate them. Later accounts revealed a serious split within the Politburo over this decision. Mao had once indicated a preference for cremation as an example of his adherence to a land-usage, land-conservation program, and it was perhaps in response to this policy that Kang Sheng, the Politburo member who died in 1976, Zhou Enlai, and Zhu De had been cremated. As stated previously, however, Mao's thoughts on the subject of the disposition of his remains were unclear, and some members of the leadership believed that he had once indicated a desire for a simple burial in his home province of Hunan instead of cremation. For other reasons which still remain unclear, Jiang Qing and the radicals reportedly preferred that Mao be cremated. Hua Guofeng, however, realizing that he owed his present eminence to Mao, insisted that the chairman's remains be preserved so that China's masses could pay their last respects to him. According to one account, Hua decided the issue by declaring that "the remains are to be preserved. Mao's remains, like his glory, will be everlasting." Hua's decision was potentially risky for him in a political sense; he left himself open to charges by the radicals that he had disregarded Mao's instructions, if Jiang Qing could ever prove that Mao preferred a cremation. Perhaps for that reason, Hua arranged that his decision not be announced publicly at that time. Upon the premier's instructions, however, the PRC hierarchy subsequently arranged for embalmers from North Vietnam, reportedly those who had prepared Ho Chi Minh's remains, to come to Peking and embalm Mao's body for mummification, and the body was soon taken to the Great Hall of the People where the late chairman lay in state.[17]

On September 11, with Mao Zedong's body on public view in the Great Hall of the People, hundreds of thousands of Chinese began to line up to enter the Hall and pay their final respects. In organizing the mourning activities, the Chinese authorities had closed off all the approaches to the Great Hall of the People for pedestrian and bicycle traffic, but motor vehicles were still permitted to proceed along Changan Avenue. Throughout the mourning period, the PLA was much in evidence, and increased its visibility as the week progressed. In Tienanmen Square, just east of the Great Hall, various civilian and military units, arriving in buses and following a procession, formed ranks of mourners. Many Chinese were visibly moved by the experience; one female mourner wailed repeatedly, "It's finished, it's finished, it's all over now."[18] Others, from the very young to the very old, with their eyes obviously puffy and red, sobbed noticeably. Many simply gazed at the huge portrait of Chairman Mao atop Tienanmen Square without showing any sorrow.

Between September 10 and September 12, the *People's Daily* began publishing condolence messages to the Central Committee from China's twenty-nine provinces and eleven military regions. These messages must have proven disconcerting to Jiang Qing; only six provinces (Liaoning, Gansu, Guanxi, Henan, Guangdong, and Qinghai) and five military regions (Shenyang, Tsinan, Nanjing, Chengtu, and Kunming) specifically offered their condolences to her.[19] Nor did Jiang Qing succeed in presenting herself as the grieving widow during the formal mourning period for her late, estranged husband. When the leadership released televised footage of the Politburo membership filing into the Great Hall of the People to pay their last respects to Mao, Jiang was shown only in her position as the fifth-ranking Politburo member. More important, unlike Deng Yingchao who received public expressions of sympathy from the leadership at the time of Zhou Enlai's death, Jiang was not pictured accepting any condolences from the other Chinese leaders.[20] The PRC media appeared to take the view that Jiang was independent of Mao, not his honored and esteemed widow.

Jiang Qing herself appeared noticeably subdued and restrained through-

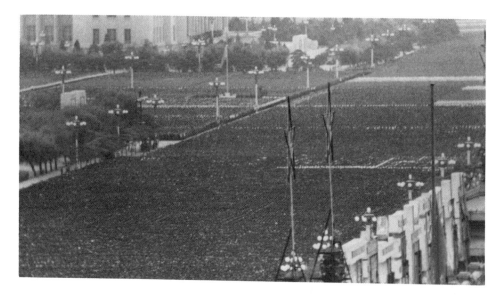

Scene in Peking during the memorial service for Mao Zedong, September 18, 1976.

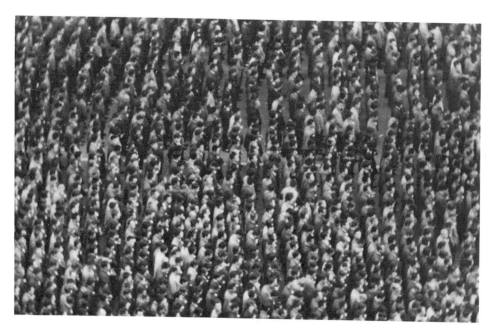

Close-up of Chinese observing the memorial service for Mao, September 18, 1976.

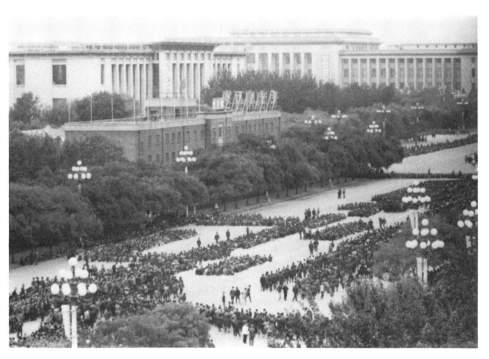

Chinese in process of assembling for the memorial service for Mao Zedong, September 18, 1976.

out the week of September 11–17. For example, she placed a wreath at Mao's bier which only bore the simple inscription, "Deeply mourn the esteemed great teacher, Chairman Mao Zedong, from your student and comrade-in-arms, Jiang Qing."[21] That simple inscription, however, which failed to mention that Jiang was Mao's widow, provoked a bitter, behind-the-scenes confrontation between Jiang and Wang Hairong in the days leading up to the memorial rally on September 18. During a private meeting of the leadership, Wang apparently flew into a rage at Jiang Qing after reading the inscription. As Harrison Salisbury has reported, "Jiang . . . and Wang . . . flew at each other [after Wang read the inscription]. Before anyone could intervene, they were scratching and clawing [at each other]. Wang grabbed Jiang by her black, bobbed hair and nearly fell backward as the hair came off in her hands—a wig! Somehow the combatants were pulled apart and their clothing readjusted and the Party made its way into public."[22]

IV

An especially critical facet of the American diplomats' China-watching exercise was observing the order in which the Chinese scheduled the various national delegations who wished to pay respects to the late Mao Zedong. The Chinese waited until the morning of September 13 before releasing an official schedule, which divided the delegations into four groups: close friends of the Chinese such as North Korea, Romania, Pakistan, and "special" foreign visitors; then Third World countries; then "Second World" countries such as the United States, Japan, and the European industrial democracies; and finally the countries of the Soviet Bloc, who were scheduled to pay their respects last. In the absence of official diplomatic relations between America and China, Tom and his colleagues interpreted the Chinese positioning of the United States with its allies as a positive sign for continued improvement in Chinese-American relations.

Tom Gates led a twelve-member USLO delegation to the Great Hall of the People at 5 P.M. on the afternoon of September 13 to offer the official condolences of the United States government to the People's Republic. The atmosphere in the Great Hall that afternoon was appropriately solemn, with long lines of mourners stretching across Tienanmen Square patiently waiting for their turn to file by Mao's body. In the receiving line stood the members of the PRC hierarchy: Premier Hua Guofeng, Wang Hongwen, Zhang Chunqiao, Chen Xilian, Wang Dongxing, plus Qiao Guanhua, Wang Hairong, and Yu Chan from the Foreign Ministry.

Of particular interest to Tom Gates during the official mourning period was the treatment which the Chinese afforded former Secretary of Defense James Schlesinger, who was visiting the PRC during the first two weeks of

September, and the way they responded to the expression of condolence sent by the Soviet Union. Schlesinger was in China at the time by invitation of Mao himself, who nine months earlier had expressed a desire for the former defense secretary to visit China. The purpose of Schlesinger's visit ostensibly was to review the PRC's military capability and defense policy. It was difficult, however, for USLO officials not to interpret Schlesinger's visit as a rebuff to the Ford administration. Schlesinger's reputation as a critic of detente, as well as his celebrated dismissal by Gerald Ford the previous year, served him well with the Chinese, who were continuously encouraging the Americans to take a stronger stand publicly against the Soviets. During his visit to China, Schlesinger attended meetings with both Qiao Guanhua and Ye Jianying in early September. Afterward, the Chinese arranged for him to tour several important military installations in the provinces. More important from the USLO's standpoint, however, the Chinese invited Schlesinger and his delegation to pay their respects to Mao with the first scheduled group of mourners, about ninety minutes before the USLO delegation was permitted to enter the Great Hall of the People. The Chinese also allowed Schlesinger to lay a wreath at Mao's bier, the only foreigner permitted such a gesture.[23]

More surprising, however, than China's treatment of Schlesinger was the rebuke it delivered to the Soviet Union and the other East European Communist parties (with the exception of Romania and Albania). On September 14, the Soviet Union, Poland, East Germany, Hungary, and Czechoslovakia all sent condolence messages, which the Chinese authorities immediately rejected. According to the Foreign Ministry, the "Chinese have no party-to-party relations" with these nations, and for that reason, the PRC regarded the messages as unacceptable and returned them to their senders. In truth, the Chinese judged these messages as highly provocative since neither the Soviets nor their Eastern Bloc satellites had offered any expressions of sympathy upon the deaths of Zhou Enlai and Zhu De. The meaning behind the messages was unmistakable, however; both the Soviets and their allies were probing for any easing in the anti-Soviet stance or any conciliatory sentiment on the part of the post-Mao leadership. When the Chinese rejected these messages, they also made it more understandable why they scheduled the Soviets and their Warsaw Pact allies for the last place in the receiving line for paying respects to the late chairman.

Nor were the Chinese satisfied with merely arranging for the Soviets to follow the other national delegations in paying their respects. In the subsequent televised reports, the Chinese devoted ninety seconds to the scene of the USLO delegation entering the Great Hall and paying its respects but showed the Soviet delegation for only forty-five seconds. The Americans in China knew that the PRC leadership gave great attention to the images which it presented to its people by television, and therefore that particular impression helped to reinforce the American view that the Chinese had certainly not altered their policies toward the Soviet Union and were, at the same time, still committed to improving relations with the United States.[24]

Since his arrival in China, Tom Gates had become acquainted with Vasily Tolstikov, the Soviet ambassador to China. To the Americans' great interest, Tom subsequently learned that Tolstikov and the officials at the Soviet Embassy deplored the fact that their brethren in Moscow chose to send a message of condolence to the PRC's Central Committee, at least so soon after Mao's death. Among Soviet officials, especially those who hoped for a thaw in Sino-Soviet relations following Mao's death, the opinion seemed to be that the Russians had overplayed their hand, forcing the Chinese to reject the messages categorically or else admit that a change had taken place in the PRC's foreign policy. Moreover, the Soviets in Peking reasoned that the Chinese leadership, strongly desirous of projecting an image of continuity and stability to its people, was required to reject such early messages. Needless to say, the Soviets in Peking felt wronged by their counterparts in Moscow, believing that an anti-China faction within the Soviet Politburo had ruined any immediate attempts at a possible rapprochement between the two nations.

V

By September 16, the Chinese in Peking were heavily involved in preparing for the huge Mao memorial rally scheduled for September 18, the largest gathering of Chinese in Peking since the 1960s. As the day of the rally drew near, Peking's urban militia began cordoning off the area around Tienanmen Square to pedestrians and bicyclists. Above the entrance to the Forbidden City stood a huge black-and-white placard which carried the inscription, "Mournfully commemorate our great leader and teacher Chairman Mao." Across the square, another large placard over one hundred meters long dominated the scene, this one inscribed "Carry out the proletarian cause left by Chairman Mao and carry through the proletarian tasks to the end." In the area several blocks east and west of Tienanmen Square, workers marked streets with paint to designate areas for the mourners to stand, installed outdoor fountains, constructed numerous outdoor latrines (all festooned in black), and assembled iron frameworks to accommodate bicycles.

When September 18 arrived, Peking was ready for one of the great spectacles in the history of the People's Republic. Just as Mao's triumph over the Nationalists on October 1, 1949, inaugurated a new era in Chinese history, so also did his funeral inaugurate another. The Chinese had continued their preparations for the rally well into the night of September 17. The Chinese had previously informed the USLO's officers that after 9 A.M. on September 18, the streets around Tienanmen Square would be closed and, once one was in the enclosed area, there would be no exit until after the memorial service concluded in the afternoon. For that reason, several USLO officers, including Richard Mueller, journeyed to the Peking Hotel in the early morning on September 18 in order to acquire a vantage point on the hotel's upper balconies. Even earlier in the morning (perhaps as early as 3 or 4 o'clock) on September 18, Chinese marshals began marching people into Tienanmen Square. Group after group, almost in military formation, filed into the square, filling it completely as well as two "filler" streets nearby. Rows in the streets were probably thirty deep with people as the mourners lined up, shoulder to shoulder, and stood waiting for hours in anticipation of the start of the rally.[25] The marshals who were interspersed throughout the throng attended to the many people for whom such physical discipline was impossible, and who had fainted under the strain.

By the time Peking television began its coverage of the memorial rally at 2:50, the USLO's officers estimated the crowd in Tienanmen Square to number somewhere between 1 and 1.5 million. At 2:59, the Politburo's funeral committee filed onto the rostrum, led by Premier Hua Guofeng, followed by Wang Hongwen and the other leaders in the appropriate protocol rank order. Wang Hongwen presided over the rally and began the proceedings exactly at 3 P.M. by calling for three minutes of silence in honor of the late chairman. Richard Mueller recalled those moments as a time when he "never heard anything as silent; all these people were out in the Square and you could literally hear not one sound." Once the moments of silence ended, Mueller remembered hearing a strange sound rushing up from the crowd down below and suddenly realized it was the noise of the Chinese sobbing, hundreds of thousands of Chinese apparently overcome with emotion. And then, almost instantly, the sobbing ceased and the PLA band played the PRC's national anthem and the "Internationale," after which Wang Hongwen introduced Premier Hua Guofeng, who was assigned to give the eulogy.[26]

Hua Guofeng's twenty-one-minute eulogy to Mao Zedong was undoubtedly the single most important address given in China during the Year of the Dragon, despite Hua's shortcomings as an orator. Certainly Tom Gates and the other USLO officers, as well as the rest of the diplomatic community, waited in great anticipation to learn the contents of Hua's address and what his remarks portended for the PRC. In his excellent book *Coming Alive: China After Mao*, Roger Garside provided a superb first-person account of Hua's speech and its application to the PRC's current political situation.

[It] was evident that [Hua] knew what he was doing. And some of what he was doing caused Wang Hongwen, who stood beside him, visible discomfort for reasons that were not far to seek. First, Hua failed to utter some words the left-controlled press was claiming to have been Mao's death bed injunction to his successors: "Act according to the principles laid down." It was not immediately clear why Hua omitted them: surely he was not signalling any intention to go against the principles laid down (whatever they might be). Unless he was a very unusual political leader, he would proclaim his predecessor's principles all the more fervently if he were about to contravene them. But I assumed the deathbed injunction was seen as aiding the Jiang Qing faction in some way we could not yet fathom. The second feature of the speech that caused Wang Hongwen to arch his eyebrows even more anxiously, and to peer over Hua's shoulder at the text of the eulogy, even more intently, was a passage in which Hua issued a warning against plotting. He gave no clues as to the identity of the plotters, but as it later transpired, he couched his warning in the very words Mao had used to reprimand the Shanghai Gang for factional maneuvering on 3 May 1975. Wang Hongwen and his friends would have no doubt whom Hua had in mind.[27]

In fact, many of Hua Guofeng's remarks in the eulogy to Mao Zedong were confusing. Certainly the tone of his speech was not especially reassuring to the moderates, even if it may have been disquieting to the radicals. Hua's usage of Mao's quotation, "You are making the socialist revolution, and yet don't know where the bourgeoisie is. It is right in the Communist Party, those in power taking the capitalist road," constituted a warning to Deng Xiaoping's allies not to count the premier in their camp (at least not yet). The radicals, however, could quickly ascertain that Hua intended to stand firm against any of their intrigues. Quoting from Mao, Hua spoke of the "Three Dos and the Three Don'ts": practice Marxism and not revisionism; unite, and don't split; be open and aboveboard, don't intrigue and conspire—the instructions which the chairman gave the leftists on May 3, 1975. Furthermore, Hua emphasized Mao's instruction that "the Party holds the gun," a cryptic reference to his support within the ranks of the PLA. Hua's warning to the radicals was unmistakable, even if he had not swung completely to the side of the moderates. Prior to the speech, Jiang Qing and the radicals even attempted unsuccessfully to edit out certain portions of the address which they found objectionable, saying that Hua's remarks were "already too long."[28]

As Hua Guofeng spoke, the television camera remained primarily focused on him but also settled in occasionally on Wang Hongwen, Ye Jianying, and Zhang Chunqiao. At 3:27 P.M., the premier concluded his eulogy, the funeral group made three farewell bows in the direction of Mao's portrait, and the PLA band played "The East Is Red." At precisely 3:30, Wang Hongwen stepped forward to declare the service ended. And then, most important, the leadership failed to step forward to clasp the hand of the widow as they had when Zhou Enlai died. The rumor which circulated within the diplomatic community that Mao had ordered that Jiang Qing not be treated as his wife, nor mentioned at his funeral, apparently was accurate.[29] Certainly the PRC hierarchy made every effort to minimize her role in the memorial activities.

After the adjournment of the rally, Tienanmen Square, which had taken over four hours to fill with mourners, emptied its crowd in two hours. Some of the groups returning from the rally took care to maintain their ranks until they were well removed from the square. For several hours after the rally, Peking remained quiet, as quiet as the observing Americans ever encountered it. By early evening, however, the Chinese who had witnessed the ceremony on their small television sets emerged into the streets, smiling and behaving playfully in apparent release from the formal requirements of mourning for seven days. By nightfall, the capital had returned to normal as though it were untouched by the day's activities.

VI

After the memorial rally for Mao Zedong, the Chinese leadership declared that the formal mourning period would be extended until the end of September. Furthermore, the leadership canceled any scheduled observance of National Day on October 1 in 1976. Having handled the immediate details and problems presented by Mao's death, the leadership appeared determined to adopt a low profile and refrain from any public appearances for the rest of September. The members of the PRC hierarchy declined all invitations to official functions in the diplomatic community, explaining that "our hearts are still heavy for Chairman Mao."[30] The vast majority of Chinese continued to wear black armbands as they went about their daily affairs.

Tom Gates and his American colleagues reasoned that the observance of such an extended mourning period provided the PRC leadership with an opportunity to escape the public limelight and hold discussions about the future of post-Mao China. While recognizing that such official absences served definite purposes, the Americans naturally wondered about what was happening in China behind the political scenes. One curious development occurred in late September when the Chinese re-routed the visit of Senator Mike Mansfield's delegation to China. The majority leader and his group, upon their arrival, were taken on a tour of several provinces, rather than going first to Peking. The Chinese almost never adopted this practice as an itinerary for foreign visitors, nor were they usually in the habit of changing itineraries. Why did they choose to alter the scheduled visit of this important American?

In fact, the acrimonious power struggle between the rival factions in the People's Republic was approaching a crisis point while Mansfield's delegation was touring the Chinese countryside. The direction of the struggle in the last two weeks of September centered on the behavior of Jiang Qing. During Mao's final weeks, many China-watchers suspected that Jiang had conspired to have Mao proclaim her as his successor before he lapsed into unconsciousness. "I am the natural successor," Jiang reportedly declared. "It only takes the chairman to say so." To that end, Jiang Qing (and her radical sup-porters) repeatedly petitioned the dying Mao to put into writing a statement designating her as his successor.[31]

Mao Zedong refused, however, to designate his estranged wife as his successor, an action which apparently infuriated her. Disgusted, disheart-ened, and disconcerted, Jiang Qing reportedly spent Mao's final weeks with her cronies, refusing to acknowledge the extent of her husband's infirmities. "The man must abdicate and let the woman take over," she again reportedly proclaimed. "Even under communism, there can be an empress."[32]

After failing in their attempt to gain Mao's authorization for a radical takeover while he lived, the leftists turned, after his death, once again to the media in their attempt to assume control of the PRC's political apparatus. On September 16, *People's Daily*, *Red Flag*, and *Liberation Army Daily* pub-lished a joint editorial in the form of a eulogy to Mao. "There are worthy successors to the proletarian revolutionary cause [which] Chairman Mao pioneered in China. Chairman Mao adjured us: 'Act according to the prin-ciples laid down,'" meaning act according to Chairman Mao's proletarian revolutionary line and policies. In that fashion, the celebrated controversy ensued between the radicals and their foes over Mao's alleged "deathbed ad-juration," the statement "Act according to the principles laid down." At issue was the person whom Mao supposedly acknowledged as his successor. Jiang Qing maintained that Mao had decided the issue at a Politburo meeting on June 3 when he allegedly told his comrades, Hua Guofeng, Ye Jianying, Li Xiannian, Wang Hongwen, Zhang Chunqiao, and others: "From now on, you should help Jiang Qing carry the Red Banner. Don't let it fall. You should alert her against committing the errors she has committed." Thus, the radicals seized the instruction to "Act according to the principles laid down" as a genuine statement by Mao Zedong designed to bolster Jiang's position.

The exact nature of this meeting, however, remains a mystery. Hua Guofeng, for instance, was not in Peking on June 3, having left for official business in Sichuan on June 2.[33] Not unexpectedly, therefore, he held a view different from Jiang Qing's on the matter of Mao's thoughts about the suc-cession question. To strengthen his position, Hua repeatedly informed the Politburo of a conversation which *he* had with Mao after the chairman's meeting with New Zealand's Prime Minister Robert Muldoon on April 30. After the meeting, Hua reportedly remained with Mao to discuss the status of the anti-Deng campaign in the provinces. According to the premier, Mao instructed him, "Take your time, don't be anxious; act according to past prin-ciples," and, "With you in charge, I am at ease." Curiously, Hua informed the Politburo of only the first two instructions, not the third, which he later claimed as proof that Mao had selected him to lead China after the chair-man's death.

The political drama heightened when, within just a short time after Mao's death and during the official mourning period, Jiang Qing allegedly went to the archives of the Party Central Committee and demanded to receive a collection of Mao's documents, including the April 30 statement in which Mao supposedly placed his confidence in Hua Guofeng as his successor. After Jiang Qing removed these documents, Zhang Yufeng, the Party's archivist, informed Wang Dongxing, the late chairman's bodyguard and the individual responsible for the archives, about Jiang's action. In response, Wang Dongxing ordered Zhang to contact Jiang Qing and demand the return of the documents. Zhang Yufeng followed Wang's instructions, but Jiang Qing refused to return the documents and instead lashed out at the archivist. She then telephoned Wang Dongxing and claimed that Zhang Yufeng had stolen some of Mao's personal papers, demanding in turn that Wang arrest the archivist. For his part, Wang refused to arrest Zhang Yufeng but instead went to Hua Guofeng and informed him of Jiang Qing's action.

Sensing a serious problem, Hua Guofeng telephoned Jiang Qing and ordered her to return the documents immediately. She complied, but only after unleashing a torrent of verbal abuse at Hua. "You want to throw me out when Chairman Mao's remains have not yet grown cold! Is this the way you show your gratitude for the kindnesses rendered to you by Chairman Mao who promoted you?" she demanded. In reply, Hua explained that he would "never forget Chairman Mao's kindness. I want to repay Chairman Mao's kindness, to enable everybody to unite together and forever implement Chairman Mao's behests. As to throwing you out, I have no such intention. You live peacefully in your own house and no one will dare throw you out."[34]

Exactly what purposes Jiang Qing had in mind for the removal of these documents remains mysterious. Some have maintained that she was searching for any material which she considered damaging to herself and the other leftists. Or she may have attempted to "fabricate" or "forge" the phrase "Act according to the principles laid down" in place of the phrase, "Act according to past principles," which appeared in the original version of Mao's instructions. But was Jiang capable of duplicating Mao's unique calligraphy? On that point, some disagreement also exists among China scholars; the possibility that she might have *attempted* to duplicate the chairman's writing certainly should not be disregarded. After recovering the documents, however, Hua Guofeng and Wang Dongxing concluded that Jiang had indeed altered two of them (perhaps the one that included Mao's so-called instructions to Hua, "With you in charge, I am at ease") and determined that Mao's widow was attempting to use the late chairman's papers in some unknown way in order to improve her own prospects for power.

Much confusion, and controversy, continues to exist over this entire sequence of events as well as the means whereby Mao supposedly tried to select Hua Guofeng as his successor. For example, many of the USLO officers considered that Mao's notice to Hua, "With you in charge, I am at ease," referred to a specific matter, perhaps the anti-Deng campaign, and was not a means of advancing Hua as his successor. Others felt that the remark may never have been uttered and that it was manufactured later by Hua and his supporters.[35] Furthermore, it remains difficult to believe that Jiang could have successfully duplicated Mao's calligraphy, although she may have tried. A further consideration is whether Mao's physical condition would have allowed him to write anything on April 30.[36]

Regardless of the circumstances, the fact remained that the radicals, working largely through Yao Wenyuan, used the national media to bombard the Chinese with "Act according to the principles laid down" propaganda during the last two weeks of September 1976. In response, Hua and his supporters attempted to counteract that barrage by making certain that Mao's "Three Dos and Three Don'ts" instruction made its way frequently into national reporting.

The propaganda war eventually led to an acrimonious Politburo meeting in Peking on September 29. By that time, Hua Guofeng apparently had grown restive over the radicals' disruptive tactics and indicated his displeasure directly to them. "Some leading comrades seriously pointed out to the radicals that their propaganda policy was wrong in playing up 'Act according to the principles laid down' and omitting the 'Three Dos and Three Don'ts,'" one account of the meeting explained. For her part, Jiang Qing took this occasion to propose herself formally for the chairmanship of the Party, claiming at the same time that Hua Guofeng was "incompetent." In reply, Hua responded by defending himself as a competent individual who knew "how to solve problems." Later events were to prove that Hua's remark at this meeting was one of Chinese history's great understatements.[37] The meeting, however, broke up with no resolution of the succession issue.

On the next day, September 30, the Politburo held another meeting which concluded with Hua Guofeng leading the hierarchy out for its traditional National Day photograph. Once again, the radicals attempted to undermine Hua, this time by taking a photograph of Jiang in a more exalted and central position than the premier. On October 1, the photograph of Jiang Qing was distributed in newspapers throughout China, once again apparently the work of Yao Wenyuan.[38]

During the first week of October, Hua Guofeng and the radicals continued to wage their propaganda battles against each other. The radicals succeeded frequently in publishing the "Act according to principles laid down" adjuration in both the *People's Daily* and the provincial media. For his part, Hua countered with an editorial on October 1 in the *People's Daily*, which urged the Chinese to study the September 9 announcement of Mao's death and also his eulogy to the late chairman on September 18. Since Hua undoubtedly took a leading role in drafting both the September 9 and September 18 statements, the USLO officers presumed that the premier considered them an effective counter to the radicals' propaganda.[39]

On October 4, however, the radicals made their most assertive challenge to Hua Guofeng's leadership of the People's Republic of China. On that day, an article published by Liang Xiao (a pseudonym for a writing group comprised of students from the radical-controlled Peking and Qinghua universities) appeared in the *Guangming Daily*, praising the adjuration and threatening grave consequences for those who tampered with Mao's thoughts and instructions.

The article, "Forever Act According to the Principles Laid Down By Chairman Mao," pointed out that "all chieftains of the revisionist line who attempt to tamper with Marxist-Leninist-Mao Zedong thought" had suffered serious political consequences. It continued by mentioning the "revisionists" deposed by Mao in the past, Liu Shaoqui, Chen Boda, and Deng Xiaoping. Hua must have considered this article as pressure upon him to share power with the radicals or risk confronting their wrath. Certainly the article's firm, almost strident, tone constituted a radical program for post-Mao China: "relentless struggles against capitalist roaders in the Party" domestically and "struggle against the two hegemonists, the United States and the Soviet Union, plus the liberation of Taiwan" internationally. The article reaffirmed the linkage in the radicals' view between domestic revisionism and foreign imperialism.[40] Without a doubt, Mao's death had led to a sharpening of the contention among China's leaders. By the first week in October 1976, the rival factions whose differences had intensified after Mao's death, faced each other at swords' point.

VII

In assessing the impact of Mao's death upon China during the Year of the Dragon, one must note three factors. First, even at the time of his death, Mao's stature and power in China were so enormous that a power vacuum inevitably developed almost instantly after he died. As Michel Oksenberg and Richard Bush have written,

[Mao] shaped the Chinese communist system so it could be responsive to him. Mao's power was not totally unconstrained; he had to cajole, threaten, and bargain to attain his ends. Occasionally, he was on the defensive and had to acquiesce to the initiative of others. [But Mao] was the dominant voice; opposition to him carried the risk of political oblivion or worse. . . . To the end of his life, [Mao was] a revolutionary and totalitarian ruler. He believed that the only way to transform China was rapidly, violently, comprehensively; its elites and its institutions would have to be subjected to continual change. . . . In his view, to transform China required vision and extraordinary confidence that a politically motivated Chinese populace, given no respite to cultivate its individual pursuits, could overcome weakness and poverty.[41]

Second, the point appeared indisputable that Mao's death created feelings of deep sorrow, as well as deep anxiety, within China. True, his death did not come unexpectedly. True, Mao was a feared and even hated ruler to millions of Chinese who had felt the sting of his wrath during the Cultural Revolution. Even so, his death in September symbolized the latest in a series of national traumas which afflicted the Chinese in 1976. After the earthquake in July, the PRC hierarchy had gone to considerable lengths to staunch the flow of rumors that Mao's death was imminent. Millions of Chinese, superstitious that an earthquake foretold the end of a regime, were convinced that Mao would soon die. When Mao did die within such a short time of the earthquake, it became more difficult for the Chinese to resist an intense foreboding about their future. As Ross Terrill noted, Mao's death was a visible demonstration that the dragon had indeed taken China by the throat in 1976.[42]

Finally, Mao's death provided the foes of the radicals with the opportunity which they had long awaited. On that point, one must note that the unique nature of that opportunity was not lost on either Deng Xiaoping or his supporters within the senior ranks of the PLA. After being dismissed from his posts in April, Deng apparently found refuge in Guangdong under the protection of General Xu Shiyou, the military commander in the region, and Wei Guoqing, the Party's provincial first secretary in Guangdong. Occasionally, Marshal Ye Jianying also visited Guangdong during the summer of 1976 to confer with Deng about plans to prevent a radical takeover of the PRC in the months after Mao's death.[43] Deng and his generation clearly would not surrender to the radicals without contesting them for power, violently if necessary. According to published accounts, Deng and his allies planned to form a military alliance with the Fuzhou and Nanjing military regions, and should Jiang assume power, this alliance would serve as a provisional Central Committee. If these accounts are true, one can only conclude that Deng and his supporters were willing to risk civil war in China rather than see the radicals inherit Mao's legacy. After Mao's death, again according to published accounts, Deng returned secretly to Peking to await the next developments in China's political drama.[44]

Deng Xiaoping's supporters within the ranks of the PLA were also only too willing to help with an effort to purge the radicals. Xu Shiyou, Deng's protector, had attended a leadership meeting in Peking shortly after Mao's death where he announced to the Party Center, "If you don't arrest that woman [Jiang Qing], I shall march north!"[45] In addition, one may safely assume that both Xu Shiyou and Ye Jianying, understanding the struggle about to occur, were actively enlisting the support of other PLA leaders in their effort to prevent Jiang Qing, the woman labeled as "the tragedy of Mao's life" by one of his former close associates, from taking control of the Chinese Communist Party. The PLA and the radicals had been at odds since the early days of the Cultural Revolution; now events were unfolding in a fashion designed to allow them to resolve their dispute. "For a gentleman, a decade is not too long to wait for revenge," one PLA officer reportedly remarked at the time.[46] The month of October 1976, like the preceding months that year, promised to have more than its share of drama and tension.

Notes

1. Thomas Gates's condolence message to Foreign Minister Qiao Guanhua read in part: "I am deeply saddened to hear the news of the death of Chairman Mao Tse-tung. I share the sorrow of the Chinese people over this tragic loss." United States Department of State, Official Files, Condolence Message from Ambassador Gates to Foreign Minister Qiao Guanhua, 9 September 1976. Hereafter cited as OF, date.

2. Fox Butterfield, "The Intriguing Matter of Mao's Successor."

3. OF, Peking to Washington, 24 June 1976; see also Fox Butterfield, "Mao's Seclusion and His Health," *New York Times*, 18 June 1976; White, "Burnout of a Revolution," pp. 30–31.

4. OF, Peking to Washington, 16 July 1976; Terrill, *Mao*, pp. 417–20.

5. Butterfield, "Intriguing Matter."

6. Terrill, *Mao*, p. 420.

7. Domes, "The 'Gang of Four' and Hua Kuo-feng," pp. 486–87.

8. Ibid.

9. Andres D. Onate, "Hua Kuo-feng and the Arrest of the 'Gang of Four,'" *China Quarterly* 75 (September 1978): 542–43.

10. OF, Peking to Washington, 13 September 1976; Garside, *Coming Alive*, pp. 139–40; Terrill, *Mao*, pp. 421–24.

11. Interview, David Dean, 14 December 1982; interview, Richard Mueller, 17 February 1983.

12. Terrill, *Mao*, pp. 421–24.

13. OF, Peking to Washington, 9 September 1976. The Chinese decision to exclude all foreigners from attending Mao's memorial service saved the Ford administration from having to make a difficult protocol decision. Both the administration and the State Department faced a potential problem in designating a representative to attend Mao's funeral, should such representation be appropriate. After the president, the most logical person to represent the United States was Vice President Nelson Rockefeller. Just the previous year, however, Rockefeller had represented the United States at the funeral of Chiang K'ai Sh'ek, and his presence may not have been welcomed by the PRC hierarchy for that reason. Eventually, after discussing many other prospective representatives (including former President Nixon) the administration concluded that Secretary of State Kissinger would represent the United States at Mao's funeral, despite any irregularities in protocol which might be evident, should the PRC ever request such representation.

14. OF, Peking to Washington, 9 September 1976.

15. OF, Peking to Washington, 13 September 1976.

16. Onate, "Hua Kuo-feng," pp. 542–43.

17. OF, Peking to Washington, 23 September 1976; see also Onate, "Hua Kuo-feng," pp. 542–43; Terrill, *Mao*, pp. 421–23; idem, *White-Boned Demon*, p. 373.

18. OF, Peking to Washington, 11 September 1976; *New York Times*, 12 September 1976.

19. Onate, "Hua Kuo-feng," pp. 544–45.

20. OF, Peking to Washington, 13 September 1976; OF, Peking to Washington, 17 September 1976.

21. OF, Peking to Washington, 13 September 1976.

22. Harrison E. Salisbury, *China: 100 Years of Revolution* (New York: Holt, Rinehart, and Winston, 1983), p. 248; Terrill, *White-Boned Demon*, p. 368.

23. OF, Peking to Washington, 14 September 1976; *Washington Post*, 13 September 1976.

24. OF, Peking to Washington, 14 September 1976; OF, 17 September 1976.

25. Interview, Richard Mueller, 17 February 1983.

26. OF, Peking to Washington, 18 September 1976.

27. Garside, *Coming Alive*, pp. 148–49.

28. OF, Peking to Washington, 18 September 1976; Onate, "Hua Kuo-feng," pp. 546–47; Hsu, *China Without Mao*, p. 18.

29. Fox Butterfield, "Moderate Policies Indicated for China in the Wake of the Anti-Leftist Campaign," *New York Times*, 22 October 1976, p. 8.

30. OF, Peking to Washington, 22 September 1976.

31. OF, Peking to Washington, 10 February 1977; OF, Peking to Washington, 19 January 1977.

32. Ibid.; Terrill, *White-Boned Demon*, p. 311.

33. Onate, "Hua Kuo-feng," pp. 545–48; Terrill, *White-Boned Demon*, p. 363. See also the interesting account in Jay Mathews and Linda Mathews, *One Billion: A China Chronicle* (New York: Random House, 1983), pp. 178–79.

34. OF, Peking to Washington, 26 October 1976.

35. Ibid.; interview, David Dean, 7 December 1982.

36. Onate, "Hua Kuo-feng," p. 549.

37. Ibid., pp. 550–51; this report was issued in the *People's Daily* on 17 December 1976.

38. Ibid., pp. 553–54.

39. OF, Peking to Washington, 6 October 1976; see also Onate, "Hua Kuo-feng," pp. 553–54.

40. OF, Peking to Washington, 6 October 1976; according to one USLO officer, the October 4 article written by Liang Xiao "turned out to be the radicals' swan song"; see OF, Peking to Washington, 12 October 1976.

41. Michel Oksenberg and Richard Bush, "China's Political Evolution," *Problems of Communism*, 2–3.

42. Terrill, *Future of China*, p. 8.

43. Garside, *Coming Alive*, pp. 140–41.

44. Ibid.; Hsu, *China Without Mao*, p. 14.

45. Garside, *Coming Alive*, p. 144; Terrill, *White-Boned Demon*, p. 371.

46. Butterfield, "Moderate Policies"; White, "Burnout of a Revolution," pp. 34–35.

CHAPTER 5

The Purges of October

On the afternoon of October 9, 1976, David Dean, the deputy chief of the United States Liaison Office in Peking, escorted Senator Mike Mansfield, the majority leader of the United States Senate, and Senator John Glenn to an important meeting at the Great Hall of the People. The Mansfield/Glenn delegation had arrived in China on September 21 and spent the next two weeks touring several provinces before coming to Peking in the first week of October for scheduled discussions with the PRC leadership. The significance of the October 9 meeting was clear to both Dean and the two senators; this session marked the first occasion since the death of Mao Zedong that any American was to meet officially with a member of the PRC's post-Mao hierarchy.

The meeting also held a special importance for David Dean. Several days earlier, Thomas Gates had returned to New York in order to be present at the opening of the United Nations General Assembly, an event which also provided an opportunity for him to participate in bilateral negotiations between Secretary of State Henry Kissinger and Foreign Minister Qiao Guanhua. In Tom's absence, Dean was the senior American official in Peking and thereby responsible for reporting and analyzing the discussions which took place between the Chinese and the two United States senators.

In preparing for the October 9 meeting, Dean assumed that the Chinese would select Vice Premier Zhang Chunqiao as their representative at the session. Zhang Chunqiao had met with Senate Minority Leader Hugh Scott and the members of his delegation when they visited China the previous

July. The memory of that prickly session with Zhang Chunqiao made Dean somewhat apprehensive about the outcome of the forthcoming session on October 9, particularly if Zhang continued to demonstrate his apparent unwillingness to establish any rapport with the Americans. Indeed, considering the sensitive state of the PRC's internal political situation during that period, Dean was even more anxious about the manner in which the Chinese might choose to conduct the meeting.[1]

When the Americans arrived at the Great Hall of the People that afternoon, however, they were surprised to be greeted by Li Xiannian, a veteran civilian member of the Politburo known more for his work in economic planning than for his experience in foreign affairs. Dean realized that Li Xiannian had represented the PRC leadership in several visits with other foreign dignitaries, but his presence always seemed to be more an example of correct protocol than an indication of any responsibility which he may have acquired in the field of foreign policy. Despite his initial surprise, Dean was considerably relieved to be meeting with Li Xiannian instead of Zhang Chunqiao. Li, who was then in his early seventies, had developed a remarkable reputation within the Chinese leadership. He was not considered a member of either the radical or the moderate faction, and his age tended to disqualify him from direct association with the neo-Maoist group assumed to be led by Hua Guofeng. He was in fact known within the PRC as a survivor, an able economic planner whose technical expertise and political savvy separated him (to an extent) from the ideological fury which had swept across China throughout the previous decade.

The meeting between Dean and the senators and Li Xiannian proceeded quite smoothly. Li discussed his views on the status of Sino-American relations, emphasizing the importance of the Shanghai Communique and the PRC's standard displeasure with the Helsinki Agreement. His comments on the status of Sino-Soviet relations also left no doubt that the PRC's attitude toward the Soviet Union had not changed in the brief time since Mao Zedong's death. "We cannot do like the Soviet Union, going around the world, begging aid and incurring debts," Li explained. "[The Soviets] sow grain in the U.S.S.R. and reap it in the United States and Canada."[2]

When the time was appropriate for the Americans to enter the discussions, Mansfield and Glenn took the occasion to express their sympathy to the Chinese leadership over the death of Chairman Mao. In responding to this gesture, Li Xiannian grew especially serious, choosing his words extremely carefully before answering the Americans. "The deaths of Zhou Enlai, Zhu De, and Chairman Mao are great losses, but unfortunately a natural inevitable development that we were unable to stop. But under the leadership of the Central Committee, *led by Premier Hua Guofeng who has succeeded Chairman Mao*, we are confident that we can manage our country. Chairman Mao's thought lives forever in our heads," Li explained (emphasis added).[3]

After the meeting, Dean, Mansfield, and Glenn understood that they had witnessed an exceptional performance by Li Xiannian, although they did not fully comprehend the degree of the session's significance until several weeks later. The October 9 meeting with Li Xiannian at the Great Hall of the People took place against the backdrop of a series of critical events which occurred in the PRC between October 4 and October 13. Dean suspected that Li's presence at the meeting, rather than Zhang's, was a visible demonstration of a change in the PRC hierarchy. Furthermore, Dean noticed that Li Xiannian had been painstakingly careful in his choice of words with the Americans on October 9; he was talking not only to his foreign visitors but also to his Chinese interpreters and the numerous junior officers in the Foreign Ministry who would read the official minutes of the meeting.

The meeting between the Americans and Li Xiannian also occurred during one of the most event-laden days of Tom Gates's tenure in China. On October 8, the USLO's officers received word that the PRC's central authorities had broadcast a bulletin to the students at Peking University, ordering them to await "an important announcement" scheduled for 6:30 P.M. on October 9. Because of this forthcoming announcement and the meeting scheduled with a member of the leadership at the Great Hall, the USLO community approached October 9 with an unusual degree of expectation.[4] Early in the morning on October 9, Peking awoke to the rhythmic pounding of drums by several hundred demonstrators, some carrying placards encouraging the Chinese to "greet the appointment of Comrade Hua Guofeng as Chairman of the Communist Party." At 11:30 A.M., several USLO officers reported a large number of official limousines streaming away from the Great Hall of the People, perhaps a signal that an important leadership meeting had just adjourned. Then, at 3 P.M., Dean and Senators Mansfield and Glenn met with Li Xiannian at the Great Hall. At 4 P.M., several members of the diplomatic community reported the sighting of numerous wall posters around the city, calling upon the Chinese to "support the decision to appoint Hua Guofeng as Chairman of the Party Central Committee and Chairman of the Military Commission" and also to "Rally Round the Party Politburo Headed by Comrade Hua." The contents of these posters sent the resident foreign journalists in Peking scurrying to the Foreign Ministry, asking for a clarification of what appeared to be a change in Hua Guofeng's status. The PRC's spokesman at the Foreign Ministry avoided a direct response to these queries, saying that he "could say no more, now," but added that another important announcement was forthcoming. Then, at 6:30 P.M., the Party Center announced to the students at Peking University that the Central Committee had decided to construct a Memorial Hall in honor of Mao

Zedong and also that Hua Guofeng was to serve as the editor of the fifth and succeeding volumes of Mao's writings. The announcement contained no official confirmation of any change in Hua Guofeng's official status. Without question, however, the Party Center had "wrapped the [new] leadership in a mantle of loyalty to Mao and it established Hua as the supreme interpreter of Mao's thought, a role that would surely go to the highest political figure in China," in the words of Roger Garside. Finally, before October 9 drew to a close, USLO officers heard the startling rumor that four leading radicals under Hua had been purged, and that Wang Hongwen was one of the four.[5]

The USLO's China-watchers had to wait for several more days before completely placing the events of October 9 into the proper perspective, as well as understanding the precise meaning of Li Xiannian's words, "under the leadership of the Party Central Committee led by Premier Hua Guofeng who has succeeded Chairman Mao." On October 10, the members of the diplomatic community began noticing considerably more poster activity in Peking than usual, and with a wider variety of messages. Numerous posters warned against "conspirators" and "splittists," and urged the masses to support the Party's two decisions of October 8. But *who* specifically were the conspirators and splittists? A possible answer to that question came later on October 10 when the USLO received further information about Wang Hongwen's situation. The four deposed leftists, according to this confidential report, were Jiang Qing, Zhang Chunqiao, Yao Wenyuan, and Wang Hongwen, all of whom were arrested for alleged complicity in a coup attempt on the Hua regime.[6] That astonishing information gained greater credence after the publication of a strongly worded editorial on October 10 in the *People's Daily*. The editorial vigorously repeated the importance of Mao's "Three Dos and Three Don'ts" instruction, language which the moderates had used earlier in the month in their propaganda battle against the radicals. Whatever the political changes then occurring in the PRC, the radicals seemed to have suffered a decisive setback.[7]

On October 11, evidence of the PLA's role in any recent political shake-up in China came into sharp focus. USLO officers received word that posters put up inside the compound of a PLA unit in Peking read: "Warmly welcome the Central Committee's brilliant resolutions. Firmly support the appointment of Hua Guofeng as Chairman of the Chinese Communist Party. Closely unite around the Party Central Committee headed by Comrade Hua Guofeng." Other posters sighted in Peking, at such locations as the Ministry of Agriculture and even at Peking University, called upon the Chinese to "Love the Army" and "Support the Army" and claimed that "Comrade Hua Guofeng's appointment was made according to the wishes of Chairman Mao."[8]

On October 12, Peking appeared outwardly normal although the diplomatic community noticed an ever-increasing number of posters appearing throughout the city. The Party media continued its practice of introducing every broadcast with the content of the October 10 editorial from the *People's Daily*, and its emphasis on Mao's "Three Dos and Three Don'ts" instructions. Such attention to a single editorial seemed particularly strange in the PRC. But on October 12, the Center published another article in the *People's Daily*, entitled "Rally Most Closely Around the Party Central Committee Headed By Comrade Hua Guofeng." This one again dealt with Mao's instructions on the subject of Party unity. The article recalled a Central Committee meeting in 1938 when Mao criticized Zhang Guotao's actions in attempting to split the Party and the Army during the Long March. In particular, the article quoted Mao's speech on Party discipline at that meeting. "In view of Zhang Guotao's serious violations of discipline, we must affirm anew the discipline of the Party," Mao reportedly declared. Specifically, Mao then went on to emphasize the importance of four tenets of Party discipline, namely, that the individual was subordinate to the organization, the minority was subordinate to the majority, the lower levels of the Party were subordinate to the upper levels (e.g., the provincial organizations were subordinate to the Party Center), and the entire membership was subordinate to the Central Committee. "Whoever violates these articles of discipline disrupts Party unity," the article concluded.[9] Clearly, the Party Center was not looking favorably upon those whom it considered violators of Party unity.

More important, however, than the publication of this article on Party discipline on October 12 was the news that the diplomatic community received which reported that celebrations were then under way throughout China, praising Hua Guofeng's elevation and also apparently rejoicing in the downfall of the four radicals. Provincial broadcasts from Hangzhou and Wuhan reported that thousands of people were parading through the streets, banging gongs and acclaiming Hua's appointment as Party chairman.[10]

Despite these broadcasts, editorials, and rumors, the fact remained that the Chinese leadership still had not officially announced Hua Guofeng's appointment as the chairman of the Chinese Communist Party by October 13. Nor had the Party Center released any word about the status (or whereabouts) of the four radicals. At the various diplomatic receptions then occurring in Peking, Chinese officials did, however, appear noticeably buoyant and cheerful, although no PRC diplomats would provide any authoritative word on the political changes which most observers believed had already taken place. One USLO officer inquired of one beaming Chinese diplomat at a reception on October 12 if he had any further information about Hua's appointment. "Oh, you know, really, I couldn't possibly comment on *that*," he grinned.[11] Finally, on October 13, the Chinese officially released the news that Hua Guofeng had in fact succeeded Mao Zedong as chairman of the

Chinese Communist Party. At a state banquet held for Prime Minister Michael Somare of Papua New Guinea, several resident journalists approached Ji Mingcong, a spokesman for the Ministry of Foreign Affairs, and asked him how long the Chinese expected to take before officially announcing Hua's elevation. Completely ready to respond, Ji said that he could "now confirm that [Hua] is Chairman of the Central Committee of the Chinese Communist Party. This information has been internally circulated and the people know about it." [12] Hua Guofeng himself even gave substance to this information at a reception for Somare held prior to the dinner. "It is an open secret that I am Chairman," he informed a group of diplomats. [13] The news of the arrests of the four radicals, by then branded as the Gang of Four, was not officially confirmed, however, until October 17.

By mid-October, David Dean and the other American China-watchers in Peking understood why Li Xiannian had so carefully chosen his words during his meeting with the Americans on October 9. On the night of October 6–7, the Hua regime apprehended Jiang Qing, Zhang Chunqiao, Wang Hongwen, and Yao Wenyuan, along with dozens of their supporters both in Peking and throughout China. Zhang Chunqiao did not meet with the Mansfield/Glenn delegation on October 9 because, by that time, he had been purged and imprisoned. The arrests of the Gang of Four and their supporters, combined with Jiang, Zhang, Wang, and Yao's being stripped of their titles, offices, and staffs by the Hua regime, served as the opening stage of a campaign by China's post-Mao leadership to deny the extreme leftists any future voice in the PRC's political affairs. More important to American foreign policy and Chinese-American relations at that time, Tom Gates, David Dean, and the USLO's other analysts considered that Li Xiannian's comment on October 9 that "Premier Hua . . . has succeeded Chairman Mao" may well have been the PRC's first notification to a foreign government that a change in China's leadership had indeed taken place. If Li sought to leave such an impression with Dean, Mansfield, and Glenn, he admittedly did so in an indirect and subtle fashion. Nevertheless, the diplomatic community received no official notice of Hua Guofeng's elevation to the chairmanship until October 13, and no news of the radicals' purge until October 17. By "informing" Dean, Mansfield, and Glenn on October 9, Li Xiannian had indicated that the Chinese continued to value its new relationship with the United States. If that were not so, Li almost certainly would have responded differently to the American delegation.

II

The purge of the Gang of Four, much more than the elevation of Hua Guofeng to the chairmanship of the Central Committee of the Chinese Communist Party, occupied China's attention in October 1976 and, in many respects, for the next six months as well. When the Hua regime arrested and deposed Jiang Qing, Zhang Chunqiao, Wang Hongwen, Yao Wenyuan, and numerous other of their leftist supporters on October 6, it set off a period of prolonged national celebration. With the radical high command now under confinement, the Chinese people appeared confident that at last its government had proclaimed an end to the Cultural Revolution. Just as the Tangshan earthquake in July diverted attention from the anti-Deng campaign, and Mao's death in September eclipsed the national importance of the earthquake relief, so also did the Gang's arrest command the interest of the Chinese people until the end of 1976.

In Tom Gates's discussions with both Chinese and foreign diplomats in the days and weeks after the arrest of the Gang of Four, he received the impression that China's masses considered the purge of the radicals long overdue; certainly the PRC's officials became much more relaxed and approachable in their dealings with American and foreign diplomats after the events of early October. To quote one Chinese intellectual at that time, "A new wind is now blowing" in China.[14] The effect of the Gang's arrest upon the atmosphere in Peking was also instantly noticeable. The loudspeakers broadcast enjoyable music instead of the vicious radical propaganda. People smiled and laughed on the streets. Color even reappeared in their clothing. Tom later described the feeling as though "one could hear a deep sigh of relief as it echoed across the vast spaces of China."[15] With the radicals detained, Tom hoped that the developments of October would provide a way for the United States and China to pursue a more constructive relationship.

Few events in recent Chinese history have received as much attention from scholars as the purge of the Gang of Four. Even so, there are still many unanswered questions, and published accounts of the purge differ considerably; a single, totally authentic and accurate account of the event may never emerge.[16] Interpretations of the "smashing of the Gang of Four" disagree on four critical points: (1) the protagonist behind the move to purge the radicals; (2) the intentions of the radicals with respect to the Hua regime (e.g., did the Gang plan to overthrow the Party Center, under Hua Guofeng's nominal leadership, by force or simply to use its propaganda apparatus as a means of turning the Chinese masses against their political foes?); (3) the circumstances involved in the actual arrests of the radicals; and (4) the means by which Hua and his anti-radical colleagues defused a potentially explosive situation in Shanghai in the aftermath of the Gang's arrest.

An analysis of the source of the move against the Gang of Four must begin with the concession that the arrest of the Gang of Four was the work of three individuals, Defense Minister Ye Jianying, Premier Hua Guofeng, and Wang Dongxing, Mao's former bodyguard and the man who commanded the Central Committee's elite 8341 unit which guarded the members of the Politburo. Wang Dongxing was a pivotal character in this episode since he was also responsible for the Party's General Office and the disposition of the secret documents in the Party archives. After the concession that Ye, Hua, and Wang engineered the overthrow of the radicals, however, the entire matter becomes somewhat confusing. Specifically, who was the protagonist for the ouster, Ye, Hua, or perhaps Deng Xiaoping? Initially, many published accounts of the arrests viewed Hua as the protagonist, the individual who assiduously cultivated the support of the PLA during the summer months and then waited for the appropriate time in which to enlist the military's support in deposing his enemies.[17] Since such accounts are well documented, one cannot reasonably deny their validity.

Even so, some problems remain when one attempts to view Hua Guofeng in such a determined, decisive fashion. Without a doubt, Hua considered the radicals (and certainly Jiang Qing) as an obstacle to his attempt to unify the PRC behind his leadership; whether he thought the best method of dealing with them was through a purge is another matter. As late as the beginning of October 1976, Tom believed that Hua and some of the radicals were still searching for a modus vivendi, a compromise whereby Hua and possibly a member of the radical faction (but not Jiang Qing) could share power in a post-Mao alignment. In such a compromise, the key individual for the radicals was Zhang Chunqiao, not Jiang Qing. In several ways, Hua and Zhang were antagonists, with neither having much respect for the talents of the other. Both were practical politicians, however. Hua realized that Zhang held a potentially secure power base in Shanghai by virtue of his years as the leader of that city's Communist Party. In addition, Zhang was also the head of the PLA's General Political Department, a post which (on the surface at least) seemed to guarantee him some support within the ranks of the military.

For his part, Zhang Chunqiao certainly realized that the events of 1976 had provided Hua Guofeng with an opportunity for assuming the leadership of post-Mao China. Even so, Hua lacked a strong political power base, and Mao's death in September deprived him of valuable time to undertake any further consolidation of his position. Because Hua was the compromise choice for premier in February, his hold on the reins of power depended to a large extent on his ability to avoid making powerful enemies on either the Left or the Right. With the exception of his prompt response to the earthquake emergency in August, Hua had not shown himself to be a particularly forceful leader over the course of his first eight months in high office. For those reasons, Tom and the other American China-watchers in Peking formed the opinion that China's post-Mao leadership may well have coalesced around Hua's assuming the chairmanship of the Party with Zhang assuming Hua's former post as premier. That opinion was not mere idle diplomatic conversation; the possibility of such an arrangement had been widely discussed and analyzed within the diplomatic community since the previous April. Such a compromise would then have led to a Center-Left coalition gaining the political ascendancy in China, with the Maoists and neo-Maoists firmly in control.[18]

In the days and weeks immediately before and after Mao's death, however, the radicals ruined any possibility for a compromise with Hua Guofeng. Not surprisingly, Jiang Qing once again became the culprit in this regard, proving her late husband correct when he warned several of his colleagues before he died, "Jiang Qing has wild ambitions. She wants Wang Hongwen to be Chairman of the Standing Committee of the National People's Congress and herself to be Chairman of the Party Central Committee. After my death, she will make trouble."[19] Desperately wishing to become the chairman of the Party, Jiang traveled extensively throughout China during the summer of 1976, attempting to build up her support for a putsch against Hua, a campaign which increased in earnestness as Mao drew closer to death. Reportedly, one favorite technique which Jiang devised involved rallying support for the radicals among younger cadres, encouraging a generation-gap mentality on their part. "Don't trust anyone over 45," she allegedly said. "Suspect anyone over 45." Zhang Chunqiao and Wang Hongwen apparently assisted Jiang in her effort to consolidate radical support around the country, with each of them spending several days in Shanghai during the last two weeks of September to make certain that the Party organization in China's largest city remained loyal to them. Such intrigues did not escape Hua's attention and probably convinced him that the leftists had no intention of sharing future power with him but were determined to wrest control of the PRC government for themselves.[20]

Tom Gates and the USLO officers therefore believed that the radicals betrayed Hua, who repeatedly kept the door open for a compromise with them. To the best of their understandings, however, Defense Minister Ye Jianying entertained no such illusions about the radicals. Ye and several of the other senior PLA officers, along with an array of strategically placed civilians such as Wei Guoqing, the first secretary of Guangdong province, Zhao Ziyang, the first secretary of Sichuan province, and probably Deng Xiaoping as well, devised a plan during September to arrest Jiang and her radical followers. Furthermore, in addition to whatever ideological differences Ye and Deng may have had with the radicals (and these were considerable), both men had personal scores to settle with the leftists. Theodore H. White has recorded that the sons of Ye Jianying and Deng Xiaoping suffered crippling injuries during the Cultural Revolution, both apparently the result of leftist-inflicted "accidents." Ye's son, a promising aviator, was forced to do exhausting agricultural labor on a commune and, one night, apparently overcome with fatigue, "put his hand into the gears of a threshing machine

[and] the hand was mangled," ending the young man's flying career. Deng Xiaoping's son, Deng Pufang, suffered permanent paralysis from the waist down after being pushed out of his fourth-floor dormitory room during the Cultural Revolution. As White observed, neither Deng nor Ye forgot the tragedies which the radicals inflicted upon their children, nor as subsequent events proved, did they ever forgive their enemies.[21]

Ye Jianying made no attempt to hide his intentions of moving against the radicals from Hua Guofeng; after Mao's death, he even went to some lengths to warn the premier of the leftists' desire to undermine him. Hua initially hesitated to support Ye's plan, however, although one truly wonders about his fate had he tried to restrain the defense minister from carrying out his effort to purge the radicals. In Hua's defense, though, one must note that he was not totally unwilling to risk a showdown with the radicals. To that end, he successfully secured the support of Wang Dongxing for a continuation of his leadership, rather than allowing Wang to fall in with the radicals, who were also presumably interested in garnering his support. Wang's support was essential to Hua and, when one considered that Wang had faithfully served Mao for over two decades, it was somewhat surprising (given the time period involved) that Wang chose to side with the neo-Maoists instead of joining the extreme leftists.

In the last months of Mao Zedong's life, however, two developments apparently soured Wang Dongxing on his future prospects with the radicals. These factors ultimately constituted the reasons behind his eventual alliance with Hua Guofeng and Ye Jianying, an alliance which permanently altered the direction of modern Chinese history. First, Wang believed that the radicals had attempted to reduce his contact with Mao when he lay hopelessly ill. Wang reportedly was especially concerned about the close relationship between Jiang Qing and Mao Yuanxin, and possibly concluded that Mao's nephew represented a potential political rival to him once the chairman died. Second, Wang Hongwen had made extensive plans to arm the Shanghai urban militia and develop the militia throughout China as a counter to the PLA. Such actions also probably convinced Wang that he was more useful to Hua and Ye than to the radicals, especially if both Mao Yuanxin and Wang Hongwen were actively trying to build up the radicals' military support without his assistance. In addition, Wang Dongxing realized the extent of the leftists' unpopularity throughout China, and should they fail in their attempt to gain control of the PRC, no one who supported them would benefit. Wang Dongxing therefore became a quiet ally of Hua and Ye by the middle of September, keeping them informed on the information which he acquired about the radicals' intrigues.[22]

The loss of Wang Dongxing proved to be a critical blow to the prospects of the radicals. Almost without question, the close cooperation between

Wang Dongxing and Hua Guofeng, both men with long experience in directing the Party's internal security forces, allowed the radicals' enemies to keep them under close surveillance. By the beginning of September, Jiang Qing undoubtedly sensed that she was being watched and lived in a constant state of anxiety. Shortly before Mao's death, she was heard to slander the Central Committee for dispatching "special agents" to collect "intelligence" against her. At various times, she reportedly asked her allies, "Have you heard anything said against me. You must have heard something said against me." Then, in a show of bravado, she exclaimed, "I am not scared. What do I fear? I fear nothing."[23]

By the first week in October, therefore, the trio of Ye Jianying, Hua Guofeng, and Wang Dongxing had lined up, more or less, against the leftists. Thus, a second question emerged: What circumstance or event provided the reason for the arrest of the Gang of Four on the night of October 6. This question has provoked serious differences of opinion. One source of dispute is the issue of whether the radicals planned to overthrow the Hua regime by the force of a civil insurrection, or whether they were simply engaged in a propaganda campaign designed to turn the Chinese masses against Hua's leadership. More dramatically, did the radicals plan to assassinate Hua, Ye, perhaps Deng Xiaoping, or even General Xu Shiyou, and certain of their other political foes? Even more dramatically, did the Gang of Four ever attempt to kill Hua or Ye? Respected scholars of Chinese history have differed considerably in their answers to these questions.[24]

In the autumn of 1976, Tom Gates and the other USLO officers believed that the radicals would resort to any means they considered necessary to gain power. Tom considered it entirely possible that the radicals mounted their propaganda effort against the Hua regime in the last weeks of September as the first stage in a campaign designed to discredit Hua Guofeng and drive him from office. In similar fashion, no USLO officer discounted the possibility that the radicals would *not* resort to violence if that was the only way to accomplish their purposes. According to accounts of this episode published since 1978, Wang Hongwen *had* succeeded in arming the thirty-thousand-member urban militia in Shanghai. In addition, Mao Yuanxin was busily involved in building up support for the leftists within the ranks of the Shenyang military region.[25] More important, Jiang Qing had approached Chen Xilian, commander of the Peking military region, shortly after Mao's death and said, "I need your troops."[26] Such evidence points to the conclusion that the radicals had calculated that the PLA was also split into its leftist and moderate factions, and if the Gang could build support within the PLA units stationed in north China, it could stage a takeover of Peking.

The Gang of Four seriously miscalculated, however, in its attempt to build military support for its plans. Marshal Ye Jianying had already received the cooperation of eight of China's ten military region commanders in his plans to depose the leftists. Moreover, Chen Xilian despised Jiang Qing and kept Ye (and presumably Hua Guofeng as well) informed about the scheming intrigues of Mao's widow. Jiang had earlier incurred Chen's wrath when she attempted to force the marriage of Chen's son to her daughter Li Na, who was then pregnant after a liaison with a regular PLA soldier. Chen's son had also been romantically linked with Li Na, but his father was adamantly opposed to marriage between the two. The prospect of becoming related through marriage to Jiang Qing apparently was too much to bear for the sturdy PLA commander.[27]

Related to the question of whether the radicals planned to use violence in their attempt to seize power is what plans they may have had to assassinate Hua Guofeng, Ye Jianying, and perhaps some of their other enemies. Toward the end of October, with the Gang of Four then in confinement, a published report indicated that a poster campaign had broken out in Peking, claiming that the radicals may have attempted to murder Hua Guofeng. According to this report, the failed attempt on his life convinced Hua that he needed to take strong action against the radicals.[28] The American China-watching contingent in Peking discounted these reports, believing that the Center's knowledge of Jiang Qing's and Wang Hongwen's actions, combined with the inflammatory tone of the Liang Xiao article on October 4, precipitated the action against the radicals.

These developments ultimately led to a third area of disagreement among China scholars, that concerning the circumstances under which the arrests of the Gang of Four occurred. Ross Terrill has written that the four radicals were arrested "while they caucused with their supporters" after leaving a Politburo meeting on the evening of October 6.[29] Roger Garside has explained that Wang Dongxing implemented a plan whereby members of the 8341 unit arrested Jiang Qing and Yao Wenyuan separately at their homes while Zhang Chunqiao and Wang Hongwen were apprehended at the Western Hills after being lured to what they believed was a special meeting of the Politburo's Standing Committee. Since each member of the Politburo was assigned its own special security detail, the arrests were carried out by those soldiers known to be loyal to the Party Center. As the arrests of Wang and Zhang took place, Hua and Ye watched the action on closed circuit television from the safety of a nearby room.[30] Immanuel Hsu's account records an even different story. Hsu wrote that only Jiang Qing was arrested at her home while Zhang, Wang, and Yao were taken captive *in Hua's presence* at the Western Hills.[31] To cite one final version, Theodore H. White has declared that one PRC official explained to him in 1983 that the Party Center "rounded up the leftists, one by one, in their homes" on the night of October 6.[32]

With such a wide variety of accounts about the actual arrests of the Gang of Four, it is not surprising that USLO officials formed their own impressions, at the time, of the purge of the Gang of Four. In essence, the USLO's China-watchers pieced together two possible explanations of the means by which Hua, Ye, and Wang deposed their leftist enemies. The first account was accepted within several weeks of the Gang's overthrow; the second took the better part of the next six months to gain credibility among the USLO's officers. The American China-watchers in Peking assembled each account only after careful analysis of the PRC media and poster sightings around Peking, conversations with other members of the diplomatic community, and the acquisition of confidential information from various sources throughout Peking.

As Tom Gates and his colleagues pieced together their first account of the arrest of the Gang of Four in the weeks immediately after the leftists downfall, they showed the drama beginning on the morning of October 6. Finally convinced that strong measures against the radicals were necessary, Hua Guofeng authorized Ye Jianying and Wang Dongxing to organize the arrests of the leftists. Such as it was, Ye's plan called for the apprehension of the radicals at a special Politburo meeting scheduled for 6 o'clock that evening at his residence (appropriately enough) in the Western Hills. At this meeting, attended by several of China's military region commanders, Hua and his anti-Gang, PLA collaborators carried out the purge of· the radical high command.

At the beginning of the meeting, Jiang Qing immediately spoke up and produced a statement which she claimed had been written by Mao, supporting her desire to be the chairman's successor. Jiang's other three radical comrades, Zhang Chunqiao, Wang Hongwen, and Yao Wenyuan, were also present at the meeting in addition to Mao Yuanxin and two members of the Liang Xiao writing team. To a person, the leftists voiced their support of Jiang's claim about the authenticity of the document which she displayed before the Politburo. Premier Hua Guofeng, however, not to be outdone, responded by displaying a tape recording (presumably of Mao's April 30 meeting with him) stating that the chairman had designated him as the next supreme leader of the CCP. Hua continued to press his claim for the chairmanship, explaining that he had spoken with Mao before his death and that the chairman had informed him, "Don't be impatient or nervous, act as you have done so far. If you are Chairman, I will die in peace." After concluding his remarks, Hua asked for a vote of the Politburo to decide the question of the succession. Every member of the Politburo subsequently supported Hua Guofeng for the chairmanship, with the exception of the four leftists, who voted for Jiang Qing.

Sensing yet another deadlock within the leadership over the succession issue, in still another Politburo meeting, Marshall Ye Jianying then signalled for security forces to enter the room and arrest all seven of the radicals—the Gang of Four, Mao Yuanxin, and the two members of the Liang Xiao writing team. Both Wang Hongwen and Mao Yuanxin resisted arrest, took out revolvers, and engaged in a shootout with their captors, wounding one officer and killing three others before being subdued. Afterward, Hua and Ye placed Jiang Qing under house arrest; the other radicals were jailed elsewhere in Peking. Leaving as little to chance as possible, Hua and Ye also ordered loyal troops to surround Peking and Shanghai that same evening and also to move in and occupy Peking and Qinghua universities. Hua and Ye also dispatched Geng Biao, another of their allies, to take control of the *People's Daily*, the New China News Agency, and Peking's radio and television stations. In addition to the arrests made in Peking on the night of October 6, Tom later heard that the PLA arrested over five hundred other radical supporters throughout China that evening. The radicals' enemies had gone a considerable distance, within a relatively brief period of time, in locking up China against them.[33]

After the arrest of the Gang of Four in October, the USLO continued to receive information for the next several months about the circumstances surrounding the arrest of the Gang of Four. As a result, by early 1977, Tom Gates and his colleagues assembled a second version of the events of October 6–7 which differed in some respects from the earlier account. The second account accepted the fact that the radicals were arrested on the night of October 6–7 but not that the arrest took place at the Politburo meeting scheduled for early that evening. At this early meeting, the members of the Politburo did indeed vote to support Hua Guofeng as the successor to Mao Zedong as the chairman of the Central Committee of the Chinese Communist Party, but the arrests of the four radicals did not occur until several hours later. After the Politburo meeting, Hua had informed those of his colleagues who were members of the Standing Committee of the National People's Congress that he had scheduled a meeting of that group later that evening, perhaps as late as midnight. Therefore, between the time of the adjournment of the early meeting of the Politburo and the later meeting of the Standing Committee, Hua and Ye made their final preparations for the arrest of the radicals. At the appointed time, Hua and Ye summoned Zhang, Wang, and Yao to the later meeting in the Western Hills. Wang Hongwen arrived first and Hua read out the arrest order to him. Wang tried to reach for his pistol but he was grabbed by four officers who were loyal to Hua and Ye and who had previously been guards for Zhou Enlai. Four other officers stood hidden behind a nearby screen in the room to render assistance, if necessary. Zhang Chunqiao arrived at the Western Hills next and he was arrested with no trouble; the same applied to Yao Wenyuan. For Jiang Qing, however, security forces went to her home in the Western Hills and arrested her. After a struggle, she was brought to Hua and Ye, who formally charged her with "usurping the power of the state and the Party" and placed her in confinement. Mao Yuanxin was apprehended by PLA troops after an effort to flee the country.[34]

The question which Tom Gates and his fellow American China-watchers faced after assembling these two accounts involve the reliability and accuracy of each version. On that point, no simple answer existed, although USLO's officers did notice that, in the weeks following the arrest of the Gang of Four, the Hua regime repeatedly emphasized that it "had smashed the Gang [of Four] in one blow." Such an assertion tended to give more weight to the first account since it provided that the Hua regime had arrested all four of the leftists at one time during the first Politburo meeting on the night of October 6. But, in fairness to the cloudiness of the historical record, one must admit that a *single* correct version may never emerge, especially since the full story remains in the minds of a small number of Chinese leaders.

In any event, Hua Guofeng convened the full Politburo again on the morning of October 7 to report on the arrests of the four radicals. Present at this meeting were Hua Guofeng, Ye Jianying, Li Xiannian, Wang Dongxing, Chen Xilian, Ji Dengkui, Chen Yonggui, Su Zhenhua, an alternate Politburo member and PLA officer who commanded the PLA Navy, and Wu Kuixian, in addition to several provincial first secretaries and military region commanders.[35] According to published reports of this meeting, Hua and Wang each delivered two reports, and Ye delivered one, to the assemblage. Each of the reports detailed the schemes of the Gang of Four and outlined the reasons for prompt action by the Party Center against the leftists.[36] In response, the Politburo then agreed to appoint Hua to two positions of great authority, chairman of the Party Central Committee and also chairman of the Military Commission. Whether Hua believed that this extra-constitutional grant of power was intended as a permanent, or merely temporary, circumstance remains a matter of conjecture.[37] Without question, however, the Politburo defied its constitutional powers by naming Hua Guofeng as the successor to Mao Zedong without first convening a plenum of the Chinese Communist Party and then securing a vote of the CCP's Central Committee on the leadership question.

The arrest of the Gang of Four on the night of October 6, and the Politburo's action in conferring extraordinary powers upon Hua Guofeng on October 7, hardly solved all the problems which the Hua-Ye coalition faced in consolidating its power. The main concern of the moderate and neo-Maoist group which took power in China on October 6–7 involved the reaction in Shanghai to the overthrow of the leftists. How would the radicals' supporters in Shanghai respond when they learned about the imprisonment of their leaders in Peking? Would the Gang of Four's municipal supporters in Shanghai passively accept the Hua regime's actions? On good authority, both Hua and Ye knew that the members of the Gang of Four had established an elaborate code designed to alert their Shanghainese colleagues should trouble befall them in the capital. Ma Tianshui, Xu Jiangxian, and Wang Xiuzhen, the leaders of Shanghai's Party organization and the Gang's closest associates in the city, had all been urged to "be prepared for fighting" if events in the capital turned against the leftists.

The method devised by Hua Guofeng and Ye Jianying to defuse a potentially explosive situation in Shanghai between October 8 and October 15 inevitably leads to a fourth question regarding the purge of the Gang of Four. Specifically, how did the Hua regime isolate the radicals' supporters in Shanghai and thereby avert what might have become outright civil war in China? In retrospect, it has now become clear that Hua and Ye skillfully avoided a civil insurrection in Shanghai by implementing three measures. First, Ye dispatched the loyal General Xu Shiyou to Shanghai on the night of October 8 to assume command of the Nanjing military region (of which Shanghai was a part) from General Ding Sheng, whose loyalty to the Center was considered questionable. Xu Shiyou was one of China's acknowledged military strongmen, as well as a man of considerable physical ferocity who was an acknowledged foe of the leftists. When Xu arrived at the headquarters of the Nanjing military region, he and Ding reportedly quarreled over the nature of his orders. Ding apparently insisted on his right to remain in military command of the region and resisted Xu's efforts to take away his authority. A quarrel between the two men followed, and one account of the dispute claimed that Xu shot and killed Ding as a result of their disagreement. The USLO's officers, however, later received information that while Ding had been stripped of his command, he was still alive in another region of China. Whatever the actual circumstances, neither Xu Shiyou, nor the anti-radical leadership in Peking, was taking any chances when they moved on Shanghai that evening. On the night of October 6, the Center had posted six PLA divisions around Shanghai, in the event that the Shanghai militia attempted to occupy the city.[38]

Second, Hua Guofeng and Ye Jianying adopted another measure designed to isolate the three Shanghai leaders, Ma Tianshui, Xu Jiangxian, and Wang Xiuzhen, from their followers in the belief that the best way to prevent violence in the city was to keep their enemies divided and uncertain. Both Roger Garside and Ross Terrill have written excellent accounts of how Hua and Ye summoned first Ma, and then Xu and Wang, to Peking between October 8 and October 12 and informed the three Shanghainese of the moderate takeover of the PRC. In addition, they also wrung from the three leftists the information about the preparations which the radicals had made in

Shanghai to resist the moderates in Peking. Such information was well known to both Ye Jianying and Hua Guofeng. In fact, Hua appeared unconcerned about these preparations but emphasized that the three Shanghainese must now return to their city and follow the dictates of the Party Center. "We have trust in you," Hua observed to Ma, Xu, and Wang.[39]

Leaderless, the leftist supporters of Ma Tianshui, Xu Jiangxian, and Wang Xiuzhen who remained behind in Shanghai could not decide whether to mobilize the urban militia in a violent challenge to the Party Center or simply admit to being outmaneuvered in a political showdown. Finally, Ma, Xu, and Wang returned to Shanghai from Peking on October 13 and informed their colleagues of the futility of resisting the Hua-Ye coalition in the capital. In return for their own freedom, the three Shanghai leaders had assured Hua and Ye that their city would not oppose the arrests of the Gang of Four: "We've switched sides, you might want to do the same."[40]

Third, the arrest of the Gang of Four in Peking also spelled the end of the political careers of their Shanghainese colleagues. Between October 8 and October 12, the Hua-Ye coalition had effectively preshrunk Ma, Xu, and Wang, and on October 21, it dispatched three of its supporters, Su Zhenhua, the commander of the PLA Navy who also attended the October 7 meeting in Peking; Ni Zhifu, another alternate Politburo member; and Peng Chong, the Party's first secretary in Jiangsu province, to assume control of Shanghai's Party operations. Su Zhenhua was the pivotal figure for the Party Center in Shanghai, an individual like Marshall Ye who possessed few illusions about the leftists and the lengths to which they might go to prevent their demise. Like Chen Xilian and Wang Dongxing, Su had also been courted by the leftists, and they hoped to bring him into their camp before undertaking the coup attempt against the Hua regime. Su realized that radical influence in Shanghai extended well beyond Mao Tianshui, Xu Jiangxian, and Wang Xiuzhen and their immediate supporters. In that regard, he bluntly informed the three Shanghainese leaders that he would guarantee their safety only if they submitted exactly to the Center's directives. Facing a hopeless situation and realizing their own unpopularity with Shanghai's urban masses, Ma, Xu, and Wang quietly accepted Su's instructions. As Tom later learned, however, Xu Jiangxian and Wang Xiuzhen did encounter harassment from the masses in China once they appeared in public after the overthrow of the Gang. Ma Tianshui's misdeeds as a radical supporter cost him his office and status in Shanghai but not his membership in the Party.[41]

Finally, Roger Garside has written that the putative leftist rebellion to the moderates in Peking ended "not with a bang, but with a whimper."[42] Undoubtedly the fact that Shanghai had not erupted in full-scale revolt came as a relief to the Party Center, although it may also have been something of a surprise. Before the Party Center's takeover of Shanghai, Su Zhenhua had calculated that the odds strongly favored a large-scale disturbance in the city. He considered it certain that the Party Center would encounter at least some organized resistance to its actions. Indeed, he was astonished that the Center succeeded in overwhelming its radical opponents in Shanghai with so little difficulty. The Gang of Four's power base in Shanghai was not as secure as the leftists believed, and as a result, the leftists and their supporters acted in a confused and tentative way when confronted with a prompt assertion of authority by the Center. For that reason, Su later reported to the Politburo that (fortunately for China), Shanghai had submitted to the Party Center without the loss of a single drop of blood.[43] Virtually none of the radicals' sympathizers in Shanghai, nor any of its presumed supporters in the PLA and the municipal Party organization, had sprung to their defense.[44]

Instead of protesting the arrest of the radicals, the Chinese in Shanghai went on a week-long celebration of the leftists' misfortunes, beginning on October 15 and ending on October 21 with a giant rally in the center of the city. With official word of Hua's elevation, the Shanghainese now enjoyed the sanction to revel in the Gang's downfall. Ordinary Chinese paraded through the streets in a great release of emotional energy. The streets were choked with people; vehicles were unable to move through the crowds. Posters and banners appeared by the hundreds all over Shanghai, including ones which were plastered to the walls on the Bund, some reaching up several stories in height. Many of the posters were especially strident in tone, including one memorable production which depicted an image repeated in dozens of other posters—that of a fist crushing opponents. The image revealed a fist with the Gang of Four, one face to a knuckle, being pounded into the ground. Foreigners in Shanghai recalled witnessing a carnival-like atmosphere in the city as the jubilant Shanghainese rejoiced over the purge of the leftists. As one Chinese remarked to a foreign journalist: "This [purge] is not at all a bad thing; it is a good phenomenon. In a communist society, there is always class struggle."[45] In the same vein, Tom later heard a Chinese diplomat describe his lack of surprise at the failure of the masses in Shanghai to rush to the support of the Gang of Four. In fact, the citizens of Shanghai welcomed the overthrow of the four radicals at least as much as did the rest of the Chinese people.[46]

III

On October 17, after completing the imprisonment of the Gang of Four and subduing the leftist leadership in Shanghai, the regime of Hua Guofeng took its anti-leftist campaign to the PRC media. On that day, two extremely strong-worded articles appeared in the *People's Daily*, both calling for the "utter eradication of 'pests' and 'vermin' within the Party." While the authors of the articles did not identify the names of the "pests" and "vermin," few of their readers were confused about the targets of the two pieces.[47] The same day, an article also appeared in the *Liberation Army Daily* which called upon the Chinese to "Persist in the Principle of the Three Dos and Three Don'ts." In a tone reminiscent of future charges brought against the Gang of Four, the author of this article referred to the radicals as "capitalist roaders [a charge which astonished the diplomatic community] who practiced revisionism, splittism, intrigues, and conspiracy." The writer of the article, Xie Zhunping (a pseudonym) also charged the Gang with fomenting a plot to split the loyalties of the PLA, a charge almost certainly true.[48]

The poster activity and the spontaneous celebrations in Peking, Shanghai, and China's other cities, combined with the sense of relief which the Chinese felt over the purge of the Gang of Four, led up to a giant rally which the Hua regime scheduled in the capital for the four days beginning on October 21. One report from Shanxi province characterized the exuberance then experienced by the Chinese people.

The whole country is in fervent celebration and the people are in great joy. In the past few days, the people of our province have fervently celebrated the appointment of Comrade Hua Guofeng as Chairman of the Central Committee of the Chinese Communist Party and Chairman of the Military Commission and fervently hailed the smashing of the conspiracy of the Gang of Four, the anti-Party clique, to usurp the Party and seize power. Some 19,000,000 [people] have staged rallies and processions. The scale is grand and unprecedented, fully proving that the Party Centre with Chairman Hua Guofeng as the head is connected in heart with the people, that the masses infinitely trust and wholeheartedly love Chairman Hua Guofeng, the Party's own leader, that Wang, Zhang, Jiang, and Yao, the Gang of Four, are harmful pests, and the elimination of the four pests makes everyone happy.[49]

On October 21, the Chinese in Peking began preparing for a four-day festival celebrating the downfall of the Gang of Four. In a year noted for its great rallies, this anti-Gang festival promised to be a particular highlight of the Year of the Dragon. The rally was designed to culminate on October 24 when the Party Center intended to reveal the formal charges against the Gang of Four and continue its effort to organize the Chinese people against leftist cadres and supporters within the Party. By 11 o'clock on the morning of October 21, tens of thousands of Chinese began marching by units into Tienanmen Square. Several of the USLO's officers who had been in Peking during the previous spring remarked that the scene in Tienanmen Square reminded them of the large rally in April organized by the leftists to confirm the purge of Deng Xiaoping. One striking difference, however, was apparent between the October rally and the one in April. Instead of a coercive, somber atmosphere in the city, Peking was alive with exuberance, verve, and genuine enthusiasm. Animatedly pounding their drums and waving enormous red banners, the marchers snake-danced around the square. Foreigners who ventured near the area of the demonstrations received smiles and friendly waves of greeting from the obviously jubilant Chinese.

Numerous stories also circulated in Peking regarding countless victims of the Cultural Revolution who had committed themselves to mental institutions during the early 1970s to escape the radicals' wrath and who now, after the arrest of the Gang of Four, found themselves miraculously cured. One story was told of Yu Jiuli, a major Party official targeted by the Gang, who entered a sanitarium in Peking in the early 1970s and then was transferred to a similar institution in Guangdong shortly thereafter. Upon learning that the Gang was imprisoned, he immediately doffed his hospital gown and returned to Peking to join in the celebration. "The Gang is in prison. I am recovered!" Yu exclaimed.[50]

As one gazed out over the spectacle, it became apparent that virtually every organization in Peking had selected a contingent to represent it at Tienanmen Square. PLA units continued to pour into the city on October 21 while schoolchildren were bused and factory workers marched into the center of the city. Each unit carried an identifying banner: groups from the Foreign Ministry, Peking University, and the Bureau of Public Security were all observed at the center of the action. Each also carried a picture of Mao Zedong; some held brightly colored banners hailing Hua's appointment to the two chairmanships. Other banners were more direct, condemning by name the "four-person, anti-Party clique of Wang, Zhang, Jiang, and Yao" for their "criminal" acts. Peking was obviously preparing for a long rally since, as with Mao's funeral, workers were observed installing portable public latrines.[51]

On October 21, the first day of the formal anti-Gang demonstrations, the Party Center again took its case against the radicals to the media as the means to explain the official, accepted rationale for the purge of the radicals. That day, the New China News Agency formally identified Hua Guofeng as the chairman of the Party Central Committee and also the Military Commission. The report described Hua's appointments as a "wise decision" made by Chairman Mao himself before his death. By contrast, the same report identified the Gang of Four as a group of plotters who "tried to usurp Party and state power," and confirmed the necessity for their arrests.[52] This charge, that the Gang had plotted to usurp Party and state power, became the centerpiece of the Hua regime's attempt to discredit the leftists, an accusation which the Chinese people were to hear continuously for the next six months.

By October 22, Tom Gates and his fellow American China-watchers estimated that approximately 1.5 million celebrants had crowded into Tienanmen Square. A steady drizzle throughout the day failed to dampen the spirits of the enormous throng of people; smiles, horseplay, vigorous drumming, and flag waving all continued uninterrupted. More and more posters appeared throughout the city, condemning the Gang for "scheming to seize the highest power in the Party" as well as "opposing Chairman Mao's revolutionary line in foreign and domestic affairs."[53] Tom detected a clearly ominous and menacing change in the tone of the anti-Gang posters and banners, however, as each day seemed to produce ever more threatening messages. Few observers could doubt that the posters and banners represented a signal by the Hua regime to its leftist enemies that "the rage of the masses" (as the Center informed Ma Tianshui, Xu Jiangxian, and Wang Xiuzhen on October 21) was directed against them.[54]

On October 24, Peking completed its plans for the huge anti-Gang rally. A crowd estimated at one million people gathered in Tienanmen Square to continue the denunciation of the radicals. The PRC hierarchy gathered in public to acknowledge the cheers of its people. Despite the fact that Hua Guofeng was now undeniably the supreme authority in the PRC, he failed to behave at the rally as one who was fully in control of his environment. He wore a military uniform, for the first time that anyone could recall, but the uniform signalled the degree of importance which he attributed to the PLA in the events of the past two months and, specifically, the past two weeks. Moreover, as Hua walked along the balcony of the Gate of Heavenly Peace to receive the acclaim of the people, he was followed in close step by Ye Jianying and Li Xiannian, two individuals definitely not associated with the neo-Maoist faction. As Roger Garside has noted, the "moves of Ye and Li were planned in China and signal messages that no one is prepared to put into print."[55] The message conveyed by Ye and Li appeared to leave the impression that China was entering a period of collective leadership despite the fact that Hua held the major posts in the state and Party.

More important, Hua Guofeng not only did not present the major address at the rally as he had on the occasion of Mao's funeral six weeks earlier, but he did not speak at all. The responsibility for presenting the Party Center's official condemnation of the Gang of Four fell to Wu De, the mayor of Peking and a vice premier and member of the Politburo, and considered one of Hua's fellow neo-Maoists. In his address, Wu De clearly minced no words in excoriating the leftists.

[China] lost our great leader and teacher Chairman Mao Zedong one and a half months ago. The whole Party, the whole Army, and the people of all nationalities were plunged into tremendous grief, anxious about the future and destiny of the Party and of the state, anxious about whether the Chinese Communist Party could carry out Chairman Mao's wishes. At that time, there was indeed a dark cloud in the sky over our country. While Chairman Mao was seriously ill and after he passed away, the anti-Party clique of Wang Hongwen, Zhang Chunqiao, Jiang Qing, and Yao Wenyuan hastily grasped at opportunities and attempted to usurp top Party and

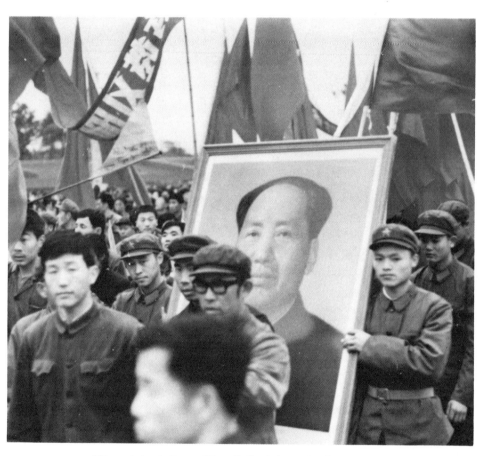

Chinese at anti–Gang of Four Rally, Peking, October 24, 1976.

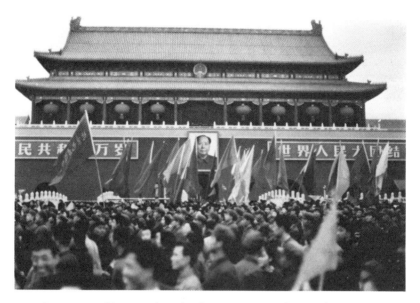

Chinese assembling in Peking for the anti–Gang Rally, October 24, 1976.

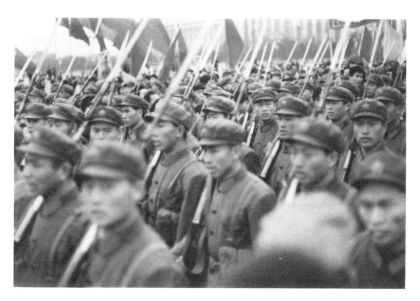

PLA soldiers marching in anti–Gang Rally, Peking, October 24, 1976.

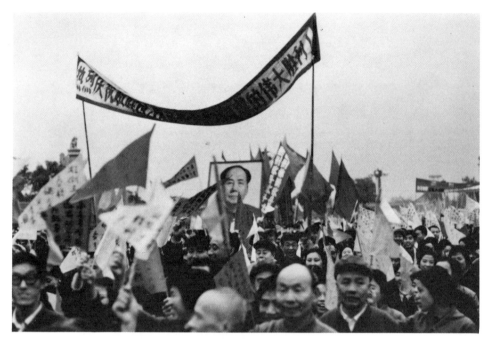

Chinese marching with flags and banners at the anti–Gang Rally, Peking, October 24, 1976.

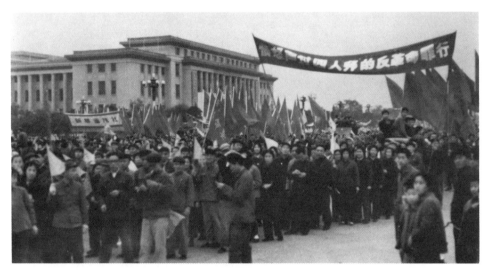

Chinese assembling in Peking for the anti–Gang Rally, October 24, 1976.

state leadership. We were confronted with the real danger of our Party turning revisionist and our country changing its political color. Our Party was in a moment of grave difficulty. In this life and death struggle between the two classes, the two roads, and two lines, our Party has emerged triumphant, the proletariat has emerged triumphant, and the people have emerged triumphant. [The people must] firmly support the October 7, 1976 resolution of the Central Committee of the Chinese Communist Party on the appointment of Comrade Hua Guofeng as Chairman of the Chinese Communist Party and the Military Commission. Comrade Hua Guofeng was selected by our great leader Chairman Mao himself as his successor. Chairman Mao himself personally proposed Comrade Hua Guofeng for the post of first vice premier of the Chinese Communist Party and Premier of the State Council in April, 1976. Then on April 30, Chairman Mao wrote to Comrade Hua Guofeng in his own handwriting, "With you in charge, I'm at ease," which expressed his boundless trust in Comrade Hua Guofeng. The course of events in the struggle against the Gang of Four shows what a wise decision Chairman Mao made.[56]

After his speech extolling Hua Guofeng, Wu De continued with the standard castigation of the Gang. According to Wu, the radicals had "wantonly tampered with Marxist-Leninist-Mao Zedong thought," they "plotted and conspired tirelessly," and tried to "usurp the supreme leadership of the Party and state."[57] Then with no small irony, Wu tarred the radicals with the same brush which they used on Deng Xiaoping.

Chairman Mao pointed out "You are making the socialist revolution and yet don't know where the bourgeoisie is. It is right in the Communist Party—those in power taking the capitalist road. The capitalist roaders are still on the capitalist road." The actions of the Wang-Zhang-Jiang-Yao clique proved that they are typical representatives of the bourgeoisie inside the Party, unrepentant capitalist roaders still traveling on the capitalist road and a gang of bourgeois conspirators and careerists. We must thoroughly expose and repudiate the anti-Party clique of Wang Hongwen, Zhang Chunqiao, Jiang Qing, and Yao Wenyuan.[58]

The castigation of the Gang of Four as "capitalist roaders" created no small amount of confusion in the minds of many foreign observers, although the Chinese seemed not at all concerned about such an obvious contradiction. One American businessman who was visiting a trade exhibition in China during the time of the Gang's arrest and criticism asked one Chinese official to explain the fact that, since the "four pests" had attacked Deng Xiaoping as a rightist and they were acknowledged leftists, how could it be that they themselves were now accused of being "capitalist roaders"? The official blandly replied that the answer was simple: "Deng Xiaoping was openly a rightist whereas the Gang of Four were secretly rightist." Such an answer did little, presumably, to clarify the situation.[59]

After Wu De's speech, various other speakers addressed the throng including representatives from the peasants and the workers, a member of the Red Guards(!), and a PLA soldier. Without a doubt, if the Hua regime intended the day to be a celebration of the Gang's errors and crimes, it succeeded fabulously in finding a crowd willing to rejoice with it. Watching these festivities, however, we were reminded of humorist Russell Baker's comment that "The election campaign now being held in China is quite different" from the Ford-Carter presidential campaign. Unlike the Americans, the Chinese seemed to have held the election first and saved the campaign for later.[60]

IV

In summarizing the impact of the purges of October upon China during the Year of the Dragon, one must note several points. First, the arrests were not simply the Hua regime's method of dealing forcefully with four of its political enemies. The arrests which occurred on the night of October 6–7 revealed the intense dislike within China of both the Gang of Four and their supporters throughout the country. The arrests, in fact, signalled the beginning of a national campaign to purge the extreme leftists from a future role in the Party. Ye Jianying, Hua Guofeng, and Wang Dongxing moved not only against the members of the Gang of Four but also against a dozen of their close followers in Peking and at least five hundred of their provincial supporters. Furthermore, the PLA took effective control of both Peking and Qinghua universities in another obvious attempt to forestall any resistance to the Center's roundup of the radicals.

Second, Hua Guofeng obviously sought to use the arrests of the Gang of Four as a means of legitimizing himself with the Chinese masses. After the Hua regime had "used" Mao's instructions as the device to bring down its enemies, so also it invoked the chairman's name in advancing its own interests by promoting a new theme of unity within the PRC. Hua's propaganda always presented his elevation as a part of Mao's specific behests and identified the four radicals as conspirators against the policies of the late chairman. On October 25, for example, a joint editorial appeared in the *People's Daily, Red Flag,* and *Liberation Army Daily* which affirmed Hua's elevation as a conscious effort by Mao himself and also attacked the "conspiratorial" activities of the Gang of Four. Citing Mao's warnings to the radicals which occurred as early as 1974, the editorial maintained that Mao had repeatedly admonished the four leftists to mend their ways. Interestingly enough, Mao himself coined the term "Gang of Four" by warning Jiang Qing and her three Shanghainese cohorts not to "act as a Gang of Four." Apparently they disregarded his advice, and before his death, Mao warned Jiang Qing about the tragedy which awaited her. "In the last ten years, I tried to teach the Chinese about revolution, but I was not successful," Mao allegedly wrote his estranged wife. "If you reach for the top and fail, you will fall into an abyss. Your body will shatter, and your bones will break."[61]

Third, the arrest of the Gang of Four in October appeared to bring about a new spirit of optimism within China. At last, the Chinese must have reasoned, someone of sufficient power had effectively disposed of the four "pests." The USLO received one report that over nineteen million people participated in organized, anti-leftist demonstrations in the PRC between October 21 and October 24. Tom noticed a great feeling of relief on the part of many Chinese diplomats in Peking as well. He also heard reports that several PRC embassies throughout the Far East had thrown their own parties when they learned of the radicals' purge from Peking. Many Chinese officials in Peking could not contain their elation. Certainly the American China-watchers in Peking had not witnessed such a phenomenon before in China. Normally uncommunicative employees and acquaintances were bursting with unflattering opinions about the Gang, and some were freely expressing their respect for Deng Xiaoping.[62] The Chinese seemed to sense that the PRC had at last buried the Cultural Revolution and could look forward to a period of security, stability, and even sanity. Some Chinese even expressed the thought they had not felt so relaxed since 1964.[63]

Fourth, the arrest of the Gang of Four still did not resolve the doubts which Tom and his USLO colleagues still held about the leadership capacity of Hua Guofeng. True, Hua had revealed himself as a sensitive politician whose talents the Gang considerably underestimated. True, at a critical point in his fortunes during the first week of October, Hua had shown himself to be both tough and decisive, even ruthless. And true, Hua had revealed himself as one who could build a consensus for his continued leadership of the PRC, even if that consensus centered chiefly on deposing the Gang of Four.

After one conceded those points, however, making an assessment of Hua Guofeng's ability became more difficult. With the Gang of Four in prison, the PRC appeared ready to embark upon a national program similar to the Four Modernizations outlined by Zhou Enlai, with economic modernization and political stability as key ingredients of that policy. A program of Zhou-ization, however, meant that Deng Xiaoping might possibly return to power, a prospect which Hua must have found unsettling. But Hua himself lacked a political program, except to present himself as the heir of the departed Mao Zedong.

Furthermore, in the weeks immediately after the Gang's purge, USLO officials noticed some subtle hints that Hua Guofeng's popular following may have shrunk considerably since Mao Zedong's death. For example, the fact that Hua did not address the Chinese people at the anti-Gang rally on October 24 seemed peculiar, especially since he clearly occupied center stage at Mao's funeral. No cheers of "Long Live Chairman Hua" emanated from the crowds, either, although he did receive polite cheers from the masses as he greeted them. More important, virtually all the Chinese diplomats with whom Tom and other USLO officials spoke regarding Mao's succession invariably referred to a power-sharing arrangement involving the Central Committee and Hua Guofeng, a definite signal that the Party had sharply limited Hua's authority. Since at least October 9, for instance, Li Xiannian always spoke of "the Central Committee led by Comrade Hua Guofeng" in referring to the current leadership situation in China. Hua Guofeng clearly was Mao's immediate successor; Hua clearly did not inherit Mao's immense powers.[64]

Fifth, how then does one make an accurate interpretation of the manner in which Ye Jianying, Hua Guofeng, Wang Dongxing, and their supporters deposed the Gang of Four? Tom Gates interpreted the purges primarily as a preemptive military coup staged by Ye and his supporters, supported by moderate civilians, against their common enemy, the radicals. Almost a month after the arrest of the Gang, one PLA officer was asked to speculate on the army's role in the purge of the leftists. "The PLA is totally obedient to the leadership of the Communist Party and the leadership of the Party directed the arrest of the Shanghai Four," the officer declared. Then when asked what the army would have done if the Gang had attempted to seize control of the leadership, the officer responded immediately that "the Army would have arrested them anyhow. The Shanghai Four were revisionists according to Mao's correct line."[65]

In that fashion, Hua Guofeng served as a willing collaborator with the PLA in the ouster of the radicals but hardly as the behind-the-scenes manipulator of the purge. Quite clearly, Ye Jianying, Xu Shiyou (and probably Deng Xiaoping), and other leading military commanders had planned the action against the leftists for some time and launched it before the Gang could gather its full strength throughout the country. Seen in that way, both Hua and the PLA had something the other wanted. Hua needed the support of the military in order to counter the challenge of the leftists. For the PLA, Hua represented legitimacy and, in a sense, continuity with the Maoist tradition that "the Party controls the gun." To the military, however, Hua was probably little more than a cosmetic necessity, the civilian leader necessary to keep their action from being viewed simply as a naked grab for power. No doubt, Hua's past experience with the PLA and the Party's internal security apparatus served him well when the moment for decision arrived in early October. What remains unclear is the price which the PLA exacted from Hua in return for his cooperation with their plans. For example, the PLA later showed its strength in early November when Hua announced that Ye would head the commission appointed to examine the crimes of the Gang of Four. With its prizes well in hand, the PLA seemed to want to make certain that they would not lose them.

Thus, with the arrests of the radicals, Hua Guofeng's place in the PRC's political environment changed abruptly. No longer did he serve as the balance wheel between the moderate and radical civilian factions in the hierarchy but instead as the mediator between the civilian survivors of October and the PLA.[66] After the purges of October, however, civilian influence in the hierarchy had declined considerably.

Finally, how does one account for the Gang of Four's swift descent from the pinnacle of authority in the People's Republic? Mao's death certainly deprived the leftists of the protection necessary to maintain their status against the concerted efforts of their enemies. Beyond that fact, however, lay several other reasons. First, the Gang proved to be no match politically for their foes. They clearly underestimated Hua Guofeng's determination to remain in power, and obsessed as they were by power and revenge, they seriously miscalculated in believing that their control of the media, a modest level of PLA support in north China, and the urban militia in Shanghai were any match for the armed might of PLA forces opposed to them. In particular, Zhang Chunqiao failed to exploit his leadership of the PLA's General Political Department (GPD) into a political base within the military. After becoming director of the GPD in January, 1975, for example, Zhang moved very cautiously in placing any of his protégés into key positions, thereby forfeiting an opportunity to gain effective control of the organization. In fact, most of the individuals which Zhang appointed, such as Liang Biye who became the GPD's deputy director, were rehabilitated military officers and civilians. Moreover, it became clear in hindsight that moderate PLA officers were wary of Zhang and blocked any attempts on his part to control the GPD's security apparatus. These moderate officers within the GPD gravitated quickly to the support of Hua Guofeng after the death of Zhou, the ouster of Deng, and the death of Mao.[67]

Indeed, the radicals' control of the media may have deceived them and millions of other people in China that the Gang of Four's strength was considerably greater than it was in fact. The radicals may also have believed that they deserved the right to govern China since they represented the most sophisticated and economically advanced region in China, a fact which mattered not a bit to their enemies.[68]

In conclusion, the purges of October represented the logical end to the efforts by Jiang Qing and her Shanghainese cohorts to preserve radical rule in China. By November 1976, political events in China had come almost full circle from those of the previous year. At the beginning of 1976, the leftists had gained access to a sick and apparently manipulable Mao Zedong, only to misuse their influence by attempting to banish Deng Xiaoping to the political wilderness. Instead, Mao surprised his followers and critics in the Politburo by appointing Hua Guofeng as Zhou Enlai's successor. In March, the leftists pressed the campaign against Zhou's memory. That action led to the Tienanmen riots during the Qing Ming festival in April, which proved to be a decisive setback for the radicals as anger against them spread throughout China. Not only did the leftists fail to remove Deng Xiaoping from his membership in the Party, but they also discovered that pragmatist influence in the Politburo, characterized principally by Ye Jianying and Li Xiannian, grew steadily throughout the spring and early summer. By mid-summer, it became apparent to the radicals that Hua Guofeng held the upper hand, and the PLA the balance of power. By the end of the summer, Hua had strengthened himself even further by his decisive action during the earthquake emergency and his leadership of the national observation for Mao's funeral and mourning period.[69]

In the final analysis, it was somewhat irrelevant whether the Gang of Four attempted a coup against the Hua regime or simply got trapped in a political showdown. As Tom later explained, "Hua moved and arrested the Gang of Four. It was his coup against theirs. [Hua's] action averted civil war, which came closer to being a reality than most people would ever know, maybe within hours."[70] Hua Guofeng was Mao's political successor, regardless of the political processes, or lack thereof, involved in his selection. Once the action started on the night of October 6–7, Hua and the leadership of the PLA acted with resolve and dispatch. The purges of October thereby eliminated the leading members of the Cultural Revolutionary left from the PRC's leadership elite, a development which contributed to a certain measure of political stability in the country during the last two months of 1976. Certainly the outburst of popular enthusiasm in China which greeted the arrest of the "four pests" confirmed Tom's belief that the Chinese would never have accepted radical rule after Mao's death. In fact, these arrests showed how delicate China's political environment had been before October since it required the combined efforts of the military-bureaucratic complex and the secret police Left to end the radicals' careers.[71]

Once Hua Guofeng had disposed of the radical threat, however, he discovered that he still had no time for relaxation. If anything, a more complex set of political challenges awaited him once the anti-Gang of Four rally ended in Tienanmen Square on October 24.

Notes

1. Interview, David Dean, 9 February 1983.
2. United States Department of State, Official Files, September–October, 1976 (hereafter cited as OF, date); OF, Peking to Washington, 9 October 1976.
3. Ibid.; see also interview, David Dean, 9 February 1983.
4. OF, Peking to Washington, 9 October 1976.
5. OF, Peking to Washington, 10 October 1976.
6. OF, Peking to Washington, 10 October 1976.

7. Ibid.

8. OF, Peking to Washington, 11 October 1976; OF, Peking to Washington, 12 October 1976.

9. OF, Peking to Washington, 14 October 1976.

10. OF, Peking to Washington, 12 October 1976.

11. OF, Peking to Washington, 13 October 1976.

12. OF, Peking to Washington, 13 October 1976.

13. OF, Peking to Washington, 13 October 1976; OF, Peking to Washington, 20 October 1976.

14. OF, Peking to Washington, 22 October 1976.

15. Thomas S. Gates Oral History, 1 January 1979. Hereafter cited as Gates OH, date.

16. See, for example, Garside, *Coming Alive,* pp. 142–67; Hsu, *China Without Mao,* pp. 3–25; Terrill, *Future of China,* pp. 110–40; and Roxane Witke, *Comrade Chiang Ching* (Boston: Little, Brown, 1977), pp. 471–77.

17. Interview, David Dean, 9 February 1983; White, "Burnout of a Revolution," pp. 32–33; Domes, "The 'Gang of Four' and Hua Kuo-feng," pp. 486–88.

18. OF, Peking to Washington, September–October, 1976; OF, Peking to Washington, 22 October 1976; OF, Peking to Washington, 28 October 1976; Peking to Washington, 19 January 1977; Terrill, *White-Boned Demon,* p. 363.

19. OF, Peking to Washington, 22 December 1976.

20. OF, Peking to Washington, 14 February 1977; Hsu, *China Without Mao,* p. 14; Terrill, *White-Boned Demon,* p. 364.

21. OF, Peking to Washington, 22 October 1976; White, "Six Who Rule—and Remember," *Time,* 26 September 1983, pp. 42–43. See also Harrison E. Salisbury, "The Little Man Who Could Never Be Put Down," *Time,* September 30, 1985, pp. 54–57. This article is excerpted from Salisbury's *The Long March: The Untold Story* (New York: Harper and Row, 1985).

22. Parris Chang, "The Rise of Wang Tung-hsing: Head of China's Security Apparatus," *China Quarterly* 73 (March 1978): 122–36.

23. OF, Peking to Washington, 10 February; Terrill, *White-Boned Demon,* pp. 366–67.

24. OF, Peking to Washington, 10 October 1976; OF, Peking to Washington, 25 March 1977.

25. Garside, *Coming Alive,* pp. 155–61; Hsu, *China Without Mao,* pp. 16–19; Terrill, *Future of China,* pp. 114–17.

26. OF, Peking to Washington, 22 October 1976.

27. Ibid.

28. Fox Butterfield, "China Posters Link Left to Killing Plot," *New York Times,* 31 October 1976, p. 7.

29. Terrill, *Future of China,* p. 112; *White-Boned Demon,* p. 371.

30. Garside, *Coming Alive,* p. 153.

31. Hsu, *China Without Mao,* p. 153. See also Salisbury, *100 Years of Revolution,* pp. 249–51.

32. White, "Burnout of a Revolution," pp. 32–33.

33. OF, Peking to Washington, 22 October 1976; OF, Peking to Washington, 1976–77; OF, Peking to Washington, 20 December 1976; OF, Peking to Washington, 19 January 1977.

34. OF, Peking to Washington, 19 January 1977.

35. OF, Peking to Washington, 21 October 1976; Hsu, *China Without Mao,* p. 14; Onate, "Hua Kuo-feng," pp. 561–65.

36. Onate, "Hua Kuo-feng," pp. 561–65.

37. OF, Tokyo to Peking, 17 November 1976.

38. OF, Peking to Washington, 8 March 1977; OF, Peking to Washington, 22 October 1976; OF, Peking to Washington, 12 January 1977; Garside, *Coming Alive,* p. 164; Domes, "Hua Kuo-feng," pp. 556–57. Because Ding Sheng apparently survived his quarrel with Xu Shiyou on October 8 does not necessarily mean that a physical confrontation did not occur between the two men. Xu was noted for being a particularly volatile and violent man, yet an

individual who loved his troops and was idolized by them. As a youth, Xu had mastered the martial arts and his displays of physical strength and prowess were admired by his soldiers. See Yin Zhihui, "The 'Wushu General,'" *China Reconstructs* 32, no. 12 (December 1983): 55–58.

39. Garside, *Coming Alive*, p. 163.

40. OF, Peking to Washington, 3 November 1976.

41. OF, Peking to Washington, 21 October 1976.

42. OF, Peking to Washington, 3 November 1976; Garside, *Coming Alive*, pp. 157–63; Salisbury, *100 Years of Revolution*, pp. 248–51.

43. OF, Peking to Washington, 2 November 1976; OF, Peking to Washington, 26 October 1976; OF, Peking to Washington, 23 May 1977.

44. Fox Butterfield, "Inheritor of Mao's Title," *New York Times*, 13 October 1976, pp. 1, 11, 12.

45. OF, Peking to Washington, 16 October 1976; OF, Peking to Washington, 29 November 1976.

46. OF, Peking to Washington, September–October, 1976.

47. OF, Peking to Washington, 18 October 1976.

48. OF, Peking to Washington, 21 October 1976.

49. OF, Peking to Washington, 27 October 1976.

50. OF, Peking to Washington, 25 January 1977.

51. Ibid.

52. OF, Peking to Washington, 22 October 1976.

53. Ibid.

54. Garside, *Coming Alive*, p. 171.

55. Ibid.

56. OF, Peking to Washington, 24 October 1976.

57. Ibid.

58. Ibid.

59. OF, USLO-Peking, W. W. Thomas to T. S. Brooks, 4 November 1976.

60. Russell Baker, "Campaign Upside Down," *New York Times*, 19 October 1976, p. 35.

61. OF, Peking to Washington, 26 October 1976; Terrill, *Future of China*, p. 121; idem, *White-Boned Demon*, p. 363.

62. OF, Peking to Washington, 1976–77.

63. Ibid.

64. OF, Peking to Washington, 26 October 1976.

65. OF, Peking to Washington, 1976–77; OF, Peking to Washington, 3 November 1976.

66. OF, Peking to Washington, 3 November 1976.

67. OF, Peking to Washington, December 1976.

68. OF, Peking to Washington, 1976–77.

69. Ibid.; OF, Peking to Washington, 20 December 1976.

70. Gates OH, 1 January 1979.

71. Domes, "The 'Gang of Four' and Hua Kuo-feng," pp. 486–88.

CHAPTER **6**

A New Environment

Following the arrest of the Gang of Four in October, the People's Republic of China underwent a crucial six-month period which tested its political stability. Between November 1976 and May 1977, the Chinese leadership, nominally headed by Hua Guofeng, faced the enormous task of unifying the nation and consolidating its power within a completely different political environment, one without the strong voice of the extreme Left. Complicating the Party Center's work was the bitter factionalism which had existed in China's provinces throughout most of 1975–76, a tension which increased after Mao's death and the arrest of the Gang of Four. Indeed, as the events of the winter of 1976–77 proved, these factional struggles resulted in a serious breakdown of law and order and a paralysis of local Party structures in at least one-third to one-half of China's provinces, as well as a serious challenge to the Party Center's ability to govern the country.

The events of the end of the Year of the Dragon and the first months of the Year of the Snake continued to fascinate Thomas Gates and his fellow American China-watchers in Peking. How specifically did the Chinese intend to make the transition to a nation not governed by the strong hand of Mao Zedong and the radicals? Indeed, Charles Cross, the American consul general in Hong Kong, expressed this expectancy about the future in a year-end poem which he sent to the American diplomats in Peking.

Funerals, earthquakes, and the Gang of Four,
What China-watcher could ask for more?

Will Ye and Li and possibly Deng,
Be able to "rest easy" with Hua Guofeng?
Remember: a snake is just a small dragon.[1]

China's new political environment dramatically changed the circumstances confronting Hua Guofeng as he attempted to govern China during the first months of the post-Mao era. Hua had succeeded in raising the expectations of the Chinese people, not only because he had participated in the overthrow of the Gang of Four, but also because he had served as a symbol of unity during the earthquake relief effort and the mourning period for Mao. Even so, Hua was a leader who lacked both a substantial following and a specific political program. For those reasons, the PRC media went to great lengths in the last months of 1976 to present him as a worthy successor to Mao and even as representative of a continuing tradition of great Chinese leaders. Leading the chorus of praise for Hua Guofeng was the PLA who acclaimed the new chairman as "selfless, loyal, and independent," fully capable of carrying on in the tradition of Zhou Enlai and Mao Zedong.[2] Nonetheless, Hua Guofeng faced an immense task in November 1976. The Chinese desperately needed a period of unity and stability after so much prolonged internal division and strife. As Li Xiannian said at an important meeting of the State Council on November 5, "Now it is unite to win victory. In the past, it was split to strive for failure."[3]

Despite such concerns, the fact remained that the purge of the Gang of Four did not eliminate every strong challenge to Hua Guofeng's continued leadership of the PRC. With the Gang of Four imprisoned, Hua had to contend with the moderate politicians of the Long March Generation who sought a return to power after the dark days of the Cultural Revolution. These moderate politicians longed for the second rehabilitation of Deng Xiaoping, certainly not a welcome prospect for Hua. In addition, the PLA under the leadership of Marshal Ye Jianying sought (as it had throughout 1976) to preserve its role as a mediator between the civilian factions. In such a way, the PLA held the balance of power in China and its political influence continued to grow in the six months after Mao's death. After the purge of the Gang of Four, therefore, a central task of the Hua regime was to develop a program broad enough not to provoke the opposition of the military-bureaucratic complex, thereby avoiding another political showdown.

Between November 1976 and May 1977, the Party Center attempted to develop such a broad program and immediately confronted the difficulty of initiating any new policies in an environment of internal turmoil. In late December, Hua Guofeng delivered an important speech to a Party conference in which he outlined what he considered the nation's "main fighting tasks" for the immediate future. These tasks included "deepening the great mass movement to expose and criticize the Gang of Four," "strengthening Party building" (in effect, neutralizing or purging leftist influence at the provincial levels), "deepening the mass movement to learn from Dazhai in agriculture and Daqing in industry and push the national economy forward," and finally, "studying works by Marx, Engels, Lenin, and Stalin."[4] The tone and direction of that speech convinced Tom that, not only had Hua taken considerable time and effort to prepare this address, but also the speech represented his strategy for rallying China to his support. He clearly intended to portray himself as a forward-looking leader who placed a high priority on economic modernization (in the tradition of Zhou Enlai and even Deng Xiaoping) while also continuing his claim as Mao's chosen successor. The pivotal question about the success of this strategy was whether the Chinese people, and the Chinese Communist Party, would accept that particular brand of leadership.

For USLO's China-watchers in the autumn of 1976, finding an answer to that critical question proved elusive. Did Hua possess the charisma and ability to lead China over the long term? Tom could not help noticing the rising influence of both Li Xiannian and Ye Jianying after Mao's death and the purge of the Gang of Four. The prominence accorded both Li and Ye indicated that, while Hua held on paper an unprecedented amount of power, other leaders were at least as involved as he in administering the policies of the Party and the state.[5] The Chinese themselves did not appear at all reluctant to refer to the existence of a "collective leadership" (Hua, Ye, Li) in power at the time.

Faced with these circumstances, Hua Guofeng and the Party Center set about to create a new political alignment in China in the six months after the purge of the Gang of Four which might prove capable of implementing the policies of the new regime. The obstacles in the path of constructing such an alignment were considerable, however. First, the Hua regime faced a potentially explosive and violent situation in many provinces after it deposed the Gang. Opponents of the Gang of Four's supporters at the provincial level not unsurprisingly leaped at the opportunity to "reckon the account" with their enemies, who in many instances had humiliated them and threatened both their lives and careers during the Cultural Revolution. More than any lingering disputes over ideology, the desire for revenge (and retaliation) drove the foes of the leftists in an effort to settle some old scores.[6]

Second, the Party Center's inevitable campaign to neutralize leftist influence in China also unleashed another round of political maneuvering whereby Hua and his supporters, the Long March moderates, and the leaders of the PLA attempted to place their provincial supporters in offices vacated by the purge of the leftists. On this matter, one must understand that the political stakes were high. All three factions realized that the next session of the National Party Congress would decide the composition of the Central Committee, and ultimately the leadership of the Party and state. Each faction wanted as many of its supporters as possible in positions where they might affect the outcome of the decisions made by the next Party Congress.

Third, Hua Guofeng fully realized that his support stemmed from a coalition of leaders from the PLA as well as some moderate civilians who preferred him to the radicals. In dealing with provincial factionalism, Hua needed to exercise appropriate caution so as not to upset this fragile coalition. Even so, Hua and other moderate civilians completely understood that they might have to rely on the PLA to restore order in some provinces where factional violence threatened to get out of control. In so doing, they ran the risk of contributing to a further increase in the PLA's authority at a time when the military's power was growing steadily.

As a result, Hua and the Party Center tended to move with considerable caution in the last months of 1976. The "rectification" campaign against provincial leftists proceeded deliberately, not in Cultural Revolutionary-fashion. The Center announced plans for economic modernization and "political liveliness." It spoke of a possible need to lower defense spending in order to concentrate more resources on the domestic economy (a policy initiative later blocked completely by Ye Jianying, Xu Shiyou, and the leadership of the PLA).

By mid-December, however, the Center had apparently concluded that its cautious approach was not working, and it therefore moved with greater alacrity in the pursuit of its goals. It dispatched PLA troops into Fujian, Yunnan, and Jiangxi to stem factional violence in those provinces. In early 1977, the Center took steps to centralize its control over China's Railway Ministry and again used the PLA as its instrument in enforcing discipline there. Hua, realizing that control of the media was essential to his success as a leader, brought his supporters into positions of authority with the *People's Daily*, *Red Flag*, and Peking's radio and television stations. Long considered a fiefdom of the radical Left, the PRC media was overdue for a shake-up. Shortly after the arrest of the Gang of Four, Hua deposed Yu Ling, the editor of the *People's Daily*, and replaced him with Hu Jiwei, a correspondent for the publication who had been its assistant editor during the 1950s. According to rumors which circulated throughout Peking, Yu Ling suffered the fate of "self-criticism" and "re-education" after being replaced. Hua also added Li Lianzheng, deputy political commissar of the Peking military region, to the *People's Daily*'s editorial staff. In addition, Hua gave control of *Red Flag* to Wang Shu, then the PRC's ambassador to West Germany, who had previously been a correspondent for the New China News Agency. Finally, the regime appointed Zhang Tianzheng as editor of Peking's radio and television broadcasts.[7]

The winter and spring of 1976–77 therefore proved to be a critical period for the PRC as it strived to move forward progressively under the leadership of "wise" Chairman Hua. Certainly the three interrelated problems of purging the influence of the leftists throughout the country, maintaining and in some instances restoring national order, and establishing an effective political alignment called for a considerable amount of wisdom on the part of the Chinese leadership.

II

The first task confronting the Hua regime in November and December 1976 was to develop a plan to deal with the radicals and their provincial supporters. In that respect, the arrest of the Gang of Four presented the Center with a host of new problems. Hua Guofeng appeared to be completely aware of the challenges facing the Party in the aftermath of the radical purge. As he informed the members of the State Council on November 5:

Now that the problem of the Gang of Four is solved, all [the other] problems can be solved accordingly. The shattering of the Gang of Four is a preliminary victory. But we must not believe the struggle is finished. Organizationally, they have been toppled. We have extirpated them from the higher level. But to eradicate their pernicious influence ideologically and politically, we must conduct exposure and criticism throughout the country. We must conduct propaganda and mass criticism in order to provide materials for everyone. What the masses know [about the Gang of Four] is limited.[8]

Specifically, now that the Gang was under arrest, what was the future status of its members? How did the Center plan to implement a policy of neutralizing the Gang's provincial supporters without unleashing a vicious season of political retaliation and possibly bloodshed? In response, the Center generally and Hua specifically announced the intention of using Mao's dictum to "cure the illness to save the patient" as a guide for keeping the "rectification" campaign in the provinces from running out of control. As early as mid-October, the Center established an investigatory committee consisting primarily of Hua, Ye, Li, Chen Xilian, the commander of the Peking Military region, and Li Desheng, commander of the Shenyang military region and the de facto strong man of north China, to review the crimes of the Gang of Four. By late October, the Center had also instructed the provincial authorities to establish their own investigatory committees responsible for gathering materials and organizing campaigns against local supporters of the Gang. The Center's instructions to its local provincial supporters, however, called for keeping the target "narrow" and showing leniency toward any cadres who confessed their past association with the purged radicals. Provincial authorities also received warnings against allowing any physical punishment or torture of provincial leftists, and instructions to permit the rehabilitation of those who admitted their past mistakes.

In keeping with its desire for economic progress, the Center also instructed its provincial supporters to make calls for increased production a partner with criticism of the Left. Indeed, at the meeting of the State Council on November 5, Hua Guofeng appeared as concerned about the dismal condition of the Chinese economy as with the national campaign to criticize the leftists. "Despite our difficulties, we must pay attention to the masses' standard of living and improve the markets," Hua informed his colleagues. "The ministries of commerce and finance must repeatedly consider what I just asked you. We must pay attention to [the] positive factors and must not have the ministry concerned exercise direct and exclusive control of enterprises. A large province must have flexibility." [9]

Throughout the month of November, therefore, the national and provincial media urged conciliation in dealing with supporters of the Gang of Four as well as increased attention to economic production. On November 28, an editorial in the *People's Daily* reminded the Chinese that criticism of the radicals in provincial organs should be confined only to charges against the Gang of Four, and that local leftists should be given "the opportunity to reform." Hua Guofeng reportedly went to considerable lengths himself to enforce this editorial policy, even instructing the media not to refer to the Gang of Four as "the Shanghai Gang" since that epithet was unfair to what the Center considered were the great majority of Shanghainese, who were not leftist supporters. [10]

Mao's doctrine of "curing the illness to save the patient," however, found little receptivity among provincial opponents of the radicals who had suffered at their hands for more than a decade. In truth, China's provinces were historically difficult to govern and had been torn by strife since the mid-1960s because of labor dissatisfaction, the anti-Deng campaign, and the succession struggle of 1975–76. Keeping the effort to criticize the Gang and its supporters "narrow" proved to be much more difficult in practice than in theory as the leftists were nowhere near as "isolated" as the Center's propaganda had claimed in October. In fact, the radicals had placed their supporters in key positions throughout local and provincial organizations and these individuals could hardly be expected to "rally around the Central Committee led by Comrade Hua Guofeng." After the anti-Gang festivities of late October, one could visualize the potential for an exceptionally harsh campaign of recrimination against local leftists.

Throughout November and December, therefore, the Party Center faced the potential not only for violence, but also for frequent occurrences of bloodshed throughout China. In Fujian, Zhejiang, and Jiangxi, the strife was serious enough to warrant the dispatch of PLA troops to restore order. In

Henan, Hubei, Guizhou, Sichuan, and Yunnan, work slowdowns and poster attacks on local leftist officials resulted after the arrest of the Gang of Four. In Guangdong, Guangxi, Hebei, Shaahxi, and Shanxi, the possibility for violence existed but serious difficulties did not immediately result from the purge of the radical leaders.

Probably the most worrisome situation for the Party Center occurred in Sichuan, a province which encountered virtual civil war following the overthrow of the Gang of Four. Sichuan's provincial leadership had expressed its support of Hua Guofeng in mid-October whereupon it immediately confronted a campaign by local leftists to undermine its authority. In Sichuan, the strife led to violence and the "sacrifice of the precious lives of many class brothers." On October 19, for example, a group of radicals employed at one of the large provincial factory complexes assaulted the local police, ransacked the Party Office, and apparently escaped with stolen weapons and secret files. On October 22, workers from another factory occupied and burned down one of its buildings, an act of violence which killed or wounded 34 people. On October 25, another group of radicals attacked or wounded 120 people during an anti-Gang rally in the province. When PLA troops intervened, they too found themselves under attack, but with support from Sichuan's provincial authorities, they managed to stabilize the situation.[11]

Other provincial reports revealed the existence of other harsh anti-leftist campaigns. On November 14, the USLO's officials received word that in Jiangxi, "a very small number of stubborn enemies will be driven to a narrow corner for us to encircle and annihilate."[12] Worse situations developed, however, in Fujian and Zhejiang, with potential unrest clearly evident in Shaahxi, Guangdong, and Henan.[13] In Fujian, a state of near-anarchy had existed since the previous summer, and the clashes between leftists and moderates caused the Center to send twelve thousand PLA troops to the province in order to "promote revolution and production" while "solving problems" associated with "splittists and revisionists."[14] Factional strife in Fujian represented a chronic problem for the Hua leadership and, by acting with dispatch and PLA intervention in November, the Center hoped to reduce the potential for discord in other provinces. Indeed, the Hua leadership probably concluded that PLA intervention in Fujian served as both a reminder and a warning to other provincial leaders that compliance with Peking's instructions was essential.[15]

Other sections of China nevertheless continued to experience their own share of factional strife in late 1976. On November 11, the USLO's officers learned that an extensive poster campaign was under way in Wuhan, calling for the "rectification" of the provincial and revolutionary committees there. Wuhan had apparently been the scene of considerable violence in the aftermath of the Gang's arrests. Travelers from the city reported that most of

Wuhan's buses were windowless, the result of urban riots and rock-throwing incidents. Other reports even spoke of some executions. At first, local security officials appeared to have the province under control, although PLA intervention could not be ruled out. A similar situation had also developed in Changsha, where violence and executions were also rumored.[16]

Struggling with the various outbreaks of factional strife occupied a great deal of the Center's attention in November. In Shanghai, for example, a vigorous poster campaign broke out, centering not only upon Ma Tianshui, Xu Jiangxian, and Wang Xiuzhien but also upon their colleagues on the city's municipal revolutionary committee. Posters identifying and denouncing such leftists as the Ten Big Henchmen, the Four Dragons, and the Four Rogues of the Writing Group appeared throughout the city. Based on such reports, Tom concluded that Su Zhenhua, Ni Zhifu, and Peng Chong were carrying out a full-fledged purge of the leftist political machine in Shanghai.[17]

In addition to the officially sponsored campaign to criticize the Gang of Four which gained increasing momentum in the last months of 1976, PLA troops were visible everywhere in Shanghai, and posters and caricatures of the Gang of Four appeared throughout the city. In one art gallery in Shanghai, one enterprising exhibitor had arranged a display of 360 of the "best" anti-Gang caricatures. The crimes of the Gang of Four were also the only constant theme of the song and dance routines of Shanghai's schoolchildren.[18]

By the beginning of December, therefore, the Hua regime had discovered the difficulty of governing China in the midst of turmoil as the strife in the provinces continued. An especially serious problem for the Center involved the situation in Baoding, a city approximately one hundred miles south of Peking. Long a leftist stronghold and the headquarters of the radical dominated 38th Army, Baoding exploded in violence during December. The USLO's officers learned of reports about leftist raids on military arsenals, sabotage of factories, looting of grain stores and shops, murders, and rapes. Once again, the Center dispatched units of the PLA to the area as a way of quelling the resistance.[19]

By mid-December, disorder was also prevalent in other parts of China. In Yunnan, for example, a broadcast in early December spoke of giving "free rein to the masses [in fighting] a People's War against Gang supporters," a certain indication that local leftists had not submitted to the Center's authority. Reports of similar incidents emanated from Hubei, where radicals had apparently carried out an "armed insurrection," including beatings of local Party officials considered to be supporters of the Center. The situation in Hubei was again so serious that the Center dispatched PLA troops under the authority of Yang Tejin, the regional military commander, to support Xiao Xinzhu, the provincial first secretary.[20]

In the midst of this internal turmoil, the Hua regime searched for a means of rallying the nation to its support. During late November and December, therefore, Hua Guofeng and the other members of the PRC hierarchy actively showcased and highlighted a series of Party functions designed to show progress in resolving some critical national problems. First, on November 24, the hierarchy assembled at the ground-breaking ceremony for the construction of the memorial mausoleum for the late Chairman Mao. This ceremony found virtually every member of the leadership in attendance and ironically was notable for the amount of attention accorded Marshal Ye Jianying, rather than Chairman Hua. Since the ouster of the Gang of Four, Ye had received almost co-equal status with Hua in the contents of articles published in *People's Daily*. Film clips shown by Peking television of this ceremony certainly failed to dispel the impression that Ye ranked near the summit of political power in China. During the ceremony, the television camera remained fixed on Hua as he read his brief speech and then walked to the cornerstone to shovel the first symbolic bit of dirt. Once Hua returned to his place at the podium, the camera focused on Marshal Ye, who walked briskly, military-style, to the cornerstone. The camera then recorded Ye's vigorous shoveling and also scanned the faces of the other assembled leaders, all smiling proudly at this enthusiastic performance given by one of the Party's elder statesmen. After completing his shoveling, Ye returned to his place at the podium, slightly behind Hua, a position duly noted by the camera.[21]

Another important development which occurred in late November and early December involved the status of Foreign Minister Qiao Guanhua. As early as mid-November, Tom began hearing rumors circulating within the diplomatic community that Qiao may have encountered political difficulties which stemmed primarily from the speech which he delivered to the United Nations General Assembly in New York on October 2. In that speech, Qiao defied Hua's instructions to delete any reference to the phrase "Act according to the principles laid down" when he presented his address. Since Qiao's speech represented the PRC's first official statement to the international community since Mao's death, diplomatic observers in Peking could well understand the chagrin which the Party Center felt over the foreign minister's remarks, especially since Hua, Ye, and Wang Dongxing were contemplating the overthrow of the Gang of Four at the time. (In an off-the-record conversation, Tom also heard that Qiao may have expected the radicals to mount their coup against the regime while he was in New York. His speech in New York might have been part of the radical campaign to confirm their takeover of the PRC.)

For his part, however, Qiao Guanhua had placed his future and immediate prospects in the hands of the radicals, even before leaving for New York. Earlier in the summer, Qiao reportedly confided to a friend that since "Mao was ill, Ye was old, and Deng would not last long," his fortunes were safer with the radicals.[22] For their part, the radicals appeared perfectly willing to retain Qiao as foreign minister; Jiang Qing was even reportedly interested in promoting him to vice premier. Furthermore, Jiang and Zhang Hanzhi, Qiao's fashionable and sophisticated second wife, were close friends, and Mao's widow also intended to elevate her colleague to a high diplomatic post.[23]

Qiao's mistakes in New York, combined with his wife's close association with Jiang Qing, disqualified him from serving in the Hua regime. At official state functions on November 15 and 16 (involving a visiting American Congressional delegation headed by Senators Carl Curtis [R-Nebraska] and Birch Bayh [D-Indiana]), Wang Hairong substituted for Qiao, a clear indication to the diplomatic community that the foreign minister's position may have been in jeopardy. When Qiao failed to appear on November 24 at the cornerstone-laying ceremony for the Mao Memorial Mausoleum, Tom and the other Americans in Peking became convinced that the foreign minister was about to be replaced, especially after word leaked out that the Party Center had requested three prominent diplomats, Wang Shu, the ambassador to West Germany; Huang Hua, the ambassador to the United Nations; and Zhang Wenjin, the ambassador to Canada, to return to China for consultations.[24] On December 3, the Center officially confirmed that Huang Hua had replaced Qiao Guanhua as foreign minister. On the same day, it also announced the purge of Yu Huiyong, formerly the minister of culture, and Zhuang Zedong, the minister of physical sport and recreation, two other radicals who had been arrested on the night of October 6–7.[25]

The Center revealed these changes in the leadership at the conclusion of a hastily called and highly secret convocation of the Third Session of the Fourth National Party Congress in early December. The sudden convocation of the NPC represented another of Hua's attempts to show some progress toward resolving some important issues, particularly in settling the matter of appointments. In discussions with other members of the diplomatic community, however, Tom learned that the meeting failed to resolve any long-term issues involving the PRC leadership. Other than Wu De's obligatory anti-Gang speech and the announcement that Deng Yingchao, Zhou Enlai's widow, had been appointed to a vice chairman's post in the Party, the session accomplished nothing of substance. One interesting development, however, was that the session contained no criticism of Deng Xiaoping. The PRC hierarchy had, in fact, laid to rest the anti-rightist campaign.[26] But the meeting certainly failed to result in any strengthening of Hua Guofeng's assertion that he was to lead the People's Republic indefinitely as Mao's chosen successor.

If the meeting therefore proved somewhat disappointing to both Hua Guofeng and his neo-Maoist supporters, that fact partially explained why the chairman put forth such a strenuous effort in late December to build public confidence in his leadership. On December 25, at the national conference on Learning from Dazhai in Agriculture (the last major reporting event for USLO's China-watchers in 1976), Hua delivered an important address in which he comprehensively reviewed the events of 1976 and outlined the tasks which he considered important for 1977. He dwelt on an address which Mao Zedong had given during the mid-1950s entitled, "On the Ten Great Relationships," obviously hoping that his speech might have the same impact as Mao's original address. In his speech, Mao had discussed the importance of consensus as the basis for unity among the PRC leadership (ironically, just prior to Mao's launching of the Great Leap Forward). Hua also endorsed the concept of unity through consensus and deplored any recurrence of the excesses of the Cultural Revolution.

1976 is a most interesting year in the history of our Party and the dictatorship of the proletariat in China. It is a year in which the whole Party, the whole Army, and the people of all nationalities throughout the country have stood rigorous tests, a year in which we have won a great historic victory. The internal and international situation at present is excellent. It is our belief that 1977 will be a year in which we shall smash the "Gang of Four" completely and go towards great order, a year of united struggle and triumphant advance. The people of the whole country must carry on Chairman Mao's behests, take upon our shoulders the cause of proletarian revolution bequeathed to us by him and carry it through to the end. We are determined to win victory. We can certainly win victory. Let us, the 800 million people and the more than 30 million Party members, unite and wage a common struggle to win still greater victories.[27]

The speech by Mao to which Hua referred was over two decades old. More important, Hua made the same appeal to order and discipline which the late chairman had made in an effort to recapture the spirit of a more harmonious time in China. Hua undoubtedly considered order and discipline essential characteristics of political and economic stability, and therefore he was proposing a more conventional, institutionalized society in which pragmatic economic progress was likely.

For those who thought that such a vision of the PRC's future appeared uninspiring, Hua Guofeng again sought to place his leadership within the context of one which looked after the people's welfare. He wanted his leadership viewed as open-minded and nondoctrinaire but nevertheless capable of making wise policy decisions. Specifically, Hua used the address to clarify and explain his goal of an economic policy which balanced the needs of agriculture with those of industry.[28]

Finally, Hua Guofeng apparently chose Chen Yonggui, another neo-Maoist, to give the major speech at the Dazhai conference. It was a tactic similar to the one which he used in October when he selected Wu De to give the principal speech condemning the crimes of the Gang of Four. To give further weight to his remarks, Hua turned to the media one week after the conference as the vehicle for hammering home the message of the New Year. In a joint editorial entitled "Advance from Victory to Victory" published on January 1, 1977, in the *People's Daily, Red Flag,* and *Liberation Army Daily,* the regime again spelled out its goals for economic development, political stability, and steady improvement in living standards.[29] Hua's emphasis upon his control of the media increased considerably in the months ahead as he tried to steer public support in his direction.

III

As 1977 began in China, Tom Gates and his USLO colleagues naturally wondered how China's leaders would handle the residue of problems left over from the previous year. Without question, the major problem facing the Party Center involved the persistent factional strife which undermined any real political and economic progress.

In the two months which had passed since the arrest of the Gang of Four, Hua Guofeng had preferred to move slowly and cautiously in attempting to resolve the tense situation in China's provinces, although he did order PLA troops into Fujian province (as well as several others) in November and December, once it became evident that local authorities could not maintain order.[30] By the beginning of 1977, however, Hua could count only marginal success in his attempt to deal with the "remnant poison of the Gang." Factional strife continued throughout the country and the Center consciously decided to adopt stronger measures in dealing with the sources of potential unrest. In addition, the Center faced the problem of selecting new provincial first secretaries to replace deposed leftists. On this matter, other sources of conflict emerged; the forces of Hua Guofeng, Deng Xiaoping, and the leadership of the PLA each wanted to place as many of its supporters as possible into key positions in the Party before the convocation of the next Party Congress.

In early January 1977, the Hua regime made its first visible demonstration of a new assertiveness in dealing with sources of conflict within China. During early January and continuing well into February, the Center encountered a major disturbance as railway workers in the Zhengzhou region revolted against their provincial leadership. Such problems gave the Center serious difficulties; the Zhengzhou region sat astride the junction of China's north-south and east-west lines and was vital to resupplying the beleaguered residents of Tangshan. Hua and Ye met this emergency by placing the Zhengzhou Railway Bureau under de facto military control. On January 2, a provincial broadcast from the region reported on a conference held in Peking on December 30 at which "Hua, Ye, and other leading comrades" had appointed Guo Weijing, the deputy commander of the PLA Railway Corps, as the first secretary of the Zhengzhou Railway Bureau. As matters developed, several of Guo's closest aides in this new post were also PLA officers.[31]

The problems with the railroads was just one symptom of the lack of communication between the Party Center and the provinces, a difficulty prevalent throughout much of 1976. Because of poor coordination between various provincial and bureau jurisdictions, trains frequently encountered delays when other trains failed to obtain clearance to transverse different bureau jurisdictions. As another complication, the provincial bureaus occasionally hoarded rolling stock, thereby depriving the entire system of the ability to respond rapidly to an emergency in a particular area of China, such as the Tangshan region when the earthquake struck in late July.

The Center's crackdown on China's railroad administration affected both the "rectification" and economic development objectives which Hua Guofeng had outlined for 1977. In 1976, only fourteen of China's twenty railway bureaus had met their economic goals, and the Center obviously feared a continuation of economic stagnation unless the railroads improved their performance. In February, the Center announced that Tuan Zhunyi, a veteran civilian administrator for Sichuan, had been appointed to head the Central Railway Ministry in Peking. Tuan's appointment signalled two developments, an attempt by the Center to promote greater discipline on the railway operations as well as a possible change in the political environment since Tuan was widely perceived as a supporter of Deng Xiaoping.[32]

In the winter and early spring of 1977, the Party Center also moved ahead with its purges of leftist provincial leaders. Apparently convinced that the provincial "People's Congresses" had completed their work, the Center again dramatized its new assertiveness by filling important Party vacancies in the provinces, with the Hua forces, the Deng faction, and the PLA all watching anxiously for the opportunity to place one of their supporters in a key provincial position.[33]

The announcements of new provincial first secretaries occurred in rapid order, beginning in late January. On January 25, the New China News Agency reported the death of Gang Qianmian, the longtime first secretary of the Ningxia autonomous region, and identified Hua Shilian as his replacement. Formerly a leading official in Shanxi province before the Cultural Revolution, Hua was considered a member of the Dengist faction. A vigorous critic of the radicals, Hua had earlier tried to expose Zhang Chunqiao as a "renegade," even taking the drastic step of writing to Mao about Zhang.[34]

On February 12, the USLO officers received news that a provincial broadcast from Yunnan had reported that An Pingsheng, also considered another Dengist and a close associate of Wei Guoqing, had replaced Qia Qiyun as the leading Party official in that province. The Center had transferred An Pingsheng to Yunnan from Guangxi, where he had held a number of high Party positions for the past several years. The appointment was viewed as the Center's way of solving the "problem of Yunnan" where factional strife and work stoppages were frequent occurrences. Qia Qiyun, moreover, was squarely in the radical camp and soon fell into eclipse after the announcement of his replacement.[35]

Following the announcement of An Pingsheng's transfer to Yunnan, another provincial broadcast on February 15 from Guangxi reported that Jaio Xiaoguang had replaced An as the provincial first secretary in that province. Jiao had been an active Party official in Guangxi since 1952 and even held several high positions in that province between 1961 and 1966. During the Cultural Revolution, however, Jiao became a victim of the leftists, but he reemerged in 1971 to resume his place in the Party. His appointment fascinated the China-watchers at USLO; it appeared that Deng's supporters were winning all the Party's early rectification skirmishes.[36]

On March 1, another province reported a change in its leadership when Liu Guangtao was named as the new first secretary in Heilongjiang. This announcement surprised few people in the diplomatic community; Liu was an army man who reportedly had been handling day-to-day work in the province for the past two years. The appointment did demonstrate, however, the PLA's active influence in the rectification campaign.[37]

Two days later, on March 3, Radio Nanjing reported that Xu Jiadong had replaced Peng Chong (previously sent to Shanghai along with Su Zhenhua and Ni Zhifu after the purge of the Gang of Four) as the first secretary in Jiangsu province. Xu's appointment was an intriguing one. An important provincial official in Jiangsu during the 1960s, Xu was purged during the Cultural Revolution only to reappear in 1970 and find another post in the Party. Generally considered a neo-Maoist in the same faction as Hua Guofeng, Xu's appointment suggested that Hua and his supporters also possessed sufficient strength to place one of their supporters at the top of a provincial Party apparatus.[38]

On March 6, a broadcast from Hangzhou revealed another political change. Tie Ying, an officer in the PLA, had assumed the control of Zhejiang province in which Hangzhou was the major city. Good reasons existed for the Center to nominate Tie to this post. Since the purge of the Gang of Four in October, Hangzhou had experienced violent factional strife, reportedly an outgrowth of Wang Hongwen's considerable intrigues to radicalize the city's factory workers. In early March, Tom Gates visited Hangzhou and witnessed a visible demonstration of the Center's attempt to keep the city under control. Posters attacking the Gang of Four were obvious throughout the city, local armed security officers and PLA troops patrolled the city's railroad stations, and armed sentries guarded the gates of the Hangzhou Hotel. The radicals' enemies in Hangzhou had apparently passed the point of simply investigating the crimes of the leftists. A printed announcement reported that a provincial court had met on February 12 and passed down twenty sentences (seven of which resulted in executions) for "counter-revolutionary crimes." The announcement itself read: "Let this be a warning to the small handful of the counter-revolutionary element. Surrender, confess, repent, and act properly or you will be struck down by the dictatorship of the proletariat."[39]

The factional problems in Hangzhou apparently stemmed from the activities of Wang Senhe, a close friend and provincial agent of Wang Hongwen. Wang Senhe reportedly had become a master of intrigue in attempting to disrupt production in the city's factories and textile mills. So nefarious were Wang Senhe's conspiracies that Mao himself had once stripped Wang of much of his power in 1975. After Mao's death and the purge of the Gang of Four, however, Wang's position in Hangzhou became even more untenable and he was purged along with numerous other provincial leftists.[40]

The first week in March brought additional changes within the provincial Party line-up of the PRC. On March 3, a broadcast from Jiangsu announced that Xu Jiadong, a Hua supporter, had taken charge of the Party's activities there. On March 6, a provincial broadcast from Guizhou reported that Ma Li, another presumed Hua supporter, had been appointed first secretary. Ma's appointment became public knowledge in Guizhou on March 5 when the Party held an anti-Gang rally designed "to convey the important instruction of Premier Hua Guofeng." The scene of factional disturbances for several years, Guizhou (according to the Center) had "suffered under the pernicious influence of the Gang of Four." In placing Ma Li, formerly a high official in Hebei, in charge of Guizhou, Hua clearly hoped to have another of his supporters bring order to a troubled province.[41] In Qinghai on March 7, Tan Qilong, a PLA veteran considered a supporter of Deng Xiaoping, assumed the provincial Party's first secretaryship.[42] Finally, by the end of the month, the Center had largely concluded its list of new appointments when it explained that Wang Enmao, a PLA officer, had accepted the top provincial post in Jilin.[43]

By April 1, 1977, the Hua regime was therefore able to claim significant progress in its rectification effort. For the first time in six years, all of China's provinces had Party first secretaries with the exception of Hanan, where Hua Guofeng continued to retain his post as the Party's first secretary.[44] Moreover, the leadership had proven itself capable of dealing resolutely with persistent factional turmoil in such places as Fujian, Yunnan, Guizhou, and Zhejiang. One area, however, remained out of the reach of the Center's direction, the Shenyang military region in Liaoning province where Li Desheng maintained his own degree of control semi-independently of Peking. The problems in the Shenyang-Liaoning area presented the Center with a series of special circumstances apart from its conduct of the "rectification" campaign in the other provinces.

Liaoning province was a source of strength for the radicals, the home and political base of Mao Yuanxin. After the arrest of the Gang of Four, however, opponents of the radicals began conducting a vicious poster campaign against Liaoning's provincial leftists, a campaign which reached its climax in mid-December. The anti-Left posters specifically claimed that Liaoning's provincial officials were covering up their role in the anti-Deng campaign, their past links to the Gang of Four, and their present opposition to Hua Guofeng. Another charge involved the allegation that Liaoning's provincial leadership had failed to supply the Party Center with some significant documents which showed the role of Mao Yuanxin as a collaborator of the Gang of Four. In addition, Liaoning's provincial leftists may have established plans to organize and conduct an underground resistance to the Center following the purge of the four radical leaders in October. One poster in Shenyang put the case against the provincial leftists bluntly: "Provincial leaders are obstructing exposure and criticism of Mao Yuanxin's crimes in the Shenyang culture and education front and will absolutely not have a good end."[45]

The situation in Liaoning continued to remain troublesome throughout the first six weeks of 1977. Indeed, the Party Center considered the province "unsafe to enter" during that period.[46] The Hua regime's problem in Liaoning was more acute than simply the need to end the factional strife in the province, however. Many China-watchers expressed the strong belief that rightist elements in the province may have set Li Desheng as their target and, if so, the prospect for continued turmoil was certain. Li Desheng controlled the PLA forces in the region, which consisted of five hundred thousand troops believed completely loyal to him. Although the poster attacks failed to mention Li Desheng by name, the fact that he was a member of the Politburo and military region commander in north China seemed to indicate that he was one (or should have been one) of the Center's responsible individuals for "rectifying" the province.

If such was Li Desheng's responsibility, his previous career made him an unlikely candidate for such a task, especially since it had included several instances of Cultural Revolutionary-style assignments. In 1973, for example, Li was transferred to Shenyang after he had used PLA troops to restore order in Anhui province. While in Anhui, Li had praised several of Jiang Qing's cultural policies and even published newspaper articles (under a pseudonym) supporting the activities of Mao's wife. Even after his transfer to Shenyang, Li and his fellow top-ranking officers in the region continued to promote leftist policies, especially during the campaign to discredit Deng Xiaoping. For those reasons, Liaoning's provincial rightists probably considered Li Desheng "fair game" as a subject for attack.[47]

Such difficulties in Liaoning created problems not only for Li Desheng but also for the Hua regime. With over five hundred thousand troops under his command, Li was obviously one of the most powerful men in China (and in Liaoning especially, a dangerous man to bring under poster attack). While the Hua regime had emphasized the importance of eliminating the Gang's supporters at the provincial levels, such a task was easier to accomplish in the provinces where the Center had been able to install its own supporters into positions of power. In early 1977, however, the Center appeared willing to permit a "Manchurian stalemate" to exist in Liaoning; at least, it took few steps to pressure Li Desheng into conforming with any of its instructions.[48] The Center seemed to allow Li Desheng a free hand in dealing with provincial leftists, perhaps even to the point of conceding that he may have been protecting several local radical officials.

In mid-March, though, the situation in Liaoning changed dramatically, probably as a result of an important Politburo meeting, or perhaps even a series of meetings on the "Liaoning problem" (which Li Desheng attended) held in Peking during late February. Between March 11 and March 13, posters began appearing in Liaoning announcing that the supporters of the Gang of Four in the provincial hierarchy had been removed on the "order of Hua Guofeng, Ye Jianying, and the Party Central Committee." At a Party rally held in Liaoning on March 14, both Li Desheng and Zeng Shaoshan, the province's first secretary, confirmed the arrests of Li Boqin, Wei Bingkui, and Liu Shengtian, the three individuals identified as the leftist leaders in the province. Li Boqin, who was rumored to be organizing the underground resistance to the Center, was the major target of the rightists. "You must prepare to cope with a certain incident," Li reportedly informed his leftist provincial colleagues in the aftermath of the arrest of the Gang of Four. Also arrested was Zhang Tiansheng, a student radical who was a leftist favorite because of his past record of defiance to China's traditional educational authorities.[49] Thus the Center and Li Desheng apparently combined their efforts to "rectify" the political situation in Liaoning. Most likely, Hua, Ye, and Li Desheng had negotiated the Center's response to Liaoning's turmoil at their meeting in Peking during late February.

IV

In summary, where did the rectification program stand in China at the end of March 1977, after over five months of internal turmoil? Such was the vital question discussed at an important (and highly secret) Central Committee work conference held in Peking in late March. During this series of meetings, Hua and the Party leadership heard reports that the problems in Baoding and Yunnan, two particularly tense areas, had stabilized.[50] More important, perhaps, was the new power alignment in China which revealed itself at the time. Essentially, Hua and his supporters had assumed political control of China's northern provinces. Deng's supporters, however, chiefly represented by Xu Shiyou and Wei Guoqing, had created a broad political base in south China. Both Xu and Wei controlled directly, or through subordinates, a broad area south of the Yangtze River that included ten of China's twenty-nine provinces. The intense maneuvering between the neo-Maoists, the Dengists, and the PLA had resulted in a standoff; both Hua's supporters and the PLA could claim four of their supporters among the ranks of the new provincial first secretaries while Deng's forces counted five.[51]

In addition to the new geographic distribution of power, an analysis of the rectification program revealed significant changes in the PRC's Central Committee. Jurgen Domes has offered the best profile of the effect which the anti-leftist purges had upon the PRC hierarchy. In analyzing the Party-wide shifts which occurred as a result of the Center's first rectification campaign against the leftists, Domes estimated that the purges and dismissals in 1976–77 affected 26.5 percent of the mass organization Left represented on the PRC's Central Committee but only 12.3 percent of the moderate civilian cadres and only 2.7 percent of the PLA. Domes also estimated that the leftist purges affected over 30 percent of the Central Committee members who had joined the Party after 1949 but only 5.6 percent of those who joined before the establishment of the PRC. Such estimates lend support to the conclusion that not only did the Gang of Four attempt to win support from younger cadres but also that the Long March moderates succeeded in frustrating these plans and then dominated the nation's political events after carrying out the arrests of the Gang. Furthermore, Domes estimated that twenty of the cadres considered purged by the Hua regime in 1976–77 represented around 10 percent of the 195 members appointed to the Central Committee in August 1974.[52] These twenty cadres included 20 percent of the women on the Central Committee, 50 percent of those younger than 40, 33 percent of those between 40 and 49, 18 percent of those in their fifties, but only 6.7 percent of those over 60.[53]

Following the announcements of the changes in the provincial governments, as well as a partial restoration of order throughout the country, the Hua regime attempted to promote its twin goals of national unity and economic modernization in the spring of 1977. On April 11, the Center announced that "a new leap forward is taking shape" (undoubtedly an ominous thought to many Chinese) in the economy and urged the Chinese to devote the next three years to rebuilding the PRC's productive capacities.[54]

On May 1, the Chinese in Peking celebrated their national holiday. In contrast to the previous year, the May Day celebration in 1977 was relaxed and festive. Hua Guofeng and the other members of the hierarchy turned out in Peking's parks and at an evening sports event and fireworks display. Throughout the city, the Chinese were given a visual reminder of Hua's claim to political legitimacy, an idealized painting of Chairman Mao's benediction of "With you in charge, I am at ease." With considerable artistic license, the scene depicted a fully alert and benevolent Mao, hand resting paternally atop the hand of a completely attentive Hua. The Chinese media reported that the picture "attracted large crowds who had their picture taken before it." In fact, the USLO's China-watchers noticed few Chinese paying any attention at all to the picture. Most appeared more intent upon enjoying themselves during this holiday.[55]

After the May Day celebration, the PRC leadership began intensive preparations for the Party Congress meeting scheduled for two months later in July.[56] At this meeting, Deng Xiaoping was officially rehabilitated for a second time and restored to the posts in the Party and the State Council from which the radicals had stripped him sixteen months earlier. Deng's return to power, however, was decided well in advance of the gathering of the Party Congress. The story of Deng's second rehabilitation is another vital chapter, in both the Year of the Dragon and the Year of the Snake.

Notes

1. United States Department of State, Official Files, Peking to Washington, February 1977 (hereafter cited as OF, date); OF, Peking to Washington, 23 December 1976.

2. OF, Peking to Washington, 9 November 1976.

3. OF, Peking to Washington, 10 February 1977.

4. Stuart Schram, "Chairman Hua Edits Mao's Literary Heritage: 'On the Ten Great Relationships,'" *China Quarterly* 69 (March 1977): 126–35.

5. OF, Peking to Washington, 11 November 1976. One rumor which circulated often within the diplomatic community at the time held that Hua would relinquish the premiership to Li Xiannian.

6. See Terrill, *Future of China*, p. 119, for an explanation of the term, "reckon the account." See also OF, SECSTATE [Secretary of State] Washington to All East Asian and Pacific Diplomatic Posts, 20 November 19/6; OF, Peking to Washington, 12 November 1976; interview, David Dean, 9 February 1983.

7. OF, 10 February 1977; OF, SECSTATE Washington to USLO, 14 February 1977; OF, Peking to Washington, 5 March 1977.

8. OF, Peking to Washington, 5 March 1977.

9. OF, Peking to Washington, 16 November 1976; OF, SECSTATE Washington to Peking, 3 December 1976; *New York Times*, 6 December 1976, p. 18.

10. OF, Peking to Washington, 22 November 1976; OF, Peking to Washington, 26 November 1976.

11. OF, Peking·to Washington, 24 March 1977; see also *New York Times*, 30 December 1976, p. 1; *New York Times*, 1 January 1977.

12. OF, Peking to Washington, 22 November 1976.

13. OF, Peking to Washington, 16 November 1976.

14. OF, Peking to Washington, 23 November 1976; OF, Peking to Washington, November–December, 1976; OF, SECSTATE Washington to USLO, 3 December 1976.

15. OF, Peking to Washington, 23 November 1976; *New York Times*, 5 December 1976, p. 5.

16. OF, Peking to Washington, 11 November 1976; OF, Peking to Washington, 3 February 1977.

17. OF, SECSTATE Washington to USLO, 3 December 1976.

18. OF, Peking to Washington, 3 March 1977.

19. OF, Peking to Washington, 24 March 1977; *New York Times*, 30 December 1976; *New York Times*, 1 January 1977.

20. OF, Peking to Washington, 16 November 1976; OF, Peking to Washington, 15 December 1976.

21. OF, Peking to Washington, 29 November 1976; OF, Peking to Washington, 26 November 1976.

22. OF, Peking to Washington, 7 October 1976.

23. OF, 26 October, 1976; OF, Peking to Washington, 1 December 1976. Once purged in 1976, Qiao did not re-emerge until 1982. See White, "Burnout of a Revolution," p. 49.

24. OF, Peking to Washington, 11 November 1976; OF, Peking to Washington, 17 November 1976; OF, Peking to Washington, 29 November 1976.

25. *New York Times*, 4 December 1976, pp. 1, 7.

26. OF, Peking to Washington, 2 December 1976.

27. OF, Peking to Washington, 22 March 1977; Schram, "Chairman Hua Edits Mao's Literary Heritage," pp. 133–35, also explores Hua's motivations and intentions for this speech.

28. OF, Peking to Washington, 22 March 1977.

29. Schram, "Chairman Hua Edits Mao's Literary Heritage," pp. 133–35.

30. OF, Peking to Washington, 16 November 1976; OF, Peking to Washington, 15 December 1976.

31. OF, Peking to Washington, 6 January 1977.

32. Ibid.

33. OF, Peking to Washington, 30 November 1976; OF, Peking to Washington, 1 February 1977.

34. OF, "Current Scene in the PRC"; Hsu, *China Without Mao*, p. 53.

35. Ibid., see also Fox Butterfield, "China Shifts a Regional Party Chief," *New York Times*, 15 February 1977, p. 3.

36. Butterfield, "China Shifts a Regional Party Chief," p. 3.

37. Ibid.

38. OF, Peking to Washington, 3 March 1977.

39. OF, Peking to Washington, 9 March 1977; OF, Peking to Washington, 30 November 1976; Hsu, *China Without Mao*, pp. 52–53.

40. Hsu, *China Without Mao*, pp. 52–53.

41. Ibid., see also OF, Peking to Washington, 8 March 1977.

42. OF, Peking to Washington, 8 March 1977.

43. Ibid.

44. Two other appointments were revealed later in June 1977. These included Mao Zhiyong, a Hua supporter, who became the Party's first secretary in Hanan, and Song Ping, also a Hua supporter, in Gansu. See OF, Peking to Washington, 21 June 1977.

45. OF, Peking to Washington, 3 February 1977.

46. OF, Peking to Washington, 15 February 1977.

47. Ibid.; interview, David Dean, 9 February 1983.

48. Interview, David Dean, 9 February 1983; OF, Peking to Washington, 3 February 1977.

49. OF, Peking to Washington, 16 March 1977; OF, Peking to Washington, 17 March 1977; ibid.

50. OF, Hong Kong to Washington, 23 May 1977.

51. Fox Butterfield, "Provincial Leadership Changes Create Southern Power Base in China," *New York Times*, 7 March 1977, p. 3.

52. Domes, "The 'Gang of Four' and Hua Kuo-feng," p. 493. Domes's list of purged cadres included the following: Wang Hongwen, Zhang Chunqiao, Jiang Qing, Yao Wenyuan, Zhuang Zedong, Xia Bangyin, Ms. Xie Zhengyi, Xu Jiangxian, Hua Linsen, Ms. Lu Xiangping, Ma Ning, Ma Tianshui, Pan Shigao, Tang Qishan, Tang Zhongfu, Ding Sheng, Tong Minghui, Ms. Wang Xiuzhen, Yu Huiyong.

53. Ibid.

54. *Washington Post*, 12 April 1977.

55. OF, Peking to Washington, 2 May 1977.

56. OF, Peking to Washington, 5 May 1977.

CHAPTER **7**

Waiting for Deng

After the anti-radical forces of the PRC arrested the Gang of Four in October 1976 and then continued their effort to reduce the influence of the Gang's supporters at the provincial levels, all of China became attracted to the question of the future status of Deng Xiaoping. Virtually given up as a political force in China after his purge at the hands of the radicals in April 1976, Deng discovered that his fortunes improved immediately once Mao Zedong died and the Gang of Four was imprisoned. Indeed, Deng did manage a "double Lazarus" (in the words of Ross Terrill) in the summer of 1977 as the Party restored him to the posts which he held in the Party, state, and military before his second purge in the spring of 1976.[1] The Party's decision to rehabilitate Deng, confirmed at important meetings of the Party Central Committee and the Fourth National Party Congress in August 1977, effectively returned the radicals' archenemy to the upper reaches of the PRC's political hierarchy, guaranteeing once again that Deng was a force to be reckoned with in the post-Mao era.[2]

After the Chinese received the news of Deng's rehabilitation, they responded with a national display of jubilation. Even so, millions of Chinese who rejoiced over Deng's return in 1977 must also have entertained serious doubts in 1976 about whether he would ever exercise power in China again. For his part, however, Deng never retreated from his goal of wresting political authority from the radicals, as the events of 1977 so conclusively demonstrated. In Roger Garside's words, "Deng was not a man who would turn back once he set his hand to the plow."[3] While Deng remained in political exile between the time of his ouster in April and the death of Mao in September, he and his supporters were simply waiting for the most opportune time to strike back at their enemies.

Following his dismissal in April 1976, Deng Xiaoping retreated to Guangdong, where he enjoyed the protection of two close allies, General Xu Shiyou and Wei Guoqing. Occasionally, Deng also met secretly with Marshal Ye Jianying, who frequently visited the hot springs near Guangdong, ostensibly for health reasons. America's China-watchers in Peking noticed a curious circumstance about Ye's visits to Guangdong during the summer of 1976, however. Throughout much of 1976, Ye appeared to be in failing health, even to the point of often being seen in Peking assisted by attendants. After the arrest of the Gang of Four, however, Ye's physical condition improved dramatically and he appeared to be completely recovered from his previous infirmities.[4] Several of the USLO officers concluded that Ye had been faking his frailties in 1976 for the purpose of not arousing too many suspicions in Peking when he decided to visit the hot springs near Guangdong. In retrospect, it became clear that Ye's frequent visits to the hot springs provided occasions to meet with Deng and make assessments of the political situation in the capital.

Deng Xiaoping's whereabouts during the autumn of 1976 remained somewhat mysterious. Shortly after the arrest of the Gang of Four, however, Thomas Gates heard that Deng had returned to Peking and was residing ("for his own safety") in the Western Hills. Immanuel Hsu, one reputable China scholar, has also written that Deng returned to Peking following Mao's death in September.[5] The extent to which Deng may have participated in the plot to overthrow the Gang of Four likewise remains a mystery, although one may safely assume that, since Ye Jianying masterminded the arrests of the four radicals and Xu Shiyou took charge of securing Shanghai for the central authorities, Deng was well aware of the plans to depose the leftists. In fact, one cannot easily dismiss the possibility that Deng was directly involved in the plot, although proving that assertion also remains elusive.

Despite the widespread public sentiment in China favoring a strong role for Deng Xiaoping in the PRC's post-Mao, post-Gang government, his second rehabilitation proved to be far from an automatic development. Certainly Deng's contempt for the radicals knew no bounds, and he had obviously struck a responsive chord in China when he criticized their economic, cultural, and educational programs. Of the radicals' views on the economy, Deng once observed, "They sit on the lavatory but don't manage a shit." Cultural life in China was monotonous, Deng maintained. "With the model operas today, you just see a bunch of people running to and fro on the stage. No trace of art, no sense bragging about them." Furthermore, Deng also scorned the leftists' educational policies, a criticism which Mao took personally and ultimately led to the vice premier's second purge. "College students are far from being real college students," Deng said in 1975. "It is a real mess. . . . Most college students today carry nothing but a brush for writing wall posters. They can't do anything else."[6] In late summer of 1975, Deng issued a critical report of the PRC's educational system; shortly thereafter, the Gang of Four unleashed its vigorous campaign to drive him from the Politburo and even the Party.[7]

Even with the radicals deposed, however, Deng's potential rehabilitation presented a serious challenge to Hua Guofeng and the neo-Maoist faction of second-generation politicians and PLA officers who had come to prominence at the Center immediately after the vice premier's second purge. Hua Guofeng, Wu De, Wang Dongxing, Ji Dengkui, Chen Yonggui, Chen Xilian, Li Desheng, and their other supporters at the provincial level had seen their power increase dramatically as a result of Deng's purge and the arrest of the Gang of Four. The neo-Maoists, later labeled by Deng and his supporters as the "Whatever" faction since they historically supported Mao *whatever* his policies may have been, viewed Deng's possible return either as a development to be postponed for as long as possible or as an opportunity for them to extract the maximum number of concessions from the Dengists before readmitting him to the councils of power.

During the months between November 1976 and May 1977, Deng and his allies, most notably Chen Yun, Xu Shiyou, Wei Guoqing, and their supporters in the PLA and the provinces, pressed the Hua regime for a prompt rehabilitation of the deposed vice premier. Confronted with this challenge to Hua Guofeng's authority, Hua and his allies temporized, procrastinated, and otherwise sought to frustrate the designs of the Dengists. Other leading officials, most notably Li Xiannian and Ye Jianying, served as mediators in the dispute between the two factions, generally supporting Deng's restoration but attempting to manage it within a framework of transition from radical to moderate rule.

While this backstage maneuvering occurred within the PRC hierarchy, the Chinese people anxiously awaited Deng's return and endured a series of tantalizing rumors which speculated on the exact timing of his reappearance. The masses came to believe that Deng would return first by the end of 1976, then at the first anniversary of the death of Zhou Enlai in early January 1977, then at the anniversary of Hua Guofeng's appointment to the acting premiership on February 7 (also the first anniversary of Deng's failure to be named as Zhou's successor), and finally at the first anniversary of the Qing Ming festival on April 5. The Chinese people, the members of the diplomatic community, and the USLO's China-watchers all became caught up in the drama of "Waiting for Deng" in the winter and spring of 1977. As one Chinese told a USLO officer one day in response to a question about his present activity, "I'm waiting for Deng." "Deng who?" the officer inquired. "Deng Xiaoping to return as Premier," came the reply.[8]

II

Any discussion of Deng Xiaoping's drive for power in the autumn, winter, and spring of 1976–77 must begin with an assessment of the problems which his rehabilitation presented for Chairman Hua Guofeng. Despite the intense secrecy which enveloped the details of the PRC's political struggle in 1976–77, Tom Gates and his fellow China-watchers had little difficulty concluding that Hua Guofeng and Deng Xiaoping were antagonists.[9] By November of 1976, Hua had clearly associated himself with the anti-Deng movement to the extent that any attempt to reinstall the former vice premier inevitably created friction within the PRC hierarchy. Hua became personally involved in the anti-Deng campaign early in February 1976 in a speech which he gave to the Politburo shortly after being named as China's acting premier. Hua used the remarks in this speech, comments also endorsed by Mao himself, to identify himself as a critic of Deng's policies. Two months later, on April 19, Hua spoke disparagingly of Deng's alleged "counter-revolutionary" line in foreign affairs when he spoke to a foreign audience in Peking. Moreover, Hua continued to speak of "deepening the criticism of Deng Xiaoping" throughout the summer of 1976 and in his eulogies for both Zhu De in July and Mao Zedong in September. Even as late as October 24, Hua endorsed Wu De's call for a continuation of the anti-Deng movement when Wu addressed the giant anti-Gang rally in Peking.[10] If Hua permitted Deng's rehabilitation, he faced the likely prospect that the former vice premier's ambitions would be difficult to restrain, even if some basic agreement existed between the two men over the division of power within the Party and the state. Hua and Deng simply represented different political aims as well as generations; Hua had gained in power as a result of the Cultural Revolution, Deng was its primary victim.[11] Hua's interest lay in the preservation of the Maoist tradition; Deng's in its prompt and speedy repudiation. Even if one assumed that Hua's criticism of Deng in 1976 simply represented the obligatory repetition of the Party's official line at a time when the leftists controlled the national media, the fact nevertheless remained that Hua had burned many of his bridges with the Dengists by joining the campaign to discredit their leader.

The train of events leading to Deng Xiaoping's official return to the PRC hierarchy began shortly after the arrest of the Gang of Four. On October 10, 1976, Deng wrote a letter to Hua, praising his action in overthrowing the leftists and pledging his support to the new chairman. In the letter, Deng graciously complimented Hua on his wisdom and energy, although many China scholars consider that the former vice premier stopped short in this letter of actually endorsing Hua's claim for continued leadership of the CCP. (The contents of this letter, as well as another which Deng sent to Hua on April 6, 1977, were not revealed until May 1977.)[12] In any event, the letter signified a conciliatory attitude on Deng's part toward Hua, perhaps in the expectation that the new chairman could now work to provide the means for Deng to rejoin the central leadership.

In response to Deng's initiative, however, Hua Guofeng and his supporters temporized. The information which Tom Gates and his USLO colleagues acquired immediately after the arrest of the Gang of Four made them believe that Hua was willing to compromise with Dengism, but not necessarily with Deng. For example, the Party's propaganda campaign against Deng, almost silent since the days of the Tangshan earthquake, disappeared almost completely. Several of Deng's past associates, such as Wan Li at the Railroad Ministry and Zhu Muzhi of the New China News Agency, found themselves restored to office.[13] Wan Li even took on the important task of supervising the construction of Mao's memorial mausoleum, a job which began in great earnest at precisely the same time as the Hua regime started its purges of the Gang's provincial supporters. But Hua's lieutenants, chiefly Wu De and Chen Xilian, continued to oppose efforts to restore Deng himself, arguing that the campaign to discredit both the Gang of Four *and* Deng Xiaoping should proceed together.[14]

By late November and early December, however, a vigorous poster campaign had broken out throughout China, a campaign calling for Deng's rehabilitation on the grounds that he "was a warrior who opposed the Gang of Four."[15] Did such activity indicate a change in Deng's status? When Tom and other USLO officials inquired about Deng's situation in conversations with other PRC diplomats, they discovered the intractability of the neo-Maoists who still held nominal control of the country's political affairs. "Comrade Deng Xiaoping has made mistakes and must be criticized," came the standard reply. And thus, the neo-Maoists and the Deng supporters remained deadlocked in the two months following the arrest of the Gang.

The first break in resolving the Deng crisis occurred in early December 1976, at the hastily called meeting of the Party Plenum in Peking. As stated previously, Hua Guofeng apparently hoped to use this meeting as a vehicle for rallying the Party around his leadership, thereby pushing the Gang permanently out of the picture and Deng temporarily to the sidelines. The Chinese hierarchy refused to support such an initiative, however, and instead confronted Hua with the totally unorthodox means by which he had assumed the chairmanship of the Party and the leadership of the state. Mao's statement to Hua "with you in charge, I am at ease" held little water with the Dengists, and more important with such individuals as Ye Jianying and Li Xiannian, both of whom interpreted Mao's remark as a personal expression of the late chairman and certainly not the decision of the Party as a whole. The Dengists maintained that the Party constitution specified the procedures for electing a chairman, procedures which Hua (and the other enemies of the Gang of Four) had disregarded just six weeks earlier. Quite typically, Ye Jianying played the role of mediator in helping to settle this question and eventually negotiated an agreement between the neo-Maoists and Deng's supporters which provided for the eventual rehabilitation of Deng with Hua maintaining his control of both the chairmanship and the Military Commission. Deng's allies thereby managed to win an important victory; Hua Guofeng had agreed, in principle, to Deng's rehabilitation. The entire matter now involved questions of timing and procedure; it was no longer a question of *if*, but *when* and *how*. Indeed, shortly after the Party convocation adjourned in December, a PRC-sponsored journal in Hong Kong, entitled *The Seventies*, admitted that the "line on Deng is currently undergoing revision."[16]

III

Once the neo-Maoists made this concession to the Deng forces in December, they retreated to a strategy designed to circumscribe and limit the amount of authority which Deng would hold once he returned to the PRC hierarchy. Such a strategy appeared to be the best means to prevent any erosion in Hua Guofeng's authority while at the same time protecting the careers and status of the neo-Maoists. Thus, Hua and his supporters demanded that Deng examine the "mistakes" which he had made between 1973 and 1975 as a precondition to his rehabilitation. The implication was obvious to Deng: he was redeemable only after submitting to a self-criticism by the group which held the statutory power in China at that time. In discussions which Tom Gates and other USLO officers held with the PRC's officials in late 1976 and early 1977, they discovered that Deng's principal "mistake" lay in the fact that "his style and policies of negating the Cultural Revolution gave the Gang of Four an excuse to grab more political power." Deng therefore had failed to demonstrate sufficient strength in limiting the intrigues of the Gang.[17]

This preliminary verbal sparring between the two factions in late 1976 resulted in stalling the campaign to rehabilitate Deng Xiaoping until the beginning of 1977. With the dawn of a new year, however, both the movement to restore Deng to his previous posts and the efforts of his foes to frustrate that development increased in intensity. The focal point for the next round of political maneuvering between the two factions centered on the commemoration of the first anniversary of Zhou Enlai's death, a series of events planned throughout China for the period from January 6 to January 16. The first anniversary of Zhou's death was January 8, and early in January, Deng's supporters began another poster campaign in Shanghai and Guangdong, calling for the former vice premier's return and linking him to the memory of the late premier. As the PRC prepared to memorialize Zhou, millions of Chinese believed that the Center intended to use the occasion to announce Deng's rehabilitation.

Despite the earlier pledges of agreement for Deng's return, Hua Guofeng and the neo-Maoists had no intention of allowing the anniversary of Zhou Enlai's death to be turned into a national demonstration in support of the deposed former vice premier. Their resistance became evident on January 5 when the USLO's officers received an invitation from the Ministry of Foreign Affairs to attend a special screening of the film *Eternal Glory to the Respected and Beloved Premier Zhou Enlai*, scheduled for showing throughout China on January 6. The film appropriately depicted Zhou Enlai's leading role in the Chinese Revolution and his leadership of the PRC, an effective tribute to a much respected leader. Nevertheless, the USLO's officers noticed an ominous omission; the movie seriously downplayed Deng Xiaoping's career as Zhou's protégé, even to the point of removing his voice from the scene at Zhou's funeral where he delivered the eulogy. Since the Chinese masses would see the film the following day, they could not help seeing the short shrift given to Deng.[18] The film conveyed two unmistakable facts of political life in China at that time; Hua and his allies controlled the national media, and these same forces were only grudgingly yielding ground to the Dengists.

On January 6, the Chinese officially began their commemoration of the first anniversary of Zhou Enlai's death. The diplomatic community, and particularly the USLO's China-watchers, took special notice of these events in order to discern any change in Deng's status. As Roger Garside explained, "The Heroes Monument on Tienanmen Square was no longer available as a focus of [political] activity because almost the whole site had been taken over as the building for constructing the Mao Memorial Hall and was surrounded by a wooden palisade. But of course the palisade provided inexhaustible display space for posters."[19]

In that regard, slogans and posters marking the first anniversary of Zhou's death began appearing on the palisade and also along Changan Avenue early in the morning on January 6. Posters calling for the people to "Mourn Premier Zhou" and reminding them that "Premier Zhou Loved the People" found their place alongside others which encouraged the Chinese to "Rally Closely Around Comrade Hua." More important, neither Tom Gates nor any of the other USLO officers noticed any posters calling for Deng

Xiaoping's rehabilitation although several of USLO's officers received other reports claiming that pro-Deng posters had been seen in various parts of Peking.[20]

The poster situation changed dramatically on January 7, however. At 5:30 P.M. that day, one USLO officer noticed the appearance of a poster on the palisade at the Tienanmen construction site, this one definitely calling for Deng's rehabilitation. The writer of the poster acknowledged that Deng had made mistakes but casually dismissed them. Furthermore, the writer asked the Central Committee (in a tone somewhere between impatient and threatening) to make its decision on Deng's status "a bit faster" so the people might know "a bit earlier."[21] The poster clearly revealed that Deng's supporters intended to refute the neo-Maoist claim about the seriousness of the former vice premier's "mistakes."

On January 8, Peking came truly alive as huge crowds joined in the commemoration of Zhou Enlai. Crowds numbering in the tens of thousands passed in and out of Tienanmen Square during the day. By 5 P.M., more than ten thousand Chinese were milling around the Square, setting up wreaths, posing for photos, and laboriously copying down the contents of the posters, slogans, and poems which appeared throughout the area. In addition, virtually every unit in Peking, including service personnel, factory workers, school teachers and children, Party and government officials, and PLA troops, held short memorial ceremonies for Zhou at some point during the day.[22]

On January 8, Peking also witnessed an increasing number of posters calling for Deng's return, with messages such as "Deng Should Return" and "The Central Committee Should Make Its Decision." More important, however, the entire poster scene took on a foreboding character on January 8. In addition to the pro-Deng and pro-Zhou posters, the USLO's China-watchers also noticed several posters critical of Wu De. "The People of the Capital Do Not Trust Wu De," declared one such poster.[23] The significance of these posters could not have been clearer; the leadership debate over Deng's future had broken out of the confines of the Politburo and gone into the streets. Wu De was known as one of Deng's major opponents and perhaps even loosely associated with the Gang of Four before their demise. In attacking Wu, Deng's supporters selected one of their most formidable critics. Furthermore, the posters focused upon Wu De's role in disbursing the pro-Zhou (and by extension, pro-Deng) demonstrations at the Qing Ming festival in April 1976, an action which ultimately led to the Tienanmen riots.[24] On January 8, Deng's postersmiths declared, "The People Insist that the Tienanmen Verdict Be Reversed," thereby exonerating Deng (and blaming the Gang and Wu De) for the disorder which plagued China during the Qing Ming festival.[25]

On January 9, Deng's postersmiths continued to pressure the Hua regime into settling the question of their leader's return to power. More pro-Deng and anti-Wu posters appeared throughout Peking, with many of the messages calling specifically upon Hua Guofeng to restore Deng to office. "Chairman Hua Personally Decided that Deng Should Resume Work," "Chairman Hua Can Rest Easy With Comrade Deng," "Comrade Deng Has No Ambition," and "How Can It Be that a Person Dares to Work and Yet Not Make Mistakes?"

Between January 11 and January 16, the campaign to rehabilitate Deng Xiaoping replaced the commemoration for the late Premier Zhou Enlai as the Chinese took to the streets of Peking to voice their support for the twice-deposed vice premier. By this time, the PRC hierarchy had largely exited from public view and the diplomatic community came to believe that high-level meetings were taking place in the capital as the central leadership wrestled with the issue of Deng's return to office. Without any official resolution of the issue, however, Deng's supporters kept up their poster campaign, criticizing not only Wu De but also Chen Xilian and even Wang Hairong.[26]

On January 12, still another development occurred which brought the Deng issue into sharper focus. On that day, the theoretical writing group of the State Council's General Office published an article in the PRC media which explored in great detail the working relationship between Chairman Mao and Premier Zhou during the years in which they controlled the Party and state. The article praised Zhou's ability to "patiently help leading leaders who had committed mistakes to realize that they had done wrong and encourage them to continue the revolution," and "in taking the initiative in looking after the daily affairs of the Party, the government, and the Army." Had Deng's allies made strong inroads into the PRC media; were they pressuring Hua publicly to restore Deng Xiaoping? Could Hua and Deng have the same working relationship as the writers idealistically ascribed to Mao and Zhou?[27]

On January 13 and 14, large-scale meetings occurred throughout Peking, despite the sense of uncertainty about the Center's attitude concerning Deng's rehabilitation. The high degree of pro-Deng poster activity, however, appeared to indicate that the hierarchy was still deadlocked on the subject. As a result, the posters became more direct. One poster, written by the pseudonymous "Capital Workers," contained a poem which extolled Deng's virtues:

Your energy is great,
Your level [of energy] is high,
Your bones are tough,
Your blood is red.[28]

The poster also bluntly argued, "If a person is stripped of all his positions because of a few mistakes, then who among us has qualifications to be a leader?"

Suddenly on January 14, the posters which were critical of Wu De virtually disappeared, leading many of the members of the diplomatic community to believe that the PRC leadership had resolved the Deng issue.[29] That belief turned out to be erroneous, however. On January 16, scores of Peking housewives carrying brushes and buckets descended upon the wooden palisade at the Tienanmen construction site and began scraping it bare of all its posters and slogans. At the same time, other groups of Party workers began collecting the hundreds of wreaths which had been placed in front of the Forbidden City as memorials to Zhou Enlai and stacked them in trucks to be driven away and presumably discarded. In such a fashion, the week commemorating the life and career of Zhou Enlai ended, without a resolution of Deng Xiaoping's future role in the PRC hierarchy. Deng supporters had engaged the neo-Maoists in a test of wills and apparently lost.[30] The battle to restore Deng to power would have to move to a different ground.

IV

By the third week in January 1977, Tom Gates and the USLO's China-watchers were certain of two facts of political life in China. First, Deng Xiaoping and his supporters were determined to find a role for the former vice premier in China's post-Mao government. Initially, the Dengists may have assumed that Deng's letter of support to Chairman Hua Guofeng, following the arrest of the Gang of Four, may have proven to be sufficient grounds for his return. When that expectation failed to materialize, however, Deng's supporters renewed their efforts and extracted a concession from the Hua faction at the meeting of the Party Congress in December, a concession which appeared to open the way for Deng's orderly return to power.

Since that concession also protected, on the surface at least, Hua's claim to the chairmanship of the Party and the Military Commission, Deng's supporters most likely believed that the former vice premier's return to power was imminent. Hua Guofeng and his supporters delayed, however, and provided no direction about the timing of Deng's restoration. In some respects, they even resisted the efforts of Deng's followers to sway public opinion in favor of their leader, as the events surrounding the commemoration of the first anniversary of Zhou Enlai's death demonstrated. Clearly, the neo-Maoists refused to be stampeded into taking a political step which might eventually lead to their own downfall.

Second, Tom Gates and the American China-watchers in Peking realized that Hua Guofeng could not forestall Deng Xiaoping's return indefinitely.

The mass outpouring of support for Deng in January throughout China, not simply in Peking, indicated that the Chinese people demanded a favorable resolution of the issue. America's China-watching contingent in Peking concluded that Hua had therefore won a Pyrrhic victory in January. While Deng's allies possessed sufficient strength to raise the question of Deng's restoration, they lacked the power to resolve it in their favor. And yet, facing the determination of the Dengists, the Hua regime could not afford to wait for other events to crowd the Deng issue out of the political picture. Deng's supporters were certain to renew their effort to bring their leader back into the hierarchy.

Between January 21 and January 25, the Politburo held several important meetings designed to discuss the rectification campaign then occurring throughout China as well as the matter of Deng's rehabilitation. Following the pattern of the Politburo meetings of the late summer and early autumn, the hierarchy found itself at loggerheads over the positions which Deng would hold once he returned to power. As a result, the Hua regime proposed to refer the Deng question to the members of the Central Committee and assess their views of the matter before making a formal decision on the entire subject.[31]

The Hua regime had good reasons once again to procrastinate in addressing the Deng issue and hoped that its referral of the question to a lower level would help to strengthen its position against the consistent pressure then being applied by Deng's allies. Deng Xiaoping's return meant change in every sector of China's political system, not only within the Politburo but also within the state and Party bureaucracies, and the ranks of the PLA. The tug-of-war over the former vice premier's rehabilitation involved approximately fifty senior PRC officials in the Politburo, the State Council, the provinces, and the PLA. The Hua leadership apparently desired to complicate the issue by involving it in the Party's personal and generational loyalties. If enough officials feared for their own careers with Deng back in power, then perhaps Hua and his supporters might still become the beneficiaries of that fear. If not, they still would possess sufficient time to make the best possible arrangement with the Dengists before returning the former vice premier to office.[32]

In addition, Tom believed that Hua Guofeng was strongly concerned about Deng's physical safety early in 1977. The first two months of 1977 was a time of domestic turmoil and political unrest throughout China and the leadership feared that a "bad element" might attempt to harm Deng if he reappeared too quickly in a tense environment. (The term "bad element" generally referred to Nationalist Chinese or Guomintang agents but, given the unsettled nature of Chinese political life at the time, the regime could not discount the possibility that Deng may have been the target of leftist violence.) Should Deng become the victim of an act of violence, the whole nation could well have turned into a battleground, with leftists and moderates fighting against each other uncontrollably. Concerned for at least the appearance of unity and order, the Hua regime decided to postpone Deng's rehabilitation until the Party had a chance to "study" the vice premier's case further. Thus, the Politburo's meeting of late January also ended inconclusively with the leadership deciding, in effect, to do nothing immediately about Deng's return.[33]

As a result, rumors circulated extensively throughout China during February, with both the neo-Maoists and Dengists contributing to an increasingly tense situation. When news of the Politburo meeting of January 21–25 leaked out, many Chinese and even some members of the diplomatic community believed that the hierarchy had agreed upon the timing of Deng's return. The first anniversary of Hua Guofeng's elevation to acting premier was rapidly approaching on February 7, and one erroneous rumor held that the Politburo intended to restore Deng to his previous posts around that time, since that occasion also marked the first anniversary of the radicals' successful attempt to keep him from the premiership.[34] But February 7 passed, too, with still no word about Deng's rehabilitation. Instead, the American China-watchers learned that Hua Guofeng was still preoccupied with studying Deng's alleged role in the Tienanmen demonstrations of the previous year. If the former vice premier had been involved in those demonstrations, as Mao had once alleged, then the chairman could hardly restore the former vice premier to the leadership without also admitting that Mao himself had made an error. Somehow the Center needed an explanation for Deng's part in those demonstrations which absolved him while also protecting Hua's position and Mao's reputation.[35]

While Hua Guofeng continued to "study" Deng Xiaoping's role in the Tienanmen demonstrations, Deng and his supporters in south China were growing increasingly impatient. As Garside again explained correctly, "The longer [Deng's] return was delayed, the more firmly in the saddle those who had something to fear from it would be."[36] In the view of Deng's allies, the process of de-Maoification began in China with the death of the late chairman and the arrest of the Gang of Four. Since the Dengists largely intended to overturn a healthy number of Mao's policies, they hardly saw the need for any lasting preservation of Mao's personality cult. As a challenge to the neo-Maoists in Peking, Deng's supporters in Guangdong wrote a strongly worded letter to Hua Guofeng and the Central Committee in February, pointing out that "the eyes of the people are wide open. Every one of them knows in his heart where Chairman Mao succeeded and where he failed." The letter went on to press for Deng's rehabilitation and an admission from the Central Committee that the Cultural Revolution was one of Mao's mistakes.[37]

The latest round of pressure from the Deng faction placed Hua Guofeng and the neo-Maoists in a difficult position. Up until February 1977, the Hua leadership had attempted to placate the Deng forces by vigorously pursuing the discrediting of the Gang of Four and arguing that the Gang had taken advantage of Mao's failing health to deceive the late chairman about the charges against Deng as a "capitalist roader" and his role in the Tienanmen riots. Hua Guofeng and his supporters also realized, however, that danger lurked in their attachment to this position. If the neo-Maoists made too great a point about Mao's infirmities during the final months of his life, they left themselves open to the charge that Mao had acted unreliably when he told Hua, "With you in charge, I am at ease." Hua's claim to power lay almost entirely on Mao's mental competence when the chairman allegedly designated him as his successor, or that Mao remained lucid through at least April 30, 1976.[38]

Now under pressure during February, Hua Guofeng and the neo-Maoists attempted to refine their position on Deng's rehabilitation. In effect, they maintained that the full Central Committee should continue to study Deng's case with the matter being eventually resolved at a meeting of the Party Plenum. Specifically, Hua instructed the Party to study whether the radicals, and particularly Mao Yuanxin, had altered Mao's instructions and directives during his final months, possibly even to the extent of forging some of his statements and writings. Since the Party Center had already concluded that one of Jiang Qing's offenses included forging some of Mao's final instructions, particularly in regard to the succession question, Hua's proposal appeared reasonable within the charged political atmosphere in Peking at the time. Such a proposal also held open the possibility that the Party could exonerate Deng from his past "mistakes," if it concluded that the Gang had slandered him. While Hua's latest proposal undoubtedly failed to satisfy the Dengists, it at least kept the door open for continued discussion of the issue within the PRC hierarchy. Nevertheless, by mid-February, China had witnessed a solid six weeks of pro-Deng demonstrations, consisting of poster campaigns and newspaper articles calling for his rehabilitation. Hua's latest proposal permitted the country to pass over, without incident, the anniversary of Deng's denial of the premiership. Whether the scene in the capital and throughout China would stay calm much longer was the question of the moment.[39]

V

By the first week in March, everyone in Peking, both the Chinese and the members of the diplomatic community, appeared to be "waiting for Deng." Considering the outpouring of support for Deng Xiaoping at the first anniversary of Zhou Enlai's death in early January and then again in the weeks immediately thereafter, the American China-watching contingent believed that the PRC hierarchy needed to resolve the Deng issue favorably before the first anniversary of the Qing Ming festival and the Tienanmen riots (then less than a month away) or else face another, and possibly uncontrollable, outburst of pro-Deng demonstrations. In some respects, the Center had already rehabilitated Deng Xiaoping, at least indirectly, by endorsing his policies for economic modernization. Moreover, Deng's publicists within the media were regularly publishing articles which refuted the charges brought against him by the Gang of Four. On March 14, for example, an article appeared in the *People's Daily*, published by an individual writing under the pseudonym of Xiang Chun, which contained the first detailed attempt to explain away Mao's allegation that Deng "was a capitalist roader still on the capitalist road."⁴⁰ Just the fact that Deng's name once again appeared in the PRC media was an indication that he had escaped from the nonperson status to which the radicals had once relegated him.

Between March 9 and March 17, the Politburo met in Peking to hold another wide-ranging series of discussions about the political situation in the country. Since this meeting occurred against the backdrop of uncertainty about Deng's future status (although the PRC hierarchy was inching closer to his rehabilitation), the USLO's officers concluded that the Center would finally reach its decision on the one matter which truly affected most Chinese. In discussions with Chinese diplomats, Tom and his colleagues now received the answer that "Deng would re-appear at an appropriate time under suitable conditions. Deng had made mistakes but also was a victim of the machinations of the Gang of Four." But since the central authorities were then in the midst of their campaign to rectify the Party and over "4,000–5,000 sympathizers of the Gang of Four remained in positions of authority" at various levels throughout China, the USLO's sources cautioned that the leadership needed to move slowly and carefully in making *any* personnel changes.⁴¹

Despite such precautionary language, the diplomatic community understood that the Center was engaged in perhaps its most crucial leadership session since Hua Guofeng convened the Politburo to discuss the arrest of the Gang of Four on October 7. In all, approximately 70 percent of the Party's Central Committee gathered in Peking during the second and third weeks of March to discuss the possible reinstatement of Deng as well as the PRC's faltering economy. On the issue of Deng's imminent return to office, Li Xiannian opened this discussion by proposing that the former vice premier be appointed premier, first vice chairman of the Party, and chief of staff of the PLA. Li spoke passionately in advocating this position (he apparently was not simply setting the opening bid high enough to leave room for compromise after further debate), with Xu Shiyou and Wei Guoqing equally passionate in their support of his remarks. Interestingly, Marshal Ye Jianying indicated that he favored Li's proposal but endorsed it considerably less vigorously than Li, Xu, and Wei.[42]

Li Xiannian's proposal brought forth instant opposition from the neo-Maoists, led principally by Wu De, Chen Xilien, and Wang Dongxing. At this point in the debate, Hua Guofeng refrained from making any comment, apparently willing to let the other neo-Maoists engage Deng's forces. Perhaps Hua also sought to keep out of the opening rounds in order to emerge as the healer and unifier later in the meeting. At any rate, Wu De spoke for the neo-Maoists and insisted that Deng Xiaoping return to office only after making a self-criticism and agreeing to strictly defined limits on his authority. Even though only a vocal minority, Wu De, Chen Xilian, and Wang Dongxing, and their supporters managed once again to forestall the resolution of the Deng issue on the terms which they considered unacceptable. Li Xiannian then offered a compromise; Deng should be restored only to the positions which he had held prior to his dismissal in the spring of 1976. Once again, however, the neo-Maoists insisted that Deng make a self-criticism and agree to prescribed limits on his authority before returning to *any* position. With the two factions once again deadlocked, the session yet again adjourned without resolving the issue.

Hua Guofeng and the other members of the Party Center did not permit the issue of Deng Xiaoping's rehabilitation to fade away for a fourth time, however. By this time, the entire leadership apparently realized that a paramount national concern involved reaching a decision on Deng's future. On March 20, therefore, Hua convened the leaders of the Party for what he labeled a "work conference," a device (so Hua claimed) which Mao had used during the 1950s and 1960s to deal with important political issues. For the next three days, the members of the Politburo, the provincial first secretaries, and the commanders of the PRC's military regions wrestled with the case of Deng Xiaoping, realizing that the issue needed to be resolved by the end of the month or the nation might face prolonged disorder. According to the USLO's sources, Marshal Ye Jianying gave the conference's opening address; apparently the task of breaking yet another deadlock within the CCP had once again fallen to the veteran defense minister. Ingeniously searching for a suitable compromise, Marshal Ye proposed that the Party agree to restore Deng to his previous posts in the Party, the state, and military. Such a restoration meant that Deng would continue to hold a position subordinate to that of Hua Guofeng; apparently Ye was still willing to protect Hua's position in the interests of national unity and Party stability. The Party was therefore to agree that, even with Deng's return to office, Hua would continue in the same posts which he presently held. In addition, Ye expressed no opposition to the idea that Deng examine his previous record to determine if it contained any "mistakes." More important, however, Ye opposed any effort by the Party to circumscribe or limit Deng's authority once he returned to office. As a veteran comrade, Deng must have the same right as any other Party member to "move ahead on his own."[43]

Shortly after Marshal Ye Jianying's speech, Hua Guofeng addressed the conference. Hua recited a list of accomplishments achieved under his leadership of the PRC—the arrest of the Gang of Four, the conferences on industry and agriculture, the construction of the Mao Memorial Mausoleum (which the Center erected in record time), and the publication of the next volume of Mao's writings. Then turning to the subject on everyone's mind, Hua praised Deng Xiaoping as a "good comrade" and "a man of many achievements." Nevertheless, Hua continued, Deng had made mistakes, principally in his handling of the Gang of Four. His blunt style had "served to alert the Gang" and allowed them to strike him down successfully. By contrast, Hua and Ye had shown themselves more decisive by "smashing the Gang with one blow."[44] Next, Hua took the extremely important step of clearing Deng from any involvement in the Tienanmen riots, blaming Jiang Qing instead as the villain behind the instigation of the disorder. "The majority of the people had been expressing their hatred of the Gang of Four for the unjust defamation of Zhou's memory," he explained.[45] Finally, Hua also instructed that "innocents" arrested at the time of the riots should be released from prison, and any cadres wrongly accused should be cleared.[46]

The work conference finally succeeded in resolving the issue of Deng Xiaoping's rehabilitation and also in settling some of the other outstanding political business then confronting the Party. After accepting the compromise dealing with Deng's second rehabilitation, the Politburo agreed to implement this decision at the next meeting of the Party Plenum, which the leadership apparently expected to hold sometime in mid-summer. The Party nevertheless instructed its members that they could begin informing lower-level cadres of the favorable decision regarding Deng's return to the hierarchy.[47] The leadership thereby managed to meet its deadline of the end of March for settling the Deng issue. Even then, the Party Center increased its security forces substantially in Peking in late March and early April (just as it also had done in early January) and indicated that it would tolerate no unusual displays of pro-Deng activity during the Qing Ming festival. In any event, the Qing Ming anniversary passed peacefully in Peking and the nation apparently began looking forward with some relief to Deng's second rehabilitation.

VI

After the adjournment of the work conference, the Hua regime still confronted the matter of justifying the return of Mao Zedong's most vigorous critic to a government which, at that time, seemed intent upon preserving a favorable impression of the late chairman. The diplomatic community marveled, in a sense, at the way in which the Party Center explained this development to its people. Essentially, the explanation occurred in a series of two articles published in the *People's Daily*, the first on March 19 and the second on March 30. It was important to note that the first article appeared shortly after the adjournment of the Politburo's expanded meeting between March 9 and March 17, and the second after the adjournment of the work conference on March 23. The timing of the appearance of those two articles seemed to indicate that the Center reached its decision on the rationale for Deng's rehabilitation *between* the two meetings. The leadership had used the expanded Politburo meeting to identify the factional differences which prevented a resolution of Deng's case and then employed the work conference as the device to reach agreement on the final compromise which settled the issue.

Both articles in the *People's Daily* presented in allegorical form a comparison between the leadership struggle in the Soviet Union which broke out between Joseph Stalin and Leon Trotsky and their supporters following the death of Vladimir Lenin in 1924 with the power struggle in China which occurred after the death of Mao Zedong. On March 19, for example, the *People's Daily* carried an article entitled "The Trotskyists Who Ganged Up to Usurp Power," signed by a pseudonymous writer named Ku Shan. Published on page 1 of the newspaper, the article drew an explicit analogy between the Trotskyites who tried to gain political control of the Soviet Union in 1926 and the Gang of Four who made a similar effort in China in 1976. The writer depicted the Trotskyites as "splittists and schemers . . . extremely similar to the Gang of Four." Then in a style unmistakable to the Chinese reader, the writer identified the personalities of the 1920s in the Soviet Union allegorically with individuals prominent in contemporary China. For example, he described Lenin as "the great leader," an obvious comparison to Mao, and Stalin as the "individual around whom the whole Party and people closely rallied following Lenin's death," a direct reference to Hua Guofeng. Trotsky and his supporters attacked the "long-tested veterans of the Russian Revolution as bureaucratic, rigid, and conservative"; the equivalent "long-tested veterans" in the PRC were those of the Long March generation, such as Ye Jianying, Li Xiannian, and Deng Xiaoping.

Showing the influence of Deng's publicists and recognizing that the Party had failed to resolve the former vice premier's case, the March 19 article then continued with an ominous reference to a "new opposition faction" which appeared in the Soviet Union following Stalin's ouster of Trotsky. "Led by [Leo] Kamenev and [Gregory] Zinoviev," this faction "openly swung to the Trotskyite position, negating Lenin's line and disputing the possibility of establishing socialism in the Soviet Union." These charges essentially paralleled those which the Dengists were currently making against Wu De (whom the USLO's officers likened to Kamenev) and Li Desheng and Wang Dongxing (likened to Zinoviev), individuals who were then disputing the Hua regime's current economic line.[48]

The second article in the allegory, "Counter-revolutionary Activities of the Trotskyites During the Period of Lenin's Critical Illness," appeared in the *People's Daily* on March 30. Once again, the article developed the analogy between the followers of Trotsky and the Gang of Four. The writer noted that a "declining Lenin" (Mao) was for a time physically incapable of "overseeing affairs" but still had moments during which he still dictated letters and final instructions. With little subtlety, the writer also implied that Mao's final illness precluded his direct involvement in Deng Xiaoping's second purge in April 1976 but that the late chairman was capable, during "slight turns for the better," of anointing Hua as his successor. The article also contained a cryptic reference to the Trotskyites (Gang of Four) winning over a "pitiful three supporters" (Wu De, Wang Dongxing, and Li Desheng) at a crucial leadership meeting. Thus, the writer concluded, "It is not difficult for us to perceive that the activities to seize Party and state power waged in our country by the Gang of Four were in many respects a replaying of the old tricks of the Trotskyite bandit gang. In essence, the Gang of Four and the Trotskyite bandit gang have nothing at all dissimilar."[49]

Like the March 19 article, the March 30 article repeated the nature of Trotsky's struggle with Stalin in terms familiar to the Chinese readers, who were by then accustomed to reading attacks on the Gang of Four. In summary, the article claimed that Trotsky (Jiang Qing) used Lenin's final illness (Mao's last months) to wage unprincipled struggle against the "old Bolsheviks" (the Long March generation) and Lenin's successor, Stalin (Hua Guofeng). Trotsky's "press overlord," Karl Radek (Yao Wenyuan) manipulated *Pravda* (*People's Daily*) to favor Trotsky's claim to succeed Lenin. Trotsky took advantage of internal economic crises (the Tangshan earthquake?) and threatening "external foes" (the two superpowers) to make his bid for power. He also used youth, especially college students, and put "his man" (Zhang Chunqiao) in charge of the Red Army's Political Department while also plotting to establish a second Party center in Moscow (Shanghai).

Those parallels lent special significance to the declining Lenin as he entered the final stage of his life. Trotsky was able to carry out his scheme because "Lenin's illness" worsened and he was "unable to oversee affairs." Nonetheless, "under conditions of a slight turn for the better in his medical condition, Lenin orally gave his last few articles and letters."[50] To the politically astute Chinese reader, the allegory's meaning was obvious: Mao's final illness prevented his direct involvement in the purge of Deng Xiaoping but he was still capable of authoritatively proclaiming to Hua, "With you in charge, I am at ease." Thus the Center devised its rationale for restoring

Deng to his posts without unduly damaging Hua's status or Mao's prestige. By making the Gang of Four its scapegoat, the Center worked its way, verbally at least, out of what appeared to be an intractable political deadlock.

After the first week in April, both the Dengists and the neo-Maoists attempted, on the surface at least, to make conciliatory gestures in each other's direction. In accordance with the agreement reached at the Party's work conference in late March, Deng wrote a second letter to Hua Guofeng on April 6. In that letter, Deng made three points: he thanked Hua for divorcing him from the Tienanmen riots, he thanked Hua for releasing from prison those who had been unjustly accused or punished, and he pledged his continued loyalty to the Party while expressing a willingness "to assume any post, in any area, at any time," as directed by the Center.[51] Moreover, Deng admitted that, while he accomplished much in 1975, he also committed unspecified "mistakes" and "shortcomings." Such a confession seemed mild indeed and the fact that Deng admitted to no specific mistakes may have indicated his resistance to admitting *any* mistakes.[52]

For his part, Hua Guofeng chose the release of the Fifth Volume of Mao's writings to officially recognize Deng's continued importance to the Party. No less than nine passages praised Deng's work in the 1950s, including a statement (which Deng must have found amusing) acclaiming him as Mao's "comrade-in-arms" with the two men enjoying a "close working relationship."[53]

VI

The Chinese Communist Party managed to avoid another potentially divisive, and perhaps explosive, situation in China during the spring of 1977 by restoring Deng Xiaoping to his posts. The first anniversary of the Qing Ming festival passed off uneventfully and peacefully.

When the Party announced Deng's rehabilitation in early August at the session of the Fourth National Party Congress, the Chinese people reacted with relief and jubilation. As Roger Garside has explained,

When the decision [to restore Deng to his posts] was announced on radio and television at 8 P.M. firecrackers and rockets shot into the air all over Peking. The next day there were jubilant processions in Peking, and throughout the country provincial leaders acclaimed his return to office. On 12 August he made his first public appearance at a soccer match in Peking's biggest stadium. There was an outside radio broadcast of the match and thunderous applause could be heard from the crowd of eighty thousand as his arrival was announced.[54]

Once Deng returned to the front ranks of the PRC hierarchy, he wasted little time informing the Party about his attitude regarding its future course of action. "There must be less empty talk and more hard work," he declared in his closing speech to the National Party Congress.[55] Such words conveyed the impression that Deng's return meant a definite setback to the career aspirations of Hua Guofeng and the neo-Maoists whose influence had risen so rapidly during the past year and which seemed to have reached its crest. "With you back, I have worries," Ross Terrill explained in describing Hua's presumed feelings about Deng's second rehabilitation.[56] Without question, Deng enjoyed the widest base of support, in both the CCP and the state, of any Chinese politician at that time. In addition, he was a more experienced, able leader, and as one who had played a key role in the events of the Chinese Revolution, he profited from an enhanced popular image. The supporters of Hua Guofeng had managed to stop Deng short of actually assuming the de facto leadership of China in the spring of 1977; they were unable to prevent him from establishing a political beachhead from which to advance his interests and those of his supporters.

"I believe that Deng interpreted his letter of confession on April 6 more as an indignity forced upon him by the neo-Maoists than as any expression of contrition," David Dean recalled in an interview. "In his mind, Deng never made mistakes, did he?" Dean added with a twinkle. "The confession was simply the minimum device necessary to admit him to the councils of power." Later on Deng made a successful effort to remove *even* those individuals (Hua Guofeng, Wu De, Wang Dongxing, and their supporters) who forced him to make the confession. Moreover, the neo-Maoists had good reason to extract the maximum number of concessions from Deng before he was rehabilitated. "They completely realized that Deng intended to promote his policies and the careers of his supporters, which he eventually did," Dean added.[57] Peking was worth a confession of "mistakes" to Deng Xiaoping in 1977. In that fashion, Deng resumed his struggle to overturn the policies of the man who had labeled him a "monster, sham-Marxist, counter-revolutionary, and capitalist-roader."[58] The spring of 1977 witnessed the resumption of Deng's efforts to win his final victory over Mao Zedong.

Notes

1. Terrill, *Future of China*, pp. 47, 67.

2. Garside, *Coming Alive*, pp. 175–82; Hsu, *China Without Mao*, pp. 31–32; Terrill, *Future of China*, pp. 67, 216–20.

3. Garside, *Coming Alive*, p. 23.

4. United States Department of State, Official Files, Peking to Washington, 25 January 1977. Hereafter cited as OF, date.

5. OF, Peking to Washington, 5 November 1976; Garside, *Coming Alive*, pp. 140–41; Hsu, *China Without Mao*, p. 14. One cannot discount the possibility, however, that Deng re-

mained in Guangdong until after the purge of the Gang of Four. See Terrill, *White-Boned Demon*, p. 372.

6. OF, Peking to Washington, 22 October 1976; Garside, *Coming Alive*, pp. 67–70.

7. OF, Peking to Washington, 13 January 1977.

8. OF, Peking to Washington, 16 March 1977; Garside, *Coming Alive*, pp. 334–35.

9. Interview, David Dean, 9 February 1983; interview, Richard Mueller, 17 February 1983.

10. OF, Peking to Washington, 20 January 1977.

11. OF, Peking to Washington, 24 January 1977.

12. Bill Brugger, *From Radicalism to Revisionism* (Totawa, N.J.: Barnes and Noble Books, 1982), pp. 202–3.

13. OF, Peking to Washington, 22 October 1976.

14. Brugger, *From Radicalism to Revisionism*, pp. 202–3.

15. Fox Butterfield, "Teng Seen Making Comeback in China After April Purge," *New York Times*, 28 November 1976, pp. 1, 21.

16. OF, Peking to Washington, 20 December 1976; Hsu, *China Without Mao*, pp. 29–30.

17. OF, Peking to Washington, 29 November 1976.

18. OF, Peking to Washington, 5 January 1977.

19. Garside, *Coming Alive*, p. 175.

20. OF, Peking to Washington, 6 January 1977. Other observers apparently did notice some pro-Deng poster activity on January 6. See *Washington Post*, 7 January 1977.

21. OF, Peking to Washington, 7 January 1977.

22. OF, Peking to Washington, 8 January 1977.

23. OF, Peking to Washington, 8 January 1977.

24. Jay Matthews, "Attacks on Peking's Mayor Seen," *Washington Post*, 9 January 1977.

25. OF, Peking to Washington, 8 January 1977.

26. OF, Peking to Washington, 10 January 1977; Fox Butterfield, "Some Chinese Uneasy Over Peking Demonstrations," *New York Times*, 13 January 1977.

27. OF, Peking to Washington, 12 January 1977.

28. OF, Peking to Washington, 13 January 1977.

29. Ibid.; OF, Peking to Washington, 14 January 1977.

30. OF, Peking to Washington, 16 January 1977.

31. OF, Peking to Washington, 2 February 1977.

32. OF, Washington to Peking, 10 February 1977; OF, Washington to Peking, 10 March 1977.

33. OF, Peking to Washington, 2 February 1977.

34. Garside, *Coming Alive*, p. 179.

35. Peking to Washington, 11 February 1977.

36. Garside, *Coming Alive*, p. 175.

37. Ibid., pp. 179–80.

38. OF, Peking to Washington, 18 January 1977; OF, Peking to Washington, 18 January 1977.

39. OF, Peking to Washington, 15 March 1977.

40. OF, Peking to Washington, 15 March 1977.

41. OF, Peking to Washington, 5 March 1977l.

42. OF, Peking to Washington, 30 March 1977; Garside, *Coming Alive*, pp. 180–81.

43. OF, Peking to Washington, 1 April 1977; OF, Peking to Washington, 16 April 1977; OF, Peking to Washington, 23 May 1977; OF, Peking to Washington, 13 July 1977; see also Garside, *Coming Alive*, pp. 180–81, and Hsu, *China Without Mao*, pp. 30–31.

44. OF, Peking to Washington, 23 May 1977.

45. Ibid.; OF, Peking to Washington, 1976–77; see also Garside, *Coming Alive*, p. 181.

46. Ibid.

47. OF, Peking to Washington, 13 July 1977.

48. OF, Peking to Washington, 28 March 1977.

49. OF, Peking to Washington, 31 March 1977.

50. Ibid.

191 Waiting for Deng

51. OF, Peking to Washington, 23 May 1977.
52. OF, Peking to Washington, 7 June 1977.
53. OF, Peking to Washington, 27 April 1977.
54. Garside, *Coming Alive*, pp. 182–83.
55. Ibid., p. 184.
56. Terrill, *Future of China*, p. 217.
57. Interview, David Dean, 9 February 1983.
58. Domes, "Hua Kuo-feng and the 'Gang of Four,'" pp. 494–95; Terrill, *Future of China*, p. 217.

CHAPTER **8**

Waiting for Carter

Jimmy Carter's razor-thin victory over Gerald Ford in the 1976 presidential election spelled the end of the Ford presidency and also of Thomas Gates's tenure as chief of the United States Liaison Office to the People's Republic of China. With the prospect for diplomatic normalization between the United States and China clearly on the horizon, Carter certainly intended to appoint his own presidential envoy to the PRC with responsibility for promoting the new administration's interests at the working level in Peking. Moreover, since 1973, the chief of the USLO had become an increasingly important individual within America's foreign policy establishment, and Carter undoubtedly found many aspirants for this post.

In late November, Tom Gates received a message from Secretary of State Henry Kissinger outlining the procedures for submitting his resignation to the president. On December 29, Tom complied with Kissinger's instructions and wrote a letter to both President Ford and President-elect Carter asking that his resignation as chief of the United States Liaison Office be accepted, effective January 21, 1977.[1] After communicating with Ford, Tom remained in Peking, awaiting word about the timing of his return to the United States. Carter had assembled a foreign policy transition group, and Tom expected to hear from Secretary of State-designate Cyrus Vance, who also happened to be a good friend, about the turnover of his office in Peking.

Once in office, however, the Carter administration appeared to be in no particular hurry to appoint Tom's replacement. In some respects, this delay had its advantages; Tom had grown especially close to his American colleagues and also enjoyed the Peking diplomatic community. We were not looking forward to leaving China but recognized that the Carter administration needed to appoint its own chief of the USLO in order to implement its own policies in China. As a result, Tom wrote to Secretary Vance after the inauguration, requesting that his resignation be officially accepted by the administration on April 14, around the time of the first anniversary of his confirmation as chief of the USLO in 1976.[2] Vance found this proposal agreeable, although we did not actually depart from China until May 8, almost one year exactly after our arrival the previous year. Between the time of Carter's election in November 1976 and our departure in May, Tom continued to direct the USLO operation, all the while waiting for the Carter administration to name his replacement and thereby begin another chapter in Chinese-American relations.

During this five-month waiting period, Tom Gates continued his effort to promote improved relations with the Chinese at the working level in Peking while also preparing the transition of the USLO office for his successor. In several respects, Carter's election to the presidency in 1976 occurred at a fortuitous time in Chinese-American relations. After the purge of the Gang of Four, the Hua regime appeared ready to pursue a more cautiously outward-looking foreign policy. In fact, many PRC officials were not at all reluctant to declare their desire for improved relations with the United States, a fact which became clear in the more open, less formal diplomatic environment of the post-Gang period.[3] "The radicals had always favored restoration of ties with the Soviet Union and opposed better relations with the United States," one Chinese official observed shortly after the Gang's arrest. "Zhou Enlai's policy to pursue better relations with the United States had been formulated by [Chairman] Mao; Hua [Guofeng] and the present leadership will now be able to carry out the 'correct' foreign policy without interference."[4]

Tom Gates and his USLO colleagues, as well as the Ford administration's senior foreign policy officers in Washington, also realized that the purge of the radicals presented an excellent opportunity for rapid progress in the completion of normalized relations between the United States and the People's Republic. Reflecting back, years later, Gerald Ford observed:

There was no doubt in my mind, had I been re-elected in 1976, that we intended to push vigorously for normalization with the PRC on reasonable terms in 1977. I was for [normalization], Kissinger was for it, and Tom Gates was for it. I wanted Tom Gates to stay on [as chief of the USLO]. Both we and the Chinese recognized the arrangements that needed to be made and we knew that the process could not be allowed to drag on *ad infinitum*. There was obviously a change in the Chinese leadership following the death of Mao and I considered that change desirable [from the standpoint of American policy].[5]

With the advent of the Carter administration, therefore, Tom Gates discovered that his basic responsibilities in Peking did not change. He continued to assure the Chinese that improved relations with the PRC would be a priority for the Carter administration, just as it had been for Presidents Nixon and Ford. His job did become more complicated, however, especially in view of the Carter administration's different approach to the entire subject of Chinese-American relations.

II

If the purge of the Gang of Four permitted the Hua regime to make some modest gestures in the direction of the United States, the Americans in Peking did not need to wait long before encountering the PRC's renewed interest in its relationship with America, especially at the diplomatic level in Peking. Essentially, the Chinese wanted expressions of assurance from the United States that the American government understood two of their primary concerns; first, the PRC's continued suspicions about the direction of Soviet foreign policy, and second, an understanding on America's part that if the Chinese should alter their rigid economic policy of self-reliance and take a more active role in the international economy, that the United States would look favorably upon such a shift.

As mentioned previously, Tom Gates heard no theme uttered more frequently by Chinese diplomats during his tenure in the PRC than that the United States needed to take a firmer position diplomatically against the Soviet Union. Officials at the Soviet Embassy in Peking clearly understood the efforts of the Chinese in this regard and even occasionally tried to frustrate them. On June 18, 1976, for example, shortly after Tom's arrival in Peking, he paid a courtesy call on Vasily Tolstikov, the Soviet ambassador, at the Soviet Embassy. The Soviet Union's diplomatic compound in Peking was one of the largest in the city, and Tom drove a considerable distance inside the Embassy grounds before arriving at the ambassador's residence. Tom had not encountered a Soviet official publicly since May 1960, when he had accompanied President Eisenhower to the ill-fated Four Power Summit in Paris in the aftermath of the U-2 crisis when the Soviets had shot down Francis Gary Powers on a surveillance mission over the Soviet Union. For that reason, he was especially curious to see how this meeting with the Soviet ambassador would turn out. After introducing himself to Tolstikov, Tom remarked that the Soviets certainly enjoyed a sizable, impressive presence in Peking. Tolstikov responded humorously, "Why not, we're a superpower."

Despite this initial display of humor, Tolstikov proved to be an especially determined individual. During his first conversation with Tom, the Soviet ambassador expressed the opinion that he wished to become better acquainted and hoped to see more of Tom than he had of Ambassadors Bruce and Bush. Perhaps, Tolstikov suggested, the Americans might be interested in scheduling some joint meetings with the staff of the Soviet Embassy, or maybe even hold a series of seminars for a day or two where the two sides could exchange views. Tom considered these offers "pretty dangerous," which if accepted could only provoke a reaction from the Chinese, and as a result, he graciously declined the invitations. Nor did the Soviets make the offers again.[6]

By the autumn of 1976, the Chinese were consistently encouraging the United States to take a stronger anti-Soviet position in their diplomatic statements. In many ways, James Schlesinger's visit to China underscored the PRC's desire for the Americans to maintain the military balance against the Soviets.[7] Then on October 6, Tom witnessed a determined attempt by the PRC to pressure the United States into responding to the Soviet threat. On that day, Tom and Secretary Kissinger met with Foreign Minister Qiao Guanhua and Huang Hua, then the Chinese ambassador to the United Nations, at the PRC's headquarters in New York for bilateral discussions relating to the opening of the United Nations General Assembly. Although both Kissinger and Tom were unaware of it at the time, this meeting turned out to be Qiao Guanhua's swan song, since he was purged after his return to China. On this occasion, however, Qiao began the discussion by reciting the traditional Chinese view of the world situation, casting special contempt on the Soviet Union. He also spoke critically of detente and warned the United States that it faced inevitable war with the Soviets unless it displayed more resolve. In Qiao's view, the Soviets were an ascending, and the United States a declining power. Kissinger was fully equal to Qiao's challenges. Somewhat impatiently, the secretary of state explained that the Ford administration considered Qiao's views inaccurate, and certainly not new. Qiao's analysis was wrong, Kissinger declared; the United States was not weak and the administration was absolutely mindful of the need to maintain a strong defense. Moreover, Kissinger emphasized that, in his opinion, the Chinese should recognize the reality of American power; for them to simply keep reciting their traditional criticisms was growing tiresome for the administration.[8]

After returning to Peking, Tom Gates found himself cast in the role of defending American strength to the new leadership of the People's Republic. On December 31, he extended a courtesy call on Huang Hua, who had succeeded Qiao Guanhua as the PRC's foreign minister on December 3. Huang

Hua was a veteran PRC diplomat, and unlike many others in China's Foreign Ministry, he had direct experience in negotiations with the United States. In addition to serving as the first ambassador of the PRC to the United Nations, Huang had been involved in the negotiations with Secretary of State George C. Marshall in 1946 when Marshall visited China in hopes of mediating a settlement of the Chinese civil war involving the Communists and the Nationalists. He also was a member of the Chinese delegation which represented the PRC at the talks in Panmunjom which ultimately ended the Korean War. During this meeting, Tom repeated America's adherence to the Shanghai Communique as the basis for improved relations between the United States and China. For his part, Huang retreated to a traditional recitation of the PRC's foreign policy litany, apparently in recognition of the fact that since both countries were engaged in their own political transitions, little could be added to the diplomatic dialogue at that time.[9]

Following Tom's official courtesy call on Huang Hua on December 31, he followed up with a formal invitation to the foreign minister on January 20, inviting the foreign minister and Madame Huang to dinner at the USLO residence any time between January 21 and January 27. Somewhat to Tom's surprise, the Foreign Ministry responded immediately, replying that Huang would be pleased to attend a dinner on Tuesday evening, January 25. In addition to the foreign minister and his wife, the Foreign Ministry explained that Wang Hairong, Tang Wensheng, Lin Ping, and several high-ranking PRC diplomats planned to attend the dinner.[10]

In many respects, the USLO's dinner for Huang Hua on January 25 represented a high point in Tom Gates's diplomatic contacts with the PRC's officials. In the first place, the dinner raised a considerable number of eyebrows in Peking's diplomatic community since direct contacts with the PRC's senior officials were rare occasions at that time. Second, Huang Hua's acceptance of this invitation, made so quickly after Carter's inauguration, was interpreted as a signal that the Chinese continued to desire improved relations with the United States generally, and with the Carter administration specifically.[11]

On the evening of January 25, the USLO's Chinese guests and the American China-watchers engaged in an extensive discussion of the international situation, particularly as it dealt with relations between the two countries. Huang Hua expressed his concern about the state of the world economy, especially about the economic health of the Western democracies. He also indicated that the Chinese were paying close attention to policy statements made by the Carter administration and were keenly interested in the identities and background of the individuals which the new president had appointed to the key positions in the State Department and the National Security Council. Tom responded to these questions as directly as his own experience permitted, explaining that he was well-acquainted with Secretary of State Vance but was largely unfamiliar with most of the other Carter appointees. Finally, Huang referred to the subject of the Sino-Soviet rivalry, adding that the Chinese believed that they were taking the Soviet threat more seriously than was the United States. Despite assurances from both Tom and David Dean that the United States intended to remain fully prepared to meet any Soviet challenge to its interests, Huang continued to emphasize that the Chinese favored a greater degree of Western political, economic, and military unity, as well as more substantial American support for NATO. For their part, the Chinese intended to "remain vigilant" in matters affecting their own policy toward the Soviets.[12]

III

In addition to the obvious concern about the poor quality of their relations with the Soviet Union, the Chinese also began making a few tentative steps toward revising their economic doctrine of self-reliance in late 1976 and early 1977. Any change in this view implied that the Chinese were considering adopting a more active future role in the international economy. On this matter, the USLO was able to be somewhat helpful in demonstrating that the United States favored such a change in the PRC's traditional economic policies, especially by encouraging the continuation of the numerous scientific, cultural, and educational exchanges then under way between the two countries, and also by assisting in the contacts which the Chinese wished to make with American businessmen and economic officers in the Ford administration. When Tom arrived in China in May 1976, American trade with the PRC for the first quarter of that year amounted to $134.5 million, of which American exports totalled $88.5 million and imports $49.0 million, and the recent purge of Deng Xiaoping implied that the Chinese had reached a standstill as far as increasing their international trading activity was concerned.[13] After the arrest of the Gang of Four, however, the prospects for greater trade involving America and China improved considerably (even if the volume of trade still was small by later standards), especially with the prospect of Deng Xiaoping's return to office. Shortly after the arrest of the Gang, the Chinese hosted a visit to the PRC by Arthur Burns, chairman of the Federal Reserve Board, also one of Tom's former associates from the Eisenhower years. Interestingly enough, Burns's arrived in the PRC in his effort to promote better economic cooperation between the United States and China at approximately the same time as the arrest of the Gang of Four. On October 11, Burns met for three hours with Pu Ming, the deputy director of the People's Bank of China, and Lin Jixi, the deputy general manager of the Bank of China. The Chinese wished to discuss a wide variety of economic issues and particularly the matter of international exchange rates.

Arthur Burns was exceptionally knowledgeable about the entire subject of international finance and the American China-watching contingent considered his visit a successful introduction of Chinese and American central bankers. [14]

On December 17, Tom Gates met with Wang Hairong at the Foreign Ministry to discuss the continuation of the numerous scientific, cultural, and technical exchanges which then existed between the United States and China. These exchanges had grown increasingly important, not only because they provided each country with the means of learning more about the other but also as a constant reminder of the continuing relationship which existed between the two nations. During this session, Wang Hairong appeared noticeably more relaxed and considerably less ideologically oriented than during her previous meetings with Tom. Tom expressed his view that the Shanghai Communique would continue to be recognized by the United States, regardless of which administration was in office. For her part, Wang indicated her approval with the numerous exchange programs then under way between the United States and China and hoped that these programs would continue. [15]

On January 11, David Rockefeller, chairman of the Chase Manhattan Bank, arrived in Peking for a five-day visit, and the USLO arranged for him to meet several high-ranking PRC officials. On January 13, Tom hosted a luncheon for Rockefeller and his group with several Chinese diplomats, and on January 14, Huang Hua also held a luncheon for the Americans. On January 15, Rockefeller, Tom, and several other Americans met with Li Xiannian at the Great Hall of the People for two and a half hours. As China's chief economic planner, Li appeared especially interested in receiving Rockefeller's assessment of the international economic situation. For his part, Rockefeller expressed a desire to learn about the way Li viewed the possible impact of China's political upheavals upon its future economic policies. Tom recalled this conversation as one of the most memorable in which he participated with the Chinese, one certainly indicative of a serious interest on the PRC's part of advancing its relationship with the United States, particularly in view of the advent of a new administration. [16]

In 1977 the Hua regime was not prepared to make a visible break with the economic policies of the Maoist past. The discussions which the Chinese held with Arthur Burns and David Rockefeller represented only exceedingly small steps taken in the direction of economic liberalization. In early April, however, Tom received a more realistic opinion from a leading PRC diplomat that the PRC's post-Mao leadership intended to move cautiously in revising its economic policy. At this time, Tom and David Dean took an eight-day trip which covered a good portion of south China. Lin Ping, director of the Foreign Ministry's Bureau of Americas and Oceania, escorted Tom and David on this visit. Since the three men had already become well-acquainted during the previous year, this visit provided an occasion for them to converse extensively about the future of China. In fact, Tom and David probed as deeply as they felt appropriate with Lin Ping, given the still-uncertain political environment which existed at the time. On the train from Hangzhou to Shanghai, they asked Lin about the permanence of the Chinese policy of economic self-reliance. How did China expect to modernize its economy by itself? How could it develop its oil resources, expand its industrial base, create an economic infrastructure, and obtain financing and foreign exchange without international assistance? For the first time, Lin indicated (albeit in qualified fashion) that a change in economic philosophy may be forthcoming under the new leadership. "Our way is right," he explained. "It *is* slower, harder for our people—but it is best for them in the long run and they know it because we are a government that belongs to them." But then he added, importantly, "But perhaps our policy of self-reliance can no longer be so exclusive." Tom and David Dean immediately sensed the difference in tone; the China of the future would go outside slowly, reluctantly, and probably only as an act of economic necessity, but it would seek the technology and management skills which it lacked. Self-reliance would remain a doctrine, but no longer an absolute rule of economic practice. The challenge confronting the Hua regime at this time was how to adapt the ideals of the Maoist past to the demands of the present and the future.[17]

Lin Ping's private views were not pronouncements of official policy, and the Hua regime certainly gave no indication, prior to our departure in May 1977 that it was modifying its doctrine on the economics of self-reliance. Just before leaving, Tom had a final opportunity to meet with Li Xiannian, who categorically asserted that the PRC continued to adhere to Mao's economic teachings. In fact, Li lectured Tom on the subject; China intended to pursue an independent course; it would not borrow large sums from the outside, it would never rely on foreign investment as the quickest route to its own economic modernization.

Within just one year's time, however, Li was speaking quite a different story. In the spring of 1978, Tom and I received an invitation from the PRC authorities to visit China as private citizens. Several months later, in late September, we returned to China and found a country considerably different from the one we had left the previous year. During October, we made a nine-city tour of China. We visited Sian and saw the two-thousand-year-old life-size army of an ancient Chinese emperor which had recently been unearthed, and we also saw the gorges of the Yangtze, the mountains of Kweilin, and the natural beauty of Hangzhou. We traveled inland through the center of China and saw the fields, the agriculture, the textile mills, the tea plantations, and the communes. We talked with the officials in Peking and the local revolutionary vice chairmen, who met us in each city. In one particular city, we heard a local official explain that "Mao's self-reliance program could be *bent* to meet a new policy that was now needed to speed up industrialization in China" (emphasis added). On one of our visits to a tea plantation, an American member of our party asked a Chinese administrator how he determined the wage scale for the individuals who worked under him: "If two men have the same job—and one does it poorly, the other produces as he should, or even better—do they have the same salary?" The administrator responded instantly, "No, the one doing the better job gets a bonus." Such comments as these would have been unthinkable in China during the previous two years.

In Peking, Tom met with Li Xiannian on October 3, this time for a two-hour conversation which dealt largely with the visible changes in the PRC's economic policies. When Tom began to probe for the reasons behind this abrupt shift in economic philosophy, Li's response was simple: "How long did it take the United States to develop [its economy]?" "Almost 200 years, from the time of the colonial period until the Industrial Revolution," Tom replied. "We can't wait that long," said Li, and he added, "Policies [have] changed. We will now modernize and be a world power. It will take time. We will borrow, barter, and trade. We will balance self-reliance and foreign technology. We will provide incentives and bonuses. We will spend [more] for defense." Tom then asked Li about his statements of the previous year. Was he not rather dramatically altering the doctrine of self-reliance? The vice premier only laughed and replied, "Let us say I have had an emancipation of the head." [18]

IV

The beginning of a new year found both Tom Gates and the officials of the PRC anxiously awaiting either some word or some signal from the Carter administration about the direction of America's China policy under a new president. Late in 1976, Tom had written to Secretary Kissinger with some recommendations which he believed that the new administration might find useful in its future relations with the Chinese. In essence, Tom recommended that the Carter administration take three steps shortly after the inauguration to indicate its desire for continued progress in Chinese-American relations. First, he recommended that the administration include Huang Zhen, the chief of the PRCLO in Washington, as one of the first of the envoys to be received by President Carter and Secretary of State Vance. Second, he recommended that the administration reaffirm its commitment to the Shanghai Communique, both in communications to Hua Guofeng and Huang Hua and in its first foreign policy statements, as the basis for improved relations between the two countries. Third, he recommended that Carter promptly name his chief of the USLO and implement an orderly turnover of the office in Peking. Tom offered to discuss his suggestions about the background and characteristics of the next chief of the USLO with either Carter or Vance. As Tom later explained in a letter to Vance, the Chinese preferred that the chief of the Liaison Office be

someone close to the President who has already an earned reputation, not someone who is expected to earn it here. [The Chinese] will work easier with such a person and open up more personally. They also respect relative seniority. These characteristics also loom large within the close-knit international community [in Peking] where most of the ambassadors are senior respected individuals, where we share views [rather exclusively] since PRC high-level contacts are rare and [because] the Chief of USLO, although unofficial is looked upon as the most important man [in the diplomatic community]. [19]

By its own admission, however, the Carter administration did not consider normalization of relations with China an immediate priority. In many respects, a well-planned initiative by the Carter administration toward the PRC in 1977 became a casualty of several high-level, pre-inaugural evaluations of American foreign policy involving Carter, Vance, and Zbigniew Brzezinski, Carter's national security adviser. The immediate priorities of the new administration involved strengthening the NATO alliance, completing the negotiations for a SALT II treaty with the Soviet Union, making progress in the Middle East in the various disputes involving Israel, the front-line Arab states, and the Palestinians, and finally, negotiating a new treaty with Panama over the rights to the Panama Canal.

Vance preferred to delay any strong moves in the direction of normalization with the PRC until 1978; Brzezinski favored eventual normalization but had set no timetable for such an event to take place. President Carter, apparently satisfied with the priorities outlined by his advisers and perhaps wishing to show a break with the policies of his Republican predecessors while not provoking a domestic controversy on the issue of China policy early in his administration, placed the subject well down on his list of must-items. [20] As Ross Terrill observed, "The Year of the Snake turned out to be a curious one for the Washington-Peking tie. Ever since the shadow of 1976 fell over Ford in the summer of 1975, it seemed that 1977 would be the year of opportunity. [But Carter] felt no passion on China [and] was advised to put normalization to one side until late 1977." [21]

Early in 1977, Tom Gates quickly learned that China policy held a low priority with the new administration. In January, David Dean traveled to Washington for consultations and, after returning to Peking, advised Tom about some of the organizational and policy changes then being contemplated by the Carter administration. Dean confirmed that the administration was preoccupied with NATO and SALT II and, while the China policy was under review, it claimed no special attention.[22] Tom and his colleagues were pleased to learn a short time later that Carter had a successful meeting with Huang Zhen in Washington on February 8. Otherwise, it appeared that the new policymakers in Washington were paying little heed to Tom's earlier suggestions.

In March, however, the Carter administration suffered its first serious foreign policy reversal when the Soviets refused to consider the administration's opening proposal at the SALT II negotiations. Carter's speeches criticizing the Soviet Union for its approach to human rights also angered the Soviets (and because these statements angered the Soviets, they were applauded by the Chinese) and, as relations with Moscow soured, the administration began directing more attention to China. The focus of this attention quickly involved an important visit to China in mid-April by a Congressional delegation headed by Congressman John Brademas (D-Indiana) and Senator Richard Schweiker (R-Pennsylvania). As an expression of the importance which Carter attached to this visit, he asked that his son Chip accompany the delegation and express the president's personal regards to the Chinese leadership.[23]

If the Chinese were impatient about the apparent lack of attention which the Carter administration had directed toward the PRC, they failed to show it once the Brademas/Schweiker delegation arrived in China. The delegation toured Peking, Shanghai, and Hangzhou between April 11 and April 17 and also engaged in some serious discussions with Huang Hua and Li Xiannian.[24] In a particularly wide-ranging discussion with Li Xiannian on April 12, the delegation encountered a candid assessment of the PRC's attitude toward the United States and the current diplomatic environment. To his credit, Brademas took special care in eliciting the Chinese view on two major issues, normalization of relations with the United States and China's rivalry with the Soviet Union.

In regard to normalization, Brademas explained to Li Xiannian that President Carter was not "entirely free" to normalize relations with the PRC without the advice of Congress, and more important, Congress expected to play a stronger role in foreign policy in the future than it had during the Nixon and Ford administrations. Normalization, the Congressman declared, "requires efforts on both sides. We and you, we have to work for it." Li replied that the PRC continued to view the normalization issue as a problem

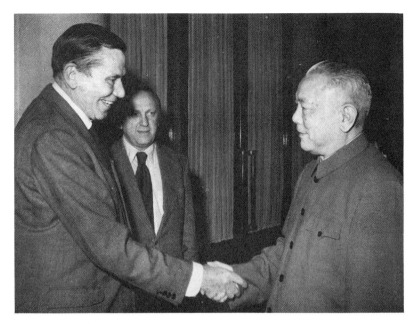

Tom Gates and Congressman John Brademas (D-Indiana) greet Vice Premier Li Xiannian, April 12, 1977.

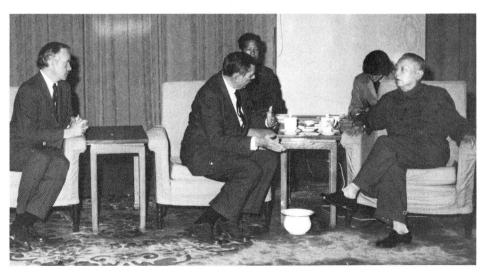

David Dean, deputy chief, USLO; Tom Gates; and Vice Premier Li Xiannian, May 5, 1977.

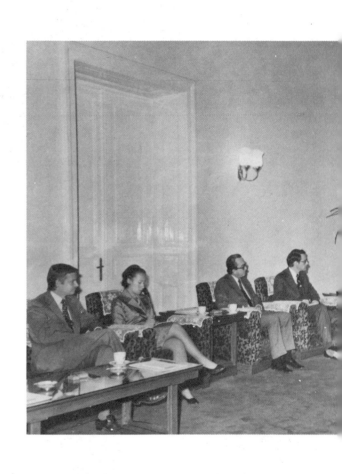

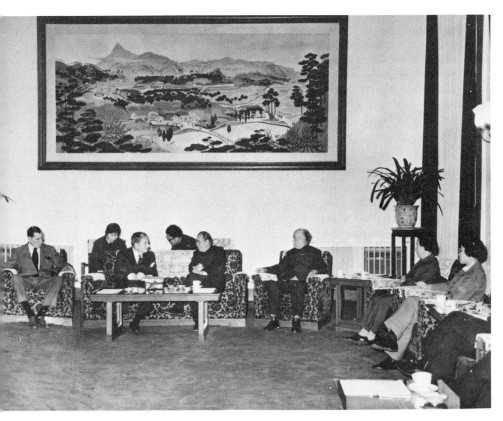

The David Rockefeller delegation meeting with the Chinese, January 1977.

for the American government, and the matter of Taiwan was strictly an internal concern of the Chinese. Thus, the new administration should not expect any change in the PRC's traditional policy.[25]

On the subject of the American response to Soviet adventurism, Brademas emphasized that both America and China recognized the dangers posed by the increasing growth of Soviet military power. He explained, however, that the United States was not appeasing the Soviet Union, especially since "the men and women in this room are the ones who have voted billions and billions of dollars for defense and weapons development." Li replied that the Chinese did not necessarily consider the size of America's defense expenditures the major issue. Instead, the PRC was equally concerned with the attitude which the United States appeared to reflect in its policy of detente with the Soviet Union, particularly in the Helsinki agreements where (in Li's view) America was unwilling to confront the Soviets' expansionist policies. Finally, Brademas inquired if the PRC planned to expand its future military capability as the means of demonstrating its resolve against the Soviets. Li responded characteristically by noting that the Chinese would never initiate military action against the Soviet Union but would defend itself vigorously if attacked. In every respect, Li's remarks corresponded with those given earlier by Huang Hua to the Americans on January 25 when he remarked that the Chinese intended to remain "vigilant" toward the Soviets.[26]

V

Coordinating the arrangements for the Brademas/Schweiker delegation was one of Thomas Gates's last official duties as chief of the United States Liaison Office to the People's Republic of China. In late April, he was notified that President Carter intended to nominate Leonard Woodcock, the former president of the United Auto Workers, as the next chief of the USLO. Woodcock had also recently chaired a commission which investigated the status of American soldiers presumed missing in action from the Vietnam War. On May 3 we opened the USLO residence for a final farewell reception for the Chinese officials with whom the USLO had had considerable contact during the past year. Li Xiannian, Huang Hua, Li Chiang, the head of the Ministry of Foreign Trade, Ding Guoyu, Wu De's principal assistant, and several dozen other Chinese diplomats attended this reception. On May 5, Li Xiannian returned the favor by inviting Tom and several members of the USLO staff to attend an informal dinner and meeting that evening. Thus our experience in China drew rapidly to a close. We found it difficult to leave our American friends and colleagues in the diplomatic community, but the prospect of returning to the United States and to our permanent home in Devon, Pennsylvania, to be reunited with our family made the homegoing more attractive. This time, Tom finally entered a permanent retirement.

Notes

1. Gates Papers, Thomas S. Gates to President Gerald R. Ford, 29 December 1976. The following day, Tom also sent a letter to President Ford which read in part: "There have been a series of great events in China during 1976. To have been here and have been a part of the changing scene has been a most rewarding and memorable experience. I am confident that the developing relationship between our two countries will continue to progress toward ultimate normalization, a goal which you have earnestly sought." Gates Papers, Thomas S. Gates to President Gerald R. Ford, 30 December 1976. Tom also received a warm letter from Secretary Kissinger on January 7, 1977, thanking him for his contributions to the administration. Kissinger's letter read in part: "You have had a brief but dramatic stay in Peking, and I did not want to leave office without telling you what a superb job I think you have done there. Your judgments, your observations, and your analysis of the last eight turbulent months in China have been invaluable to me and my colleagues. You have, once again, done a great service for our country and you have my appreciation and thanks." See Gates Papers, Secretary of State Henry Kissinger to Thomas S. Gates, 7 January 1977.

2. Gates Papers, "For Secretary of State Vance," 2 March 1977.

3. United States Department of State, Official Files, Peking to Washington, 11 November 1976. Hereafter cited as OF, date.

4. OF, Peking to Washington, 28 October 1976.

5. Interview, Gerald R. Ford.

6. Thomas S. Gates Oral History, 31 October 1982. Hereafter cited as Gates OH, date.

7. Robert L. Bartley, "New Significance to a China Trip," *Wall Street Journal*, 14 September 1976.

8. Gates OH, 1 January 1979.

9. Gates Papers, Thomas S. Gates to Anne Ponce et al., 7 February 1977.

10. OF, Peking to Washington, 20 January 1977.

11. Gates Papers, Thomas S. Gates to Anne Ponce et al., 7 February 1977.

12. OF, Peking to Washington, 26 January 1977; OF, Peking to Washington, February 1977.

13. OF, Memorandum to Ambassador Gates from William W. Thomas, 6 May 1976.

14. OF, Peking to Washington, 29 October 1976.

15. OF, Peking to Washington, 17 December 1976.

16. Gates Papers, Thomas S. Gates to Anne Ponce et al., 7 February 1977. Both Rockefeller and the Chase Manhattan Bank were active in a business relationship with the PRC at that time. See Peter Collier and David Horowitz, *The Rockefellers* (New York: Holt, Rinehart, Winston, 1976), p. 429.

17. Gates OH, 1 January 1979.

18. Ibid.; Gates Papers, Mrs. Ralph Lazarus to Thomas S. Gates, October 1978.

19. Gates Papers, "For Secretary of State Vance," 2 March 1977.

20. Jimmy Carter, *Keeping Faith: Memoirs of a President* (New York: Bantam, 1982), pp. 192–99; Cyrus Vance, *Hard Choices: Critical Years in American Foreign Policy* (New York: Simon and Schuster, 1983), pp. 75–83; Zbigniew Brzezinski, *Power and Principle: Memoirs of a National Security Adviser, 1977–1981* (New York: Farrar, Strauss, Giroux, 1983), pp. 198–202.

21. Terrill, *Future of China*, p. 170.

22. Gates Papers, Thomas S. Gates to Anne Ponce et al., 7 February 1977. See also Gates Papers, Secretary of State Vance to Ambassador Gates, 10 February 1977.

23. Carter, *Keeping Faith*, pp. 196–99; Terrill, *Future of China*, p. 170; Brzezinski, *Power and Principle*, p. 200; Vance, *Hard Choices*, pp. 75–83. See also *New York Times*, 6 April 1977, p. 9; and Bernard Gwertzman, "China Has Come Up Faster than Mr. Carter Expected," *New York Times*, 17 April 1976, p. 4. In addition to Brademas and Schweiker and several members of their staffs, the delegation included Representatives Silvio Conte, Mark Andrews, George Danielson, and Barbara Mikulski, and Senators William Roth and John Durkin.

24. OF, Peking to Washington, 19 April 1977.

25. OF, Peking to Washington, 12 April 1977.

26. Ibid.

CONCLUSION
Holding the Fort

Warren I. Cohen, a diplomatic historian who has written extensively on the history of recent Chinese-American relations, has claimed that the United States and China began an "era of respect" in their relations with each other in 1971–72, following the Nixon-Kissinger visits to the People's Republic. This new era of respect, which replaced two decades of mutual suspicion and fear between the United States and China, was characterized by significant policy changes which each nation's government adopted toward the other, by changes in the attitudes of the American and Chinese peoples toward each other, and finally, by an ever-increasing number of cultural, trade, scientific, technical, and educational exchanges which were designed to foster better communication and understanding between both countries.[1]

Since the United States and China indeed entered a historic new era during the early and mid-1970s, a proper subject with which to conclude this study is the degree to which Thomas Gates contributed to the improvement of America's relations with the People's Republic of China while serving as chief of the United States Liaison Office in 1976–77. As Tom himself explained his role during the critical twelve-month period of his appointment to the PRC,

My position was really to hold the fort until after the elections of 1976 when we could have made progress [toward normalization]. In an election year, it was obviously impossible for either side to commit itself to any new steps. A pause in the pace of the relationship was convenient to the Chinese as well because they were undergoing a great deal of turmoil in their own political affairs. So it was convenient [for both nations] to remain friendly and live under the ambiguity of the Shanghai Communique.[2]

In retrospect, Tom Gates's task of holding the fort in Peking essentially meant continuing the process of placing the chief of the USLO into the network of American foreign policy and the diplomatic community in Peking. Such a process of institutionalization became especially vital by 1976, especially since the domestic controversies in both America and China during the previous three years had made it virtually impossible to achieve the kind of progress characterized by the summit-style meetings which had involved the American and Chinese leadership just a short time earlier. Between 1973 and 1976, the focus for advancing Chinese-American relations shifted abruptly from the level of the heads-of-state in America and China to the working level in Washington and Peking. During those three years, with the exception of Gerald Ford's visit to the PRC in late 1975, the patient practice of applied diplomacy replaced the summit spectacular as the means of promoting improved understanding between the United States and the PRC. In that timely but less glamorous environment, Tom Gates and his USLO colleagues sought to preserve the American relationship with China until domestic conditions in each nation made it possible for the resumption of stronger initiatives designed to settle some of the outstanding and more complex matters which separated the two countries.

By 1976, the chief of USLO had clearly become a well-recognized personality in Peking's diplomatic community. Much of the increased visibility associated with the chief involved his diplomatic status as both a presidential envoy and a quasi-ambassador. The unique nature of this "job description" worked to great advantage for America's diplomatic interests in the Far East. Because Tom was Ford's (and later Carter's) personal representative to the PRC, he was seriously regarded by the Chinese, perhaps even more than had he been an "official" member of the diplomatic community. In that regard, both the Ford administration and the PRC authorities found the chief of USLO a particularly valuable person, especially for conveying sensitive diplomatic messages (such as when Tom personally delivered Ford's offer of humanitarian assistance to the Chinese at the time of the Tangshan earthquake) or performing particularly important diplomatic tasks. For example, shortly after Tom arrived in Peking, he presented Foreign Minister Qiao Guanhua with a personal request from President Ford that he be granted a meeting with Premier Hua Guofeng, an individual only faintly familiar to the administration. The fact that the Chinese complied with the request, and scheduled this appointment with Hua within one month of Tom's arrival, served as an indicator to the administration that the Chinese continued to desire improved relations with the United States. Indeed, the fact that Tom found numerous occasions to visit with such senior officials as Li Xiannian, Qiao Guanhua, and later Huang Hua, reinforced the American belief that the Chinese intended to use the USLO device as an effective diplomatic tool.

To repeat, the Chinese found it convenient to deal with the chief of USLO, not only with Tom Gates but also with David Bruce and George Bush. When Tom turned the position over to the Carter administration and Leonard Woodcock in 1977, he left a post which had an established place in the diplomatic community and particularly with the Chinese. The best example of how valuable the post became occurred in the summer and autumn of 1978 when Woodcock served as the Carter administration's link with the PRC and the on-the-scene negotiator in the discussions which ultimately resulted in normalized relations between America and China in 1978–79.[3] Clearly, the post of chief of the USLO grew in stature and importance between 1973 and 1978, and despite its short lifespan of five years, it should be remembered that the men who served as chiefs of the United States Liaison Office, and the foreign service professionals who served in Peking in the mid-1970s, played major roles in promoting improved Chinese-American relations. Indeed, given the internal problems which handicapped the implementation of each nation's foreign policy between 1973 and 1976, the progress which the Chinese and the Americans were able to make in the mid-1970s underscores the fact that Kissinger and Zhou acted just in time when they established the liaison offices in 1974.

The importance of the chief of the USLO to America's China policy was also evident on the quasi-ambassadorial level. The internal power struggle between China's rival political factions, the economic and social disruptions caused by the Tangshan earthquake, the death of Mao Zedong, the purge of the Gang of Four following Mao's death, and the rehabilitation of Deng Xiaoping were all developments which affected America's diplomatic understanding of China. More important from the standpoint of the formulation of an effective China policy, these events required professional reporting and analysis, supplied in large part by Tom and the other American China-watchers in Peking who occupied an unequalled vantage point from which to observe these dramatic developments. In addition, the chief of USLO's presence in Peking was a visible demonstration to the rest of the diplomatic community, particularly to the Soviet Union, that the United States took its new link with the Chinese seriously and, as Kissinger once explained, considered it part of the international political landscape.

The quasi-ambassadorial responsibilities of the chief of the USLO also placed him directly within the policy-making process as it affected America's relations with China. In 1976–77, Sino-American relations centered on three subjects, the issue of normalization, each nation's concern about the growing military power of the Soviet Union, and the efforts to broaden the relationship through cultural, scientific, trade, educational, and economic exchanges. Tom went to China specifically intending to work for the normalization of relations between America and the PRC. Achieving normalization with the PRC and determining the future status of Taiwan remained as a goal, but it had to be set aside because of domestic problems. As a result, as Tom explained, each side found it more convenient to "live under the ambiguity of the Shanghai Communique" and focus attention on other aspects of the relationship. The cultural, scientific, and trade exchanges between the United States and China, for example, continued to increase during Tom's tenure. In addition, several important Congressional delegations, such as the ones involving Senator Hugh Scott, Senators Mike Mansfield and John Glenn, and Congressman John Brademas and Senator Richard Schweiker, also visited China throughout 1976–77 in an effort to promote better relations between the two countries.

But one primary reason for the establishment of the liaison offices, according to Henry Kissinger, was that both America and China desired to have a permanent point of contact as a means of showing progress in their relationship, particularly in view of the concern which each nation felt over the growing military power of the Soviet Union. In that regard, few Americans were as qualified as Tom Gates to address the Chinese concern about the expansion of Soviet military power and the American response to it. Tom had spent almost eight years in the Defense Department during the Eisenhower administration and was thoroughly familiar with the outline of both America's strategic policy and that of the Soviet Union. As a former secretary of defense, he was well able to offer assurances to the Chinese that the United States intended to maintain its forces at a level sufficient to protect its interests. In repeated conversations with Li Xiannian, Qiao Guanhua, and Huang Hua, Tom emphasized the American determination to recognize and deal with the Soviet threat. Whether the Chinese were reassured about the strength of America's resolve was another matter. One point was certain, however; in appointing Tom Gates as chief of USLO, the Ford administration recognized the Chinese suspicions about Soviet expansionism and sent a presidential envoy who was able to discuss this concern with them intelligently and competently.

To conclude, Chinese-American relations therefore did not necessarily stagnate between 1973 and 1977, as some writers have maintained.[5] Instead, the relations simply moved from the level of the heads of state to the working level in Washington and Peking. The practice of applied, traditional diplomacy (although conducted in a nontraditional fashion) became a pragmatic substitute for the diplomatic breakthroughs of the early 1970s and the achievement of normalization in 1978–79. Between 1973 and 1977, and particularly in 1976–77, the Americans and the Chinese endured a pause in the pace of their earlier relationship, an interlude which awaited the advent of a different set of domestic conditions in each country. The pause served as a prelude to the time when America and China could initiate another period of creative diplomacy, a period which continues to this day.

Notes

1. Warren I. Cohen, "American Perceptions of China," in Michel Oksenberg and Robert B. Oxnam, eds., *Dragon and Eagle: United States-China Relations: Past and Present* (New York: Basic Books, 1978), pp. 83–85. See also Cohen, *America's Response to China* (New York: John Wiley and Sons, 1980).

2. Gates Papers, Thomas S. Gates to Anne Ponce et al., 8 August 1976; Thomas S. Gates Oral History, 31 October 1982.

3. Brzezinski, *Power and Principle,* pp. 224–26, 229–33; Carter, *Keeping Faith,* pp. 196–99; Vance, *Hard Choices,* pp. 114–18.

4. Kissinger, *Years of Upheaval,* pp. 60–63.

5. Brzezinski, *Power and Principle,* p. 198; Seymour M. Hersh, *The Price of Power: Kissinger in the Nixon White House* (New York: Simon and Schuster, 1983), p. 636.

Bibliography

The major source of materials for this study was the official files of the United States Department of State as related to the United States Liaison Office to the People's Republic of China during the period when Thomas S. Gates was chief of USLO in 1976–77. These files remain the possession of the State Department and specific references to sources are listed in the Notes following each chapter.

Thomas S. Gates also donated a collection of his personal papers to the University of Pennsylvania. This collection includes various unclassified materials from his years in the Defense Department and the State Department as well as correspondence, oral histories, photographs, and other assorted items. Where appropriate, citation of these materials is also indicated in the Notes.

Other primary materials, such as articles from the national and international press, are specifically cited in the Notes.

Published Works

Borklund, C. W. *Men of the Pentagon.* New York: Praeger, 1966.

Brugger, Bill. *From Radicalism to Revisionism.* Totowa, N.J.: Barnes and Noble, 1982.

Brzezinski, Zbigniew. *Power and Principle: Memoirs of A National Security Adviser, 1977–1981.* New York: Farrar, Straus, Giroux, 1983.

Butterfield, Fox. "The Intriguing Matter of Mao's Successor." *New York Times Magazine*, 1 August 1976, pp. 12, 37, 46, 48.

Cannon, Lou. *Reagan*. New York: G. P. Putnam's Sons, 1982.

Carter, Jimmy. *Keeping Faith: Memoirs of a President*. New York: Bantam, 1982.

Chang, Parris. "The Rise of Wang Tunghsing: Head of China's Security Apparatus." *China Quarterly* 73 (March 1978): 122–36.

Cohen, Warren I. *America's Response to China*. New York: Wiley, 1980.

———. "American Perceptions of China." *Dragon and Eagle: United States-China Relations: Past and Present*. Edited by Michel Oksenberg and Robert B. Oxnam. New York: Basic Books, 1978.

Collier, Peter, and David Horowitz. *The Rockefellers*. New York: Holt, Rinehart, and Winston, 1976.

Domes, Jurgen. "The 'Gang of Four' and Hua Kuo-feng: An Analysis of Political Events in 1975–1976." *China Quarterly* 71 (June 1977): 473–97.

Eisenhower, Dwight D. *Mandate for Change: White House Years, 1953–1956*. Garden City, N.Y.: Doubleday, 1963.

———. *Waging Peace: White House Years, 1956–1961*. Garden City, N.Y.: Doubleday, 1965.

Evans, Rowland, and Robert Novak. *The Reagan Revolution*. New York: E. P. Dutton, 1981.

Ford, Gerald R. *A Time to Heal*. New York: Harper and Row/Reader's Digest Press, 1979.

Garside, Roger. *Coming Alive: China After Mao*. New York: McGraw-Hill, 1981.

Gates, Thomas S. "On China." *Pennsylvania Gazette* 76, no. 8 (September 1978): 29–30.

Hartmann, Robert T. *Palace Politics: An Inside Account of the Ford Years*. New York: McGraw-Hill, 1980.

Hersh, Seymour M. *The Price of Power: Kissinger in the Nixon White House*. New York: Simon and Shuster, 1983.

Hsu, Immanuel C. Y. *China Without Mao: The Search for a New Order*. New York: Oxford University Press, 1983.

Kissinger, Henry A. *White House Years*. Boston: Little, Brown, 1979.

———. *Years of Upheaval*. Boston: Little, Brown, 1981.

———. *Observations*. Boston: Little, Brown, 1985.

Mathews, Jay, and Linda Mathews. *One Billion: A China Chronicle*. New York: Random House, 1983.

Nessen, Ron. *It Sure Looks Different from the Inside*. Chicago: Playboy Press, 1978.

Nixon, Richard M. *RN: The Memoirs of Richard Nixon*. New York: Warner, 1978.

———. *The Real War*. New York: Warner, 1980.

Oksenberg, Michel, and Sai-cheung Yeung. "Hua Kuo-feng's Pre-Cultural Revolution Years, 1949–1960: The Making of a Political Generalist." *China Quarterly* 69 (March 1977): 3–53.

Onate, Andres D. "Hua Kuo-feng and the Arrest of the 'Gang of Four.'" *China Quarterly* 75 (September 1978): 540–65.

Salisbury, Harrison E. *China: 100 Years of Revolution*. New York: Holt, Rinehart, and Winston, 1983.

———. *The Long March: The Untold Story*. New York: Harper and Row, 1985.

Schram, Stuart. "Chairman Hua Edits Mao's Literary Heritage: 'On the Ten Great Relationships.'" *China Quarterly* 69 (March 1977): 126–35.

Shawcross, William. *Sideshow*. New York: Simon and Schuster, 1979.

Terrill, Ross. *Mao: A Political Biography*. New York: Harper and Row, 1980.

———. *The Future of China—After Mao*. New York: Delacorte Press, 1978.

———. *The White-Boned Demon: A Biography of Madame Mao Zedong*. New York: William Morrow, 1984.

Vance, Cyrus. *Hard Choices: Critical Years in American Foreign Policy*. New York: Simon and Schuster, 1983.

Wadleigh, James. "Thomas Sovereign Gates." *American Secretaries of the Navy*, edited by Paolo Coletta, vol. 2. Annapolis, Md.: Naval Institute Press, 1980.

White, Theodore H. "Burnout of a Revolution." *Time*, September 26, 1983, pp. 30–49.

Witcover, Jules. *Marathon*. New York: Viking Press, 1977.

Witke, Roxane. *Comrade Chiang Ching*. Boston: Little, Brown, 1977.

Zhihui, Yin. "The 'Wushu General.'" *China Reconstructs*, December 1983, pp. 55–58.

Interviews by the Authors

David Dean
James H. Douglas
Gerald R. Ford
Richard W. Mueller

Index